D1162697

Food Allergy

Food Allergy

Adverse Reactions to Foods and Food Additives

EDITED BY

DEAN D. METCALFE MD
Chief, Laboratory of Allergic Diseases
National Institute of Allergy and Infectious Diseases
National Institutes of Health
Bethesda, MD, USA

HUGH A. SAMPSON MD
Kurt Hirschhorn Professor of Pediatrics
Dean for Translational Biomedical Sciences
Director, Jaffe Food Allergy Institute Department of Pediatrics
Icahn School of Medicine at Mount Sinai
New York, NY, USA

RONALD A. SIMON MD
Head, Division of Allergy, Asthma and Immunology
Scripps Clinic
San Diego, CA, USA;
Adjunct Professor
Department of Molecular and Experimental Medicine
Scripps Research Institute
La Jolla, CA, USA

GIDEON LACK MBBCh (Oxon)
MA (Oxon), FRCPCH
Professor of Paediatric Allergy
King's College London Clinical Lead for Allergy Service
Guy's and St Thomas' NHS Foundation Trust
St Thomas' Hospital
London, UK

FIFTH EDITION

WILEY Blackwell

Wiley-Blackwell is an imprint of John Wiley & Sons, formed by the merger of Wiley's global Scientific, Technical and Medical business with Blackwell Publishing.

Registered office: John Wiley & Sons, Ltd, The Atrium, Southern Gate, Chichester, West Sussex, PO19 8SQ, UK

Editorial offices: 9600 Garsington Road, Oxford, OX4 2DQ, UK
The Atrium, Southern Gate, Chichester, West Sussex, PO19 8SQ, UK
111 River Street, Hoboken, NJ 07030-5774, USA

For details of our global editorial offices, for customer services and for information about how to apply for permission to reuse the copyright material in this book please see our website at www.wiley.com/wiley-blackwell

Library of Congress Cataloging-in-Publication Data

Food allergy (John Wiley & Sons, Ltd.)
Food allergy : adverse reactions to foods and food additives / edited by Dean D. Metcalfe, Hugh A. Sampson, Ronald A. Simon, Gideon Lack. – Fifth edition.
p. ; cm.
Includes bibliographical references and index.
ISBN 978-0-470-67255-6 (cloth : alk. paper) – ISBN 978-1-118-74414-7 (ePub) – ISBN 978-1-118-74416-1 (ePdf) – ISBN 978-1-118-74417-8 (eMobi) – ISBN 978-1-118-74418-5
I. Metcalfe, Dean D., editor of compilation. II. Sampson, Hugh A., editor of compilation. III. Simon, Ronald A., editor of compilation. IV. Lack, Gideon, editor of compilation. V. Title.
[DNLM: 1. Food Hypersensitivity. 2. Food Additives–adverse effects. WD 310]
RC596
616.97′5–dc23

2013017942

A catalogue record for this book is available from the British Library.

Wiley also publishes its books in a variety of electronic formats. Some content that appears in print may not be available in electronic books.

Cover image: Generated by Christian Radauer and Heimo Breiteneder, Medical University of Vienna, Austria
Cover design by Andrew Magee Design Ltd

Set in 9.25/12pt Meridien by Aptara® Inc., New Delhi, India
Printed and bound in Singapore by Markono Print Media Pte Ltd

01 2014

Contents

Part 3 Adverse Reactions to Foods: Diagnosis

Part 4 Adverse Reactions to Food Additives

Part 5 Contemporary Topics in Adverse Reactions to Foods

List of Contributors

Maria Laura Acebal, JD
Board Director and Former CEO
FARE: Food Allergy Research and Education
(formerly The Food Allergy & Anaphylaxis
Network (FAAN))
Washington, DC, USA

Shradha Agarwal, MD
Assistant Professor of Medicine
Division of Allergy and Clinical Immunology
Icahn School of Medicine at Mount Sinai
New York, NY, USA

Katrina J. Allen, MD, PhD
Professor of Paediatrics
Murdoch Childrens Research Institute;
The University of Melbourne Department of
Paediatrics;
Department of Allergy and Immunology
Royal Children's Hospital
Melbourne, VIC, Australia

Matthew Aresery, MD
Allergist
Maine General Medical Center
Augusta, ME, USA

James L. Baldwin, MD
Associate Professor
Division of Allergy and Clinical Immunology
University of Michigan
Ann Arbor, MI, USA

Gary A. Bannon, PhD
Global Regulatory Sciences and Affairs
Monsanto
St Louis, MO, USA

Joseph L. Baumert, PhD
Assistant Professor Co-Director
Food Allergy Research and Resource Program
Department of Food Science and Technology
Food Allergy Research and Resource Program
University of Nebraska
Lincoln, NE, USA

M. Cecilia Berin, PhD
Associate Professor of Pediatric Allergy
and Immunology
Icahn School of Medicine at Mount Sinai
New York, NY, USA

Kirsten Beyer, MD
Professor of Experimental Pediatrics
Charité Universitätsmedizin Berlin
Klinik für Pädiatrie m.S. Pneumologie und
Immunologie
Berlin, Germany

Stephan C. Bischoff, MD
Professor of Medicine
Director, Institute of Nutritional Medicine and
Immunology
University of Hohenheim
Stuttgart, Germany

John V. Bosso, MD
Affiliate Faculty Member
Columbia University College of Physicians and
Surgeons;
Chief, Allergy and Immunology
Nyack Hospital
Nyack, NY, USA

Heimo Breiteneder, PhD
Professor of Medical Biotechnology
Department of Pathophysiology and Allergy
Research
Medical University of Vienna
Vienna, Austria

A. Wesley Burks, MD
Curnen Distinguished Professor and Chairman
Department of Pediatrics
University of North Carolina
Chapel Hill, NC, USA

Robert K. Bush, MD
Emeritus Professor
Division of Allergy, Immunology, Pulmonary,
Critical Care, and Sleep Medicine
Department of Medicine
University of Wisconsin School of Medicine and
Public Health
Madison, WI, USA

André Cartier, MD
Clinical Professor of Medicine
Université de Montréal
Hôpital du Sacré-Coeur de Montréal
Montreal, QC, Canada

Soheil Chegini, MD
Attending Physician
Exton Allergy and Asthma Associates
Exton, PA, USA

Leslie G. Cleland, MD, FRACP
Director of Rheumatology
Rheumatology Unit
Royal Adelaide Hospital
Adelaide, SA, Australia

Ma. Lourdes B. de Asis, MD
Allergy and Asthma Consultants of Rockland and Bergen West
Nyack, NY, USA

Raymond C. Dobert, PhD
Global Regulatory Sciences and Affairs
Monsanto, St. Louis, MO, USA

George Du Toit, MD
Consultant in Paediatric Allergy
King's College London
Clinical Lead for Allergy Service
Guy's and St Thomas'
NHS Foundation Trust
St Thomas' Hospital
London, UK

John M. Fahrenholz, MD
Division of Allergy, Pulmonary and Critical Care Medicine
Vanderbilt University Medical Center
Nashville, TN, USA

David M. Fleischer, MD
Associate Professor of Pediatrics
University of Colorado Denver School of Medicine
Division of Pediatric Allergy and Immunology
National Jewish Health

Timothy J. Franxman, MD
Fellow
Division of Allergy and Clinical Immunology
University of Michigan
Ann Arbor, MI, USA

Roy L. Fuchs, phD
Global Regulatory Sciences and Affairs
Monsanto, St. Louis, MO, USA

Matthew J. Greenhawt, MD, MBA, FAAP
Assistant Professor
Division of Allergy and Clinical Immunology
Food Allergy Center
University of Michigan Medical School
Ann Arbor, MI, USA

Marion Groetch, MS, RD, CDN
Director of Nutrition Services
The Elliot and Roslyn Jaffe Food Allergy Institute
Division of Allergy and Immunology
Department of Pediatrics
Icahn School of Medicine at Mount Sinai
New York, NY, USA

Robert G. Hamilton, PhD, D.ABMLI
Professor of Medicine and Pathology
Departments of Medicine and Pathology
Johns Hopkins University School of Medicine
Baltimore, MD, USA

Ralf G. Heine, MD, FRACP
Department of Allergy & Immunology
Royal Children's Hospital, Melbourne, VIC, Australia
Murdoch Childrens Research Institute, Melbourne, Australia
Department of Paediatrics
The University of Melbourne, Melbourne, Australia

David J. Hill, MD, FRACP
Senior Consultant Allergist
Murdoch Childrens Research Institute
Melbourne, VIC, Australia

Jonathan O'B. Hourihane, DM, FRCPI
Professor of Paediatrics and Child Health
University College Cork, Ireland

Sangeeta J. Jain, MD
Section of Clinical Immunology, Allergy and Rheumatology
Tulane University Health and Sciences Center
New Orleans, LA, USA

Stacie M. Jones, MD
Professor of Pediatrics
Chief, Division of Allergy and Immunology
University of Arkansas for Medical Sciences and Arkansas Children's Hospital
Little Rock, AR, USA

Hirsh D. Komarow, MD
Staff Clinician
Laboratory of Allergic Diseases
National Institute of Allergy and Infectious Diseases
National Institutes of Health
Bethesda, MD, USA

Jennifer J. Koplin, PhD
Postdoctoral Research Fellow
Murdoch Childrens Research Institute
Royal Children's Hospital
Melbourne, VIC, Australia

Samuel B. Lehrer, PhD
Research Professor of Medicine, Emeritus
Tulane University
New Orleans, LA, USA

Donald Y.M. Leung, MD, PhD
Professor of Pediatrics
University of Colorado Denver School of Medicine
Edelstein Family Chair of Pediatric Allergy and Immunology
National Jewish Health

Chris A. Liacouras, MD
Professor of Pediatrics
Division of Gastroenterology and Nutrition
The Children's Hospital of Philadelphia
Philadelphia, PA, USA

Jay Lieberman, MD
Assistant Professor
Department of Pediatrics
The University of Tennessee Health Sciences Center
Memphis, TN, USA

Madhan Masilamani, PhD
Assistant Professor of Pediatric Allergy and Immunology
Icahn School of Medicine at Mount Sinai
New York, NY, USA

Lloyd Mayer, MD
Professor of Medicine and Immunobiology
Division of Allergy and Clinical Immunology
Immunology Institute
Icahn School of Medicine at Mount Sinai
New York, NY, USA

E.N. Clare Mills, PhD
Professor
Manchester Institute of Biotechnology
University of Manchester
Manchester, UK

Michelle Montalbano, MD
Advanced Allergy and Asthma, PLLC
Silverdale, WA, USA

Amanda Muir, MD
Fellow, Pediatric Gastroenterology
Division of Gastroenterology and Nutrition
The Children's Hospital of Philadelphia
Philadelphia, PA, USA

Anne Muñoz-Furlong, BA
Founder and CEO
The Food Allergy and Anaphylaxis Network
Fairfax, VA, USA

Joseph A. Murray, MD
Professor of Medicine
Mayo Clinic
Rochester, MN, USA

Kari Nadeau, MD, PhD, FAAAAI
Associate Professor
Division of Immunology and Allergy
Stanford Medical School and Lucile Packard Children's Hospital
Stanford, CA, USA

Jennifer A. Namazy, MD
Division of Allergy, Asthma and Immunology
Scripps Clinic
San Diego, CA, USA

Julie A. Nordlee, MS
Clinical Studies Coordinator
Department of Food Science and Technology
Food Allergy Research and Resource Program
University of Nebraska
Lincoln, NE, USA

Anna Nowak-Węgrzyn, MD
Associate Professor of Pediatrics
Department of Pediatrics, Allergy and Immunology
Jaffe Food Allergy Institute
Icahn School of Medicine at Mount Sinai
New York, NY, USA

Raymond M. Pongonis, MD
Division of Allergy, Pulmonary and Critical Care Medicine
Vanderbilt University Medical Center
Nashville, TN, USA

Graham Roberts, DM, MA, BM BCh
Professor and Consultant in Paediatric Allergy and Respiratory Medicine
University Hospital Southampton NHS Foundation Trust
Southampton, UK

David M. Robertson, MD
Allergist/Immunologist
Hampden County Physician Associates
Springfield, MA, USA;
Clinical Assistant Professor of Pediatrics
Tufts University School of Medicine
Boston, MA, USA

Alberto Rubio-Tapia, MD
Assistant Professor of Medicine
Division of Gastroenterology and Hepatology
Mayo Clinic
Rochester, MN, USA

David R. Scott, MD
Fellow, Division of Allergy, Asthma and Immunology
Scripps Clinic
San Diego, CA, USA

Gernot Sellge, MD PhD
Clinical and Research Fellow
University Hospital Aachen
Department of Medicine III
Aachen, Germany

Scott H. Sicherer, MD
Professor of Pediatrics
The Elliot and Roslyn Jaffe Food Allergy Institute
Division of Allergy and Immunology
Department of Pediatrics
Icahn School of Medicine at Mount Sinai
New York, NY, USA

Maxcie M. Sikora, MD
Alabama Allergy and Asthma Center
Birmingham, AL, USA

Lisa K. Stamp, FRACP, PhD
Professor and Rheumatologist
University of Otago–Christchurch
Christchurch, New Zealand

Lauren Steele, BA
Doris Duke Clinical Research Fellow
Division of Allergy and Immunology Department of Pediatrics
Icahn School of Medicine at Mount Sinai
New York, NY, USA

Donald D. Stevenson, MD
Senior Consultant
Division of Allergy, Asthma and Immunology
Scripps Clinic
La Jolla, CA, USA

Von Ta, MD
Research Fellow
Division of Immunology and Allergy
Stanford Medical School and Lucile Packard Children's Hospital
Stanford, CA, USA

Steve L. Taylor, PhD
Professor
Department of Food Science and Technology
Co-Director, Food Allergy Research and Resource Program
University of Nebraska
Lincoln, NE, USA

Ashraf Uzzaman, MD
Saline Allergy Asthma Sinus Specialists
Saline, MI, USA

Julie Wang, MD
Associate Professor of Pediatrics
Jaffe Food Allergy Institute
Department of Pediatrics
Icahn School of Medicine at Mount Sinai
New York, NY, USA

Jason M. Ward, PhD
Global Regulatory Sciences and Affairs
Monsanto, St. Louis, MO, USA

Richard W. Weber, MD
Professor of Medicine
National Jewish Health
Professor of Medicine
University of Colorado Denver School of Medicine
Denver, CO, USA

Laurianne G. Wild, MD
Section of Clinical Immunology, Allergy and Rheumatology
Tulane University Health and Sciences Center
New Orleans, LA, USA

Katharine M. Woessner, MD
Program Director
Allergy, Asthma and Immunology Training Program
Scripps Clinic Medical Group
San Diego, CA, USA

Robert A. Wood, MD
Professor of Pediatrics and International Health
Director, Pediatric Allergy and Immunology
Johns Hopkins University School of Medicine
Baltimore, MD, USA

Preface to the Fifth Edition

It is the privilege of the editors to present the fifth edition of *Food Allergy: Adverse Reactions to Foods and Food Additives*. As in the first four editions, we have attempted to create a book that in one volume would cover pediatric and adult adverse reactions to foods and food additives, stress efforts to place adverse reactions to foods and food additives on a sound scientific basis, select authors to present subjects on the basis of their acknowledged expertise and reputation, and reference each contribution thoroughly. Hugh, Ron, and I as co-editors of the fifth edition are pleased to be joined by Professor Gideon Lack, Head of the Children's Allergy Service at Guy's and St Thomas' NHS Foundation Trust, and Professor of Pediatric Allergy at King's College London, who brings a unique perspective to the understanding of the evolution of the food allergic state.

The growth in knowledge in this area continues to be gratifying and is reflected in the diversity of subject matter in this edition. Again, this book is directed toward clinicians, nutritionists, and scientists interested in food reactions, but we also hope that patients and parents of patients interested in such reactions will find the book to be a valuable resource. The chapters cover basic and clinical perspectives of adverse reactions to food antigens, adverse reactions to food additives, and contemporary topics. Basic science begins with overview chapters on immunology with particular relevance to the gastrointestinal tract as a target organ in allergic reactions and the properties that govern reactions initiated at this site. Included are chapters relating to biotechnology and to thresholds of reactivity. This is followed by chapters reviewing the clinical science of adverse reactions to food antigens from the oral allergy syndrome to cutaneous disease, and from eosinophilic gastrointestinal disease to anaphylaxis. The section on diagnosis constitutes a review of the approaches available for diagnosis, and their strengths and weaknesses. Adverse reactions to food additives include chapters addressing specific clinical reactions and reactions to specific agents. The final section on contemporary topics includes discussions of the pharmacologic properties of food, the natural history and prevention of food allergy, diets and nutrition, neurologic reactions to foods and food additives, psychological considerations, and adverse reactions to seafood toxins.

Each of the chapters in this book is capable of standing alone, but when placed together they present a mosaic of the current ideas and research on adverse reactions to foods and food additives. Overlap is unavoidable but, we hope, is held to a minimum. Ideas of one author may sometimes differ from those of another, but in general there is remarkable agreement from chapter to chapter. We, the editors, thus present the fifth edition of a book that we believe represents a fair, balanced, and defensible review of adverse reactions of foods and food additives.

Dean D. Metcalfe
Hugh A. Sampson
Ronald A. Simon
Gideon Lack

About the cover: The cover picture shows the structure of the vicilin and major peanut allergen Ara h 1 (Protein Data Bank accession number 3s7i). Vicilins are a large family of seed storage proteins that contains many important allergens from legumes, tree nuts, and seeds. The picture was generated by Christian Radauer and Heimo Breiteneder, Department of Pathophysiology and Allergy Research, Medical University of Vienna, Austria.

Abbreviations

AA	Arachidonic acid
AAF	Amino acid-based formula
AAP	American Association of Pediatrics
ACCD	1-Aminocyclopropane-1-carboxylic acid deaminase
ACD	Allergic contact dermatitis
AD	Atopic dermatitis
ADA	Americans with Disabilities Act
AE	Atopic eczema
AEC	Absolute eosinophil count
AERD	Aspirin exacerbated respiratory disease
AFP	Antifreeze protein
AGA	Anti-gliadin antibodies
AI	Adequate intake
ALA	Alimentary toxic aleukia
ALDH	Aldehyde dehydrogenase
ALS	Advanced Life Support
ALSPAC	Avon Longitudinal Study of Parents and Children
AMDR	Acceptable Macronutrient Distribution Ranges
AMP	Almond major protein
APC	Antigen-presenting cell
APT	Atopy patch test
ASCA	Anti-*Saccharomyces cerevisiae*
ASHMI	Anti-asthma Herbal Medicine Intervention
ASP	Amnesic shellfish poisoning
AZA	Azaspiracid
AZP	Azaspiracid shellfish poisoning
BAL	Bronchoalveolar lavage
BAT	Basophil activation test
BCR	B-cell receptor
BER	Bioenergy regulatory
BFD	Bioelectric functions diagnosis
BHA	Butylated hydroxyanisole
BHR	Basophil histamine release
BHT	Butylated hydroxytoluene
BLG	b-lactoglobulin
BMI	Body mass index
BN	Brown–Norway
BP	Blood pressure
BPRS	Brief Psychiatric Rating Scale
BTX	Brevetoxins
CAS	Chemical Abstract Society
CAST	Cellular allergosorbent test
CCD	Cross-reactive carbohydrate determinants
CCP	Cyclic citrullinated peptide
CDC	Centers for Disease Control and Prevention
CFA	Chemotactic factor of anaphylaxis
CFR	Code of Federal Regulations
CGRP	Calcitonin gene-related peptide
CIU	Chronic idiopathic urticaria
CIUA	Chronic idiopathic urticaria/angioedema
CLA	Cutaneous lymphocyte-associated antigen
CLSI	Clinical and Laboratory Standards Institute
CM	Cow's milk
CMA	Cow's milk allergy
CMF	Cow's milk formula
CMP	Cow's milk protein
CMV	Cucumber mosaic virus
CNS	Central nervous system
COX	Cyclo-oxygense
CRH	Corticotropin-releasing hormone
CRP	C-reactive protein
CRS	Chinese restaurant syndrome
CSPI	Center for Science in the Public Interest
CSR	Class-switch recombination
CTL	Cytotoxic T-lymphocyte
CTX	Ciguatoxins
CU	Cholinergic urticaria
DAO	Diamine oxidase
DBPC	Double-blind, placebo-controlled
DBPCFC	Double-blind, placebo-controlled food challenge
DC	Dendritic cell
DHA	Docosahexaenoic acid
DMARD	Disease modifying anti-rheumatic agent
DoH	Department of Health

DRI	Dietary reference intakes
DSP	Diarrhetic shellfish poisoning
DTH	Delayed-type hypersensitivity
DTT	Dithiothreitol
DTX	Dinophysistoxins
EAR	Estimate average requirement
EAV	Electroacupuncture according to Voll
ECP	Eosinophil cationic protein
EDN	Eosinophil-derived neurotoxin
EDS	Electrodermal screening
EE	Eosinophilic esophagitis
EEG	Electroencephalogram
EER	Estimated energy requirement
EFA	Essential fatty acid
EFSA	European Food Safety Authority
EGID	Eosinophil-associated gastrointestinal disorders
EIA	Enzyme immunoassay
ELISA	Enzyme-linked immunosorbent assays
EMA	Anti-endomysial
EMT	Emergency Medical Technical
EoE	Eosinophilic esophagitis
EoG	Eosinophilic gastroenteritis
EoP	Eosinophilic proctocolitis
EPA	Eicosapentaneoic acid
EPO	Eosinophilic peroxidase
EPSPS	Enzyme 5-enolpyruvylshikimate-3-phosphate synthase
EPX	Eosinophil protein X
ESR	Erythrocyte sedimentation rate
FAAN	Food Allergy & Anaphylaxis Network
FAE	Follicle-associated epithelium
FAFD	Food-additive-free diet
FALCPA	Food Allergen Labeling and Consumer Protection Act
FAO	Food and Agricultural Organization
FASEB	Federation of American Societies for Experimental Biology
FDA	Food and Drug Administration
FDDPU	Food-dependent delayed pressure urticaria
FDEIA	Food-dependent exercise-induced anaphylaxis
FEC	Food-and-exercise challenge
FEIA	Fluorescent-enzyme immunoassay
FFQs	Food Frequency Questionnaires
FFSPTs	Fresh food skin prick tests
FPIES	Food protein-induced enterocolitis syndrome
FSIS	Food Safety Inspection Service
GALT	Gut-associated lymphoid tissue
GBM	Glomerular basement membrane
GER	Gastroesophageal reflux
GERD	Gastroesophageal reflux disease
GFD	Gluten-free diet
GH	Growth hormone
GHRH	Growth hormone releasing hormone
GI	Gastrointestinal
GINI	German Infant Nutritional Interventional
GOX	Glyphosate oxidoreductase
GrA	Granzymes A
GRAS	Generally recognized as safe
GrB	Granzymes B
GRS	Generally regarded as safe
GSH	Glutathione
GVHD	Graft-versus-host disease
HACCP	Hazard analysis and critical control point
HAQ	Health Assessment Questionnaire
HBGF	Heparin-binding growth factors
HCN	Hydrogen cyanide
HE	Hen's egg
HEL	Hen's egg lysozyme
HEV	High endothelial venules
HKE	Heat-killed *Esherichia coli*
HKL	Heat-killed *Listeria monocytogene*
HKLM	Heat-killed *Listeria monocytogenes*
HLA	Human leukocyte antigen
HMW	High molecular weight
HNL	Human neutrophil lipocalin
HPF	High-powered field
HPLC	High-performance liquid chromatography
HPP	Hydrolyzed plant protein
HRFs	Histamine releasing factors
HRP	Horseradish peroxidase
HSP	Hydrolyzed soy protein
HVP	Hydrolyzed vegetable protein
IAAs	Indispensable amino acids
ICD	Irritant contact dermatitis
IDECs	Inflammatory dendritic epidermal cells
IEC	Intestinal epithelial cells
IEI	Idiopathic environmental intolerances
IFN-γ	Interferon gamma
IgA	Immunoglobulin A
IgE	Immunoglobulin E
IgG	Immunoglobulin G
IgM	Immunoglobulin M
IL-4	Interleukin-4
ISB	Isosulfan blue
ISS	Immunostimulatory sequences
IST	Intradermal skin test
ISAC	Immuno-solid phase allergen chip
ISU	ISAC units
ITAM	Immunoreceptor tyrosine-based activation motif
ITIM	Immunoreceptor tyrosine-based inhibitory motif
IUIS	International Union of Immunological Societies
JECFA	Expert Committee on Food Additives
KA	Kainic acid
KGF	Keratinocyte growth factor
KLH	Key-hole limpet hemocyanin
kU/L	Kilo unit per liter, where 1 U = 2.4 ng of IgE

kU_A/L	Kilo allergen-specific IgE unit per liter
LA	Linoleic acid
LCPUFA	Long-chain polyunsaturated fatty acids
LCs	Langerhans cells
LFI	Lateral flow immunochromatographic
LGG	Lactobacillus rhamnosus GG
LLDC	Langerhans-like dendritic cell
LMW	Low molecular weight
LOAELs	Lowest observed adverse effect level
LOX	Lipoxygenase
LP	Lamina propria
LPL	LP lymphocytes
LPS	Lipopolysaccharide
LRTIs	Lower respiratory tract infections
LSD	Lysergic acid diethylamide
LT	Leukotrienes
LTP	Lipid-transfer protein
MALDI	Matrix-assisted laser desorption/ionization
MALT	Mucosa-associated lymphoid tissue
MAO	Monoamine oxidase
MAPK	Mitogen-activated protein kinase
MAS	Multicenter Allergy Study
MBP	Major basic protein
MC	Mast cell
MCS	Multiple chemical sensitivity
MED	Minimal eliciting dose
MFA	Multiple food allergies
MHC	Major histocompatibility complex
MIP	Macrophage inflammatory protein-1
MMP	Matrix metalloproteinase
MMPI	Minnesota Multiphasic Personality Inventory
MMR	Measles–mumps–rubella
MPO	Myeloperoxidase
MSG	Monosodium glutamate
MTX	Maitotoxins
MUFA	Monounsaturated fatty acids
MWL	Mushroom worker's lung
NADPH	Nicotinamide dinucleotide phosphate
NASN	National Association of School Nurses
NCHS	National Center for Health Statistics
NDGA	Nordihydroguaiaretic acid
NIAID	National Institute of Allergy and Infectious Diseases
NIOSHA	National Institute for Occupational Safety and Health
NK	Natural killer
NLEA	National Labeling and Education Act
NOEL	No observable effect level
NPA	Negative predictive accuracy
NPIFR	Nasal peak inspiratory flow
NPV	Negative predictive values
NSAID	Non-steroidal anti-inflammatory drugs
NSBR	Non-specific bronchial responsiveness
NSP	Neurotoxic shellfish poisoning
OAS	Oral allergy syndrome
ODN	Oligodeoxynucleotides
OFC	Oral food challenge
OPRA	Occupational Physicians Reporting Activity
OT	Oral tolerance
OVA	Ovalbumin
PAF	Platelet-activating factor
PAMP	Pathogen-associated molecular pattern
PBB	Polybrominated biphenyls
PBMC	Peripheral blood mononuclear cell
PBT	Peripheral blood T-cells
PCB	Polychlorinated biphenyls
PEF	Peak expiratory flow
PEFR	Peak expiratory flow rate
PFS	Pollen–food syndrome
PFT	Pulmonary function testing
PHA	Phytohemagglutinin
PK	Prausnitz-Küstner
PKC	Protein kinase C
PMN	Polymorphonuclear leukocytes
PPA	Positive predictive accuracy
PPI	Protein phosphatase inhibition
PPs	Peyer's patches
PPT	PP-derived T-cells
PPV	Positive predictive value
PR	Pathogenesis-related
PSP	Paralytic shellfish poisoning
PST	Prick skin test
PTX	Pectenotoxins
PUFA	Polyunsaturated fatty acids
PUVA	Psoralen + ultraviolet A radiation
RADS	Reactive airways dysfunction syndrome
RAST	Radioallergosorbent test
RBA	Receptor-binding assay
RBL	Basophilic leukemia
RDA	Recommended dietary allowances
RDBPC	Randomized double–blind, placebo-controlled
RF	Rheumatoid factor
RIA	Radioimmunoassay
ROS	Reactive oxygen species
SBPC	Single-blinded placebo-controlled
SC	Secretory component
SCF	Stem cell factor
SCIT	Subcutaneous immunotherapy
SCN	Soybean cyst nematode
SFAP	School Food Allergy Program
SGF	Simulated gastric fluid
SHM	Somatic hyper mutation
SIF	Simulated intestinal fluid
SIgA	Secretory IgA
SIgM	Secretory IgM
SIT	Specific immunotherapy
SLIT	Sublingual immunotherapy
SPECT	Single photon emission computed tomography

SPT	Skin prick test
STX	Saxitoxins
SVR	Sequential vascular response
TCM	Traditional Chinese medicine
TCR	T-cell receptor
TLP	Thaumatin-like protein
TLR	Toll-like receptor
TNF	Tumor necrosis factor
TPA	Tetradecanoylphorbol-13-acetate
TSA	Transportation Security Administration
TTG	Tissue transglutaminase
TTX	Tetrodotoxin
UGI	Upper GI
UL	Upper intake level
USDA	United States Department of Agriculture
VAR	Voice-activated audiotape recording
VIP	Vasoactive intestinal peptide
WHO	World Health Organization
YTX	Yessotoxin

1 Adverse Reactions to Food Antigens: Basic Science

1 The Mucosal Immune System

Shradha Agarwal & Lloyd Mayer

Division of Clinical Immunology, Icahn School of Medicine at Mount Sinai, New York, NY, USA

Key Concepts

- The gastrointestinal tract is the largest lymphoid organ in the body. The mucosal immune system is unique in its ability to suppress responses against commensal flora and dietary antigens.
- The mucosal immune system is characterized by unique cell populations (intraepithelial lymphocytes, lamina propria lymphocytes) and antigen-presenting cells (epithelial cells, tolerized macrophages, and dendritic cells) that contribute to the overall nonresponsive state.
- Numerous chemical (extremes of pH, proteases, bile acids) and physical (tight junctions, epithelial membranes, mucus, trefoil factors) barriers reduce antigen access to the underlying mucosal immune system (non-immune exclusion).
- Secretory IgA serves as a protective barrier against infection by preventing attachment of bacteria and viruses to the underlying epithelium (immune exclusion).
- Oral tolerance is the active nonresponse to antigen administered via the oral route. Factors affecting the induction of oral tolerance to antigens include the age and genetics of the host; the nature, form, and dose of the antigen; and the state of the mucosal barrier.

Introduction

An allergic response is thought to be an aberrant, misguided, systemic immune response to an otherwise harmless antigen. An allergic response to a food antigen then can be thought of as an aberrant mucosal immune response. The magnitude of this reaction is multiplied several fold when one looks at this response in the context of normal mucosal immune responses, that is, responses that are suppressed or downregulated. The current view of mucosal immunity is that it is the antithesis of a typical systemic immune response. In the relatively antigen pristine environment of the systemic immune system, foreign proteins, carbohydrates, or even lipids are viewed as potential pathogens. A coordinated reaction seeks to decipher, localize, and subsequently rid the host of the foreign invader. The micro- and macroenvironment of the gastrointestinal (GI) tract is quite different, with continuous exposure to commensal bacteria in the mouth, stomach, and colon and dietary substances (proteins, carbohydrates, and lipids) that, if injected subcutaneously, would surely elicit a systemic response. The complex mucosal barrier consists of the mucosa, epithelial cells, tight junctions, and the lamina propria (LP) containing Peyer's patches (PP), lymphocytes, antigen-presenting macrophages, dendritic cells (DCs), and T cells with receptors for major histocompatibility complex (MHC) class I- and II-mediated antigen presentation. Pathways have been established in the mucosa to allow such nonharmful antigens/organisms to be tolerated [1, 2]. In fact, it is thought that the failure to tolerate commensals and food antigens is at the heart of a variety of intestinal disorders (e.g., celiac disease and gluten [3, 4], inflammatory bowel disease, and normal commensals [5–7]). Those cells exist next to a lumen characterized by extremes of pH replete with digestive enzymes. Failure to maintain this barrier may result in food allergies. For example, studies in murine models demonstrated that coadministration of antacids results in breakdown of oral tolerance implying that acidity plays a role in the prevention of allergies and promotion of tolerance [8, 9]. Thus, it makes sense that some defect in mucosal immunity would predispose a person to food allergy. This chapter will lay the groundwork for the understanding of mucosal immunity. The subsequent chapters will focus on the specific pathology seen

Food Allergy: Adverse Reactions to Foods and Food Additives, Fifth Edition. Edited by Dean D Metcalfe, Hugh A Sampson, Ronald A Simon and Gideon Lack.

when the normal immunoregulatory pathways involved in this system are altered.

Mucosal immunity is associated with suppression: the phenomena of controlled inflammation and oral tolerance

As stated in the introduction, the hallmark of mucosal immunity is suppression. Two linked phenomena symbolize this state: controlled/physiologic inflammation and oral tolerance. The mechanisms governing these phenomena are not completely understood, as the dissection of factors governing mucosal immunoregulation is still evolving. It has become quite evident that the systems involved are complex and that the rules governing systemic immunity frequently do not apply in the mucosa. Unique compartmentalization, cell types, and routes of antigen trafficking all come together to produce the immunosuppressed state.

Controlled/physiologic inflammation

The anatomy of the mucosal immune system underscores its unique aspects (Figure 1.1). There is a single layer of columnar epithelium that separates a lumen replete with dietary, bacterial, and viral antigens from the lymphocyte-rich environment of the underlying loose connective tissue stroma, called the lamina propria. Histochemical staining of this region reveals an abundance of plasma cells, T cells, B cells, macrophages, and DCs [2, 10–12]. The difference between the LP and a peripheral lymph node is that there is no clear-cut organization in the LP and cells in the LP are virtually all activated memory cells. While the cells remain activated, they do not cause destruction of the tissue or severe inflammation. The cells appear to reach a stage of activation but never make it beyond that stage.

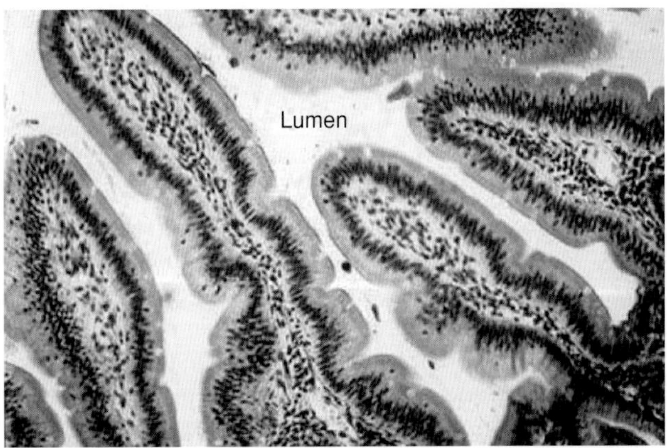

Figure 1.1 Hematoxylin and eosin stain of a section of normal small intestine (20×). Depicted is the villi lined with normal absorptive epithelium. The loose connective tissue stroma (lamina propria) is filled with lymphocytes, macrophages, and dendritic cells. This appearance has been termed controlled or physiologic inflammation.

This phenomenon has been called controlled/physiologic inflammation. The entry and activation of the cells into the LP is antigen driven. Germ-free mice have few cells in their LP. However, within hours to days following colonization with normal intestinal flora (no pathogens), there is a massive influx of cells [13–16]. Despite the persistence of an antigen drive (luminal bacteria), the cells fail to develop into aggressive, inflammation-producing lymphocytes and macrophages. Interestingly, many groups have noted that cells activated in the systemic immune system tend to migrate to the gut. It has been postulated that this occurs due to the likelihood of reexposure to a specific antigen at a mucosal rather than a systemic site. Activated T cells and B cells express the mucosal integrin $\alpha_4\beta_7$ which recognizes its ligand, MadCAM [13–20], on high endothelial venules (HEV) in the LP. They exit the venules into the stroma and remain activated in the tissue. Bacteria or their products play a role in this persistent state of activation. Conventional ovalbumin-T-cell receptor (OVA-TCR) transgenic mice have activated T cells in the LP even in the absence of antigen (OVA) while OVA-TCR transgenic mice crossed on to a RAG-2-deficient background fail to have activated T cells in the LP [21]. In the former case, the endogenous TCR can rearrange or associate with the transgenic TCR generating receptors that recognize luminal bacteria. This tells us that the drive to recognize bacteria is quite strong. In the latter case, the only TCR expressed is that which recognizes OVA and even in the presence of bacteria no activation occurs. If OVA is administered orally to such mice, activated T cells do appear in the LP. So antigen drive is clearly the important mediator. The failure to produce pathology despite the activated state of the lymphocytes is the consequence of suppressor mechanisms in play. Whether this involves regulatory cells, cytokines, or other, as yet undefined, processes is currently being pursued. It may reflect a combination of events. It is well known that LP lymphocytes (LPLs) respond poorly when activated via the TCR [22, 23]. They fail to proliferate although they still produce cytokines. This phenomenon may also contribute to controlled inflammation (i.e., cell populations cannot expand, but the cells can be activated). In the OVA-TCR transgenic mouse mentioned above, OVA feeding results in the influx of cells. However, no inflammation is seen even when the antigen is expressed on the overlying epithelium [24]. Conventional cytolytic T cells (class I restricted) are not easily identified in the mucosa and macrophages respond poorly to bacterial products such as lipopolysaccharide (LPS) because they downregulate a critical component of the LPS receptor, CD14, which associates with Toll-like receptor-4 (TLR-4) and MD2 [25]. Studies examining cellular mechanisms regulating mononuclear cell recruitment to inflamed and noninflamed intestinal mucosa demonstrate that intestinal macrophages express chemokine receptors but do not migrate to the ligands. In contrast, autologous blood monocytes expressing the same receptors do migrate to the ligands and chemokines derived from LP extracellular matrix [26]. These findings imply that monocytes are necessary in maintaining the macrophage population in noninflamed mucosa and are the source of macrophages in inflamed mucosa. All of these observations support the existence of control mechanisms that tightly regulate mucosal immune responses.

Clearly, there are situations where the inflammatory reaction is intense, such as infectious diseases or ischemia. However, even in the setting of an invasive pathogen such as *Shigella* or *Salmonella*, the inflammatory response is limited and restoration of the mucosal barrier following eradication of the pathogen is quickly followed by a return to the controlled state. Suppressor mechanisms are thought to be a key component of this process as well.

Oral tolerance

Perhaps the best-recognized phenomenon associated with mucosal immunity and equated with suppression is oral tolerance (Figure 1.2) [27–32]. Oral tolerance can be defined as the active, antigen-specific nonresponse to antigens administered orally, characterized by the secretion of interleukin (IL)-10 and transforming growth factor beta (TGF-β) by T lymphocytes. Many factors play a role in tolerance induction and there may be multiple forms of tolerance elicited by different factors. The concept of oral tolerance arose from the recognition that we do not frequently generate immune responses to foods we eat, despite the fact that they can be quite foreign to the host. Disruption in oral tolerance results in food allergies and food intolerances such as celiac disease. Part of the explanation for this observation is trivial, relating to the properties of digestion. These processes take large macromolecules and, through aggressive proteolysis and carbohydrate and lipid degradation, render potentially immunogenic substances nonimmunogenic. In the case of proteins, digestive enzymes break down large polypeptides into nonimmunogenic di- and tri-peptides, too small to bind to MHC molecules. However, several groups have reported that upwards of 2% of dietary proteins enter the draining enteric vasculature intact [33]. Two percent is not a trivial amount, given the fact that Americans eat 40–120 g of protein per day in the form of beef, chicken, or fish.

Box 1.1 Factors affecting the induction of oral tolerance.

- Age of host (reduced tolerance in the neonate)
- Genetics of the host
- Nature of the antigen (protein → carbohydrate → lipid)
- Form of the antigen (soluble → particulate)
- Dose of the antigen (low dose → regulatory T cells; high dose → clonal deletion or anergy)
- State of the barrier (decreased barrier → decreased tolerance)

The key question then is: How do we regulate the response to antigens that have bypassed complete digestion? The answer is oral tolerance. Its mechanisms are complex (Box 1.1) and depend on age, genetics, nature of

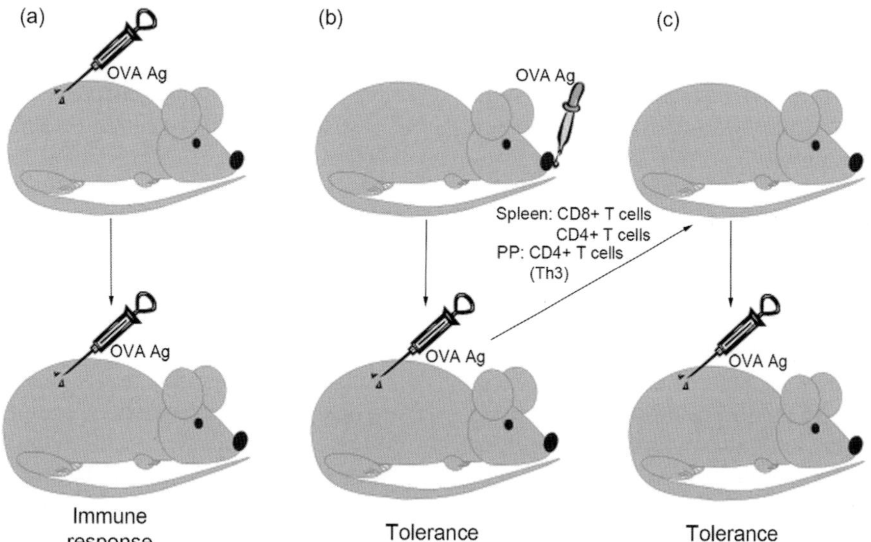

Figure 1.2 Comparison of immune responses elicited by changing the route of administration of the soluble protein antigen ovalbumin. (a) The outcome of systemic immunization. Mice generate both T-cell and antibody responses. (b) If mice are fed OVA initially, systemic immunization fails to generate a T- or B-cell response. (c) When T cells are transferred from mice initially fed OVA antigen to naïve mice, systemic immunization fails to generate a T- or B-cell response. Tolerance is an active process since it can be transferred by either PP CD4+ T cells (Strober, Weiner) or splenic CD8+ T cells (Waksman). These latter findings suggest that there are multiple mechanisms involved in tolerance induction. Adapted from Chehade M, Mayer L. Oral tolerance and its relation to food hypersensitivities. *J Allergy Clin Immunol* 2005; 115:3–12; quiz 13.

the antigen, form of the antigen, dose of the antigen, and the state of the mucosal barrier.

Several groups have noted that oral tolerance is difficult to achieve in neonates [34]. This may relate to the rather permeable barrier that exists in the newborn and/or the immaturity of the mucosal immune system. The limited diet in the newborn may serve to protect the infant from generating a vigorous response to food antigens. However, several epidemiological studies have suggested that delayed introduction may contribute to food allergies [35, 36], though these studies were retrospective and difficult to control. Thus, recent guidelines for introduction of allergenic solid foods were revised to reflect that insufficient evidence exists to support delayed weaning as a strategy to prevent allergies [37]. In contrast, early introduction may also not be the solution to prevent food allergies as there may exist a time for immune regulation to mature. Interestingly, in humans, despite the relatively early introduction of cow's milk (in comparison to other foods) it remains one of the most common food allergens in children [38]. A study by Strobel demonstrated enhancement of immunologic priming in neonatal mice fed antigen in the first week of life, whereas tolerance developed after waiting 10 days to introduce antigen [39].

The next factor involved in tolerance induction is the genetics of the host. Berin et al. examined allergic sensitization in TLR4+ and TLR4− mice on two genetic backgrounds, C3H and Balb/c, and found Th2 skewing in TLR4-deficient C3H mice compared with TLR4-sufficient C3H mice. This pattern of Th2 skewing was not observed in TLR4-deficient mice on a Balb/c background [40]. Lamont et al. [41] published a report detailing tolerance induction in various mouse strains using the same protocol. Balb/c mice tolerize easily while others failed to tolerize at all. Furthermore, some of the failures to tolerize were antigen specific; upon oral feeding, a mouse could be rendered tolerant to one antigen but not another. This finding suggested that the nature and form of the antigen also play a significant role in tolerance induction.

Protein antigens are the most tolerogenic while carbohydrates and lipids are much less effective in inducing tolerance [42]. The form of the antigen is critical; for example, a protein given in soluble form (e.g., OVA) is quite tolerogenic whereas, once aggregated, it loses its potential to induce tolerance. The mechanisms underlying these observations have not been completely defined but appear to reflect the nature of the antigen-presenting cell (APC) and the way in which the antigen trafficks to the underlying mucosal lymphoid tissue. Insolubility or aggregation may also render a luminal antigen incapable of being sampled [2]. In this setting, nonimmune exclusion of the antigen would lead to ignorance from lack of exposure of the mucosa-associated lymphoid tissue (MALT) to the antigen in question. One study examining the characteristics of milk allergens involved in sensitization and elicitation of allergic response demonstrated that pasteurization led to aggregation of whey proteins but not casein and that the formation of aggregates changed the path of antigen uptake, away from absorptive enterocytes to PP. Subsequently, pasteurized β-lactoglobulin leads to enhanced IgE as well as Th2 cytokine responses in the initial sensitization step, and in contrast only soluble milk proteins triggered anaphylaxis in mice, since transepithelial uptake across the small intestinal epithelium was not impaired [43].

Lastly, prior sensitization to an antigen through extraintestinal routes affects the development of a hypersensitivity response. For example, sensitization to peanut protein has been demonstrated by application of topical agents containing peanut oil to inflamed skin in children [44]. Similar results were obtained by Hsieh's group in epicutaneous sensitized mice to the egg protein ovalbumin [45].

The dose of antigen administered during a significant period early in life is also critical to the form of oral tolerance generated. In addition, frequent or continuous exposure to relatively low doses typically results in potent oral tolerance induction. In murine models, high-dose exposure to antigen early in life can produce lymphocyte anergy while low doses of antigen appears to activate regulatory/suppressor T cells [38, 46, 47] of both CD4 and CD8 lineages. Th3 cells were the initial regulatory/suppressor cells described in oral tolerance [47–49]. These cells appear to be activated in the PP and secrete TGF-β. This cytokine plays a dual role in mucosal immunity; it is a potent suppressor of T- and B-cell responses while promoting the production of IgA (it is the IgA switch factor) [34, 50–52]. An investigation of the adaptive immune response to cholera toxin B subunit and macrophage-activating lipopeptide-2 in mouse models lacking the TGF-βR in B cells (TGFβRII-B) demonstrated undetectable levels of antigen-specific IgA-secreting cells, serum IgA, and secretory IgA (SIgA) [53]. These results demonstrate the critical role of TGF-βR in antigen-driven stimulation of SIgA responses *in vivo*. The production of TGF-β by Th3 cells elicited by low-dose antigen administration helps explain an associated phenomenon of oral tolerance, bystander suppression. As mentioned earlier, oral tolerance is antigen specific, but if a second antigen is coadministered systemically with the tolerogen, suppression of T- and B-cell responses to that antigen will occur as well. The participation of other regulatory T cells in oral tolerance is less well defined. Tr1 cells produce IL-10 and appear to be involved in the suppression of graft-versus-host disease (GVHD) and colitis in mouse models, but their activation during oral antigen administration has not been as clear-cut [54–56]. Frossard et al. demonstrated increased antigen-induced IL-10-producing cells in PP from tolerant mice after β-lactoglobulin feeding but not in anaphylactic mice suggesting that reduced IL-10 production in PP may support food allergies [57]. There is some evidence for the activation of CD4+CD25+ regulatory T cells during oral tolerance induction protocols but the nature of their role in the process is still under investigation [58–61]. Experiments in transgenic mice expressing TCRs for OVA demonstrated increased numbers of CD4+CD25+ T cells expressing cytotoxic T-lymphocyte antigen 4 (CTLA-4) and cytokines TGF-β and IL-10 following OVA feeding. Adoptive transfer of CD4+CD25+ cells from the fed mice suppressed *in vivo* delayed-type hypersensitivity responses in recipient mice [62]. Furthermore, tolerance studies done in mice depleted of CD25+ T cells along with TGF-β neutralization failed in the induction of oral tolerance by high and low doses of oral OVA suggesting that CD4+CD25+ T cells and TGF-β together are involved in the induction of oral tolerance partly through the regulation of expansion of antigen-specific CD4+ T cells [63]. Markers such as glucocorticoid-induced TNF receptor and transcription factor FoxP3, whose genetic deficiency results in an autoimmune and inflammatory syndrome, have been shown to be expressed CD4+CD25+ Tregs [64,65]. Lastly, early studies suggested that antigen-specific CD8+ T cells were involved in tolerance induction since transfer of splenic CD8+ T cells following feeding of protein antigens could transfer the tolerant state to naïve mice [66–69]. Like the various forms of tolerance described, it is likely that the distinct regulatory T cells defined might work alone depending on the nature of the tolerogen or in concert to orchestrate the suppression associated with oral tolerance and more globally to mucosal immunity.

As mentioned, higher doses of antigen lead to a different response, either the induction of anergy or clonal deletion. Anergy can occur through T-cell receptor ligation in the absence of costimulatory signals provided by IL-2 or by interactions between receptors on T cells (CD28) and counterreceptors on APCs (CD80 and CD86) [70]. Clonal deletion occurring via FAS-mediated apoptosis [71] may be a common mechanism given the enormous antigen load in the GI tract.

The last factor affecting tolerance induction is the state of the barrier. Several states of barrier dysfunction are associated with aggressive inflammation and a lack of tolerance. In murine models the permeability of the barrier is influenced by exposures to microbial pathogens such as viruses, alcohol, and nonsteroidal anti-inflammatory drugs, which can result in changes in gene expression and phosphorylation of tight junction proteins such as occludins, claudins, and JAM-ZO1, which have been associated with changes in intestinal mast cells and allergic sensitization [72, 73]. Increased permeability throughout the intestine has been shown in animal models of anaphylaxis by the disruption of tight junctions, where antigens are able to pass through paracellular spaces [74–76]. More recently, mutations in the gene encoding filaggrin have been linked to the barrier dysfunction in patients with atopic dermatitis, which has been associated with increased prevalence of food allergy. Similarly, barrier defects associated with decreased filaggrin expression have been demonstrated in patients with eosinophilic esophagitis [77]. It is speculated that barrier disruption leads to altered pathways of antigen uptake and failure of conventional mucosal sampling and regulatory pathways. For example, treatment of mice with interferon gamma (IFN-γ) can disrupt the inter-epithelial tight junctions allowing for paracellular access by fed antigens. These mice fail to develop tolerance to OVA feeding [78, 79]. However, as IFN-γ influences many different cell types, mucosal barrier disruption may be only one of several defects induced by such treatment.

Do these phenomena relate to food allergy? There is no clear answer yet, though both allergen-specific and non-specific techniques to induce tolerance are being studied in clinical trials in food-allergic patients [80–83]. While these studies are interventional and may not provide insight into the mechanisms involved in the naturally occurring mucosal tolerance, they are valuable in determining successful treatment approaches to food-allergic patients.

The nature of antibody responses in the gut-associated lymphoid tissue

IgE is largely the antibody responsible for food allergy. In genetically predisposed individuals an environment favoring IgE production in response to an allergen is established. The generation of T-cell responses promoting a B-cell class switch to IgE has been described (i.e., Th2 lymphocytes secreting IL-4). The next question, therefore, is whether such an environment exists in the gut-associated lymphoid tissue (GALT) and what types of antibody responses predominate in this system.

Antibodies provide the first line of protection at the mucosal surface with IgA being the most abundant antibody isotype in mucosal secretions. In fact, given the surface area of the GI tract (the size of one tennis court), the cell density, and the overwhelming number of plasma cells within the GALT, IgA produced by the mucosal immune system far exceeds the quantity of any other antibody in the body. IgA is divided into two subclasses, IgA1 and IgA2, with IgA2 as the predominant form at mucosal surfaces. The production of a unique antibody isotype SIgA was the first difference noted between systemic and mucosal immunity. SIgA is a dimeric form of IgA produced in the LP and transported into the lumen by a specialized pathway through the intestinal epithelium (Figures 1.1–1.3) [84]. SIgA is unique in that it is anti-inflammatory in nature. It does not bind classical complement components but rather binds to luminal antigens, preventing their attachment to the epithelium or promoting agglutination and subsequent removal of the antigen in the mucus layer overlying the epithelium. These latter two events reflect "immune exclusion," as opposed to the nonspecific mechanisms of exclusion alluded to earlier (the epithelium, the mucus barrier, proteolytic digestion, etc.). SIgA has one additional unique aspect—its ability to bind to an epithelial cell-derived glycoprotein called secretory component (SC), the receptor for polymeric Ig (pIgR) [85–88]. SC serves two functions: it promotes the transcytosis of SIgA from the LP through the epithelium into the lumen, and, once in the lumen, it protects the antibody against proteolytic degradation. This role is critically important, because the enzymes used for protein digestion are equally effective at degrading antibody molecules. For example, pepsin and papain in the stomach digest IgG into $F(ab')_2$ and Fab fragments. Further protection against trypsin and chymotrypsin in the lumen allows SIgA to exist in a rather hostile environment.

IgM is another antibody capable of binding SC (pIgR). Like IgA, IgM uses J chain produced by plasma cells to form polymers—in the case of IgM, a pentamer. SC binds to the Fc portions of the antibody formed by the polymerization. The ability of IgM to bind SC may be important in patients with IgA deficiency. Although not directly proven, secretory IgM (SIgM) may compensate for the absence of IgA in the lumen.

What about other Ig isotypes? The focus for years in mucosal immunity was SIgA. It was estimated that upwards of 95% of antibody produced at mucosal surfaces was IgA. Initial reports ignored the fact that IgG was present not only in the LP, but also in secretions [89, 90]. These latter observations were attributed to leakage across the barrier from plasma IgG. However, recent attention has focused on the potential role of the neonatal Fc receptor, FcR_n, which might serve as a bidirectional transporter of IgG [91, 92]. FcR_n is an MHC class I-like molecule that functions to protect IgG and albumin from catabolism, mediates transport of IgG across epithelial cells, and is involved in antigen presentation by professional APCs. FcR_n is expressed early on, possibly as a mechanism to transport IgG from mother to fetus and neonate for passive immunity [93–95]. Its expression was thought to be downregulated after weaning, but studies suggest that it may still be expressed in adult lung, kidney, and possibly gut epithelium. Recent studies have explored the possibility of utilizing these unique properties of FcR_n in developing antibody-based therapeutics for autoimmune diseases [96–98].

We are left then with IgE. Given the modest amounts present in the serum, it has been even more difficult to detect IgE in mucosal tissues or secretions. Mucosal mast cells are well described in the gut tissue. The IgE Fc receptor, FcεRI, is present and mast cell degranulation is reported (although not necessarily IgE related). FcεRI is not expressed by the intestinal epithelium, so it is unlikely

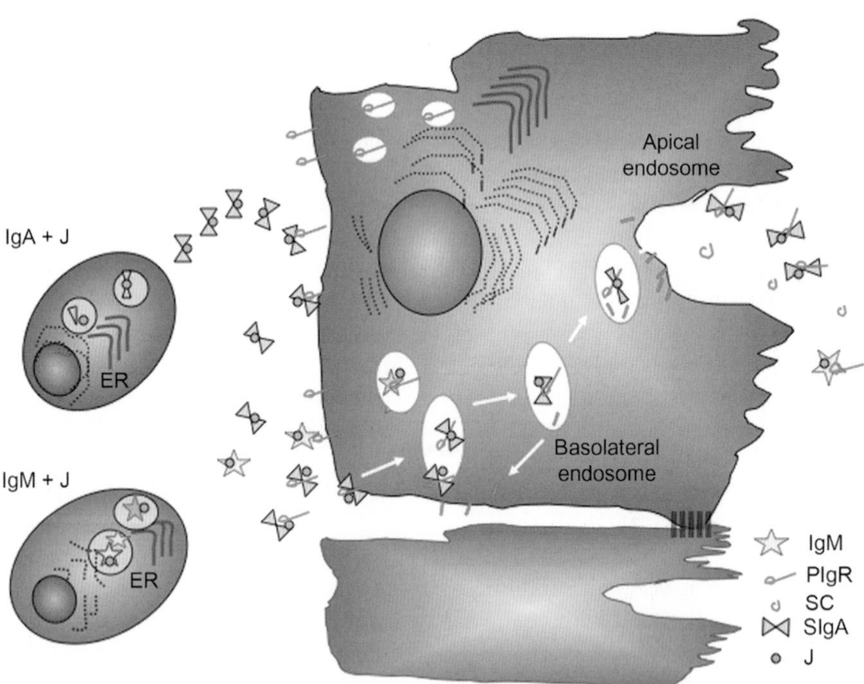

Figure 1.3 Depiction of the transport of secretory IgA (SIgA) and SIgM. Plasma cells produce monomeric IgA or IgM that polymerizes after binding to J chain. Polymeric immunoglobulins are secreted into the lamina propria and taken up by the polymeric Ig receptor (PIgR) or secretory component (SC) produced by intestinal epithelial cells and expressed on the basolateral surface. Bound SIgA or SIgM are internalized and transcytosed in vesicles across the epithelium and releases with SC into the intestinal lumen. SC protects the SIgA from degradation once in the lumen.

that this molecule would serve a transport function. CD23 (FcεRII), however, has been described on gut epithelial cells, and one model has suggested that it may play a role in facilitated antigen uptake and consequent mast cell degranulation [99–101]. In this setting, degranulation is associated with fluid and electrolyte loss into the luminal side of the epithelium, an event clearly associated with an allergic reaction in the lung and gut.

Thus, the initial concept that IgA was the be-all and end-all in the gut may be shortsighted and roles for other isotypes in health and disease require further study.

The anatomy of the gut-associated lymphoid tissue: antigen trafficking patterns

The final piece of the puzzle is probably the most critical for regulating mucosal immune responses: the cells involved in antigen uptake and presentation (Figure 1.4). As alluded to earlier, antigens in the GI tract are treated very differently than in the systemic immune system. There are additional hurdles to jump. Enzymes, detergents (bile salts), and extremes of pH can alter the nature of the antigen before it comes in contact with the GALT. If the antigen survives this onslaught, it has to deal with a thick mucous barrier, a dense epithelial membrane, and intercellular tight junctions. Mucin produced by goblet cells and trefoil factors produced by epithelial cells provide a viscous barrier to antigen passage. However, despite these obstacles antigens manage to find their way across the epithelium and immune responses are elicited.

Probably the best-defined pathway of antigen trafficking is in the GI tract through the specialized epithelium overlying the organized lymphoid tissue of the GALT, the Peyer's patches (PPs). PPs consist of germinal centers comprising switched IgA B cells. The specialized epithelial surface overlying the PPs and lymphoid follicles is called follicle-associated epithelium (FAE). Within the FAE reside specialized M (microfold) cells derived from enterocytes under the influence of Notch signaling pathways. The M cell, in contrast to the adjacent absorptive epithelium, has few microvilli, a limited mucin overlayer, a thin elongated cytoplasm, and a shape that forms a pocket around subepithelial lymphocytes, macrophages, and DCs. The initial description of the M cell documented not only its unique structure, but also its ability to take up large particulate antigens from the lumen into the subepithelial space [102–105]. M cells contain few lysosomes, so little or no processing of antigen can occur [106]. M cells protrude into the lumen, pushed up by the underlying PP. This provides a larger area for contact with luminal contents. The surface of the M cell is special in that it expresses a number of lectin-like molecules, which help promote binding to specific pathogens [107, 108]. For example, poliovirus binds to the M cell surface via a series of glycoconjugate

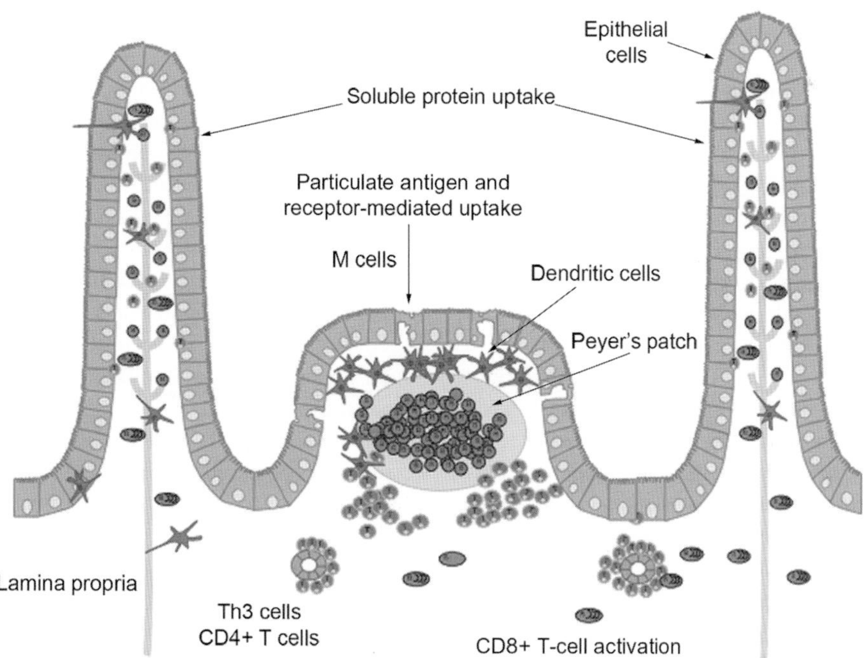

Figure 1.4 Sites of antigen uptake in the gut. Antigen taken up by M cells travel to the underlying Peyer's patch where Th3 (TGF-β-secreting) T cells are activated and isotype switching to IgA occurs (B cells). This pathway favors particulate or aggregated antigen. Antigen taken up by intestinal epithelial cells may activate CD8+ T cells that suppress local (and possibly systemic tolerance) responses. This pathway favors soluble antigen.

interactions [109]. Interestingly, antigens that bind to the M cell and get transported to the underlying PP generally elicit a positive (SIgA) response. Successful oral vaccines bind to the M cell and not to the epithelium. Thus, this part of the GALT appears to be critical for the positive aspects of mucosal immunity.

The M cell is a conduit to the PP. Antigens transcytosed across the M cell and into the subepithelial pocket are taken up by macrophages/DCs and carried into the PP. Once in the patch, TGF-β-secreting T cells promote B-cell isotype switching to IgA [52]. These cells leave the patch and migrate to the mesenteric lymph node, and eventually to other mucosal sites, where they undergo terminal maturation to dimeric IgA-producing plasma cells. In relation to food allergy and tolerance mechanisms, Frossard et al. compared antigen-specific IgA-secreting cells in PP from mice sensitized to β-lactoglobulin resulting in anaphylaxis versus tolerant mice. Tolerant mice were found to have higher numbers of β-lactoglobulin-specific IgA-secreting cells in PPs, in addition to higher fecal β-lactoglobulin-specific IgA titers compared to anaphylactic mice. The increase in antigen-specific SIgA is induced by IL-10 and TGF-β production by T cells from PPs [110].

Several groups have suggested that M cells are involved in tolerance induction as well. The same TGF-β-producing cells activated in the PP that promote IgA switching also suppress IgG and IgM production and T-cell proliferation. These are the Th3 cells described by Weiner's group initially [46]. Other observations, however, must also be considered. First, M cells are more limited in their distribution, so that antigen sampling by these cells may be modest in the context of the whole gut. Second, M cells are rather inefficient at taking up soluble proteins. As stated earlier, soluble proteins are the best tolerogens. These two factors together suggest that sites other than PPs are important for tolerance induction.

Studies have attempted to clearly define the role of M cells and the PP in tolerance induction [111–113]. Work initially performed by Kerneis et al. documented the requirement of PP for M-cell development [114]. The induction of M-cell differentiation was dependent upon direct contact between the epithelium and PP lymphocytes (B cells). In the absence of PP, there are no M cells. In B-cell-deficient animals (where there are no PP), M cells have not been identified [115]. Several groups looked at tolerance induction in manipulated animals to assess the need for M cells in this process. In most cases, there appeared to be a direct correlation between the presence of PP and tolerance; however, each manipulation (LTβ–/–, LTβR–/–, treatment with LTβ-Fc fusion protein *in utero*) [116–118] is associated with abnormalities in systemic immunity as well (e.g., no spleen, altered mesenteric LNs), so interpretation of these data is clouded. Furthermore, compared to mice with intact PPs, PP-deficient mice were found to have the same frequencies of APCs in secondary lymphoid organs after oral administration of soluble antigen [113]. More recent data demonstrate that tolerance can occur in the absence of M cells and PPs. Kraus et al. created a mouse model of surgically isolated small bowel loops (fully vascularized with intact lymphatic drainage) that either contained or were deficient in M cells and PPs. They were able to generate comparable tolerance to OVA peptides in the presence or absence of PPs. These data strongly support the concept that cells other than M cells are involved in tolerance induction [111–113].

DCs play an important role in the tolerance and immunity of the gut. They function as APCs, directly sampling antigen from the lumen through transepithelial projections; help in maintaining gut integrity through expression of tight junction proteins; and orchestrate immune responses. DCs continuously migrate within lymphoid tissues even in the absence of inflammation and present self-antigens, likely from dying apoptotic cells, to maintain self-tolerance [119]. DCs process internalized antigens slower than macrophages, allowing adequate accumulation, processing, and eventually presentation of antigens [120]. They have been found within the LP and their presence is dependent on the chemokine receptor CX3CR1 to form transepithelial dendrites, which allows for direct sampling of antigen in the lumen [121, 122]. Studies are ongoing to determine the chemokines responsible for migration of DCs to the LP. However, what has been found is that epithelial cell-expressed CCL25, the ligand for CCR9 and CCR10, may be a DC chemokine in the small bowel, and CCL28, ligand for CCR3 and CCR10, may be a DC chemokine in the colon [123–125]. DCs in the LP were found to take up the majority of orally administered protein suggesting they may be tolerogenic [126]. Mowat, Viney, and colleagues expanded DCs in the LP by treating mice with Flt-3 ligand. The increase in gut DCs directly correlated with enhanced tolerance [127]. The continuous sampling and migration by DCs is thought to be responsible for T-cell tolerance to food antigens [128]. Several studies have examined the pathways by which DCs may be tolerogenic, including their maturation status at the time of antigen presentation to T cells; downregulation of costimulatory molecules CD80 and CD86; production of suppressive cytokines IL-10, TGF-β, and IFN-α; and interaction with costimulatory molecules CD200 [122, 129, 130]. Man et al. examined DC–T-cell cross-talk in relation to IgE-mediated allergic reactions to food, specifically investigating T-cell-mediated apoptosis of myeloid DCs from spleen and PPs of mice with a cow's milk allergy. DCs from mice with milk allergy exhibited reduced apoptosis compared to DCs from control nonallergic donors. This suggests that dysregulation of DCs, both systemic and gut derived, influences the development of food allergy and is necessary for controlling immune responses [131].

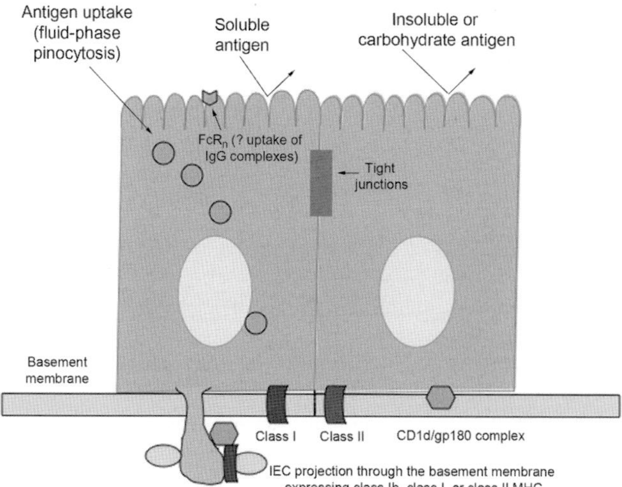

Figure 1.5 Antigen uptake by intestinal epithelial cells. Soluble proteins are taken up by fluid-phase endocytosis and pursue a transcellular pathway (endolysosomal pathway). Particulate and carbohydrate Ags are either not taken up or taken up with slower kinetics. Paracellular transport is blocked by the presence of tight junctions. In the case of antigen presentation by the intestinal epithelial cell, a complex of a nonclassical class I molecule (CD1d) and a CD8 ligand, gp180, is recognized by a subpopulation of T cells in the lamina propria (possibly intraepithelial space as well). The interaction of IEC with the LPL occurs by foot processes extruded by the IEC into the lamina propria through fenestrations in the basement membrane. Antigens can also be selectively taken up by a series of Fc receptors expressed by IEC (neonatal FcγR for IgG or CD23 for IgE). The consequences of such uptake may affect responses to food antigens (food allergy).

The other cell type potentially involved in antigen sampling is the absorptive epithelium (intestinal epithelial cells, IECs) based on its location between the lumen and a wide array of mucosal lymphocytes. The exact role of IECs in the adaptive and innate mucosal immune responses is still being investigated though it is likely the epithelium maintains homeostasis by modulating lymphocyte activation and controlling local inflammation through more than one mechanism and secreted products. This cell not only takes up soluble proteins but also expresses MHC class I, II, as well as nonclassical class I molecules to serve as restriction elements for local T-cell populations (Figure 1.5). Indeed, a number of groups have documented the capacity of IECs to serve as APCs, to both CD4+ and CD8+ T cells, recognizing and responding to bacterial and viral motifs by expression of the nucleotide-binding oligomerization domain and TLRs, and in turn producing cytokines and chemokines, which influence immune responses [132–140]. Furthermore, studies have shown that intestinal epithelial cells can influence T-regulatory cell expansion in the intestine [141]. In man, *in vitro* studies have suggested that normal IECs used as APCs selectively activate CD8+ suppressor T cells [137]. Activation of such cells could be involved in controlled inflammation and possibly oral tolerance. The studies by Kraus et al. described earlier (loop model) strongly support a role of IECs in tolerance induction. However, a role for IECs in the regulation of mucosal immunity is best demonstrated in studies of inflammatory bowel disease [142,143]. In *in vitro* coculture experiments with IECs from patients with inflammatory bowel disease, stimulated CD4+ T cells, rather than suppressive CD8+ cells, were activated by normal enterocytes [142]. Furthermore, Kraus et al. demonstrated that oral antigen administration does not result in tolerance in patients with inflammatory bowel but rather results in active immunity [144].

Once again, how does this fit into the process of food allergy? Do allergens traffic differently in predisposed individuals? Is there a Th2-dominant environment in the GALT of food-allergic patients? The real key is how the initial IgE is produced and what pathways are involved in its dominance. The answers to these questions will provide major insights into the pathogenesis and treatment of food allergy.

References

1. Kiyono H. Mucosal immune system: close encounter in the uncharted world of immunology. *Ophthalmologica* 2001; 215(Suppl. 1):22–32.
2. Mayer L, Sperber K, Chan L, Child J, Toy L. Oral tolerance to protein antigens. *Allergy* 2001; 56(Suppl. 67):12–15.
3. Farrell RJ, Kelly CP. Celiac sprue. *N Engl J Med* 2002; 346(3):180–188.
4. Freeman H, Lemoyne M, Pare P. Coeliac disease. *Best Pract Res Clin Gastroenterol* 2002; 16(1):37–49.
5. Farrell RJ, LaMont JT. Microbial factors in inflammatory bowel disease. *Gastroenterol Clin North Am* 2002; 31(1):41–62.
6. Basset C, Holton J. Inflammatory bowel disease: is the intestine a Trojan horse? *Sci Prog* 2002; 85(Pt. 1):33–56.
7. Prantera C, Scribano ML. Crohn's disease: the case for bacteria. *Ital J Gastroenterol Hepatol* 1999; 31(3):244–246.
8. Untersmayr E, Bakos N, Scholl I, et al. Anti-ulcer drugs promote IgE formation toward dietary antigens in adult patients. *FASEB J* 2005; 19(6):656–658.
9. Untersmayr E, Jensen-Jarolim E. The role of protein digestibility and antacids on food allergy outcomes. *J Allergy Clin Immunol* 2008; 121(6):1301–1308; quiz 1309–1310.
10. Geboes K. From inflammation to lesion. *Acta Gastroenterol Belg* 1994; 57(5–6):273–284.
11. Sartor RB. Current concepts of the etiology and pathogenesis of ulcerative colitis and Crohn's disease. *Gastroenterol Clin North Am* 1995; 24(3):475–507.
12. Mayer L. Mucosal immunity and gastrointestinal antigen processing. *J Pediatr Gastroenterol Nutr* 2000; 30(Suppl.):S4–S12.
13. Anderson JC. The response of gut-associated lymphoid tissue in gnotobiotic piglets to the presence of bacterial antigen in the alimentary tract. *J Anat* 1977; 124(3):555–562.

14. Ishikawa K, Satoh Y, Tanaka H, Ono K. Influence of conventionalization on small-intestinal mucosa of germ-free Wistar rats: quantitative light microscopic observations. *Acta Anat (Basel)* 1986; 127(4):296–302.
15. Cebra JJ, Periwal SB, Lee G, Lee F, Shroff KE. Development and maintenance of the gut-associated lymphoid tissue (GALT): the roles of enteric bacteria and viruses. *Dev Immunol* 1998; 6(1–2):13–18.
16. Rothkotter HJ, Ulbrich H, Pabst R. The postnatal development of gut lamina propria lymphocytes: number, proliferation, and T and B cell subsets in conventional and germ-free pigs. *Pediatr Res* 1991; 29(3):237–242.
17. Hamann A, Andrew DP, Jablonski-Westrich D, Holzmann B, Butcher EC. Role of alpha 4-integrins in lymphocyte homing to mucosal tissues in vivo. *J Immunol* 1994; 152(7):3282–3293.
18. Shyjan AM, Bertagnolli M, Kenney CJ, Briskin MJ. Human mucosal addressin cell adhesion molecule-1 (MAdCAM-1) demonstrates structural and functional similarities to the alpha 4 beta 7-integrin binding domains of murine MAdCAM-1, but extreme divergence of mucin-like sequences. *J Immunol* 1996; 156(8):2851–2857.
19. De Keyser F, Elewaut D, De Wever N, Bensbaho K, Cuvelier C. The gut associated addressins: lymphocyte homing in the gut. *Baillieres Clin Rheumatol* 1996; 10(1):25–39.
20. Viney JL, Jones S, Chiu HH, et al. Mucosal addressin cell adhesion molecule-1: a structural and functional analysis demarcates the integrin binding motif. *J Immunol* 1996; 157(6):2488–2497.
21. Saparov A, Kraus LA, Cong Y, et al. Memory/effector T cells in TCR transgenic mice develop via recognition of enteric antigens by a second, endogenous TCR. *Int Immunol* 1999; 11(8):1253–1264.
22. Qiao L, Schurmann G, Betzler M, Meuer SC. Activation and signaling status of human lamina propria T lymphocytes. *Gastroenterology* 1991; 101(6):1529–1536.
23. De Maria R, Fais S, Silvestri M, et al. Continuous in vivo activation and transient hyporesponsiveness to TcR/CD3 triggering of human gut lamina propria lymphocytes. *Eur J Immunol* 1993; 23(12):3104–3108.
24. Vezys V, Olson S, Lefrancois L. Expression of intestine-specific antigen reveals novel pathways of CD8 T cell tolerance induction. *Immunity* 2000; 12(5):505–514.
25. Smith PD, Smythies LE, Mosteller-Barnum M, et al. Intestinal macrophages lack CD14 and CD89 and consequently are down-regulated for LPS- and IgA-mediated activities. *J Immunol* 2001; 167(5):2651–2656.
26. Smythies LE, Maheshwari A, Clements R, et al. Mucosal IL-8 and TGF-beta recruit blood monocytes: evidence for cross-talk between the lamina propria stroma and myeloid cells. *J Leukoc Biol* 2006; 80(3):492–499.
27. Xiao BG, Link H. Mucosal tolerance: a two-edged sword to prevent and treat autoimmune diseases. *Clin Immunol Immunopathol* 1997; 85(2):119–128.
28. Whitacre CC, Gienapp IE, Meyer A, Cox KL, Javed N. Treatment of autoimmune disease by oral tolerance to autoantigens. *Clin Immunol Immunopathol* 1996; 80(3 Pt. 2): S31–S39.
29. Weiner HL, Mayer LF. Oral tolerance: mechanisms and applications [Introduction]. *Ann NY Acad Sci* 1996; 778:xiii–xviii.
30. Titus RG, Chiller JM. Orally induced tolerance. Definition at the cellular level. *Int Arch Allergy Appl Immunol* 1981; 65(3):323–338.
31. Strober W, Kelsall B, Marth T. Oral tolerance. *J Clin Immunol* 1998; 18(1):1–30.
32. MacDonald TT. T cell immunity to oral allergens. *Curr Opin Immunol* 1998; 10(6):620–627.
33. Webb Jr KE. Amino acid and peptide absorption from the gastrointestinal tract. *Fed Proc* 1986; 45(8):2268–2271.
34. Strobel S. Neonatal oral tolerance. *Ann NY Acad Sci* 1996; 778:88–102.
35. Du Toit G, Katz Y, Sasieni P, et al. Early consumption of peanuts in infancy is associated with a low prevalence of peanut allergy. *J Allergy Clin Immunol* 2008; 122(5):984–991.
36. Fox AT, Sasieni P, du Toit G, Syed H, Lack G. Household peanut consumption as a risk factor for the development of peanut allergy. *J Allergy Clin Immunol* 2009; 123(2): 417–423.
37. Greer FR, Sicherer SH, Burks AW. Effects of early nutritional interventions on the development of atopic disease in infants and children: the role of maternal dietary restriction, breast-feeding, timing of introduction of complementary foods, and hydrolyzed formulas. *Pediatrics* 2008; 121(1):183–191.
38. Burks AW, Laubach S, Jones SM. Oral tolerance, food allergy, and immunotherapy: implications for future treatment. *J Allergy Clin Immunol* 2008; 121(6):1344–1350.
39. Strobel S, Ferguson A. Immune responses to fed protein antigens in mice. 3. Systemic tolerance or priming is related to age at which antigen is first encountered. *Pediatr Res* 1984; 18(7):588–594.
40. Berin MC, Zheng Y, Domaradzki M, Li XM, Sampson HA. Role of TLR4 in allergic sensitization to food proteins in mice. *Allergy* 2006; 61(1):64–71.
41. Lamont AG, Mowat AM, Browning MJ, Parrott DM. Genetic control of oral tolerance to ovalbumin in mice. *Immunology* 1988; 63(4):737–739.
42. Garside P, Mowat AM. Mechanisms of oral tolerance. *Crit Rev Immunol* 1997; 17(2):119–137.
43. Roth-Walter F, Berin MC, Arnaboldi P, et al. Pasteurization of milk proteins promotes allergic sensitization by enhancing uptake through Peyer's patches. *Allergy* 2008; 63(7):882–890.
44. Lack G, Fox D, Northstone K, Golding J. Factors associated with the development of peanut allergy in childhood. *N Engl J Med* 2003; 348(11):977–985.
45. Hsieh KY, Tsai CC, Wu CH, Lin RH. Epicutaneous exposure to protein antigen and food allergy. *Clin Exp Allergy* 2003; 33(8):1067–1075.
46. Friedman A, Weiner HL. Induction of anergy or active suppression following oral tolerance is determined by antigen dosage. *Proc Natl Acad Sci USA* 1994; 91(14):6688–6692.
47. Hafler DA, Kent SC, Pietrusewicz MJ, Khoury SJ, Weiner HL, Fukaura H. Oral administration of myelin induces antigen-specific TGF-beta 1 secreting T cells in patients with multiple sclerosis. *Ann NY Acad Sci* 1997; 835:120–131.

48. Fukaura H, Kent SC, Pietrusewicz MJ, Khoury SJ, Weiner HL, Hafler DA. Induction of circulating myelin basic protein and proteolipid protein-specific transforming growth factor-beta1-secreting Th3 T cells by oral administration of myelin in multiple sclerosis patients. *J Clin Invest* 1996; 98(1):70–77.
49. Inobe J, Slavin AJ, Komagata Y, Chen Y, Liu L, Weiner HL. IL-4 is a differentiation factor for transforming growth factor-beta secreting Th3 cells and oral administration of IL-4 enhances oral tolerance in experimental allergic encephalomyelitis. *Eur J Immunol* 1998; 28(9):2780–2790.
50. Kunimoto DY, Ritzel M, Tsang M. The roles of IL-4, TGF-beta and LPS in IgA switching. *Eur Cytokine Netw* 1992; 3(4):407–415.
51. Kim PH, Kagnoff MF. Transforming growth factor beta 1 increases IgA isotype switching at the clonal level. *J Immunol* 1990; 145(11):3773–3778.
52. Coffman RL, Lebman DA, Shrader B. Transforming growth factor beta specifically enhances IgA production by lipopolysaccharide-stimulated murine B lymphocytes. *J Exp Med* 1989; 170(3):1039–1044.
53. Borsutzky S, Cazac BB, Roes J, Guzman CA. TGF-beta receptor signaling is critical for mucosal IgA responses. *J Immunol* 2004; 173(5):3305–3309.
54. Groux H, O'Garra A, Bigler M, et al. A CD4+ T-cell subset inhibits antigen-specific T-cell responses and prevents colitis. *Nature* 1997; 389(6652):737–742.
55. Levings MK, Roncarolo MG. T-regulatory 1 cells: a novel subset of CD4 T cells with immunoregulatory properties. *J Allergy Clin Immunol* 2000; 106(1 Pt. 2):S109–S112.
56. Roncarolo MG, Bacchetta R, Bordignon C, Narula S, Levings MK. Type 1 T regulatory cells. *Immunol Rev* 2001; 182:68–79.
57. Frossard CP, Tropia L, Hauser C, Eigenmann PA. Lymphocytes in Peyer patches regulate clinical tolerance in a murine model of food allergy. *J Allergy Clin Immunol* 2004; 113(5):958–964.
58. Sakaguchi S, Toda M, Asano M, Itoh M, Morse SS, Sakaguchi N. T cell-mediated maintenance of natural self-tolerance: its breakdown as a possible cause of various autoimmune diseases. *J Autoimmun* 1996; 9(2):211–220.
59. Sakaguchi S, Sakaguchi N, Shimizu J, et al. Immunologic tolerance maintained by CD25+ CD4+ regulatory T cells: their common role in controlling autoimmunity, tumor immunity, and transplantation tolerance. *Immunol Rev* 2001; 182:18–32.
60. Shevach EM, Thornton A, Suri-Payer E. T lymphocyte-mediated control of autoimmunity. *Novartis Found Symp* 1998; 215:200–211; discussion 11–30.
61. Nakamura K, Kitani A, Strober W. Cell contact-dependent immunosuppression by CD4(+)CD25(+) regulatory T cells is mediated by cell surface-bound transforming growth factor beta. *J Exp Med* 2001; 194(5):629–644.
62. Zhang X, Izikson L, Liu L, Weiner HL. Activation of CD25(+)CD4(+) regulatory T cells by oral antigen administration. *J Immunol* 2001; 167(8):4245–4253.
63. Chung Y, Lee SH, Kim DH, Kang CY. Complementary role of CD4+CD25+ regulatory T cells and TGF-beta in oral tolerance. *J Leukoc Biol* 2005; 77(6):906–913.
64. Hori S, Nomura T, Sakaguchi S. Control of regulatory T cell development by the transcription factor Foxp3. *Science* 2003; 299(5609):1057–1061.
65. McHugh RS, Shevach EM. The role of suppressor T cells in regulation of immune responses. *J Allergy Clin Immunol* 2002; 110(5):693–702.
66. Mowat AM, Lamont AG, Strobel S, Mackenzie S. The role of antigen processing and suppressor T cells in immune responses to dietary proteins in mice. *Adv Exp Med Biol* 1987; 216A:709–720.
67. Mowat AM, Lamont AG, Parrott DM. Suppressor T cells, antigen-presenting cells and the role of I-J restriction in oral tolerance to ovalbumin. *Immunology* 1988; 64(1):141–145.
68. Mowat AM. Depletion of suppressor T cells by 2'-deoxyguanosine abrogates tolerance in mice fed ovalbumin and permits the induction of intestinal delayed-type hypersensitivity. *Immunology* 1986; 58(2):179–184.
69. Mowat AM. The role of antigen recognition and suppressor cells in mice with oral tolerance to ovalbumin. *Immunology* 1985; 56(2):253–260.
70. Appleman LJ, Boussiotis VA. T cell anergy and costimulation. *Immunol Rev* 2003; 192:161–180.
71. Chen Y, Inobe J, Marks R, Gonnella P, Kuchroo VK, Weiner HL. Peripheral deletion of antigen-reactive T cells in oral tolerance. *Nature* 1995; 376(6536):177–180.
72. Forbes EE, Groschwitz K, Abonia JP, et al. IL-9- and mast cell-mediated intestinal permeability predisposes to oral antigen hypersensitivity. *J Exp Med* 2008; 205(4):897–913.
73. Groschwitz KR, Hogan SP. Intestinal barrier function: molecular regulation and disease pathogenesis. *J Allergy Clin Immunol* 2009; 124(1):3–20; quiz 21–22.
74. Brandt EB, Strait RT, Hershko D, et al. Mast cells are required for experimental oral allergen-induced diarrhea. *J Clin Invest* 2003; 112(11):1666–1677.
75. Li XM, Schofield BH, Huang CK, Kleiner GI, Sampson HA. A murine model of IgE-mediated cow's milk hypersensitivity. *J Allergy Clin Immunol* 1999; 103(2 Pt. 1):206–214.
76. Berin MC, Kiliaan AJ, Yang PC, Groot JA, Kitamura Y, Perdue MH. The influence of mast cells on pathways of transepithelial antigen transport in rat intestine. *J Immunol* 1998; 161(5):2561–2566.
77. Blanchard C, Stucke EM, Burwinkel K, et al. Coordinate interaction between IL-13 and epithelial differentiation cluster genes in eosinophilic esophagitis. *J Immunol* 2010; 184(7):4033–4041.
78. Madara JL, Stafford J. Interferon-gamma directly affects barrier function of cultured intestinal epithelial monolayers. *J Clin Invest* 1989; 83(2):724–727.
79. Zhang ZY, Michael JG. Orally inducible immune unresponsiveness is abrogated by IFN-gamma treatment. *J Immunol* 1990; 144(11):4163–4165.
80. Skripak JM, Nash SD, Rowley H, et al. A randomized, double-blind, placebo-controlled study of milk oral immunotherapy for cow's milk allergy. *J Allergy Clin Immunol* 2008; 122(6):1154–1160.
81. Clark AT, Islam S, King Y, Deighton J, Anagnostou K, Ewan PW. Successful oral tolerance induction in severe peanut allergy. *Allergy* 2009; 64(8):1218–1220.

82. Jones SM, Pons L, Roberts JL, et al. Clinical efficacy and immune regulation with peanut oral immunotherapy. *J Allergy Clin Immunol* 2009; 124(2):292–300; e1–e97.
83. Blumchen K, Ulbricht H, Staden U, et al. Oral peanut immunotherapy in children with peanut anaphylaxis. *J Allergy Clin Immunol* 2010; 126(1):83–91; e1.
84. Kagnoff MF. Immunology of the intestinal tract. *Gastroenterology* 1993; 105(5):1275–1280.
85. Brandtzaeg P, Valnes K, Scott H, Rognum TO, Bjerke K, Baklien K. The human gastrointestinal secretory immune system in health and disease. *Scand J Gastroenterol Suppl* 1985; 114:17–38.
86. Mostov KE, Kraehenbuhl JP, Blobel G. Receptor-mediated transcellular transport of immunoglobulin: synthesis of secretory component as multiple and larger transmembrane forms. *Proc Natl Acad Sci USA* 1980; 77(12):7257–7261.
87. Mostov KE, Blobel G. Transcellular transport of polymeric immunoglobulin by secretory component: a model system for studying intracellular protein sorting. *Ann NY Acad Sci* 1983; 409:441–451.
88. Mostov KE, Friedlander M, Blobel G. Structure and function of the receptor for polymeric immunoglobulins. *Biochem Soc Symp* 1986; 51:113–115.
89. Raux M, Finkielsztejn L, Salmon-Ceron D, et al. IgG subclass distribution in serum and various mucosal fluids of HIV type 1-infected subjects. *AIDS Res Hum Retroviruses* 2000; 16(6):583–594.
90. Schneider T, Zippel T, Schmidt W, et al. Increased immunoglobulin G production by short term cultured duodenal biopsy samples from HIV infected patients. *Gut* 1998; 42(3):357–361.
91. Israel EJ, Taylor S, Wu Z, et al. Expression of the neonatal Fc receptor, FcRn, on human intestinal epithelial cells. *Immunology* 1997; 92(1):69–74.
92. Dickinson BL, Badizadegan K, Wu Z, et al. Bidirectional FcRn-dependent IgG transport in a polarized human intestinal epithelial cell line. *J Clin Invest* 1999; 104(7):903–911.
93. Brambell FW. The transmission of immune globulins from the mother to the foetal and newborn young. *Proc Nutr Soc* 1969; 28(1):35–41.
94. Brambell FW, Hemmings WA, Morris IG. A theoretical model of gamma-globulin catabolism. *Nature* 1964; 203:1352–1354.
95. Simister NE, Mostov KE. An Fc receptor structurally related to MHC class I antigens. *Nature* 1989; 337(6203):184–187.
96. Roopenian DC, Sun VZ. Clinical ramifications of the MHC family Fc receptor FcRn. *J Clin Immunol* 2010; 30(6):790–797.
97. Masuda A, Yoshida M, Shiomi H, et al. Role of Fc receptors as a therapeutic target. *Inflamm Allergy Drug Targets* 2009; 8(1):80–86.
98. Sesarman A, Vidarsson G, Sitaru C. The neonatal Fc receptor as therapeutic target in IgG-mediated autoimmune diseases. *Cell Mol Life Sci* 2010; 67(15):2533–2550.
99. Berin MC, Yang PC, Ciok L, Waserman S, Perdue MH. Role for IL-4 in macromolecular transport across human intestinal epithelium. *Am J Physiol* 1999; 276(5 Pt. 1):C1046–C1052.
100. Li H, Chehade M, Liu W, Xiong H, Mayer L, Berin MC. Allergen-IgE complexes trigger CD23-dependent CCL20 release from human intestinal epithelial cells. *Gastroenterology* 2007; 133(6):1905–1915.
101. Berin MC, Mayer L. Immunophysiology of experimental food allergy. *Mucosal Immunol* 2009; 2(1):24–32.
102. Bhalla DK, Owen RL. Migration of B and T lymphocytes to M cells in Peyer's patch follicle epithelium: an autoradiographic and immunocytochemical study in mice. *Cell Immunol* 1983; 81(1):105–117.
103. Kraehenbuhl JP, Pringault E, Neutra MR. Review article: intestinal epithelia and barrier functions. *Aliment Pharmacol Ther* 1997; 11(Suppl. 3):3–8; discussion 8–9.
104. Neutra MR. Current concepts in mucosal immunity. V Role of M cells in transepithelial transport of antigens and pathogens to the mucosal immune system. *Am J Physiol* 1998; 274(5 Pt. 1):G785-G791.
105. Owen RL. Sequential uptake of horseradish peroxidase by lymphoid follicle epithelium of Peyer's patches in the normal unobstructed mouse intestine: an ultrastructural study. *Gastroenterology* 1977; 72(3):440–451.
106. Allan CH, Mendrick DL, Trier JS. Rat intestinal M cells contain acidic endosomal-lysosomal compartments and express class II major histocompatibility complex determinants. *Gastroenterology* 1993; 104(3):698–708.
107. Kraehenbuhl JP, Neutra MR. Epithelial M cells: differentiation and function. *Annu Rev Cell Dev Biol* 2000; 16:301–332.
108. Miller H, Zhang J, Kuolee R, Patel GB, Chen W. Intestinal M cells: the fallible sentinels? *World J Gastroenterol* 2007; 13(10):1477–1486.
109. Sicinski P, Rowinski J, Warchol JB, et al. Poliovirus type 1 enters the human host through intestinal M cells. *Gastroenterology* 1990; 98(1):56–58.
110. Frossard CP, Hauser C, Eigenmann PA. Antigen-specific secretory IgA antibodies in the gut are decreased in a mouse model of food allergy. *J Allergy Clin Immunol* 2004; 114(2):377–382.
111. Kraus TA, Brimnes J, Muong C, et al. Induction of mucosal tolerance in Peyer's patch-deficient, ligated small bowel loops. *J Clin Invest* 2005; 115(8):2234–2243.
112. Mowat AM. Anatomical basis of tolerance and immunity to intestinal antigens. *Nat Rev Immunol* 2003; 3(4):331–341.
113. Kunkel D, Kirchhoff D, Nishikawa S, Radbruch A, Scheffold A. Visualization of peptide presentation following oral application of antigen in normal and Peyer's patches-deficient mice. *Eur J Immunol* 2003; 33(5):1292–1301.
114. Kerneis S, Bogdanova A, Kraehenbuhl JP, Pringault E. Conversion by Peyer's patch lymphocytes of human enterocytes into M cells that transport bacteria. *Science* 1997; 277(5328):949–952.
115. Gonnella PA, Waldner HP, Weiner HL. B cell-deficient (mu MT) mice have alterations in the cytokine microenvironment of the gut-associated lymphoid tissue (GALT) and a defect in the low dose mechanism of oral tolerance. *J Immunol* 2001; 166(7):4456–4464.
116. Fujihashi K, Dohi T, Rennert PD, et al. Peyer's patches are required for oral tolerance to proteins. *Proc Natl Acad Sci USA* 2001; 98(6):3310–3315.

117. Spahn TW, Fontana A, Faria AM, et al. Induction of oral tolerance to cellular immune responses in the absence of Peyer's patches. *Eur J Immunol* 2001; 31(4):1278–1287.
118. Spahn TW, Weiner HL, Rennert PD, et al. Mesenteric lymph nodes are critical for the induction of high-dose oral tolerance in the absence of Peyer's patches. *Eur J Immunol* 2002; 32(4):1109–1113.
119. Steinman RM, Hawiger D, Nussenzweig MC. Tolerogenic dendritic cells. *Annu Rev Immunol* 2003; 21:685–711.
120. Delamarre L, Pack M, Chang H, Mellman I, Trombetta ES. Differential lysosomal proteolysis in antigen-presenting cells determines antigen fate. *Science* 2005; 307(5715):1630–1634.
121. Niess JH, Brand S, Gu X, et al. CX3CR1-mediated dendritic cell access to the intestinal lumen and bacterial clearance. *Science* 2005; 307(5707):254–258.
122. Niess JH, Reinecker HC. Lamina propria dendritic cells in the physiology and pathology of the gastrointestinal tract. *Curr Opin Gastroenterol* 2005; 21(6):687–691.
123. Kunkel EJ, Campbell DJ, Butcher EC. Chemokines in lymphocyte trafficking and intestinal immunity. *Microcirculation* 2003; 10(3–4):313–323.
124. Zhao X, Sato A, Dela Cruz CS, et al. CCL9 is secreted by the follicle-associated epithelium and recruits dome region Peyer's patch CD11b+ dendritic cells. *J Immunol* 2003; 171(6):2797–2803.
125. Caux C, Vanbervliet B, Massacrier C, et al. Regulation of dendritic cell recruitment by chemokines. *Transplantation* 2002; 73(1 Suppl.):S7–S11.
126. Chirdo FG, Millington OR, Beacock-Sharp H, Mowat AM. Immunomodulatory dendritic cells in intestinal lamina propria. *Eur J Immunol* 2005; 35(6):1831–1840.
127. Viney JL, Mowat AM, O'Malley JM, Williamson E, Fanger NA. Expanding dendritic cells in vivo enhances the induction of oral tolerance. *J Immunol* 1998; 160(12):5815–5825.
128. Mowat AM, Donachie AM, Parker LA, et al. The role of dendritic cells in regulating mucosal immunity and tolerance. *Novartis Found Symp* 2003; 252:291–302; discussion 302–305.
129. Gorczynski RM, Lee L, Boudakov I. Augmented induction of CD4+CD25+ Treg using monoclonal antibodies to CD200R. *Transplantation* 2005; 79(4):488–491.
130. Yamagiwa S, Gray JD, Hashimoto S, Horwitz DA. A role for TGF-beta in the generation and expansion of CD4+CD25+ regulatory T cells from human peripheral blood. *J Immunol* 2001; 166(12):7282–7289.
131. Man AL, Bertelli E, Regoli M, Chambers SJ, Nicoletti C. Antigen-specific T cell-mediated apoptosis of dendritic cells is impaired in a mouse model of food allergy. *J Allergy Clin Immunol* 2004; 113(5):965–972.
132. Bland PW. Antigen presentation by gut epithelial cells: secretion by rat enterocytes of a factor with IL-1-like activity. *Adv Exp Med Biol* 1987; 216A:219–225.
133. Bland PW, Kambarage DM. Antigen handling by the epithelium and lamina propria macrophages. *Gastroenterol Clin North Am* 1991; 20(3):577–596.
134. Hershberg RM, Framson PE, Cho DH, et al. Intestinal epithelial cells use two distinct pathways for HLA class II antigen processing. *J Clin Invest* 1997; 100(1):204–215.
135. Hershberg RM, Cho DH, Youakim A, et al. Highly polarized HLA class II antigen processing and presentation by human intestinal epithelial cells. *J Clin Invest* 1998; 102(4):792–803.
136. Hershberg RM, Mayer LF. Antigen processing and presentation by intestinal epithelial cells—polarity and complexity. *Immunol Today* 2000; 21(3):123–128.
137. Mayer L, Shlien R. Evidence for function of Ia molecules on gut epithelial cells in man. *J Exp Med* 1987; 166(5):1471–1483.
138. Mayer L. The role of the epithelium in mucosal immunity. *Res Immunol* 1997; 148(8–9):498–504.
139. Kaiserlian D, Vidal K, Revillard JP. Murine enterocytes can present soluble antigen to specific class II-restricted CD4+ T cells. *Eur J Immunol* 1989; 19(8):1513–1516.
140. Dahan S, Roth-Walter F, Arnaboldi P, Agarwal S, Mayer L. Epithelia: lymphocyte interactions in the gut. *Immunol Rev* 2007; 215:243–253.
141. Allez M, Brimnes J, Dotan I, Mayer L. Expansion of CD8+ T cells with regulatory function after interaction with intestinal epithelial cells. *Gastroenterology* 2002; 123(5):1516–1526.
142. Mayer L, Eisenhardt D. Lack of induction of suppressor T cells by intestinal epithelial cells from patients with inflammatory bowel disease. *J Clin Invest* 1990; 86(4):1255–1260.
143. Dotan I, Allez M, Nakazawa A, Brimnes J, Schulder-Katz M, Mayer L. Intestinal epithelial cells from inflammatory bowel disease patients preferentially stimulate CD4+ T cells to proliferate and secrete interferon-gamma. *Am J Physiol Gastrointest Liver Physiol* 2007; 292(6):G1630–G1640.
144. Kraus TA, Toy L, Chan L, Childs J, Mayer L. Failure to induce oral tolerance to a soluble protein in patients with inflammatory bowel disease. *Gastroenterology* 2004; 126(7):1771–1778.

2

The Immunological Basis of IgE-Mediated Reactions

Stephan C. Bischoff[1] & Gernot Sellge[2]
[1]Institute of Nutritional Medicine and Immunology, University of Hohenheim, Stuttgart, Germany
[2]Department of Medicine III, University Hospital Aachen, Aachen, Germany

Key Concepts

- Sensitization to food allergens resulting in synthesis of specific IgE against food occurs via the gastrointestinal tract (true food allergens) or via the pulmonary route (cross-reactive aeroallergens).
- Food allergens are not completely hydrolyzed in the stomach and may cross the mucosal barrier and be transported throughout the body in an immunologically intact form that can bind to antigen-specific IgE.
- A dysregulated immune response to food allergens, consisting of a strong Th2 and IgE response and a low regulatory T cell and IgG/IgA response, promotes the development of IgE-dependent allergic reactions to foods.
- Genetic, epigenetic, and environmental factors influence an individual immune reaction to a food allergen.
- Cross-linking of IgE on tissue mast cells is followed by the release of proinflammatory mediators and initiates the acute-phase reaction and the recruitment of eosinophils, basophils, and lymphocytes.

Introduction

Food allergy, defined as immune-mediated food intolerance, can be divided into "IgE-mediated" disorders (immediate-type gastrointestinal hypersensitivity, oral allergy syndrome, acute urticaria and angioedema, allergic rhinitis, acute bronchospasm, anaphylaxis) and "non-IgE-mediated" disorders (dietary protein-induced enterocolitis and proctitis, celiac disease, and dermatitis herpetiformis). This classification has been extended by supposing a third subgroup of "mixed IgE- and non-IgE-mediated" disorders such as allergic eosinophilic esophagitis and gastroenteritis, atopic dermatitis, and allergic asthma [1, 2].

In this chapter, the underlying immune mechanisms of IgE-mediated allergic reactions with a particular focus on food allergy and gastrointestinal reactions will be discussed. The development of food allergy is a multistep process, requiring repetitive exposure to a particular food antigen, in contrast to nonimmune-mediated reactions, which can cause symptoms even after a single food exposure. The disease is preceded by a sensitization phase without symptoms, in which allergen-specific T and B cells are primed and IgE is produced. Recurrent allergen challenge of sensitized individuals results in IgE cross-linking bound on tissue mast cells that subsequently induces the release of proinflammatory mediators and perpetuates allergic inflammation involving other cells such as basophils, eosinophils, and T cells.

Route of sensitization

Food allergy may result from sensitization to ingested food proteins or to aeroallergens through the respiratory route. Several pollen allergens can confer cross-reactivity to homologous proteins in plant foods. It has been suggested that oral sensitization only occurs when allergens are highly resistant to digestion in the gastrointestinal tract, while pollen food cross-reactive proteins are labile [2]. The route of sensitization appears, therefore, to influence the allergenic response on a molecular level and influence the clinical manifestations after challenge. This relationship has been supported by a multicenter study across Europe [3]. In the Netherlands, Austria, and northern Italy apple allergy is mild (90% present exclusively oral symptoms) and precedes birch pollen allergy. The apple allergy arises

Food Allergy: Adverse Reactions to Foods and Food Additives, Fifth Edition. Edited by Dean D Metcalfe, Hugh A Sampson, Ronald A Simon and Gideon Lack.

as a result of the cross-reactivity between the birch pollen allergen Bet v 1 and the apple allergen Mal d 1. In Spain, exposure to birch pollen is virtually absent and the main apple allergen is Mal d 3. The authors suggested that the apple allergy in Spain is a result of a primary sensitization to peach and its major allergen Pru p 3, which is cross-reactive to Mal d 3. Both proteins belong to the nonspecific lipid transfer proteins, which are resistant to proteolysis and responsible for severe anaphylactic reactions. Consequently, about 35% of the Spanish patients have systemic reactions after double-blind, placebo-controlled food challenges with apple [3].

Allergen uptake in the intestine

The gut epithelium forms a tight barrier to the enormous bulk of food and indigenous microbes present in the lumen. Innate and adoptive mechanisms have been developed to control the immune balance to food and commensals and to fend off pathogens. Gastric acid, mucus, an intact epithelial layer, digestive enzymes, and intestinal peristalsis constitute the "nonimmunological" barrier. The immunological defense mechanisms include innate (antimicrobial peptides, immune cells expressing pattern recognition molecules, etc.) and adaptive mechanisms (lymphocytes, IgA) [4]. However, antigens such as nondigested or partially digested food proteins and bacterial products (e.g., peptidoglycans) as well as whole commensal bacteria can be detected in the mucosa and draining lymph nodes, while soluble antigens can also be found in the blood and may reach other tissues. During intestinal steady-state conditions, this antigen uptake is tightly regulated and can occur via different routes, including passage through intestinal epithelial cells and M cells or through direct uptake by transepithelial dendrites of dendritic cells [4–6].

Breakdown of the intestinal barrier is associated with the development of food allergy [7]. Neutralization of gastric acid results in increased mucosal transport of ingested proteins and sensitization to allergens [8]. Intestinal permeability is increased in patients suffering from food allergy [9]. Interestingly, one study showed that intestinal permeability is increased in patients with bronchial asthma, supporting the hypothesis that a general defect of the mucosal system may facilitate the development of allergic diseases [10]. Further evidence that a barrier dysfunction is a risk factor for developing food allergy comes from the notion that IgA deficiency or retarded IgA development in infants [7, 11, 12] is associated with a higher risk of atopy.

Many food allergens are fairly stable to heat, acid, and proteases, making them resistant to digestion and allowing them to interact with the intestinal immune system. It has been demonstrated that ingested food proteins may be transported throughout the body in an immunologically intact form [2, 13]. This may explain why symptoms of food allergies are not restricted to the gastrointestinal tract, but often cause additional or even exclusive extraintestinal symptoms.

T-cell response in IgE-mediated allergy

A hallmark of IgE-mediated allergic disorders is the generation of allergen-specific CD4+ T helper (Th) 2 lymphocytes. These cells produce a characteristic Th2 cytokine profile consisting of IL-4, IL-5, IL-9, and IL-13. IL-4 and IL-13 induce IgE class-switching in B cells; IL-4 and IL-9 are important growth and activation factors for mast cells; and IL-5 promotes eosinophil development and recruitment. IL-13 additionally triggers mucus secretion in the lung and provokes airway hypersensitivity [14, 15]. In the 1990s, allergic sensitization to environmental proteins (allergens) was attributed to a dysregulation of the Th1/Th2 balance. However, the simple dichotomy of the Th1/Th2 system has been challenged by the discovery of a plethora of new helper T-cell subsets, including Th9, Th17, Th22 cells, follicular helper CD4+ T cells (TFH), nonclassical T cells such as NKT and γδ T cells, different subsets of CD8+ T cells, and regulatory T (Treg) cells [16, 17]. Studies also now show high variability in cytokine profiles of distinct subtypes and phenotypic plasticity [16]. For example, Th2 cells can develop into "noninflammatory Th2 cells" that produce the anti-inflammatory cytokine IL-10 [17]. A human study describes distinct peanut-specific Th2 subtypes in patients with IgE-dependent anaphylactic reactions to peanuts that express IL-4, but not IL-5, and in patients with IgE-independent eosinophilic gastroenteritis that express IL-4 and IL-5 [18].

The actual concept states that allergies and also autoimmune diseases result from an imbalance between a protective Treg response and a disease-inducing effector Th2 (in the case of allergy) or Th1/Th17 response (in the case of autoimmune diseases) [16]. Furthermore, different effector T-cell subsets have counter-regulatory functions, which also play a role in the immune-regulatory network. Natural Tregs (nTregs) that express the transcription factor forkhead box P3 (FoxP3) are formed in the thymus and react to self-antigens. Inducible regulatory T cells (iTreg) develop in the periphery and are specific to foreign antigens. iTreg are further subdivided into FoxP3+ T cells and FoxP3-negative regulatory T cells such as IL-10-producing Tr1 cells and TGF-β-producing Th3 cells. iTreg are triggered by host factors such as TGF-β and environmental factors such as retinoic acid and the intestinal microbiota [19, 20]. Whereas nTregs are important to suppress autoimmune disease, iTreg control the immune response to environmental antigens such as allergens [21]. Tregs act via the production of TGF-β and IL-10 or by cell–cell contact-dependent suppression. They suppress effector Th cell activation, stimulate IgG4 (indirectly induced by IL-10) and IgA (induced by TGF-β) class-switch in B cells, and inhibit mast cell and eosinophil functions through the production of IL-10 and TGF-β [20]. The function of Treg cells are impaired or dysregulated in allergic patients [22]. It is noteworthy to mention that a large number of healthy individuals are sensitized to allergens. However, these persons likely mount a balanced immune response, consisting of allergen-specific Tr1 cells and high levels of protective antigen-specific IgG4 and IgA (Figure 2.1) [22]. Evidence for the importance of Treg cells in the prevention of allergy arises also from the finding that successful specific immunotherapy (SIT) is associated with a decrease in allergen-specific Th2 cell responses and the induction of allergen-induced Tr1 and Th3 cells (Figure 2.1) [22, 23].

Why an overreacting Th2-type response occurs in allergic patients remains largely obscure. Th2 cells are protective in the course of helminth infections and are stimulated by innate immune signals that are triggered by helminth-derived factors, which are sensed by pattern recognition receptors. Also allergens have been shown to trigger the innate immune system leading to the production of a Th2-type environment (see below). Factors released by epithelial cells in response to helminths and allergens are IL-25, IL-33, and TLSP that stimulate innate immune cells such as basophils (via TLSP) and a class of immune cells exerting a lymphoid morphology (via IL-25 and IL-33). These cells secrete Th2-type cytokines like IL-4, IL-5, and IL-13, further orchestrating the priming of Th2 cells and subsequent IgE production by plasma cells. These innate lymphocytes have been named natural helper, nuocyte, and MPP type 2 cells [17, 24].

B-cell response in IgE-mediated allergy

Antigen-specific IgE produced by B cells is essential for type I allergic reactions. Apart from its pathological function in allergies, antigen-specific IgE is an important component of protective immunity against helminths [25]. Class-switch recombination (CSR) is strongly dependent on T-cell help [26], although some evidence exists that other cells, including mast cells, basophils, and eosinophils, can also provide the required signals [27]. Naïve B cells capture their specific antigen (allergen) by the B-cell receptor (BCR), process it, and present it in the context of major histocompatibility complex (MCH) class II to T cells. A number of findings provide strong evidence that T-cell help within germinal centers of lymphoid follicles is provided by specialized follicular helper CD4+ T cells (TFH) rather than by canonical Th cells. TFH cells depend on the expression of the master regulator transcription factor Bcl6 and are characterized by the expression of specific factors such as high levels of IL-21. The understanding of how the development of distinct TFH cell subsets is related to classical Th cells and how they regulate the CSR in B cells for the expression of different immunoglobulin subclasses is incomplete [26]. However, an important role of IL-4-producing TFH cells for a Th2-type immune response upon parasite infections has been shown [28].

Activated B cells subsequently expand and are subjected to affinity maturation by somatic hypermutation. It is a matter of debate whether (i) IgE+ B cells mature mainly within germinal centers comparable to IgG+ B cells and produce high-affinity IgEs [29] or whether (ii) most IgE+ B cells are only transiently present in germinal centers, producing low-affinity IgE while high-affinity IgE production occurs via IgG1+ intermediates in which somatic hypermutation and affinity maturation take place followed by a post-IgE-switching phase [30]. After CSR and affinity maturation, B cells migrate from the lymphoid organs to mucosal effector sites and undergo terminal differentiation to plasma cells [4]. However, some reports suggested that CSR might also occur at mucosal sites in allergic patients [31].

IgE plasma levels are the lowest and the biological half-life is the shortest (~12 hours in the serum [32] and ~14 days in the skin [33]) of all immunoglobulin classes. Elevated titers of antigen-specific IgE are found in

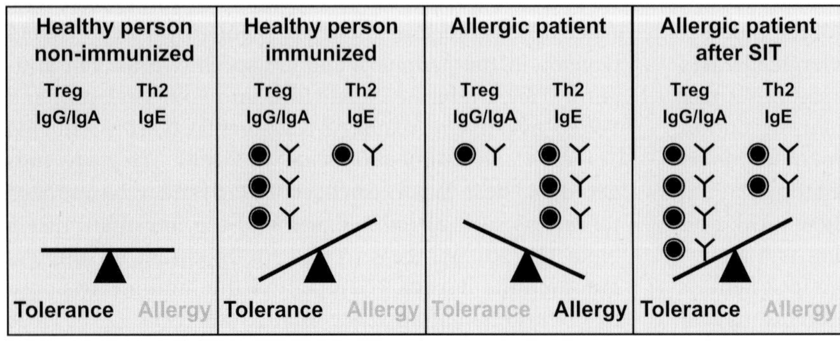

Figure 2.1 Immune response to allergens in healthy and allergic individuals.

allergic patients and after helminth infections, even in the absence of antigen for several years [25, 34]. This observation is consistent with clinical experience, since patients can develop recurrent allergic symptoms despite long-term allergen avoidance. Stable maintenance of B-cell memory can be divided into two broad categories: long-lived plasma cells and memory B cells. Three competing concepts, which are not mutually exclusive, might explain humoral memory. First, short-lived plasma cells (which do not divide) are constantly generated from memory B cells, a process that might be driven by persisting antigen. Second, long-lived plasma cells with a defined half-life of several weeks develop from cytokine-receptor or Toll-like receptor (TLR)-activated memory B cells. Third, memory arises from long-lived plasma cells that survive in appropriate survival niches, which are located in the bone marrow and possibly in secondary lymphoid organs and inflamed tissue [35]. Whether IgE is predominately produced within or outside mucosal sites is a matter of debate [35, 36]. The fact that allergen-specific IgE production can be transferred by bone marrow transplantation argues that bone marrow-derived IgE might contribute to the sensitization of effector cells at mucosal surfaces [37]. The persistence of allergen-specific IgE even under immunosuppressive therapy suggests that long-lived plasma cells (possibly located in the bone marrow) contribute substantially to IgE-mediated allergy, because long-lived plasma cells are resistant to immunosuppression [35].

Allergen-specific IgG and IgA

Allergen-specific IgG1, IgG4, and IgA are frequently detectable in allergic and nonallergic individuals. It has been proposed that these immunoglobulin subclasses prevent allergic reactions. Evidence for the protective effect of allergen-specific IgG arises from SIT and oral immunotherapy studies [38–40]. Specific IgE levels do not always decrease upon successful SIT or even increase at the beginning of the therapy [41]. However, many studies show that allergen-specific IgG1 and, in particular, IgG4 levels largely increase [38–41] (Figure 2.1). Allergen-specific IgG/IgE ratios rather than total allergen-specific IgE levels have been linked to allergen tolerance and the effectiveness of immunotherapy (Figure 2.1). For example, allergen-specific IgG4/IgE ratios were found to be about 1000 times higher in nonallergic beekeepers compared with bee venom-allergic individuals [42].

IgG acts as "blocking antibody" while competing with IgE for the binding of allergen epitopes and, therefore, inhibits high-affinity Fc receptor (FcεRI) cross-linking on mast cells and basophils [38, 39, 43, 44]. Furthermore, allergen-specific IgG co-aggregates FcγRIIB with FcεRI. FcγRIIB contains an intracytoplasmatic immunoreceptor tyrosine-based inhibitory motif (ITIM) and has been reported to inhibit IgE-induced mast cell and basophil activation [44, 45]. Co-cross-linking of FcγRIIB and FcεRI might also be exploited for the engineering of safe therapeutic agents for SIT that maintain all B- and T-cell epitopes. A human IgG1 Fc fragment fused to the cat allergen Fel d 1 was reported to inhibit Fel d 1-induced activation of human mast cells and basophils sensitized with serum from patients allergic to Fel d 1 and also Fel d 1-induced anaphylaxis in human FcεRIa transgenic mice [46].

The relationship between the efficacy of SIT and the induction of allergen-specific IgG has also been questioned, because some studies failed to demonstrate a correlation [47]. One study showed that long-term effectiveness after allergen immunotherapy is associated with the presence of high-affinity allergen-specific IgG with strong inhibitory bioactivity, although overall allergen-specific IgG levels decreased nearly to pre-immunotherapy levels during discontinuation of the therapy [48].

The conflicting data might also be explained by the fact that allergen-specific IgG can have immune-enhancing effects. For example, IgG can stimulate immune cells such as mast cells and eosinophils through binding to activating Fcγ receptors (Table 2.1). Allergen-specific IgG may enhance allergic reactions by the formation of larger allergen aggregates (super-cross-linking) [50] or by activating complement (IgG1–3, not IgG4). Furthermore, the binding of certain IgG to allergens can enhance IgE affinity, which may be due to changes of the three-dimensional allergen structure [51]. However, IgG4 seems to be of particular importance to prevent allergic reactions. It binds only with low affinity to Fcγ receptors and does not activate complement. Furthermore, it has been shown that IgG4 antibodies are dynamic molecules that exchange Fab arms by swapping a heavy chain and attached light chain (half-molecule) with a heavy–light chain pair from another molecule, which results in bispecific antibodies. IgG4 molecules thereby lose their ability to cross-link antigen and to form immune complexes under most conditions. This mechanism might provide the basis for the anti-inflammatory activity attributed to IgG4 [52].

Obviously, the clinical consequences of an allergen exposure are influenced by several factors: (i) allergen structure, (ii) dose and duration of exposure, (iii) epitope specificity and affinity of the antibodies, (iv) absolute and relative amounts of immunoglobulin subclasses, (v) expression profiles of Fc receptors on effector cells, (vi) composition and activation status of immune cells in the exposed tissue, and (vii) profile of allergen-specific effector T cells. This demonstrates that monitoring of SIT by measurement of antigen-specific immunoglobulins can sometimes be misleading and that complex biological systems are required to analyze the immunological effects of SIT.

Table 2.1 Fc receptors on mast cells, eosinophils, and basophils.

Receptor (CD)	Chains	Binding affinity	Ligands	Expression MC, E, Ba	Other cells
FcγRI(CD64)	α, γ	Ig1: 10^8 M^{-1}	(1) IgG1 = IgG3, (2) IgG4, (3) IgG2	MC, E[a]	M, N[a], DC
FcγRII-A(CD32)	α	Ig1: 2×10^6 M^{-1}	(1) IgG1, (2) IgG2[b] = IgG3, (3) IgG4	MC, E, Ba[c]	M, N, LC, P
FcγRII-B(CD32)	α[d]	Ig1: 2×10^6 M^{-1}	(1) IgG1 = IgG3, (2) IgG4, (3) IgG2	MC, E, Ba[c]	M, N, B
FcγRIII(CD16)	α, β, γ	Ig1: 5×10^5 M^{-1}	(1) IgG1 = IgG3, (2) IgG4, (3) IgG2	E	M, N, B
FcαRI(CD89)	α, γ	IgA1, IgA2:	IgA1 = IgA2	E	M, N
FcεRI	α, β, γ	IgE: 10^{10} M^{-1}	IgE	MC, Ba, E[a,e]	M[e],DC[e],LC[e]
FcεRII[f](CD23)	Single	IgE: 10^8 M^{-1},	IgE, others[g]	E	B, T, M, LC, P

Source: Modified from Reference 49.

MC, mast cells; E, eosinophils; Ba, basophils; M, monocytes; N, neutrophils; B, B cells; T, T cells; DC, dendritic cells; LC, Langerhans cells; P, platelets.

[a]Inducible.

[b]Only some allotypes of FcγRII-A bind IgG2.

[c]CD32 expression has been shown, but to date it is not clear whether FcγRII-A or FcγRII-B is expressed.

[d]Contains an ITIM motif (inhibitory).

[e]β-Chain is not expressed.

[f]Two isoforms (a and b) exist. FcεRIIa is mainly expressed on B cells; FcεRIIb also on other cells.

[g]See text (IgE receptors).

Genes and environment

It is generally acknowledged that risk factors for the development of allergic diseases include genetic and environmental factors. More recently, epigenetic factors have experienced increasing attention in allergology.

Sibling and family studies have revealed that the genetic background affects the risk of developing allergy. These observations can be related to several gene polymorphisms. Not surprisingly, many of these genes encode for key factors of Th2-type and IgE-related immune reactions, such as FcεRI b chain, IL-4R, IL-13, and STAT6 [53, 54]. For certain atopic diseases, particular mutations have been identified. For example, loss-of-function mutations in filaggrin have been described in patients with atopic eczema and are associated with an increased risk of atopic sensitization in these individuals [55]. In contrast, for other diseases such as food allergy, data are limited and can be only extrapolated from inhalant allergies and asthma to food allergy. Interestingly, genes encoding for innate immune receptors that recognize bacteria or bacterial products, such as CD14 and NOD1, are associated with allergy [56]. These analyses suggest that the threshold of the immune system to environmental stimuli is controlled by natural genetic variation and gene–environment interaction, as well as by pathogenic or commensal bacteria.

In the last few years, the role of the commensal intestinal microbiota has drawn attention. The microbiota interacts with the innate and adaptive arms of the host's intestinal mucosal immune system and through these mechanisms drives regulatory cell differentiation in the gut that is critically involved in maintaining immune tolerance. Specifically, the microbiota can activate distinct tolerogenic dendritic cells in the gut and through this interaction can drive regulatory T-cell differentiation. In addition, the microbiota is important in driving Th1 cell differentiation, which corrects the Th2 immune skewing that is thought to occur at birth. If appropriate immune tolerance is not established in early life and maintained throughout life, this represents a risk factor for the development of IgE-dependent allergic diseases and other immune-mediated disorders [57].

Prevalence of allergic diseases is considerably lower in developing countries and in rural areas in comparison to urban areas within one country. Furthermore, the number of allergic patients has increased within the last few decades, further arguing that environmental factors are substantially responsible for atopy [58]. However, there is little consistent evidence to suggest that obvious risk factors, such as increased exposure to indoor allergens, pollution, or changes in diet and breast-feeding, could account for the rise in allergic diseases. Another category of environmental factors that show some inverse association with atopy are infections, vaccinations, absence of antibiotic treatment, traditional farming environments, older siblings, day care attendance, and pet ownership [58, 59]. Most relevant in this context is the finding that children living on farms were exposed to a wider range of microbes than were other children in other living areas, and this exposure explains a substantial fraction of the inverse relation between asthma and growing up on a farm [60].

These findings lead to the "hygiene hypothesis," which is now not only based on epidemiologic association studies [61]. The hypothesis is thus strengthened by findings indicating particular microbiological stimuli are needed for the transfer of protection such as *Bacteroides fragilis*-derived polysaccharide [62] or *Acinetobacter lwoffii* and *Lactococcus lactis* [63]. Such findings could become the basis not only of novel prevention strategies but also for the development of new preventive drugs like bacterial polysaccharides or probiotic-like substances [64]. However, such new findings are not easily transferred to clinical practice just by using existing probiotics developed for other purposes than allergy protection as evidenced by the conflicting results on allergy and eczema protection by maternal treatment with *Lactobacillus rhamnosus* GG [65].

Tolerance induction might involve both the innate and the adaptive immune systems. Animal studies show protective effects of certain TLR ligands in allergen-induced inflammation [56]. Furthermore, microbial components such as CpG-containing immunostimulatory DNA, a TLR9 agonist, or the bacterial cell wall component monophosphoryl lipid A have been used successfully as adjuvants in clinical studies for SIT. These compounds considerably improve immunological surrogate markers and clinical outcome [66, 67]. Chronic infections might induce Treg cells that provide nonspecific bystander suppression [68]. Moreover, it has been suggested that cross-reactive IgE and IgG-binding structures exist in allergens and parasite antigens [68]. Interestingly, parasite-specific IgG4 antibodies can inhibit IgE-mediated degranulation of effector cells isolated from allergic patients, suggesting that chronic parasite infections induce allergen-cross-reactive "blocking antibodies" [69].

Environmental factors might influence IgE-dependent allergic reactions via epigenetic mechanisms as revealed by studies showing that early environmental exposures play a key role in activating or silencing genes by altering DNA and histone methylation, histone acetylation, and chromatin structure. These modifications determine the degree of DNA compaction and accessibility for gene transcription, altering gene expression, phenotype, and disease susceptibility. While there is evidence that a number of early environmental exposures are associated with an increased risk of IgE-dependent allergic disease, several studies indicate *in utero* microbial and dietary exposures can modify gene expression and allergic disease propensity through epigenetic modification [70]. Novel data indicate that epigenetic mechanisms contribute to the development of Th cell function including the pattern of Th1/Th2 cell differentiation, regulatory T-cell differentiation, and Th17 development [59, 70]. Environmental factors, including diesel exhaust particles, vitamins, tobacco smoke, and microbes operate through such mechanisms [71]. Indeed, a recent study confirmed that the epigenetic patterns in asthma candidate genes are influenced by farm exposure. In cord blood, regions in ORMDL1 and STAT6 were hypomethylated in DNA from farmers' as compared to nonfarmers' children, while regions in RAD50 and IL-13 were hypermethylated. Changes in methylation over time occurred in 15 gene regions and clustered in the genes highly associated with asthma (ORMDL family) and IgE regulation (RAD50, IL13, and IL4), but not in the T-regulatory genes such as FOXP3 or RUNX3 [72].

Innate immune recognition of allergens

The driving force for the induction of an adaptive immune response is the innate immune recognition system in hematopoietic and non-hematopoietic cells. Sensing occurs mainly through innate immune receptors such as TLRs, NOD-like receptors, or glycan-sensing C-type lectin receptors (CLRs). In light of this model, it is interesting to note that many allergens contain immune stimulatory properties that target the innate immune system. Although allergens represent a heterogeneous group of proteins, it has been noted that some structural features are commonly overrepresented, which may account for their resistance against proteolytic digestion and for their recognition by the innate immune system [73].

Many (food) allergens are glycoproteins and protein glycosylation may contribute to the binding by CLRs. For example, glycosylated, but not de-glycosylated, Ara h 1 (the major peanut allergen) is recognized by the CLR DC-SIGN, leading to dendritic cell activation and subsequent priming of a Th2-skewed T-cell response [73, 74]. Ara h 1 is an N-glycan that shares structural similarities to N-glycans from *Schistosoma mansoni* egg antigens, which are well-studied Th2 pathogen-associated molecular patterns (PAMPs). Several respiratory allergens, including the house dust mite allergen Der p 2, share structural and functional homology with MD-2, the LPS-binding component of the TLR4 signaling complex. Der p 2 together with low doses of LPS, which is commonly present in house dust mite extracts, stimulates pro-allergic cytokines such as GM-CSF, TSLP, IL-25, and IL-33 in lung epithelial cells, leading to allergic asthma in mice [75]. Several allergens have enzymatic functions, frequently protease activities, that facilitate transepithelial allergen delivery and spreading, but also cleavage of cellular receptors such as CD40 ligand on monocytes, CD25 on T cells, or protease-activated receptors (PARs) on cell types including epithelial, stromal, and immune cells. The consequences are decreased production of the Th2-antagonistic cytokine IL-12 in monocytes, enhanced Th2-type cytokine production in T cells, and the production of proinflammatory and Th2-skewing cytokines in PAR-activated cells such as TSLP and IL-33 in epithelial/stromal cells and IL-4 in basophils [73, 76].

In most cases, protein allergens do not directly promote innate immune receptor-dependent stimulation. However, most allergens derive from complexes that may include other distinct molecules that trigger innate immune functions. For example, whole peanut extracts have stronger immune-activating capacities than the isolated allergens, which can be attributed to proteins that by themselves are not major allergens but stimulate innate immune cells or activate complement. These functions may facilitate adaptive immune responses and/or act synergistically with IgE-dependent effector cell activation and exacerbate anaphylactic reactions [73]. Furthermore, cow's milk sphingolipids can activate invariant natural killer cells to produce IL-4 and IL-13 [77] and pollens contain intrinsic NADPH oxidase activity, generating reactive oxygen species (ROS) [78] and/or bioactive lipids (phytoprostanes) [79]. The pollen intrinsic bioactivities have been shown to instruct a Th2 cell polarization and allergic airway inflammation. These data strongly suggest that allergens provoke allergies by a two-signal strategy, in which signal 1 triggers the innate response and signal 2 is the specific antigen interacting with B- and T-cell receptors.

Allergic inflammation

Once an individual is sensitized and allergen-specific IgE has been formed, recurrent antigen exposure readily induces the manifestations of allergic inflammation and atopic disease. Allergic inflammation is due to a complex interplay between several inflammatory cells, including mast cells, basophils, lymphocytes, dendritic cells, eosinophils, and tissue cells, orchestrated by several transcription factors, particularly NF-κB and GATA3 [80]. The response has been categorized into three phases: (i) acute or immediate-phase reaction, (ii) late-phase reaction, and (iii) chronic allergic inflammation (Figure 2.2).

An acute reaction occurs when the allergen, after crossing the mucosa, binds to antigen-specific IgE on the surface of mast cells and basophils. This induces cross-linking of FcεRI, resulting in the release of proinflammatory mediators, such as histamine, eicosanoids, and cytokines. Clinical signs of the acute response (weal and flare) develop within seconds to minutes. A particular characteristic of intestinal food allergy might be a delayed "acute reaction" because of the passage time of dietary antigens through the esophagus and the stomach. The immediate reaction may be followed by a late-phase reaction starting after 4–48 hours. Mast cell-derived mediators induce expression of adhesion molecules on endothelial cells, which bind ligand on the surface of eosinophils, basophils, Th2 cells, and NKT cells [81]. This leads to the preferential extravasation of these cells through vessel walls into sites of inflammation. Their recruitment to the target organ depends on the production of a number of chemokines [82]. Within the tissue, infiltrating cells are further activated by the inflammatory environment and allergens via antigen-specific recognition (IgE on basophils and MHC class II-dependent antigen presentation to Th2 cells). Late-phase reactions may develop independent of IgE. It has been reported that birch

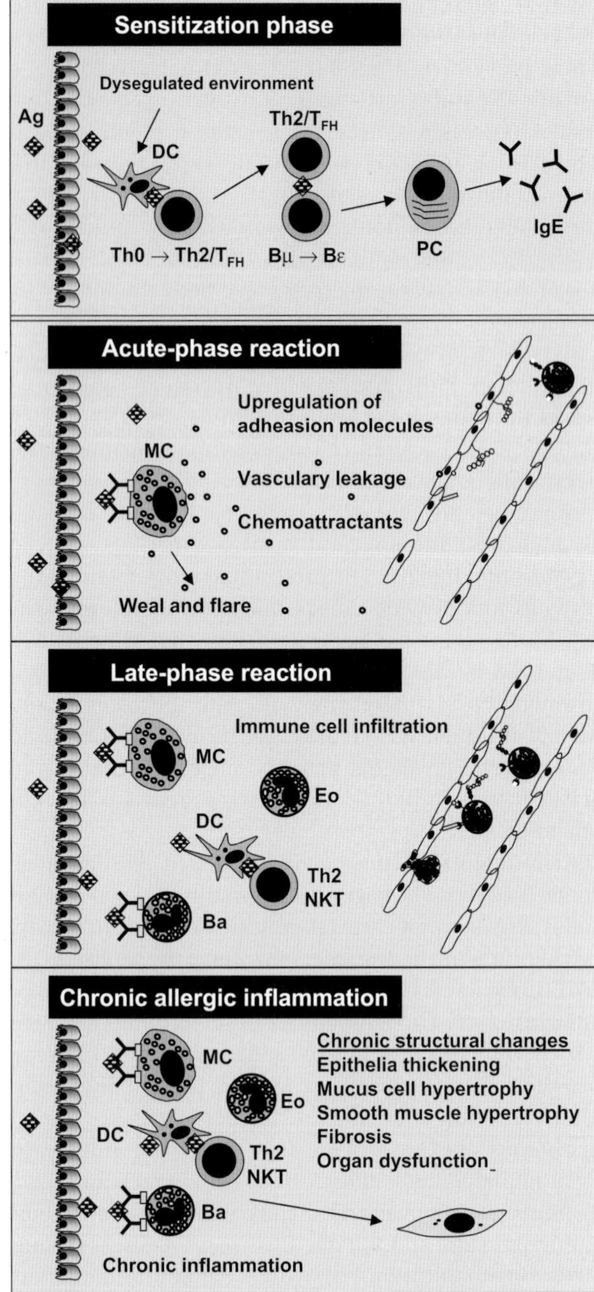

Ag, antigen; DC, dendritic cell; Th0, naïve CD4 + lymphocyte; Th2, Th2 lymphocyte; T_{FH}, T follicular helper cells; Bμ, naïve B cell; Bε, primed B cell after IgE class-switch; PC, plasma cell; MC, mast cell; Eo, eosinophil; Ba, basophil; NKT, NKT cell

Figure 2.2 Phases of allergic disease. For details see text.

pollen-related food allergen that lost its capacity to bind to IgE because of cooking, but retained its T -cell stimulatory potency, does not induce an acute-phase reaction such as the oral allergy syndrome but can still induce a late-phase response like atopic eczema [81]. Repeated allergen exposure may lead to a chronic inflammatory response causing persistent infiltration of mast cells, eosinophils, basophils, lymphocytes, and dendritic cells. Moreover, allergic inflammation affects tissue cells, such as epithelial cells, fibroblasts, vascular cells, and airway smooth muscle cells, resulting in chronic structural changes of the tissue, such as goblet cell and smooth muscle hypertrophy, fibrosis, and organ dysfunction. Sensory nerves are sensitized and activated during allergic inflammation and produce symptoms. There are several endogenous anti-inflammatory mechanisms, including anti-inflammatory lipids and cytokines, which may be defective in allergic disease, thus amplifying and perpetuating the inflammation. The specific clinical features of each of the different phases vary according to the anatomical site affected (Figure 2.2).

IgE receptors

Most IgE is bound to FcεRI expressed on mast cells, basophils, monocytes, dendritic cells, Langerhans cells, eosinophils, and platelets (Table 2.1). Monomeric IgE binds to FcεRI with high affinity and has a slow dissociation rate (half-life of about 20 hours). The FcεRI is composed of an IgE-binding α chain, a tetraspanning transmembrane β chain, and a homodimeric disulfide-linked γ chain. The β chain, which is only expressed in mast cells and basophils, functions as an amplifier and in its absence the receptor initiates only weak signals. Cross-linking of FcεRI initiates signaling mediated through the immunoreceptor tyrosine-based activation motifs (ITAMs) encoded in the cytoplasmic tails of the β and γ chains. For a detailed description of the signaling events via FcεRI, the reader is referred to comprehensive reviews [83–85]. In brief, downstream signaling results in intracellular calcium release and activation of protein kinase C (PKC), mitogen-activated protein kinase (MAPK) pathways, nuclear factor-kappaB (NF-κB), phosphoinositide-3 kinase (PI3K), and phospholipase A_2 (PLA_2). In mast cells and basophils, these events result in degranulation, generation of arachidonic acid metabolites, and enhanced expression of genes encoding for proinflammatory cytokines and chemokines. IgE binding in the absence of antigen increases receptor expression, induces anti-apoptotic signals, and triggers low-level cytokine production in the mast cells [86, 87]. The downstream signaling induced by monomeric IgE binding remains elusive. In antigen-presenting cells, FcεRI has been shown to facilitate antigen presentation by IgE-dependent capture of antigens [36,88].

The low-affinity IgE receptor (FcεRII/CD23) is not a member of the Ig superfamily. CD23 is a type II integral membrane protein with a C-lectin domain at the distal C-terminal end of the extracellular sequence. The lectin domain contains the binding sites for all known ligands of CD23 including IgE, complement receptors CR2, CR3, and CR4 (also termed CD21, CD18-CD11b, CD18-CD11c, respectively), and vitronectin. CD23 facilitates antigen presentation to B cells and acts as a negative feedback regulator of the IgE class-switch. In enterocytes, CD23 facilitates the bidirectional transport of IgE–antigen complexes and thus may participate in antigen sampling from the intestinal lumen [36].

Mast cells

Mast cells are widely distributed throughout the body, frequently found around blood vessels, adjacent to nerves and at mucosal surfaces. Bone marrow-derived mast cell progenitors migrate via the peripheral blood into tissues, where they undergo final maturation under the influence of local, microenvironmental factors. Stem cell factor (SCF), produced either in a soluble or membrane-bound form by fibroblasts, endothelial cells, and stromal cells, is the essential factor for both mast cell maturation and survival of mature mast cells [89]. The importance of SCF and its receptor KIT is stressed by the fact that KIT-deficient mice basically lack mast cells. Mature mast cells are long-living cells that maintain the capability to grow. In particular IL-4, but also IL-3 and IL-9, induce proliferation of tissue mast cells in an SCF-dependent manner [90–92].

Human mast cells are commonly classified according to their protease content and related ultrastructural signatures of their granules. Mast cells containing only tryptase (MC_T) predominate in the lung and intestinal mucosa. Tryptase and chymase-positive mast cells (MC_{TC}) are mainly located in the skin and the intestinal submucosa. It has been suggested that these subtypes can be further classified according to their responsiveness to certain IgE-independent agonists. This heterogeneity might reflect that mast cells exhibit differences in biochemical and functional properties, depending on the anatomical site in which the cells reside and/or the biological process in which they participate.

Mast cells exert their biological functions mainly by the release of humoral mediators. Mast cell, as well as eosinophil and basophil, mediators can be categorized into three groups: (i) preformed secretory granule-associated mediators, (ii) *de novo*-synthesized eicosanoid metabolites, and (iii) cytokines and chemokines which are mainly *de novo* synthesized but are also sometimes found to be stored within secretory granules (Table 2.2). Secretory granule-associated mediators of mast cells are mainly histamine, proteases, and proteoglycans. Histamine exerts its wide-ranging biological activities via binding to four histamine receptors (H1–4). With regard to allergic inflammation, the H1 receptor seems to be of particular importance. Its activation affects the function of blood vessels (dilation

Table 2.2 Mediators of mast cells, eosinophils, and basophils.

Mast cells	
Granule associated	Histamine, tryptase, chymase, carboxypeptidase A, heparin, chondroitin sulfate E, many acid hydrolases, cathepsin G
De novo synthesized	LTC_4, LTB_4, PGD_2, PAF
Cytokines/chemokines	IL-1β, IL-3, IL-5, IL-6, IL-8, IL-9, IL-10, IL-11, IL-13, IL-16, IL-18, IL-25, TNF-α, TGF-β, GM-CSF, CCL3/MIP-1α, bFGF, VPF/VEGF, and others
Eosinophils	
Granule associated	ECP, EDN (formerly called EPX), MBP, EPO, CLC
De novo synthesized	LTC_4, LTB_4, PAF, PGE_1/E_2, thromboxane B_2, oxygen metabolites (H_2O_2, O_2^-)
Cytokines/chemokines	IL-2, IL-3, IL-4, IL-5, IL-6, IL-8, IL-10, IL-12, IL-13, IL-16, IL-18, TNF-α, TGF-α, TGF-β, GM-CSF, CCL2/MCP-1, CCL3/MIP-1α, CCL5/RANTES, CCL11/eotaxin-1, VPF/VEGF, PDGF-B
Basophils	
Granule associated	Histamine, chondroitin sulfate A, neutral protease with bradykinin-generating activity, β-glucuronidase, elastase, cathepsin G-like enzyme, MBP, CLC, granzyme B (induced by IL-3)
De novo synthesized	LTC_4
Cytokines/chemokines	IL-4, IL-13, CCL3/MIP-1α

and increased permeability), smooth muscles (contraction), epithelial cells (mucus production), and Th2 lymphocytes (recruitment) [93]. Mast cell proteases cleave several host proteins, including protease-activating receptors, and have been linked to immune as well as non-immune functions of mast cells, such as tissue repair and fibrinolysis. For example, mast cell-derived proteases cleave endogenous (endothelin-1, induced by bacterial infection) and exogenous (snake and honeybee venoms) toxins and subsequently limit pathology [94, 95]. Moreover, mast cell proteases mediate cleavage of allergens. This might be an important negative feedback loop terminating or weakening allergic inflammation [96]. The main mast cell-produced metabolites of arachidonic acid (and their prominent function) are PGD_2 (smooth muscle contraction, chemoattractant for eosinophils, and Th2 cells), LTC_4 (increase of vascular permeability, mucus production, and smooth muscle contraction), and LTB_4 (chemoattractant for neutrophils, eosinophils, and T cells) [97]. A significant amount of cytokines and chemokines are produced by mast cells. Among them, IL-3, IL-5, and IL-13 seem to be specifically important in allergic reactions [98]. They mediate basophil (IL-3) and eosinophil (IL-5) recruitment, IgE class-switching, mucus production, and airway hyperreactivity (all IL-13). Although detectable in rodent mast cells [99], human mast cells produce no or only small amounts of IL-4 [100].

Cross-linking of the FcεRI is the most potent trigger to activate mast cells for the release of all three classes of mediators, and therefore, mast cells play a central role as effector cells in IgE-dependent allergic reactions (Table 2.1) [89, 98]. Degranulation and eicosanoid production occur within minutes. Cytokines, if not stored within the granules, are mainly transcriptionally regulated and produced within 2–6 hours [100]. IL-3, IL-4, and IL-5 enhance FcεRI-mediated reactions [91, 100, 101], ensuring an autocrine- and paracrine-positive feedback loop, because the main producers of these cytokines are mast cells (IL-3, IL-5) and, after recruitment, basophils (IL-4), eosinophils (IL-3, IL-5), and Th2 cells (IL-4, IL-5) (Table 2.2). IL-4 induces IL-5 production by mast cells even in the absence of IgE cross-linking [93]. On the other hand, the central modulatory cytokines of Treg cells, IL-10 and TGF-β, have been shown to induce apoptosis in mast cells (TGF-β) and decrease FcεRI-induced mediator production (IL-10 and TGF-β) [102]. Several IgE-independent mast cell triggers have been described. SCF, complement factors (C5a), neuropeptides (substance P), adenosine, IgG cross-linking of FcγRI, and several TLR ligands stimulate mast cell effector functions, but are substantially less effective than FcεRI-mediated signals [50].

Considering the multiple biological effects of mast cell mediators, one can propose several possible functions of mast cells *in vivo*. A mouse mast cell "knock-in" model has considerably contributed to the understanding of the role of mast cells in several pathologies. Apart from allergies, recent studies point out that mast cells are important effector cells in immune complex-induced autoimmune models (mediated via Fcγ on mast cells) [103] and confer protection against acute bacterial infections [104–106]. Using this mast cell knock-in model, it has been shown that mast cells contribute to all stages of immunopathology in allergic asthma, which are the immediate-phase, late-phase, and chronic allergic reactions. Mast cell effector functions were mainly, but not exclusively, dependent on FcεRI/FcγRIII expression [107].

An exciting field of mast cell research concerns the questions whether and how mast cells contribute to the instruction of the adaptive immune response. Several lines of evidence now indicate that mast cells deliver signals important for dendritic cell activation and T-/B-cell priming, such as cytokines (e.g., TNF-α) and co-stimulatory molecules (CD40L, OX40 ligand). In an allograft model, mast cells were absolutely essential in Treg cell-dependent peripheral tolerance. IL-9 represented the functional link through which Treg recruited and activated mast cells to mediate regional immune suppression [108]. However, it remains elusive as to whether mast cells play a role (either activating or tolerizing) during the sensitization phase of allergies.

Despite the new enthusiasm about the multiple functions of mast cells in immune diseases and immune regulation, one should consider that most of the data derived from the murine system, in particular with regard to mast cell functions, may not always reflect the human situation [81]. Moreover, many data on *in vivo* mast cell functions are based on mast cell-deficient Kit mutant mice, while recent work in new mouse mutants with unperturbed Kit function could not confirm such functions [109]. These findings indicate that key physiological functions of mast cells have to be reconsidered.

Basophils

Basophils were once considered as the circulating progenitor of tissue mast cells, because of their similar morphology and staining characteristics (due to the basophilic granule contents) and their overlapping functional properties. It is now generally accepted that mast cells and basophils originate from separate lineages [110–112]. Basophils fully mature within the bone marrow and are subsequently released to the peripheral blood, where they form the smallest population of leukocytes (0.5–1% of total leukocytes, considerably increased in allergic patients). IL-3 is the most important basophil growth factor, but other growth factors such as IL-5, GM-CSF, NGF, and TGF-β have been identified [111, 112]. Basophils enter the tissue at sites of inflammation, being directed by adhesion molecules and chemoattractants [81, 113]. This array of growth factors and chemoattractants largely overlaps with factors promoting eosinophil development and recruitment. This may explain the combined involvement of both cell types in many diseases. In contrast to mast cells, both basophils and eosinophils are short-lived cells, surviving in the tissue only for several days [111, 114]. Basophils have been detected particularly in allergic late-phase reactions within the skin and the lung, whereas their involvement in gastrointestinal pathologies is largely unknown.

Similar to mast cells, basophils release large amounts of histamine and LTC_4, but no PGD_2, which is specifically mast cell derived. Basophils are a major source of IL-4 and IL-13 [114, 115] that can be released upon IgE-dependent and IgE-independent stimulation. On a per cell basis, activated basophils produce more IL-4 and IL-13 than any other cell type. Basophils produce a much more limited cytokine profile than mast cells and eosinophils (Table 2.1). However, the specific expression of IL-4, which is questionably produced by mast cells and eosinophils, suggests a particular role for basophils in the antigen-specific priming of T cells to Th2 cells [116], although the data are controversial in this respect [117]. The interaction between basophils and T cells is not restricted to priming of T cells by cytokines, since basophils can also act as antigen-presenting cells for an allergen-induced Th type 2 response [118].

After cross-linking of FcεRI, the release of histamine and eicosanoid is nearly complete by 20 minutes, whereas IL-4 and IL-13 production follows a time course with a maximal response after 4 and 20 hours, respectively. Small amounts of IL-4 (10 pg/10^6 basophils) become detectable within 5–10 minutes after stimulation, suggesting that preformed IL-4 is released [115]. IgE-independent secretagogues are the anaphylatoxins C3a and C5a, platelet-activating factor (PAF), eosinophil-derived major basic protein (MBP), cytokines (IL-3, IL-5, GM-CSF), and chemokines (MCP-1, -3, eotaxin, RANTES, MIP-1α, IL-8). Of particular interest is the observation that IL-3, IL-5, and GM-CSF only induce small amounts of mediator release, but substantially enhance the effects of almost all IgE-dependent and IgE-independent agonists. The latter seems to be of greater importance, particularly in the allergic late-phase reaction characterized by enhanced cytokine production, and has been named "basophil priming." Similar observations could be made for other inflammatory cells such as eosinophils, suggesting a rather general way of inflammatory cell regulation [114, 115]. IL-33, an IL-1 family member, is a basophil/eosinophil priming agent that promotes IgE-dependent allergic inflammation and Th2 polarization likely by the selective activation of these two granulocyte types [119]. In the rodent system, another regulator of basophil proliferation and function has been identified, the cytokine thymic stromal lymphopoietin (TSLP), for which gene polymorphisms had been described earlier that are associated with atopic diseases in humans. TSLP promotes systemic basophilia and elicits basophil subtypes, promoting Th2-mediated inflammation [120].

A growing body of evidence suggests that basophils are involved in the defense against helminth infections [121]. However, *in vivo* basophil studies are limited, because a basophil-deficient mouse strain does not exist. Mukai et al. have demonstrated in a series of elegant transfer studies that basophils, in the absence of T cells and reacting mast cells, induce an IgE-dependent delayed-onset allergic inflammation, whereas mast cells were necessary for the immediate-phase response [122].

The role of the intestinal microbiota for the control of IgE-dependent allergic reactions has been discussed [57]. In turn, alteration of commensal bacterial populations, for example, via oral antibiotic treatment, can result in elevated serum IgE concentrations, increased basophil populations, and exaggerated basophil-mediated Th2 cell responses, as shown by Artis and coworkers [123]. This is an impressive example showing the central role of the intestinal commensal bacteria in controlling IgE-dependent allergic reactions. In mice as well as in human subjects with hyperimmunoglobulinemia E syndrome, elevated serum IgE levels correlated with increased circulating basophil populations. Yet unknown bacterial signals likely regulate basophil development as well as B-cell functions. These results identify a previously unrecognized pathway through which commensal-derived signals influence susceptibility to IgE-dependent inflammation and allergic disease [123].

Eosinophils

Eosinophils fully mature within the bone marrow, from which they enter the bloodstream. IL-3, IL-5, and GM-CSF are particularly effective in regulating eosinophil growth and maturation. Of these three, IL-5 is the most specific and potent [112]. Eosinophils normally account for only 1–3% of peripheral blood leukocytes, and under physiological conditions their presence in tissue is primarily limited to the gastrointestinal mucosa, which forms the largest eosinophil reservoir of the body. In the course of several diseases, including allergy, eosinophilic gastroenteritis, and helminth infection, eosinophils can selectively accumulate in the peripheral blood or any tissue [124, 125]. Recruitment of eosinophils depends on the production of a number of chemokines (e.g., CCL5/RANTES and CCL11/eotaxin-1, CCL24/eotaxin-2, and CCL26/eotaxin-3). Only IL-5 and the eotaxins selectively regulate eosinophil trafficking [125]. Anti-IL-5 treatment reduced tissue eosinophilia in asthma patients by 55%, however, without affecting symptoms [126].

Eosinophils secrete an array of cytotoxic granule cationic proteins that are present in large quantities in the cells: eosinophil cationic protein (ECP), eosinophil-derived neurotoxin (EDN), MBP, and eosinophilic peroxidase (EPO). The enzymatic activities and several functions of these proteins have been defined and have been reviewed in detail [127]. Apart from their toxic effects and antiviral activity, these proteins activate mast cells (EPO, MBP) and suppress T-cell proliferation (ECP) and immunoglobulin synthesis (ECP). Eosinophils produce several eicosanoid metabolites, oxygen radicals, and multiple cytokines/chemokines (Table 2.2).

C5a, C3a, and PAF cause degranulation in eosinophils, whereas other stimuli, such as the cytokines IL-3, IL-5, and GM-CSF, have a weak or no direct effect. However, this set of cytokines "prime" eosinophils for enhanced mediator release to other stimuli, including otherwise ineffective agonists [128]. Interestingly, PAF produced by eosinophils has been considered as an autocrine secretagogue [126]. Furthermore, chemokines, such as the CCR3 ligands, CCL7, CCL13, and CCL11, induce degranulation in eosinophils [127]. Eosinophils express FcαRI, FcγRII, and FcγRI (inducible, Table 2.1) and secretory IgA and IgG are strong signals for degranulation [129] mediating, for example, antibody (or complement)-dependent cellular toxicity against helminths. The role of FcεRI on the eosinophil is still a matter of controversy [129]. Eosinophil activation by cytokines and immunoglobulins is critically dependent on β2-integrins, especially on Mac-1 binding to ICAM-1 [130], suggesting that their activity is silenced in the bloodstream.

There is strong evidence that eosinophils play a considerable role in the defense against helminths. This is supported by the findings in both humans and animal models [127, 131]. Moreover, they are key effector cells in a number of obviously IgE-independent, helminth-independent, idiopathic gastrointestinal diseases. These eosinophil gastrointestinal diseases (EGID) can manifest at any site of the digestive tract and are clearly separated from the hypereosinophilic syndrome that can also involve the gastrointestinal tract. The underlying mechanisms of EGID are not fully understood, thus causal therapy is lacking [132].

Conclusion

The allergen-specific Th2 and B-cell priming, the function of IgE and FcεRI, and the biology of allergic effector cells have been intensively studied during the last few decades. The current advances in understanding these fundamental immunological mechanisms led to the design of new treatment approaches, of which some have reached the level of clinical trials or approval [14, 126, 133]. We are only beginning to understand the regulatory network of the immune system, in particular the function of Treg cells and "blocking" allergen-specific antibodies. Therefore, we still need to learn how we can direct the immune system toward a tolerizing response to introduce more rational and safer vaccine strategies [14]. The link between environmental stimuli and allergy has made substantial progress during the last few years. In particular, the role of the commensal bacterial microbiota in the intestine seems to be an underestimated regulator of mast cells, basophils, and IgE responses.

A specific problem concerning food allergy lies in the fact that the general pathophysiological concepts of allergy have mainly been developed in model systems of nonfood-related atopy. This applies also to this chapter, which reviews in some part data generated in studies of nonfood allergy. This is further reflected by the fact that new drugs are often designed for the treatment of asthma, rhinoconjunctivitis, atopic dermatitis, or insect allergy, but rarely for food allergy. The pathophysiology and the clinical management of food allergy might be considered more complex in comparison to other allergic disorders, in particular, as the gastrointestinal tract is difficult to access for investigation and the symptoms are often variable and unspecific. Therefore, a better understanding of the specific immunopathology of food allergy and an improvement in the organ-specific diagnostic approach are necessary to provide improved treatment options.

References

1. Bischoff S, Crowe SE. Gastrointestinal food allergy: new insights into pathophysiology and clinical perspectives. *Gastroenterology* 2005; 128:1089–1113.
2. Sampson HA. Update on food allergy. *J Allergy Clin Immunol* 2004; 113:805–819.
3. Fernandez-Rivas M, Bolhaar S, Gonzalez-Mancebo E, et al. Apple allergy across Europe: how allergen sensitization profiles determine the clinical expression of allergies to plant foods. *J Allergy Clin Immunol* 2006; 118:481–488.
4. Brandtzaeg P. Food allergy: separating the science from the mythology. *Nat Rev Gastroenterol Hepatol* 2010; 7:380–400.
5. Sansonetti PJ. War and peace at mucosal surfaces. *Nat Rev Immunol* 2004; 4:953–964.
6. Sellge G, Schnupf P, Sansonetti PJ. Anatomy of the gut barrier and establishment of intestinal homeostasis. In: Sansonetti PJ (ed.) *Bacterial Virulence: Basic Principles, Models and Global Approaches*. Wiley-VCH, 2010.
7. Perrier C, Corthesy B. Gut permeability and food allergies. *Clin Exp Allergy* 2010; 41:20–28.
8. Untersmayr E, Jensen-Jarolim E. The effect of gastric digestion on food allergy. *Curr Opin Allergy Clin Immunol* 2006; 6:214–219.
9. Ventura MT, Polimeno L, Amoruso AC, et al. Intestinal permeability in patients with adverse reactions to food. *Dig Liver Dis* 2006; 38:732–736.
10. Benard A, Desreumeaux P, Huglo D, et al. Increased intestinal permeability in bronchial asthma. *J Allergy Clin Immunol* 1996; 97:1173–1178.
11. Zeiger RS, Heller S, Mellon MH, et al. Effect of combined maternal and infant food-allergen avoidance on development of atopy in early infancy: a randomized study. *J Allergy Clin Immunol* 1989; 84:72–89.
12. Taylor B, Norman AP, Orgel HA, et al. Transient IgA deficiency and pathogenesis of infantile atopy. *Lancet* 1973; 2:111–113.
13. Husby S, Foged N, Host A, Svehag SE. Passage of dietary antigens into the blood of children with coeliac disease. Quantification and size distribution of absorbed antigens. *Gut* 1987; 28:1062–1072.
14. Larche M, Akdis CA, Valenta R. Immunological mechanisms of allergen-specific immunotherapy. *Nat Rev Immunol* 2006; 6:761–771.
15. Akdis CA. Allergy and hypersensitivity mechanisms of allergic disease. *Curr Opin Immunol* 2006; 18:718–726.
16. Zhou L, Mark MW, Chong A, Littman DR. Plasticity of CD4+ T cell lineage differentiation. *Immunity* 2009; 30:646–655.
17. Pulendran B, David Artis D. New paradigms in type 2 immunity. *Science* 2012; 337:431–435.
18. DeLong JH, Simpson KH, Wambre E, James EA, Robinson D, Kwok WW. Ara h 1-reactive T cells in individuals with peanut allergy. *J Allergy Clin Immunol* 2011; 127:1211–1218.
19. Atarashi K, Tanoue T, Shima T, et al. Induction of colonic regulatory T cells by indigenous Clostridium species. *Science* 2011; 331:337–341.
20. Mucida D, Park Y, Cheroutre H. From the diet to the nucleus: vitamin A and TGF-beta join efforts at the mucosal interface of the intestine. *Semin Immunol* 2009; 21:14–21.
21. Josefowicz SZ, Niec RE, Kim HY, et al. Extrathymically generated regulatory T cells control mucosal TH2 inflammation. *Nature* 2012; 482:395–400.
22. Akdis M. Healthy immune response to allergens: T regulatory cells and more. *Curr Opin Immunol* 2006; 18:738–744.
23. Jutel M, Akdis M, Budak F, et al. IL-10 and TGF-beta cooperate in the regulatory T cell response to mucosal allergens in normal immunity and specific immunotherapy. *Eur J Immunol* 2003; 33:1205–1214.
24. Coffman RL. The origin of TH2 responses. *Science* 2010; 328:1116–1117.
25. Mitre E, Nutman TB. IgE memory: persistence of antigen-specific IgE responses years after treatment of human filarial infections. *J Allergy Clin Immunol* 2006; 117:939–945.
26. Shane C. Follicular helper CD4 T cells (TFH). *Annu Rev Immunol* 2011; 29:621–663.
27. Reinhardt R, Liang H, Locksley R. Cytokine-secreting follicular T cells shape the antibody repertoire. *Nat Immunol* 2009; 10:385–393.
28. Wynn TA. Basophils trump dendritic cells as APCs for TH2 responses. *Nat Immunol* 2009; 10:679–681.
29. Talay O, Yan D, Brightbill HD, et al. IgE memory B cells and plasma cells generated through a germinal-center pathway. *Nat Immunol* 2012; 13:396–404.
30. Yang Z, Sullivan BM, Allen CD. Fluorescent in vivo detection reveals that IgE(+) B cells are restrained by an intrinsic cell fate predisposition. *Immunity* 2012; 36:857–872.
31. Coker HA, Durham SR, Gould HJ. Local somatic hypermutation and class switch recombination in the nasal mucosa of allergic rhinitis patients. *J Immunol* 2003; 171:5602–5610.
32. Vieira P, Rajewsky K. The half-lives of serum immunoglobulins in adult mice. *Eur J Immunol* 1988; 18:313–316.
33. Tada T, Okumura K, Platteau B, et al. Half-lives of two types of rat homocytotropic antibodies in circulation and in the skin. *Int Arch Allergy Appl Immunol* 1975; 48:116–131.
34. Golden DB, Kagey-Sobotka A, Norman PS, et al. Outcomes of allergy to insect stings in children, with and without venom immunotherapy. *N Engl J Med* 2004; 351:668–674.
35. Radbruch A, Muehlinghaus G, Luger EO, et al. Competence and competition: the challenge of becoming a long-lived plasma cell. *Nat Rev Immunol* 2006; 6:741–750.
36. Gould HJ, Sutton BJ, Beavil AJ, et al. The biology of IgE and the basis of allergic disease. *Annu Rev Immunol* 2003; 21:579–628.

37. Hallstrand TS, Sprenger JD, Agosti JM, et al. Long-term acquisition of allergen-specific IgE and asthma following allogeneic bone marrow transplantation from allergic donors. *Blood* 2004; 104:3086–3090.
38. Rachid R, Umetsu DT. Immunological mechanisms for desensitization and tolerance in food allergy. *Semin Immunopathol* 2012; 34:689–702.
39. Linhart B, Rudolf Valenta R. Vaccines for allergy. *Curr Opin Immunol* 2012; 24:354–336.
40. Burks AW, Jones SM, Wood RA, et al. Consortium of Food Allergy Research (CoFAR). Oral immunotherapy for treatment of egg allergy in children. *N Engl J Med* 2012; 367:233–243.
41. Jones SM, Pons L, Roberts JL, et al. Clinical efficacy and immune regulation with peanut oral immunotherapy. *J Allergy Clin Immunol* 2009; 124:e1–e97.
42. Carballido JM, Carballido-Perrig N, Kagi MK, et al. T cell epitope specificity in human allergic and nonallergic subjects to bee venom phospholipase A2. *J Immunol* 1993; 150:3582–3591.
43. Ejrnaes AM, Svenson M, Lund G, et al. Inhibition of rBet v 1-induced basophil histamine release with specific immunotherapy-induced serum immunoglobulin G: no evidence that FcgammaRIIB signalling is important. *Clin Exp Allergy* 2006; 36:73–82.
44. Strait RT, Morris SC, Finkelman FD. IgG-blocking antibodies inhibit IgE-mediated anaphylaxis in vivo through both antigen interception and Fc gamma RIIb cross-linking. *J Clin Invest* 2006; 116:833–841.
45. Bruhns P, Fremont S, Daeron M. Regulation of allergy by Fc receptors. *Curr Opin Immunol* 2005; 17:662–669.
46. Zhu D, Kepley CL, Zhang K, et al. A chimeric human–cat fusion protein blocks cat-induced allergy. *Nat Med* 2005; 11:446–449.
47. Djurup R, Malling HJ. High IgG4 antibody level is associated with failure of immunotherapy with inhalant allergens. *Clin Allergy* 1987; 17:459–468.
48. James LK, Shamji MH, Walker SM, et al. Long-term tolerance after allergen immunotherapy is accompanied by selective persistence of blocking antibodies. *J Allergy Clin Immunol* 2011; 127:509–516.
49. Janeway CA, Travers P, Walport M, Shlomchik M. *Immunobiology: The Immune System in Health and Disease*, 5th edn. New York: Garland Publishing, a member of the Taylor & Francis Group, 2001.
50. Sellge G, Laffer S, Mierke C, et al. Development of an in vitro system for the study of allergens and allergen-specific immunoglobulin E and immunoglobulin G: Fc epsilon receptor I supercross-linking is a possible new mechanism of immunoglobulin G-dependent enhancement of type I allergic reactions. *Clin Exp Allergy* 2005; 35:774–781.
51. Denepoux S, Eibensteiner PB, Steinberger P, et al. Molecular characterization of human IgG monoclonal antibodies specific for the major birch pollen allergen Bet v 1. Anti-allergen IgG can enhance the anaphylactic reaction. *FEBS Lett* 2000; 465:39–46.
52. van der Neut Kolfschoten M, Schuurman J, Losen M, et al. Anti-inflammatory activity of human IgG4 antibodies by dynamic Fab arm exchange. *Science* 2007; 317:1554–1557.
53. Barnes KC. Genomewide association studies in allergy and the influence of ethnicity. *Curr Opin Allergy Clin Immunol* 2010; 10:427–433.
54. Vercelli D. Advances in asthma and allergy genetics in 2007. *J Allergy Clin Immunol* 2008; 122:267–271.
55. Palmer CN, Irvine AD, Terron-Kwiatkowski A, et al. Common loss-of-function variants of the epidermal barrier protein filaggrin are a major predisposing factor for atopic dermatitis. *Nat Genet* 2006; 38:441–446.
56. Vercelli D. Gene–environment interactions in asthma and allergy: the end of the beginning? *Curr Opin Allergy Clin Immunol* 2010; 10:145–148.
57. McLoughlin RM, Mills KH. Influence of gastrointestinal commensal bacteria on the immune responses that mediate allergy and asthma. *J Allergy Clin Immunol* 2011; 127:1097–1107.
58. Custovic A, Marinho S, Simpson A. Gene–environment interactions in the development of asthma and atopy. *Expert Rev Respir Med* 2012; 6:301–308.
59. Antó JM, Pinart M, Akdis M, et al. WHO Collaborating Centre on Asthma and Rhinitis (Montpellier). Understanding the complexity of IgE-related phenotypes from childhood to young adulthood: a Mechanisms of the Development of Allergy (MeDALL) seminar. *J Allergy Clin Immunol* 2012; 129:943–954.
60. Ege MJ, Mayer M, Normand AC, et al.; GABRIELA Transregio 22 Study Group. Exposure to environmental microorganisms and childhood asthma. *N Engl J Med* 2011; 364:701–709.
61. Renz H, von Mutius E, Brandtzaeg P, Cookson WO, Autenrieth IB, Haller D. Gene–environment interactions in chronic inflammatory disease. *Nat Immunol* 2011; 12:273–277.
62. Mazmanian SK, Liu CH, Tzianabos AO, Kasper DL. An immunomodulatory molecule of symbiotic bacteria directs maturation of the host immune system. *Cell* 2005; 122:107–118.
63. Debarry J, Garn H, Hanuszkiewicz A, et al. Acinetobacter lwoffii and Lactococcus lactis strains isolated from farm cowsheds possess strong allergy-protective properties. *J Allergy Clin Immunol* 2007; 119:1514–1521.
64. Khosravi A, Mazmanian SK. Breathe easy: microbes protect from allergies. *Nat Med* 2012; 18:492–494.
65. Boyle RJ, Ismail IH, Kivivuori S, et al. *Lactobacillus* GG treatment during pregnancy for the prevention of eczema: a randomized controlled trial. *Allergy* 2011; 66:509–516.
66. Simons FE, Shikishima Y, Van Nest G, et al. Selective immune redirection in humans with ragweed allergy by injecting Amb a 1 linked to immunostimulatory DNA. *J Allergy Clin Immunol* 2004; 113:1144–1151.
67. von BV, Hermes A, von BR, et al. Allergoid-specific T-cell reaction as a measure of the immunological response to specific immunotherapy (SIT) with a Th1-adjuvanted allergy vaccine. *J Investig Allergol Clin Immunol* 2005; 15:234–241.
68. Yazdanbakhsh M, Kremsner PG, van Ree R. Allergy, parasites, and the hygiene hypothesis. *Science* 2002; 296:490–494.

69. Hussain R, Poindexter RW, Ottesen EA. Control of allergic reactivity in human filariasis. Predominant localization of blocking antibody to the IgG4 subclass. *J Immunol* 1992; 148:2731–2737.
70. Martino DJ, Prescott SL. Silent mysteries: epigenetic paradigms could hold the key to conquering the epidemic of allergy and immune disease. *Allergy* 2010; 65:7–15.
71. Marsh LM, Pfefferle PI, Pinkenburg O, Renz H. Maternal signals for progeny prevention against allergy and asthma. *Cell Mol Life Sci* 2011; 68:1851–1862.
72. Michel S, Busato F, Genuneit J, et al.; PASTURE study group. Farm exposure and time trends in early childhood may influence DNA methylation in genes related to asthma and allergy. *Allergy* 2013; 68:355–364.
73. Ruiter B, Shreffler WG. Innate immunostimulatory properties of allergens and their relevance to food allergy. *Semin Immunopathol* 2012; 34:617–632.
74. Shreffler WG, Castro RR, Kucuk ZY, et al. The major glycoprotein allergen from Arachis hypogaea, Ara h 1, is a ligand of dendritic cell-specific ICAM-grabbing nonintegrin and acts as a Th2 adjuvant in vitro. *J Immunol* 2006; 177:3677–3685.
75. Trompette A, Divanovic S, Visintin A, et al. Allergenicity resulting from functional mimicry of a Toll-like receptor complex protein. *Nature* 2009; 457:585–589.
76. Sokol CL, Barton GM, Farrr AG, Medzhitov R. A mechanism for the initiation of allergen-induced T helper type 2 responses. *Nat Immunol* 2008; 9:310–318.
77. Jyonouchi S, Abraham V, Orange JS, et al. Invariant natural killer T cells from children with versus without food allergy exhibit differential responsiveness to milk-derived sphingomyelin. *J Allergy Clin Immunol* 2011; 128:e13.
78. Boldogh I, Bacsi A, Choudhury BK, et al. ROS generated by pollen NADPH oxidase provide a signal that augments antigen-induced allergic airway inflammation. *J Clin Invest* 2005; 115:2169–2179.
79. Traidl-Hoffmann C, Mariani V, Hochrein H, et al. Pollen-associated phytoprostanes inhibit dendritic cell interleukin-12 production and augment T helper type 2 cell polarization. *J Exp Med* 2005; 201:627–636.
80. Barnes PJ. Pathophysiology of allergic inflammation. *Immunol Rev* 2011; 242:31–50.
81. Bohle B, Zwolfer B, Heratizadeh A, et al. Cooking birch pollen-related food: divergent consequences for IgE- and T cell-mediated reactivity in vitro and in vivo. *J Allergy Clin Immunol* 2006; 118:242–249.
82. Bochner BS, Schleimer RP. Mast cells, basophils, and eosinophils: distinct but overlapping pathways for recruitment. *Immunol Rev* 2001; 179:5–15.
83. Rivera J, Fierro NA, Olivera A, Suzuki R. New insights on mast cell activation via the high affinity receptor for IgE. *Adv Immunol* 2008; 98:85–120.
84. Wu LC. Immunoglobulin E receptor signaling and asthma. *J Biol Chem* 2011; 286:32891–32897.
85. MacGlashan Jr DW. IgE-dependent signaling as a therapeutic target for allergies. *Trends Pharmacol Sci* 2012; 33:502–509.
86. Matsuda K, Piliponsky AM, Iikura M, et al. Monomeric IgE enhances human mast cell chemokine production: IL-4 augments and dexamethasone suppresses the response. *J Allergy Clin Immunol* 2005; 116:1357–1363.
87. Kalesnikoff J, Huber M, Lam V, et al. Monomeric IgE stimulates signaling pathways in mast cells that lead to cytokine production and cell survival. *Immunity* 2001; 14: 801–811.
88. Würtzen PA, Lund G, Lund K, Arvidsson M, Rak S, Ipsen H. A double-blind placebo-controlled birch allergy vaccination study II: correlation between inhibition of IgE binding, histamine release and facilitated allergen presentation. *Clin Exp Allergy* 2008; 38:1290–1301.
89. Bischoff SC. Role of mast cells in allergic and non-allergic immune responses: comparison of human and murine data. *Nat Rev Immunol* 2007; 7:93–104.
90. Bischoff SC, Sellge G, Lorentz A, et al. IL-4 enhances proliferation and mediator release in mature human mast cells. *Proc Natl Acad Sci USA* 1999; 96:8080–8085.
91. Gebhardt T, Sellge G, Lorentz A, et al. Cultured human intestinal mast cells express functional IL-3 receptors and respond to IL-3 by enhancing growth and IgE receptor-dependent mediator release. *Eur J Immunol* 2002; 32:2308–2316.
92. Kearley J, Erjefalt JS, Andersson C, et al. IL-9 governs allergen-induced mast cell numbers in the lung and chronic remodeling of the airways. *Am J Respir Crit Care Med* 2011; 183:865–875.
93. Akdis CA, Jutel M, Akdis M. Regulatory effects of histamine and histamine receptor expression in human allergic immune responses. *Chem Immunol Allergy* 2008; 94:67–82.
94. Maurer M, Wedemeyer J, Metz M, et al. Mast cells promote homeostasis by limiting endothelin-1-induced toxicity. *Nature* 2004; 432:512–516.
95. Metz M, Piliponsky AM, Chen CC, et al. Mast cells can enhance resistance to snake and honeybee venoms. *Science* 2006; 313:526–530.
96. Rauter I, Krauth MT, Flicker S, et al. Allergen cleavage by effector cell-derived proteases regulates allergic inflammation. *FASEB J* 2006; 20:967–969.
97. Boyce JA. Mast cells and eicosanoid mediators: a system of reciprocal paracrine and autocrine regulation. *Immunol Rev* 2007; 217:168–185.
98. Galli SJ, Tsai M. IgE and mast cells in allergic disease. *Nat Med* 2012; 18:693–704.
99. Plaut M, Pierce JH, Watson CJ, et al. Mast cell lines produce lymphokines in response to cross-linkage of Fc epsilon RI or to calcium ionophores. *Nature* 1989; 339:64–67.
100. Lorentz A, Schwengberg S, Sellge G, et al. Human intestinal mast cells are capable of producing different cytokine profiles: role of IgE receptor cross-linking and IL-4. *J Immunol* 2000; 164:43–48.
101. Ochi H, De Jesus NH, Hsieh FH, et al. IL-4 and -5 prime human mast cells for different profiles of IgE-dependent cytokine production. *Proc Natl Acad Sci USA* 2000; 97:10509–10513.
102. Gebhardt T, Lorentz A, Detmer F, et al. Growth, phenotype, and function of human intestinal mast cells are tightly regulated by transforming growth factor beta1. *Gut* 2005; 54:928–934.

103. Benoist C, Mathis D. Mast cells in autoimmune disease. *Nature* 2002; 420:875–878.
104. Bischoff SC. Physiological and pathophysiological functions of intestinal mast cells. *Semin Immunopathol* 2009; 31:185–205.
105. Moon TC, St Laurent CD, Morris KE, et al. Advances in mast cell biology: new understanding of heterogeneity and function. *Mucosal Immunol* 2010; 3:111–128.
106. Hofmann AM, Abraham SN. New roles for mast cells in pathogen defense and allergic disease. *Discov Med* 2010; 9:79–83.
107. Yu M, Tsai M, Tam SY, et al. Mast cells can promote the development of multiple features of chronic asthma in mice. *J Clin Invest* 2006; 116:1633–1641.
108. Lu LF, Lind EF, Gondek DC, et al. Mast cells are essential intermediaries in regulatory T-cell tolerance. *Nature* 2006; 442:997–1002.
109. Rodewald HR, Feyerabend TB. Widespread immunological functions of mast cells: fact or fiction? *Immunity* 2012; 37:13–24.
110. Falcone FH, Knol EF, Gibbs BF. The role of basophils in the pathogenesis of allergic disease. *Clin Exp Allergy* 2011; 41:939–947.
111. Siracusa MC, Perrigoue JG, Comeau MR, Artis D. New paradigms in basophil development, regulation and function. *Immunol Cell Biol* 2010; 88:275–284.
112. Gauvreau GM, Ellis AK, Denburg JA. Haemopoietic processes in allergic disease: eosinophil/basophil development. *Clin Exp Allergy* 2009; 39:1297–1306.
113. Lim LH, Burdick MM, Hudson SA, et al. Stimulation of human endothelium with IL-3 induces selective basophil accumulation in vitro. *J Immunol* 2006; 176:5346–5353.
114. Schroeder JT. Basophils: emerging roles in the pathogenesis of allergic disease. *Immunol Rev* 2011; 242:144–160.
115. Ochensberger B, Tassera L, Bifrare D, Rihs S, Dahinden CA. Regulation of cytokine expression and leukotriene formation in human basophils by growth factors, chemokines and chemotactic agonists. *Eur J Immunol* 1999; 29:11–22.
116. Oh K, Shen T, Le GG, Min B. Induction of Th2 type immunity in a mouse system reveals a novel immunoregulatory role of basophils. *Blood* 2007; 109:2921–2927.
117. Sullivan BM, Liang HE, Bando JK, et al. Genetic analysis of basophil function in vivo. *Nat Immunol* 2011; 12:527–535.
118. Sokol CL, Chu NQ, Yu S, Nish SA, Laufer TM, Medzhitov R. Basophils function as antigen-presenting cells for an allergen-induced T helper type 2 response. *Nat Immunol* 2009; 10:713–720.
119. Pecaric-Petkovic T, Didichenko SA, Kaempfer S, Spiegl N, Dahinden CA. Human basophils and eosinophils are the direct target leukocytes of the novel IL-1 family member IL-33. *Blood* 2009; 113:1526–1534.
120. Siracusa MC, Saenz SA, Hill DA, et al. TSLP promotes interleukin-3-independent basophil haematopoiesis and type 2 inflammation. *Nature* 2011; 477:229–233.
121. Mitre E, Nutman TB. Basophils, basophilia and helminth infections. *Chem Immunol Allergy* 2006; 90:141–156.
122. Mukai K, Matsuoka K, Taya C, et al. Basophils play a critical role in the development of IgE-mediated chronic allergic inflammation independently of T cells and mast cells. *Immunity* 2005; 23:191–202.
123. Hill DA, Siracusa MC, Abt MC, et al. Commensal bacteria-derived signals regulate basophil hematopoiesis and allergic inflammation. *Nat Med* 2012; 18:538–546.
124. Kato M, Kephart GM, Morikawa A, Gleich GJ. Eosinophil infiltration and degranulation in normal human tissues: evidence for eosinophil degranulation in normal gastrointestinal tract. *Int Arch Allergy Immunol* 2001; 125: 55–58.
125. Blanchard C, Rothenberg ME. Biology of the eosinophil. *Adv Immunol* 2009; 101:81–121.
126. Leckie MJ, ten Brinke A, Khan J, et al. Effects of an interleukin-5 blocking monoclonal antibody on eosinophils, airway hyper-responsiveness, and the late asthmatic response. *Lancet* 2000; 356:2144–2148.
127. Rosenberg HF, Dyer KD, Foster PS. Eosinophils: changing perspectives in health and disease. *Nat Rev Immunol* 2013; 13:9–22.
128. Gleich GJ. Mechanisms of eosinophil-associated inflammation. *J Allergy Clin Immunol* 2000; 105:651–663.
129. Muraki M, Gleich GJ, Kita H. Antigen-specific IgG and IgA, but not IgE, activate the effector functions of eosinophils in the presence of antigen. *Int Arch Allergy Immunol* 2011; 154:119–127.
130. Horie S, Kita H. CD11b/CD18 (Mac-1) is required for degranulation of human eosinophils induced by human recombinant granulocyte-macrophage colony-stimulating factor and platelet-activating factor. *J Immunol* 1994; 152:5457–5467.
131. Klion AD, Nutman TB. The role of eosinophils in host defense against helminth parasites. *J Allergy Clin Immunol* 2004; 113:30–37.
132. Powell N, Walker MM, Talley NJ. Gastrointestinal eosinophils in health, disease and functional disorders. *Nat Rev Gastroenterol Hepatol* 2010; 7:146–156.
133. Busse W, Corren J, Lanier BQ, et al. Omalizumab, anti-IgE recombinant humanized monoclonal antibody, for the treatment of severe allergic asthma. *J Allergy Clin Immunol* 2001; 108:184–190.

3 The Immunological Basis of Non-IgE-Mediated Reactions

Ashraf Uzzaman[1] & Hirsh D. Komarow[2]

[1]Saline Allergy Asthma Sinus Specialists, Saline, MI, USA
[2]Laboratory of Allergic Diseases, National Institute of Allergy and Infectious Diseases, National Institutes of Health, Bethesda, MD, USA

Key Concepts

- Genetic, environmental, and developmental factors as well as antigenic properties of food proteins influence the development of food allergy.
- The mucosal barrier together with the innate and adaptive arms of the immune system comprise the defense of the gastrointestinal tract against luminal antigens.
- The uptake and transport of luminal antigens is facilitated by intestinal epithelial cells, M cells, and dendritic cells where they are subsequently presented to T cells in association with MHC class II molecules.
- Oral tolerance is a physiologic, "active" non-response to an encountered antigen and a failure of oral tolerance leads to immunologic reactions to foods.
- Celiac disease is the result of an aberrant immune response to dietary gliadin mediated by non-IgE mechanisms.
- Food protein-induced enterocolitis, food protein-induced enteropathy, and allergic proctocolitis represent a spectrum of non-IgE-mediated diseases that range from potentially life threatening to benign.
- Eosinophilic esophagitis is a mixed, non-IgE- and IgE-mediated, chronic disease thought to be driven by an aberrant immune response that manifests clinically as esophageal dysfunction and histologically as eosinophil-dominant tissue inflammation.

Introduction

The first authentic report of food hypersensitivity more than 2300 years ago is attributed to Hippocrates for his observation that there exist individual differences in reactions to milk [1, 2]. Quantitatively, food proteins account for one of the largest antigenic challenges confronting the human immune system [3]. Nonetheless, only a small number of foods instigate the majority of abnormal immune responses. These abnormal responses to foods may be classified as toxic, such as to food contaminants which are not dependent on individual susceptibility, and nontoxic, which are dependent on individual susceptibility. Nontoxic responses may be separated into nonimmune mediated, such as food intolerance to lactose, and immune mediated, such as food allergy. The mechanisms of immune-mediated adverse reactions may be further divided into IgE-mediated or immediate-in-time and non-IgE-mediated or delayed-in-time responses [4, 5]. Furthermore, a number of diseases have a mixed IgE and non-IgE immune-mediated pathogenesis, hereafter referred to as mixed IgE-mediated, such as eosinophilic esophagitis (EoE). Consistent with the global increase in the prevalence of atopic diseases, there has been a significant rise in mixed IgE-mediated food allergies [6, 7].

This chapter provides a comprehensive overview of the immunologic basis of non-IgE-mediated, as well as mixed IgE-mediated mechanisms of food allergy. We elaborate on factors affecting the development of food allergy, the immunologic anatomy and defense mechanisms of the gut that avert the development of food allergy, the processing of enteral food antigens and their presentation to immune-competent cells of the gastrointestinal tract, and the effector cells and inflammatory mediators critical to the propagation and consequences of abnormal reactions to foods.

Development of food allergy

Genetic, environmental, and developmental factors, as well as a number of antigenic characteristics of food

Food Allergy: Adverse Reactions to Foods and Food Additives, Fifth Edition. Edited by Dean D Metcalfe, Hugh A Sampson, Ronald A Simon and Gideon Lack.

proteins, influence the development of food allergy. Genetic factors, such as a family history of atopic disease [8], and genetic polymorphisms [9] have been implicated. Early infectious exposure [10, 11], rural upbringing with exposure to animals [12, 13] and commensal [14], and pathogenic microorganisms within the GI tract are environmental factors that correlate with reduced atopic sensitization [15–18]. Developmental factors, including immaturity of the gut mucosa and the gut immune system in infants and children, appear to contribute to the development of food allergy [19]. In addition, the antigenic characteristics of food proteins also impact on the occurrence of food allergy.

The genetic basis of IgE-mediated food allergies has been more thoroughly characterized [20–25] than for mixed and non-IgE-mediated food allergies [26–28]. Studies of familial clustering, twin studies, and isolation of genetic polymorphisms illustrate the genetic influences on non-IgE-mediated diseases. For example, celiac disease (CD), a prototypical non-IgE-mediated food allergy, shows familial clustering [29, 30] and a high concordance rate of approximately 75% among monozygotic twins [31, 32]. This disease has also been shown to be associated with two conventional DQ molecules, HLA-DQ2 and HLA-DQ8 [27, 28, 33, 34]. Studies showing the genetic contribution of the HLA region on the familial clustering of CD suggest that HLA haplotypes are an important feature of the genetic background to the development of CD [35]. More recently genome-wide association studies have identified new loci associated with disease risk [36]. Genetic associations with disease have also been made in EoE where familial clustering occurs, and observation of a single nucleotide polymorphism in the human eotaxin-3 gene has been reported [26]. Furthermore, genome-wide analyses have implicated chromosome 5q22 in the pathogenesis of EoE and have identified thymic stromal lymphopoietin (TSLP) as the most likely candidate gene. TSLP is a cytokine involved in Th2 cell differentiation and is overexpressed in esophageal biopsies from individuals with EoE [37]. A common filaggrin gene deletion variant (2282del4) has also been found to be overexpressed in individuals with EoE as compared to controls and appears to be independent of the presence of atopic dermatitis [38]. Individuals with certain genetic variants in the TGF-β1 promoter region have been shown to be better responders to topical corticosteroid therapy [39]. These findings in EoE help identify genetics risk and susceptibility [8].

A number of environmental factors influence the development of allergy [40]. Studies show that improved social conditions lead to a more "sanitary" living environment, which may increase the risk for developing allergies, including those to foods [41, 42]. A dominant role of early environmental exposures in the development of immune tolerance has also been reported. A farm upbringing, particularly with exposure to animals and livestock, appears relatively protective against the development of allergies [43, 44]. One study documented a decreased prevalence of allergic sensitization in children growing up on farms compared to their counterparts residing in the same geographic regions [45], and the possible protective effect of these exposures during pregnancy [46]. Exposure to infection may also increase allergic manifestations [47, 48]. These observations are the basis of the "hygiene hypothesis." The inheritance of primary eosinophilic disorders thus appears to be multifactorial, with interplay between genetic and environmental factors and where a majority of individuals are atopic [49] and demonstrate symptomatic improvement when the offending foods are eliminated from the diet [50].

Both commensal and pathogenic microorganisms in the gut stimulate local B cells and T cells to induce normal development of the GI mucosal immune system. Animals reared in a germ-free environment have an underdeveloped GI mucosal immune system [51, 52]. Intestinal epithelial cells (IECs) contain lectins, adhesins, nucleotide-binding oligomerization domain (NOD) family proteins and toll-like receptors (TLRs), which recognize and respond to viral and bacterial motifs and secrete chemokines, such as IL-8, epithelial neutrophil-activating protein 78, and macrophage inflammatory protein 3α (MIP3α); and cytokines such as IL-18, IL-7, IL-15, granulocyte-macrophage colony-stimulating factor, IL-6, and transforming growth factor β (TGF-β). This process appears critical to the development of the innate as well as the adaptive arm of the mucosal immune system [53, 54].

Upregulation of cytokines has been shown in inflammatory bowel diseases [55] and aberrant secretion of chemokines such as IL-15 in response to the gliadin peptide plays a critical role in the pathogenesis of CD. There is also evidence that TH17 as well as TH1 responses occur during active CD [56]. It has been proposed that disturbances in the gut flora, along with disruption of the gut barrier and breakdown of the innate mucosal immunity caused by enteral pathogenic microorganisms, all contribute to the development of food allergy. GI microorganisms similarly contribute to the pathogenesis of reflux esophagitis [57], gastritis, gastric ulcers [58], and infectious diarrhea [59]. These conditions are all characterized by disruptions of the gut barrier resulting in irregularities in permeability and antigen transport across the GI epithelium, perhaps fostering the development of food allergy.

In infants, the relative immaturity of the GI mucosal immune system and mucosal barrier functions contribute to the pathogenesis of food allergy [1]. The mucosal immune system immaturity is associated with a low basal acid output in the stomach and relatively low levels of proteolytic activity. These conditions result in decreased luminal breakdown of antigen which leads to increased antigen absorption, as well as absorption of large antigenic molecules that interact with the mucosal immune system [60].

The age at which a particular food is introduced in the diet may relate to the development of a food allergy. It is unclear as to the most appropriate time for introducing allergenic foods such as peanuts. Recent studies suggest early consumption of peanuts in high doses during childhood may lead to a lower incidence of peanut allergy [61]. Antigenic characteristics of food proteins may also contribute to specific food allergies [62]. Physical characteristics of food proteins, such as their size, relative abundance [63], and resistance to acidic and enzymatic denaturation and digestion [64], their immunogenicity, and the method by which they are presented to T cells, are key determinants of antigenic potential [65]. Food proteins that are allergenic also tend to be resistant to food processing including heating and to acidic degradation and digestion within the GI tract [66].

Gut anatomy

The primary anatomical constituents that relate to immunological responses in the GI tract include mucus, glycocalyx, microvilli, the epithelial layer, the lamina propria, the muscularis mucosa, and gut-associated lymphoid tissue (GALT) (Figure 3.1). The mucus layer is composed of mucin, free protein, and dialyzable salts and is 95% water. It forms an adherent mucus gel layer over epithelial cells and creates a near-neutral pH at the epithelial surface. It is resistant to acidic and proteolytic digestion,

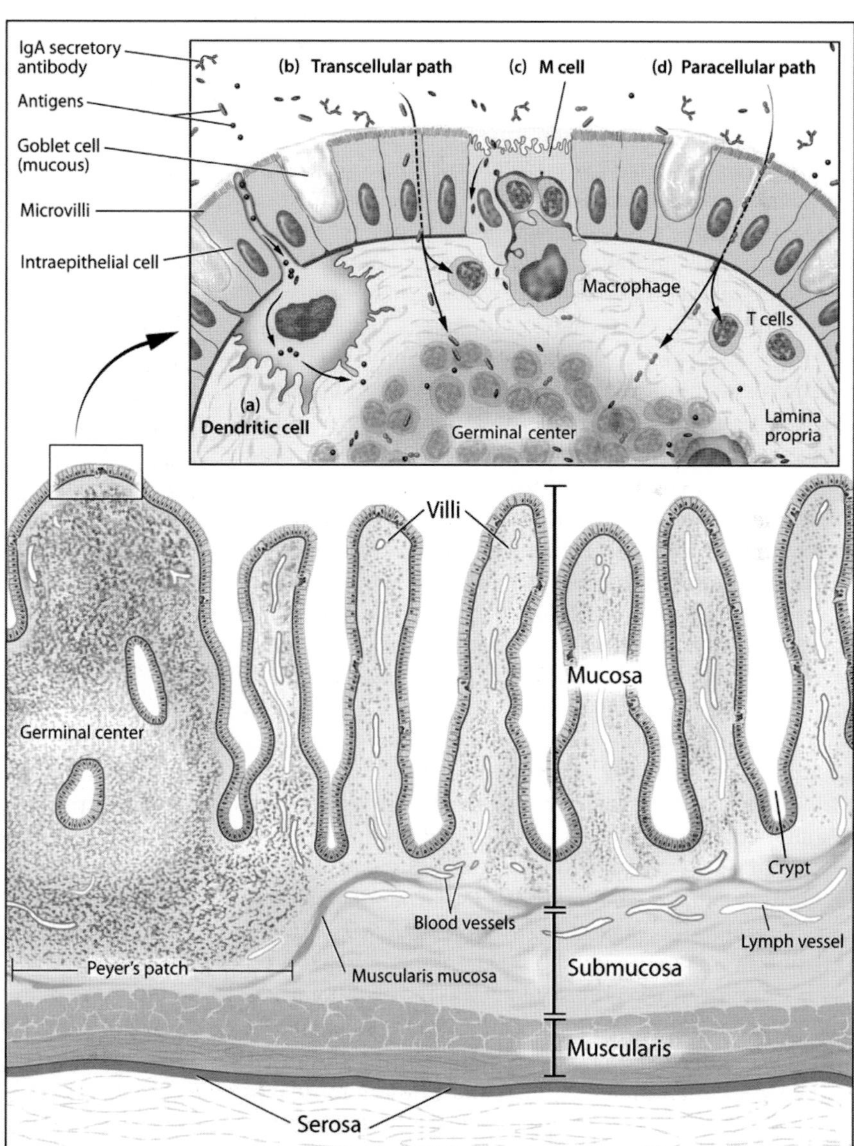

Figure 3.1 Ultrastructure of the GI wall illustrating some of its physical characteristics, which comprises the intrinsic factors of the defense mechanisms. (Inset) Pathways of antigen uptake in the gut: (a) dendritic cells extend foot processes to sample luminal antigens; (b) antigen uptake across the apical surface of the IECs; (c) uptake of antigens by M cells, which subsequently deliver them to the germinal centers; (d) uptake of antigen via the tight junctions of the IECs.

thereby protecting the underlying mucosa [67]. Internal to the mucus layer is the cell surface coat, the glycocalyx, which is composed primarily of carbohydrates and contains various enzymes such as enteropeptidases, dipeptidases, and disaccharidases; and nonenzymatic proteins that are essential for terminal digestion of food and absorption of nutrients [68, 69]. Luminal to the epithelial cells and beneath the glycocalyx are dense microvilli, which increase the absorptive surface area [70]. The epithelial layer is singular and composed of columnar cells. Together with the luminal mucus, this layer functions as the primary separation between the gastrointestinal mucosal immune system and the microbiota and enteral food proteins [71]. The epithelium also contains mucus goblet cells, undifferentiated crypt epithelial cells, and intra-epithelial lymphocytes, each of which performs a unique and integrated function (Figure 3.1a). IECs are bound by tight junctions at their apical surfaces, which function as a selective barrier to prevent the ingress of harmful viruses, bacteria, and antigens while allowing the transport of essential nutrients [72].

The lamina propria is a connective and supportive tissue layer between the basement membrane upon which the epithelium rests and the underlying muscularis mucosa. The lamina propria contains significant numbers of adaptive and innate immunocompetent cells: dendritic cells, T cells (predominantly CD4 and TCRαβ+ cells), plasma cells (mostly IgA producing), eosinophils, macrophages, and mast cells [73]. Gut microbiota contribute to intestinal digestion, stimulate gut mucosal immunity, and provide nutrient substrate for the host. Invading pathogens compete for these nutrients, which leads to changes in the composition of commensal bacteria and susceptibility to infection. Short-chain fatty acids influence gut pathogenicity and their makeup is determined by microbiota [74].

The immune system of the GI tract which resides within the mucosal layer is considered to be the largest immunologic organ in the body [71]. Humans have a well-developed gut immune system by 19 weeks' gestation, similar to most lymphoid tissues. The GALT is larger in children than in adults and consists of lymphoid follicles and lymphoid cells. The lymphoid follicles are distributed within the wall of the GI tract as Peyer's patches and also as solitary lymphoid follicles in the small intestine [75, 76]. Lymphoid cells are present diffusely within the epithelium as intra-epithelial lymphocytes, within the lamina propria, and in the Peyer's patches [77]. Peyer's patches serve as antigen-sampling sites for the gut immune system. Each Peyer's patch consists of many follicles, and each follicle is made up of a central germinal center. The germinal center develops following antigenic exposure at birth [78] and is composed of B lymphocytes surrounded by a number of T lymphocytes [79]. Overlying the follicle is a dome region consisting of the follicle-associated epithelium (Figure 3.1), which contains the specialized microfold cells (M cells) [80, 81]. M cells are derived from IECs and have microfolds on their luminal surface unlike epithelial cells which possess microvilli [82]. M cells facilitate the uptake of antigens from the gut lumen and present them to dendritic cells and macrophages contained beneath the follicle-associated epithelium. In the small intestine, additional lymphoid tissue aggregates have been described, which include isolated mucosal lymphoid follicles and submucosal lymphoid aggregations that are thought to be solitary Peyer's patch follicles [83]. The appendix is a prominent constituent of the GALT. It is organized into a large number of repeating lymphoid follicles which are morphologically similar to those present in the Peyer's patches [84].

Within the colon, lymphoid follicles may be present as lymphoglandular complexes which are organized lymphoid structures [85] and appear to be intimately associated with the luminal epithelium. These complexes are located at the points of defects in the muscularis mucosa and consist of compact spherical aggregates of lymphocytes situated below the muscularis mucosa. Such complexes are also in continuity with a less clearly circumscribed collection of lymphocytes located within the colonic lamina propria. Individual lymphoid follicles may be found within the colonic submucosa and lamina propria and are most common in the rectum [86]. The cell types present in these lymphoglandular complexes, such as dendritic cells, T and B lymphocytes, macrophages, and epithelial cells, have ultrastructural characteristics similar to M cells and appear to be similar to cells that exist in the lymphoepithelial complexes of the small intestine [85].

Defense mechanisms

The GI epithelium functions, in essence, as a gatekeeper, allowing the passage of essential nutrients necessary for growth and development, while maintaining an effective barrier against food proteins, and commensal and pathogenic microorganisms. The mucosal barrier in conjunction with the innate and adaptive immune systems comprises the primary host defense of the GI tract. The innate immune system provides protection by barrier mechanisms, while the adaptive immune system prevents indiscriminate immune responses to innocuous antigens [87].

An abnormal immune response may be observed when there are perturbations in these defense mechanisms, which in certain disease processes may be triggered by small amounts of absorbed residual, nondegraded dietary enteral proteins [88]. The GI defense system may also be divided into extrinsic factors, which are features that restrict the quantity of antigen that is able to reach the epithelial surface, and intrinsic factors, which are characteristics of the physical barriers of the GI wall. These extrinsic and intrinsic factors appear to act synergistically to limit the absorption of food antigens.

The extrinsic factors consist of proteolysis of food proteins, GI acidity, mucus production, peristalsis, and secretory IgA. The stomach produces proteolytic enzymes, such as pepsin and papain, while the small intestine harbors trypsin, chymotrypsin, and pancreatic proteases that lead to protein denaturation and degradation and alters the epitopes necessary for immunologic recognition [62, 64]. A number of diseases and the effects of some medications lead to reduced gastric acidity, which may promote increased antigen absorption [89]. Patients with cystic fibrosis that are deficient in pancreatic enzymes may have increased antigen absorption [90]. Mucus in unison with the peristaltic activity of the gut impedes the access of food antigens. Peristaltic waves result in mixing of mucus with food antigens, which limits the interaction with the absorptive epithelial surface and subsequent uptake [91]. Large intestine peristaltic waves are fewer and less vigorous compared to the small intestine and may promote absorption of food antigens [92]. Secretory antibodies provide the immunologic barrier within the gut lumen. Breast milk, especially colostrum, appears to provide, as well as enhance, secretory IgA production, a majority of which remains within the gut lumen [93, 94]. Luminal IgA binds to food antigens which hastens their transport within the GI tract [95]. IgA may also act as a cell surface receptor and attach to food antigens, which facilitate their transport into epithelial cells where these antigens are digested within phagolysosomes [96, 97].

The intrinsic barrier consists of the microvillus and IECs with their tight junctions, intracellular organelles, and proteolytic enzymes. Food antigen must maneuver across the components of the extrinsic barrier prior to coming in contact with the intrinsic barrier. The abundant microvilli, which cover the epithelial cell surface, constitute a significant barrier due to their size, close apposition to each other [98], and negative charge [99]. The IECs appear to be more than just passive barriers to the luminal contents, given the presence of a selectively permeable membrane at the base of the microvilli [100]. These IECs are also hyperpolarized and joined together by tight junctions which further augment barrier function [101]. Food proteins are ultimately endocytosed into vesicles where they are acidified and degraded by proteases and delivered to lysosomes where most antigens are eventually destroyed.

Oral tolerance

Immune responses against foods may lead to decreased absorption of food constituents and essential nutrients. Abnormal responses to foods may result in intestinal pathology, as exemplified by CD and other food-sensitive enteropathies. Under physiologic conditions, when a novel antigen is ingested, IgA antibodies are secreted in the mucosa, which is followed by a systemic humoral and/or a cell-mediated immune response. Subsequently, a systemic and local immune hyporesponsiveness may develop, which prevents a deleterious immune response with subsequent encounter of the specific antigen. This is referred to as oral tolerance [102, 103].

Although the mechanisms of oral tolerance have been primarily elucidated in animal models [104, 105], there does exist clinical and experimental evidence of oral tolerance in humans [106, 107]. Studies have suggested that at least two mechanisms are responsible for the development of oral tolerance: (1) induction of clonal anergy (or deletion) of antigen-specific T cells and (2) stimulation of regulatory T cells (Treg) which mediate active suppression of the immune response to food antigens. Clonal anergy results from a lack of costimulatory molecules on the antigen-presenting cells (CD80 and CD86) or interaction with inhibitory costimulatory molecules such as CD152 or cytotoxic T-lymphocyte-associated antigen-4 (CTLA4) and PD-1 [108–112]. Clonal anergy is an outcome of the activation of apoptotic pathways, which permanently remove antigen-specific T cells [113]. Further, a single high dose of food antigen is more likely to induce tolerance by clonal anergy whereas repeated intake of low doses may stimulate Treg cell activity [114–116]. Stimulation of Treg cells is the other mechanism by which oral tolerance may be induced. However, studies show that clonal anergy and active regulation by Treg cells are not necessarily distinct aspects of T-cell function [111]. Current research suggests that Treg cells are more likely to be CD4+ cells than the earlier believed CD8+ T cells. Several subsets of CD4+ Treg cells have been identified, which include TGF-β-producing Th3 cells, IL-10-producing Tr1, and CD4+CD25+ Treg cells. Th3 cells are formed in the GALT and appear to be pivotal in the mediation of tolerance to dietary antigens and inhibit the activation of all lymphocytes in close proximity. This is often referred to as bystander tolerance. Th3 cells then migrate to lymphoid organs where they suppress immune responses by hindering the generation of effector cells and to target organs where they suppress disease by releasing antigen-nonspecific cytokines [117]. Studies have shown that compared to normal individuals, children suffering from food allergies may have reduced numbers of Th3 cells in their duodenal mucosa, which supports the finding that TGF-β is an important regulator of intestinal immunity [118]. Antigen and naïve T-cell interactions lead to a preferential induction of Treg cells, which secrete downregulatory cytokines such as IL-10 and TGF-β. IL-10 appears to downregulate inflammatory cytokines such as IL-1, IL-6, and TNF-α, which are secreted by gut wall macrophages upon interacting with luminal bacteria [119]. Thymus-dependent CD4+CD25+ Treg cells have been shown in experimental studies to prevent colitis, possibly relating to increased levels of TGF-β [120]. Oral tolerance, once induced, suppresses T-cell allergic responses, the basis of most non-IgE-mediated food-allergic diseases. A breakdown of oral tolerance may lead to CD and cow's milk protein allergy in which aberrant CD4+ T-cell responses to gliadin and milk protein antigens, respectively, lead to mucosal injury [121].

Antigen transport

Nutrients and antigens from enteral food are primarily absorbed by IECs across their apical surface or through their tight junctions or by M cells. IECs absorb antigens in a fluid phase as well as soluble antigens, whereas M cells primarily deliver samples of large particulate antigens to the lymphoid tissues via an active vesicular transport [122,123]. Studies have suggested that this membrane traffic is charge dependent, as is seen in polarized epithelial cells [124]. The M cells have a limited number of cytoplasmic lysosomes, which makes intracellular processing of antigenic foods unlikely. The large particulate antigens which are absorbed across M cells are more likely to be of bacterial and viral origin [125].

Antigens are transported at the apical surface via a transcellular pathway or through tight junctions by means of the paracellular pathway. Across the apical surface, antigens are transported in membrane-bound vesicles by pinocytosis [126]. The tight junctions, under physiologic conditions, make paracellular transport of antigens and other macromolecules almost unachievable. Tight junctions appear to be dynamic structures. Activation of certain transport systems embedded within the apical membrane of the IEC may lead to transient and reversible increases in permeability. For example, activation of the Na+-coupled transport of glucose and amino acids dilates tight junctions and allows for increased absorption of food antigens [127, 128]. Similarly, TNF-α, IFN-γ, IL-4, and IL-13 increase epithelial permeability, but TGF-β appears to enhance barrier functions [129–132].

Antigen processing and presentation

The uptake, processing, and presentation of food antigens to naïve T cells are necessary for the mounting of an immune response by immune-competent cells of the GI tract. The uptake of antigens peaks during the neonatal period and decreases as the gut matures. In the adult GI tract, minute quantities of ingested food antigens may be absorbed and transported to the portal venous and systemic circulations in immunologically intact forms [133]. Subsequent to uptake, the processing of antigenic food proteins by IECs is achieved by proteolysis within endosomes. The antigens may then be presented to T cells by dendritic cells, macrophages, and B cells, the professional antigen-presenting cells that constitutively express class II MHC molecules; and eosinophils and mast cells, the nonprofessional antigen-presenting cells which express class II MHC molecules on their cell surface when activated. However, IECs appear to be the only nonprofessional antigen-presenting cells that constitutively express MHC class II molecules on their surface [134]. The antigen-presenting cells may take up the antigen by endocytosis, which is nonspecific and less efficient, than by receptor-mediated methods, which appear to be more efficient [135, 136]. Only professional antigen-presenting cells with the following three key characteristics are able to activate normally naïve T cells to become memory and effector cells [137]. First, there must be expression of specific surface glycoproteins. Second, absorption of antigens must occur by either receptor-mediated or fluid-phase endocytosis. Finally, there must be processing of the absorbed antigens within intracytoplasmic organelles, forming a complex with products of class II MHC molecules for presentation to T cells.

In addition to their role in barrier function and as nonprofessional antigen-presenting cells, IECs may also play a role in the regulation of regional immunologic function. These cells absorb and process antigens and may present them directly to T cells in an MHC-dependent manner [138]. The IECs express class II MHC molecules, mostly on their basolateral surface, where they interact with lymphocytes in the intra-epithelial spaces and in the lamina propria. The expression of MHC molecules appears to be enhanced during gut inflammation [139]. Absorbed luminal antigens may be processed by dissimilar proteolytic enzymes contained in different phagolysosomes that generate a diversity of antigenic epitopes that ultimately interact with T cells [140]. An antigen absorbed at the apical surface may not elicit an immune response, but may if it is absorbed at the basolateral surface [141]. In contrast to professional antigen-presenting cells, IECs may selectively activate CD8+ suppressor T cells, which enhance the suppression of the gut immune response [142]. This process appears to be regulated by the nonclassical MHC class I molecule CD1d and an IEC membrane glycoprotein, the CD8 ligand gp180 [143–146]. The precise mechanisms implicated and the roles played in downregulating the mucosal immune responses, however, remain incompletely understood.

Dendritic cells are derived from circulating monocytes, which originate from bone-marrow-derived myeloid precursors [147–149]. Dendritic cells are specialized for the uptake, processing, transport, and presentation of antigens, as well as the priming of naïve T cells. During differentiation, dendritic cells upregulate expression of MHC class II molecules, which increases their antigen-presenting efficiency. They also alter their expression of chemokine receptors and production of cytokines, which are vital to T-cell differentiation [150, 151]. Microbes within the intestinal lumen also appear to stimulate dendritic cells to secrete immunostimulatory cytokines, including IL-12, which upregulate the expression of MHC class II molecules, as well as produce costimulatory molecules [150]. Within gut lymphoid follicles, dendritic cells may be classified as follicular and nonfollicular cells. Follicular dendritic cells express antigen, which is vital for the maintenance of memory B cells. The nonfollicular dendritic cells are preferentially localized within the dome regions of Peyer's patches, the lamina propria, in T-cell zones and in certain other parts of the GALT.

The uptake of antigens by dendritic cells may be achieved by macropinocytosis and by receptor-dependent mechanisms [152, 153]. Dendritic cells may also send foot processes between IECs [154] or they may become lodged between adjacent IECs and endocytose luminal antigens before migrating to the lamina propria [155]. Subsequently, these cells reach secondary lymphoid organs, such as mesenteric lymph nodes where they interact with and activate naïve T cells [156]. Occasionally, antigens may also reach dendritic cells within secondary lymphoid organs by direct dissemination through draining gastrointestinal lymphatics or via the bloodstream.

T cells

The production of food-antigen-specific IgE antibodies is facilitated by cytokines produced by T cells, such as IL-4 and IL-13. Non-IgE-mediated food allergies result in part from an imbalance between inflammatory cytokines secreted by T cells, such as IFN-γ, TNF-α, and IL-15, and regulatory cytokines such as IL-10 [157]. Antigenic stimulation of naïve T cells leads to priming, followed by proliferation into memory T cells and subsequent entrance into the circulation. From the vasculature, memory T cells may return to the GI tract to function as effector cells in disease pathogenesis. Increased expression of α4β7 on memory T-cell subsets correlates with enhanced recruitment into Peyer's patches. Naïve T cells that are α4β7low and the subset of memory T cells that are α4β7high are equally well recruited to Peyer's patches. However, the subset of memory T cells which are α4β7low is excluded [158]. The specific ligand for α4β7 on vascular endothelial cells within the high endothelial venules is mucosal addressin-cell adhesion molecule-1 (MAdCAM-1), which facilitates the migration of T cells. Stimulation of peripheral T cells by β lactoglobulin present in cow's milk results in the selective increased expression of α4β7, which suggests that allergen exposure enhances the migration of memory T cells [159]. Patients with subclinical CD have increased numbers of T cells within the gut mucosa, which proliferate further when the individual becomes symptomatic [160, 161].

CD is characterized by the presence of gluten-specific CD4+ T cells in the lamina propria and increased numbers of intra-epithelial lymphocytes of the TCRαβ+ CD8+CD4– and TCRγδ+ CD8–CD4– lineage [162]. Cytokines secreted by CD4+ cells, intra-epithelial lymphocytes, and IECs are the primary effectors of mucosal injury in CD. Gluten-activated mucosal CD4+ cells secrete IFN-γ, which together with TNF-α secreted by macrophages leads to increased permeability and direct cytotoxic effects on the small IECs [163, 164]. Activated stromal cells within the lamina propria are induced by TNF-α to produce keratinocyte growth factor (KGF), an epithelial mitogen, which stimulates small IEC proliferation and results in crypt cell hyperplasia [165]. IECs, dendritic cells, and macrophages produce IL-15, which is upregulated within the lamina propria and the intestinal epithelium during active disease and plays a critical role in the pathogenesis of CD [166]. Gliadin may act independently or in concert with IL-15 to activate IECs and induce the expression of the nonconventional HLA I molecule, MHC class I chain A related molecule (MICA). Expression of MICA leads to direct cytotoxicity of IECs in an antigen-nonspecific manner [167]. IL-15 may also upregulate the expression of NKG2D, an activating receptor that is normally expressed on most natural killer (NK) cells, as well as on CD8+ TCRαβ+ and TCRγδ+ cells [168–170]. MICA serves as a ligand for NKG2D, which may result in lymphocyte-mediated cytotoxicity of IECs and in villus atrophy and small intestinal mucosal injury [171].

Food protein-induced enterocolitis is a non-IgE-mediated disease. However, there is evidence to suggest the involvement of antigen-specific T cells and production of proinflammatory cytokines which dysregulate the permeability of the intestinal barrier [172, 173]. Humoral-specific antibody responses have also been shown to contribute to pathogenesis [174]. It has been postulated that an antigen-specific T-cell response in food protein-induced enterocolitis syndrome (FPIES) resulting in the secretion of proinflammatory cytokines disrupts intestinal permeability and that activated T cells secrete high levels of TNF-α which increases intestinal permeability [175]. Furthermore, increased fecal levels of TNF-α have been shown in individuals with cow's milk allergy with intestinal manifestations during a milk challenge. Significantly greater levels of TNF-α have been reported in duodenal epithelial cells in individuals with FPIES who had villous atrophy compared to those who did not [173]. These data support a critical role for TNF-α in disease pathogenesis. TGF-β1 is known to induce T-cell suppression and contribute to intestinal barrier integrity. Decreased TGF-β1 levels have been shown in the intestinal mucosa of less than 3-month-old infants [176]. Reduced levels of type 1 but not type 2 receptors for TGF-β have been reported in duodenal biopsy specimens from individuals with FPIES, consistent with a role for TGF-β in disease pathogenesis [173].

In some individuals, the underlying mechanism of cow's milk allergy may be non-IgE mediated. Individuals with cow's milk allergy, in contrast to individuals with CD, usually do not develop villous atrophy or an increased mononuclear cell infiltrate within the lamina propria. However, TCRγδ+ CD8–CD4– cells may occur as the majority of intra-epithelial lymphocytes, which suggests that a cytokine imbalance leads to the disease phenotype [177]. CD is primarily Th1 biased, whereas cow's milk protein allergy in individuals with an atopic predisposition appears to be predominantly Th2 biased. This is evidenced by a high production of IL-4, IL-5, and IL-13 and a low production of IFN-γ [178, 179]. However, non-atopic individuals may exhibit a Th0-like cytokine phenotype [180]. One study has demonstrated differences in an immune activation profile between individuals with non-IgE-mediated cow's milk allergy and CD. This group with cow's milk allergy demonstrated an upregulation of CCR4 and IL-6 mRNA and downregulation of IL-18 and IL-2 mRNA within the gut mucosal tissue, suggesting a Th-2-biased immune response. In contrast, individuals with CD showed upregulation of IFN-γ and downregulation of IL-12p35-, IL-12p40-, and IL-18-specific mRNA [181].

In patients with FPIES and sensitivity to soy and milk, tolerance to milk tends to occur more frequently than to soy within several years of the initial adverse reaction [182]. A higher frequency of CD4+CD25+ T regulatory cells has been shown in individuals who had outgrown non-IgE-mediated allergy to cow's milk protein in comparison to those with active ongoing disease [183]. In addition, the suppressive effect of T regulatory cells was mediated in this study by direct cell-to-cell contact and by secretion of TGF-β, thus highlighting the role of T regulatory cells in the development of immune tolerance.

Eosinophils

Mixed IgE- and non-IgE-based reactions to foods is a feature of eosinophil-associated gastrointestinal disorders (EGID) [1, 184, 185]. Individuals with EGID have an eosinophil-rich infiltrate within the wall of the esophagus, stomach, and/or small and large intestines [186]. They may be allergic to multiple foods, have an elevated serum IgE, and exhibit a peripheral eosinophilia [187, 188].

Numerous inflammatory mediators have been implicated in the recruitment of eosinophils to tissues. Of these, eotaxin, constitutively expressed by the GI epithelium, and IL-5 appear to be relatively specific eosinophil chemoattractants [189]. Eotaxin appears to modulate the recruitment of eosinophils by selectively binding and signaling through the chemokine receptor, CCR3, found primarily on eosinophils [190]. Eotaxin also appears to facilitate the movement of eosinophils from blood vessels to gut tissue, which is dependent on the interaction of α4β7 present on eosinophils with MAdCAM-1 [191]. Basic fibroblast growth factor (bFGF) has also been shown to be involved in the pathogenesis of EoE. It may act synergistically to increase the activation and half-life of esophageal eosinophils in individuals with EoE [192].

In a physiologic state, eosinophils exist in small numbers within the GI wall and the presence of relatively large numbers denotes an underlying disease process. The esophageal wall, however, lacks eosinophils and the presence of eosinophils which are unresponsive to acid suppression therapy indicates a pathologic course [193]. The mere presence of tissue eosinophils is not diagnostic of a specific disease since it may occur in diseases such as EoE, eosinophilic gastroenteritis, gastroesophageal reflux disease (GERD), chronic noneosinophilic esophagitis, fungal and parasitic infections, and inflammatory bowel disease.

IL-5 has also been shown to be involved in eosinophil differentiation, proliferation, survival, recruitment, and trafficking within the GI tract. IL-5, along with eotaxin, has been established to be essential in the pathogenesis of EoE [194]. Furthermore, increased levels of IL-13 in tissue biopsies from individuals with EoE indicate a key role of adaptive Th2 immunity in its pathogenesis [195]. A stepwise interaction between endothelial cells of the blood vessels and eosinophils then promotes their migration to the mucosal tissues. The rolling of an eosinophil over the endothelial cell surface is assisted primarily by P-selectin, the adhesion molecule present on endothelial cells [196]. Rolling is followed by adherence which is facilitated by molecules of the integrin family [197]. Within the mucosal tissues, eosinophil survival is cytokine dependent. Granulocyte–macrophage colony-stimulating factor (GM-CSF) increases the survival of tissue eosinophils and IL-12 appears to increase apoptosis [198].

Studies have demonstrated that, in addition to eosinophils, the cellular component of the inflammatory infiltrate in EGID also consists of increased numbers of activated CD4+ T cells and mast cells [199]. Monocytes and neutrophils are other cell types that are associated with the disease [200]. Eosinophils propagate disease pathogenesis and instigate mucosal injury by release of inflammatory mediators, eosinophilic cytotoxic granule proteins, cytokines, and reactive oxygen intermediates. Cytokines,

Table 3.1 An overview of immune mechanisms and symptoms of non-IgE-mediated and mixed food allergies.

Disease	Immune mechanism	Symptoms
Food-protein-induced enterocolitis	Cell-mediated	Profuse vomiting, diarrhea (± microscopic blood); severe symptoms may lead to lethargy, dehydration, and shock
Food-protein-induced proctocolitis	Cell-mediated	Gradual onset bleeding progressing to streaks of blood; infant typically thriving and usually well
Food-protein-induced enteropathy (gluten-sensitive enteropathy)	Cell-mediated	Dyspepsia, reflux, diarrhea abdominal distension, flatulence, failure to thrive; other symptoms depend on extraintestinal manifestations
Allergic eosinophilic esophagitis	Cell-mediated and/or IgE-mediated	Difficulty feeding, failure to thrive, gastroesophageal reflux, vomiting, dysphagia, and food impaction
Allergic eosinophilic gastroenteritis	Cell-mediated and/or IgE-mediated	Recurrent abdominal pain and vomiting, failure to thrive, peripheral blood eosinophilia (50%)

immunoglobulins, and complement components may activate eosinophils to generate inflammatory mediators such as IL-1, IL-3, IL-4, IL-5, IL-13, GM-CSF, TNF-α, MIP 1α, and vascular endothelial cell growth factor. This suggests that eosinophils may modulate the many features of the immune response [201]. Furthermore, epithelial growth, fibrosis, and tissue remodeling may be influenced by eosinophil-derived TGF-β and the eosinophilic cytotoxic granule proteins including eosinophilic cationic protein [202], major basic protein [203], and eosinophil peroxidase [204]. Eosinophilic cationic protein may insert toxic pores into the IEC membrane, which leads to the entry of other toxic molecules [205]. Major basic protein induces smooth muscle reactivity and may initiate degranulation of mast cells and basophils [206].

Respiratory burst enzyme pathways in eosinophils generate superoxide that may cause mucosal damage [207]. Eosinophil peroxidase generates toxic hydrogen peroxide and halic acids that may trigger further injury [208]. Neutrophils also generate lipid mediators such as LTB4, LTC4, LTD4, and LTE4 which lead to increased vascular permeability, mucin secretion, and smooth muscle contraction [209]. Moreover, the extent of GI wall eosinophil infiltration and the quantity of eosinophilic cytotoxic proteins correlate with disease severity [210,211]. Table 3.1 lists diseases with non-IgE- and mixed immune-mediated mechanisms and a summary of their clinical features [212–216].

Food protein-induced enterocolitis and proctocolitis

FPIES and proctocolitis occur predominantly in infants and are characterized by severe small and large intestine mucosal injury. The common dietary culprits implicated in pathogenesis are cow's milk and soybean. Cereal grains (rice, oat, barley), fish, poultry, and vegetables are infrequent offenders [217]. The diagnosis is chiefly made by clinical symptoms and challenge testing, but may also be supported by resolution of symptoms after dietary elimination of the perpetrator protein. Typical symptoms include vomiting and diarrhea which are associated with the presence of blood, leukocytes, eosinophils, and increased carbohydrate content in the stool [218]. Histologic studies of endoscopic biopsy specimens in symptomatic patients reveal an increase in eosinophils and plasma cells, presence of crypt abscesses, and mild villous injury. A few infants may show evidence of gastritis and esophagitis [219].

Celiac disease

CD is often categorized as an autoimmune disorder affecting the small intestines, induced by the intake of gluten in wheat and analogous proteins present in barley and rye. CD is closely associated with genes that code HLA-II antigens, mainly of the DQ2 and DQ8 classes [220, 221]. CD may manifest early in life following the introduction of gluten in the diet or may develop later in life. The clinical manifestations include abdominal pain with distension, dyspepsia, presence of gastroesophageal reflux (GERD), recurrent episodes of diarrhea and/or constipation, weight loss, bone disease, anemia, and weakness. Symptoms tend to remit upon strict compliance to a gluten-free diet. The demonstration of circulatory IgA antibodies to transglutaminase (tTG-IgA) is supportive of the diagnosis. Histologic examination of endoscopic samples is confirmatory [222]. However, patchy involvement of the mucosa may lead to a false-negative diagnosis. Histologic changes within the mucosa include villus atrophy, crypt hyperplasia, thickening of the epithelial basement membrane, and reduced numbers of goblet cells. Evidence of mucosal inflammation is manifested by an increase in intra-epithelial lymphocytes and an influx of immune cells within the small intestinal lamina propria and loss of basal nuclear orientation as well as a change of the IECs to a cuboidal morphology.

Allergic eosinophilic esophagitis and gastroenteritis

Primary eosinophilic gastrointestinal disorders include EoE, gastritis, gastroenteritis, enteritis, and eosinophilic colitis. These diseases are occurring with increasing frequency and are mediated by mixed immune mechanisms [223]. They are characterized by an eosinophil-rich infiltrate within the gut wall in the absence of other causes of gut wall eosinophilia, such as drug reactions, parasitic infections, and malignancy. The constellation of symptoms includes abdominal pain, dysphagia, vomiting, diarrhea, gastric dysmotility, irritability, and failure to thrive [224]. The diagnosis of primary eosinophilic gastrointestinal disorders is contingent upon the histologic assessment of endoscopic biopsy samples with vigilant consideration of the quantity, location, and characteristics of the eosinophilic infiltration [185].

Conclusions

We have reviewed the non-IgE-mediated mechanisms associated with adverse reactions to foods. We have detailed the barrier functions of the gut; the processing, absorption, and presentation of antigens to the immune-competent cells; the mounting of a response; and the inflammatory changes and mucosal damage as propagated by infiltrating cells within the gut mucosa. It is apparent that non-IgE-mediated gastrointestinal allergic diseases may be associated with gastrointestinal epithelial barrier dysfunction. It is not clear if barrier dysfunction is an outcome or a contributing factor to the development of food allergies. Intertwined in disease pathogenesis are T cells, which are pivotal to the induction of oral tolerance as well as the propagation of disease, and eosinophils, which are central in the pathogenesis and modulation of eosinophilic gastrointestinal disorders. An appreciation of the immune mechanisms involved in food hypersensitivities and its associated diseases and the counseling of genetically susceptible individuals will facilitate the development of new and novel approaches to treating patients with these diseases.

Acknowledgment

This work was partially supported by the Division of Intramural Research, NIAID, NIH.

References

1. Sampson HA. Food allergy. Part 1: immunopathogenesis and clinical disorders. *J Allergy Clin Immunol* 1999; 103(5 Pt. 1):717–728.
2. Hippocrates. *The Medical Works of Hippocrates*. Oxford Press, 1950.
3. Buckley RH, Metcalfe D. Food allergy. *J Am Med Assoc* 1982; 248(20):2627–2631.
4. Johansson SG, Bieber T, Dahl R, et al. Revised nomenclature for allergy for global use: report of the Nomenclature Review Committee of the World Allergy Organization, October 2003. *J Allergy Clin Immunol* 2004; 113(5):832–836.
5. Johansson SG, Hourihane JO, Bousquet J, et al. A revised nomenclature for allergy. An EAACI position statement from the EAACI Nomenclature Task Force. *Allergy* 2001; 56(9):813–824.
6. Grundy J, Matthews S, Bateman B, Dean T, Arshad SH. Rising prevalence of allergy to peanut in children: data from 2 sequential cohorts. *J Allergy Clin Immunol* 2002; 110(5):784–789.
7. Cherian S, Smith NM, Forbes DA. Rapidly increasing prevalence of eosinophilic oesophagitis in Western Australia. *Arch Dis Child* 2006; 91(12):1000–1004.
8. Tan TH, Ellis JA, Saffery R, Allen KJ. The role of genetics and environment in the rise of childhood food allergy. *Clin Exp Allergy* 2012; 42(1):20–29.
9. Hong X, Wang G, Liu X, et al. Gene polymorphisms, breast-feeding, and development of food sensitization in early childhood. *J Allergy Clin Immunol* 2011; 128(2):374–381; e2.
10. Rook GA. Hygiene and other early childhood influences on the subsequent function of the immune system. *Dig Dis* 2011; 29(2):144–153.
11. Ruemmele FM, Bier D, Marteau P, et al. Clinical evidence for immunomodulatory effects of probiotic bacteria. *J Pediatr Gastroenterol Nutr* 2009; 48(2):126–141.
12. von Mutius E, Vercelli D. Farm living: effects on childhood asthma and allergy. *Nat Rev Immunol* 2010; 10(12):861–868.
13. Dimich-Ward H, Chow Y, Chung J, Trask C. Contact with livestock—a protective effect against allergies and asthma? *Clin Exp Allergy* 2006; 36(9):1122–1129.
14. Tlaskalova-Hogenova H, Stepankova R, Hudcovic T, et al. Commensal bacteria (normal microflora), mucosal immunity and chronic inflammatory and autoimmune diseases. *Immunol Lett* 2004; 93(2–3):97–108.
15. Loss G, Apprich S, Waser M, et al. The protective effect of farm milk consumption on childhood asthma and atopy: the GABRIELA study. *J Allergy Clin Immunol* 2011; 128(4):766–773; e4.

16. Ege MJ, Herzum I, Buchele G, et al. Prenatal exposure to a farm environment modifies atopic sensitization at birth. *J Allergy Clin Immunol* 2008; 122(2):407–412; e1–e4.
17. Radon K, Schulze A. Adult obesity, farm childhood, and their effect on allergic sensitization. *J Allergy Clin Immunol* 2006; 118(6):1279–1283.
18. Perkin MR, Strachan DP. Which aspects of the farming lifestyle explain the inverse association with childhood allergy? *J Allergy Clin Immunol* 2006; 117(6):1374–1381.
19. Strobel S. Neonatal oral tolerance. *Ann NY Acad Sci* 1996; 778:88–102.
20. Krogulska A, Borowiec M, Polakowska E, Dynowski J, Mlynarski W, Wasowska-Krolikowska K. FOXP3, IL-10, and TGF-beta genes expression in children with IgE-dependent food allergy. *J Clin Immunol* 2011; 31(2):205–215.
21. Dreskin SC, Tripputi MT, Aubrey MT, et al. Peanut-allergic subjects and their peanut-tolerant siblings have large differences in peanut-specific IgG that are independent of HLA class II. *Clin Immunol* 2010; 137(3):366–373.
22. Behnecke A, Li W, Chen L, Saxon A, Zhang K. IgE-mediated allergen gene vaccine platform targeting human antigen-presenting cells through the high-affinity IgE receptor. *J Allergy Clin Immunol* 2009; 124(1):108–113.
23. Sicherer SH, Furlong TJ, Maes HH, Desnick RJ, Sampson HA, Gelb BD. Genetics of peanut allergy: a twin study. *J Allergy Clin Immunol* 2000; 106(1 Pt. 1):53–56.
24. Liu X, Beaty TH, Deindl P, et al. Associations between specific serum IgE response and 6 variants within the genes IL4, IL13, and IL4RA in German children: the German Multicenter Atopy Study. *J Allergy Clin Immunol* 2004; 113(3):489–495.
25. Matsuo H, Kohno K, Morita E. Molecular cloning, recombinant expression and IgE-binding epitope of omega-5 gliadin, a major allergen in wheat-dependent exercise-induced anaphylaxis. *FEBS J* 2005; 272(17):4431–4438.
26. Blanchard C, Wang N, Rothenberg ME. Eosinophilic esophagitis: pathogenesis, genetics, and therapy. *J Allergy Clin Immunol* 2006; 118(5):1054–1059.
27. Hovhannisyan Z, Weiss A, Martin A, et al. The role of HLA-DQ8 beta57 polymorphism in the anti-gluten T-cell response in coeliac disease. *Nature* 2008; 456(7221):534–538.
28. Tollefsen S, Arentz-Hansen H, Fleckenstein B, et al. HLA-DQ2 and -DQ8 signatures of gluten T cell epitopes in celiac disease. *J Clin Invest* 2006; 116(8):2226–2236.
29. Macdonald WC, Dobbins III WO, Rubin CE. Studies of the familial nature of celiac sprue using biopsy of the small intestine. *N Engl J Med* 1965; 272:448–456.
30. Rich N. Assessing the role of HLA-linked and unlinked determinants of disease. *Am J Hum Genet* 1987; 40(1):1–14.
31. Greco L, Romino R, Coto I, et al. The first large population based twin study of coeliac disease. *Gut* 2002; 50(5):624–628.
32. Bardella MT, Fredella C, Prampolini L, Marino R, Conte D, Giunta AM. Gluten sensitivity in monozygous twins: a long-term follow-up of five pairs. *Am J Gastroenterol* 2000; 95(6):1503–1505.
33. Bodd M, Tollefsen S, Bergseng E, Lundin KE, Sollid LM. Evidence that HLA-DQ9 confers risk to celiac disease by presence of DQ9-restricted gluten-specific T cells. *Hum Immunol* 2012; 73(4):376–381.
34. Clouzeau-Girard H, Rebouissoux L, Taupin JL, et al. HLA-DQ genotyping combined with serological markers for the diagnosis of celiac disease: is intestinal biopsy still mandatory? *J Pediatr Gastroenterol Nutr* 2011; 52(6):729–733.
35. Petronzelli F, Bonamico M, Ferrante P, et al. Genetic contribution of the HLA region to the familial clustering of coeliac disease. *Ann Hum Genet* 1997; 61(Pt. 4):307–317.
36. Trynka G, Hunt KA, Bockett NA, et al. Dense genotyping identifies and localizes multiple common and rare variant association signals in celiac disease. *Nat Genet* 2011; *43*(12):1193–1201.
37. Sherrill JD, Gao PS, Stucke EM, et al. Variants of thymic stromal lymphopoietin and its receptor associate with eosinophilic esophagitis. *J Allergy Clin Immunol* 2010; 126(1):160–165; e3.
38. Blanchard C, Stucke EM, Burwinkel K, et al. Coordinate interaction between IL-13 and epithelial differentiation cluster genes in eosinophilic esophagitis. *J Immunol* 2010; 184(7):4033–4041.
39. Aceves SS, Newbury RO, Chen D, et al. Resolution of remodeling in eosinophilic esophagitis correlates with epithelial response to topical corticosteroids. *Allergy* 2010; 65(1):109–116.
40. Svanes C, Jarvis D, Chinn S, Burney P. Childhood environment and adult atopy: results from the European Community Respiratory Health Survey. *J Allergy Clin Immunol* 1999; 103(3 Pt. 1):415–420.
41. Linneberg A, Ostergaard C, Tvede M, et al. IgG antibodies against microorganisms and atopic disease in Danish adults: the Copenhagen Allergy Study. *J Allergy Clin Immunol* 2003; 111(4):847–853.
42. von Mutius E, Weiland SK, Fritzsch C, Duhme H, Keil U. Increasing prevalence of hay fever and atopy among children in Leipzig, East Germany. *Lancet* 1998; 351(9106):862–866.
43. Ege MJ, Bieli C, Frei R, et al. Prenatal farm exposure is related to the expression of receptors of the innate immunity and to atopic sensitization in school-age children. *J Allergy Clin Immunol* 2006; 117(4):817–823.
44. Ege MJ, Mayer M, Normand AC, et al. Exposure to environmental microorganisms and childhood asthma. *N Engl J Med* 2011; 364(8):701–709.
45. Alfven T, Braun-Fahrlander C, Brunekreef B, et al. Allergic diseases and atopic sensitization in children related to farming and anthroposophic lifestyle–the PARSIFAL study. *Allergy* 2006; 61(4):414–421.
46. Roduit C, Wohlgensinger J, Frei R, et al. Prenatal animal contact and gene expression of innate immunity receptors at birth are associated with atopic dermatitis. *J Allergy Clin Immunol* 2011; 127(1):179–185; 85 e1.
47. Hogg JC. Childhood viral infection and the pathogenesis of asthma and chronic obstructive lung disease. *Am J Respir Crit Care Med* 1999; 160(5 Pt. 2):S26–S28.
48. Denlinger LC, Sorkness RL, Lee WM, et al. Lower airway rhinovirus burden and the seasonal risk of asthma exacerbation. *Am J Respir Crit Care Med* 2011; 184(9):1007–1014.

49. Rothenberg ME. Biology and treatment of eosinophilic esophagitis. *Gastroenterology* 2009; 137(4):1238–1249.
50. Markowitz JE, Spergel JM, Ruchelli E, Liacouras CA. Elemental diet is an effective treatment for eosinophilic esophagitis in children and adolescents. *Am J Gastroenterol* 2003; 98(4):777–782.
51. MacPherson GG, Liu LM. Dendritic cells and Langerhans cells in the uptake of mucosal antigens. *Curr Top Microbiol Immunol* 1999; 236:33–53.
52. Cebra JJ. Influences of microbiota on intestinal immune system development. *Am J Clin Nutr* 1999; 69(5):1046S–1051S.
53. Kelly D, Conway S. Bacterial modulation of mucosal innate immunity. *Mol Immunol* 2005; 42(8):895–901.
54. Abreu MT, Fukata M, Arditi M. TLR signaling in the gut in health and disease. *J Immunol* 2005; 174(8):4453–4460.
55. Zahn A, Giese T, Karner M, et al. Transcript levels of different cytokines and chemokines correlate with clinical and endoscopic activity in ulcerative colitis. *BMC Gastroenterol* 2009; 9:13.
56. Castellanos-Rubio A, Santin I, Irastorza I, Castano L, Carlos Vitoria J, Ramon Bilbao J. TH17 (and TH1) signatures of intestinal biopsies of CD patients in response to gliadin. *Autoimmunity* 2009; 42(1):69–73.
57. Nordenstedt H, Nilsson M, Johnsen R, Lagergren J, Hveem K. Helicobacter pylori infection and gastroesophageal reflux in a population-based study (The HUNT Study). *Helicobacter* 2007; 12(1):16–22.
58. Figura N, Perrone A, Gennari C, et al. CagA-positive Helicobacter pylori infection may increase the risk of food allergy development. *J Physiol Pharmacol* 1999; 50(5):827–831.
59. Zuckerman MJ, Watts MT, Bhatt BD, Ho H. Intestinal permeability to [51Cr]EDTA in infectious diarrhea. *Dig Dis Sci* 1993; 38(9):1651–1657.
60. Kaczmarski M, Kurzatkowska B. The contribution of some environmental factors to the development of cow's milk and gluten intolerance in children. *Rocz Akad Med Bialymst* 1988–1989; 33–34:151–165.
61. Du Toit G, Katz Y, Sasieni P, et al. Early consumption of peanuts in infancy is associated with a low prevalence of peanut allergy. *J Allergy Clin Immunol* 2008; 122(5):984–991.
62. Bannon GA. What makes a food protein an allergen? *Curr Allergy Asthma Rep* 2004; 4(1):43–46.
63. Metcalfe DD, Astwood JD, Townsend R, Sampson HA, Taylor SL, Fuchs RL. Assessment of the allergenic potential of foods derived from genetically engineered crop plants. *Crit Rev Food Sci Nutr* 1996; 36(Suppl.):S165–S186.
64. Untersmayr E, Jensen-Jarolim E. The effect of gastric digestion on food allergy. *Curr Opin Allergy Clin Immunol* 2006; 6(3):214–219.
65. Sen M, Kopper R, Pons L, Abraham EC, Burks AW, Bannon GA. Protein structure plays a critical role in peanut allergen stability and may determine immunodominant IgE-binding epitopes. *J Immunol* 2002; 169(2):882–887.
66. Astwood JD, Leach JN, Fuchs RL. Stability of food allergens to digestion in vitro. *Nat Biotechnol* 1996; 14(10):1269–1273.
67. Allen A, Flemstrom G. Gastroduodenal mucus bicarbonate barrier: protection against acid and pepsin. *Am J Physiol Cell Physiol* 2005; 288(1):C1–C19.
68. Poley JR. Loss of the glycocalyx of enterocytes in small intestine: a feature detected by scanning electron microscopy in children with gastrointestinal intolerance to dietary protein. *J Pediatr Gastroenterol Nutr* 1988; 7(3):386–394.
69. Ito S. Structure and function of the glycocalyx. *Fed Proc* 1969; 28(1):12–25.
70. Danielsen EM, Hansen GH. Lipid raft organization and function in brush borders of epithelial cells. *Mol Membr Biol* 2006; 23(1):71–79.
71. Chehade M, Mayer L. Oral tolerance and its relation to food hypersensitivities. *J Allergy Clin Immunol* 2005; 115(1):3–12; quiz 3.
72. Guttman JA, Li Y, Wickham ME, Deng W, Vogl AW, Finlay BB. Attaching and effacing pathogen-induced tight junction disruption in vivo. *Cell Microbiol* 2006; 8(4):634–645.
73. MacDonald TT. The mucosal immune system. *Parasite Immunol* 2003; 25(5):235–246.
74. Keeney KM, Finlay BB. Enteric pathogen exploitation of the microbiota-generated nutrient environment of the gut. *Curr Opin Microbiol* 2011; 14(1):92–98.
75. Lugering A, Kucharzik T. Induction of intestinal lymphoid tissue: the role of cryptopatches. *Ann NY Acad Sci* 2006; 1072:210–217.
76. Moghaddami M, Cummins A, Mayrhofer G. Lymphocyte-filled villi: comparison with other lymphoid aggregations in the mucosa of the human small intestine. *Gastroenterology* 1998; 115(6):1414–1425.
77. Van Kruiningen HJ, West AB, Freda BJ, Holmes KA. Distribution of Peyer's patches in the distal ileum. *Inflamm Bowel Dis* 2002; 8(3):180–185.
78. Bridges RA, Condie RM, Zak SJ, Good RA. The morphologic basis of antibody formation development during the neonatal period. *J Lab Clin Med* 1959; 53(3):331–357.
79. Strobel S. Mechanisms of mucosal immunology and gastrointestinal damage. *Pediatr Allergy Immunol* 1993; 4(3 Suppl.):25–32.
80. Spahn TW, Kucharzik T. Modulating the intestinal immune system: the role of lymphotoxin and GALT organs. *Gut* 2004; 53(3):456–465.
81. Fujimura Y, Kihara T, Ohtani K, et al. Distribution of microfold cells (M cells) in human follicle-associated epithelium. *Gastroenterol Jpn* 1990; 25(1):130.
82. Owen RL, Jones AL. Epithelial cell specialization within human Peyer's patches: an ultrastructural study of intestinal lymphoid follicles. *Gastroenterology* 1974; 66(2):189–203.
83. Velaga S, Herbrand H, Friedrichsen M, et al. Chemokine receptor CXCR5 supports solitary intestinal lymphoid tissue formation, B cell homing, and induction of intestinal IgA responses. *J Immunol* 2009; 182(5):2610–2619.
84. Bockman DE. Functional histology of appendix. *Arch Histol Jpn* 1983; 46(3):271–292.
85. O'Leary AD, Sweeney EC. Lymphoglandular complexes of the colon: structure and distribution. *Histopathology* 1986; 10(3):267–283.
86. Langman JM, Rowland R. The number and distribution of lymphoid follicles in the human large intestine. *J Anat* 1986; 149:189–194.

87. Seibold F. Food-induced immune responses as origin of bowel disease? *Digestion* 2005; 71(4):251–260.
88. Mahe S, Messing B, Thuillier F, Tome D. Digestion of bovine milk proteins in patients with a high jejunostomy. *Am J Clin Nutr* 1991; 54(3):534–538.
89. Untersmayr E, Bakos N, Scholl I, et al. Anti-ulcer drugs promote IgE formation toward dietary antigens in adult patients. *FASEB J* 2005; 19(6):656–658.
90. Walker WA, Wu M, Isselbacher KJ, Bloch KJ. Intestinal uptake of macromolecules. IV.—the effect of pancreatic duct ligation on the breakdown of antigen and antigen-antibody complexes on the intestinal surface. *Gastroenterology* 1975; 69(6):1223–1229.
91. Reinhardt MC. Macromolecular absorption of food antigens in health and disease. *Ann Allergy* 1984; 53(6 Pt. 2):597–601.
92. Walker WA, Bloch KJ. Gastrointestinal transport of macromolecules in the pathogenesis of food allergy. *Ann Allergy* 1983; 51(2 Pt. 2):240–245.
93. Roberts SA, Freed DL. Neonatal IgA secretion enhanced by breast feeding. *Lancet* 1977; 2(8048):1131.
94. Weaver LT, Arthur HM, Bunn JE, Thomas JE. Human milk IgA concentrations during the first year of lactation. *Arch Dis Child* 1998; 78(3):235–239.
95. Levinsky RJ. Factors influencing intestinal uptake of food antigens. *Proc Nutr Soc* 1985; 44(1):81–86.
96. Matthews DM. Absorption of amino acids and peptides from the intestine. *Clin Endocrinol Metab* 1974; 3(1):3–16.
97. Kraehenbuhl JP, Neutra MR. Molecular and cellular basis of immune protection of mucosal surfaces. *Physiol Rev* 1992; 72(4):853–879.
98. Phillips AD, France NE, Walker-Smith JA. The structure of the enterocyte in relation to its position on the villus in childhood: an electron microscopical study. *Histopathology* 1979; 3(2):117–130.
99. Snoeck V, Goddeeris B, Cox E. The role of enterocytes in the intestinal barrier function and antigen uptake. *Microbes Infect* 2005; 7(7–8):997–1004.
100. Schindler J, Nothwang HG. Aqueous polymer two-phase systems: effective tools for plasma membrane proteomics. *Proteomics* 2006; 6(20):5409–5417.
101. Massey-Harroche D. Epithelial cell polarity as reflected in enterocytes. *Microsc Res Tech* 2000; 49(4):353–362.
102. Ko J, Mayer L. Oral tolerance: lessons on treatment of food allergy. *Eur J Gastroenterol Hepatol* 2005; 17(12):1299–1303.
103. Strober W, Kelsall B, Marth T. Oral tolerance. *J Clin Immunol* 1998; 18(1):1–30.
104. Strobel S, Ferguson A. Modulation of intestinal and systemic immune responses to a fed protein antigen, in mice. *Gut* 1986; 27(7):829–837.
105. Strobel S, Ferguson A. Immune responses to fed protein antigens in mice. 3. Systemic tolerance or priming is related to age at which antigen is first encountered. *Pediatr Res* 1984; 18(7):588–594.
106. Kopac P, Rudin M, Gentinetta T, et al. Continuous apple consumption induces oral tolerance in birch-pollen-associated apple allergy. *Allergy* 2012; 67(2):280–285.
107. Blumchen K, Ulbricht H, Staden U, et al. Oral peanut immunotherapy in children with peanut anaphylaxis. *J Allergy Clin Immunol* 2010; 126(1):83–91; e1.
108. Nakada M, Nishizaki K, Yoshino T, et al. CD80 (B7-1) and CD86 (B7-2) antigens on house dust mite-specific T cells in atopic disease function through T–T cell interactions. *J Allergy Clin Immunol* 1999; 104(1):222–227.
109. Teft WA, Kirchhof MG, Madrenas J. A molecular perspective of CTLA-4 function. *Annu Rev Immunol* 2006; 24:65–97.
110. Greenwald RJ, Freeman GJ, Sharpe AH. The B7 family revisited. *Annu Rev Immunol* 2005; 23:515–548.
111. von Boehmer H. Mechanisms of suppression by suppressor T cells. *Nat Immunol* 2005; 6(4):338–344.
112. Leibson PJ. The regulation of lymphocyte activation by inhibitory receptors. *Curr Opin Immunol* 2004; 16(3):328–336.
113. Kaufman M, Andris F, Leo O. A logical analysis of T cell activation and anergy. *Proc Natl Acad Sci USA* 1999; 96(7):3894–3899.
114. Friedman A, Weiner HL. Induction of anergy or active suppression following oral tolerance is determined by antigen dosage. *Proc Natl Acad Sci USA* 1994; 91(14):6688–6692.
115. Melamed D, Fishman-Lovell J, Uni Z, Weiner HL, Friedman A. Peripheral tolerance of Th2 lymphocytes induced by continuous feeding of ovalbumin. *Int Immunol* 1996; 8(5):717–724.
116. Melamed D, Friedman A. In vivo tolerization of Th1 lymphocytes following a single feeding with ovalbumin: anergy in the absence of suppression. *Eur J Immunol* 1994; 24(9):1974–1981.
117. Faria AM, Weiner HL. Oral tolerance. *Immunol Rev* 2005; 206:232–259.
118. Perez-Machado MA, Ashwood P, Thomson MA, et al. Reduced transforming growth factor-beta1-producing T cells in the duodenal mucosa of children with food allergy. *Eur J Immunol* 2003; 33(8):2307–2315.
119. Fiorentino DF, Zlotnik A, Mosmann TR, Howard M, O'Garra A. IL-10 inhibits cytokine production by activated macrophages. *J Immunol* 1991; 147(11):3815–3822.
120. Duchmann R, Zeitz M. T regulatory cell suppression of colitis: the role of TGF-beta. *Gut* 2006; 55(5):604–606.
121. Kagnoff MF. Celiac disease: pathogenesis of a model immunogenetic disease. *J Clin Invest* 2007; 117(1):41–49.
122. Wolf JL, Bye WA. The membranous epithelial (M) cell and the mucosal immune system. *Annu Rev Med* 1984; 35:95–112.
123. Neutra MR, Pringault E, Kraehenbuhl JP. Antigen sampling across epithelial barriers and induction of mucosal immune responses. *Annu Rev Immunol* 1996; 14:275–300.
124. Neutra MR. M cells in antigen sampling in mucosal tissues. *Curr Top Microbiol Immunol* 1999; 236:17–32.
125. Niedergang F, Kweon MN. New trends in antigen uptake in the gut mucosa. *Trends Microbiol* 2005; 13(10):485–490.
126. Snoeck V, Goddeeris B, Cox E. The role of enterocytes in the intestinal barrier function and antigen uptake. *Microbes Infect* 2005; 7(7–8):997–1004.

127. Pappenheimer JR, Volpp K. Transmucosal impedance of small intestine: correlation with transport of sugars and amino acids. *Am J Physiol* 1992; 263(2 Pt. 1):C480–C493.
128. Madara JL, Pappenheimer JR. Structural basis for physiological regulation of paracellular pathways in intestinal epithelia. *J Membr Biol* 1987; 100(2):149–164.
129. Planchon SM, Martins CA, Guerrant RL, Roche JK. Regulation of intestinal epithelial barrier function by TGF-beta 1. Evidence for its role in abrogating the effect of a T cell cytokine. *J Immunol* 1994; 153(12):5730–5739.
130. Resta-Lenert S, Barrett KE. Probiotics and commensals reverse TNF-alpha- and IFN-gamma-induced dysfunction in human intestinal epithelial cells. *Gastroenterology* 2006; 130(3):731–746.
131. Colgan SP, Resnick MB, Parkos CA, et al. IL-4 directly modulates function of a model human intestinal epithelium. *J Immunol* 1994; 153(5):2122–2129.
132. Madden KB, Whitman L, Sullivan C, et al. Role of STAT6 and mast cells in IL-4- and IL-13-induced alterations in murine intestinal epithelial cell function. *J Immunol* 2002; 169(8):4417–4422.
133. Husby S, Jensenius JC, Svehag SE. Passage of undegraded dietary antigen into the blood of healthy adults. Quantification, estimation of size distribution, and relation of uptake to levels of specific antibodies. *Scand J Immunol* 1985; 22(1):83–92.
134. Mayer L. Epithelial cell antigen presentation. *Curr Opin Gastroenterol* 2000; 16(6):531–535.
135. Bajtay Z, Csomor E, Sandor N, Erdei A. Expression and role of Fc- and complement-receptors on human dendritic cells. *Immunol Lett* 2006; 104(1–2):46–52.
136. Giodini A, Rahner C, Cresswell P. Receptor-mediated phagocytosis elicits cross-presentation in nonprofessional antigen-presenting cells. *Proc Natl Acad Sci USA* 2009; 106(9):3324–3329.
137. Brandtzaeg P. Nature and function of gastrointestinal antigen-presenting cells. *Allergy* 2001; 56(Suppl. 67):16–20.
138. Hershberg RM, Framson PE, Cho DH, et al. Intestinal epithelial cells use two distinct pathways for HLA class II antigen processing. *J Clin Invest* 1997; 100(1):204–215.
139. Mayer L, Eisenhardt D, Salomon P, Bauer W, Plous R, Piccinini L. Expression of class II molecules on intestinal epithelial cells in humans. Differences between normal and inflammatory bowel disease. *Gastroenterology* 1991; 100(1):3–12.
140. Hershberg RM, Cho DH, Youakim A, et al. Highly polarized HLA class II antigen processing and presentation by human intestinal epithelial cells. *J Clin Invest* 1998; 102(4):792–803.
141. Hershberg RM, Mayer LF. Antigen processing and presentation by intestinal epithelial cells—polarity and complexity. *Immunol Today* 2000; 21(3):123–128.
142. Mayer L, Shlien R. Evidence for function of Ia molecules on gut epithelial cells in man. *J Exp Med* 1987; 166(5):1471–1483.
143. Panja A, Blumberg RS, Balk SP, Mayer L. CD1d is involved in T cell-intestinal epithelial cell interactions. *J Exp Med* 1993; 178(3):1115–1119.
144. Campbell NA, Park MS, Toy LS, et al. A non-class I MHC intestinal epithelial surface glycoprotein, gp180, binds to CD8. *Clin Immunol* 2002; 102(3):267–274.
145. Yio XY, Mayer L. Characterization of a 180-kDa intestinal epithelial cell membrane glycoprotein, gp180. A candidate molecule mediating t cell-epithelial cell interactions. *J Biol Chem* 1997; 272(19):12786–12792.
146. Perera L, Shao L, Patel A, et al. Expression of nonclassical class I molecules by intestinal epithelial cells. *Inflamm Bowel Dis* 2007; 13(3):298–307.
147. Banchereau J, Steinman RM. Dendritic cells and the control of immunity. *Nature* 1998; 392(6673):245–252.
148. Tacke F, Randolph GJ. Migratory fate and differentiation of blood monocyte subsets. *Immunobiology* 2006; 211(6–8):609–618.
149. Iwamoto S, Iwai S, Tsujiyama K, et al. TNF-alpha drives human CD14+ monocytes to differentiate into CD70+ dendritic cells evoking Th1 and Th17 responses. *J Immunol* 2007; 179(3):1449–1457.
150. Thoma-Uszynski S, Kiertscher SM, Ochoa MT, et al. Activation of toll-like receptor 2 on human dendritic cells triggers induction of IL-12, but not IL-10. *J Immunol* 2000; 165(7):3804–3810.
151. Wu L, Dakic A. Development of dendritic cell system. *Cell Mol Immunol* 2004; 1(2):112–118.
152. Inaba K, Inaba M, Naito M, Steinman RM. Dendritic cell progenitors phagocytose particulates, including bacillus Calmette-Guerin organisms, and sensitize mice to mycobacterial antigens in vivo. *J Exp Med* 1993; 178(2):479–488.
153. Jiang W, Swiggard WJ, Heufler C, et al. The receptor DEC-205 expressed by dendritic cells and thymic epithelial cells is involved in antigen processing. *Nature* 1995; 375(6527):151–155.
154. Niess JH, Brand S, Gu X, et al. CX3CR1-mediated dendritic cell access to the intestinal lumen and bacterial clearance. *Science* 2005; 307(5707):254–258.
155. Rescigno M, Urbano M, Valzasina B, et al. Dendritic cells express tight junction proteins and penetrate gut epithelial monolayers to sample bacteria. *Nat Immunol* 2001; 2(4):361–367.
156. Chirdo FG, Millington OR, Beacock-Sharp H, Mowat AM. Immunomodulatory dendritic cells in intestinal lamina propria. *Eur J Immunol* 2005; 35(6):1831–1840.
157. Eigenmann PA, Frossard CP. The T lymphocyte in food-allergy disorders. *Curr Opin Allergy Clin Immunol* 2003; 3(3):199–203.
158. Williams MB, Butcher EC. Homing of naive and memory T lymphocyte subsets to Peyer's patches, lymph nodes, and spleen. *J Immunol* 1997; 159(4):1746–1752.
159. Eigenmann PA, Tropia L, Hauser C. The mucosal adhesion receptor alpha4beta7 integrin is selectively increased in lymphocytes stimulated with beta-lactoglobulin in children allergic to cow's milk. *J Allergy Clin Immunol* 1999; 103(5 Pt. 1):931–936.
160. Veres G, Helin T, Arato A, et al. Increased expression of intercellular adhesion molecule-1 and mucosal adhesion molecule alpha4beta7 integrin in small intestinal mucosa

of adult patients with food allergy. *Clin Immunol* 2001; 99(3):353–359.

161. Vandezande LM, Wallaert B, Desreumaux P, et al. Interleukin-5 immunoreactivity and mRNA expression in gut mucosa from patients with food allergy. *Clin Exp Allergy* 1999; 29(5):652–659.
162. Rust C, Kooy Y, Pena S, Mearin ML, Kluin P, Koning F. Phenotypical and functional characterization of small intestinal TcR gamma delta + T cells in coeliac disease. *Scand J Immunol* 1992; 35(4):459–468.
163. Madara JL, Stafford J. Interferon-gamma directly affects barrier function of cultured intestinal epithelial monolayers. *J Clin Invest* 1989; 83(2):724–727.
164. Deem RL, Shanahan F, Targan SR. Triggered human mucosal T cells release tumour necrosis factor-alpha and interferon-gamma which kill human colonic epithelial cells. *Clin Exp Immunol* 1991; 83(1):79–84.
165. Bajaj-Elliott M, Poulsom R, Pender SL, Wathen NC, MacDonald TT. Interactions between stromal cell-derived keratinocyte growth factor and epithelial transforming growth factor in immune-mediated crypt cell hyperplasia. *J Clin Invest* 1998; 102(8):1473–1480.
166. Mention JJ, Ben Ahmed M, Begue B, et al. Interleukin 15: a key to disrupted intraepithelial lymphocyte homeostasis and lymphomagenesis in celiac disease. *Gastroenterology* 2003; 125(3):730–745.
167. Hue S, Mention JJ, Monteiro RC, et al. A direct role for NKG2D/MICA interaction in villous atrophy during celiac disease. *Immunity* 2004; 21(3):367–377.
168. Reinecker HC, MacDermott RP, Mirau S, Dignass A, Podolsky DK. Intestinal epithelial cells both express and respond to interleukin 15. *Gastroenterology* 1996; 111(6):1706–1713.
169. Ebert EC. Interleukin 15 is a potent stimulant of intraepithelial lymphocytes. *Gastroenterology* 1998; 115(6):1439–1445.
170. Bauer S, Groh V, Wu J, et al. Activation of NK cells and T cells by NKG2D, a receptor for stress-inducible MICA. *Science* 1999; 285(5428):727–729.
171. Meresse B, Chen Z, Ciszewski C, et al. Coordinated induction by IL15 of a TCR-independent NKG2D signaling pathway converts CTL into lymphokine-activated killer cells in celiac disease. *Immunity* 2004; 21(3):357–366.
172. Mori F, Barni S, Cianferoni A, Pucci N, de Martino M, Novembre E. Cytokine expression in CD3 +cells in an infant with food protein-induced enterocolitis syndrome (FPIES): case report. *Clin Dev Immunol* 2009; 2009:679381.
173. Chung HL, Hwang JB, Park JJ, Kim SG. Expression of transforming growth factor beta1, transforming growth factor type I and II receptors, and TNF-alpha in the mucosa of the small intestine in infants with food protein-induced enterocolitis syndrome. *J Allergy Clin Immunol* 2002; 109(1):150–154.
174. Shek LP, Bardina L, Castro R, Sampson HA, Beyer K. Humoral and cellular responses to cow milk proteins in patients with milk-induced IgE-mediated and non-IgE-mediated disorders. *Allergy* 2005; 60(7):912–919.
175. Heyman M, Darmon N, Dupont C, et al. Mononuclear cells from infants allergic to cow's milk secrete tumor necrosis factor alpha, altering intestinal function. *Gastroenterology* 1994; 106(6):1514–1523.
176. Penttila IA, van Spriel AB, Zhang MF, et al. Transforming growth factor-beta levels in maternal milk and expression in postnatal rat duodenum and ileum. *Pediatr Res* 1998; 44(4):524–531.
177. Kokkonen J, Holm K, Karttunen TJ, Maki M. Children with untreated food allergy express a relative increment in the density of duodenal gammadelta+ T cells. *Scand J Gastroenterol* 2000; 35(11):1137–1142.
178. Nilsen EM, Lundin KE, Krajci P, Scott H, Sollid LM, Brandtzaeg P. Gluten specific, HLA-DQ restricted T cells from coeliac mucosa produce cytokines with Th1 or Th0 profile dominated by interferon gamma. *Gut* 1995; 37(6):766–776.
179. Schade RP, Van Ieperen-Van Dijk AG, Van Reijsen FC, et al. Differences in antigen-specific T-cell responses between infants with atopic dermatitis with and without cow's milk allergy: relevance of TH2 cytokines. *J Allergy Clin Immunol* 2000; 106(6):1155–1162.
180. Schade RP, Tiemessen MM, Knol EF, Bruijnzeel-Koomen CA, van Hoffen E. The cow's milk protein-specific T cell response in infancy and childhood. *Clin Exp Allergy* 2003; 33(6):725–730.
181. Paajanen L, Kokkonen J, Karttunen TJ, Tuure T, Korpela R, Vaarala O. Intestinal cytokine mRNA expression in delayed-type cow's milk allergy. *J Pediatr Gastroenterol Nutr* 2006; 43(4):470–476.
182. Sicherer SH. Food protein-induced enterocolitis syndrome: clinical perspectives. *J Pediatr Gastroenterol Nutr* 2000; 30(Suppl.):S45–S49.
183. Karlsson MR, Rugtveit J, Brandtzaeg P. Allergen-responsive CD4+CD25+ regulatory T cells in children who have outgrown cow's milk allergy. *J Exp Med* 2004; 199(12):1679–1688.
184. Weller PF. The immunobiology of eosinophils. *N Engl J Med* 1991; 324(16):1110–1118.
185. Rothenberg ME. Eosinophilic gastrointestinal disorders (EGID). *J Allergy Clin Immunol* 2004; 113(1):11–28; quiz 9.
186. Kelly KJ. Eosinophilic gastroenteritis. *J Pediatr Gastroenterol Nutr* 2000; 30(Suppl.):S28–S35.
187. Jaffe JS, Metcalfe DD. Cytokines and their role in the pathogenesis of severe food hypersensitivity reactions. *Ann Allergy* 1993; 71(4):362–364.
188. Johnstone JM, Morson BC. Eosinophilic gastroenteritis. *Histopathology* 1978; 2(5):335–348.
189. Rothenberg ME, Zimmermann N, Mishra A, et al. Chemokines and chemokine receptors: their role in allergic airway disease. *J Clin Immunol* 1999; 19(5):250–265.
190. Shinagawa K, Trifilieff A, Anderson GP. Involvement of CCR3-reactive chemokines in eosinophil survival. *Int Arch Allergy Immunol* 2003; 130(2):150–157.
191. Mishra A, Hogan SP, Brandt EB, et al. Enterocyte expression of the eotaxin and interleukin-5 transgenes induces compartmentalized dysregulation of eosinophil trafficking. *J Biol Chem* 2002; 277(6):4406–4412.
192. Huang JJ, Joh JW, Fuentebella J, et al. Eotaxin and FGF enhance signaling through an extracellular signal-related kinase (ERK)-dependent pathway in the pathogenesis of

eosinophilic esophagitis. *Allergy Asthma Clin Immunol* 2010; 6(1):25.

193. Fox VL, Nurko S, Furuta GT. Eosinophilic esophagitis: it's not just kid's stuff. *Gastrointest Endosc* 2002; 56(2):260–270.
194. Stein ML, Collins MH, Villanueva JM, et al. Anti-IL-5 (mepolizumab) therapy for eosinophilic esophagitis. *J Allergy Clin Immunol* 2006; 118(6):1312–1319.
195. Blanchard C, Stucke EM, Rodriguez-Jimenez B, et al. A striking local esophageal cytokine expression profile in eosinophilic esophagitis. *J Allergy Clin Immunol* 2011; 127(1):208–217; e1–e7.
196. Symon FA, Walsh GM, Watson SR, Wardlaw AJ. Eosinophil adhesion to nasal polyp endothelium is P-selectin-dependent. *J Exp Med* 1994; 180(1):371–376.
197. Wardlaw AJ, Walsh GM, Symon FA. Adhesion interactions involved in eosinophil migration through vascular endothelium. *Ann NY Acad Sci* 1996; 796:124–137.
198. Rothenberg ME. Eosinophilia. *N Engl J Med* 1998; 338(22):1592–1600.
199. Hogan SP, Rothenberg ME. Eosinophil function in eosinophil-associated gastrointestinal disorders. *Curr Allergy Asthma Rep* 2006; 6(1):65–71.
200. Hogan SP, Rothenberg ME, Forbes E, Smart VE, Matthaei KI, Foster PS. Chemokines in eosinophil-associated gastrointestinal disorders. *Curr Allergy Asthma Rep* 2004; 4(1):74–82.
201. Miike S, Kita H. Human eosinophils are activated by cysteine proteases and release inflammatory mediators. *J Allergy Clin Immunol* 2003; 111(4):704–713.
202. Venge P, Bystrom J, Carlson M, et al. Eosinophil cationic protein (ECP): molecular and biological properties and the use of ECP as a marker of eosinophil activation in disease. *Clin Exp Allergy* 1999; 29(9):1172–1186.
203. Furuta GT, Nieuwenhuis EE, Karhausen J, et al. Eosinophils alter colonic epithelial barrier function: role for major basic protein. *Am J Physiol Gastrointest Liver Physiol* 2005; 289(5):G890–G897.
204. Wang J, Slungaard A. Role of eosinophil peroxidase in host defense and disease pathology. *Arch Biochem Biophys* 2006; 445(2):256–260.
205. Young JD, Peterson CG, Venge P, Cohn ZA. Mechanism of membrane damage mediated by human eosinophil cationic protein. *Nature* 1986; 321(6070):613–616.
206. O'Donnell MC, Ackerman SJ, Gleich GJ, Thomas LL. Activation of basophil and mast cell histamine release by eosinophil granule major basic protein. *J Exp Med* 1983; 157(6):1981–1991.
207. Otamiri T, Sjodahl R. Oxygen radicals: their role in selected gastrointestinal disorders. *Dig Dis* 1991; 9(3):133–141.
208. Spalteholz H, Panasenko OM, Arnhold J. Formation of reactive halide species by myeloperoxidase and eosinophil peroxidase. *Arch Biochem Biophys* 2006; 445(2):225–234.
209. Nielsen OH, Ahnfelt-Ronne I, Elmgreen J. Abnormal metabolism of arachidonic acid in chronic inflammatory bowel disease: enhanced release of leucotriene B4 from activated neutrophils. *Gut* 1987; 28(2):181–185.
210. Rothenberg ME, Mishra A, Brandt EB, Hogan SP. Gastrointestinal eosinophils. *Immunol Rev* 2001; 179:139–155.
211. Talley NJ, Shorter RG, Phillips SF, Zinsmeister AR. Eosinophilic gastroenteritis: a clinicopathological study of patients with disease of the mucosa, muscle layer, and subserosal tissues. *Gut* 1990; 31(1):54–58.
212. Powell GK. Milk- and soy-induced enterocolitis of infancy. Clinical features and standardization of challenge. *J Pediatr* 1978; 93(4):553–560.
213. Lake AM. Food-induced eosinophilic proctocolitis. *J Pediatr Gastroenterol Nutr* 2000; 30(Suppl.):S58–S60.
214. Green PH, Jabri B. Celiac disease. *Annu Rev Med* 2006; 57:207–221.
215. Walsh SV, Antonioli DA, Goldman H, et al. Allergic esophagitis in children: a clinicopathological entity. *Am J Surg Pathol* 1999; 23(4):390–396.
216. Sampson HA. 9. Food allergy. *J Allergy Clin Immunol* 2003; 111(2 Suppl.):S540–S547.
217. Nowak-Wegrzyn A, Sampson HA, Wood RA, Sicherer SH. Food protein-induced enterocolitis syndrome caused by solid food proteins. *Pediatrics* 2003; 111(4 Pt. 1):829–835.
218. Sicherer SH. Food protein-induced enterocolitis syndrome: clinical perspectives. *J Pediatr Gastroenterol Nutr* 2000; 30(Suppl.):S45–S49.
219. Odze RD, Wershil BK, Leichtner AM, Antonioli DA. Allergic colitis in infants. *J Pediatr* 1995; 126(2):163–170.
220. Sollid LM, Jabri B. Is celiac disease an autoimmune disorder? *Curr Opin Immunol* 2005; 17(6):595–600.
221. Stepniak D, Koning F. Celiac disease—sandwiched between innate and adaptive immunity. *Hum Immunol* 2006; 67(6):460–468.
222. Rostom A, Dube C, Cranney A, et al. The diagnostic accuracy of serologic tests for celiac disease: a systematic review. *Gastroenterology* 2005; 128(4 Suppl. 1):S38–S46.
223. Furuta GT. Emerging questions regarding eosinophil's role in the esophago-gastrointestinal tract. *Curr Opin Gastroenterol* 2006; 22(6):658–663.
224. Guajardo JR, Plotnick LM, Fende JM, Collins MH, Putnam PE, Rothenberg Me. Eosinophil-associated gastrointestinal disorders: a world-wide-web based registry. *J Pediatr* 2002; 141(4):576–581.

4 Food Allergens—Molecular and Immunological Characteristics

Heimo Breiteneder[1] & E.N. Clare Mills[2]

[1]Department of Pathophysiology and Allergy Research, Medical University of Vienna, Vienna, Austria
[2]Manchester Institute of Biotechnology, University of Manchester, Manchester, UK

Key Concepts

- Food allergens belong to a limited number of protein families with different molecular properties that may mean routes of sensitization differ for different allergen families.
- Food allergens that sensitize via the gastrointestinal tract have molecular features that enhance stability to thermal and proteolytical denaturation.
- Two allergen families (caseins and cupins) thought to sensitize via the gastrointestinal tract retain their allergenicity even after digestion for reasons that are not understood.
- Plant food allergens related to pollen allergens generally have no stability-enhancing characteristics and only induce oral allergy syndrome as a secondary reaction to primary sensitization to pollen.

Introduction

The postgenomic era, with its explosion of information about protein and genome sequences, is allowing us to study molecular relationships in new ways and, notably, within the context of protein evolution. Allergenic proteins did not suddenly appear in the protein landscape but are the result of a long chain of formative processes that resulted in the creation of protein architectures that are treated as allergenic by the immune system of certain individuals. A growing body of literature shows that allergens bias the immune response by interacting with conserved innate immune receptors [1, 2]. Allergens are restricted to a very small number of protein families with characteristic three-dimensional structures or scaffolds, as has been shown for plant food [3] and pollen allergens [4]. The AllFam database (http://www.meduniwien.ac.at/allergens/allfam/; last accessed August 2013) lists all protein families that contain allergens [5]. The origins of some of these protein scaffolds can be traced back to Archaea, as has been done for the cupin superfamily [6] or the Bet v 1 superfamily [7]. However, the most prominent allergen-containing superfamily is the prolamin superfamily, which seems to have arisen only after plants conquered land. Most members of the prolamin superfamily seem to be restricted to the seeds of dicotyledonous plants [8], yet proteins related to 2S albumins have been identified in the spores of the ostrich fern [9]. The common ancestors of ferns and angiosperms lived more than 300 million years ago. Some of the evolved protein structures have proven so successful that they are conserved between plants and animals, as is the case for thaumatin-like proteins [10]. In summary, allergenicity seems to be linked to certain structural features of molecules that are members of a limited number of protein families. In general, within a given protein family allergens represent only a fraction of its members, which has been well demonstrated for the Bet v 1 family of proteins [7, 11]. In addition to any intrinsic allergenicity of a protein scaffold, sensitization to a given protein also relates to issues of exposure, with some proteins not being found in edible tissues or only transiently expressed during development such that levels in the exposing agent are low. It is well-accepted that the allergenic potential of a protein also has to be realized within the context of a host immune system which is predisposed toward being atopic. In this chapter, the most important animal and plant food allergen families are discussed.

Food Allergy: Adverse Reactions to Foods and Food Additives, Fifth Edition. Edited by Dean D Metcalfe, Hugh A Sampson, Ronald A Simon and Gideon Lack.

Food allergen protein families

Based on shared amino acid sequences and conserved three-dimensional structures proteins can be classified into families using various bioinformatics tools which form the basis of several protein family databases, one of which is Pfam [12]. Over the past 15 years the numbers of well-characterized allergens that have been sequenced has increased rapidly and they are now being collected into a number of databases to facilitate bioinformatic analysis (Table 4.1); [18, 19]. We have undertaken this analysis for both plant [3] and animal food allergens [20] along with pollen allergens [4]. The current AllFam version of September 9, 2011, illustrates similar distributions of animal and plant food allergens into protein families with the majority of allergens falling into just three or four families with a tail of between 20 and 30 families comprising between one and three allergens each. With regard to food allergens, around 60% of those from plants belong to just four protein families: the prolamin, cupin, Bet v 1-related, and profilin families [3], supporting molecular and structural approaches to the classification of plant food allergens [8, 21]. Similarly, animal food allergens can be classified into three main families: the EF-hand domain, tropomyosins, and caseins [5, 20]. Such patterns of distribution beg the question why certain protein scaffolds dominate the landscape of allergen structures? Are there structural features that predispose certain proteins to becoming allergens? Certainly, detailed analyses of the secondary structure elements in proteins have not shown any relationship with allergenicity [22] but protein structure–function relationships can be very subtle. Using the food allergen family classification we will summarize the properties of known food allergens and discuss how their structures and properties might result in their allergenic potential.

Food allergens of animal origin (Table 4.2)

Tropomyosins

Tropomyosins are a family of closely related proteins present in muscle and nonmuscle cells [36]. Together with actin and myosin, they play a key regulatory role in muscle contraction, containing 40 uninterrupted heptapeptide repeats and are two-stranded proteins that occur as α-helical coiled coils [37]. Tropomyosins form head-to-tail polymers along the length of an actin filament [38] and are the major allergens of two invertebrate groups, Crustacea and Mollusca, which are generally referred to as shellfish. Various species of shrimp, crab, squid, and abalone are assumed to be especially responsible for seafood allergies. Tropomyosins were originally identified as major shrimp allergens by several laboratories [39–41] and today they are recognized as invertebrate pan-allergens [42]. The first two residues of the IgE-binding region (epitope) in the C-terminal portion of the protein appear to be crucial for IgE binding and are not found in vertebrate tropomyosins. As a consequence of the lack of homology in the IgE epitopes there is no cross-reactivity between IgE from shellfish-allergic individuals and animal muscle tropomyosins. Allergenic tropomyosins are heat-stable and cross-reactive between the various crustacean and molluscan species [43]. Extracts from boiled *Penaeus indicus* shrimp contained Pen i 1 with unaltered allergenicity [44]. Water-soluble shrimp allergens were also detected in the cooking water after boiling [45].

Parvalbumins

Parvalbumins, the major fish allergens, belong to the wide range of calcium-binding proteins that are extremely abundant and cross-reactive in many fish species [46]. Present in high levels in the white muscle of many fish species, parvalbumins are characterized by the possession of a widely found calcium-binding domain which is known as the EF-hand [47]. The EF-hand is a motif that consists of a loop of 12 amino acid residues that is flanked on either side by a 12-residue α-helical domain. Parvalbumins comprise three such domains [48], two of which are able to bind calcium [49]. Parvalbumins are important for the relaxation of muscle fibers by binding free intracellular calcium [50]. The binding of the calcium ligands is necessary for the correct parvalbumin conformation and loss of calcium results in a large change in conformation with an associated loss of IgE-binding capacity [45, 51, 52]. Parvalbumins with bound calcium ions possess a remarkable stability to denaturation by heat [53–55]. The ability to act as major fish allergens is obviously linked to the stability of parvalbumins to heat, denaturing chemicals, and proteolytic enzymes [56]. Parvalbumins can be subdivided into two distinct evolutionary lineages, the α- and the β-parvalbumins, although their overall architectures are very similar. The β-parvalbumins are generally allergenic. Gad c 1, a codfish allergen, was the first allergenic fish parvalbumin that was purified and characterized [57, 58]. Today, allergenic β-parvalbumins have been characterized from many different bony fish species and are considered as pan-allergens in fish [59]. Recently, two allergenic parvalbumins were also described from red stingray [60]. The cross-reactivity of fish and frog muscle in fish-allergic individuals has been attributed to the structural similarities between their parvalbumins [61]. An α-parvalbumin of frog has also been described as allergenic [62].

Caseins

Structurally mobile proteins, caseins are found in mammalian milk at a concentration of around 15 mg/mL and are responsible for binding calcium through clusters of phosphoserine and/or phosphothreonine residues in α_{s1}-,

Table 4.1 Allergen databases.

Database	Host	Database type	Curation	Citations	URL
Allergen Online	University of Nebraska, Food Allergy Research and Resource Programme (FARRP), USA	Repository of allergen sequences which can be readily downloaded for subsequent sequence analysis	Review by a panel with annual database updates	N/A	http://allergenonline.com; last accessed August 2013.
WHO-International Union of Immunological Societies (IUIS)	University of Nebraska Lincoln, USA	Repository of allergen sequences with links; organized by phylogeny	Expert panel reviews submissions of new allergens; the only body officially able to give allergen designations	13	http://www.allergen.org/; last accessed August 2013.
The Allergen Database	The Food and Environment Research Agency	Information on allergens and epitopes	Not defined	N/A	http://allergen.csl.gov.uk/; last accessed August 2013.
Structural Database of Allergen Proteins (SDAP)	University of Texas, USA	Repository of allergen sequences, structures, and models. Organization by allergen families	Curated by host scientists with oversight by a review panel	14	http://fermi.utmb.edu/SDAP/sdap_ver.html; last accessed August 2013.
AllFam	Medical University of Vienna, Austria	Classifies selected allergen sequences from the Allergome database	Curated by host scientists	5	http://www.meduniwien.ac.at/allergens/allfam/; last accessed August 2013.
Allergen Database for Food Safety (ADFS)	National Institute of Health Sciences, Japan	Contains information on allergens from AllergenOnline, supplemented with information from UniProt together with other allergenic compounds from AllAllergy	Not defined	N/A	http://allergen.nihs.go.jp/ADFS/; last accessed August 2013.
AllerMatch	Collaboration between RIKILT—Institute of Food Safety and Plant Research International, The Netherlands	Three linked databases of allergen sequences derived from UNIPROT, IUIS and a combination of the two databases	Not defined	15	http://www.allermatch.org/; last accessed August 2013.
Allergome	Allergy Data Laboratories sc (ADL), Italy	Information on allergenic molecules and sources	Not defined	16	http://www.allergome.org/; last accessed August 2013.
Informall	Institute of Food Research, UK	Information on allergenic foods and allergen molecules	Curated by host scientists with oversight by a review panel	17	http://www.foodallergens.info/; last accessed August 2013.

Table 4.2 Exemplar animal food allergens.

Animal food allergen— family	Function	Source	Allergen name	Sequence accession	Reference
Tropomyosin family	Tropomyosins bind to actin in muscle increasing thin filament stability and rigidity. They may play an important role with troponins in controlling muscle contraction	Black tiger shrimp (*Penaeus monodon*)	Pen m 1	A1KYZ2	23
		North Sea shrimp (*Crangon crangon*)	Cra c 1	D7F1J4	24
		American lobster (*Homarus americanus*)	Hom a 1	O44119	25
		Squid (*Todarodes pacificus*)	Tod p 1	Peptides only	26
		Oyster (*Crassostrea gigas*)	Cra g 1, Cra g 2, Cra g 1.03	Q95WY0	27
		Abalone (*Haliotis diversicolor*)	Hal d 1	Q9GZ71	28
Parvalbumin family	Parvalbumins control the flow of calcium from troponin C back to membrane-bound pumps after a muscle contraction	Cod (*Gadus morhua*)	Gad m 1	Q90YK9, Q90YL0	29
		Carp (*Cyprinus carpio*)	Cyp c 1.01, Cyp c 1.02	Q8UUS3, Q8UUS2	30
Caseins	Caseins form stable micellar calcium phosphate protein complexes in mammalian milks	Domestic cow (*Bos taurus*)	Bos d 8: total casein fraction		31
			Bos d 9: α_{s1}-casein	P02662	32
			Bos d 10: α_{s2}-casein	P02663	33
			Bos d 11: β-casein	P02666	34
			Bos d 12: κ-casein	P02668	35

α_{s2}-, and β-caseins. The casein polypeptides form a shell around amorphous calcium phosphate to form microstructures called nanoclusters, allowing calcium levels in milk to exceed the solubility limit of calcium phosphate. The nanoclusters are assembled into the casein micelles found in milk, which are in turn stabilized by κ-casein [63]. The α- and β-caseins are related to the secretory calcium-binding phosphoprotein family together with proteins involved in mineralization and salivary proteins while κ-caseins may be distantly related to the fibrinogen γ-chain [64]. Caseins are major food allergens involved in cow's milk allergy, which affect predominantly young children. Studies on the IgE cross-reactivity between different types of caseins in a group of cow's milk allergic infants found that 90% had serum IgE against α_{s2}-casein, 55% had serum IgE against α_{s1}-casein, while only 15% had IgE against β-casein [65]. This pattern of reactivity appears to be related to the degree of similarity between bovine and human caseins, with caseins least like human caseins being more reactive. Thus, bovine β-casein appears to be the least reactive and has the highest identity to human casein of 53%, while bovine α_{s2}-caseins were the most reactive, being least similar with only ~16% identity to the closest human homologue, α_{s1}-casein, the α_{s2}-casein gene not being expressed in humans. There is considerable similarity in the caseins from different mammalian milks used for human consumption, which explains their IgE cross-reactivity. It has been observed that cow's milk allergic patients generally react to goat's milk on oral challenge [66] as caseins from domestic cattle and goats have sequence identities of over 90%. However, it appears that when this sequence identity drops to between 22% and 66%, as is the case between mare's and cow's milk caseins, it is associated with tolerance, since individuals with cow's milk can tolerate mare's milk [67] and do not show IgE cross-reactivity to milk proteins from species such as camel [68]. Bovine and human κ-caseins share around 50% homology and efforts to epitope map bovine κ-casein have shown the presence of shared IgE epitopes [69], as does β-casein [70]. These similarities may explain the rare allergic reactions to human milk which have been reported [71]. Recent studies using a combination of recombinant α_{s1}-casein expressed in *Escherichia coli* and synthetic peptides showed the presence of IgE epitopes spanning the protein sequence [72]. However, such data need to be treated cautiously since such recombinant proteins lack the significant post-translational modifications of casein, notably phosphorylation of up to nine serine residues that span the protein sequence, the loss of which has been shown to affect IgE reactivity [73].

Minor families

Lipocalins

The lipocalins are a group of diverse proteins sharing about 20% sequence identity with conserved three-dimensional structures characterized by a central tunnel, which can often accommodate a diversity of lipophilic ligands [74]. They are thought to function as carriers of odorants, steroids, lipids, and pheromones among others and are being implicated in a host of biological functions from regulating glucose metabolism [75] to moderating innate immune functioning [76]. The majority of lipocalin allergens are respiratory, having been identified as the major allergens in rodent urine, animal dander, and saliva as well as in insects such as cockroaches; the only lipocalin which acts as a food allergen is the cow's milk allergen, β-lactoglobulin [77]. The lipocalin-interacting membrane receptor (LIMR) has recently been shown to mediate uptake of β-lactoglobulin in a model neurocarcinoma cell line [78] and may explain uptake by the intestine.

Lysozyme family

Lysozyme type C and α-lactalbumins belong to the glycoside hydrolase family 22 clan of the *O*-glycosyl hydrolase superfamily and have probably evolved from a common ancestral protein. However, they have distinctly different functions as α-lactalbumin is involved in lactose synthesis in milk, lysozyme acting as a muramidase, hydrolyzing peptidoglycans found in bacterial cell walls. Furthermore α-lactalbumin, unlike hen's egg lysozyme, binds calcium. Two food allergens belong to this clan: the minor hen's egg allergen lysozyme (Gal d 4), and the minor cow's milk allergen α-lactalbumin. These proteins share little sequence homology but have superimposable three-dimensional structures [79].

Transferrin family

Transferrins are eukaryotic sulfur-rich iron-binding glycoproteins that function *in vivo* to control the level of free iron. Members of the family that have been identified as minor food allergens include milk lactotransferrin (lactoferrin) and hen's egg white ovotransferrin [80, 81].

Serpins

Serpins, a class of serine protease inhibitors, are found in all types of organisms with the exception of fungi and are involved in a variety of physiological processes. Many of the family members have lost their inhibitory activity [82]. Only one food allergen has been identified as belonging to this family, the hen's egg allergen, ovalbumin [83].

Arginine kinases

Arginine kinases belong to a family of structurally and functionally related ATP:guanido phosphotransferases that reversibly catalyze the transfer of phosphate between ATP and various phosphogens. Arginine kinases have been identified as allergens in invertebrates including food allergen sources such as shrimp [24, 84] and as cross-reactive allergens from the Indian meal moth, king prawn, lobster, and mussel [85].

Ovomucoids

Kazal inhibitors, which inhibit a number of serine proteases, belong to a family of proteins that includes pancreatic secretory trypsin inhibitor, avian ovomucoid, and elastase inhibitors. These proteins contain between 1 and 7 Kazal-type inhibitor repeats [86]. Avian ovomucoids contain three Kazal-like inhibitory domains [87]. Chicken ovomucoid has been shown to be the dominant hen's egg white allergen Gal d 1 [66]. Gal d 1 comprises 186 amino acid residues that are arranged in three tandem domains (Gal d 1.1, Gal d 1.2, Ga1.3). Each domain contains three intradomain disulfide bonds. Gal d 1.1 and Gal d 1.2 contain two carbohydrate chains each, and about 50% of the Gal d 1.3 domains contain one carbohydrate chain, which may act to stabilize the protein against proteolysis [88]. Another Kazal inhibitor has been implicated as the allergenic component of bird's nest used to make the Chinese delicacy bird's nest soup [89].

Food allergens of plant origin (Table 4.3)

The prolamin superfamily

The prolamin superfamily derives its name from the alcohol-soluble proline- and glutamine-rich storage proteins of cereals. This superfamily was initially defined in 1985 by Kreis and coworkers [105], who observed that three groups of apparently unrelated seed proteins contained a conserved pattern of cysteine residues. These included two types of cereal seed proteins, namely the sulfur-rich prolamins and the α-amylase/trypsin inhibitors of monocotyledonous cereal seeds, together with the 2S storage albumins (Figure 4.1a) found in a variety of dicotyledonous seeds including castor bean and oilseed rape. Subsequently, other low molecular weight allergenic proteins were identified as belonging to this superfamily including soybean hydrophobic protein (Figure 4.1b), nonspecific lipid transfer proteins (nsLTPs, Figure. 4.1c), and α-globulins. Apart from the conserved cysteine pattern, little sequence similarities exist between the members of different subfamilies. The conserved cysteine pattern comprises a core of eight cysteine residues which includes a characteristic Cys–Cys and Cys–X–Cys motifs (X representing any other residue). Two additional cysteine residues are found in the α-amylase/trypsin inhibitors. In the cereal seed storage prolamins the disulfide skeleton has been disrupted by the insertion of a repetitive domain

Table 4.3 Exemplar plant food allergens.

Plant food allergen—family	Function	Source	Allergen name	Sequence accession	Reference
Prolamins	Seed storage proteins	Wheat (*Triticum aestivum*)	Tri a 19: omega-5 gliadin	P08453	90
			Tri a 21: αβ-gliadin	D2T2K3	91
			Tri a 26: high molecular weight glutenin	P10388	92
			Tri a 36: low molecular weight glutenin	JF776367	NA
Nonspecific lipid transfer proteins	Function uncertain; maybe involved in transport of suberin monomers and plant defense	Peach (*Prunus persica*)	Pru p 3	P81402	93
		Hazelnut (*Corylus avellana*)	Cor a 8	AF329829	94
2S albumins	Seed storage protein	Walnut (*Juglans regia*)	Jug r 1	JRU66866	95
		Peanut (*Arachis hypogea*)	Ara h 2	L77197	96
			Ara h 6	AF091737	97
			Ara h 7	AF092846	98
Bet v 1 family	Possibly plant hormone or lipid transporters	Apple (*Malus domestica*)	Mal d 1	P43211	99
		Celery root (*Apium graveolens*)	Api g 1.0101	P49372	100
		Hazelnut (*Corylus avellana*)	Cor a 1.0401	Q9SWR4	101
Cupin superfamily: 7S (vicilin-like) globulins	Seed storage protein	Peanut (*Arachis hypogea*)	Ara h 1	L34402	102
11S (legumin-like) globulins	Seed storage protein	Peanut (*Arachis hypogea*)	Ara h 3.0101	082580	103
Cysteine protease C 1 family	Cysteine proteases	Kiwi (*Actinidia deliciosa*)	Actinidin	Q43367	104

comprising motifs rich in proline and glutamine. While the way in which the disulfide connectivities formed by the cysteine residues varies in the different types of prolamin superfamily members, they share a common three-dimensional structure, examples of which are shown in Figure 4.1. This figure illustrates the three-dimensional structures shared by these proteins, which consist of bundles of four α-helices stabilized by disulfide bonds and which are arranged in such a way as to create a lipid-binding tunnel in the nsLTPs which is collapsed in the 2S albumin structures. As yet no ancestral type has been identified, and consequently this scaffold appears to have evolved when plants conquered land [106].

The lipid-binding tunnel of the nsLTPs shows considerable flexibility, being able to accommodate a diverse range of lipids including prostaglandins [107] and up to two fatty acids lying side-by-side [108]. Apart from the seed storage prolamins, whose properties are dominated by the inserted repetitive domain, the physicochemical properties of prolamin superfamily members are dominated by their intramolecular disulfide bonds. Compact proteins, the disulfide bonds in the prolamin superfamily members, are responsible for maintaining the three-dimensional structure even after heating, which is associated with their retaining their allergenic properties after cooking [109]. Their structure and IgE-binding properties are only altered if severe heating results in hydrolysis of these bonds [110]. These same structural attributes underlie their resistance to proteolysis, with several members, including the 2S albumins [111] and nsLTP allergens [112], being highly resistant to gastric and duodenal digestion. Any degradation that does occur appears to leave the major IgE-binding sites intact, explaining the fact that simulated gastrointestinal digestions do not alter their ability to elicit skin reactions *in vivo* as has been observed for the grape nsLTP [113].

Cereal prolamins

As a consequence of the inserted repetitive domain, the α-helical structure has been disrupted in the seed storage prolamins. Their properties are dominated by the repetitive domain, which is thought to adopt an ensemble of unfolded and secondary structures comprising overlapping β-turns or poly-L-proline II structures that may form a loose spiral structure [114]. They comprise around half of the protein found in grain from the related cereals, wheat, barley, and rye, those from wheat being able to form large disulfide-linked polymers, which comprise the viscoelastic protein fraction known as gluten. These proteins are characteristically insoluble in dilute salt solutions, either in the native state or after reduction of interchain disulfide bonds, being soluble instead in aqueous alcohols. In addition to their role in triggering celiac disease, several types of cereal storage prolamins have been identified as triggering IgE-mediated allergies including γ-, α-, and ω-5

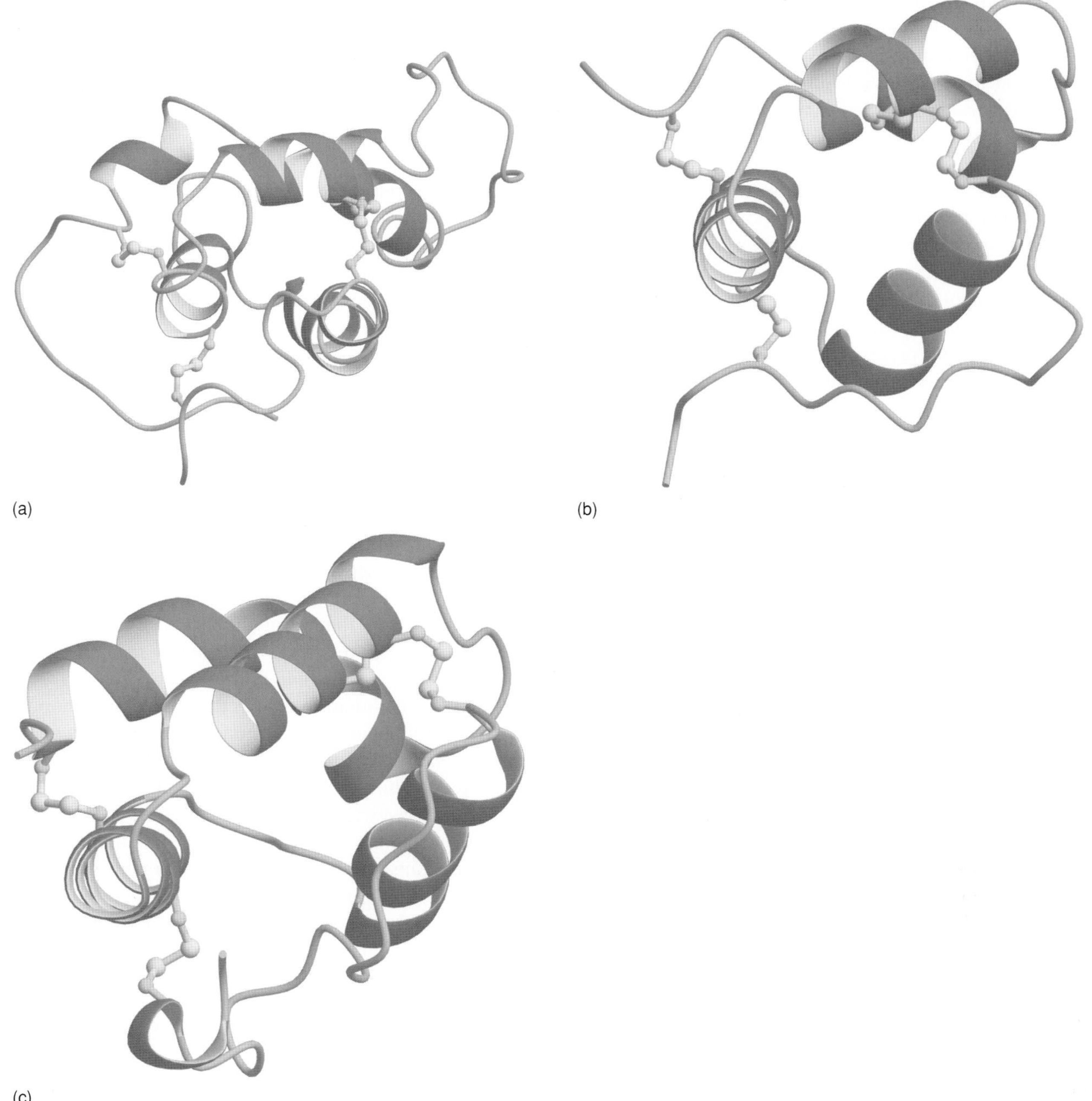

Figure 4.1 Typical structures of various members of the prolamin superfamily that have been identified as allergens, shown as ribbon cartoons with ball-and-stick disulfide bridges. PDB codes are given in parentheses. (a) Typical single-chain 2S albumin from sunflower SFA-8 (1S6D). (b) Soybean hydrophobic protein (1HYP). (c) Nonspecific lipid transfer protein (nsLTP) from peach, Pru p 3 (2B5S).

gliadins [115–117] in addition to the polymeric HMW and LMW subunits of glutenin [118–121]. Cooking appears to affect allergenicity and one study suggested that baking may be essential for allergenicity of cereal prolamins [122]. A recent study has shown that deamidated gluten proteins, found in certain types of wheat isolate, which have been treated with alkali, appear to be responsible for triggering allergic reactions in individuals who can tolerate native gluten proteins. In these patients, IgE responses toward ω-2 and γ-gliadins predominated with deamidation being essential for IgE binding [123]. This condition appears to be quite distinct to allergy to native wheat proteins, where there are indications that deamidation removes IgE epitopes [124].

Bifunctional inhibitors

The other group of prolamin superfamily allergens unique to cereals is the α-amylase/trypsin inhibitors, which have been found to sensitize individuals via the lungs resulting in occupational allergies to wheat flour such as bakers' asthma or via the gastrointestinal tract for cereal-containing foods including wheat, barley, and rice. They were initially identified in extracts made with chloroform/methanol mixtures (and hence called CM proteins) but are also soluble in water, dilute saline, or alcohol/water mixtures. More detailed studies have revealed a range of monomeric, dimeric, and tetrameric forms, many of the subunits being glycosylated [125]. The individual subunits are either inactive or inhibitory to trypsin (and sometimes other proteinases), α-amylases from insects (including pests), or both enzymes (i.e., the inhibitors are bifunctional). The best characterized allergens are the α-amylase inhibitors of rice grains [126], while there is one report of a M_r ~15 000 subunit being involved in wheat allergy [127, 128]. Allergens with M_r of 16 000 have also been characterized in corn and beer (originating from barley), which appear to belong to the α-amylase inhibitor family [129, 130].

2S albumins

The 2S albumins are a major family of seed storage proteins [131] widely distributed in both mono- and dicotyledonous plants where they may accompany the cupin globulin seed storage proteins (see The cupin superfamily). Most 2S albumins are synthesized as single chains of M_r 10 000–15 000 which, depending on the plant species, may be posttranslationally processed to give small and large subunits, which usually remain joined by disulfide bonds. In some plant species, such as peanut and sunflower, the precursors are unprocessed and remain as a single polypeptide chain (Figure 4.1a). Although the main biological role of 2S albumins is thought to be storage, several other physiological functions have been attributed to these proteins [132]. In recent years, an increasing number of 2S albumins have been described as major food allergens [133]. They can act as both occupational (sensitizing through inhalation of dusts) and food allergens, having been identified as the major allergenic components of many foods, including the peanut allergens Ara h 2, 6, 7 [96, 97], oriental and yellow mustard allergens Bra j 1 and Sin a 1 [134, 135], the walnut allergen Jug r 1 [95], Ses i 1 and 2 from sesame [136, 137], Ber e 1 from Brazil nut [138], Ana o 1 from cashew [139], and 2S albumins from almond [140] and sunflower seeds [141]. Ber e 1, being one of the richest food sources of sulfur-containing amino acids, remains an important target for nutritional studies [142]. There is some evidence that the 2S albumins of soy [143] and chickpea [144] are also allergenic.

Nonspecific lipid transfer proteins

One of the most important family of allergens to have been identified within the prolamin superfamily are the type 1 nsLTPs, which are involved in severe allergies to fresh fruits such as peach in the south of Europe around the Mediterranean area. They have been termed "pan-allergens" [145] and are the most widely distributed type of prolamin found in a variety of plant organs including seeds, fruit, and vegetative tissues. In addition to being identified in many different fruits and seeds, they have also been characterized in pollen of plant species such as *Parietaria judaica* and olive [146, 147], thus establishing them as important pan-allergens of plants. nsLTPs have been identified as major allergens in fruits such Pru p 3 (Figure 4.1c) in peach [148], Mal d 3 in apple [145], and Vit v 1 in grape [149]. Allergenic nsLTPs have also been characterized in vegetables such as asparagus [150], cereals such as maize [130], and in a number of nuts including hazelnut [151]. While there is extensive IgE cross-reactivity between nsLTPs from closely related plant species, once sequence similarities drop below a certain level, this cross-reactivity decreases significantly with the nsLTP from kiwi Act d 3 not being cross-reactive with the peach nsLTP Pru p 3 [152]. As their name implies, nsLTPs were originally defined on the basis of their ability *in vitro* to transfer a range of phospholipid types from liposomes to various types of membranes, such as those from mitochondria. However, this is not their *in vivo* function, and it is emerging that plants have used the nsLTP scaffold in a wide range of contexts. Those involved in food allergies are found in epidermal tissues. This observation, along with their lipid-binding characteristics, has led to the view that they play a role in transporting lipids involved in the synthesis of waxy cutin and suberin layers in outer plant tissues in seeds and pollen. Nevertheless, their exact biological role *in vivo* remains unclear but several possible functions have been proposed [106].

The cupin superfamily

The cupins are a functionally diverse protein superfamily which has probably evolved from a prokaryotic ancestor but has not found its way into the animal kingdom. They possess a characteristic β-barrel structure, the name "cupin" being derived from Latin for barrel [6]. This basic scaffold has been utilized for a diverse range of functions including sporulation proteins in fungi, sucrose-binding activities, and enzymatic activities found in germins where manganese is bound in the center of the barrel. The cupin motif has been duplicated in cupin storage proteins of flowering plants to give rise to the bicupin motif that is used by the 7S and 11S globulin storage proteins. The three-dimensional structure of the 11S globulin of soya, proglycinin, is an example of a cupin storage protein containing the bicupin motif (Figure 4.2b). The 11S–12S

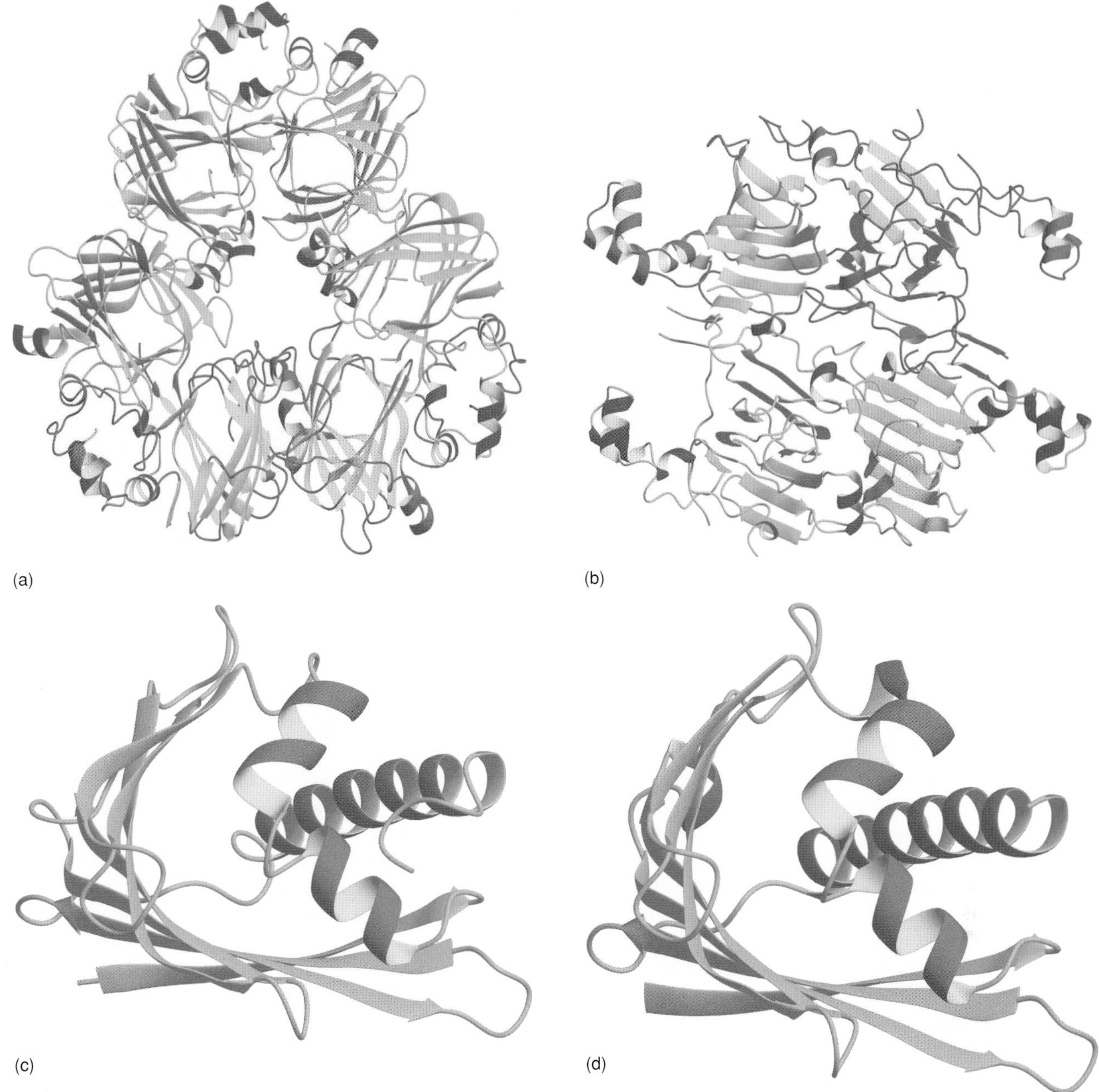

Figure 4.2 Typical structures of the cupin and Bet v 1 superfamily allergens shown as ribbon cartoons. PDB codes are given in parentheses. (a) Trimeric structure of soybean 7S globulin β-conglycinin comprising solely β-subunits (1UIJ). (b) Edge-on view of soybean 11S globulin showing the way in which individual subunits are stacked within the hexamer (2D5H). (c) Major birch pollen allergen Bet v 1 (1BV1). (d) Allergenic Bet v 1 homologue from celery root, Api g 1 (2BK0).

globulins are found in the seeds of many monocotyledonous and dicotyledonous plants with homologues having been identified in gymnosperms (including conifers). They are sometimes termed legumins because they are particularly found in legume seeds and are oligomers of M_r ~300 000–450 000. Each oligomer consists of six subunits of M_r about 60 000, the products of a multigene family, noncovalently associated by intertwining α-helical regions. Each subunit is posttranslationally processed to give rise to acidic (M_r about 40 000) and basic (M_r about 20 000) chains, linked by a single disulfide bond and are rarely, if ever, glycosylated [153]. In contrast, the 7/8S globulins are usually trimeric proteins of M_r about 150 000–190 000, comprising subunits of M_r ~40 000–80 000, but typically about 50 000. They are also termed vicilins since they are particularly found in the Viciae group of legumes. The subunits are again the products of a multigene family and also undergo proteolytic processing and glycosylation, the extent of which varies depending on the plant species [153].

Major allergens include the 7S (Figure 4.2a) and 11S globulins (Figure 4.2b) of soybean [154–156], Ara h 1 and Ara h 3 of peanut [96, 102, 157], Ana c 1 and Ana c 2 of cashew nut [158, 159], the 7S globulins Jug r 2 of walnut [160], Len c 1 of lentil [161], and the 7S globulins of sesame [137] and hazelnut [151]. The 11S globulins have also been shown to be allergens in almond, also known as AMP [162], and in hazelnut [163]. In general, these vicilin-like and legumin-like seed globulins exhibit a high degree of thermostability, requiring temperatures in excess of 70°C for denaturation and have a propensity to form large aggregates on heating which still retain, to a large degree, their native secondary structure [164–166]. At high protein concentrations these proteins can form heat-set gels [166]. The type of heating affects the denaturation and impacts on allergenicity. Thus, boiling Ara h 1 results in the formation of branched aggregates with reduced IgE-binding capacity although the T-cell reactivity of the allergen is unaltered [167]. In contrast, Ara h 1 purified from roasted nuts was highly denatured, lacked a branched structure but retained the IgE-binding capacity of the native protein.

Since the globulins are partially or fully insoluble between pH 3.5 and 6.5 it is likely that only limited solubilization of globulins would occur when they enter the stomach. However, the 7S globulins seem to be highly susceptible to pepsinolysis, although several lower molecular weight polypeptides seem to persist following digestion of the peanut 7S globulin allergen Ara h 1, [168, 169] and there is evidence that they still possess IgE-binding sites following proteolysis [170]. Similarly *in vitro*-simulated gastrointestinal digestion results in rapid and almost complete degradation of the protein to relatively small polypeptides although these retain their allergenic properties [99].

The Bet v 1 family

The association of plant food allergies with birch pollen allergy is the most frequently observed of the cross-reactivity syndromes [171]. The clinical symptoms of the birch-pollen-allergy-related OAS are caused by cross-reactive IgE between the major birch pollen allergen Bet v 1 (Figure 4.2c) and its homologues in a wide range of fruits and vegetables, including apple [172], celery (Figure 4.2d) [100], peanut [173], mung bean [174], Sharon fruit [175], and even jackfruit [176]. However, systemic reactions can also be caused in certain patients by Bet v 1 homologous allergens present in celery [177, 178], carrot [179], and soybean [180, 181]. Bet v 1 is a member of the Bet v 1-like superfamily of proteins that contains 23 609 sequences from 4418 species (http://pfam.sanger.ac.uk/clan/CL0209; accessed August 2013). The origin of the Bet v 1 architecture can be traced back to the beginnings of life [7].

Bet v 1 was the first allergen identified to possess similarities to family 10 of the pathogenesis-related proteins [182, 183]. The PR-10 family is a subfamily of the Bet v 1 family, which is one of the 14 member families of the Bet v 1-like superfamily [7]. As a possible biological function in plants, a general plant-steroid carrier function for Bet v 1 and related PR-10 proteins was suggested [184]. A broader range of amphiphilic and lipid molecules also seemed to be potential Bet v 1 ligands [185]. The known structures of Bet v 1 [184, 186] and its homologues in cherry [187], celery [188], carrot [189], and soybean [190] illustrate the high identity of the molecular surfaces that are accessible to IgE and thus offer a molecular explanation for the observed clinical cross-reactivities. A structural bioinformatic analysis of Bet v 1 and its homologous allergens from apple, soybean, and celery showed that conservation of three-dimensional structure plays an important role in the conservation of IgE-binding epitopes and underlies the birch pollen—plant food syndrome [3]. There is evidence on the T-cell level that Bet v 1 is the relevant sensitizing agent [191]. Moreover, exposure of dendritic cells from birch pollen-allergic donors to Bet v 1 resulted in a robust Th2 skewing whereas Api g 1, the homologous food allergen from celery, significantly enhanced the production of the Th1 cytokine INF-γ and downregulated IL-13 [192]. It has been shown that a subpopulation of patients with birch pollen allergy and atopic dermatitis reacted with worsening of eczema after oral challenge with foods harboring Bet v 1 homologous proteins [193]. Bet v 1-specific T cells could be found in the lesional skin of these patients [193]. T-cell cross-reactivity between Bet v 1 and related food allergens occurs independently of IgE cross-reactivity. Gastrointestinal or heat degradation destroyed the histamine-releasing but not the T-cell-activating properties of Bet v 1 homologous food allergens [194, 195]. Thus, ingestion of cooked birch-pollen-allergy-related foods did not induce OAS but caused atopic eczema to worsen [195].

Minor families

Chitinases

Chitinases are enzymes that catalyze the hydrolysis of chitin polymers. Chitinases are members of the glycoside hydrolase families 18 or 19 [196]. Endochitinases from plants belong to family 19 (also known as classes IA or I and IB or II) and are able to degrade chitin, a major structural component of the exoskeleton of insects and of the cell walls of many pathogenic fungi [197]. Class I chitinases contain an N-terminal so-called hevein-like domain with putative chitin-binding properties [198]. This hevein-like domain shares high sequence identity with the major *Hevea brasiliensis* latex allergen Hev b 6.02, hevein [199]. Class I chitinases from fruits such as avocado [200], banana [201], and chestnut [202] have been identified as major allergens that cross-react with Hev b 6.02. Although the IgE response to hevein-like domains is elicited by hevein as sensitizing allergen in most cases, no correlation between latex-associated plant food allergy and sensitization to hevein or hevein-like domains was found [203]. Pers a 1, an allergenic class I chitinase from avocado, was extensively degraded when subjected to simulated gastric fluid digestion. The resulting peptides, particularly those corresponding to the hevein-like domain, were clearly reactive both *in vitro* and *in vivo* [204]. The 43-residue polypeptide chain of hevein-like domains contains four disulfide bonds to which it owes its stability [205]. Class III chitinases do not possess a hevein domain and belong to the family 18 of glycoside hydrolases. Class III chitinases from Indian jujube [206] and from raspberry have been described as allergens [207].

Cysteine protease superfamily

Cysteine proteases of the C1, or papain-like, family were originally characterized by having a cysteine residue as part of their catalytic site, which has now been extended to include conserved glutamine, cysteine, histidine, and asparagine residues [208]. While sharing the fold of the C1 protease family, some members may have lost the capacity to act as proteases, a notable example being the soybean P34 protein, in which a glycine has replaced the active site cysteine residue [209]. Two major food allergens belong to this superfamily, actinidin (Act d 1) from kiwi fruit [104] and a soybean allergen involved in soybean-induced atopic dermatitis known as Gly m Bd 30K, Gly m 1, or P34 [210]. The cysteine protease superfamily also includes several inhalant allergens such as the mite allergens Der p 1 and Der f 1 [211]. Studies in model systems suggest that the proteolytic activity of certain of these allergens may play a role in determining their allergenic properties by affecting intestinal barrier function [212] or by interacting with immune cells through protease-activated receptors to drive Th2 immune reactions [213].

Profilins

Profilins from higher plants constitute a family of highly conserved proteins with sequence identities of at least 75% even between members of distantly related organisms [214]. Profilins are cytosolic proteins of 12–15 kDa in size that are found in all eukaryotic cells. Profilins bind to monomeric actin and a number of other proteins, thus regulating the actin polymerization and depolymerization during processes such as cell movement, cytokinesis, and signaling [215]. Originally, plant profilins were discovered as cross-reactive pollen allergens, eliciting IgE responses in 10–20% of pollen-allergic patients. Later, they were also described as allergens in plant foods and *Hevea* latex [216]. Structures of three plant profilins have been elucidated so far, those from *Arabidopsis thaliana* pollen [217], birch pollen [218] and *H. brasiliensis* latex. Since profilin-specific IgE cross-reacts with homologues from virtually every plant source, sensitization to these allergens has been considered a risk factor for allergic reactions to multiple pollen sources [219] and for pollen-associated food allergy [220]. However, the clinical relevance of plant food profilin-specific IgE is still under debate [221, 222]. As a plant food allergen, profilin elicits mild reactions. Its clinical relevance has been shown in a study by Asero and colleagues for melon, watermelon, tomato, banana, pineapple, and orange [223]. Additional studies support the clinical relevance of profilin as a major allergen for individuals with melon [224] and persimmon [225] allergy. Despite sequence identities of below 30%, plant profilin structures are highly similar to the structures of profilins from mammals, fungi, and amoeba. IgE directed to plant profilins weakly binds to the human homologue as well [226]. However, no profilins from sources other than plants have been shown to elicit allergic reactions.

Protease inhibitors and lectins

The Kunitz/bovine pancreatic trypsin inhibitor family members are active against serine, thiol, aspartic, and subtilisin proteases. They are generally small (~50 residues) with three disulfide bonds constraining the proteins' three-dimensional structure and belong to a superfamily of structurally related proteins, which share no sequence similarity and include such diverse proteins as interleukin-1 proteins, HBGF, and histactophilin. In plants they probably play a role in defense against pests and pathogens. Minor allergens have been identified belonging to the Kunitz inhibitor family in soybean [227, 228] and potato [229] with a related protein being the major IgE-binding protein in the fish parasite, Ani s 1 [230]. It is thought that their stability to processing and digestion is important for their allergenic activity. In addition agglutinin, a lectin found in peanut as well as in red kidney bean [231], has been identified as a minor allergen [228].

Thaumatin-like proteins

Thaumatin-like proteins (TLPs) derive their name from their sequence similarities to thaumatin, an intensely sweet-tasting protein isolated from the fruits of the West African rain forest shrub *Thaumatococcus daniellii*. TLPs accumulate in plants in response to pathogen challenge and belong to the PR-5 family of proteins that also includes thaumatin and osmotin [232]. Phylogenetic and structural studies revealed that PR-5 proteins constitute an ancient protein superfamily that is conserved between plants, insects, and nematodes and that appears to have originated in early eukaryotes [10, 233]. Several allergenic TLPs from fruits have been described. These include Mal d 2 from apple [234], Cap a 1 from bell pepper [235], Pru av 2 from sweet cherry [236, 237], Act c 2 from kiwi [238], and an allergenic TLP from grape [149]. The confirmation of TLPs is stabilized by eight disulfide bonds. This extensive disulfide cross-linking confers high stability to proteolysis to the TLP scaffold as has been shown for zeamatin, a TLP from corn [239]. This is also the reason why the allergenic TLPs produced by grape berries persist during the entire vinification process and are among the major proteins present in wine [240].

Allergen databases

While the majority of allergen sequences can be found in large sequence depositories, such as UniProt (Universal Protein Resource; http://www.uniprot.org/; last accessed August 2013), information on properties, such as allergenicity, does not use controlled ontology (a generic term used in information science for the structural frameworks used for organizing information). The general need of the molecular allergology community for well-curated sets of allergen sequences to support *in silico* assessments of allergenic potential of genetically modified organisms has led to the development of a number of databases (Table 4.1); [19, 241].However, the development of effective allergen ontologies will be crucial to facilitate the development of the semantic web [242] and realize its power to enable users to find, share, and combine information more easily. As part of efforts to drive it, some years ago it was noted that a markup language (ML) for allergens was required, which could be used to annotate information in a consistent manner, in the same way that publishers "mark up" manuscripts using symbols [243]. Subsequently an ML for allergens has been proposed [244] but such ontological frameworks will require the input, acceptance, and adoption by the whole community if their potential to promote more effective data linking is to be realized.

Another crucial aspect of relying increasingly on database searching for information and hence the potential of the semantic web is the need to ensure that data accessed are valid. There is a value in the immediacy that comes from having databases which are rapidly updated with allergen information, since this helps ensure speedy application of new knowledge. However, where such databases are used for regulatory purposes or safety assessments, well-curated databases are more appropriate, where content is peer reviewed by experts drawn from the community as a whole, including both molecular scientists and clinicians and updating is done in a more considered fashion. Lastly, such repositories will need to be set within a sustainable framework with institutional support, and—especially when used for regulatory purposes—independence and credibility are important for ensuring transparency in regulatory decisions which might rest on such databases. For example, one resource that was developed as a comprehensive repository of curated allergen sequences called Allergen Atlas [245] can now only be accessed in an archival form.

What does this mean?

Many of the proteins that have been described as allergens in plant foods function as seed storage proteins, providing the nutrients for a developing plant, with the cow's milk caseins functioning in a similar fashion to provide essential nutrition to young mammals. This relationship may not be so surprising since these are the proteins predominantly found in nuts and seeds and as a consequence exposure in the human diet, especially to the abundant storage proteins, is considerable. Extent of exposure to a given protein probably plays a role in determining its allergenicity, with extensive exposure now thought to be important for tolerization, total exclusion precluding an individual from developing an allergy, with low levels of exposure possibly being more effective at sensitizing [246,247]. However, it is emerging that there is a complex dialogue between different routes of exposure with evidence from animal models that cutaneous exposure may prevent the development of oral tolerance [248].

There are a number of allergens which are less abundant in foods, notably the nsLTPs where the prolamin superfamily fold may play a role in potentiating the allergenicity of these proteins. Intriguingly, many of the allergens that are less abundant in plant-derived foods have a role in plant protection. Others have alluded to the fact that many plant food allergens are involved in defense [249], with many of them being classified as pathogenesis-related proteins according to the criteria defined by van Loon and van Strien [250]. These include for example the PR-10 proteins from the Bet v 1 family of allergens, the PR14 nsLTPs, while others, such as the cereal α-amylase inhibitors although they have not been classified as PR proteins are thought to have a protective function. In addition, certain minor animal food allergens also have an imputed protective function. Many PR proteins are resistant to the effects of extremes in pH and highly resistant to proteolysis, possibly to evade the degradative environment created by pests and pathogens infecting plant tissues [8].

It has been hypothesized that resistance to digestion is important in allowing sufficient immunologically active fragments to come into contact with the immune system, particularly with regard to sensitization via the gastrointestinal tract. However, it is evident that some allergen families, notably the caseins and the cupins, are readily degraded in the gastrointestinal tract. Nevertheless, for the cupins at least there is evidence that degradation does not affect the ability of these proteins to elicit histamine release *in vitro* [99], although the impact of digestion on the sensitization potential of these proteins is not clear. For animal allergens there may also be the need to consider the evolutionary distance from man, since animal food allergens, notably the tropomyosins, lie at the borders of self–nonself recognition. Thus, it may be that in addition to the routes and extent of exposure, the mechanisms whereby different scaffolds sensitize and elicit allergic reactions may differ. Such complex interacting factors underlie the reasons why we still do not understand why some food proteins, and not others, cause allergic reactions in man. Other factors, such as food processing and modification of allergens, or adjuvant effects of other food components, may also play a role in stimulating IgE, rather than IgG responses in foods such as peanuts. Only an improved understanding of these factors and the mechanisms underlying the generation of aberrant IgE responses will enable us to understand what makes a protein become an allergen.

Acknowledgment

Author Heimo Breiteneder wishes to thank the Austrian Science Fund Grant SFB F4608 for support.

References

1. Wills-Karp M. Allergen-specific pattern recognition receptor pathways. *Curr Opin Immunol* 2010; 22(6):777–782.
2. Oliphant CJ, Barlow JL, McKenzie AN. Insights into the initiation of type 2 immune responses. *Immunology* 2011; 134(4):378–385.
3. Jenkins JA, Griffiths-Jones S, Shewry PR, Breiteneder H, Mills EN. Structural relatedness of plant food allergens with specific reference to cross-reactive allergens: an in silico analysis. *J Allergy Clin Immunol* 2005; 115(1): 163–170.
4. Radauer C, Breiteneder H. Pollen allergens are restricted to few protein families and show distinct patterns of species distribution. *J Allergy Clin Immunol* 2006; 117(1):141–147.
5. Radauer C, Bublin M, Wagner S, Mari A, Breiteneder H. Allergens are distributed into few protein families and possess a restricted number of biochemical functions. *J Allergy Clin Immunol* 2008; 121:847–852.
6. Dunwell JM, Purvis A, Khuri S. Cupins: the most functionally diverse protein superfamily? *Phytochemistry* 2004; 65(1):7–17.
7. Radauer C, Lackner P, Breiteneder H. The Bet v 1 fold: an ancient, versatile scaffold for binding of large, hydrophobic ligands. *BMC Evol Biol* 2008; 8:286.
8. Mills EN, Jenkins JA, Alcocer MJ, Shewry PR. Structural, biological, and evolutionary relationships of plant food allergens sensitizing via the gastrointestinal tract. *Crit Rev Food Sci Nutr* 2004; 44(5):379–407.
9. Rodin J, Rask L. Characterization of matteuccin, the 2.2S storage protein of the ostrich fern. Evolutionary relationship to angiosperm seed storage proteins. *Eur J Biochem* 1990; 192(1):101–107.
10. Shatters Jr RG, Boykin LM, Lapointe SL, Hunter WB, Weathersbee III AA. Phylogenetic and structural relationships of the PR5 gene family reveal an ancient multigene family conserved in plants and select animal taxa. *J Mol Evol* 2006; 63(1):12–29.
11. Liscombe DK, MacLeod BP, Loukanina N, Nandi OI, Facchini PJ. Evidence for the monophyletic evolution of benzylisoquinoline alkaloid biosynthesis in angiosperms. *Phytochemistry* 2005; 66(20):2501–2520.
12. Punta M, Coggill PC, Eberhardt RY, et al. The Pfam protein families database. *Nucleic Acids Res* 2012; 40(Database Issue):D290–D301.
13. Chapman MD, Pomés A, Breiteneder H, Ferreira F. Nomenclature and structural biology of allergens. *J Allergy Clin Immunol* 2007; 119:414–420.
14. Ivanciuc O, Mathura V, Midoro-Horiuti T, Braun W, Goldblum RM, Schein CH. Detecting potential IgE-reactive sites on food proteins using a sequence and structure database, SDAP-Food. *J Agric Food Chem* 2003; 51(16): 4830–4837.
15. Fiers MWEJ, Kleter GA, Nijland H, Peijnenburg AACM, Nap J-P, Van Ham RCHJ. AllermatchTM, a webtool for the prediction of potential allergenicity according to current FAO/WHO Codex alimentarius guidelines. *BMC Bioinf* 2004; 5:133.
16. Mari A, Scala E, Palazzo P, Ridolfi S, Zennaro D, Carabella G. Bioinformatics applied to allergy: allergen databases, from collecting sequence information to data integration. The Allergome platform as a model. *Cell Immunol* 2007; 244:97–100.
17. Mills EN, Jenkins JA, Sancho AI, et al. Food allergy information resources for consumers, industry and regulators. *Arb Paul Ehrlich Inst Bundesamt Sera Impfstoffe Frankf A M* 2006; (95):17–25; discussion 25–27.
18. Gendel SM, Jenkins JA. Allergen sequence databases. *Mol Nutr Food Res* 2006; 50(7):633–637.
19. Mari A, Rasi C, Palazzo P, Scala E. Allergen databases: current status and perspectives. *Curr Allergy Asthma Rep* 2009; 9(5):376–383.
20. Jenkins JA, Breiteneder H, Mills ENC. Evolutionary distance from human homologs reflects allergenicity of animal food proteins. *J Allergy Clin Immunol* 2007; 120(6):1399–1405.
21. Breiteneder H, Radauer C. A classification of plant food allergens. *J Allergy Clin Immunol* 2004; 113(5):821–830.
22. Aalberse RC. Structural biology of allergens. *J Allergy Clin Immunol* 2000; 106(2):228–238.
23. Motoyama K, Suma Y, Ishizaki S, Nagashima Y, Shiomi K. Molecular cloning of tropomyosins identified as allergens in six species of crustaceans. *J Agric Food Chem* 2007; 55:985–991.
24. Bauermeister K, Wangorsch A, Garoffo LP, et al. Generation of a comprehensive panel of crustacean allergens from the North Sea shrimp *Crangon crangon*. *Mol Immunol* 2011; 48(15–16):1983–1992.

25. Mykles DL, Cotton JL, Taniguchi H, Sano K, Maeda Y. Cloning of tropomyosins from lobster (*Homarus americanus*) striated muscles: fast and slow isoforms may be generated from the same transcript. *J Muscle Res Cell Motil* 1998; 19(2):105–115.
26. Miyazawa H, Fukamachi H, Inagaki Y, et al. Identification of the first major allergen of a squid (*Todarodes pacificus*). *J Allergy Clin Immunol* 1996; 98(5 Pt. 1):948–953.
27. Leung PS, Chu KH. cDNA cloning and molecular identification of the major oyster allergen from the Pacific oyster *Crassostrea gigas*. *Clin Exp Allergy* 2001; 31(8):1287–1294.
28. Chu KH, Wong SH, Leung PS. Tropomyosin is the major mollusk allergen: reverse transcriptase polymerase chain reaction, expression and IgE reactivity. *Mar Biotechnol (NY)* 2000; 2(5):499–509.
29. Van Do T, Hordvik I, Endresen C, Elsayed S. The major allergen (parvalbumin) of codfish is encoded by at least two isotypic genes: cDNA cloning, expression and antibody binding of the recombinant allergens. *Mol Immunol* 2003; 39(10):595–602.
30. Swoboda I, Bugajska-Schretter A, Verdino P, et al. Recombinant carp parvalbumin, the major cross-reactive fish allergen: a tool for diagnosis and therapy of fish allergy. *J Immunol* 2002; 168(9):4576–4584.
31. Bernard H, Creminon C, Yvon M, Wal JM. Specificity of the human IgE response to the different purified caseins in allergy to cow's milk proteins. *Int Arch Allergy Immunol* 1998; 115(3):235–244.
32. Nagao M, Maki M, Sasaki R, Chiba R. Isolation and sequence analysis of bovine alpha-S1-casein cDNA clone. *Agric Biol Chem* 1984; 48:1663–1667.
33. Stewart AF, Bonsing J, Beattie CW, Shah F, Willis IM, Mackinlay AG. Complete nucleotide sequences of bovine alpha S2- and beta-casein cDNAs: comparisons with related sequences in other species. *Mol Biol Evol* 1987; 4(3):231–241.
34. Bonsing J, Ring JM, Stewart AF, Mackinlay AG. Complete nucleotide sequence of the bovine beta-casein gene. *Aust J Biol Sci* 1988; 41(4):527–537.
35. Stewart AF, Willis IM, Mackinlay AG. Nucleotide sequences of bovine alpha S1- and kappa-casein cDNAs. *Nucleic Acids Res* 1984; 12(9):3895–3907.
36. MacLeod AR. Genetic origin of diversity of human cytoskeletal tropomyosins. *Bioessays* 1987; 6(5):208–212.
37. Li Y, Mui S, Brown JH, et al. The crystal structure of the C-terminal fragment of striated-muscle alpha-tropomyosin reveals a key troponin T recognition site. *Proc Natl Acad Sci USA* 2002; 99(11):7378–7383.
38. Gunning PW, Schevzov G, Kee AJ, Hardeman EC. Tropomyosin isoforms: divining rods for actin cytoskeleton function. *Trends Cell Biol* 2005; 15(6):333–341.
39. Shanti KN, Martin BM, Nagpal S, Metcalfe DD, Rao PV. Identification of tropomyosin as the major shrimp allergen and characterization of its IgE-binding epitopes. *J Immunol* 1993; 151(10):5354–5363.
40. Daul CB, Slattery M, Reese G, Lehrer SB. Identification of the major brown shrimp (*Penaeus aztecus*) allergen as the muscle protein tropomyosin. *Int Arch Allergy Immunol* 1994; 105(1):49–55.
41. Leung PS, Chu KH, Chow WK, et al. Cloning, expression, and primary structure of *Metapenaeus ensis* tropomyosin, the major heat-stable shrimp allergen. *J Allergy Clin Immunol* 1994; 94(5):882–890.
42. Reese G, Ayuso R, Lehrer SB. Tropomyosin: an invertebrate pan-allergen. *Int Arch Allergy Immunol* 1999; 119(4):247–258.
43. Motoyama K, Ishizaki S, Nagashima Y, Shiomi K. Cephalopod tropomyosins: identification as major allergens and molecular cloning. *Food Chem Toxicol* 2006; 44(12):1997–2002.
44. Naqpal S, Rajappa L, Metcalfe DD, Rao PV. Isolation and characterization of heat-stable allergens from shrimp (*Penaeus indicus*). *J Allergy Clin Immunol* 1989; 83(1):26–36.
45. Lehrer SB, Ibanez MD, McCants ML, Daul CB, Morgan JE. Characterization of water-soluble shrimp allergens released during boiling. *J Allergy Clin Immunol* 1990; 85(6):1005–1013.
46. Lee PW, Nordlee JA, Koppelman SJ, Baumert JL, Taylor SL. Evaluation and comparison of the species-specificity of 3 antiparvalbumin IgG antibodies. *J Agric Food Chem* 2011; 59(23):12309–12316.
47. Lewit-Bentley A, Rety S. EF-hand calcium-binding proteins. *Curr Opin Struct Biol* 2000; 10(6):637–643.
48. Ikura M. Calcium binding and conformational response in EF-hand proteins. *Trends Biochem Sci* 1996; 21(1):14–17.
49. Declercq JP, Tinant B, Parello J, Rambaud J. Ionic interactions with parvalbumins. Crystal structure determination of pike 4.10 parvalbumin in four different ionic environments. *J Mol Biol* 1991; 220(4):1017–1039.
50. Pauls TL, Cox JA, Berchtold MW. The Ca2+(-)binding proteins parvalbumin and oncomodulin and their genes: new structural and functional findings. *Biochim Biophys Acta* 1996; 1306(1):39–54.
51. Bugajska-Schretter A, Elfman L, Fuchs T, et al. Parvalbumin, a cross-reactive fish allergen, contains IgE-binding epitopes sensitive to periodate treatment and Ca2+ depletion. *J Allergy Clin Immunol* 1998; 101(1 Pt. 1):67–74.
52. Bugajska-Schretter A, Grote M, Vangelista L, et al. Purification, biochemical, and immunological characterisation of a major food allergen: different immunoglobulin E recognition of the apo- and calcium-bound forms of carp parvalbumin. *Gut* 2000; 46(5):661–669.
53. Filimonov VV, Pfeil W, Tsalkova TN, Privalov PL. Thermodynamic investigations of proteins. IV. Calcium binding protein parvalbumin. *Biophys Chem* 1978; 8(2):117–122.
54. Somkuti J, Bublin M, Breiteneder H, Smeller L. Pressure-temperature stability, Ca2+-binding and p-T phase diagram of cod parvalbumin: Gad m 1. *Biochemistry* 2012; 51(30):5903–5911.
55. Griesmeier U, Bublin M, Radauer C, et al. Physicochemical properties and thermal stability of Lep w 1, the major allergen of whiff. *Mol Nutr Food Res* 2010; 54(6):861–869.
56. Elsayed S, Aas K. Characterization of a major allergen (cod). Observations on effect of denaturation on the allergenic activity. *J Allergy* 1971; 47(5):283–291.
57. Aas K, Jebsen JW. Studies of hypersensitivity to fish. Partial purification and crystallization of a major allergenic component of cod. *Int Arch Allergy Appl Immunol* 1967; 32(1):1–20.

58. Elsayed S, Bennich H. The primary structure of allergen M from cod *Scand J Immunol* 1975; 4(2):203–208.
59. Hajeb P, Selamat J. A contemporary review of seafood allergy. *Clin Rev Allergy Immunol* 2012; 42(3):365–385.
60. Cai QF, Liu GM, Li T, et al. Purification and characterization of parvalbumins, the major allergens in red stingray (*Dasyatis akajei*). *J Agric Food Chem* 2010; 58(24):12964–12969.
61. Hilger C, Thill L, Grigioni F, et al. IgE antibodies of fish allergic patients cross-react with frog parvalbumin. *Allergy* 2004; 59(6):653–660.
62. Hilger C, Grigioni F, Thill L, Mertens L, Hentges F. Severe IgE-mediated anaphylaxis following consumption of fried frog legs: definition of alpha-parvalbumin as the allergen in cause. *Allergy* 2002; 57(11):1053–1058.
63. Tuinier R, de Kruif CG. Stability of casein micelles in milk. *J Chem Phys* 2002; 117(3):1290–1295.
64. Kawasaki K, Weiss KM. Mineralized tissue and vertebrate evolution: the secretory calcium-binding phosphoprotein gene cluster. *Proc Natl Acad Sci USA* 2003; 100(7):4060–4065.
65. Natale M, Bisson C, Monti G, et al. Cow's milk allergens identification by two-dimensional immunoblotting and mass spectrometry. *Mol Nutr Food Res* 2004; 48(5):363–369.
66. Bellioni-Businco B, Paganelli R, Lucenti P, Giampietro PG, Perborn H, Businco L. Allergenicity of goat's milk in children with cow's milk allergy. *J Allergy Clin Immunol* 1999; 103(6):1191–1194.
67. Businco L, Giampietro PG, Lucenti P, et al. Allergenicity of mare's milk in children with cow's milk allergy. *J Allergy Clin Immunol* 2000; 105(5):1031–1034.
68. Restani P, Gaiaschi A, Plebani A, et al. Cross-reactivity between milk proteins from different animal species. *Clin Exp Allergy* 1999; 29(7):997–1004.
69. Han N, Järvinen KM, Cocco RR, Busse PJ, Sampson HA, Beyer K. Identification of amino acids critical for IgE-binding to sequential epitopes of bovine kappa-casein and the similarity of these epitopes to the corresponding human kappa-casein sequence. *Allergy* 2008; 63(2):198–204.
70. Bernard H, Negroni L, Chatel JM, et al. Molecular basis of IgE cross-reactivity between human beta-casein and bovine beta-casein, a major allergen of milk. *Mol Immunol* 2000; 37(3–4):161–167.
71. Makinen-Kiljunen S, Plosila M. A fathers' IgE-mediated contact urticaria from mothers' milk. *J Allergy Clin Immunol* 2004; 113:353–354.
72. Schulmeister U, Hochwallner H, Swoboda I, et al. Cloning, expression, and mapping of allergenic determinants of alphaS1-casein, a major cow's milk allergen. *J Immunol* 2009; 182(11):7019–7029.
73. Bernard H, Meisel H, Creminon C, Wal JM. Post-translational phosphorylation affects the IgE binding capacity of caseins. *FEBS Lett* 2000; 467(2–3):239–244.
74. Flower DR. The lipocalin protein family: structure and function. *Biochem J* 1996; 318(Pt. 1):1–14.
75. Cho KW, Zhou Y, Sheng L, Rui L. Lipocalin-13 regulates glucose metabolism by both insulin-dependent and insulin-independent mechanisms. *Mol Cell Biol* 2011; 31(3):450–457.
76. Clifton MC, Corrent C, Strong RK. Siderocalins: siderophore-binding proteins of the innate immune system. *Biometals* 2009; 22(4):557–564.
77. Virtanen T. Lipocalin allergens. *Allergy* 2001; 56(Suppl. 67):48–51.
78. Fluckinger M, Merschak P, Hermann M, Haertlé T, Redl B. Lipocalin-interacting-membrane-receptor (LIMR) mediates cellular internalization of β-lactoglobulin. *Biochim Biophys Acta* 2008; 1778(1):342–347.
79. Nitta K, Sugai S. The evolution of lysozyme and alpha-lactalbumin. *Eur J Biochem* 1989; 182(1):111–118.
80. Aabin B, Poulsen LK, Ebbehoj K, et al. Identification of IgE-binding egg white proteins: comparison of results obtained by different methods. *Int Arch Allergy Immunol* 1996; 109(1):50–57.
81. Holen E, Elsayed S. Characterization of four major allergens of hen egg-white by IEF/SDS-PAGE combined with electrophoretic transfer and IgE-immunoautoradiography. *Int Arch Allergy Appl Immunol* 1990; 91(2):136–141.
82. van Gent D, Sharp P, Morgan K, Kalsheker N. Serpins: structure, function and molecular evolution. *Int J Biochem Cell Biol* 2003; 35(11):1536–1547.
83. Bernhisel-Broadbent J, Dintzis HM, Dintzis RZ, Sampson HA. Allergenicity and antigenicity of chicken egg ovomucoid (Gal d III) compared with ovalbumin (Gal d I) in children with egg allergy and in mice. *J Allergy Clin Immunol* 1994; 93(6):1047–1059.
84. García-Orozco KD, Aispuro-Hernández E, Yepiz-Plascencia G, Calderón-de-la-Barca AM, Sotelo-Mundo RR. Molecular characterization of arginine kinase, an allergen from the shrimp *Litopenaeus vannamei*. *Int Arch Allergy Immunol* 2007; 144(1):23–28.
85. Binder M, Mahler V, Hayek B, et al. Molecular and immunological characterization of arginine kinase from the Indianmeal moth, *Plodia interpunctella*, a novel cross-reactive invertebrate pan-allergen. *J Immunol* 2001; 167(9):5470–5477.
86. Laskowski Jr M, Kato I, Ardelt W, et al. Ovomucoid third domains from 100 avian species: isolation, sequences, and hypervariability of enzyme-inhibitor contact residues. *Biochemistry* 1987; 26(1):202–221.
87. Kato I, Schrode J, Kohr WJ, Laskowski Jr M. Chicken ovomucoid: determination of its amino acid sequence, determination of the trypsin reactive site, and preparation of all three of its domains. *Biochemistry* 1987; 26(1):193–201.
88. Cooke SK, Sampson HA. Allergenic properties of ovomucoid in man. *J Immunol* 1997; 159(4):2026–2032.
89. Ou K, Seow TK, Liang RC, et al. Identification of a serine protease inhibitor homologue in Bird's Nest by an integrated proteomics approach. *Electrophoresis* 2001; 22(16):3589–3595.
90. Sugiyama T, Rafalski A, Soell D. The nucleotide sequence of a wheat gamma-gliadin genomic clone. *Plant Sci* 1986; 44:205–209.
91. Sander I, Rozynek P, Rihs HP, et al. Multiple wheat flour allergens and cross-reactive carbohydrate determinants bind IgE in baker's asthma. *Allergy* 2011; 66:1208–1215.
92. Anderson OD, Greene FC, Yip RE, Halford N.G., Shewry P.R., Malpica-Romero J.M. Nucleotide sequences of the two high-molecular-weight glutenin genes from the D-genome of a hexaploid bread wheat, *Triticum aestivum* L. cv Cheyenne. *Nucleic Acids Res* 1989; 17:461–462.

93. Pastorello EA, Farioli L, Pravettoni V, et al. The major allergen of peach (*Prunus persica*) is a lipid transfer protein. *J Allergy Clin Immunol* 1999; 103(3 Pt. 1):520–526.
94. Schocker F, Luttkopf D, Scheurer S, et al. Recombinant lipid transfer protein Cor a 8 from hazelnut: a new tool for in vitro diagnosis of potentially severe hazelnut allergy. *J Allergy Clin Immunol* 2004; 113(1):141–147.
95. Teuber SS, Dandekar AM, Peterson WR, Sellers CL. Cloning and sequencing of a gene encoding a 2S albumin seed storage protein precursor from English walnut (*Juglans regia*), a major food allergen. *J Allergy Clin Immunol* 1998; 101(6 Pt. 1):807–814.
96. Burks AW, Williams LW, Connaughton C, Cockrell G, O'Brien TJ, Helm RM. Identification and characterization of a second major peanut allergen, Ara h II, with use of the sera of patients with atopic dermatitis and positive peanut challenge. *J Allergy Clin Immunol* 1992; 90(6 Pt. 1):962–969.
97. Kleber-Janke T, Crameri R, Appenzeller U, Schlaak M, Becker WM. Selective cloning of peanut allergens, including profilin and 2S albumins, by phage display technology. *Int Arch Allergy Immunol* 1999; 119(4):265–274.
98. Stanley JS, King N, Burks AW, et al. Identification and mutational analysis of the immunodominant IgE binding epitopes of the major peanut allergen Ara h 2. *Arch Biochem Biophys* 1997; 342(2):244–253.
99. Eiwegger T, Rigby N, Mondoulet L, et al. Gastro-duodenal digestion products of the major peanut allergen Ara h 1 retain an allergenic potential. *Clin Exp Allergy* 2006; 36(10):1281–1288.
100. Breiteneder H, Hoffmann-Sommergruber K, O'Riordain G, et al. Molecular characterization of Api g 1, the major allergen of celery (*Apium graveolens*), and its immunological and structural relationships to a group of 17-kDa tree pollen allergens. *Eur J Biochem* 1995; 233(2):484–489.
101. Luttkopf D, Muller U, Skov PS, et al. Comparison of four variants of a major allergen in hazelnut (*Corylus avellana*) Cor a 1.04 with the major hazel pollen allergen Cor a 1.01. *Mol Immunol* 2002; 38(7):515–525.
102. Burks AW, Williams LW, Helm RM, Connaughton C, Cockrell G, O'Brien T. Identification of a major peanut allergen, Ara h I, in patients with atopic dermatitis and positive peanut challenges. *J Allergy Clin Immunol* 1991; 88(2):172–179.
103. Rabjohn P, Helm EM, Stanley JS, et al. Molecular cloning and epitope analysis of the peanut allergen Ara h 3. *J Clin Invest* 1999; 103(4):535–542.
104. Pastorello EA, Conti A, Pravettoni V, et al. Identification of actinidin as the major allergen of kiwi fruit. *J Allergy Clin Immunol* 1998; 101(4 Pt. 1):531–537.
105. Kreis M, Forde BG, Rahman S, Miflin BJ, Shewry PR. Molecular evolution of the seed storage proteins of barley, rye and wheat. *J Mol Biol* 1985; 183(3):499–502.
106. Edstam MM, Viitanen L, Salminen TA, Edqvist J. Evolutionary history of the non-specific lipid transfer proteins. *Mol Plant* 2011; 4(6):947–964.
107. Tassin-Moindrot S, Caille A, Douliez JP, Marion D, Vovelle F. The wide binding properties of a wheat nonspecific lipid transfer protein. Solution structure of a complex with prostaglandin B2. *Eur J Biochem* 2000; 267(4):1117–1124.
108. Douliez JP, Jegou S, Pato C, Molle D, Tran V, Marion D. Binding of two mono-acylated lipid monomers by the barley lipid transfer protein, LTP1, as viewed by fluorescence, isothermal titration calorimetry and molecular modelling. *Eur J Biochem* 2001; 268(2):384–388.
109. Pastorello EA, Pompei C, Pravettoni V, et al. Lipid-transfer protein is the major maize allergen maintaining IgE-binding activity after cooking at 100 degrees C, as demonstrated in anaphylactic patients and patients with positive double-blind, placebo-controlled food challenge results. *J Allergy Clin Immunol* 2003; 112(4):775–783.
110. Sancho AI, Rigby NM, Zuidmeer L, et al. The effect of thermal processing on the IgE reactivity of the non-specific lipid transfer protein from apple, Mal d 3. *Allergy* 2005; 60(10):1262–1268.
111. Moreno FJ, Mellon FA, Wickham MS, Bottrill AR, Mills EN. Stability of the major allergen Brazil nut 2S albumin (Ber e 1) to physiologically relevant in vitro gastrointestinal digestion. *FEBS J* 2005; 272(2):341–352.
112. Asero R, Mistrello G, Roncarolo D, et al. Lipid transfer protein: a pan-allergen in plant-derived foods that is highly resistant to pepsin digestion. *Int Arch Allergy Immunol* 2000; 122(1):20–32.
113. Vassilopoulou E, Rigby N, Moreno FJ, et al. Effect of in vitro gastric and duodenal digestion on the allergenicity of grape lipid transfer protein. *J Allergy Clin Immunol* 2006; 118(2):473–480.
114. Shewry PR, Halford NG, Belton PS, Tatham AS. The structure and properties of gluten: an elastic protein from wheat grain. *Philos Trans R Soc Lond B Biol Sci* 2002; 357(1418):133–142.
115. Palosuo K, Alenius H, Varjonen E, et al. A novel wheat gliadin as a cause of exercise-induced anaphylaxis. *J Allergy Clin Immunol* 1999; 103(5 Pt. 1):912–917.
116. Palosuo K, Varjonen E, Kekki OM, et al. Wheat omega-5 gliadin is a major allergen in children with immediate allergy to ingested wheat. *J Allergy Clin Immunol* 2001; 108(4):634–638.
117. Matsuo H, Morita E, Tatham AS, et al. Identification of the IgE-binding epitope in omega-5 gliadin, a major allergen in wheat-dependent exercise-induced anaphylaxis. *J Biol Chem* 2004; 279(13):12135–12140.
118. Watanabe M, Tanabe S, Suzuki T, Ikezawa Z, Arai S. Primary structure of an allergenic peptide occurring in the chymotryptic hydrolysate of gluten. *Biosci Biotechnol Biochem* 1995; 59(8):1596–1597.
119. Tanabe S, Arai S, Yanagihara Y, Mita H, Takahashi K, Watanabe M. A major wheat allergen has a Gln-Gln-Gln-Pro-Pro motif identified as an IgE-binding epitope. *Biochem Biophys Res Commun* 1996; 219(2):290–293.
120. Maruyama N, Ichise K, Katsube T, et al. Identification of major wheat allergens by means of the *Escherichia coli* expression system. *Eur J Biochem* 1998; 255(3): 739–745.
121. Simonato B, Pasini G, Giannattasio M, Peruffo AD, De Lazzari F, Curioni A. Food allergy to wheat products: the effect

of bread baking and in vitro digestion on wheat allergenic proteins. A study with bread dough, crumb, and crust. *J Agric Food Chem* 2001; 49(11):5668–5673.
122. Simonato B, De Lazzari F, Pasini G, et al. IgE binding to soluble and insoluble wheat flour proteins in atopic and non-atopic patients suffering from gastrointestinal symptoms after wheat ingestion. *Clin Exp Allergy* 2001; 31(11):1771–1778.
123. Denery-Papini S, Bodinier M, Larré C, et al. Allergy to deamidated gluten in patients tolerant to wheat: specific epitopes linked to deamidation. *Allergy* 2012; 67(8):1023–1032.
124. Kumagai H, Suda A, Sakurai H, et al. Improvement of digestibility, reduction in allergenicity, and induction of oral tolerance of wheat gliadin by deamidation. *Biosci Biotechnol Biochem* 2007; 71(4):977–985.
125. Carbonero P, García-Olmedo F. *A Multigene Family of Trypsin/Alpha-Amylase Inhibitors from Cereals*. Dordrecht, The Netherlands: Kluwer Academic Publishers, 1999.
126. Nakase M, Adachi T, Urisu A, et al. Rice (*Oryza sativa* L.) alpha amylase inhibitors of 14-16 kDa are potential allergens and products of a multi gene family. *J Agric Food Chem* 1996; 44:2624–2628.
127. James JM, Sixbey JP, Helm RM, Bannon GA, Burks AW. Wheat alpha-amylase inhibitor: a second route of allergic sensitization. *J Allergy Clin Immunol* 1997; 99(2):239–244.
128. Pastorello EA, Farioli L, Conti A, et al. Wheat IgE-mediated food allergy in European patients: alpha-amylase inhibitors, lipid transfer proteins and low-molecular-weight glutenins. Allergenic molecules recognized by double-blind, placebo-controlled food challenge. *Int Arch Allergy Immunol* 2007; 144(1):10–22.
129. Curioni A, Santucci B, Cristaudo A, et al. Urticaria from beer: an immediate hypersensitivity reaction due to a 10-kDa protein derived from barley. *Clin Exp Allergy* 1999; 29(3):407–413.
130. Pastorello EA, Farioli L, Pravettoni V, et al. The maize major allergen, which is responsible for food-induced allergic reactions, is a lipid transfer protein. *J Allergy Clin Immunol* 2000; 106(4):744–751.
131. Shewry PR, Pandya MJ. *The 2S Albumin Storage Proteins*. Dordrecht, The Netherlands: Kluwer Academic Publishers, 1999.
132. Maria-Neto S, Honorato RV, Costa FT, et al. Bactericidal activity identified in 2S albumin from sesame seeds and in silico studies of structure-function relations. *Protein J* 2011; 30(5):340–350.
133. Moreno FJ, Clemente A. 2S albumin storage proteins: what makes them food allergens? *Open Biochem J* 2008; 2:16–28.
134. Menendez-Arias L, Moneo I, Dominguez J, Rodriguez R. Primary structure of the major allergen of yellow mustard (*Sinapis alba* L.) seed, Sin a I. *Eur J Biochem* 1988; 177(1):159–166.
135. Monsalve RI, Gonzalez de la Pena MA, Menendez-Arias L, Lopez-Otin C, Villalba M, Rodriguez R. Characterization of a new oriental-mustard (*Brassica juncea*) allergen, Bra j IE: detection of an allergenic epitope. *Biochem J* 1993; 293(Pt. 3):625–632.
136. Pastorello EA, Varin E, Farioli L, et al. The major allergen of sesame seeds (*Sesamum indicum*) is a 2S albumin. *J Chromatogr B Biomed Sci Appl* 2001; 756(1–2):85–93.
137. Beyer K, Bardina L, Grishina G, Sampson HA. Identification of sesame seed allergens by 2-dimensional proteomics and Edman sequencing: seed storage proteins as common food allergens. *J Allergy Clin Immunol* 2002; 110(1):154–159.
138. Pastorello EA, Farioli L, Pravettoni V, et al. Sensitization to the major allergen of Brazil nut is correlated with the clinical expression of allergy. *J Allergy Clin Immunol* 1998; 102(6 Pt. 1):1021–1027.
139. Robotham JM, Wang F, Seamon V, et al. Ana o 3, an important cashew nut (*Anacardium occidentale* L.) allergen of the 2S albumin family. *J Allergy Clin Immunol* 2005; 115(6):1284–1290.
140. Poltronieri P, Cappello MS, Dohmae N, et al. Identification and characterisation of the IgE-binding proteins 2S albumin and conglutin gamma in almond (*Prunus dulcis*) seeds. *Int Arch Allergy Immunol* 2002; 128(2):97–104.
141. Kelly JD, Hlywka JJ, Hefle SL. Identification of sunflower seed IgE-binding proteins. *Int Arch Allergy Immunol* 2000; 121(1):19–24.
142. Alcocer M, Rundqvist L, Larsson G. Ber e 1 protein: the versatile major allergen from Brazil nut seeds. *Biotechnol Lett* 2012; 34(4):597–610.
143. Shibasaki M, Suzuki S, Tajima S, Nemoto H, Kuroume T. Allergenicity of major component proteins of soybean. *Int Arch Allergy Appl Immunol* 1980; 61(4):441–448.
144. Vioque J, Sanchez-Vioque R, Clemente A, Pedroche J, Bautista J, Millan F. Purification and partial characterization of chickpea 2S albumin. *J Agric Food Chem* 1999; 47(4):1405–1409.
145. Salcedo G, Sánchez-Monge R, Barber D, Díaz-Perales A. Plant non-specific lipid transfer proteins: an interface between plant defence and human allergy. *Biochim Biophys Acta* 2007; 1771(6):781–791.
146. Duro G, Colombo P, Costa MA, et al. cDNA cloning, sequence analysis and allergological characterization of Par j 2.0101, a new major allergen of the *Parietaria judaica* pollen. *FEBS Lett* 1996; 399(3):295–298.
147. Tejera ML, Villalba M, Batanero E, Rodriguez R. Identification, isolation, and characterization of Ole e 7, a new allergen of olive tree pollen. *J Allergy Clin Immunol* 1999; 104(4 Pt. 1):797–802.
148. Pastorello EA, Farioli L, Pravettoni V, et al. The major allergen of peach (Prunus persica) is a lipid transfer protein. *J Allergy Clin Immunol* 1999; 103(3 Pt. 1):520–526.
149. Pastorello EA, Farioli L, Pravettoni V, et al. Identification of grape and wine allergens as an endochitinase 4, a lipid-transfer protein, and a thaumatin. *J Allergy Clin Immunol* 2003; 111(2):350–359.
150. Diaz-Perales A, Tabar AI, Sanchez-Monge R, et al. Characterization of asparagus allergens: a relevant role of lipid transfer proteins. *J Allergy Clin Immunol* 2002; 110(5):790–796.
151. Pastorello EA, Vieths S, Pravettoni V, et al. Identification of hazelnut major allergens in sensitive patients with

positive double-blind, placebo-controlled food challenge results. *J Allergy Clin Immunol* 2002; 109(3):563–570.
152. Bernardi ML, Giangrieco I, Camardella L, et al. Allergenic lipid transfer proteins from plant-derived foods do not immunologically and clinically behave homogeneously: the kiwifruit LTP as a model. *PLoS One* 2011; 6(11):e27856.
153. Mills ENC, Jenkins JA, Bannon GA. *Plant Seed Globulin Allergens*. Oxford: Blackwell Publishing, 2004.
154. Burks Jr AW, Brooks JR, Sampson HA. Allergenicity of major component proteins of soybean determined by enzyme-linked immunosorbent assay (ELISA) and immunoblotting in children with atopic dermatitis and positive soy challenges. *J Allergy Clin Immunol* 1988; 81(6):1135–1142.
155. Ogawa T, Bando N, Tsuji H, Nishikawa K, Kitamura K. Alpha-subunit of beta-conglycinin, an allergenic protein recognized by IgE antibodies of soybean-sensitive patients with atopic dermatitis. *Biosci Biotechnol Biochem* 1995; 59(5):831–833.
156. Beardslee TA, Zeece MG, Sarath G, Markwell JP. Soybean glycinin G1 acidic chain shares IgE epitopes with peanut allergen Ara h 3. *Int Arch Allergy Immunol* 2000; 123(4):299–307.
157. Rabjohn P, Helm EM, Stanley JS, et al. Molecular cloning and epitope analysis of the peanut allergen Ara h 3. *J Clin Invest* 1999; 103(4):535–542.
158. Wang F, Robotham JM, Teuber SS, Tawde P, Sathe SK, Roux KH. Ana o 1, a cashew (Anacardium occidental) allergen of the vicilin seed storage protein family. *J Allergy Clin Immunol* 2002; 110(1):160–166.
159. Wang F, Robotham JM, Teuber SS, Sathe SK, Roux KH. Ana o 2, a major cashew (Anacardium occidentale L.) nut allergen of the legumin family. *Int Arch Allergy Immunol* 2003; 132(1):27–39.
160. Teuber SS, Jarvis KC, Dandekar AM, Peterson WR, Ansari AA. Identification and cloning of a complementary DNA encoding a vicilin-like proprotein, jug r 2, from English walnut kernel *(Juglans regia)*, a major food allergen. *J Allergy Clin Immunol* 1999; 104(6):1311–1320.
161. Lopez-Torrejon G, Salcedo G, Martin-Esteban M, Diaz-Perales A, Pascual CY, Sanchez-Monge R. Len c 1, a major allergen and vicilin from lentil seeds: protein isolation and cDNA cloning. *J Allergy Clin Immunol* 2003; 112(6):1208–1215.
162. Roux KH, Teuber SS, Sathe SK. Tree nut allergens. *Int Arch Allergy Immunol* 2003; 131(4):234–244.
163. Beyer K, Grishina G, Bardina L, Grishin A, Sampson HA. Identification of an 11S globulin as a major hazelnut food allergen in hazelnut-induced systemic reactions. *J Allergy Clin Immunol* 2002; 110(3):517–523.
164. Mills EN, Huang L, Noel TR, Gunning AP, Morris VJ. Formation of thermally induced aggregates of the soya globulin beta-conglycinin. *Biochim Biophys Acta* 2001; 1547(2):339–350.
165. Mills EN, Marigheto NA, Wellner N, et al. Thermally induced structural changes in glycinin, the 11S globulin of soya bean (Glycine max)—an in situ spectroscopic study. *Biochim Biophys Acta* 2003; 1648(1–2):105–114.
166. Yamauchi F, Yamagishi T, Iwabuchi S. Molecular understanding of heat-induced phenomena of soybean protein. *Food Rev Int* 1991; 7:283–322.
167. Blanc F, Vissers YM, Adel-Patient K, et al. Boiling peanut Ara h 1 results in the formation of aggregates with reduced allergenicity. *Mol Nutr Food Res* 2011; 55:1887–1894.
168. Maleki SJ, Kopper RA, Shin DS, et al. Structure of the major peanut allergen Ara h 1 may protect IgE-binding epitopes from degradation. *J Immunol* 2000; 164(11):5844–5849.
169. Kopper RA, Odum NJ, Sen M, Helm RM, Steve Stanley J, Wesley Burks A. Peanut protein allergens: gastric digestion is carried out exclusively by pepsin. *J Allergy Clin Immunol* 2004; 114(3):614–618.
170. Shin DS, Compadre CM, Maleki SJ, et al. Biochemical and structural analysis of the IgE binding sites on ara h1, an abundant and highly allergenic peanut protein. *J Biol Chem* 1998; 273(22):13753–13759.
171. Vieths S, Scheurer S, Ballmer-Weber B. Current understanding of cross-reactivity of food allergens and pollen. *Ann NY Acad Sci* 2002; 964:47–68.
172. Vanek-Krebitz M, Hoffmann-Sommergruber K, Laimer da Camara Machado M, et al. Cloning and sequencing of Mal d 1, the major allergen from apple (*Malus domestica*), and its immunological relationship to Bet v 1, the major birch pollen allergen. *Biochem Biophys Res Commun* 1995; 214(2):538–551.
173. Mittag D, Akkerdaas J, Ballmer-Weber BK, et al. Ara h 8, a Bet v 1-homologous allergen from peanut, is a major allergen in patients with combined birch pollen and peanut allergy. *J Allergy Clin Immunol* 2004; 114(6):1410–1417.
174. Mittag D, Vieths S, Vogel L, et al. Birch pollen-related food allergy to legumes: identification and characterization of the Bet v 1 homologue in mungbean (*Vigna radiata*), Vig r 1. *Clin Exp Allergy* 2005; 35(8):1049–1055.
175. Bolhaar ST, van Ree R, Ma Y, et al. Severe allergy to sharon fruit caused by birch pollen. *Int Arch Allergy Immunol* 2005; 136(1):45–52.
176. Bolhaar ST, Ree R, Bruijnzeel-Koomen CA, Knulst AC, Zuidmeer L. Allergy to jackfruit: a novel example of Bet v 1-related food allergy. *Allergy* 2004; 59(11):1187–1192.
177. Ballmer-Weber BK, Vieths S, Lüttkopf D, Heuschmann P, Wüthrich B. Celery allergy confirmed by double-blind, placebo-controlled food challenge: a clinical study in 32 subjects with a history of adverse reactions to celery root. *J Allergy Clin Immunol* 2000; 106(2):373–378.
178. Lüttkopf D, Ballmer-Weber BK, Wüthrich B, Vieths S. Celery allergens in patients with positive double-blind placebo-controlled food challenge. *J Allergy Clin Immunol* 2000; 106(2):390–399.
179. Ballmer-Weber BK, Wüthrich B, Wangorsch A, Fötisch K, Altmann F, Vieths S. Carrot allergy: double-blinded, placebo-controlled food challenge and identification of allergens. *J Allergy Clin Immunol* 2001; 108(2):301–307.
180. Kleine-Tebbe J, Vogel L, Crowell DN, Haustein UF, Vieths S. Severe oral allergy syndrome and anaphylactic reactions caused by a Bet v 1- related PR-10 protein in soybean, SAM22. *J Allergy Clin Immunol* 2002; 110(5):797–804.

181. Mittag D, Vieths S, Vogel L, et al. Soybean allergy in patients allergic to birch pollen: clinical investigation and molecular characterization of allergens. *J Allergy Clin Immunol* 2004; 113(1):148–154.
182. Breiteneder H, Pettenburger K, Bito A, et al. The gene coding for the major birch pollen allergen Betv1, is highly homologous to a pea disease resistance response gene. *EMBO J* 1989; 8(7):1935–1938.
183. Hoffmann-Sommergruber K. Plant allergens and pathogenesis-related proteins. What do they have in common? *Int Arch Allergy Immunol* 2000; 122(3):155–166.
184. Markovic-Housley Z, Degano M, Lamba D, et al. Crystal structure of a hypoallergenic isoform of the major birch pollen allergen Bet v 1 and its likely biological function as a plant steroid carrier. *J Mol Biol* 2003; 325(1):123–133.
185. Mattila K, Renkonen R. Modelling of Bet v 1 binding to lipids. *Scand J Immunol* 2009; 70(2):116–124.
186. Gajhede M, Osmark P, Poulsen FM, et al. X-ray and NMR structure of Bet v 1, the origin of birch pollen allergy. *Nat Struct Biol* 1996; 3(12):1040–1045.
187. Neudecker P, Schweimer K, Nerkamp J, et al. Allergic cross-reactivity made visible: solution structure of the major cherry allergen Pru av 1. *J Biol Chem* 2001; 276(25):22756–22763.
188. Schirmer T, Hoffimann-Sommergrube K, Susani M, Breiteneder H, Markovic-Housley Z. Crystal structure of the major celery allergen Api g 1: molecular analysis of cross-reactivity. *J Mol Biol* 2005; 351(5):1101–1109.
189. Marković-Housley Z, Basle A, Padavattan S, Maderegger B, Schirmer T, Hoffmann-Sommergruber K. Structure of the major carrot allergen Dau c 1. *Acta Crystallogr D Biol Crystallogr* 2009; 65(Pt. 11):1206–1212.
190. Berkner H, Neudecker P, Mittag D, et al. Cross-reactivity of pollen and food allergens: soybean Gly m 4 is a member of the Bet v 1 superfamily and closely resembles yellow lupine proteins. *Biosci Rep* 2009; 29(3):183–192.
191. Bohle B, Radakovics A, Jahn-Schmid B, Hoffmann-Sommergruber K, Fischer GF, Ebner C. Bet v 1, the major birch pollen allergen, initiates sensitization to Api g 1, the major allergen in celery: evidence at the T cell level. *Eur J Immunol* 2003; 33(12):3303–3310.
192. Smole U, Wagner S, Balazs N, et al. Bet v 1 and its homologous food allergen Api g 1 stimulate dendritic cells from birch pollen-allergic individuals to induce different Th-cell polarization. *Allergy* 2010; 65(11):1388–1396.
193. Reekers R, Busche M, Wittmann M, Kapp A, Werfel T. Birch pollen-related foods trigger atopic dermatitis in patients with specific cutaneous T-cell responses to birch pollen antigens. *J Allergy Clin Immunol* 1999; 104(2 Pt. 1):466–472.
194. Schimek EM, Zwolfer B, Briza P, et al. Gastrointestinal digestion of Bet v 1-homologous food allergens destroys their mediator-releasing, but not T cell-activating, capacity. *J Allergy Clin Immunol* 2005; 116(6):1327–1333.
195. Bohle B, Zwolfer B, Heratizadeh A, et al. Cooking birch pollen-related food: divergent consequences for IgE- and T cell-mediated reactivity in vitro and in vivo. *J Allergy Clin Immunol* 2006; 118(1):242–249.
196. Henrissat B. A classification of glycosyl hydrolases based on amino acid sequence similarities. *Biochem J* 1991; 280(Pt. 2):309–316.
197. Kasprzewska A. Plant chitinases—regulation and function. *Cell Mol Biol Lett* 2003; 8(3):809–824.
198. Beintema JJ. Structural features of plant chitinases and chitin-binding proteins. *FEBS Lett* 1994; 350(2–3):159–163.
199. Salcedo G, Diaz-Perales A, Sanchez-Monge R. The role of plant panallergens in sensitization to natural rubber latex. *Curr Opin Allergy Clin Immunol* 2001; 1(2):177–183.
200. Sowka S, Hsieh LS, Krebitz M, et al. Identification and cloning of prs a 1, a 32-kDa endochitinase and major allergen of avocado, and its expression in the yeast *Pichia pastoris*. *J Biol Chem* 1998; 273(43):28091–28097.
201. Sanchez-Monge R, Blanco C, Diaz-Perales A, et al. Isolation and characterization of major banana allergens: identification as fruit class I chitinases. *Clin Exp Allergy* 1999; 29(5):673–680.
202. Diaz-Perales A, Collada C, Blanco C, et al. Class I chitinases with hevein-like domain, but not class II enzymes, are relevant chestnut and avocado allergens. *J Allergy Clin Immunol* 1998; 102(1):127–133.
203. Radauer C, Adhami F, Fürtler I, et al. Latex-allergic patients sensitized to the major allergen hevein and hevein-like domains of class I chitinases show no increased frequency of latex-associated plant food allergy. *Mol Immunol* 2011; 48(4):600–609.
204. Diaz-Perales A, Blanco C, Sanchez-Monge R, Varela J, Carrillo T, Salcedo G. Analysis of avocado allergen (Prs a 1) IgE-binding peptides generated by simulated gastric fluid digestion. *J Allergy Clin Immunol* 2003; 112(5):1002–1007.
205. Breiteneder H, Mills EN. Molecular properties of food allergens. *J Allergy Clin Immunol* 2005; 115(1):14–23.
206. Lee MF, Hwang GY, Chen YH, Lin HC, Wu CH. Molecular cloning of Indian jujube (*Zizyphus mauritiana*) allergen Ziz m 1 with sequence similarity to plant class III chitinases. *Mol Immunol* 2006; 43(8):1144–1151.
207. Marzban G, Herndl A, Kolarich D, et al. Identification of four IgE-reactive proteins in raspberry (*Rubus ideaeus* L.). *Mol Nutr Food Res* 2008; 52(12):1497–1506.
208. Rawlings ND, Barrett AJ. Evolutionary families of peptidases. *Biochem J* 1993; 290(Pt. 1):205–218.
209. Kalinski A, Weisemann JM, Matthews BF, Herman EM. Molecular cloning of a protein associated with soybean seed oil bodies that is similar to thiol proteases of the papain family. *J Biol Chem* 1990; 265(23):13843–13848.
210. Ogawa T, Tsuji H, Bando N, et al. Identification of the soybean allergenic protein, Gly m Bd 30K, with the soybean seed 34-kDa oil-body-associated protein. *Biosci Biotechnol Biochem* 1993; 57(6):1030–1033.
211. Chruszcz M, Pomés A, Glesner J, et al. Molecular determinants for antibody binding on group 1 house dust mite allergens. *J Biol Chem* 2012; 287(10):7388–7398.
212. Čavić M, Grozdanović M, Bajić A, Srdić-Rajić T, Anđjus PR, Gavrović-Jankulović M. (2012). Actinidin, a protease from kiwifruit, induces changes in morphology and adhesion of T84 intestinal epithelial cells. *Phytochemistry* 2012; 77:46–52.

213. Liang G, Barker T, Xie Z, Charles N, Rivera J, Druey KM. Naive T cells sense the cysteine protease allergen papain through protease-activated receptor 2 and propel TH2 immunity. *J Allergy Clin Immunol* 2012; 129(5):1377–1386.
214. Radauer C, Willerroider M, Fuchs H, et al. Cross-reactive and species-specific immunoglobulin E epitopes of plant profilins: an experimental and structure-based analysis. *Clin Exp Allergy* 2006; 36(7):920–929.
215. Witke W. The role of profilin complexes in cell motility and other cellular processes. *Trends Cell Biol* 2004; 14(8):461–469.
216. Radauer C, Hoffimann-Sommergrube K. *Profilins*. Oxford: Blackwell Publishing, 2004.
217. Thorn KS, Christensen HE, Shigeta R, et al. The crystal structure of a major allergen from plants. *Structure* 1997; 5(1):19–32.
218. Fedorov AA, Ball T, Mahoney NM, Valenta R, Almo SC. The molecular basis for allergen cross-reactivity: crystal structure and IgE-epitope mapping of birch pollen profilin. *Structure* 1997; 5(1):33–45.
219. Mari A. Multiple pollen sensitization: a molecular approach to the diagnosis. *Int Arch Allergy Immunol* 2001; 125(1):57–65.
220. Asero R, Mistrello G, Roncarolo D, et al. Detection of clinical markers of sensitization to profilin in patients allergic to plant-derived foods. *J Allergy Clin Immunol* 2003; 112(2):427–432.
221. Wensing M, Akkerdaas JH, van Leeuwen WA, et al. IgE to Bet v 1 and profilin: cross-reactivity patterns and clinical relevance. *J Allergy Clin Immunol* 2002; 110(3):435–442.
222. Santos A, Van Ree R. Profilins: mimickers of allergy or relevant allergens? *Int Arch Allergy Immunol* 2011; 155(3):191–204.
223. Asero R, Monsalve R, Barber D. Profilin sensitization detected in the office by skin prick test: a study of prevalence and clinical relevance of profilin as a plant food allergen. *Clin Exp Allergy* 2008; 38(6):1033–1037.
224. López-Torrejón G, Crespo JF, Sánchez-Monge R, et al. Allergenic reactivity of the melon profilin Cuc m 2 and its identification as major allergen. *Clin Exp Allergy* 2005; 35(8):1065–1072.
225. Anliker MD, Reindl J, Vieths S, Wüthrich B. Allergy caused by ingestion of persimmon (*Diospyros kaki*): detection of specific IgE and cross-reactivity to profilin and carbohydrate determinants. *J Allergy Clin Immunol* 2001; 107(4):718–723.
226. Valenta R, Duchene M, Pettenburger K, et al. Identification of profilin as a novel pollen allergen; IgE autoreactivity in sensitized individuals. *Science* 1991; 253(5019):557–560.
227. Moroz LA, Yang WH. Kunitz soybean trypsin inhibitor: a specific allergen in food anaphylaxis. *N Engl J Med* 1980; 302(20):1126–1128.
228. Burks AW, Cockrell G, Connaughton C, Guin J, Allen W, Helm RM. Identification of peanut agglutinin and soybean trypsin inhibitor as minor legume allergens. *Int Arch Allergy Immunol* 1994; 105(2):143–149.
229. Seppala U, Majamaa H, Turjanmaa K, et al. Identification of four novel potato (*Solanum tuberosum*) allergens belonging to the family of soybean trypsin inhibitors. *Allergy* 2001; 56(7):619–626.
230. Kobayashi Y, Ishizaki S, Nagashima Y, Shiomi K. Ani s 1, the major allergen of Anisakis simplex: purification by affinity chromatography and functional expression in *Escherichia coli*. *Parasitol Int* 2008; 57(3):314–319.
231. Kasera R, Singh BP, Lavasa S, Prasad KN, Sahoo RC, Singh AB. Kidney bean: a major sensitizer among legumes in asthma and rhinitis patients from India. *PLoS One* 2011; 6(11):e27193.
232. van Loon LC, Rep M, Pieterse CM. Significance of inducible defense-related proteins in infected plants. *Annu Rev Phytopathol* 2006; 44:135–162.
233. Liu JJ, Sturrock R, Ekramoddoullah AK. The superfamily of thaumatin-like proteins: its origin, evolution, and expression towards biological function. *Plant Cell Rep* 2010; 29(5):419–436.
234. Krebitz M, Wagner B, Ferreira F, et al. Plant-based heterologous expression of Mal d 2, a thaumatin-like protein and allergen of apple (Malus domestica), and its characterization as an antifungal protein. *J Mol Biol* 2003; 329(4):721–730.
235. Fuchs HC, Hoffmann-Sommergrube K, Wagner B, Krebitz M, Scheiner O, Breiteneder H. Heterologous expression in Nicotiana benthamiana of Cap a 1, a thaumatin-like protein and major allergen from bell pepper (*Capsicum annuum*). *J Allergy Clin Immunol* 2002; 109(S):134–135.
236. Inschlag C, Hoffmann-Sommergruber K, O'Riordain G, et al. Biochemical characterization of Pru a 2, a 23-kD thaumatin-like protein representing a potential major allergen in cherry (*Prunus avium*). *Int Arch Allergy Immunol* 1998; 116(1):22–28.
237. Fuchs HC, Bohle B, Dall'Antonia Y, et al. Natural and recombinant molecules of the cherry allergen Pru av 2 show diverse structural and B cell characteristics but similar T cell reactivity. *Clin Exp Allergy* 2006; 36(3):359–368.
238. Gavrovic-Jankulovic M, cIrkovic T, Vuckovic O, et al. Isolation and biochemical characterization of a thaumatin-like kiwi allergen. *J Allergy Clin Immunol* 2002; 110(5):805–810.
239. Roberts WK, Selitrennikoff CP. Zeamatin, an antifungal protein from maize with membrane-permeabilizing activity. *J Gen Microbiol* 1990; 136:1771–1778.
240. Flamini R, De Rosso M. Mass spectrometry in the analysis of grape and wine proteins. *Expert Rev Proteomics* 2006; 3(3):321–331.
241. Gendel SM. Allergen databases and allergen semantics. *Regul Toxicol Pharmacol* 2009; 54(3 Suppl.):S7–S10.
242. Berners-Lee T, Hendler J, Lassila O. The semantic web. *Sci Am* 2001; 284:34–43.
243. Valarakos AG, Karkaletsis V, Alexopoulou D, Papadimitriou E, Spyropoulos CD, Vouros G. Building an allergens ontology and maintaining it using machine learning techniques. *Comput Biol Med* 2006; 36(10):1155–1184.
244. Ivanciuc O, Gendel SM, Power TD, Schein CH, Braun W. AllerML: markup language for allergens. *Regul Toxicol Pharmacol* 2011; 60(1):151–160.

245. Tong JC, Lim SJ, Muh HC, Chew FT, Tammi MT. Allergen Atlas: a comprehensive knowledge center and analysis resource for allergen information. *Bioinformatics* 2009; 25(7):979–980.
246. Lack G, Golding J. Peanut and nut allergy. Reduced exposure might increase allergic sensitisation. *BMJ* 1996; 313(7052):300.
247. Strid J, Thomson M, Hourihane J, Kimber I, Strobel S. A novel model of sensitization and oral tolerance to peanut protein. *Immunology* 2004; 113(3):293–303.
248. Strid J, Hourihane J, Kimber I, Callard R, Strobel S. Epicutaneous exposure to peanut protein prevents oral tolerance and enhances allergic sensitization. *Clin Exp Allergy* 2005; 35(6):757–766.
249. Hoffmann-Sommergruber K. Pathogenesis-related (PR)-proteins identified as allergens. *Biochem Soc Trans* 2002; 30(Pt. 6):930–935.
250. Van Loon LC, Van Strien EA. The families of pathogenesis related proteins, their activities, and comparative analysis of PR-1-type proteins. *Physiol Mol Plant Pathol* 1999; 5:85–97.

5 Biotechnology and Genetic Engineering

Gary A. Bannon, Jason M. Ward, Raymond C. Dobert, & Roy L. Fuchs
Global Regulatory Sciences and Affairs, Monsanto, St. Louis, MO, USA

Key Concepts

- All agricultural biotechnology products are assessed for safety according to international guidelines to ensure the risk of allergy is appropriately addressed prior to their commercialization, and that a consistent assessment approach is used around the world.
- The current allergy assessment process identifies the potential risks associated with the introduced protein as well as the overall allergenic risks associated with a transformed food crop.
- No single, predictive assay is capable of assessing the allergenic potential of all proteins introduced into food crops and, therefore, all aspects of the current safety assessment testing strategy need to be considered in a "weight of evidence" approach rather than relying too heavily on one test to determine protein safety.
- The protective value of current allergy testing approaches and future approaches that adopt sound risk assessment principles and new methods as they become validated, have in the past and will continue to provide robust assurances to risk managers and consumers alike for present and future biotech products.

Introduction

The population of the world is expected to increase by 2.5 billion people in the next 25 years. Food requirements for this growing population are expected to double by the year 2025. In contrast, there has been a decline in the annual rate of increase in cereal yield such that the annual rate of yield increase is below the rate of population increase [1]. In order to feed this growing population, crop yield will have to be increased and some of the increase in yield will be due to genetic engineering of foods. In addition, the incidence of food allergies appears to be on the rise, particularly in developed countries [2, 3]. Genetic engineering of food crops should have little practical consequence for the occurrence, frequency, and natural history of food allergy if simple precautions are observed. Essential aspects of the health safety assessment for products derived from this technology are discussed in this chapter; and the accepted strategy for addressing any potential impact on food allergy will be reviewed in detail. It should be noted that no single, predictive assay appears to be capable of assessing the allergenic potential of all the proteins introduced into food crops [4]. However, through the use of *in vivo* and *in vitro* immunological assays in combination with a comparative evaluation relative to the characteristics of known food allergens, a sound scientific basis for allergenicity assessment has evolved. The biochemical properties of common food allergens have been described in this book and elsewhere [5, 6]; allergens tend to be stable to proteolysis, tend to be abundant, tend to be resistant to heat (cooking or processing), and all have multiple IgE-binding epitopes. Thus, these factors have been used to discriminate potentially harmful allergens from safe proteins entering the food supply.

This chapter will briefly summarize the development and commercialization of food biotechnology products, the internationally recognized approach to food safety assessment for these foods, and will provide a comprehensive review of food allergy considerations in this context.

Plant biotechnology

Twenty years ago, the improvement of crop productivity was a sophisticated process, albeit dependent on trial

Food Allergy: Adverse Reactions to Foods and Food Additives, Fifth Edition. Edited by Dean D Metcalfe, Hugh A Sampson, Ronald A Simon and Gideon Lack.

and error. Many years of meticulous observations were required to determine whether desired traits were stable in the new varieties and cultivars of food crops created by this process. Crop improvement and the science of plant breeding depended on existing intraspecies genetic variation of plants, interspecies introgression of traits from "wild" or taxonomically similar plants, and on the creation of new genetic variability by chemical or irradiation mutagenesis. While there are limitations to these approaches, crop scientists and geneticists were nevertheless able to improve crop yield and food production per unit area of agricultural land several fold by creating new and more productive crops, and by improving agronomic practices.

With the advent of molecular biology and biotechnology, it became possible not only to identify a desirable phenotypic trait but also to identify the precise genetic material responsible for that genetic trait. Recombinant DNA and plant transformation techniques have made it possible to alter the composition of individual plant components (lipids, carbohydrates, proteins) beyond what is easily possible through traditional breeding practices. Direct and stable gene transfer into plants was first reported in 1984 [7, 8]. Since then, at least 88 different plant species and many economically important crops have been genetically engineered [9], usually via *Agrobacterium* [10, 11] or particle gun technologies [12, 13].

The thrust of most first-generation biotech crops has been to improve resistance to insect predation, increase resistance to pesticides for easier weed control, confer immunity to viral pathogens, and improve the ripening characteristics of fresh fruits and vegetables. These crops are essentially unchanged from the nontransformed parental crops and have no significant changes in key nutrients. To a lesser extent, products with enhanced functional or nutritional properties have appeared as a result of intended alteration of specific metabolites such as oil (lipid) profiles, amino acid composition, and starch (carbohydrate) content. However, the majority of current products have had their biggest impact on agricultural practices of producers (i.e., by reducing pesticide use, improving soil conservation practices, and reducing energy inputs on farms). The availability of these so-called "agronomic" traits has driven the adoption of biotech crops since the introduction of the first product, Flavr Savr tomato, in 1994 (Figure 5.1). Today, over 90% of the worldwide acreage of biotech crops have agronomic traits, as shown in Table 5.1 [14]. Of the principal food crops grown worldwide in 2011, biotech soybean occupied 75.4 million hectares and maize occupied 37.3 million hectares. Herbicide tolerance has consistently been the dominant trait planted in the field followed by insect resistance and then products containing both of these traits in a stacked combination. In 2011, herbicide tolerance deployed in soybean, maize, canola, cotton, and alfalfa occupied 93.9 million hectares (59%) of the global biotech 160 million hectares, with 42.2 million hectares (26%) planted to the stacked traits of *Bacillus thuringiensis* and herbicide tolerance. The accumulated hectarage from 1996 to 2011 exceeded a billion hectares, with an unprecedented 94-fold increase between 1996 and 2010, making biotech crops the fastest adopted crop technology in the history of modern agriculture [14]. Over the next 5–10 years, it is expected that the proportion of food biotechnology products that have been developed for nutritional and functional benefits will increase significantly [16].

Below we describe the development of Roundup Ready soybeans to illustrate the application of agricultural biotechnology. We then briefly summarize the safety assessment procedures for food biotechnology illustrated by reference to the data developed for Roundup Ready

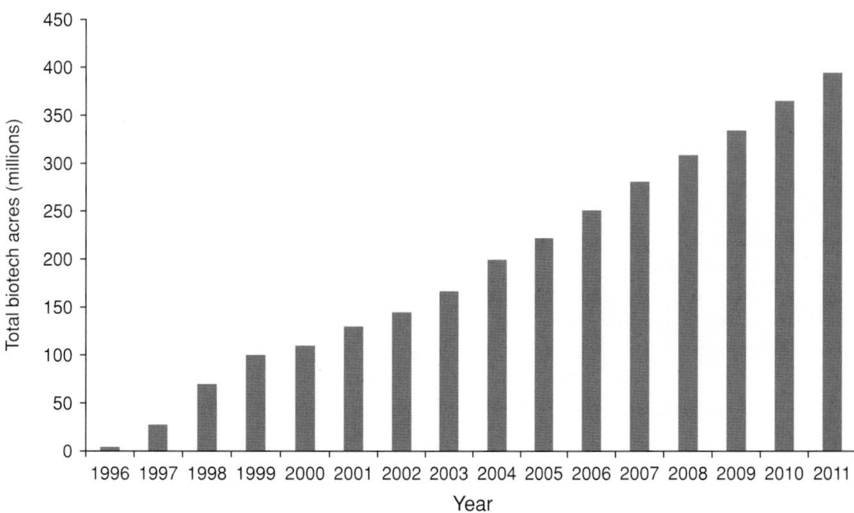

Figure 5.1 Worldwide acreage of biotech crops since introduction in 1996. Based on data reported in References 14 and 15, and literature cited therein.

Table 5.1 Current biotechnology food crops where FDA consultations have been completed through November 2011 (www.cfsan.fda.gov).

Crop	Introduced gene(s)	Source of gene(s)	Trait
Corn	Cry3A	*Bacillus thuringiensis*	Resistance to corn rootworm
	cDHDPS	*Corynebacterium glutamicum*	Increase lysine level for use in animal feed
	Cry3Bb1	*Bacillus thuringiensis*	Resistance to Coleopteran insects, including corn rootworm
	Cry34Ab1, Cry35Ab1/PAT	*Bacillus thuringiensis/Streptomyces viridochromogenes*	Resistance to Coleopteran insects/tolerance to the herbicide glufosinate ammonium
	Cry1F/PAT	*Bacillus thuringiensis/Streptomyces viridochromogenes*	Resistance to certain lepidopteran insects/tolerance to the herbicide glufosinate
	EPSPS	*Agrobacterium*	Tolerance to the herbicide glyphosate
	Barnase	*Bacillus amyloliquefaciens*	Male sterility
	Modified EPSPS	Corn	Tolerance to the herbicide glyphosate
	Cry9C protein/PAT	*Bacillus thuringiensis/Streptomyces hygroscopicus*	Resistance to several lepidopteran insects/tolerance to the herbicide glufosinate
	DAM/PAT	*Escherichia coli/Streptomyces viridochromogenes*	Male sterility/tolerance to glufosinate
	CrylAc	*Bacillus thuringiensis*	Resistance to European corn borer
	CrylAb/EPSPS	*Bacillus thuringiensis/Agrobacterium*	Resistance to European corn borer; tolerance to the herbicide glyphosate
	CrylAb	*Bacillus thuringiensis*	Resistance to European corn borer
	Barnase/PAT	*Bacillus amyloliquefaciens/Streptomyces hygroscopicus*	Male sterility/tolerance to glufosinate
	PAT	*Streptomyces hygroscopicus*	Tolerance to glufosinate
	CspB	*Bacillus subtilis*	Reduction to yield loss under water limiting conditions
	aad1	*Sphingobium herbicidovorans*	Confer tolerance to the herbicide 2,4-dichlorophenoxyacetic acid (or "2,4-D") and certain aryloxyphenoxypropionate herbicides (e.g., quizalofop, cyhalofop, haloxyfop).
Canola	Nitrilase	*Klebsiella ozaenae*	Tolerance to the herbicide bromoxynil
	Phytase	*Aspergillus niger*	Degradation of phytate in animal feed
	Barnase/PAT	*Bacillus amyloliquefaciens/Streptomyces hygroscopicus*	Male sterility/tolerance to glufosinate
	Barstar/PAT	*Bacillus amyloliquefaciens/Streptomyces hygroscopicus*	Fertility restorer/tolerance to glufosinate
	PAT	*Streptomyces hygroscopicus*	Tolerance to glufosinate
	12:0 Acyl carrier protein thioesterase	*Umbellularia californica*	High laurate canola oil
	EPSPS/GOX	*Agrobacterium* sp. strain CP4, *Achromobacter*	Tolerance to the herbicide glyphosate
Soybean	PAT	*Streptomyces hygroscopicus*	Tolerance to glufosinate
	GmFad2-1 gene	Soybean	High oleic acid soybean oil
	EPSPS	*Agrobacterium* sp. strain CP4	Tolerance to the herbicide glyphosate
	Cry1Ac	*Bacillus thuringiensis*	Resistance to lepidopteran insects
	dmo	*Stenotrophomonas maltophilia*	Tolerance to the herbicide dicamba
	AAD-12	*Delftia acidovorans*	Tolerance to the herbicide 2,4-D
	csr1-2	*Arabidopsis thaliana*	Tolerance to imidizolinone herbicides
	RNA-based suppression of the palmitoyl acyl carrier protein thioesterase and delta-12 desaturase		Increased levels of oleic acid, and decreased levels of linoleic, palmitic, and stearic acid
Cotton	Nitrilase/Cry1Ac protein	*Klebsiella pneumoniae/Bacillus thuringiensis*	Tolerance to bromoxynil/resistance to certain lepidopteran insects
	Cry2ab; Cry1ac	*Bacillus thuringiensis*	Resistance to lepidopteran insects
	ALS	*Nicotiana tabacum*	Tolerance to the herbicide sulfonylurea
	EPSPS	*Agrobacterium* sp. strain CP4	Tolerance to the herbicide glyphosate
	Cry1F/PAT	*Bacillus thuringiensis/Streptomyces viridochromogenes*	Resistance to lepidopteran insects/tolerance to the herbicide glufosinate ammonium
	VIP3A protein	*Bacillus thuringiensis*	Resistance to lepidopteran insects
	CrylAc protein	*Bacillus thuringiensis*	Resistance to cotton bollworm, pink bollworm, and tobacco budworm
	Nitrilase	*Klebsiella ozaenae*	Tolerance to the herbicide bromoxynil

Table 5.1 *(Continued)*

Crop	Introduced gene(s)	Source of gene(s)	Trait
Sugar beet	EPSPS	*Agrobacterium* sp. strain CP4	Tolerance to the herbicide glyphosate
	PAT	*Streptomyces hygroscopicus*	Tolerance to glufosinate
Tomato	CryIAc protein	*Bacillus thuringiensis*	Resistance to certain lepidopteran insects
	S-adenosylmethionine hydrolase	*E. coli* bacteriophage T3	Delayed fruit ripening due to reduced ethylene synthesis
	ACCS gene fragment	Tomato	Delayed ripening due to reduced ethylene synthesis
	PG	Tomato	Delayed softening due to reduced pectin degradation
	ACCD	*Pseudomonas chloraphis*	Delayed softening due to reduced ethylene synthesis
	PG antisense gene	Tomato	Delayed softening due to reduced pectin degradation
Potato	CryIIIA/PVY coat protein	*Bacillus thuringiensis*/PVY	Resistance to Colorado potato beetle and PVY
	CryIIIA/PLRV replicase	*Bacillus thuringiensis*/Potato Leafroll virus	Resistance to Colorado potato beetle and PLRV
	CryIIIA	*Bacillus thuringiensis*	Resistance to Colorado potato beetle
Rice	PAT	*Streptomyces hygroscopicus*	Tolerance to glufosinate
Cantaloupe	*S*-adenosylmethionine hydrolase	*E. coli* bacteriophage T3	Delayed fruit ripening due to reduced ethylene synthesis
Radicchio	Barnase/PAT	*Bacillus amyloliquefaciens*/*Streptomyces hygroscopicus*	Male sterility/tolerance to glufosinate
Squash	Coat proteins from CMV, ZYMV, and WMV2	CMV, ZYMV, and WMV2	Resistance to the viruses CMV, ZYMV, and WMV2
	ZYMV and WMV2 coat proteins	ZYMV and WMV2	Resistance to the viruses ZYMV and WMV2
Papaya	PRV coat protein	PRSV	Resistance to PRSV
Flax	ALS (csr-1)	*Arabidopsis*	Tolerance to the herbicide sulfonylurea

ACCD, 1-aminocyclopropane-1-carboxylic acid deaminase; ALS, acetolactate synthase; cDHDPS, dihydrodipicolinate synthase; CMV, cucumber mosaic virus; DAM, DNA adenine methylase; GOX, glyphosate oxidoreductase; PAT, phosphinothricin acetyl transferase; PG, polygalacturonase; PRSV, papaya ringspot virus; PVY, potato virus Y; WMV2, watermelon mosaic virus 2; ZYMV, zucchini yellow mosaic virus.

soybeans. Following this general discussion, we provide a detailed account of current approaches and issues in allergy assessment for these products, also illustrated by the data developed for Roundup Ready soybeans.

Roundup Ready soybeans: a case study in food safety assessment

Soybean (*Glycine max*) ranks fifth in world production of major crops after wheat, maize, rice, and potato. In the United States, soybeans represent $5.6 billion in farm gate receipts [14, 17]. Soybeans represent approximately one-third of all crops grown in the United States. The major food use of soybeans is the oil, whereas 96% of soybean meal is used for animal feed. Approximately 75% of vegetable food-grade oil used in foods such as shortenings, margarines, and salad/cooking oils is from soybeans. Soybean flour (meal) is used in foods such as soups, stews, beverages, desserts, bakery goods, cereals, and meat products and extenders [18]. Soybeans were the most common transgenic crop planted in 2006, representing 57% of the total acres planted with biotech traits, followed by maize (25%), cotton (13%), and canola (5%) [14]. The most common biotechnology trait was herbicide tolerance, followed by insect protection [14].

Development and benefits of Roundup Ready soybeans

The genetically engineered soybean line GTS 40-3-2 was developed to allow the use of glyphosate, the active ingredient in the wide-spectrum herbicide Roundup®, as a weed control option for soybean. This genetically engineered soybean line contains a glyphosate tolerant form of the plant enzyme 5-enolpyruvylshikimate-3-phosphate synthase (EPSPS) isolated from the common soil bacterium, *Agrobacterium tumefaciens* strain CP4 (CP4 EPSPS). The EPSPS enzyme is part of the shikimate pathway that is involved in the production of aromatic amino acids and other aromatic compounds in plants [19]. When conventional plants are treated with glyphosate, the plants cannot produce the aromatic amino acids needed to survive. GTS 40-3-2 was developed by introducing the CP4 EPSPS coding sequence into the soybean variety A5403, a commercial soybean variety of Asgrow Seed Company, using particle-acceleration (biolistic) transformation. A5403 is a maturity group V cultivar that combines consistently high-yield potential with resistance to races 3 and 4 of the soybean cyst nematode (SCN). It also possesses good standability, excellent seedling emergence, and tolerance to many leaf and stem diseases.

Weed control in soybeans represents a major financial and labor input by growers. Since soybeans are dicots, grassy weeds are controlled by one class of herbicides, and dicot (broadleaf) weeds are controlled by a second class of herbicides. Since soybeans are also broadleaf plants, their physiology and biochemistry are similar to broadleaf weeds. Therefore, in conventional soybeans, it is technically challenging to control both grassy and broadleaf weeds without harming the soybean plants themselves [17].

Glyphosate is used as a foliar-applied, nonselective herbicide and is effective against the majority of grasses and broadleaf weeds. Glyphosate has no preemergence or residual soil activity [19]. Furthermore, glyphosate is not prone to leaching, degrades rapidly in soil, and is essentially nontoxic to mammals, birds, and fish [20–22].

Roundup Ready soybeans offer growers an additional tool for improved weed control. Control of weeds in the soybean crop is essential, as weeds compete with the crop for sunlight, water, and nutrients. Failure to control weeds within the crop results in decreased yields and reduced crop quality. In addition, weeds reduce the efficiency of the mechanical harvest of the crop.

Roundup Ready soybeans have been produced commercially in the United States, Argentina, and Canada beginning in 1996 and provide the following environmental and economic benefits:

• Improved efficacy in weed control compared with herbicide programs used in conventional soybeans, as specific preemergent herbicides that are used for prevention are replaced by a broad-spectrum postemergent herbicide that can be used on an "as needed" basis [23]. The introduction of Roundup Ready soybeans in the United States has resulted in a 12% reduction in the number of herbicide applications from 1996 to 1999, even though the total soybean acres increased by 18% [17]. The decrease in herbicide applications means that growers make fewer trips over the field to apply herbicides and translates into ease of management.

• A reduction in herbicide costs for the farmer. It has been estimated that United States soybean growers spent $216 million less in 1999 for weed control (including a technology fee for Roundup Ready soybean), compared with 1995, the year before Roundup Ready soybeans were introduced [17].

• Less labor required due to the elimination of hand weeding and high-cost, early post-directed sprays, which require special equipment.

• High compatibility with integrated pest management and soil conservation techniques [24], resulting in a number of important environmental benefits including reduced soil erosion and improved water quality [25–27], improved soil structure with higher organic matter [28, 29], improved wildlife habitat and improved carbon sequestration [30, 31], and reduced CO_2 emissions [28, 32].

Safety assessment of Roundup Ready soybeans

Safety assessment principles

In 1996, a joint report from an expert consultation sponsored by the World Health Organization (WHO) and the Food and Agricultural Organization (FAO) of the United Nations concluded that "biotechnology provides new and powerful tools for research and for accelerating the development of new and better foods" [33]. The FAO/WHO expert consultation also concluded that it is vitally important to develop and apply appropriate strategies and safety assessment criteria for food biotechnology to ensure the long-term safety and wholesomeness of the food supply.

Following these criteria, foods derived from biotechnology have been extensively assessed to ensure they are as safe and nutritious as traditional foods. All foods, independent of whether they are derived from biotech crops or traditionally bred plants, must meet the same rigorous food safety standard. Numerous national and international organizations have considered the safety of foods derived from biotech crops. They have concluded that the food safety considerations are basically of the same nature for food derived from biotech crops as for those foods derived using other methods like traditional breeding.

This concept of comparing the safety of the food from a biotech crop with that of a food with an established history of safe use is referred to as "substantial equivalence" [34, 35]. The process of substantial equivalence involves comparing the characteristics, including the levels of key nutrients and other components, of the food derived from a biotech crop to the food derived from conventional plant breeding. When a food is shown to be substantially equivalent to a food with a history of safe use, then "the food is regarded to be as safe as its conventional counterpart" [33]. An FAO/WHO expert consultation in 1995 concluded "this approach provides equal or greater assurance of the safety of food derived from genetically modified organisms as compared to foods or food components derived by conventional methods" [33]. As a practical matter, this evaluation brings together an evaluation of the introduced proteins and accounts for unexpected effects due to the protein *per se*, or due to pleiotropic effects created by gene insertion as assessed at the level of phenotype: the agronomic and compositional parameters of the biotech crop in comparison with traditional counterparts [36].

CP4 5-enolpyruvylshikimate-3-phosphate synthase protein safety

Usually, when a gene is chosen for transformation into a crop, the encoded protein has been well characterized in terms of function (mechanism of action, evolutionary heritage, physicochemical properties, etc.). This information has been extensively evaluated during the development of biotech crops such as NewLeaf™ potato,

[37] RoundupReady™ soybeans [38], and YieldGard™ corn [39]. An important consideration in protein safety is whether or not the protein can be established to have been used or eaten previously—is there a history of safe use?

The CP4 EPSP synthase protein produced in Roundup Ready soybeans is functionally similar to a diverse family of EPSPS proteins typically present in food and feed derived from plant and microbial sources [40]. The EPSPS proteins are required for the production of aromatic amino acids in plants and microbes. The enzymology and known function of EPSPS proteins generally, and CP4 EPSPS specifically, indicate that this class of enzymes performs a well-described and understood biochemical role in plants. From the perspective of safety, this characterization indicates that metabolic effects owing to the expression of the CP4 EPSPS gene are limited to conferring the Roundup Ready trait alone. Part of this evaluation includes the known structural relationship between CP4 EPSPS and other EPSPS proteins found in food as is demonstrated by comparison of the amino acid sequences with conserved identity of the active site residues, and the expected conserved three-dimensional structure based on similarity of the amino acid sequence. With respect to amino acid sequence, there is considerable divergence among known EPSPSs. For instance, the amino acid sequence of CP4 EPSPS is 41% identical at the amino acid level to *Bacillus subtilis* EPSPS, whereas the soybean EPSPS is 30% identical to *Bacillus subtilis* EPSPS. Thus, the divergence of the CP4 EPSPS amino acid sequence from typical food EPSPS sequences is on the same order as the divergence among food EPSPSs themselves [38].

The detailed enzymology [38] and subsequent biochemical composition evaluations [41, 42] confirm and demonstrate that CP4 EPSPS, as expressed in line 40-3-2, has the predicted and expected metabolic effects on soybeans: the production of aromatic amino acids via the shikimic acid biosynthetic pathway.

Another aspect used for the assessment of potential toxic effects of proteins introduced into plants is to compare the amino acid sequence of the protein to known toxic proteins. Homologous proteins derived from a common ancestor have similar amino acid sequences, are structurally similar, and often share common function. Therefore, it is undesirable to introduce DNA that encodes for a protein that is homologous to a protein that is toxic to animals and people. Homology is determined by comparing the degree of amino acid similarity between proteins using published criteria [43]. The CP4 EPSPS protein does not show meaningful amino acid sequence similarity when compared to known protein toxins.

Lack of protein toxicity is confirmed by evaluating acute oral toxicity in mice or rats [44]. This study is typically a 2-week program in which the pure protein is fed to animals at doses that should be 100–1000 times higher than the highest anticipated exposure via consumption of the whole food product containing that protein. Table 5.2 summarizes the data from several acute oral toxicity studies. Although these studies were designed to obtain LD_{50}s, in fact no lethal dose has been achieved for these proteins [40, 44–47]. For CP4 EPSPS, there were no treatment-related adverse effects in mice, administered CP4 EPSPS protein by oral gavage, at dosages up to 572 mg/kg, the highest dose tested. This dose represents a significant (approximately 1300-fold) safety margin relative to the highest potential human consumption of CP4 EPSPS and assumes that the protein is expressed in multiple crops in addition to soybeans [40].

Table 5.2 Summary of the data from standardized acute oral toxicity LD_{50} studies in mice. The no observable effect level (NOEL) was the highest dose tested for each protein.

Protein	Crop	NOEL[a] (mg/kg)
Cry1Ac	Cotton, tomato	4200
Cry1Ab	Corn	4000
Cry2Aa	Cotton	3000
Cry2Ab	Corn, cotton	3700
Cry3A	Potato	5200
Cry3Bb1	Corn	3780
CP4 EPSPS	Soybean, cotton, canola, sugar beet	572
NPTII	Cotton, potato, tomato	5000
GUS	Soybean, sugar beet	100
GOX	Canola, cotton, corn, sugar beet	100

When accounting for the level of these proteins in the crops in which they are found (Table 5.1), these doses represent between 10^4 and 10^6 times the levels typically consumed as food.

[a]No observed effect level.

Cry1Ac, Cry1Ab, Cry2Aa, Cry2Ab, Cry3A, Cry3Bb1 are all "crystal" proteins from *Bacillus thuringiensis*.

CP4 EPSPS, CP4 5-enolpyruvylshikimate-3-phosphate synthase; GOX, glyphosate oxidoreductase; GUS, b-glucuronidase; NPTII, neomycin phosphotransferase II.

Phenotype evaluation (substantial equivalence)

Compositional analyses are a critical component of the safety assessment process that integrates with the evaluation of the trait (e.g., CP4 EPSP synthase) described above. Each of the measured parameters provides an assessment of the cumulative result of numerous biochemical pathways and hence provides an assessment of a wide range of metabolic pathways. Comparisons of various nutrients and anti-nutrients are made to both a closely related traditional counterpart and the established published range for the specific component within that crop to compare the observed levels to the natural variation of that component in current plant varieties. The composition of Roundup Ready soybeans has been thoroughly characterized and the results of these studies have been published [41, 42]. Over 1400 individual analyses have been conducted and they establish that the composition of Roundup Ready soybeans is substantially equivalent to the nontransgenic parental soybean variety and other commercial soybean varieties. Table 5.3 summarizes the composition of Roundup Ready soybeans and traditional soybeans, which include:

• *Proximate analysis*: protein, fat, fiber, ash, carbohydrates, and moisture.
• *Anti-nutrients*: trypsin inhibitors, lectins, phytoestrogens (genistein and daidzein), stachyose, raffinose, and phytate.
• *Fatty acid profile*: percentage of individual fatty acids.
• *Amino acid composition*: levels of individual amino acids.

In addition to a demonstration of substantially equivalent composition, further agronomic evaluation of the biotech crop is necessary to establish that there are no unexpected biological effects of the introduced trait. While compositional assessments provide good assurance that no untoward metabolic, nutritional, or anti-nutritional effects have occurred, an additional and very sensitive measure has been to compare a wide variety of biological characteristics at the whole plant level. The basic question asked is, does the biotech crop fit within the usual definition of that crop? For example, do Roundup Ready soybeans still possess the expected plant performance of traditional soybeans? Agronomic and yield characteristics are very sensitive to untoward perturbations in metabolism and in genetic pleiotropy.

Wholesomeness (nutrition) of Roundup Ready soybeans

Farm animal nutrition studies have provided supplementary confirmation of the substantial equivalence and safety of crop biotechnology. Currently there are many options for animal studies; the choice, of which, depends on the crop being engineered and its intended use. In over 65 farm animal studies completed to date, the factors evaluated include feed intake, body weight, carcass yield, feed conversion, milk yield, milk composition, digestibility, and nutrient composition of the resulting animal-derived foods [57].

A series of animal-feeding studies has been completed using diets incorporating raw or processed Roundup Ready soybeans. The animal-feeding studies included two separate 4-week studies in rats (one with unprocessed soybean meal and one with processed soybean meal), a 4-week dairy cow study, a 6-week chicken study, a 10-week catfish study, and a 5-day quail study. Animals were fed either raw soybean, unprocessed or processed soybean meal (dehulled, defatted, toasted). Included in these studies were control groups fed a nonmodified parental soybean line from which both events were derived. Results from all groups were compared using conventional statistical methods to detect differences between groups in measured parameters.

All soybean samples tested provided similar growth and feed efficiency for rats, chickens, catfish, and quail [58]. Milk production, composition, and rumen fermentation parameters for dairy cows were also comparable across all groups [58]. Results for other parameters measured in each feeding study were also similar across all groups. When compared to the US population as a whole, the levels of soybean consumption (in mg/kg of body weight) in these animal-feeding studies were 100-fold or more, higher than the average human daily consumption of soybean-derived foods in the United States. All these studies confirmed the food and feed safety and nutritional equivalence of diets from Roundup Ready soybeans.

General assessment strategy for food allergy

The consumer marketplace reflects widespread interest and concern about adverse reactions to certain foods and food additives. A consumer survey indicated that 30% of the people interviewed reported that they or some family member had an allergy to a food product [59]. This survey also found that 22% avoided particular foods on the mere possibility that the food may contain an allergen. In reality, food-allergic reactions affect only about 6% of children and 4% of the adult population [60–62]. The most common food allergies known to affect children are IgE-mediated reactions to cow's milk, eggs, peanuts, soybeans, wheat, fish, and tree nuts. Approximately 80% of all reported food allergies in children are due to peanuts, milk, or eggs. While most childhood food allergies are outgrown, allergies to peanuts, tree nuts, and fish are rarely resolved in adulthood. In adults, the most common food allergies are to peanuts, tree nuts, fish, and shellfish. The incidence of IgE-mediated reactions to specific food crops is increasing, particularly in developed countries, likely due to increased levels of protein consumption. Allergic reactions are typically elicited by a defined subset of proteins that are found in abundance in the food.

Identification and purification of allergens have been essential for the structural and immunological studies necessary to understand how these molecules stimulate IgE antibody formation [63]. In the past several years, a number of allergens have been identified that stimulate IgE production and cause IgE-mediated disease in man. Significant information now exists on the identification and purification of allergens from a wide variety of sources, including foods, pollens, dust mites, animal dander, insects, and fungi [63]. However, despite increasing knowledge of the structure and amino acid sequences of the identified allergens, specific features associated with IgE antibody formation have not been fully determined [63].

Table 5.3 Summary of historical and literature ranges for the nutritional composition of Roundup Ready soybeans

Component	Historical Roundup Ready soybean range[a]	Literature soybean range[b]
Proximates (% dw)		
Moisture (% fw)	5.32–8.85	5.30–11 [48–50]
Protein	37.0–45.0	36.9–46.4 [49]
Fat	13.27–23.31	13.2–22.5 [49, 51]
Ash	4.45–5.87	4.29–5.88 [48]
Carbohydrates	27.6–40.74	29.3–41.3 [48]
Fiber (% dw)		
Acid detergent fiber	9.76–12.46	Not available
Neutral detergent fiber	11.02–11.81	Not available
Crude fiber	5.45–9.82	5.74–8.10 [48, 52]
Amino acid (g/100 g dw)		
Alanine	1.48–1.88	1.49–1.87 [53, 54]
Arginine	2.20–3.57	2.45–3.49 [53, 54]
Aspartic acid	3.85–5.25	3.87–4.98 [53, 54]
Cystine	0.54–0.69	0.50–0.66 [48, 52]
Glutamic acid	6.00–8.34	6.10–8.72 [53, 54]
Glycine	1.48–1.90	1.60–2.02 [48, 53, 54]
Histidine	0.91–1.18	0.89–1.16 [1, 53, 54]
Isoleucine	1.51–1.95	1.46–2.12 [53, 54]
Leucine	2.60–3.37	2.71–3.37 [53, 54]
Lysine	2.30–2.88	2.35–2.86 [53, 54]
Methionine	0.50–0.62	0.49–0.66 [53, 54]
Phenylalanine	1.64–2.20	1.70–2.19 [48, 53, 54]
Proline	1.76–2.30	1.88–2.61 [53, 54]
Serine	1.80–2.60	1.81–2.32 [53, 54]
Threonine	1.39–1.74	1.33–1.79 [53, 54]
Tryptophan	0.42–0.64	0.48–0.63 [48, 52]
Tyrosine	1.23–1.58	1.12–1.62 [53, 54]
Valine	1.58–2.02	1.52–2.24 [53, 54]
Fatty acids (% of total FA)[c]		
12:0 Lauric acid	,0.01% fw to 0.40	Not available
14:0 Myristic acid	,0.01 fw to 0.17	Not available
16:0 Palmitic acid	10.63–12.75	7–12 [55], 9.63–13.09 [56]
16:1 Palmitoleic acid	0.11–0.17	Not available
17:0 Heptadecanoic acid	0.10–0.17	0.11–0.14 [48]
17:1 Heptadecenoic acid	,0.01% fw	Not available
18:0 Stearic acid	4.01–5.93	2–5.5 [55], 2.69–4.40 [56]
18:1 Oleic acid	15.56–32.52	20–50 [55], 19.63–36.58 [56]
18:2 Linoleic acid	42.41–54.48	35–60 [55], 42.61–58.16 [56]
18:3 Linolenic acid	4.99–10.37	2–13 [55], 5.66–8.58 [56]
20:0 Arachidic acid	0.30–0.51	0.31–0.43 [48]
20:1 Eicosenoic acid	0.14–0.28	0.14–0.26 [48]
22:0 Behenic acid	0.49–0.62	0.46–0.59 [48]

(*continued*)

Table 5.3 *(Continued)*

Component	Historical Roundup Ready soybean range[a]	Literature soybean range[b]
Isoflavones (Total as aglycones)		
Daidzein (mg/g dw)	90.5–1260	161–1190 [48, 52]
Genistein (mg/g dw)	106–1243	230–1380 [48, 52]
Glycitein (mg/g dw)	10.8–184	Not available
Miscellaneous		
Vitamin E mg/100g dw	1.85–4.26	1.95 [57]
Trypsin inhibitor (TIU/mg dw)	35.5–59.5	26.4–93.2 [58]
Lectin (HU/mg fw)	0.5–1.6	0.8–2.4 [48]

[a]Range of values from Roundup Ready soybean event: 40-3-2 [41, 42].
[b]Commercial/nontransgenic control values: [1](40); [2](47); [3](48); [4](49); [5](50); [6](51); [7](41); [8](52); [9](53); [10](54): units in mg/100 g edible portion); [11](55).
[c]",0.01% fw" is below the lower limit of quantitation.

Because potential allergens cannot at present be accurately identified based on a single characteristic, the allergy assessment testing strategy, as originally proposed by the US Food and Drug Administration (FDA) [64] and further modified by FAO/WHO scientific panels [65, 66], proposes that all proteins introduced into crops be assessed for their similarity to a variety of structural and biochemical characteristics of known allergens. As the primary method of disease management for food-allergic people is avoidance, a core principle of these recommended strategies is to experimentally determine whether candidate proteins for genetic engineering into foods represent known food allergens currently. Prevention of unwanted exposures to food allergens is addressed by accurate labeling of food ingredients—labeling is seen as a central tool in food protection policy in the United States.

The current allergy assessment process is designed to identify the potential risks associated with the introduced protein as well as the overall allergenic risks associated with a transformed food crop. The current allergy assessment process follows recommendations made by Codex (http://www.codexalimentarius.net/web/index_en.jsp). Codex is an intergovernmental body representing 168 member states responsible for protecting the health of consumers and facilitating trade by setting international safety standards. The Codex recommendations for allergy assessment include evaluation of the introduced protein with respect to origin (from a known allergenic source or not), sequence homology to known allergens, stability in *in vitro* digestion assays, and when appropriate, IgE-binding capacity in *in vitro* and *in vivo* clinical tests.

Analyzing the sources of introduced genes

The source of the introduced gene is the first variable to consider in the allergy assessment process. If a gene transferred into a food crop is obtained from a source known to be allergenic, the assessment process calls for *in vitro* diagnostic tests to determine if the target protein binds IgE from patients allergic to the source of the protein. In addition, *in vivo* diagnostic tests such as skin prick tests and double-blind, placebo-controlled food challenges (DBPCFCs) may be required if the protein is to be introduced into a commodity crop. The FDA recognizes this need and realizes that such risks to consumers can be avoided [64]. In addition to tests to determine potential allergenicity, the use of labels that clearly indicate the presence of ingredients that may cause harmful effects, such as allergies, gives consumers the opportunity to avoid these foods or food ingredients. For example, to assist people who suffer from celiac disease, the FDA has determined that products containing gluten should be identified as to the source, that is, wheat versus corn gluten (wheat gluten cannot be safely consumed by these patients, unlike corn gluten). In the case of food allergy, voluntary labeling already occurs for certain snack foods that do not ordinarily contain peanuts, but that may come into contact with peanuts during preparation. This type of labeling provides protection for peanut allergy sufferers and helps prevent accidental and unwanted exposure. The FDA has also stated that, if known allergens are genetically engineered into food crops, the resulting foods must be labeled disclosing the source of the introduced genes [64, 67]. Moreover, proteins derived from known allergenic sources should be treated as allergens until demonstrated otherwise. The methodology to assess whether the transferred protein is allergenic is described below.

Different approaches can be taken to assess the potential allergenicity of a protein that originates from a nonallergenic source. As described below, a search for amino acid sequence homology of the introduced protein with all known allergens can be performed. In addition, the physicochemical properties of the introduced protein can be compared with the biochemical properties of known food allergens. From biochemical analysis of a limited number of allergens, certain characteristics shared by most but not necessarily all can be identified. For example, food allergens are typically relatively abundant in the food source, have multiple, linear IgE-binding epitopes, and are resistant to denaturation and digestion [68]. These characteristics are purported to be important to the allergenicity of a protein for various reasons. The observation that most food allergens are relatively abundant in the food source was explained by the idea that the immune system was more likely to encounter these proteins than one that was present as a small percentage of the total protein ingested. Resistance to denaturation and digestion of an allergen is thought to be an important characteristic because the longer a significant portion of the protein remains intact, the more likely it is to trigger an immune response. Finally, most food allergens have multiple, linear binding epitopes so that even when they are partially digested or denatured, they are still capable of interacting with IgE and causing an allergic reaction [69].

Amino acid sequence comparisons to known allergens

The proteins introduced into all genetically engineered plants that have been put into commerce in the United States have been screened by comparing their amino acid sequence to those of known allergens and gliadins as one of many assessments performed to evaluate product safety [4, 70]. The purpose of bioinformatic analyses is to describe the biological and taxonomical relatedness of a query sequence to other functionally related proteins. In the context of allergy, the goal is to identify the level of amino acid similarity and structural relatedness between a protein of interest and sequences from known allergens in order to determine whether the query protein is similar to known allergens or has the potential to cross-react with IgE directed against known allergens. Because candidate genes for transfer into commodity crops could be from a variety of sources, most allergen databases contain all known allergens including aeroallergens, food allergens, and proteins implicated in celiac disease. For example, the FARRP allergen database (www.allergenonline.com) contains all known allergen, gliadin, and glutenin protein sequences. The protein sequences in the FARRP allergen database were assembled and evaluated for evidence of allergenicity by an international panel of allergy experts, making this one of the more highly curated, publicly available allergen databases. High percentage matches between a query sequence and a sequence in the allergen database suggests that the query sequence could cross-react with IgE directed against that allergen. This is because homologous proteins share secondary structure and common three-dimensional folds [71] and are more likely to share allergenic cross-reactive conformational and linear epitopes than unrelated proteins; however, the degree of similarity between homologs varies widely and homologous allergens do not always share epitopes [72]. To distinguish among many matches, criteria can be used to judge the ranked scores produced by programs such as FASTA. For example, the Codex Alimentarius (http://www.codexalimentarius.net/web/index_en.jsp) recommended a percentage identity score of at least 35% matched amino acid residues of at least 80 residues as being the lowest identity criteria for proteins derived from biotechnology that could suggest IgE cross-reactivity with a known allergen. However, Aalberse [73] has noted that proteins sharing less than 50% identity across the full length of the protein sequence are unlikely to be cross-reactive, and immunological cross-reactivity may not occur unless the proteins share at least 70% identity. Recent published work has led to the harmonization of the methods used for bioinformatic searches and a better understanding of the data generated [74, 75] from such studies.

An additional bioinformatics approach can be taken by searching for 100% identity matches along short sequences contained in the query sequence as they are compared to sequences in a database. These regions of short amino acid sequence homologies are intended to represent the smallest sequence that could function as an IgE-binding epitope [76]. If any exact matches between a known allergen and a transgenic sequence were found using this strategy, it could represent the most conservative approach to predicting potential for a peptide fragment to act as an allergen. Critical to this type of search algorithm is the selection of the overlapping sequence length (i.e., the sliding window). As the length of this window of overlapping amino acids to search with is shortened, the chance for random, false-positive matches becomes higher. Although different window lengths have been recommended, a length of eight amino acids has been shown to be informative without acquiring a majority of matches based on random chance [74, 77, 78].

There exist clear limits to the utility of performing sequence searches based on potential epitopes, with a major limitation being the lack of a comprehensive database of confirmed IgE-binding sequential epitopes for existing allergens. Development of this type of database represents a challenging task due to the fact that many allergens that bind IgE in patient sera and are known to cause clinical allergy symptoms do not have B- and T-cells epitopes described for them in the scientific literature [76]. At this time, there is no database of epitope sequences that can fully describe epitopes for all of the known protein allergens. This makes assessments of biotechnology food protein sequences with an epitope database impractical at this time and is not recommended as a safety assessment strategy [74]. Thus, further research regarding epitope identity and sequence length is required in order to make short amino acid search strategies informative beyond the theoretical identity matching strategy currently available [74]. Moreover, it must also be noted that many IgE-binding epitopes are conformational in nature [76], not just a string of primary amino acid sequences. The analysis of conformational IgE epitopes is difficult and involves methods such as site-directed mutagenesis of the full length allergen, mimicking conformational IgE-binding sites by short phage displayed peptides, or even structural analysis of allergen immune complexes [79, 80].

It should also be recognized that two IgE-binding epitopes on the same molecule are required to cross-link high-affinity IgE receptors on mast cells and induce an intracellular signal. If sufficient numbers of receptors are stimulated, the mast cell will degranulate, releasing histamine and leukotrienes. Therefore, a single match in this analysis may or may not be clinically significant and must be assessed by a second tier of studies such as *in vitro* and *in vivo* IgE assays discussed below.

Protein stability

One biophysical property shared by many but not all food allergens is resistance to degradation. The idea that this biophysical aspect of some food proteins can be used to predict potential allergenicity is based on the premise that the longer significant portions of the protein remain intact, the more likely it is to trigger an immune response. There also appears to be a correlation between protein stability and allergenic potential [81], but this correlation is not absolute [82]. This property is not a predominant characteristic of aeroallergens, primarily because their route of sensitization is through the respiratory tract where they would not be expected to encounter the harsh conditions of the gastrointestinal (GI) tract.

Initially, investigators [83, 84] tested the correlation between protein stability and allergenicity by disrupting the secondary and tertiary structures of the major allergens from milk and wheat and showed that the allergens were strikingly sensitive to pepsin digestion and lost their ability to elicit allergic reactions. Another food allergen, peanut allergen, Ara h 2, is stabilized by disulfide linkages that, when intact, protect a portion of the protein from degradation. Amino acid sequence analysis of the resistant protein fragments indicated that they contained most of the immunodominant IgE-binding epitopes. These results provide a link between allergen structure and the most allergenic portions of the protein [85, 86].

Models of digestion are commonly used to assess the stability of dietary proteins [87–89]. A digestion model using simulated gastric fluid (SGF) was adapted to evaluate the allergenic potential of dietary proteins [81]. In this model, stability to digestion by pepsin has been used as a criterion for distinguishing food allergens from safe, nonallergenic dietary proteins. Although these digestibility models are representative of human digestion, they are not designed to predict the $t_{1/2}$ of proteins *in vivo*, even though some investigators have attempted to measure protein half-life in this qualitative *in vitro* assay [90]. Thomas et al. [91] assessed changes to enzyme concentration, pH, protein purity, and method of detection in this SGF assay and proposed a standardized process so that results from different laboratories can be directly compared.

In addition to the SGF assay, simulated intestinal fluid (SIF) is also used for *in vitro* studies to assess the digestibility of food components [92]. SIF is an *in vitro* digestion model where proteins undergo digestion at neutral pH by a mixture of enzymes collectively known as pancreatin. However, the relationship between protein allergenicity and protein stability in the *in vitro* SIF study is limited because the protein has not been first exposed to the acidic, denaturing conditions of the stomach, as would be the case *in vivo* [93]. For this reason, we recommend that the SGF and SIF assays be done sequentially to fully assess a protein's potential allergenicity.

in vitro immunoassays of allergenicity

For transgenic proteins from allergenic sources or with significant sequence homology with known allergens, it is recommended that *in vitro* assays such as radioallergosorbent tests (RAST) [94, 95], enzyme-linked immunosorbent assays (ELISA) [96], or immunoblotting assays should be undertaken to determine if an allergen or protein that is cross-reactive with an allergen has been transferred to the target plant. These assays use IgE fractions of serum from appropriately sensitized individuals who are allergic to the food, from which the transferred gene was derived. Serum donors should meet clinically relevant criteria, including a convincing history or positive responses in DBPCFCs [94, 97, 98]. An FAO/WHO scientific panel [66] has recommended that, in addition to using serum IgE from individuals who are allergic to the food from which the transferred gene was derived, the serum IgE from patients allergic to plants in the same botanical family also be used in these assays (targeted serum screening). However, the current Codex allergy assessment guidelines (http://www.codexalimentarius.net/web/index_en.jsp) do not appear to support the recommendations for targeted serum screening because its usefulness has not been practically demonstrated [99]. Furthermore, the utility of serum screening in the absence of sufficient structural similarity between the protein of interest and a known allergen as recommended by Thomas et al. [74] (e.g., at a level of 35%

over 80 or greater amino acids), has not been rigorously tested.

in vivo assays of allergenicity

For transgenic proteins from allergenic sources or with significant sequence homology with known allergens, further evaluation may be required to determine if the introduced protein could precipitate IgE-mediated reactions. In addition to *in vitro* immunoassays, *in vivo* skin prick testing may be required for some proteins. Skin prick testing is an excellent negative predictor of allergenicity but is only 50–60% predictive if a positive result is obtained [100]. The best *in vivo* test of allergenicity is the DBPCFC. This procedure involves testing with sensitive and nonsensitive patients under controlled clinical conditions. Patients who are known to be allergic to proteins from the source would be tested directly for hypersensitivity to food containing the protein encoded by the gene from the allergenic source. The ethical considerations for this type of assessment would include factors such as the likelihood of inducing anaphylactic shock in test subjects, potential value to test subjects, availability of appropriate safety precautions, and approval of local institutional review boards. If sensitive patients underwent a reaction in these tests, food derived from crops containing the protein would require labeling. In practice, however, such a discovery has led to the discontinuation of product development for brazil-nut allergen containing soybeans.

Changes in endogenous allergens (substantial equivalence)

In the context of substantial equivalence, it is important to establish that the expression of new genes or effects due to the insertion of genes into plant genomes does not alter the levels of endogenous (existing) allergens in food crops. This is likely to be especially true for crops that are commonly allergenic, such as soybeans, wheat, or tree nuts. From the perspective of human health risk, it is generally agreed that substantive changes in the allergenicity of allergenic foods leading to increased incidence or severity of food allergy should be evaluated and considered in safety assessment [39]. To date, evaluations of endogenous allergens have typically been performed for crops that fall into the top eight "commonly" allergenic food groups. Experimentally, these evaluations involve *in vitro* IgE immunoassays by western blot, ELISA, ELISA inhibition, or a combination of these techniques. Examples utilizing each of these different techniques to determine the IgE-binding capacity of transgenic versus nontransgenic foods and biotech proteins have appeared in the literature [101–105]. All studies conducted to date have concluded that there were no meaningful differences between genetically modified and traditional food crops.

Allergy assessment summary: Roundup Ready soybeans

Source of CP4 EPSPS: The gene encoding CP4 EPSPS was isolated from the common soil bacterium *Agrobacterium tumefaciens* strain CP4. *Agrobacterium tumefaciens* is not an allergen. Furthermore, this enzyme is present in all plants, bacteria, and fungi. However, animals do not synthesize their own aromatic amino acids and, therefore, lack this enzyme. Because the aromatic amino acid biosynthetic pathway is not present in mammalian, avian, or aquatic life forms, glyphosate has little if any toxicity for these organisms. In addition, the EPSPS enzyme is normally present in food for human consumption derived from plant and microbial sources indicating that the protein has a long history of safe use.

Bioinformatic analysis of CP4 EPSPS: A search for amino acid sequence similarity between the CP4 EPSPS protein and known allergens was conducted according to the methods described in this chapter. The search revealed no significant amino acid sequence homologies with known allergens either by the FASTA alignment or the short amino acid identity search. In addition, analysis of the amino acid sequence of the inserted CP4 EPSPS enzyme did not show homologies with known mammalian protein toxins and was not judged to have any potential for human toxicity.

In vitro digestibility of CP4 EPSPS: An *in vitro* pepsin digestion assay was performed using *Escherichia coli* produced CP4 EPSPS that had previously been shown to be biochemically identical to that produced in plants. The intact CP4 EPSPS protein was digested rapidly and no stable fragments were detected after 15 seconds exposure to the enzyme. These results indicate that the CP4 EPSPS protein is unlikely to be an allergen.

These data, taken together with the comprehensive characterization data for the CP4 EPSPS protein and very low expression level of the CP4 EPSPS gene (protein accumulates to less than 0.05% of total soybean meal protein), suggest that CP4 EPSPS is neither currently a known food allergen nor likely to become a food allergen as consumed in Roundup Ready soybeans.

Trends in the science of risk assessment

Animal models for predicting allergenicity

The potential for animal models to mimic the human disease process makes them an invaluable tool for potentially predicting allergenicity of nutritionally enhanced crops. Most of the allergy animal models developed to date have been designed to test reagents for immunotherapeutic treatment of allergic disease and to predict the potential allergenicity of proteins [106]. These two disparate goals, identifying effective treatment regimens and predicting potential human allergenicity, require many of the same variables to be considered in the development of an effective animal model. To date, animal models of food allergy developed to test immunotherapeutic reagents have seen some success [107–109]. On the other hand, animal models developed to predict allergenicity are not as prevalent [110, 111] and are yet to be widely accepted.

There has been considerable interest in the development of animal models that would permit a more direct evaluation of the sensitizing potential of novel proteins. The development of a predictive animal model could help to address the third category of public health risk posed by introduction of GM proteins into food crops—that of a novel protein becoming an allergen. In this context, attention has focused on the production of IgE in response to the novel protein and a wide variety of organisms are being developed for this purpose including rodents [112–114], dogs [115], and swine [116]. Many variables are being tested in the development of each model organism including route of sensitization, dose, use of adjuvant, age of organism, diet, and genetics. Unfortunately, there are currently no validated models available for assessing the allergenic potential of specific proteins in naïve subjects. This is due in part to the extremely complex nature of the immune response to foods and proteins and also in part due to the fact that most animal models of food allergy were originally developed to understand the mechanisms of allergenicity rather than assessing the allergenic potential of novel proteins. The development of an animal model that can accurately predict human allergenicity would be an invaluable tool for assessing the allergenicity of nutritionally enhanced food crops. However, while some progress is being made in select models [117, 118], there remains much work to be done before there is confidence that any one model will provide positive predictive value with regard to protein allergenicity in humans.

Refinements of *in vitro* pepsin digestion assay

As described above, the pepsin digestion assay can be a reasonable contributor to an overall allergy assessment of specific proteins. However, even more enlightening information may be obtained if the underlying structural basis for an allergen's ability to resist pepsin digestion was known. It is with this in mind that the sequence specificity of the pepsin substrate and the minimum peptide size required for eliciting the clinical symptoms of allergy are discussed.

Pepsin is an aspartic endopeptidase obtained from the gastric mucosa of vertebrates. However, all mammalian pepsins have similar specificities. Pepsin preferentially cleaves the peptide bond between any large hydrophobic residue (L, F, W, or Y) and most other hydrophobic or neutral residues except P [119]. In order to cleave the peptide bond between two hydrophobic residues, the active site groove of pepsin binds to a segment of the protein containing the sessile peptide bond and four amino acids on either side of the cleavage site. There have been a number of studies evaluating the efficiency of pepsin cleavage and the effect of various amino acids around the sessile peptide bond. To facilitate discussion, the positions have been assigned identification labels such that the amino acid (aa) residues located on the amino-terminal side of the sessile bond are labeled P_1, P_2, P_3, or P_4, and on the carboxyl-side labeled P_1', P_2', and so on. The bond between P_1 and P_1' is the sessile bond. The most efficiently cleaved peptides have aromatic or hydrophobic residues at both the P_1 and P_1' positions. The rate of pepsin cleavage is slowed if a proline is at amino acid position P_2' or if arginines are in the P_2, P_3, or P_4 positions [120, 121].

The resistance of a protein to pepsin digestion raises the possibility that it will be taken up by antigen-processing cells at the mucosal surface of the small intestine and could sensitize susceptible individuals who have consumed the protein, leading to the production of antigen-specific IgE. In addition there is the possibility that a pepsin-resistant peptide could provoke an IgE-mediated allergic response in those who are already sensitized. IgE plays a pivotal role during the induction of an allergic response by triggering effecter cells such as the tissue mast cells (and possibly blood basophils) to release histamine, leukotrienes, and inflammatory proteases. This is accomplished when two or more IgE molecules are bound to a single peptide fragment while the antibody is bound to the high-affinity IgE receptors (FcεRI) on these effecter cells. Studies of rat basophilic leukemia (RBL) cells indicate that it probably requires the cross-linking of well over 1000 of the 200 000 or so FcεRI receptors on a single cell to cause degranulation of that cell [122]. IgE antibody cross-linking occurs through the binding of multivalent antigens by IgE molecules bound to the surface of mast cells. While various IgE-antigen binding arrangements are possible, only certain ones will lead to the productive signaling and degranulation of the mast cells [123, 124]. The binding is only effective if it is maintained long enough (by a high-affinity interaction) and if the spatial relationship and rigidity of the antigen are sufficient to cross-link and induce intracellular signaling. Baird, Holowka, and colleagues used haptens with linkers of various sizes to determine the effective spacing for degranulation and to study intracellular signaling. Results demonstrated that oligomerization of the FceRI-IgE-antigen molecules was more effective at inducing degranulation. Further, minimum spatial distances were identified using the artificial hapten-spacer constructs indicating that while tight IgE binding can occur with bivalent haptens spanning 30 Å (angstroms), the RBL cells were not induced to degranulate. Bivalent haptens of 50 Å were required to obtain modest degranulation while similar haptens spaced between 80 and 240 Å apart seemed to provide optimum degranulation [123, 124]. These results may be used to provide guidance on the sizes of peptides that might be required to cause an allergic reaction upon challenge.

In order to evaluate the minimum peptide size that might effectively cross-link receptors on mast cells, the maximum overall spacing (length) may be calculated, but various assumptions must be made regarding epitope size and peptide conformation. The first assumption regards the size of a typical IgE-binding epitope observed in a food allergen. Most food allergen IgE-binding epitopes are reported to range in size from 6 to 15 amino acids in length [76]. Therefore the absolute minimum size of a peptide would have to be 12–30 amino acids long and contain two IgE-binding epitopes. However, this does not take into account the data of Kane et al. [125, 126], which shows the IgE-binding epitopes must be at least 80–240 Å apart to provide optimum degranulation. Assuming the two IgE-binding epitopes are separated by the minimum length of 80 Å and that the diameter size for an amino acid such as alanine is 5 Å, the minimum size for a peptide that would be expected to elicit the clinical symptoms of an allergic reaction would be 29 amino acids long or a peptide of about 3190 Da (29 amino acids with an average molecular weight of each amino acid of 110 Da). These calculations do not take into account the secondary structure of the peptide. For example, the peptide could be in an α-helical arrangement, a β-pleated sheet, or a random coil depending on its amino acid sequence. Depending on the secondary structure of the peptide, mast cell degranulation would only be possible if each end of the fragment represents a strong IgE-binding epitope and if the peptide is in a β-strand conformation. Based on this rationale, it appears improbable that the presence of a protease-resistant fragment of 3 kDa in the *in vitro* pepsin digestion assay would have the ability to degranulate mast cells and therefore would not be likely to pose a risk to consumers.

While the discussion above is theoretical, there is recent evidence that pepsin-resistant allergen fragments produced in an *in vitro* pepsin digestion assay were 0.3 kDa and contained multiple IgE-binding epitopes. The major peanut allergen Ara h 2 is a 17-kDa protein that has eight cysteine residues that could form up to four disulfide bonds. Upon treatment with pepsin, a 10-kDa fragment was produced that was resistant to further enzymatic digestion. The resistant Ara h 2 peptide fragment contained intact IgE-binding epitopes and several potential enzyme cut sites that were protected from the enzyme by the compact structure of the protein. Amino acid sequence analysis of the resistant protein fragments indicates that they contained most of the immunodominant IgE-binding epitopes. These results provide a link between allergen structure and the immunodominant IgE-binding epitopes within a population of food-allergic individuals and lend additional biological relevance to the *in vitro* pepsin digestion assay [127].

The link between food allergenicity and protein stability appears to have been confirmed, at least for milk and wheat allergy. Buchanan and colleagues have shown that when stability of the major allergens from these foods is disrupted by reduction of disulfide bonds, the allergens were strikingly sensitive to pepsin digestion and lost their allergenicity as determined by their ability to provoke skin test and GI symptoms in previously sensitized dogs [128, 129]. Other food allergens will have to be tested in this same manner in order to determine if this is a general characteristic of food allergens.

In an attempt to assess the positive and negative predictive values (PPV and NPV, respectively) for the pepsin digestion assay in identifying potential food allergens, Bannon et al. [130] compared the stability of 20 known food allergens and 10 nonfood allergens and calculated a PPV for these proteins of 0.95 and an NPV of 0.80. This analysis indicates that the pepsin digestion assay is a good positive and negative predictor of the potential of a protein to be an allergen. However, the results should be interpreted with some caution as food allergens associated with oral allergy syndrome (OAS) were not included in this analysis and only 30 proteins were tested in this manner. In any event, assay standardization and the study of the biochemical properties of many proteins (allergens and nonallergens) will inform the allergy assessment strategy with respect to the robustness and predictive power of this physicochemical property of proteins.

Value of measuring allergen expression levels as part of the allergy risk assessment of biotech crops

The comparative measurement of total IgE reactivity or total allergen levels has been a part of the allergy safety assessment for biotech crops that are commonly allergenic, such as soybean. The measurement of total allergen levels is the most appropriate safety assessment of endogenous allergenicity given that soy allergic disease is manifested by a polyclonal IgE response to numerous soy proteins unique to the susceptible individual [131–133].

Even though the etiology of soybean allergic disease varies with each susceptible individual, it has typically been manifested by a polyclonal IgE response to numerous soy proteins. The measurement of individual allergens as part of the safety assessment of biotech crops has been recommended by EFSA [134]. To date, 10 soybean allergens, which include glycinin, β-conglycinin, gly m 1, gly m 2, gly m 4, gly m 4, gly m Bd 28K, gly m Bd 30K, gly 50K, and Kunitz trypsin inhibitor, are known to cause soybean allergic disease. Only eight of these allergens have been identified and have full sequence information available [135]. Although significant advances have been made in the identification of allergenic proteins, little is known about the allergenic epitopes of these proteins or the threshold levels required for allergic sensitization or elicitation [131, 136]. Because the soybean allergic response is a polyclonal IgE response and the threshold levels of soybean allergens are largely unknown, it is unclear what added safety value is gained from the measurement of individual allergen levels as part of the allergy safety assessment of biotech soybean varieties, especially when an assessment of total IgE reactivity (measurement of total allergen levels) is already performed. Despite the lack of clear safety information that would be gained from such an analysis, methods to measure individual allergen levels in GM and non-GM soybeans are being developed.

In addition to human IgE serological methods that have already been discussed above, it is possible to measure individual allergens using monoclonal or polyclonal IgG antibodies raised to each allergen in an ELISA or Western blot assay, gel-based comparisons, or mass spectrometry (MS) based comparisons. Protein expression analyses that use IgG antibodies from the serum of an immunized animal could be used in the safety assessment. ELISA-based approaches using these allergen-specific IgG antibodies are commonly used to detect and quantify allergens in food products to ensure that allergen labeling requirements are met by the food industry [137]. These types of methods are reliable and sensitive, enabling the detection of small amounts of allergen. IgG-based ELISAs are appropriate for measurement of individual allergen levels as part of the safety assessment of biotech soybean varieties. However, these assays have not been developed for most soybean allergens. Some of the allergens, namely glycinin and β-conglycinin, consist of multiple protein subunits that have high degrees of sequence similarity meaning that it may not be possible to develop antibodies that can distinguish each of these protein subunits [138]. However, measurement of each glycinin or β-conglycinin subunit separately provides limited safety information since it is not clear that IgE differentially recognizes and binds one subunit over the other. Taken together, the use of IgG antibodies to develop quantitative ELISA-based assays that are sensitive and reproducible is a viable approach to measure individual allergen levels as part of the safety assessment of biotech soybeans; however, a significant amount of effort will be needed to develop these assays for each allergen.

Protein separation methods, such as two-dimensional electrophoresis (2DE), have been instrumental in the identification of a number of allergens. 2DE has also been used as a proteomic tool to measure the expression levels of a large number of proteins and has recently been used to compare allergen levels in wild type and transgenic plants [139–141]. Using this method, biotech and control soybean extracts are run on separate gels. These proteins are separated in two dimensions, first by isoelectric point and then by molecular weight. The gels are stained with Coomassie Blue or a fluorescent stain and protein spot intensities are compared between gels. Another protein separation technique, called difference gel electrophoresis (DIGE), allows comparison of two protein extracts on the same gel. Using this method, protein extracts are labeled with different fluorescent dyes, mixed, and then separated by 2DE. Protein spot intensities are measured for each fluorescent dye and then comparisons are made between individual protein spots from each extract. For both 2DE and DIGE, individual protein spots can be identified using MS. Taken together, these two protein separation techniques can provide a comparative analysis between two protein extracts (i.e., biotech and conventional soybean extracts) and the allergen spots can be identified, meaning these techniques could be used for the endogenous allergen assessment as part of the safety assessment of biotech crops. MS can be used to quantify proteins, including allergens. In fact there are a number of MS-based methods that have been developed to measure allergen expression levels [142–144]. MS-based methods typically quantify a protein level relative to a known standard, which can be an isotopically labeled version of the protein being measured or a labeled peptide that matches an enzymatically digested fragment of the protein being measured. It is also possible to use a label-free method to quantify proteins, in which the relative quantification of a protein relies on spectral counting or on the ion signal intensity. A detailed description of each of these methods and a discussion of how they can be used to measure allergen levels have been provided in other review articles [142, 144]. Studies have shown that these MS-based methods can be applied to measure allergen levels to compare conventional and transgenic plants [144]. Like the IgG-antibody-based ELISAs, these MS-based methods have been shown to be capable of measuring allergen levels. However, in most cases the methods have not been developed to measure each soybean allergen. Some work has been completed to develop both a label-free method and an isotope-labeled peptide absolute quantitation method for some of the soybean allergens [145]. In this work, the amounts of eight soybean allergens were measured in 20 different conventional soybean varieties by both spectral counting and absolute quantitation using AQUA peptides, demonstrating that these methods could be used to compare allergen levels between conventional soybean varieties. This study also provided some information about the range of allergen levels present in commercially available conventional soybean varieties, which is needed to put the measurement of individual allergen levels in biotech soybean varieties within a context of safety.

In addition to the lack of clear safety information that would be gained from a comparative analysis of individual allergens as part of the allergy safety assessment of GM soybeans, another key challenge limiting the routine application of this technology to the allergy assessment process is the need to define the natural variability of allergen abundance in food crops with different genetic backgrounds and grown in different environments. Since protein abundance is a characteristic of known allergens, before informed decisions on whether a protein's abundance has significantly increased can be made, we must first know the normal range of protein abundance that is seen in nature. Without this point of reference, it is impossible to interpret the effect of any changes that are detected in protein abundance. Another key point to keep in mind is that having the ability to detect a change, especially given the ongoing improvements in the sensitivity of the equipment, does not immediately imply that the change will have any biological effect on allergenicity.

Removing allergens from foods

Genetic engineering can be used to (1) reduce the levels of known allergens by post-transcriptional gene silencing using an RNA antisense approach, (2) reduce their allergenicity by reducing disulfide bonds that are critical for allergenicity using thioredoxin, or (3) by directly modifying the genes encoding the allergen(s).

The RNA antisense approach has been successfully applied to reduce the allergenic potential of rice. Most rice allergens have been found in the globulin fraction of rice seed [146–150]. The globulins and albumins have been estimated to comprise about 80–90% of the total protein in rice seeds. From this fraction, a 16 kDa a-amylase/trypsin inhibitor-like protein was identified as the major allergen involved in hypersensitivity reactions to rice [146, 147].

Using this antisense RNA approach, Nakamura and Matsuda [150] generated several rice lines that contained transgenes producing antisense RNA for the 16 kDa rice allergen. These authors successfully lowered the allergen content in rice by as much as 80% without a concomitant change in the amount of other major seed storage proteins (Figure 5.2).

The concept of reducing disulfide bonds to reduce allergenicity has been tested on allergens in wheat and milk by

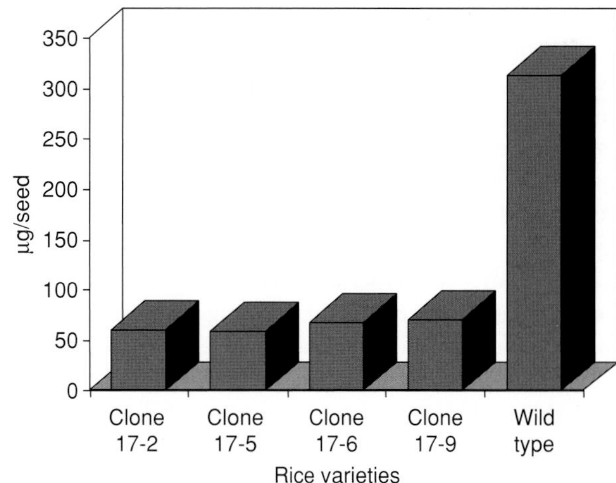

Figure 5.2 Suppression of a 16-kDa rice allergen using antisense technology. Rice allergen levels were quantified by ELISA from each genetically engineered rice variety (clones 17-2, 17-5, 17-6, and 17-9) and were compared with wild-type rice seeds. From Reference 152, with permission from Matsuda.

Buchanan and colleagues and has been shown to significantly reduce the allergic symptoms elicited from sensitized dogs [128, 129, 151]. Briefly, the authors exposed either the purified allergens or an extract from the food source containing the allergens to thioredoxin purified from *E. coli* and then performed skin tests and monitored GI symptoms in a sensitized dog model. Allergens that had their disulfide bonds reduced by thioredoxin showed greatly reduced skin reactions and GI symptoms (Figure 5.3). These results provide a critical proof-of-concept for this approach before constructing transgenic wheat lines that overproduce thioredoxin.

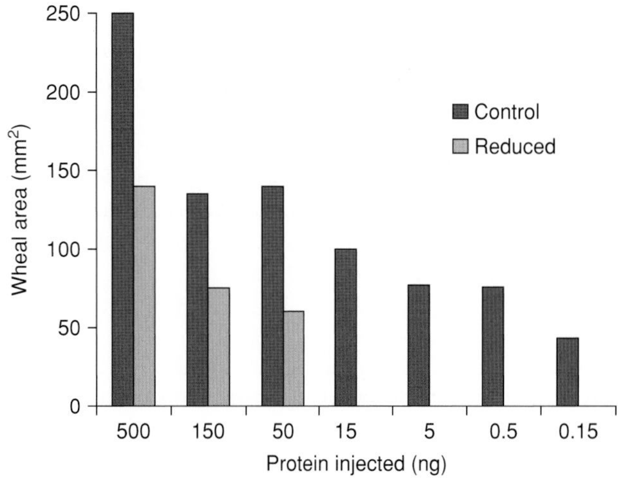

Figure 5.3 Thioredoxin mitigation of milk allergen reactivity in dogs sensitized to milk. Milk was incubated in physiological buffered saline containing 5 mL of 100 mmol/L dithiothreitol (DTT) and boiled for 5 minutes prior to skin testing in milk-allergic dogs. Reproduced from Reference 129.

One of the more ambitious approaches to reducing allergenicity of food crops is by modification of the genes encoding the allergens so that they produce hypoallergenic forms of these proteins [153, 154]. This approach is based on the observation that most food allergens have linear IgE-binding epitopes that can be readily defined using overlapping peptides representing the entire amino acid sequence of the allergen and serum IgE from a population of individuals with hypersensitivity reactions to the food in question [76]. Once the IgE-binding epitopes are determined, critical amino acids can be identified that, when changed to another amino acid, result in loss of IgE binding to that epitope without modification of the function of that protein. Any changes that result in loss of IgE binding can then be introduced into the gene by site-directed mutagenesis.

Serum IgE from patients with documented peanut hypersensitivity and overlapping peptides were used to identify the IgE-binding epitopes of the major peanut allergens Ara h 1, Ara h 2, and Ara h 3. At least 23 different linear IgE-binding epitopes located throughout the length of the Ara h 1 molecule were identified [155]. In a similar fashion, 10 IgE-binding epitopes and 4 IgE-binding epitopes were identified in Ara h 2 and Ara h 3, respectively [156, 157]. Mutational analysis of each of the IgE-binding epitopes revealed that single amino acid changes within these peptides had dramatic effects on IgE-binding characteristics. Substitution of a single amino acid led to loss of IgE binding [156–159]. Analysis of the type and position of amino acids within the IgE-binding epitopes that had this effect indicated that substitution of hydrophobic residues in the center of the epitopes was more likely to lead to loss of IgE binding [155]. Site-directed mutagenesis of the cDNA encoding each of these allergens was then used to change a single amino acid within each IgE-binding epitope. The hypoallergenic versions of these allergens were produced in *E. coli* and tested for their ability to bind IgE and to stimulate proliferation of T cells from peanut-allergic patients. The results of these studies indicated that it is possible to produce hypoallergenic forms of the peanut allergens that bind less allergen-specific IgE, interact with T cells from peanut-sensitive patients, and release significantly lower amounts of mediators from passively sensitized mast cells [160, 161].

International consensus: a common strategy

The development of national and international regulations, guidelines, and policies to assess the safety of food products derived from genetically engineered plants has led to broad discussions and a general consensus on the types of information that are appropriate to assess the potential allergenicity of such foods. Gaining international consensus on allergy assessment is critical because many genetically engineered plant products are commodity products (e.g., corn, soybean, wheat) grown and traded globally. A consensus approach provides producers, regulators, and consumers with the assurance that the risk of allergy to these products is appropriately addressed prior to their marketing, and that a consistent assessment approach is used around the world.

Conclusion and future considerations

The allergy assessment testing strategy, as it is presently formulated, is a tiered, hazard identification approach that utilizes currently available scientific data regarding allergens and the allergic response. It is extremely important to emphasize that all aspects of the current safety assessment testing strategy need to be considered when assessing a novel protein, not just the results from a single arm of this strategy. While a hazard assessment approach has served the public interest well, it may not be adequate in the assessment of future products, which may have proteins that may have unknown or unpredictable mechanisms of action or which may share one or more properties with food allergens while concomitantly providing significant nutritional and human health benefits. Considering the advances in the science of allergy assessment detailed in this chapter, the allergy assessment strategies proposed by Metcalfe et al., and the most recent recommendations by the scientific advisory panel of the FAO/WHO, we have described the current practices and issues in allergy assessment. This strategy takes advantage of the past assessments but, by its tiered design, attempts to place more importance on the "weight of evidence" from each test rather than relying too heavily on one test to determine whether a protein is likely to have allergenic potential.

We conclude that the current testing strategy will need to be integrated into a risk assessment model where risk is defined as a function of the level of the hazard and the level of exposure to the hazard. This strategy consists of four steps: hazard assessment, dose-response evaluation, exposure assessment, and risk characterization [162]. To apply risk assessment principles to the issue of the allergenicity of proteins and food biotechnology, new scientific data must be collected for each step in this process. This review of scientific progress on these issues indicates that this process of integration has already begun. For example, the issue of dose-response evaluation is beginning to be addressed by a variety of investigators exploring threshold doses for traditional allergenic foods in clinically allergic patients [163, 164]. The issue of exposure assessment consists of three parts: the abundance of the protein in the food, the stability of the protein in the GI tract, and the amount of the GM crop consumed in the diet. We believe that the protective value of current testing approaches and future approaches that adopt sound risk assessment principles, have provided and will continue to provide robust assurances to risk managers and consumers alike for present and future biotech products [15].

References

1. Somerville C, Briscoe J. Genetic engineering and water. *Science* 2001; 292:2217.
2. Sicherer SH, Burks AW, Sampson HA. Clinical features of acute allergic reactions to peanut and tree nuts in children. *Pediatrics* 1998; 102:e6.
3. Taylor SL, Lemanske Jr RF, Bush RK, Busse, WW. Chemistry of food allergens. Food allergy. In: Chandra RK (ed.) *Food Allergy*. St John's Nutrition Research Education Foundation, 1987; pp. 21–44.
4. Fuchs RL, Astwood JD. Allergenicity assessment of foods derived from genetically modified plants. *Food Tech* 1996; 50:83–88.
5. Taylor SL. Chemistry and detection of food allergens. *Food Tech* 1992; 46:146–152.
6. Stanley JS, Bannon GA. Biochemistry of food allergens. *Clin Rev Allergy Immunol* 1999; 17:279–291.
7. Horsch RB, Fraley RT, Rogers SG, et al. Inheritance of functional foreign genes in plants. *Science* 1984; 223:496–498.
8. De Block M, Herrera-Estrella L, Van Montagu M, et al. Expression of foreign genes in regenerated plants and their progeny. *EMBO J* 1984; 3:1681–1689.
9. Fiske HJ, Dandekar AM. The introduction and expression of transgenes in plants. *Sci Hort* 1993; 55:5–36.
10. Van Larebeke N, Engler G, Holsters M, et al. Large plasmid in *Agrobacterium tumafaciens* is essential for crown gall inducing activity. *Nature* 1974; 252:169.
11. Zambryski PC. Chronicles from the *Agrobacterium*-plant cell transfer story. *Annu Rev Plant Physiol Plant Mol Biol* 1992; 43:465–490.
12. Sanford JC, Klein TM, Wolf ED, Allen N. Delivery of substances into cells and tissues using a particle bombardment process. *J Part Sci Technol* 1987; 5:27–37.
13. Sanford JC, Smith FD, Russell JA. Optimizing the biolistic process for different biological application. *Methods Enzymol* 1992; 217:483–509.
14. James C. *Global Status of Commercialized Biotech/GM Crops 2011*. ISAAA Brief No 43-2011. Ithaca, NY: ISAAA, 2011.
15. Brookes G, Barfoot P. *GM Crops: The First Ten Years—Global Socio-Economic and Environmental Impacts*. ISAAA Brief No 36. Ithaca, NY: ISAAA, 2006.
16. GAO (2002) *Report on Biotechnology*. Available at http://www.gao.gov/new.items/d02566.pdf (Last accessed June 28, 2013).
17. Carpenter J, Gianessi L. Herbicide use on roundup ready crops. *Science* 2000; 287:803–804.
18. Liu K. *Soybeans: Chemistry, Technology and Utilization*. Chapman and Hall, 1997.
19. Steinrucken HC, Amrhein N. The herbicide glyphosate is a potent inhibitor of 5-enolpyruvyl-shikimate-3-phosphate synthase. *Biochem Biophys Res Commun* 2001; 94:1207–1212.
20. EPA. *Reregistration Eligibility Decision (RED): Glyphosate*. Washington, DC: Office of Prevention, Pesticides and Toxic Substances, US Environmental Protection Agency, 1993.
21. WHO. *Glyphosate. Environmental Health Criteria No 159*. Geneva, Switzerland: World Health Organization (WHO), International Programme of Chemical Safety (IPCS), 1994.
22. Williams GM, Kroes R, Munro IC. Safety evaluation and risk assessment of the herbicide roundup and its active ingredient, glyphosate, for humans. *Regul Toxicol Pharmacol* 2000; 31:117–165.
23. Culpepper AS, York AC. Weed management in glyphosate-tolerant cotton. *J Cotton Sci* 1998; 2:174–185.
24. Keeling JW, Dotray PA, Osborn TS, Asher BS. Postemergence weed management with Roundup Ultra, Buctril and Staple in Texas High Plains cotton. *Proc Beltwide Cotton Conf*, 1998; 1:861–862.
25. Baker JL, Laflen JM. Runoff losses of surface-applied herbicides as affected by wheel tracks and incorporation. *J Environ Qual* 1979; 8:602–607.
26. Hebblethewaite JF. *The Contribution of No-Till to Sustainable and Environmentally Beneficial Crop Production: A Global Perspective*. West Lafayette, IN: Conservation Technology Information Center, 1995.
27. CTIC. *Crop Residue Management Survey*. West Lafayette, IN: Conservation Technology Information Center, 1998.
28. Kay BD. Soil quality: impact of tillage on the structure of tilth of soil. In: *Farming for a Better Environment*. Ankeny, IA: Soil and Water Conservation Society, 1995; www.swcs.org/en/publications/books/index.cfm?nodeID=7035&audienceID=1.
29. CTIC. *Top Ten Benefits*. West Lafayette, IN: Conservation Technology Information Center, 2000; www.swcs.org/en/publications/books/index.cfm?nodeID=7035&audienceID=1.
30. Reicosky DC. Impact of tillage on soil as a carbon sink. In: *Farming for a Better Environment*. Ankeny, IA: Soil and Water Conservation Society, 1995.
31. Reicosky DC, Lindstrom MJ. Impact of fall tillage on short-term carbon dioxide flux. In: Lal R, Kimble J, Levine E, Stewart BA (eds), *Soils and Global Change*. Chelsea, MI: Lewis Publishers, 1995; pp. 177–187.
32. Kern JS, Johnson MG. Conservation tillage impacts on national soil and atmospheric carbon levels. *Soil Sci Soc Am J* 1993; 57:200–210.
33. FAO/WHO. *Biotechnology and Food Safety*. Geneva, Switzerland: FAO/WHO, 1996; pp. 1–27.
34. FAO/WHO. *Strategies for Assessing the Safety of Foods Produced by Biotechnology*. Geneva, Switzerland: FAO/WHO, 1991; pp. iii–59.
35. OECD. *Safety Evaluation of Foods Derived by Modern Biotechnology: Concepts and Principles*. Paris: Organization for Economic Cooperation and Development (OECD), 1993.
36. Astwood JD, Fuchs RL. Status and safety of biotech crops. In: Baker DR, Umetsu NK (eds), *Agrochemical Discovery. Insect, Weed and Fungal Control*. ACS Symposium Series 774. Washington, DC: American Chemical Society, 2001; pp. 152–164.

37. Lavrik PB, Bartnicki DE, Feldman J, et al. Safety assessment of potatoes resistant to colorado potato beetle. In: Engel KH, Takeoka GR, Teranishi R (eds), *Genetically Modified Foods. Safety Issues*. ACS Symposium Series 605. Washington, DC: American Chemical Society, 1995; pp. 148–158.
38. Padgette SR, Re DB, Barry GF, et al. New weed control opportunities: development of soybeans with a Roundup Ready™ gene. In: Duke SO (ed.) *Herbicide-Resistant Crops. Agricultural, Environmental, Economic, Regulatory, and Technical Aspects*. CRC Lewis Publishers, 1996; pp. 53–84.
39. Sanders P, Lee TC, Groth ME, et al. Safety assessment of insect-protected corn. In: Thomas JA (ed.) *Biotechnology and Safety Assessment*, 2nd edn. Taylor & Francis, 1998; pp. 241–256.
40. Harrison LA, Bailey MR, Naylor MW, et al. The expressed protein in glyphosate-tolerant soybean, 5-enolpyruvylshikimate-3-phosphate synthase from *Agrobacterium* sp. strain CP4, is rapidly digested in vitro and is not toxic to acutely gavaged mice. *J Nutr* 1996; 126: 728–740.
41. Padgette SR, Taylor NB, Nida DL, et al. The composition of glyphosate-tolerant soybean seeds is equivalent to that of conventional soybeans. *J Nutr* 1996; 126:702–716.
42. Taylor NB, Fuchs RL, MacDonald J, et al. Compositional analysis of glyphosate-tolerant soybeans treated with glyphosate. *J Agric Food Chem* 1999; 47:4469–4473.
43. Doolitltle RF. Searching through sequence databases. *Meth Enzymol* 1990; 183:99–110.
44. McClintock JT, Schaffer CR, Sjoblad RD. A comparative review of the mammalian toxicity of *Bacillus thuringiensis*-based pesticides. *Pest Sci* 1995; 45:95–105.
45. Fuchs RL, Ream JE, Hammond BG, et al. Safety assessment of the neomycin phosphotransferase II (NPTII) protein. *Biotechnology* 1993; 11:1543–1547.
46. Gilissen LJ, Metz W, Stiekema W, Nap JP. Biosafety of *E. coli* beta-glucuronidase (GUS) in plants. *Transgenic Res* 1998; 7:157–163.
47. Hammond BG, Fuchs RL. Safety evaluation for new varieties of food crops developed through biotechnology. In: Thomas JA (ed.) *Biotechnology and Safety Assessment*. Philadelphia, PA: Taylor &Francis, 1998; pp. 61–79.
48. Smith AK, Circle SJ. Chemical composition of the seed. In: Smith AK, Circle SJ (eds), *Soybeans: Chemistry and Technology*, vol 1. Westport, CT: Avi Publishing, 1972; pp. 61–92.
49. Perkins EG. Composition of soybeans and soybean products. In: Erickson DR (ed.) *Practical Handbook of Soybean Processing and Utilization*. Champaign, IL and St. Louis, MO: AOCS Press and United Soybean Board, 1995; pp. 9–28.
50. Wilcox JR. Breeding soybean for improved oil quantity and quality. In: Shible R (ed.) *World Soybean Research Conference III: Proceedings*. Boulder, CO: Westview Press, 1985; pp. 380–386.
51. Han Y, Parsons CM, Hymowitz T. Nutritional evaluation of soybeans varying in trypsin inhibitor content. *Poultry Sci* 1991; 70:896–906.
52. Visentainer JV, Laguila JE, Matsushita M, et al. Fatty acid composition in several lines of soybean recommended for cultivation in Brazil. *Arg Biol Tecnol* 1991; 34:1–6.
53. Orthoefer FT. Processing and utilization. In: Norman AG (ed.) *Soybean Physiology, Agronomy, and Utilization*. New York: Academic Press, 1978; pp. 219–246.
54. Pryde EH. Composition of soybean oil. In: Erickson DR, Pryde EH, Brekke OL, Mounts, RTL, Falb, RA (eds) *Handbook of Soy Oil Processing and Utilization*. St. Louis, MO and Champaign, IL: American Soybean Association and American Oil Chemists' Society, 1990.
55. USDA (2001) *Subtopic: Soybeans, Mature Seeds, Raw*. Available at http://www.nal.usda.gov/fnic/cgi-bin/nut_search.pl ?soybean (Last accessed June 28, 2013).
56. Kakade ML, Simons NR, Liener IE, Lambert JW. Biochemical and nutritional assessment of different lines of soybeans. *J Agric Food Chem* 1972; 20:87–90.
57. Faust MA. New feeds from genetically modified plants: the US approach to safety for animals in the food chain. *Livest Prod Sci* 2002; 74:239–254.
58. Hammond BG, Vicini JL, Hartnell GF, et al. The feeding value of soybeans fed to rats, chickens, catfish and dairy cattle is not altered by genetic incorporation of glyphosate tolerance. *J Nutr* 1996; 126:717–727.
59. Sloan AE, Powers ME. A perspective on popular perceptions of adverse reactions to foods. *J Allergy Clin Immunol* 1986; 78:127–133.
60. AAAAI. Overview of allergic disease. *Allergy Rep* 2000; 1:1–3.
61. Sicherer SH, Sampson HA. Food allergy. *J Allergy Clin Immunol* 2006; 117:S470–S475.
62. Woods RK, Stoney RM, Raven J, et al. Reported adverse food reactions overestimate true food allergy in the community. *Eur J Clin Nutr* 2002; 56:31–36.
63. Anderson JA, Sogn DD. *Adverse Reactions to Foods*. NIH Publication No. 84-2442, 1984; pp. 1–6.
64. US Food and Drug Administration, Department of Health and Human Services. Statement of policy: food derived from new plant varieties. *Fed Regist* 1992; 57:22984–23005.
65. FAO/WHO. Safety aspects of genetically modified foods of plant origin. *Report of a Joint FAO/WHO Expert Consultation on Allergenicity of Foods Derived from Biotechnology*. May 29–June 2, 2000. Geneva, Switzerland.
66. FAO/WHO. Evaluation of allergenicity of genetically modified foods. *Report of a Joint FAO/WHO Expert Consultation on Allergenicity of Foods Derived from Biotechnology*. January 22–25, 2001. Rome, Italy.
67. US Food and Drug Administration, Department of Health and Human Services. Secondary direct food additives permitted in food for human consumption; food additives permitted in feed and drinking water of animals; aminoglycoside 3′-phosphotransferase II. *Fed Regist* 1994; 59:26700–26711.
68. Bannon GA. What makes a food protein an allergen? *Curr Allergy Asthma Rep* 2004; 4:43–46.
69. Burks W, Helm R, Stanley S, Bannon GA. Food allergens. *Curr Opin Allergy Clin Immunol* 2001; 1:243–248.
70. Metcalfe DD, Astwood JD, Townsend R, et al. Assessment of the allergenic potential of foods derived from genetically engineered crop plants. *Crit Rev Food Sci Nutr* 1996; 36:S165–S186.
71. Pearson WR. Effective protein sequence comparison. *Meth Enzymol* 1996; 266:227–258.

72. Astwood JD, Silvanovich A, Bannon GA. Vicilins: a case study in allergen pedigrees. *J Allergy Clin Immunol* 2002; 110:26–27.
73. Aalberse RC. Structural biology of allergens. *J Allergy Clin Immunol* 2000; 106:228–238.
74. Thomas K, Bannon G, Hefle S, et al. In silico methods for evaluating human allergenicity to novel proteins. Bioinformatics workshop meeting report, February 23–24, 2005. *Toxicol Sci* 2005; 88:307–310.
75. Ladics GS, Bannon GA, Silvanovich A, Cressman, RF. Comparison of conventional FASTA identity searches with the 80 amino acid sliding window FASTA search for the elucidation of potential identities to known allergens. *Mol Nutr Food Res* 2007; 51:985–998.
76. Bannon G, Ogawa T. Evaluation of available IgE-binding epitope data and its utility in bioinformatics. *Mol Nutr Food Res* 2006; 50:638–644.
77. Hileman RE, Silvanovich A, Goodman RE, et al. Bioinformatic methods for allergenicity assessment using a comprehensive allergen database. *Int Archives Allergy Immunol* 2002; 128:280–291.
78. Silvanovich A, Nemeth MA, Song P, et al. The value of short amino acid sequence matches for prediction of protein allergenicity. *Toxicol Sci* 2005; 90:252–258.
79. Neudecker P, Lehmann K, Nerkamp J, et al. Mutational epitope analysis of Pru av 1 and Api g 1, the major allergens of cherry (*Prunus avium*) and celery (*Apium graveolens*): correlating IgE reactivity with three-dimensional structure. *Biochem J* 2003; 376:97–107.
80. Mittag D, Batori V, Neudecker P, et al. A novel approach for investigation of specific and cross-reactive IgE epitopes on Bet v 1 and homologous food allergens in individual patients. *Mol Immunol* 2006; 43:268–278.
81. Astwood JD, Leach JN, Fuchs RL. Stability of food allergens to digestion in vitro. *Nat Biotechnol* 1996; 14:1269–1273.
82. Fu T-J, Abbott UR, Hatzos C. Digestibility of food allergens and non-allergenic proteins in simulated gastric fluid and simulated intestinal fluid—a comparative study. *J Agric Food Chem* 2002; 50:7154–7160.
83. Buchanan BB, Adamidi C, Lozano RM, et al. Thioredoxin-linked mitigation of allergic responses to wheat. *Proc Natl Acad Sci USA* 1997; 94:5372–5377.
84. del Val G, Yee BC, Lozano RM, et al. Thioredoxin treatment increases digestibility and lowers allergenicity of milk. *J Allergy Clin Immunol* 1999; 103:690–697.
85. Sen MM, Kopper R, Pons L, et al. Protein structure plays a critical role in peanut allergen stability and may determine immunodominant IgE-binding epitopes. *J Immunol* 2002; 169:882–887.
86. Lehmann K, Schweimer K, Reese G, et al. Structure and stability of 2S albumin-type peanut allergens: implications for the severity of peanut allergic reactions. *Biochem J* 2006; 395:463–472.
87. Petschow BW, Talbott RD. Reduction in virus-neutralizing activity of a bovine colostrum immunoglobulin concentrate by gastric acid and digestive enzymes. *J Pediatr Gastroenterol Nutr* 1994; 19:228–235.
88. Silano M, De Vincenzi M. In vitro screening of food peptides toxic for coeliac and other gluten-sensitive patients: a review. *Toxicology* 1999; 132:99–110.
89. Besler M, Steinhart H, Paschke A. Stability of food allergens and allergenicity of processed foods. *J Chromatogr B Biomed Sci Appl* 2001; 756:207–228.
90. Herman RA, Woolhiser MM, Ladics GS, et al. Stability of a set of allergens and non-allergens in simulated gastric fluid. *Int J Food Sci Nutr* 2007; 58:125–141.
91. Thomas K, Aalbers M, Bannon GA, et al. A multi-laboratory evaluation of a common in vitro pepsin digestion assay protocol used in assessing the safety of novel proteins. *Regul Toxicol Pharmacol* 2004; 39:87–98.
92. Okunuki H, Techima R, Shigeta T, et al. Increased digestibility of two products in genetically modified food (CP4-EPSPS and Cry1Ab) after preheating. *J Food Hyg Soc Japan* 2002; 43:68–73.
93. Yagami T, Haishima Y, Nakamura A, et al. Digestibility of allergens extracted from natural rubber latex and vegetable foods. *J Allergy Clin Immunol* 2000; 106:752–762.
94. Sampson HA, Albergo R. Comparison of results of skin test, RAST, and double blind, placebo-controlled food challenges in children with atopic dermatitis. *J Allergy Clin Immunol* 1984; 74:26–33.
95. Yunginger JW, Adolphson CR. *Standardization of Allergens*. Washington, DC: American Society of Microbiology, 1992; pp. 678–684.
96. Burks AW, Brooks JR, Sampson HA. Allergenicity of major component proteins of soybean determined by enzyme-linked immunosorbent assay (ELISA) and immunoblotting in children with atopic dermatitis and positive soy challenges. *J Allergy Clin Immunol* 1988; 81:1135–1142.
97. Sampson HA, Scanion SM. Natural history of food hypersensitivity in children with atopic dermatitis. *J Pediatr* 1989; 115:23–27.
98. Bock SA, Sampson HA, Atkins FM, et al. Double-blind, placebo-controlled food challenges (DBPCFC) as an office procedure. *J Allergy Clin Immunol* 1988; 82:986–997.
99. Thomas K, Bannon G, Herouet-Guicheney C, et al. The utility of a global sera bank for use in evaluating human allergenicity to novel proteins. *Toxicol Sci* 2007; 97:27–31.
100. Hill DJ, Hosking CS, Reyes-Benito V. Reducing the need for food allergen challenges in young children: a comparison of in vitro with in vivo tests. *Clin Exp Allergy* 2001; 31:1031–1035.
101. Kim SH, Kim HM, Ye YM, et al. Evaluating the allergic risk of genetically modified soybean. *Yonsei Med J* 2006; 47:505–512.
102. Batista R, Nunes B, Carmo M, et al. Lack of detectable allergenicity of transgenic maize and soya samples. *J Allergy Clin Immunol* 2005; 116:403–410.
103. Burks AW, Fuchs RL. Assessment of the endogenous allergens in glyphosate-tolerant and commercial soybean varieties. *J Allergy Clin Immunol* 1996; 96:1008–1010.
104. Park JH, Chung TC, Kim JH, et al. Comparison of allergens in genetically modified soybean with conventional soybean. *Yakhak Hoeji* 2001; 45:293–301.

105. Hoff M, Son D-Y, Gubesch M, et al. Serum testing of genetically modified soybeans with special emphasis on potential allergenicity of the heterologous protein CP4 EPSPS. *Mol Nutr Food Res* 2007; 51:946–955.
106. Knippels LM, van Wijk F, Penninks AH. Food allergy: what do we learn from animal models? *Curr Opin Allergy Clin Immunol* 2004; 4:205–209.
107. Morafo V, Srivastava K, Huang CK, et al. Genetic susceptibility to food allergy is linked to differential TH2-TH1 responses in C3H/HeJ and BALB/c mice. *J Allergy Clin Immunol* 2003; 111:1122–1128.
108. Pons L, Ponnappan U, Hall RA, et al. Soy immunotherapy for peanut-allergic mice: modulation of the peanut-allergic response. *J Allergy Clin Immunol* 2004; 114:915–921.
109. Srivastava KD, Kattan JD, Zou ZM, et al. The Chinese herbal medicine formula FAHF-2 completely blocks anaphylactic reactions in a murine model of peanut allergy. *J Allergy Clin Immunol* 2005; 115:171–178.
110. Buchanan BB, Frick OL. The dog as a model for food allergy. *Ann NY Acad Sci* 2002; 964:173–183.
111. Dearman RJ, Stone S, Caddick HT, et al. Evaluation of protein allergenic potential in mice: dose–response analyses. *Clin Exp Allergy* 2003; 33:1586–1594.
112. Li XM, Schofield BH, Huang CK, et al. A murine model of IgE-mediated cow's milk hypersensitivity. *J Allergy Clin Immunol* 1999; 103:206–214.
113. Dearman RJ, Kimber I. Determination of protein allergenicity: studies in mice. *Toxicol Lett* 2001; 120:181–186.
114. Akiyama H, Teshima R, Sakushima JI, et al. Examination of oral sensitization with ovalbumin in Brown Norway rats and three strains of mice. *Immunol Lett* 2001; 78:1–5.
115. Frick OL. Food allergy in atopic dogs. *Adv Exp Med Biol* 1996; 409:1–7.
116. Helm RM, Furuta GT, Stanley JS, et al. A neonatal swine model for peanut allergy. *J Allergy Clin Immunol* 2002; 109:136–142.
117. Ermel RW, Kock M, Griffey SM, et al. The atopic dog: a model for food allergy. *Lab Anim Sci* 1997; 47:40–49.
118. Li XM, Serebrisky D, Lee SY, et al. A murine model of peanut anaphylaxis: T- and B-cell responses to a major peanut allergen mimic human responses. *J Allergy Clin Immunol* 2000; 106:150–158.
119. Voet D, Voet JG. *Biochemistry*, 2nd edn. New York: John Wiley & Sons Inc, 1995; p. 112.
120. Shintani T, Nomura K, Ichishima E. Engineering of porcine pepsin. Alteration of S1 substrate specificity of pepsin to those of fungal aspartic proteinases by site-directed mutagenesis. *J Biol Chem* 1997; 272:18855–18861.
121. Dunn BM, Hung SH. The two sides of enzyme-substrate specificity: lessons from the aspartic proteinases. *Biochim Biophys Acta* 2000; 1477:231–240.
122. Holowka D, Baird B. Antigen-mediated IGE receptor aggregation and signaling: a window on cell surface structure and dynamics. *Annu Rev Biophys Biomol Struct* 1996; 25:79–112.
123. Schweitzer-Stenner R, Licht A, Pecht I. Dimerization kinetics of the IgE-class antibodies by divalent haptens. I. The Fab-hapten interactions. *Biophys J* 1992; 63:551–562.
124. Schweitzer-Stenner R, Licht A, Pecht I. Dimerization kinetics of the IgE-class antibodies by divalent haptens. II. The interactions between intact IgE and haptens. *Biophys J* 1992; 63:563–568.
125. Kane P, Erickson J, Fewtrell C, et al. Cross-linking of IgE-receptor complexes at the cell surface: synthesis and characterization of a long bivalent hapten that is capable of triggering mast cells and rat basophilic leukemia cells. *Mol Immunol* 1986; 23:783–790.
126. Kane PM, Holowka D, Baird B. Cross-linking of IgE-receptor complexes by rigid bivalent antigens greater than 200 A in length triggers cellular degranulation. *J Cell Biol* 1988; 107:969–980.
127. Sen MM, Kopper R, Pons L, et al. Protein structure plays a critical role in peanut allergen stability and may determine immunodominant IgE-binding epitopes. *J Immunol* 2002; 169:882–887.
128. Buchanan B, Adamidi C, Lozano RM, et al. Thioredoxin-linked mitigation of allergic responses to wheat. *Proc Natl Acad Sci USA* 1997; 94:5372–5377.
129. de Val G, Yee BC, Lozano RM, et al. Thioredoxin treatment increases digestibility and lowers allergenicity of milk. *J Allergy Clin Immunol* 1999; 103:690–697.
130. Bannon GA, Goodman RE, Leach JN, et al. Digestive stability in the context of assessing the potential allergenicity of food proteins. *Comments Toxicol* 2002; 8; 271–285.
131. L'Hocine L, Boye JJ. Allergenicity of soybean: new developments in identification of allergenic proteins, cross-reactivities and hypoallergenization technologies. *Crit Rev Food Sci Nutr* 2007; 47(2):127–143.
132. Batista R, Martins I, Jeno P, Ricardo CP, Oliveira MM. A proteomic study to identify soya allergens—the human response to transgenic versus non-transgenic soya samples. *Int Arch Allergy Immunol* 2007; 144(1):29–38.
133. Ballmer-Weber BK, Holzhauser T, Scibilia J, et al. Clinical characteristics of soybean allergy in Europe: a double-blind, placebo-controlled food challenge study. *J Allergy Clin Immunol* 2007; 119(6):1489–1496.
134. EFSA. Scientific opinion on the assessment of allergenicity of GM plants and microorganisms and derived food and feed. *EFSA J* 2010; 8:1700.
135. FARRP *Allergen Database*. Lincoln, NE: University of Nebraska, Food Allergy Research and Resource Program, 2012.
136. Taylor SL, Hefle SL, Bindslev-Jensen C, et al. Factors affecting the determination of threshold doses for allergenic foods: how much is too much?. *J Allergy Clin Immunol* 2002; 109:24–30.
137. Schubert-Ullrich P, Rudolf J, Ansari P, et al. Commercialized rapid immunoanalytical tests for determination of allergenic food proteins: an overview. *Anal Bioanal Chem* 2009; 395(1):69–81.
138. Nielsen NC, Dickinson CD, Cho TJ, et al. Characterization of the glycinin gene family in soybean. *Plant Cell* 1989; 1(3):313–328.
139. Batista R, Oliveira M. Plant natural variability may affect safety assessment data. *Regul Toxicol Pharmacol* 2010; 58(3 Suppl.):S8–S12.

140. Rouquie D, Capt A, Eby WH, et al. Investigation of endogenous soybean food allergens by using a 2-dimensional gel electrophoresis approach. *Regul Toxicol Pharmacol* 2010, 58(3 Suppl.):S47–S53.
141. Ruebelt MC, Leimgruber NK, Lipp M, et al. Application of two-dimensional gel electrophoresis to interrogate alterations in the proteome of genetically modified crops. 1. Assessing analytical validation. *J Agric Food Chem* 2006, 54(6):2154–2161.
142. Kirsch S, Fourdrilis S, Dobson R, et al. Quantitative methods for food allergens: a review. *Anal Bioanal Chem* 2009; 395(1):57–67.
143. Sancho AI, Mills EN. Proteomic approaches for qualitative and quantitative characterisation of food allergens. *Regul Toxicol Pharmacol* 2010; 58(3 Suppl.):S42–S46.
144. Stevenson SE, Houston NL, Thelen JJ. Evolution of seed allergen quantification—from antibodies to mass spectrometry. *Regul Toxicol Pharmacol* 2010; 58(3 Suppl.):S36–S41.
145. Houston NL, Lee DG, Stevenson SE, et al. Quantitation of soybean allergens using tandem mass spectrometry. *J Proteome Res* 2011; 10(2):763–773.
146. Shibasaki M, Suzuki S, Nemoto H, Kuroume T. Allergenicity and lymphocyte-stimulating property of rice protein. *J Allergy Clin Immunol* 1979; 64:259–265.
147. Matsuda T, Sugiyama M, Nakamura R, Torii S. Purification and properties of an allergenic protein in rice grains. *Agric Biol Chem* 1988; 52:1465–1470.
148. Matsuda T, Nomura R, Sugiyama M, Nakamura R. Immunochemical studies on rice allergenic proteins. *Agric Biol Chem* 1991; 55:509–513.
149. Nakase M, Alvarez AM, Adachi T, et al. Immunochemical and biochemical identification of the rice seed protein encoded by cDNA clone A3-12. *Biosci Biotechnol Biochem* 1996; 60:1031–1042.
150. Nakamura R, Matsuda T. Rice allergenic protein and molecular-genetic approach for hypoallergenic rice. *Biosci Biotech Biochem* 1996; 60:1215–1221.
151. Buchanan BB, Schurmann P, Decottignies P, Lozano RM. Thioredoxin: a multifunctional regulatory protein with a bright future in technology and medicine. *Arch Biochem Biophys* 1994; 314:257–260.
152. Matsuda T, Nakase M, Adachi T, et al. *Allergenic proteins in rice: strategies for reduction and evaluation.* Presented at the Symposium of Food Allergies and Intolerances, May 10–13, 1995, Bonn, Germany.
153. Bannon GA, Shin D, Maleki S, et al. Tertiary structure and biophysical properties of a major peanut allergen, implications for the production of a hypoallergenic protein. *Int Arch Allergy Immunol* 1999; 118:315–316.
154. Burks AW, King N, Bannon GA. Modification of a major peanut allergen leads to loss of IgE binding. *Int Arch Allergy Immunol* 1999; 118:313–314.
155. Burks AW, Shin D, Cockrell G, et al. Mapping and mutational analysis of the IgE-binding epitopes on Ara h 1, a legume vicilin protein and a major allergen in peanut hypersensitivity. *Eur J Biochem* 1997; 245:334–339.
156. Stanley JS, King N, Burks AW, et al. Identification and mutational analysis of the immunodominant IgE binding epitopes of the major peanut allergen Ara h 2. *Arch Biochem Biophys* 1997; 342:244–253.
157. Bannon GA, Cockrell G, Connaughton C, et al. Engineering, characterization and in vitro efficacy of the major peanut allergens for use in immunotherapy. *Int Arch Allergy Immunol* 2001; 124:70–72.
158. Rabjohn P, Helm EM, Stanley JS, et al. Molecular cloning and epitope analysis of the peanut allergen Ara h 3. *J Clin Invest* 1999; 103:535–542.
159. Rabjohn P, West CM, Connaughton C, et al. Modification of peanut allergen Ara h 3: effects on IgE binding and T cell stimulation. *Int Arch Allergy Immunol* 2002; 128:15–23.
160. King N, Helm R, Stanley JS, et al. Allergenic characteristics of a modified peanut allergen. *Mol Nutr Food Res* 2005; 49:963–971.
161. Hodgson E, Levi PE. *A Textbook of Modern Toxicology*, 2nd edn. Stamford, CT:Appleton and Lange, 1997.
162. Taylor S, Hefle SL, Bindslev-Jensen C, et al. Factors affecting the determination of threshold doses for allergenic foods: how much is too much? *J Allergy Clin Immunol* 2002; 109:24–30.
163. Taylor SL, Hefle SL, Bindslev-Jensen C, et al. A consensus protocol for the determination of the threshold doses for allergenic foods: how much is too much? *Clin Exp Allergy* 2004; 34:689–695.
164. Bannon GA, Martino-Catt S. Application of current allergy assessment guidelines to next generation biotechnology derived crops. *J AOAC Int* 2007; 90:1492–1499.

6 Food Allergen Thresholds of Reactivity*

Steve L. Taylor[1], Jonathan O'B. Hourihane[2], & Joseph L. Baumert[1]

[1]Department of Food Science and Technology and Food Allergy Research and Resource Program, University of Nebraska, Lincoln, NE, USA

[2]Department of Pediatrics and Child Health, University College Cork, Cork, Ireland

Key Concepts

- Threshold doses of food allergens do exist below which patients will not react adversely to residues of an allergenic food.
- Threshold doses vary considerably from one patient to another.
- Clinical determination of threshold doses is best done through specifically designed double-blind placebo-controlled food challenges.
- Knowledge of individual threshold doses can provide guidance to patients in the successful implementation of avoidance diets.

Food-allergic individuals must adhere to specific food-avoidance diets. Most allergists in clinical practice advise food-allergic patients to avoid completely the specific allergenic food(s) and all ingredients made from those food(s). The presumption is made that the threshold dose for the offending food is zero and thus complete avoidance is a necessity. From a practical perspective, this advice is probably prudent, but it poses restrictions on patients that can be a major burden. Food-allergic individuals can react adversely to exposure to small quantities of the offending food [1, 2], but it is now well documented that food-allergic individuals have threshold doses below which they will not experience adverse reactions [3, 4]. Thus, the absolute avoidance of the allergenic food may not be so critical for many patients, though the judgments they might need to make in carrying on their day-to-day lives may be very difficult.

Ultimately, individualized assessments of threshold could be helpful to allergic individuals, their physicians, the food industry, and governmental regulatory agencies in protecting the health of these consumers. However, the determination of individual threshold doses is not yet a common clinical procedure, and no consensus exists on the establishment of regulatory threshold doses below which the vast majority of a population of patients allergic to a specific food, for example, peanut, would not be expected to react.

Definition of threshold

A good discussion about the usefulness of threshold presupposes that there is a universally held definition for the term "threshold." In much of the existing clinical literature, the threshold dose is operationally defined as the lowest dose capable of eliciting an allergic reaction. From the toxicology and risk assessment perspective, this dose would be known as the lowest observed adverse effect level (LOAEL) or the minimal eliciting dose (MED) [3]. However, from a risk assessment perspective, the threshold dose should actually be defined as the highest amount of the allergenic food that will not cause a reaction in individuals allergic to that food. This dose would be known as the no observed adverse effect level (NOAEL). Unfortunately, in much of the clinical literature on dose–response relationships for allergenic foods, the NOAEL is not clearly reported.

Clearly, NOAELs and LOAELs can be defined on either an individual basis or a population basis. For an individual, the NOAEL or LOAEL can be experimentally determined by challenge trials conducted in a clinical setting on a particular day. Individual NOAELs or LOAELs might vary from one day to another or from one season to another based on many factors that are not

*This chapter is dedicated to the memory of Susan L. Hefle, PhD, who provided inspiration to us over many years in debates and discussions about allergic reactions to foods and threshold doses.

Food Allergy: Adverse Reactions to Foods and Food Additives, Fifth Edition. Edited by Dean D Metcalfe, Hugh A Sampson, Ronald A Simon and Gideon Lack.

completely understood. Few studies have been done comparing individual NOAELs or LOAELs from one occasion to another, although it is well described that children who are outgrowing their food allergy [5] and patients undergoing successful immunotherapy [6] can become more tolerant of an allergenic food. Certainly, considerable variation occurs in the NOAELs and LOAELs between individuals with a given food allergy. Individual NOAELs for peanut, for example, in controlled clinical challenges can range from 0.4 mg to perhaps 10 g [7].

The population threshold can be defined as the largest amount of the allergenic food which will not cause a reaction when tested experimentally in a defined population of allergic individuals. Of course, this definition presumes that a representative population can be identified and tested experimentally that would include some of the most highly sensitive (as defined by dose) individuals. Clinically, concerns are raised about population threshold estimates if some patients, such as those with histories of severe reactions, are excluded from the clinical threshold trial. However, some clinical evidence indicates that peanut-allergic patients with histories of severe reactions do not have lower threshold doses than patients with histories of less serious reactions [7]. The derivation of the population threshold can be approached using such data through statistical modeling of the dose–response relationship with individual thresholds ideally from a large number of patients. In this case, the threshold is defined as the amount of the allergenic food that will not cause a reaction in a specified proportion of an allergic population. These different definitions imply the use of different approaches to the determination of thresholds that would have different uses in advising patients, labeling of foods, and regulating the food industry.

Thresholds for sensitization versus elicitation

Allergic responses occur in two phases: sensitization and elicitation. Thresholds may apply to both phases [8]. In the sensitization phase, the susceptible individual develops allergen-specific IgE antibodies in response to allergen exposure. Because allergic reactions have not yet occurred, the level of exposure to the allergenic food can be quite high, for example, feeding of milk-based formula to an infant. However, clinical experience suggests, but does not prove, that some infants are sensitized by exposure to much lower doses of the allergenic foods via breast milk, where the level of the allergens is presumably restricted to the small amounts that can transfer from the mother's digestive tract to the breast milk [9]. Cutaneous exposure to food allergens has been implicated in sensitization in retrospective case-control series [10] and animal studies have confirmed this is possible, especially through inflamed skin [11]. The presence of peanut in the household is a risk factor for allergic sensitization to peanuts even when peanuts are being excluded from the diet, suggesting that sensitization can occur to small doses through the skin [12]. Very little information is known about threshold doses for sensitization, and gathering clinical evidence about thresholds for sensitization to common food allergens in humans is likely unethical.

Therefore, this chapter will be devoted to a discussion of the threshold dose for elicitation. The MED is the lowest amount of the allergenic food needed to elicit an allergic reaction in a previously sensitized individual. These food-allergic individuals are the ones who implement specific avoidance diets and must be reasonably protected by food industry practices and labeling standards.

Clinical determination of individual threshold doses

Double blind placebo controlled food challenge (DBPCFC) remains the gold standard for diagnosis of food allergy [13, 14]. The inclusion of extremely low doses of allergenic foods in challenges has been common in research practice for more than a decade [3, 15]. Starting with lower doses means a longer challenge, as challenges must continue until the equivalent of a reasonable serving of the food has been consumed. As noted, no correlation has yet been found between patients who react on challenge to very low doses and patients with histories of severe reactions. Indeed severe reactions to the lowest doses used during the challenge have not been reported in any of the most cited studies where low starting doses were used, and inclusion of low doses, for example, 1 mg or even less of peanut protein, is becoming the norm, particularly since the onset of studies of induction of tolerance to food allergens. In these studies, the clinical end point of a challenge threshold during DBPCFC is relatively easily demonstrated, compared to proof that exposure to higher amounts in an uncontrolled setting in the community are tolerated (or even just survived). It appears therefore that the inclusion of very low doses in DBPCFCs has further increased the safety of food challenges for research and clinical interests.

DBPCFCs that include low doses are now commonplace and most adhere to consensus protocols developed with input from stakeholders from the medical, industrial, and regulatory communities [16]. These challenges proceed in exactly the same fashion as "normal" food challenges. A major consideration has been how to set criteria for a definitive result. Subjective symptoms such as noncooperation (in children particularly), abdominal pain, or itch are easily elicited but are then difficult to quantify on a consistent basis between clinical investigators. Thresholds for subjective symptoms appear to be lower than for objective symptoms [15, 17]. Comparison of apparently similar patients in similar or identical studies in different countries would be difficult if criteria for stopping a challenge were not standardized. It has been agreed that most low-dose challenges, especially in adults, should continue until objective signs are elicited, such as urticaria or angioedema. Subjective symptoms should be carefully recorded and more significant subjective symptoms such as abdominal pain in infants and children, in particular, are frequently considered as an adequate basis to stop the challenge trial [16]. However, as with other diagnostic food challenges, low-dose challenges should be stopped before more significant signs are elicited, such as wheezing. Put simply, low-dose challenge studies add up to three or four extra doses at the start of the challenge, but after the low doses have been safely consumed, there is nothing more complex about a low-dose challenge than there is for any other diagnostic food challenge.

There will always be concerns that volunteers for research studies are self-selected and that there are likely to be more sensitive subjects who do not wish to volunteer. Furthermore, subjects who agree to undergo a challenge, whether clinically motivated or for research studies, must be in optimal health at the time of challenge, so the effects of asthma, reactivity to pollen, or use of medications such as angiotensin-converting enzyme (ACE) inhibitors are eliminated from the challenge in a way that they cannot be eliminated from exposures to allergens in the community [18]. Airway stability must be assessed before challenge by assessment of Peak Expiratory Flow Rate, FEV1 measurement, or formal spirometry. Regular medications that may affect elicitation of an allergic reaction during challenge, such as antihistamines, must be stopped appropriately before the challenge [16].

The severity of previous reactions by history was not an exclusion criterion for the first threshold study of 14 peanut-allergic patients [15] and published data now exist on more than 450 low dose peanut challenges in subjects, including 40 individuals classified as "severe reactors" [7, 15, 18]. Taylor et al. [7] reported low-dose challenges of patients with a spectrum of clinical reactivity so it therefore appears that, within the constraints of research-motivated challenges in volunteers, both adult and children, a spectrum of clinical reactivity has been fully represented in low-dose challenges to date.

The use of standardized protocols is critical for direct comparison of challenge studies, as the outcome of challenges can be affected by considerations such as use of different vehicles for challenges [19] or different types of allergen, for example, raw egg versus cooked egg, defatted peanut flour versus roasted peanut, and so on. [3]. While such factors should be considered, statistical dose–distribution relationships for the peanut-allergic population have been successfully developed for patients from multiple challenge studies by normalizing the challenge doses on a consistent basis, either whole peanut or peanut protein [7, 20]. The form of the processed food used in the challenge may be a bigger factor with milk and egg as compared to peanut. Recent clinical studies have documented that many milk- and egg-allergic patients become tolerant of baked milk or egg before they develop a tolerance for these foods in forms that are subjected to lesser degrees of heat processing [21, 22]. While these clinical studies were not designed to delineate comparative thresholds, the threshold dose for baked milk or egg was clearly higher than the threshold dose for less-heated forms of these foods.

Repeated food challenge is often necessary in children to ascertain persistence or resolution of food allergy. Clinical experience in pediatric practice suggests that increasing amounts of allergen can be tolerated as oral tolerance is achieved, suggesting a change in individual threshold doses, but this has not been formally evaluated. Changes in thresholds over time have not been extensively investigated, with isolated reports suggesting there is no substantial change in adults [15, 23]. Certainly, increased individual threshold doses are predicted to occur more frequently in children to some foods (milk, egg, and soybean) than to others (peanut and tree nuts).

Clinical correlates of thresholds of reactivity

Allergen-specific IgE levels in serum and skin prick test wheal size are now widely used in clinical practice to assess the progress of oral tolerance acquisition in pediatric patients and determine appropriate times for confirmatory challenge trials [24, 25]. Furthermore, a Dutch study [26] reported that nine subjects with the lowest eliciting dose of peanut (0.1–1.0 mg peanut flour) had a higher median peanut-specific IgE value (44 KU_A/L) than three subjects with a higher threshold (>10 mg, peanut-specific IgE values 4.7 KU_A/L, $p = 0.018$). Thus, some correlation seems to exist between the levels of allergen-specific IgE levels in serum and individual threshold doses. However, it has not been possible to strongly correlate serum allergen-specific IgE levels or skin prick test wheal sizes with the severity of both reported reactions and more importantly of future exposures, possibly because many other factors are in play in community exposures [18]. Studies designed to specifically examine low-dose reactivity have begun to alter this perception. A British study has shown a moderate inverse correlation between peanut-specific IgE levels and challenge-induced reaction score, which is stronger in adults than in children [18, 27]. Wensing et al. [28] reported that subjects who reported moderate to severe reactions during exposures to peanut in the community reacted (with mainly subjective symptoms) to significantly lower doses of peanut during low-dose DBPCFC than did subjects whose previous reactions had been mild (p = 0.027). In contrast, Hourihane et al. [29] found little correlation between "community" and "challenge" severity when an estimate of the dose of allergen was considered in the assessment of reaction severity. It appears possible that the inclusion of very low doses in challenges can improve the information that can be gathered from a challenge and that the use of allergen-specific IgE levels could be developed for the prediction of the severity of reactions in challenges with peanut. This association remains to be demonstrated for other food allergens and it is possible that the significance of allergen-specific IgE levels will remain confined to interpretation of low-dose challenge studies, rather than replacing them. To our knowledge, there are insufficient data available to date to examine relationships of MEDs and individual protein components of the major allergenic foods studied, such as Ara h 2 in peanut or Gal d 1 in egg.

MEDs for specific foods

Oral challenges, often DBPCFCs, are often conducted as part of the clinical diagnostic procedure for patients suspected to have a food allergy [13]. In the recommended clinical procedure, the initial dose for diagnostic challenges is described as less than that estimated by the patient to be required to produce symptoms [13]. Thus, considerable physician discretion and experience is involved in the selection of the initial dose in diagnostic DBPCFC. In routine clinical practice, challenge doses historically often started at 500 mg of the specific food [30]. First-dose reactions were reported to range from 17% for fish to 55% for milk [30], so clearly the MED was at an undefined dose somewhere below 500 mg. Furthermore, 11% of patients had experienced severe reactions to the initial dose of 500 mg [30], perhaps suggesting that the initial dose was considerably higher than the patient's MED. Others have similarly reported severe reactions occurring to the initial dose in a diagnostic DBPCFC when starting at higher doses [31]. More recently, a few patients were reported to experience severe reactions at first challenge doses of 0.1 mL for cow's milk protein, 5 mg egg protein, and 28 mg for wheat protein [32] and as low as 20 mg for peanut [33].

In contrast, half or more of allergic individuals had MEDs of 600 mg or more, ranging up to 8 g [30]. Similar results were reported by other clinical groups [7, 34] in sharing clinical experiences with large numbers of patients involved in diagnostic DBPCFC and in results from several immunotherapy trials for peanut allergy [35–37]. This can be interpreted as suggesting that the majority of food-allergic individuals are likely to experience anything more than mild symptoms only when exposed to food that has been rather seriously contaminated or mislabeled.

Very importantly, some exceptionally sensitive patients exist. Individual patients with MEDs of less than 1 mg have been described for milk, peanut, and egg, especially among infants [7]. The percentage of patients with individual MEDs that are well below the typical initial dose used in diagnostic DBPCFC (<100 mg) is unknown for many food allergens. For peanut, threshold values for 489 peanut-allergic individuals are available in the published clinical literature, of which approximately 20–30% react with objective reactions at doses below the typical 100 mg starting dose. The identification of such patients may be quite important as these are predicted to be the individuals who would be at greatest risk from exposure to foods contaminated with trace levels of the offending food.

Clinical trials using low-dose challenges have been conducted on peanut [7, 15, 17, 27, 28, 33, 35–44], milk [34, 45–59], egg [34, 38, 45, 46, 49, 57, 60–64], hazelnut [65, 66], soybean [54, 67–69], wheat [70–72], mustard [73–75], shrimp [38, 76], sesame seed [34, 77–79], fish [80, 81], celery [82], and lupine [83–85] for multiple purposes including diagnosis, the determination of thresholds, or the evaluation of various therapeutic treatments. Sufficient numbers of patients have been included in these various published trials to allow the determination of a population-based threshold dose with a reasonable degree of certainty. Table 6.1 lists the number of subjects whose individual threshold doses are available from various published low-dose challenge studies for all of these foods. From Table 6.1, individual MEDs appear to be quite variable, with the lowest dose observed to trigger an objective reaction in any patient for the allergenic foods ranging from 0.1 mg for peanut protein to a high of 4600 mg for shrimp protein. The population thresholds for these various foods, except celery and fish where insufficient data existed, are to be published [86].

The interpretation of these data to determine population-based thresholds is complicated by numerous factors. The use of a study population that is representative of the entire cross-section of individuals allergic to a particular food should be an essential feature in the determination of population-based thresholds. The compilations of diagnostic challenge experiences indicate that the majority of food-allergic patients have individual threshold doses above the typical 100 mg initial dose used in diagnostic challenges [7, 30, 31]. An examination of the studies reviewed in Table 6.1 indicates that low-dose challenge trials seem to include a preponderance of patients who have lower individual threshold doses. This observation is not surprising since the use of low doses in diagnostic challenges is typically predicated on the patient's historical accounts of reactions to ingestion of small amounts [13, 30] but suggests that these individuals may not be representative of the entire population allergic to a particular food. However, this factor will likely

Table 6.1 Range of individual threshold doses for food-allergic individuals.

Allergenic food	Total no. of patients with objective symptoms	Lowest MED (mg protein)	Highest MED (mg protein)	References
Peanut	489	0.1	7900	7, 15, 17, 27, 28, 33, 35–44
Cows' milk	222	3.3	13 000	34, 45–59
Egg	110	0.21	7700	34, 38, 45, 46, 49, 57, 60–64
Hazelnut	41	1.0	1400	65, 66
Soybean	43	88.0	27 000	54, 67–69
Wheat	37	2.6	2500	70–72
Mustard	33	0.26	240	73–75
Shrimp	25	4600	74 000	38, 76
Sesame seed	21	1.0	3100	34, 77–79
Fish	15	10.2	1300	80, 81
Celery	12	14.0	560	82
Lupine	9	50.0	3150	83–85

MED, minimal eliciting dose (LOAEL) expressed in mg total protein from the allergenic source.

assume less importance when individual threshold data become available from larger groups of patients, studied in internationally standardized DBPCFCs.

Several other factors complicate the search for data on individual threshold doses that are needed to build a robust population database for the establishment of population-based thresholds from existing published data. In many cases, the LOAELs are reported but NOAELs are not or must be inferred. The doses are reported as discrete doses in some cases and as cumulative doses in others. More importantly, the challenge materials are not consistent and need to be normalized. For example, peanuts are approximately 25% protein while peanut flour is about 50% protein. In some studies, subjective responses such as the oral allergy syndrome were used as the criterion for a positive response [28, 65] while in other studies, LOAELs were reported on the basis of objective reactions [7, 27]. Typically, population threshold estimates have been based upon the NOAELs and LOAELs for objective symptoms [7].

A deterministic safety assessment approach based upon binomial probability distributions has been considered as another approach to estimating the population-based threshold [8]. In this approach, 29 patients allergic to a particular food are challenged in a low-dose manner to identify a dose below which none of the 29 patients experiences an adverse reaction. Binomial probability theory then allows the conclusion that there is 95% certainty that fewer than 10% of this food-allergic population will react to ingestion of this dose of the particular food [8]. If a higher number of patients is studied, the power increases; for example, 58 subjects give a 95% probability that <5% will react [87]. Of course, the group of 29 subjects must be representative of the entire allergic population. This approach allows for the possibility that a small, defined percentage of patients allergic to that food will react to ingestion of that dose and this possibility may be considered as too high by regulators, manufacturers, and patients. Quantitative risk assessment based upon statistical dose distribution modeling of collective data from several studies is becoming the preferred approach to determine the population-based threshold [8]. It is important to note that in dose distribution modeling of peanut threshold data, the choice of the statistical dose distribution model was not an important factor when data were available from a large number of subjects [7]. Currently, there is no biological justification to favor one dose distribution model over another, so careful examination of the distribution curve in relation to the individual MEDs is important for selection of the best-fit dose distribution model. An example of a statistical dose-distribution relationship using data from 450 peanut-allergic individuals [7] is provided in Figure 6.1.

Usefulness of individual thresholds for reactivity

Knowledge of an individual patient's threshold dose allows the allergist to provide the patient with more useful advice. While all food-allergic patients should employ avoidance diets, patients with comparatively low threshold doses are thought to be at greater risk because exposure to small residual amounts of allergenic foods is more likely to provoke an adverse reaction. These individuals must be extremely vigilant because shared utensils, cooking vessels, and frying oil might be expected to transfer milligram quantities of the allergenic food. Even kissing someone who has consumed the allergenic food may pose a risk [88, 89].

Low-dose oral challenges allow determination of an individual's threshold dose for reactivity via ingestion. Anecdotally, food-allergic individuals have also reacted

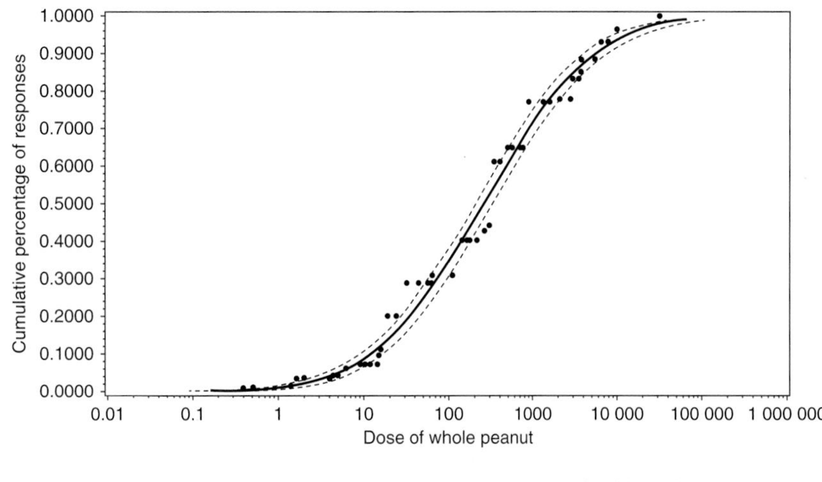

Figure 6.1 Log-normal dose–distribution relationship using 450 individual peanut thresholds with associated 95% confidence intervals. Note: Peanuts contain approximately 25% peanut protein.

to exposure to very small quantities of allergenic foods through other routes such as skin contact with food residues on kitchen surfaces, inhalation of vapors from cooking of the food, and exposure to dust in airplane cabins [3, 90, 91]. Routes of exposure other than the oral route, for example, inhalation or skin contact, may be comparatively more sensitive, although this has not been carefully studied. Thus, knowledge of the oral threshold dose may be of limited value in providing advice regarding other routes of exposure. However, it is known that minor skin contact with peanut rarely causes more than mild cutaneous reactions [92], but if fish-allergic individuals inhale fish steam during cooking, they often wheeze, possibly due to the direct bronchial exposure.

Infants and children are sometimes able to outgrow their food allergies, apparently through the development of oral tolerance [93]. That is particularly true for milk, egg, soybean, and wheat allergies [93]. The individual thresholds of these children appear to increase until they can tolerate typical servings of these foods. Thus, it is tempting to speculate that those individuals with very low individual threshold doses would be less likely to outgrow their food allergy or it would require a longer time period for that to occur.

In at least one study [28], individuals with histories of severe food allergies had significantly lower individual threshold doses. Perhaps this observation should not be surprising because exposure to small amounts of the allergenic food is likely to elicit reactions in such individuals and inadvertent exposure to large doses seems likely to provoke more serious manifestations. Because of their vulnerability to small doses of hidden allergens, individuals with comparatively low threshold doses should probably be among the patients who would benefit the most from carrying an emergency epinephrine kit. In Europe, where epinephrine prescription is not the default outcome of a medical review, as it appears to be in North America, low-dose reactivity is indeed a supporting consideration for epinephrine prescription [94]. However, in other studies [29], the correlation between the severity of reactions suffered in the community and the severity of reactions elicited during low-dose challenges was poor. The doses involved in reactions occurring in the community are certainly not controlled and could affect attempts to make such correlations. Such observations do indicate the value of clinical conservatism in decisions about access to epinephrine.

Anecdotally, families appreciate knowing their child's MED as it helps them in their task of risk assessment every day. Food allergy-related quality of life is significantly affected adversely by uncertainty. It has been shown that even children who fail a food challenge (by reacting during the challenge) have a significant improvement in their food allergy quality of life (FAQL) after the challenge. Despite having to maintain their precautions, the emotional and social impacts of their food allergy diminish [95, 96]. Some allergists are starting to stratify their advice about the relative stringency of food allergen avoidance based on MED identification. However, this approach has not been studied systematically and we cannot recommend adoption of this approach at present on a more widespread basis.

Food industry and regulatory uses of threshold information

Unfortunately, scientific and regulatory consensus does not yet exist to allow the establishment of population-based threshold levels. The key reason for the lack of consensus is the general lack of data due to the relatively low numbers of patients with known and published individual threshold doses generated in low-dose blinded challenge trials. However, considerable progress has been made opportunistically in this regard in recent years, in part due to the use of low-dose challenges in oral immunotherapy trials. Sufficient data now exist, especially for peanut, milk, egg, and hazelnut, and the consensus discussions have begun, especially in Australia and Europe.

Governmental regulatory agencies could make effective use of population-based thresholds. Regulatory agencies have the responsibility to assure the safety of the food supply in their country or region. Certainly, undeclared major allergens in packaged foods should be considered as a potential health hazard for consumers with that food allergy. Recalls of products from the marketplace are common in some countries (the United States, Canada, and Australia) as a result of undeclared allergens. Currently, any level of an undeclared allergen can be the basis for a recall, which may in some cases be considered an overresponse. With the establishment of population-based thresholds, enforcement could be focused on products with undeclared allergens at levels likely to exceed these thresholds.

The food industry has the responsibility for maintaining effective allergen control in their manufacturing facilities to assure the safety of food-allergic consumers. However, economic efficiencies mandate the use of shared equipment and shared facilities between more allergenic and less allergenic formulations. The establishment of population-based thresholds would allow the food industry to establish uniform and appropriate guidelines for evaluation of the effectiveness of their allergen control programs. Methods currently exist that allow the detection of residues of many commonly allergenic foods at parts per million (ppm) or micrograms per gram levels [97]. The effectiveness of factory sanitation is often confirmed with these methods. However, the establishment and adoption of population-based thresholds would assure that these existing methods are sufficient to mitigate any possible hazards from allergen cross-contact.

The use of advisory labeling (e.g., "may contain peanut") has proliferated on packaged foods in recent years. Many foods have such labels even though allergen residues cannot be detected in those foods [98]. Food-allergic consumers should be advised to avoid products bearing such advisory statements, but evidence indicates that these consumers (and possibly their clinicians) are increasingly ignoring these statements [98]. These advisory labeling statements are voluntary and companies have widely differing criteria for the use of such statements on packages. The establishment of population-based thresholds could be used by regulatory agencies as the basis for criteria for the use of advisory labeling statements. Such action would likely curtail the rampant use of such labeling and improve the quality of life of consumers with restricted avoidance diets.

"Allergen-free" products are also appearing on the market in many countries. The use of such labeling is voluntary and not well regulated in most circumstances. While consumers probably believe that no residues of the allergenic food are present in such products, that belief is not documented as fact in the case of most of these products. The establishment of population-based thresholds could provide the basis for "allergen-free" products. The use of gluten-free labeling on products for the benefit of patients with celiac disease is a good example of the use of such labeling and regulation. While the regulatory standards for gluten-free are somewhat variable around the world, consensus appears to be developing that <20 ppm gluten is reasonable and safe for the vast majority of celiac patients [99]. Thus, the establishment of a regulatory, population-based threshold based on clinical science has allowed the prudent development of a gluten-free market category that benefits these patients. Whether this can be adapted to the more immediately life-threatening condition of IgE-mediated food allergy remains to be seen, although, dairy-free, peanut-free, and even allergen-free products are presently marketed in some countries with little regulatory oversight.

Conclusions

Diagnostic challenge procedures for food allergy allow physicians to determine the individual threshold doses for patients. As it stands, most food-allergic patients do not know their individual threshold dose because so few allergy clinics can make this assessment. The knowledge of individual threshold doses could allow physicians to offer more complete advice to food-allergic patients in terms of their comparative vulnerability to hidden residues of allergenic foods, but this clinical approach remains to be tested systematically. The clinical determination of large numbers of individual threshold doses is now starting to allow estimates of population-based thresholds for some allergenic foods, using appropriate statistical modeling approaches. The food industry and regulatory agencies could also make effective use of information on population-based threshold doses to establish improved labeling regulations and practices and allergen-control programs.

References

1. Gern JE, Yang E, Evrard HM, Sampson HA. Allergic reactions to milk-contaminated "nondairy" products. *N Engl J Med* 1991; 324:976–979.
2. Yman IM. Detection of inadequate labelling and contamination as causes of allergic reactions to food. *Acta Aliment Hung* 2004; 33:347–357.

3. Taylor SL, Hefle SL, Bindslev-Jensen C, et al. Factors affecting the determination of threshold doses for allergenic foods: how much is too much? *J Allergy Clin Immunol* 2002; 109:24–30.
4. Hefle SL, Taylor SL. How much food is too much? Threshold doses for allergenic foods. *Curr Allergy Asthma Rep* 2002; 2:63–66.
5. Savage JH, Kaeding AJ, Matsui EC, Wood RA. The natural history of soy allergy. *J Allergy Clin Immunol* 2010; 125:683–686.
6. Nowak-Wegrzyn A, Sampson HA. Future therapies for food allergies. *J Allergy Clin Immunol* 2011; 127:558–573.
7. Taylor SL, Moneret-Vautrin DA, Crevel RWR, et al. Threshold dose for peanut: risk characterization based upon diagnostic oral challenge of a series of 286 peanut-allergic individuals. *Food Chem Toxicol* 2010; 48:814–819.
8. Crevel RWR, Briggs D, Hefle SL, Knulst AC, Taylor SL. Hazard characterisation in food allergen risk assessment: the application of statistical approaches and the use of clinical data. *Food Chem Toxicol* 2007; 45:691–701.
9. Lack G, Fox D, Northstone K, Golding J. Factors associated with the development of peanut allergy in childhood. *N Engl J Med* 2003; 348:977–985.
10. Strid J, Hourihane J, Kimber I, Callard R, Strobel S. Disruption of the stratum corneum allows potent epicutaneous immunization with protein antigens resulting in a dominant systemic Th2 response. *Eur J Immunol* 2004; 34:2100–2109.
11. Adel-Patient K, Ah-Leung S, Bernard H, Durieux-Alexandrenne C, Créminon C, Wal J-M. Oral sensitization to peanut is highly enhanced by application of peanut extracts to intact skin, but is prevented when CpG and cholera toxin are added. *Int Arch Allergy Immunol* 2007; 143:10–20.
12. Fox AT, Sasieni P, du Toit G, Syed H, Lack G. Household peanut consumption as a risk factor for the development of peanut allergy. *J Allergy Clin Immunol* 2009; 123:417–423.
13. Bock SA, Sampson HA, Atkins FM, et al. Double-blind, placebo-controlled food challenge (DBPCFC) as an office procedure: a manual. *J Allergy Clin Immunol* 1988; 82:986–997.
14. Bindslev-Jensen C, Ballmer-Weber BK, Bengtsson U, et al. Standardization of food challenges in patients with immediate reactions to foods—position paper from the European Academy of Allergology and Clinical Immunology. *Allergy* 2004; 59:690–697.
15. Hourihane JO'B, Kilburn SA, Nordlee JA, Hefle SL, Taylor SL, Warner JO. An evaluation of the sensitivity of subjects with peanut allergy to very low doses of peanut protein: a randomized, double-blind, placebo-controlled food challenge study. *J Allergy Clin Immunol* 1997; 100:596–600.
16. Taylor SL, Hefle SL, Bindslev-Jensen C, et al. A consensus protocol for the determination of the threshold doses for allergenic foods: how much is too much? *Clin Exp Allergy* 2004; 34:689–695.
17. Flinterman AE, Pasmans SG, Hoekstra MO, et al. Determination of no-observed-adverse-effect levels and eliciting doses in a representative group of peanut-sensitized children. *J Allergy Clin Immunol* 2006; 117:448–454.
18. Hourihane JO'B, Knulst AC. Thresholds of allergenic proteins in foods. *Toxicol Appl Pharmacol* 2005; 207:S152–S156.
19. Grimshaw KEC, King RM, Nordlee JA, Hefle SL, Warner JO, Hourihane JO'B. Presentation of allergen in different food preparations affects the nature of the allergic reaction—a case series. *Clin Exp Allergy* 2003; 33:1581–1585.
20. Taylor SL, Crevel RWR, Sheffield D, Kabourek J, Baumert J. Threshold dose for peanut: risk characterization based upon published results from challenges of peanut-allergic individuals. *Food Chem Toxicol* 2009; 47:1198–1204.
21. Nowak-Wegrzyn A, Bloom KA, Sicherer SH, et al. Tolerance to extensively heated milk in children with cow's milk allergy. *J Allergy Clin Immunol* 2008; 122:342–347.
22. Lemon-Mule H, Sampson HA, Sicherer SH, Shreffler WG, Noone S, Nowak-Wegrzyn A. Immunologic changes in children with egg allergy ingesting extensively heated egg. *J Allergy Clin Immunol* 2008; 122:977-983.
23. van der Zee JA, Wensing M, Penninks AH, Bruijnzeel-Koomen CAF, Knulst AC (eds) (2003) *Threshold Levels in Peanut and Hazelnut Allergic Patients do not Change Over Time*. Proceedings of XXII Congress of European Academy of Allergology and Clinical Immunology, Paris.
24. Sampson HA. Update on food allergy. *J Allergy Clin Immunol* 2004; 113:805–819.
25. Roberts G, Lack G. Diagnosing peanut allergy with skin prick and specific IgE testing. *J Allergy Clin Immunol* 2005; 115:1291–1296.
26. Peeters KA, Koppelman SJ, van Hoffen E, et al. Does skin prick test reactivity to purified allergens correlate with clinical severity of peanut allergy? *Clin Exp Allergy* 2007; 37:108–115.
27. Lewis SA, Grimshaw KEC, Warner JO, Hourihane JO'B. The promiscuity of immunoglobulin E binding to peanut allergens, as determined by Western blotting, correlates with the severity of clinical symptoms. *Clin Exp Allergy* 2005; 35:767–773.
28. Wensing M, Penninks AH, Hefle SL, Koppelman SJ, Bruijnzeel-Koomen CAFM, Knulst AC. The distribution of individual threshold doses eliciting allergic reactions in a population with peanut allergy. *J Allergy Clin Immunol* 2002; 110:915–920.
29. Hourihane JO'B, Grimshaw KEC, Lewis SA, et al. Does severity of low-dose, double-blind, placebo-controlled food challenges reflect severity of allergic reactions to peanut in the community? *Clin Exp Allergy* 2005; 35:1227–1233.
30. Sicherer SH, Morrow EH, Sampson HA. Dose-response in double-blind, placebo-controlled oral food challenges in children with atopic dermatitis. *J Allergy Clin Immunol* 2000; 105:582–586.
31. Perry TT, Matsui EC, Conover-Walker MK, Wood RA. Risk of oral food challenges. *J Allergy Clin Immunol* 2004; 114:1164–1168.
32. Rolinck-Werninghaus C, Niggemann B, Grabenhenrich L, Wahn U, Beyer K. Outcome of oral food challenges in children in relation to symptom-eliciting allergen dose and allergen-specific IgE. *Allergy* 2012; 67:951–957.
33. Wainstein BK, Studdert J, Ziegler M, Ziegler JB. Prediction of anaphylaxis during peanut food challenge: usefulness of the peanut skin prick test (SPT) and specific IgE level. *Pediatr Allergy Immunol* 2010; 21:603–611.
34. Morisset M, Moneret-Vautrin DA, Kanny G, et al. Thresholds of clinical reactivity to milk, egg, peanut and sesame

in immunoglobulin E-dependent allergies: evaluation by double-blind or single-blind placebo-controlled oral challenges. *Clin Exp Allergy* 2003; 33:1046–1051.
35. Leung DYM, Sampson HA, Yunginger JW, et al. Effect of anti-IgE therapy in patients with peanut allergy. *N Engl J Med* 2003; 348:986–993.
36. Oppenheimer JJ, Nelson HS, Bock SA, Christensen F, Leung DYM. Treatment of peanut allergy with rush immunotherapy. *J Allergy Clin Immunol* 1992; 90:256–262.
37. Nelson HS, Lahr J, Rule R, Bock A, Leung D. Treatment of anaphylactic sensitivity to peanuts by immunotherapy with injections of aqueous peanut extract. *J Allergy Clin Immunol* 1997; 99:744–751.
38. Atkins FM, Steinberg SS, Metcalfe DD. Evaluation of immediate adverse reactions to foods in adult patients II. A detailed analysis of reaction patterns during oral food challenge. *J Allergy Clin Immunol* 1985; 75:356–363.
39. Anagnostou K, Islam S, King Y, Deighton J, Clark AT, Ewan PW. Induction of tolerance in severe peanut allergy. *Clin Exp Allergy* 2009; 39:1954.
40. Clark AT, Islam S, King Y, Deighton J, Anagnostou K, Ewan PW. Successful oral tolerance induction in severe peanut allergy. *Allergy* 2009; 64:1218–1220.
41. Clark AT, King Y, Islam S, Anagnostou K, Deighton J, Ewan PW. The study of tolerance to oral peanut (STOP). *Clin Exp Allergy* 2008; 38:1995.
42. Nicolaou N, Poorafshar M, Murray C, et al. Allergy or tolerance in children sensitized to peanut: prevalence and differentiation using component-resolved diagnostics. *J Allergy Clin Immunol* 2010; 125:191–197.
43. Blumchen K, Ulbricht H, Staden U, et al. Oral peanut immunotherapy in children with peanut anaphylaxis. *J Allergy Clin Immunol* 2010; 126:83–91.
44. Patriarca G, Nucera E, Pollastrini E, et al. Oral rush desensitization in peanut allergy: a case report. *Dig Dis Sci* 2006; 51:471–473.
45. Staden U, Rolinck-Werninghaus C, Brewe F, Wahn U, Niggemann B, Beyer K. Specific oral tolerance induction in food allergy in children: efficacy and clinical patterns of reaction. *Allergy* 2007; 62:1261–1269.
46. Norgaard A, Bindslev-Jensen C. Egg and milk allergy in adults: diagnosis and characterization. *Allergy* 1992; 47:503–509.
47. Caminiti L, Passalacqua G, Barberi S, et al. A new protocol for specific oral tolerance induction in children with IgE-mediated cow's milk allergy. *Allergy Asthma Proc* 2009; 30:443–448.
48. Patriarca G, Buonomo A, Roncallo C, et al. Oral desensitisation in cow milk allergy: immunological findings. *Int J Immunopathol Pharmacol* 2002; 15:53–58.
49. Morisset M, Moneret-Vautrin DA, Guenard L, et al. Oral desensitization in children with milk and egg allergies obtains recovery in a significant proportion of cases. A randomized study in 60 children with cow's milk allergy and 90 children with egg allergy. *Eur Ann Allergy Clin Immunol* 2007; 39: 12–19.
50. Longo G, Barbi E, Berti I, et al. Specific oral tolerance induction in children with very severe cow's milk-induced reactions. *J Allergy Clin Immunol* 2008; 121:343–347.
51. Skripak JM, Nash SD, Rowley H, et al. A randomized, double-blind, placebo-controlled study of milk oral immunotherapy for cow's milk allergy. *J Allergy Clin Immunol* 2008; 122:1154–1160.
52. Lam HY, van Hoffen E, Michelsen A, et al. Cow's milk allergy in adults is rare but severe: both casein and whey proteins are involved. *Clin Exp Allergy* 2008; 38:995–1002.
53. Hill DJ, Ford RPK, Shelton MJ, Hosking CS. A study of 100 infants and young children with cow's milk allergy. *Clin Rev Allergy* 1984; 2:125–142.
54. Fiocchi A, Travaini M, D'Auria E, Banderali G, Bernardo L, Riva E. Tolerance to a rice hydrolysate formula in children allergic to cow's milk and soy. *Clin Exp Allergy* 2003; 33:1576–1580.
55. Baehler P, Chad Z, Gurbindo C, Bonin AP, Bouthillier L, Seidman EG. Distinct patterns of cow's milk allergy in infancy defined by prolonged, two-stage double-blind, placebo-controlled food challenges. *Clin Exp Allergy* 1996; 26:254–261.
56. Flinterman AE, Knulst AC, Meijer Y, Bruijnzeel-Koomen CAFM, Pasmans SGMA. Acute allergic reactions in children with AEDS after prolonged cow's milk elimination diets. *Allergy* 2006; 61:370–374.
57. Orhan F, Karakas T, Cakir M, Aksoy A, Baki A, Gedik Y. Prevalence of immunoglobulin E-mediated food allergy in 6–9-year-old urban schoolchildren in the eastern Black Sea region of Turkey. *Clin Exp Allergy* 2009; 39:1027–1035.
58. Devenney I, Norrman G, Oldæus G, Strömberg L, Fälth-Magnusson K. A new model for low-dose food challenge in children with allergy to milk or egg. *Acta Paediatr* 2006; 95:1133–1139.
59. Høst A, Samuelsson E-G. Allergic reactions to raw, pasteurized, and homogenized/pasteurized cow milk: a comparison. *Allergy* 1988; 43:113–118.
60. Benhamou AH, Zamora SA, Eigenmann PA. Correlation between specific immunoglobulin E levels and the severity of reactions in egg allergic patients. *Pediatr Allergy Immunol* 2008; 19:173–179.
61. Caffarelli C, Cavagni G, Giordano S, Stapane I, Rossi C. Relationship between oral challenges with previously uningested egg and egg-specific IgE antibodies and skin prick tests in infants with food allergy. *J Allergy Clin Immunol* 1995; 95:1215–1220.
62. Knight AK, Shreffler WG, Sampson HA, et al. Skin prick test to egg white provides additional diagnostic utility to serum egg white-specific IgE antibody concentration in children. *J Allergy Clin Immunol* 2006; 117:842–847.
63. Unsel M, Sin AZ, Ardeniz O, et al. New onset egg allergy in an adult. *J Investig Allergol Clin Immunol* 2007; 17:55–58.
64. Eggesbø M, Botten G, Halvorsen R, Magnus P. The prevalence of allergy to egg: a population-based study in young children. *Allergy* 2001; 56:403–411.
65. Wensing M, Penninks AH, Hefle SL, et al. The range of minimum provoking doses in hazelnut-allergic patients as determined by double-blind, placebo-controlled food challenges. *Clin Exp Allergy* 2002; 32:1757–1762.
66. Flinterman AE, Hoekstra MO, Meijer Y, et al. Clinical reactivity to hazelnut in children: association with sensitization to

birch pollen or nuts? *J Allergy Clin Immunol* 2006; 118:1186–1189.

67. Ballmer-Weber BK, Holzhauser T, Scibilia J, et al. Clinical characteristics of soybean allergy in Europe: a double-blind, placebo-controlled food challenge study. *J Allergy Clin Immunol* 2007; 119:1489–1496.
68. Zeiger RS, Sampson HA, Bock SA, et al. Soy allergy in infants and children with IgE-associated cow's milk allergy. *J Pediatr* 1999; 134:614–622.
69. Magnolfi CF, Zani G, Lacava L, Patria MF, Bardare M. Soy allergy in atopic children. *Ann Allergy Asthma Immunol* 1996; 77:197–201.
70. Ito K, Futamura M, Borres MP, et al. IgE antibodies to v-5 gliadin associate with immediate symptoms on oral wheat challenge in Japanese children. *Allergy* 2008; 63:1536–1542.
71. Pastorello EA, Farioli L, Conti A, et al. Wheat IgE-mediated food allergy in European patients: alpha-amylase inhibitors, lipid transfer proteins and low-molecular-weight glutenins. Allergenic molecules recognized by double-blind, placebo-controlled food challenge. *Int Arch Allergy Immunol* 2007; 144:10–22.
72. Scibilia J, Pastorello EA, Zisa G, et al. Wheat allergy: a double-blind, placebo-controlled study in adults. *J Allergy Clin Immunol* 2006; 117:433–439.
73. Figueroa J, Blanco C, Dumpierrez AG, et al. Mustard allergy confirmed by double-blind placebo-controlled food challenges: clinical features and cross-reactivity with mugwort pollen and plant-derived foods. *Allergy* 2005; 60:48–55.
74. Morisset M, Moneret-Vautrin DA, Maadi F, et al. Prospective study of mustard allergy: first study with double-blind placebo-controlled food challenge trials (24 cases). *Allergy* 2003; 58:295–299.
75. Rancé F, Dutau G, Abbal M. Mustard allergy in children. *Allergy* 2000; 55:496–500.
76. Daul CB, Morgan JE, Hughes J, Lehrer SB. Provocation-challenge studies in shrimp-sensitive individuals. *J Allergy Clin Immunol* 1988; 81:1180–1186.
77. Leduc V, Moneret-Vautrin DA, Tzen JTC, Morisset M, Guerin L, Kanny G. Identification of oleosins as major allergens in sesame seed allergic patients. *Allergy* 2006; 61:349–356.
78. Kolopp-Sarda MN, Moneret-Vautrin DA, Gobert B, et al. Specific humoral immune responses in 12 cases of food sensitization to sesame seed. *Clin Exp Allergy* 1998; 27:1285–1291.
79. Kanny G, De Hauteclocque C, Moneret-Vautrin DA. Sesame seed and sesame seed oil contain masked allergens of growing importance. *Allergy* 1996; 51:952–957.
80. Helbling A, Haydel R Jr, McCants ML, Musmand JJ, El-Dahr J, Lehrer SB. Fish allergy: is cross-reactivity among fish species relevant? Double-blind placebo-controlled food challenge studies of fish allergic adults. *Ann Allergy Asthma Immunol* 1999; 83:517–523.
81. Hansen TK, Bindslev-Jensen C. Codfish allergy in adults: identification and diagnosis. *Allergy* 1992; 47:610–617.
82. Ballmer-Weber BK, Vieths S, Lüttkopf D, Heuschmann P, Wüthrich B. Celery allergy confirmed by double-blind, placebo-controlled food challenge: a clinical study in 32 subjects with a history of adverse reactions to celery root. *J Allergy Clin Immunol* 2000; 106:373–378.
83. Moneret-Vautrin DA, Guérin L, Kanny G, Flabbee J, Frémont S, Morisset M. Cross-allergenicity of peanut and lupine: the risk of lupine allergy in patients allergic to peanuts. *J Allergy Clin Immunol* 1999; 104:883–888.
84. Fiocchi A, Sarratud P, Terracciano L, et al. Assessment of the tolerance to lupine-enriched pasta in peanut-allergic children. *Clin Exp Allergy* 2009; 39:1045–1051.
85. Shaw J, Roberts G, Grimshaw K, White S, Hourihane J. Lupin allergy in peanut-allergic children and teenagers. *Allergy* 2008; 63:370–373.
86. Taylor SL, Baumert JL, Houben G, et al. Establishment of action levels for allergenic food residues based upon individual threshold doses for food-allergic individuals. *Food Chem Toxicol* 2012; in preparation.
87. Hourihane JOB, Bedwani SJ, Dean TP, Warner JO. Randomised, double blind, crossover challenge study of allergenicity of peanut oils in subjects allergic to peanuts. *Br Med J (Clin Res Ed)* 1997; 314:1084–1088.
88. Eriksson NE, Möller C, Werner S, Magnusson J, Bengtsson U. The hazards of kissing when you are food allergic. *J Investig Allergol Clin Immunol* 2003; 13:149–154.
89. Hallett R, Haapanen LAD, Teuber SS. Food allergies and kissing. *N Engl J Med* 2002; 346:1833–1834.
90. Sicherer SH, Furlong TJ, DeSimone J, Sampson HA. Self-reported allergic reactions to peanut on commercial airliners. *J Allergy Clin Immunol* 1999; 104:186–189.
91. Perry TT, Conover Walker MK, Pomés A, Chapman MD, Wood RA. Distribution of peanut allergen in the environment. *J Allergy Clin Immunol* 2004; 113:973–976.
92. Simonte SJ, Ma S, Mofidi S, Sicherer SH. Relevance of casual contact with peanut butter in children with peanut allergy. *J Allergy Clin Immunol* 2003; 112:180–182.
93. Sampson HA. Epidemiology of food allergy. *Pediatr Allergy Immunol* 1996; 7 Suppl. 9:42–50.
94. Muraro A, Roberts G, Clark A, et al. The management of anaphylaxis in childhood: position paper of the European academy of allergology and clinical immunology. *Allergy* 2007; 62:857–871.
95. DunnGalvin A, Cullinane C, Daly DA, Flokstra-de Blok BM, Dubois AE, Hourihane JO. Longitudinal validity and responsiveness of the Food Allergy Quality of Life Questionnaire—Parent Form in children 0–12 years following positive and negative food challenges. *Clin Exp Allergy* 2010; 40:476–485.
96. Knibb RC, Ibrahim NF, Stiefel G, et al. The psychological impact of diagnostic food challenges to confirm the resolution of peanut or tree nut allergy. *Clin Exp Allergy* 2012; 42:451–459.
97. Koppelman SJ, Hefle SL. *Detecting Allergens in Food*. Cambridge, UK: Woodhead Publishing Ltd, 2006; 422 p.
98. Hefle SL, Furlong TJ, Niemann L, Lemon-Mule H, Sicherer S, Taylor SL. Consumer attitudes and risks associated with packaged foods having advisory labeling regarding the presence of peanuts. *J Allergy Clin Immunol* 2007; 120:171–176.
99. Catassi C, Fasano A. Celiac disease. *Curr Opin Gastroenterol* 2008; 24:687–691.

7 Immunological Tolerance

Lauren Steele[1] & M. Cecilia Berin[2]

[1]Department of Medical Education, Icahn School of Medicine at Mount Sinai, New York, NY, USA
[2]Pediatric Allergy and Immunology, Icahn School of Medicine at Mount Sinai, New York, NY, USA

Key Concepts

- Oral tolerance is an active immune response to ingested antigen and is mediated through anergy or deletion of reactive T cells and induction of regulatory T cells.
- Antigen form, dose, and timing are important modifiers of oral tolerance induction, as are host characteristics such as age and the gastrointestinal milieu.
- Dendritic cells play a crucial role in directing the gastrointestinal immune response to ingested antigen and commensal bacteria.
- Development of immune tolerance in infants is affected by immunologic interactions between the mother and fetus during pregnancy and between the mother and child through breast-feeding.

Introduction

The gut-associated lymphoid tissue is the largest immune organ in the body and plays a crucial role in coordinating two opposing immune reactions: protection from pathogens and suppression of inappropriate immune response toward harmless antigens derived from food and commensal bacteria. Oral tolerance to food protein was first described by Wells and Osborne in 1911 by experiments that showed that anaphylaxis in guinea pigs could not be induced to proteins that were already present in their diet [1,2]. Oral tolerance is defined as active systemic suppression of cellular or humoral immune responses to an antigen following prior administration of the antigen by the oral route [3]. In the absence of danger signals, tolerance is the default immune response to protein antigens in the gastrointestinal tract. Multiple factors can influence the development of oral tolerance. These include antigen-specific elements as well as host factors such as age, genetics, and the intestinal microbial environment. This chapter will focus on the underlying mechanisms governing oral tolerance. At present, the majority of research studies on oral tolerance have been performed in animal models, although data from human studies are included where possible.

Organization of the gastrointestinal immune system

The digestive tract is variably populated with a population of cells that participate in innate and adaptive immunity against foreign antigens. These include intraepithelial lymphocytes and a dense population of resident immune cells in the lamina propria, as well as organized lymphoid structures such as Peyer's patches (PPs), isolated lymphoid follicles, and mesenteric lymph nodes (MLNs) that drain the small and large intestine. The mucosal immune system can be further divided into effector and inductive sites. The resident population of cells in the lamina propria forms the effector arm of the mucosal immune system and consists of phagocytes that engulf and kill microbes, cytotoxic T cells that kill infected cells, B cells that produce neutralizing antibodies, and helper T cells that support these effector functions through production of cytokines.

Inductive sites of the gastrointestinal tract are organized lymphoid structures that bring together naïve T cells, B cells, and antigen-presenting cells (APC). These include the draining lymph nodes and specialized lymphoid structures within the gastrointestinal mucosa; the latter include PPs

Food Allergy: Adverse Reactions to Foods and Food Additives, Fifth Edition. Edited by Dean D Metcalfe, Hugh A Sampson, Ronald A Simon and Gideon Lack.

in the small intestine and structurally similar lymphoid tissues in the rectum, as well as smaller isolated lymphoid follicles and cryptopatches (precursors to intestinal lymphoid follicles), which are scattered throughout the intestine. After activation in these organized tissues, antigen-specific T and B cells home to the effector sites of the gastrointestinal mucosa.

Gastrointestinal antigen uptake

The gastrointestinal mucosa is exposed to approximately 50–90 g of dietary protein daily [4]. The mucosal immune system is separated from the contents of the lumen by a single layer of columnar epithelial cells that are joined by tight junctions, preventing the passive entry of macromolecules into the lamina propria. As food proteins pass through the stomach and duodenum, gastric acid and digestive enzymes destroy their conformational and linear epitopes and break them down into di- and tripeptides, rendering them less immunogenic while simultaneously permitting absorption of peptides and amino acids as nutrients [5]. In addition to digestion, other barriers to entry of intact food antigens into the mucosa include secretory IgA (sIgA) and a hydrophobic layer of mucin oligosaccharides that trap antigen and prevent absorption of antigenic macromolecules across the intestinal epithelium [6]. Despite these barriers, small but immunologically relevant quantities of food antigen do reach the systemic circulation under normal conditions [7, 8].

Specialized epithelial cells called microfold (M) cells are found in the dome epithelium overlying PPs and lymphoid follicles. These are the main cells that take up particulate antigen (bacteria, viruses, or insoluble food antigens) due to their limited glycocalyx and microvilli [9]. Their sparse cytoplasm and their high endocytic activity allow for efficient delivery to the underlying dendritic cells (DCs), which then transport and present antigen to naïve T cells in the PPs. $CD11c^+$ mononuclear phagocytes also directly sample antigen by extending dendrites across epithelial cells and into the intestinal lumen [10, 11]. In mice, these mononuclear phagocytes express the chemokine receptor CX_3CR1 that is necessary for dendrite formation, are derived from blood monocytes, and do not migrate to the lymph nodes in the steady state [12, 13]. They are considered to be more similar to macrophages than to DCs, despite their expression of CD11c. Soluble antigens do not require specialized antigen-sampling mechanisms to reach the lamina propria. Walker and colleagues showed that antigen was transported across the epithelium of rats by an active endocytic uptake that delivered intact antigen to the basolateral spaces between epithelial cells [14–16]. This transcellular uptake of macromolecules across enterocytes has been confirmed in intestinal resections from human subjects [17]. Once antigen has breached the epithelial barrier, the default immune response is tolerance.

Assessment of oral tolerance

Oral tolerance is defined as systemic nonresponsiveness to antigens after initial exposure by the oral route. In order to measure the extent of this nonresponsiveness, mice are immunized to antigen and compared to immunized mice that were not fed with antigen. Outcome measures can include purely immunologic measures, such as suppression of antigen-specific recall responses from T cells or serum antibody levels [18]. Alternatively, functional outcomes such as suppression of a delayed-type hypersensitivity response [19] or antigen-driven disease (experimental food allergy [20] or experimental autoimmune encephalomyelitis [21]) are used. Experimental oral tolerance can be induced in humans by feeding a non-dietary neo-antigen such as keyhole limpet hemocyanin (KLH), followed by immunization with KLH. Prior oral exposure to antigen results in a suppression of T-cell recall responses in healthy individuals [22, 23].

Site of tolerance induction

The PP was initially thought to be the site of induction of tolerance to food antigens, given its specialized antigen uptake mechanisms. Induction of suppressor cells within the PP could be detected in response to antigen feeding [24, 25]. When tools became available to mechanistically address the role of different gastrointestinal lymphoid compartments, it became clear that PP was not necessary for the development of tolerance. Treatment of pregnant mice with lymphotoxin beta (LTβ) receptor–IgG fusion protein (to neutralize LTβ) abolishes PP in the offspring but leaves the MLN intact. Treatment of pregnant mice with LTβ receptor–IgG fusion protein plus tumor necrosis factor (TNF) receptor–IgG fusion protein abolishes both PP and MLN in the offspring. Offspring lacking PP could be tolerized, whereas mice lacking both PP and MLN could not be tolerized [26, 27]. Tolerance can be induced in exteriorized loops of small intestine that are removed from the flow of luminal contents but that retain their mesenteric connections. This tolerance is not dependent on the presence of a PP in the loop [18]. In contrast, surgical removal of the MLN was found to abolish the tolerance response to orally administered ovalbumin [28]. There is evidence that the liver can also participate in the induction of oral tolerance [29]. The relative role of different sites in the induction of tolerance may be dependent on the nature of the antigen and how it is handled after breaching the intestinal epithelial barrier. It should be noted that immune tolerance can also be induced through the sublingual route [30], indicating that multiple sites along the gastrointestinal tract likely contribute to the development of clinical tolerance to food antigens. However, only the MLNs have been shown to be necessary for the development of tolerance to soluble antigens.

Effector mechanisms of oral tolerance

Anergy, deletion, and suppression

Once antigen has access to the mucosal immune system, it is presented to T cells and generates an adaptive immune response. In oral tolerance, presentation of antigen to naïve T cells results in one of three responses: (1) anergy of antigen-specific T cells, (2) deletion of antigen-specific T cells, and (3) suppression of T effector responses through regulatory T cells (Tregs). Early studies showed that these pathways of tolerance to ingested antigen are dose-dependent. For example, administration of relatively high doses (>5 mg) of fed antigen causes functional disabling of antigen-specific T cells through anergy [31] and deletion [32] of reactive T cells. T cells that become anergic maintain surface Ag receptors but lose the capacity to clonally expand or secrete effector T-cell cytokines (except IL-10), most likely via aberrant antigen presentation by MHC class II lacking key co-stimulators CD80/86 [33]. Anergic cells are capable of mediating active suppression [34], although this requires close cell–cell contact between APC, anergic T cells, and responder T cells, and only occurred when the epitope recognized by the anergic T cell was present [35].

In contrast to high-dose antigen, ingestion of low doses of antigen modulates the immune response through antigen-specific Tregs [32, 36], which actively suppress effector responses. In response to low-dose antigen feeding, both $CD4^+$ and $CD8^+$ T cells have been observed to mediate tolerance as Tregs: feeding antigen was shown to induce regulatory or suppressive $CD4^+$ or $CD8^+$ T cells that can transfer tolerance to a naïve animal [32, 37, 38].

It should be noted, however, that this generalization about the impact of antigen dose on mechanism of tolerance does not always hold. Antigen-specific Tregs have been shown to develop (and transfer) tolerance in the face of high doses (50 mg) of fed antigen [20, 39]. Furthermore, deletion of effector cells and generation of Tregs can coexist as tolerance mechanisms [40]. However, the demonstration of anergy and deletion shows that other tolerance mechanisms exist outside of the generation of Tregs.

Regulatory T cells

Tregs can have many different phenotypes. As mentioned above, tolerance can be transferred to naïve animals with either $CD4^+$ or $CD8^+$ T cells, although oral tolerance occurs normally in the absence of CD8 [32, 36, 41].

One of the first Tregs to be identified as playing a role in both mouse and human oral tolerance was called the Th3 cell [42–44]. Th3 cells were discovered as mucosally derived $CD4^+$ T cells that exhibited both mucosal T helper function and downregulatory properties for Th1 cells via TGF-β [42]. Th3 cells secrete high amounts of TGF-β and low amounts of IL-4 and IL-10. They induce immune tolerance in the periphery and are TGF-β-dependent; treatment with anti-TGF-β abrogated the development of Th3 differentiation [45]. One of the important markers of Th3 cells is their expression of latency-associated peptide (LAP) on the cell surface. LAP is noncovalently attached to TGF-β and forms a latent TGF-β complex. Th3 cells can be distinguished from other regulatory and effector cells by their phenotype of $CD4^+CD25^-Foxp3^-LAP^+$ [46].

Another mucosal Treg has been termed the Tr1 cell. Tr1 cells produce high levels of IL-10 in the absence of IL-2 or IL-4 and can suppress colitis *in vivo* [47]. Although IL-10 is critical for the suppression of (microbial-induced) colitis [48, 49] and is involved in the function of regulatory cells in the airways [50, 51], there is conflicting data on a role for IL-10 and Tr1 cells in the development of oral tolerance [39, 52–54].

Mutations in the transcription factor Foxp3 were identified in 2001 as the basis of disease in scurfy mouse and in immune dysregulation, polyendocrinopathy, enteropathy, X-linked syndrome (IPEX) in humans [55, 56]. Foxp3 was subsequently shown to be expressed in naturally arising thymic-derived Tregs and to control Treg development [57]. Natural Tregs are $CD4^+CD25^+$ and $Foxp3^+$, and their absence results in systemic autoimmunity. Antigen-specific induced Tregs (iTregs) are also $CD4^+CD25^+Foxp3^+$, but they are induced in the periphery from $Foxp3^-$ cells. Using a transgenic T- and B-cell mouse model, it was demonstrated that natural Tregs are not required for the development of oral tolerance, while induced Tregs are essential [39]. $Foxp3^+$ Tregs are necessary for the development of oral tolerance; tolerance was abolished in DEREG mice in which deletion of $Foxp3^+$ T cells is accomplished *in vivo* by treatment with diphtheria toxin [20, 58]. Although deletion of Tregs was transient after antigen feeding (so that at the time of antigen challenge the total number of $Foxp3^+$ Tregs had normalized), antigen-specific Tregs induced by feeding would have been abolished. These data support the concept that iTregs mediate oral tolerance *in vivo*.

A function for one subset of Tregs in the induction of oral tolerance does not preclude the contribution of other subsets. Different subsets may contribute to tolerance in a multistep process; for example, Th3 cells induce the development of $Foxp3^+$ iTregs through a TGF-β-dependent mechanism [45].

Gastrointestinal antigen presentation: the role of dendritic cells

Antigen-specific T cells, whether regulatory or effector cells, are generated from naïve T cells in the periphery through interaction with APC. Of the APC found in the gastrointestinal tract, DCs are the only antigen-capturing cells with the capacity to activate naïve T cells [59]. DCs are found densely packed in the lamina propria and the subepithelial dome of PP. These cells can acquire antigen and migrate to T-cell areas of the PP [60] or the MLN [13].

DCs were shown to contribute to oral tolerance in studies using Flt3 ligand, a growth factor that expands DCs in peripheral lymphoid tissues [61]. Expansion of DCs by Flt3L was associated with a lowered threshold of oral tolerance induction in mice; those that were treated with Flt3L to expand DCs and subsequently fed OVA exhibited a greater degree of tolerance at lower doses of antigen than the control mice. Moreover, lamina propria DCs from antigen-fed mice can transfer tolerance in a manner similar to that induced by transferring Tregs [62].

As discussed previously, the MLN is thought to be the primary site of tolerance induction to fed protein antigens. A subset of DCs within the MLN bearing the marker CD103 is specialized for the induction of Tregs from naïve precursors. CD103$^+$ DCs induce Foxp3$^+$CD4$^+$CD25$^+$ Treg production through a TGF-β and retinoic acid-dependent mechanism in mice and humans [63,64]. CD103$^+$ DCs also express the enzyme indoleamine 2,3-dioxygenase (IDO) which contributes to their ability to induce Foxp3$^+$ Tregs, resulting in the induction of oral tolerance *in vivo* [65]. Retinoic acid and TGF-β production by CD103$^+$ DCs also induce gut-homing IgA plasma cells [66], which may contribute to tolerance through immune exclusion.

CD103$^+$ DCs are the only migratory population of DC in the intestinal lamina propria under steady-state conditions [12, 13]. They migrate to the MLN in a manner dependent on the chemokine receptor CCR7; CCR7–/–mice are deficient in CD103$^+$ DCs in the MLN [67, 68]. These mice are also resistant to development of oral tolerance [69]. Induction of Tregs in the MLN is thought to be the first in a multistep process leading to tolerance. CD103$^+$ DCs imprint gut-homing markers on Tregs, and homing to the lamina propria is required for optimal Treg function [58]. In the LP, these Tregs are expanded by the resident CD11c$^+$ mononuclear phagocytes in a CX$_3$CR1-dependent manner [20].

Mechanisms of tolerance induction may involve different pathways at different sites. For example, induction of tolerance by the sublingual route was mediated by CD11b$^+$CD11c$^-$ macrophage-like cells that express the enzyme for retinoic acid production [30]. In a model of allergic contact dermatitis to a hapten, plasmacytoid DCs in the liver and MLN induce depletion of antigen-specific CD8$^+$ T cells [29]. There is also an associated systemic induction of CD4$^+$ Tregs following initiation of oral tolerance by plasmacytoid DCs in gut-associated lymphoid tissues that contributes to tolerance, but the direct role of plasmacytoid DCs in Treg induction was not determined [40].

Factors affecting development of oral tolerance

Age

Timing of exposure to antigen to optimize tolerance is a matter currently under debate. Several studies have suggested that there may exist a "window of exposure" to antigen that reflects a critical period in developing oral tolerance, both in animals and in humans. This is thought to be related to both the maturity of the infant's immune system and the permeability of the gut barrier. Prospective birth cohort studies have shown that a Th2-dominant immune profile and production of IgE to egg, milk, and peanut are common even in nonatopic infants who do not develop food allergy [70, 71]. However, in these children, the Th2 profile is transient and IgE levels decrease past infancy, while these responses persist and strengthen in allergic children [72]. There is some indication that delayed introduction to foods confer higher risks of allergies in humans, shown in studies on wheat and peanut [73, 74], although it is difficult to draw definitive conclusions based on retrospective studies. In mice, exposure to antigens in the first few days of life resulted in sensitization, whereas tolerance developed when antigen was introduced at 7–10 days of life [75, 76]. In contrast, early oral antigen exposure in neonatal pigs demonstrates that they have a normal capacity for tolerance induction [77].

Barrier function

Intestinal barrier function is provided by the epithelial cells lining the intestinal tract, secreted factors such as mucins and IgA, and digestion of proteins by digestive enzymes. Encapsulation of antigen within liposomes to protect from digestion can transform a tolerance response into a priming response [78]. Administration of antacids has been shown to result in a disruption of oral tolerance induction [79]. Treatment of mice with antacids given either orally or systemically promotes allergic sensitization to digestion-labile allergens such as hazelnut and fish proteins [80, 81]. Some of this adjuvant activity was shown to be due to the alum component of antacids; proton pump inhibitors had a less pronounced effect on immune tolerance [82]. Human studies, although more limited, have shown that long-term antiulcer treatment promotes the development of IgE toward normal digestion-labile dietary compounds such as milk, potato, celery, carrots, apple, orange, wheat, and rye flour [83]. Similarly, in a subset of patients who followed a 3-month course of antiulcer treatment, an increase of hazelnut-specific IgE, hazelnut-specific skin reactivity, and positive oral challenge to hazelnut was observed [80].

A lack of immune exclusion provided by IgA antibodies may also contribute to a defect in tolerance induction. IgA deficiency in children has been reported to be associated with elevated frequency of food allergy [84]. However, IgA deficiency can be found in otherwise healthy individuals, although it is associated with higher levels of systemic antibody responses to food antigens [85, 86].

Immune status

Oral tolerance is the default response to feeding of a neo-antigen, but when adaptive immunity already exists to an antigen it is more difficult to reestablish tolerance and antigen feeding can boost immune responses rather than induce tolerance. This has been a major challenge for the use of oral tolerance as a therapeutic mechanism. The local immune milieu may be a critical factor in the development of tolerance or immunity to fed antigens. In a murine model of celiac disease, it was demonstrated that elevated expression of the cytokine IL-15 in the intestinal mucosa transformed the influence of retinoic acid from regulatory to pro-inflammatory [87] and resulted in a pathogenic response to dietary antigen. In one of the few human trials of oral tolerance induction, subjects with inflammatory bowel disease could not be tolerized by the oral route to a protein neo-antigen [23]. Therefore the existing immune status—either immunity to antigens or the inflammatory milieu in the intestine—may have a profound influence on the development of tolerance.

Microbial influence

Enteric bacteria are an important influence on the GI mucosal immune response to antigen. There are an estimated 1000 species of bacteria and approximately 10^{14} organisms in the healthy human intestinal tract. This flora is readily affected by diet, host genotype, antibiotic use, and infection, among others [88]. Foxp3$^+$ Tregs and IL-17-producing CD4$^+$ cells are particularly abundant in the intestinal mucosa, and their function and numbers are markedly affected by the presence of intestinal microbiota [88]. The intestinal microbiome may act as the primary stimulus for postnatal immune development. Germ-free mice exhibit decreased activation of PP immune cells [89] and absent intestinal IgA secretion [90], and may fail to develop oral tolerance, although evidence to date has been controversial [91, 92]. It is clear, however, that colonization of the gastrointestinal tract is required for normal immunologic development. *Bacteroides thetaiotaomicron*, a commensal bacterium, was shown to modulate expression of genes involved in nutrient absorption, mucosal barrier fortification, xenobiotic metabolism, angiogenesis, and postnatal intestinal maturation in germ-free mice [93]. Signaling by commensal bacteria through TLR9 has been shown to favor increased development of T effector cells over T regulatory cells in the small intestine [94]. The presence of certain microbial species, such as segmented filamentous bacteria, can promote the development of Th17 cells in the small intestine [95, 96]. In contrast to these effector cell-promoting effects of microbial constituents, polysaccharide A from *Bacteroides fragilis* interacts with innate immune Toll-like receptors and promotes downstream induction of Foxp3$^+$ Tregs that produce IL-10 during colonization in germ-free animals [97]. A loss of pro-tolerogenic microbial species, or a gain of anti-tolerogenic species, may hinder the development of normal tolerance to dietary antigens. Although extensive studies of the microbiome of food-allergic individuals have not yet been performed, it has been shown that allergic children are colonized with less enterococci and bifidobacteria during the first year of life compared to nonallergic children [98]. Other examples of dysbiosis in food allergy have also been reported [99]. Colonization of germ-free mice with flora derived from healthy infants showed a protective effect on the development of experimental food allergy [100]. It has not yet been determined if flora from allergic individuals would be less protective.

Maternal influence in the breast-feeding infant

The relationship between exposure to antigen during pregnancy and breast-feeding and development of tolerance is a matter of continued debate. Exposure to antigen during pregnancy and lactation has been shown to be protective in animal models [101–103], although most of the studies have been performed in OVA-induced asthma models using inhalation exposure. The ability to draw conclusions about human tolerance induction from these animal studies is limited; studies employing food allergy models have used rodent mothers that are either antigen-naïve or antigen-sensitized, whereas most pregnant or lactating mothers are often antigen-tolerant and will have normal physiologic production of food-specific IgA and IgG. The data presented below are drawn largely from animal studies, although human studies are discussed when possible.

Dose of antigen exposure during pregnancy and lactation can influence the development of tolerance [104]. Low-dose OVA during pregnancy induced a lasting tolerance in pups and was associated with high levels of TGF-β in breast milk, whereas high-dose exposure early in pregnancy and/or the perinatal period induced transient inhibition of IgE followed by higher IgE production. TGF-β has been shown to be active at the intestinal mucosa and promote oral tolerance in mice that were fed with antigen plus TGF-β [105]. Mechanistic studies have shown that antigen exposure through the breast milk results in immune tolerance and protection from experimental asthma in the

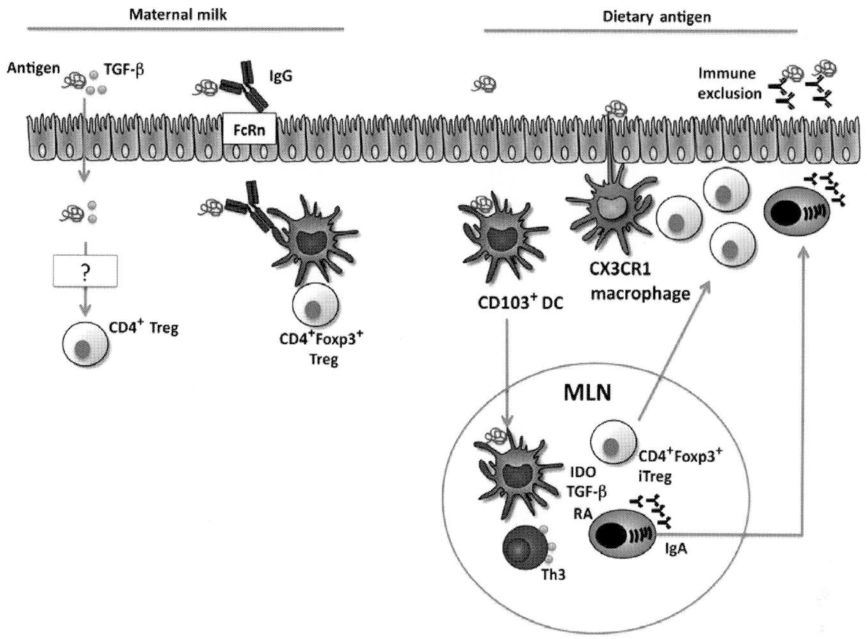

Figure 7.1 Mechanisms of tolerance induction. In the neonate, exposure to antigens in breast milk that contains TGF-β can induce immune tolerance mediated by regulatory T cells (Tregs). This induction of Tregs is dependent on TGF-β signaling on the T cell. When IgG antibodies are present in the breast milk, facilitated antigen uptake through FcRn leads to TGF-β-independent tolerance induction. DCs stimulated with antigen–IgG complexes induce Foxp3$^+$CD4$^+$ Tregs. In the adult, dietary antigens induce immune tolerance by default. Migratory CD103$^+$ DCs capture antigen and migrate to the MLN, where they induce gut-homing Tregs through IDO, TGF-β, and retinoic acid (RA). These Tregs migrate back to the lamina propria where they are expanded by resident macrophages. CD103$^+$ DCs also promote the development of IgA-secreting gut-homing plasma cells that can contribute to tolerance through immune exclusion.

offspring. Tolerance induced in the offspring is mediated by CD4$^+$ Tregs whose generation is dependent on milk-derived TGF-β but is independent of IL-10 [106].

Studies on the impact of maternal immune status have shown that antigen-exposed sensitized or immunized mothers transfer a more profound tolerance to their offspring than naïve mothers [54]. Mothers immunized with a Th1 adjuvant were found to induce a greater level of tolerance in their offspring compared to mothers immunized with a Th2 adjuvant [107]. Mothers immunized to a bystander antigen did not transmit tolerance to their offspring, indicating that there is antigen specificity to the tolerance response. This tolerance in sensitized or immunized mice was subsequently found to be due to the presence of IgG–antigen complexes in the breast milk, and tolerance induction was dependent on the epithelial IgG receptor FcRn [54, 108]. FcRn on epithelial cells functions as an antigen-sampling mechanism to draw antigen–IgG complexes across the epithelial barrier [109]. DCs exposed to antigen in the context of immune complexes with IgG preferentially induced CD4$^+$CD25$^+$Foxp3$^+$ Tregs [54]. These studies show that antibodies present in maternal milk can play a profound role in shaping the resulting immune response of the infant. Human studies have shown that antigen-specific and total IgA levels in maternal milk were significantly lower in mothers whose children developed cow's milk allergy, indicating that IgA may play a critical role in preventing early sensitization to food allergens [110].

In addition to TGF-β and antibodies, human breast milk contains growth factors that promote cell maturation in the intestine and intestinal colonization by bacterial flora, as well as bioactive cytokines, sIgA, lactoferrin, lysozyme, and platelet-activating factor acetylhydrolase, which have varied roles in enhancing the maturation of the infant's immune system [111]. TGF-β, IL-6, and IL-10 are involved in IgA synthesis and were found to correlate with total colostrum IgA; it is possible that this association may explain a stimulatory effect on IgA production in breast-fed infants [112]. Other immunomodulatory agents including prostaglandin E2 and IL-10 have been identified at physiologically active levels in breast milk [112, 113].

Finally, in humans there is conflicting data on the impact of maternal peanut consumption during pregnancy or lactation. Peanut consumption has been reported to have no effect on child sensitization to peanut in one study [114], while another study found a dose-dependent positive association of maternal peanut consumption with sensitization of the infants to peanut [115]. The LEAP (*Learning Early About Peanut allergy*) study and the EAT (*Enquiring About Tolerance*) study are underway and have been designed specifically to address whether early introduction of peanut into the infant diet will promote the development of immune tolerance to peanut.

Conclusion

Development of oral tolerance to ingested antigens is a multistep process influenced by immune and environmental factors. The immunological milieu of the mucosal immune system facilitates tolerance based on the coordinated interactions between antigen, DCs, and T cells. We know that the normal response of the mucosal immune system, one of active immune tolerance to food antigen, is mediated largely by a specialized subset of gastrointestinal DCs that induce Tregs in response to orally ingested antigen. Local immune factors, including the production of TGF-β and retinoic acid by gastrointestinal DCs, promote this tolerance response. Multiple environmental factors including commensal microbiota and factors in breast milk may influence the development of tolerance in children. A summary of these mucosal tolerance mechanisms is shown in Figure 7.1. In the context of food allergy, a comprehensive understanding of these tolerance mechanisms may lead to the development of new prevention strategies to avoid sensitization to foods as well as therapeutic strategies to reestablish tolerance to foods.

References

1. Wells HG. Studies on the chemistry of anaphylaxis (III). Experiments with isolated proteins, especially those of the hen's egg.*J Infect Dis* 1911; 9(2):147–171.
2. Wells HG, Osborne TB. The biological reactions of the vegetable proteins. *J Infect Dis* 1911; 8:66–124.
3. Chase MW. Inhibition of experimental drug allergy by prior feeding of the sensitizing agent. *Proc Soc Exp Biol Med* 1946; 61:257–259.
4. Fulgoni III VL. Current protein intake in America: analysis of the National Health and Nutrition Examination Survey, 2003–2004. *Am J Clin Nutr* 2008; 87(5):1554S–1557S.
5. Michael JG. The role of digestive enzymes in orally induced immune tolerance. *Immunol Invest* 1989; 18(9–10):1049–1054.
6. Perrier C, Corthesy B. Gut permeability and food allergies. *Clin Exp Allergy* 2011; 41(1):20–28.
7. Husby S, Jensenius JC, Svehag SE. Passage of undegraded dietary antigen into the blood of healthy adults. Quantification, estimation of size distribution, and relation of uptake to levels of specific antibodies. *Scand J Immunol* 1985; 22(1):83–92.
8. Husby S, Jensenius JC, Svehag SE. Passage of undegraded dietary antigen into the blood of healthy adults. Further characterization of the kinetics of uptake and the size distribution of the antigen. *Scand J Immunol* 1986; 24(4):447–455.
9. Frey A, Giannasca KT, Weltzin R, et al. Role of the glycocalyx in regulating access of microparticles to apical plasma membranes of intestinal epithelial cells: implications for microbial attachment and oral vaccine targeting. *J Exp Med* 1996; 184(3):1045–1059.
10. Rescigno M, Urbano M, Valzasina B, et al. Dendritic cells express tight junction proteins and penetrate gut epithelial monolayers to sample bacteria. *Nat Immunol* 2001; 2(4):361–367.
11. Niess JH, Brand S, Gu X, et al. CX3CR1-mediated dendritic cell access to the intestinal lumen and bacterial clearance. *Science* 2005; 307(5707):254–258.
12. Bogunovic M, Ginhoux F, Helft J, et al. Origin of the lamina propria dendritic cell network. *Immunity* 2009; 31(3):513–525.
13. Schulz O, Jaensson E, Persson EK, et al. Intestinal CD103+, but not CX3CR1+, antigen sampling cells migrate in lymph and serve classical dendritic cell functions.*J Exp Med* 2009; 206(13):3101–3114.
14. Walker WA, Cornell R, Davenport LM, Isselbacher KJ. Macromolecular absorption. Mechanism of horseradish peroxidase uptake and transport in adult and neonatal rat intestine. *J Cell Biol* 1972; 54(2):195–205.
15. Cornell R, Walker WA, Isselbacher KJ. Small intestinal absorption of horseradish peroxidase. A cytochemical study. *Lab Invest* 1971; 25(1):42–48.
16. Warshaw AL, Walker WA, Cornell R, Isselbacher KJ. Small intestinal permeability to macromolecules. Transmission of horseradish peroxidase into mesenteric lymph and portal blood. *Lab Invest* 1971; 25(6):675–684.
17. Soderholm JD, Streutker C, Yang PC, et al. Increased epithelial uptake of protein antigens in the ileum of Crohn's disease mediated by tumour necrosis factor alpha. *Gut* 2004; 53(12):1817–1824.
18. Kraus TA, Brimnes J, Muong C, et al. Induction of mucosal tolerance in Peyer's patch-deficient, ligated small bowel loops.*J Clin Invest* 2005; 115(8):2234–2243.
19. Blazquez AB, Mayer L, Berin MC. Thymic stromal lymphopoietin is required for gastrointestinal allergy but not oral tolerance. *Gastroenterology* 2010; 139(4):1301–1309.
20. Hadis U, Wahl B, Schulz O, et al. Intestinal tolerance requires gut homing and expansion of FoxP3+ regulatory T cells in the lamina propria. *Immunity* 2011; 34(2):237–246.
21. Gonnella PA, Chen YH, Waldner H, Weiner HL. Induction of oral tolerization in CD86 deficient mice: a role for CD86 and B cells in the up-regulation of TGF-beta. *J Autoimmun* 2006; 26(2):73–81.
22. Husby S, Mestecky J, Moldoveanu Z, Holland S, Elson CO. Oral tolerance in humans. T cell but not B cell tolerance after antigen feeding. *J Immunol* 1994; 152(9):4663–4670.
23. Kraus TA, Toy L, Chan L, Childs J, Mayer L. Failure to induce oral tolerance to a soluble protein in patients with inflammatory bowel disease. *Gastroenterology* 2004; 126(7):1771–1778.
24. Ngan J, Kind LS. Suppressor T cells for IgE and IgG in Peyer's patches of mice made tolerant by the oral administration of ovalbumin. *J Immunol* 1978; 120(3):861–865.
25. MacDonald TT. Immunosuppression caused by antigen feeding II. Suppressor T cells mask Peyer's patch B cell priming to orally administered antigen. *Eur J Immunol* 1983; 13(2):138–142.
26. Spahn TW, Fontana A, Faria AM, et al. Induction of oral tolerance to cellular immune responses in the absence of Peyer's patches. *Eur J Immunol* 2001; 31(4):1278–1287.
27. Spahn TW, Weiner HL, Rennert PD, et al. Mesenteric lymph nodes are critical for the induction of high-dose oral tolerance in the absence of Peyer's patches. *Eur J Immunol* 2002; 32(4):1109–1113.
28. Worbs T, Bode U, Yan S, et al. Oral tolerance originates in the intestinal immune system and relies on antigen carriage by dendritic cells. *J Exp Med* 2006; 203(3):519–527.

29. Goubier A, Dubois B, Gheit H, et al. Plasmacytoid dendritic cells mediate oral tolerance. *Immunity* 2008; 29(3):464–475.
30. Mascarell L, Saint-Lu N, Moussu H, et al. Oral macrophage-like cells play a key role in tolerance induction following sublingual immunotherapy of asthmatic mice. *Mucosal Immunol* 2011; 4(6):638–647.
31. Whitacre CC, Gienapp IE, Orosz CG, Bitar DM. Oral tolerance in experimental autoimmune encephalomyelitis. III. Evidence for clonal anergy. *J Immunol* 1991; 147(7):2155–2163.
32. Chen Y, Inobe J, Weiner HL. Induction of oral tolerance to myelin basic protein in CD8-depleted mice: both CD4+ and CD8+ cells mediate active suppression. *J Immunol* 1995; 155(2):910–916.
33. Schwartz RH. T cell anergy. *Annu Rev Immunol* 2003; 21:305–334.
34. Jordan MS, Riley MP, von Boehmer H, Caton AJ. Anergy and suppression regulate CD4(+) T cell responses to a self peptide. *Eur J Immunol* 2000; 30(1):136–144.
35. Taams LS, van Rensen AJ, Poelen MC, et al. Anergic T cells actively suppress T cell responses via the antigen-presenting cell. *Eur J Immunol* 1998; 28(9):2902–2912.
36. Garside P, Steel M, Liew FY, Mowat AM. CD4+ but not CD8+ T cells are required for the induction of oral tolerance. *Int Immunol* 1995; 7(3):501–504.
37. Zhang X, Izikson L, Liu L,Weiner HL. Activation of CD25(+)CD4(+) regulatory T cells by oral antigen administration. *J Immunol* 2001; 167(8):4245–4253.
38. Arnaboldi PM, Roth-Walter F, Mayer L. Suppression of Th1 and Th17, but not Th2, responses in a CD8(+) T cell-mediated model of oral tolerance. *Mucosal Immunol* 2009; 2(5):427–438.
39. Mucida D, Kutchukhidze N, Erazo A, Russo M, Lafaille JJ, Curotto de Lafaille MA. Oral tolerance in the absence of naturally occurring Tregs. *J Clin Invest* 2005; 115(7):1923–1933.
40. Dubois B, Joubert G, Gomez de Aguero M, Gouanvic M, Goubier A, Kaiserlian D. Sequential role of plasmacytoid dendritic cells and regulatory T cells in oral tolerance. *Gastroenterology* 2009; 137(3):1019–1028.
41. Lider O, Santos LM, Lee CS, Higgins PJ, Weiner HL. Suppression of experimental autoimmune encephalomyelitis by oral administration of myelin basic protein. II. Suppression of disease and in vitro immune responses is mediated by antigen-specific CD8+ T lymphocytes. *J Immunol* 1989; 142(3):748–752.
42. Chen Y, Kuchroo VK, Inobe J, Hafler DA, Weiner HL. Regulatory T cell clones induced by oral tolerance: suppression of autoimmune encephalomyelitis. *Science* 1994; 265(5176):1237–1240.
43. Fukaura H, Kent SC, Pietrusewicz MJ, Khoury SJ, Weiner HL, Hafler DA. Induction of circulating myelin basic protein and proteolipid protein-specific transforming growth factor-beta1-secreting Th3 T cells by oral administration of myelin in multiple sclerosis patients. *J Clin Invest* 1996; 98(1):70–77.
44. Inobe J, Slavin AJ, Komagata Y, Chen Y, Liu L, Weiner HL. IL-4 is a differentiation factor for transforming growth factor-beta secreting Th3 cells and oral administration of IL-4 enhances oral tolerance in experimental allergic encephalomyelitis. *Eur J Immunol* 1998; 28(9):2780–2790.
45. Carrier Y, Yuan J, Kuchroo VK, Weiner HL. Th3 cells in peripheral tolerance. I. Induction of Foxp3-positive regulatory T cells by Th3 cells derived from TGF-beta T cell-transgenic mice. *J Immunol* 2007; 178(1):179–185.
46. Weiner HL, da Cunha AP, Quintana F, Wu H. Oral tolerance. *Immunol Rev* 2011; 241(1):241-259.
47. Groux H, O'Garra A, Bigler M, et al. A CD4+ T-cell subset inhibits antigen-specific T-cell responses and prevents colitis. *Nature* 1997; 389(6652):737–742.
48. Kuhn R, Lohler J, Rennick D, Rajewsky K, Muller W. Interleukin-10-deficient mice develop chronic enterocolitis. *Cell* 1993; 75(2):263–274.
49. Rakoff-Nahoum S, Paglino J, Eslami-Varzaneh F, Edberg S, Medzhitov R. Recognition of commensal microflora by toll-like receptors is required for intestinal homeostasis. *Cell* 2004; 118(2):229–241.
50. Akbari O, DeKruyff RH, Umetsu DT. Pulmonary dendritic cells producing IL-10 mediate tolerance induced by respiratory exposure to antigen. *Nat Immunol* 2001; 2(8):725–731.
51. Akbari O, Freeman GJ, Meyer EH, et al. Antigen-specific regulatory T cells develop via the ICOS-ICOS-ligand pathway and inhibit allergen-induced airway hyperreactivity. *Nat Med* 2002; 8(9):1024–1032.
52. Gonnella PA, Waldner HP, Kodali D, Weiner HL. Induction of low dose oral tolerance in IL-10 deficient mice with experimental autoimmune encephalomyelitis. *J Autoimmun* 2004; 23(3):193–200.
53. Zhou Y, Kawasaki H, Hsu SC, et al. Oral tolerance to food-induced systemic anaphylaxis mediated by the C-type lectin SIGNR1. *Nat Med* 2010; 16(10):1128–1133.
54. Mosconi E, Rekima A, Seitz-Polski B, et al. Breast milk immune complexes are potent inducers of oral tolerance in neonates and prevent asthma development. *Mucosal Immunol* 2010; 3(5):461–474.
55. Bennett CL, Christie J, Ramsdell F, et al. The immune dysregulation, polyendocrinopathy, enteropathy, X-linked syndrome (IPEX) is caused by mutations of FOXP3. *Nat Genet* 2001; 27(1):20–21.
56. Brunkow ME, Jeffery EW, Hjerrild KA, et al. Disruption of a new forkhead/winged-helix protein, scurfin, results in the fatal lymphoproliferative disorder of the scurfy mouse. *Nat Genet* 2001; 27(1):68–73.
57. Hori S, Nomura T, Sakaguchi S. Control of regulatory T cell development by the transcription factor Foxp3. *Science* 2003; 299(5609):1057–1061.
58. Cassani B, Villablanca EJ, Quintana FJ, et al. Gut-tropic T cells that express integrin alpha4beta7 and CCR9 are required for induction of oral immune tolerance in mice. *Gastroenterology* 2011; 141(6):2109–2118.
59. Liu LM, MacPherson GG. Antigen acquisition by dendritic cells: intestinal dendritic cells acquire antigen administered orally and can prime naive T cells in vivo. *J Exp Med* 1993; 177(5):1299–1307.
60. Shreedhar VK, Kelsall BL, Neutra MR. Cholera toxin induces migration of dendritic cells from the subepithelial dome region to T- and B-cell areas of Peyer's patches. *Infect Immun* 2003; 71(1):504–509.

61. Viney JL, Mowat AM, O'Malley JM, Williamson E, Fanger NA. Expanding dendritic cells in vivo enhances the induction of oral tolerance. *J Immunol* 1998; 160(12):5815–5825.
62. Chirdo FG, Millington OR, Beacock-Sharp H, Mowat AM. Immunomodulatory dendritic cells in intestinal lamina propria. *Eur J Immunol* 2005; 35(6):1831–1840.
63. Coombes JL, Siddiqui KR, Arancibia-Carcamo CV, et al. A functionally specialized population of mucosal CD103+ DCs induces Foxp3+ regulatory T cells via a TGF-beta and retinoic acid-dependent mechanism. *J Exp Med* 2007; 204(8):1757–1764.
64. Jaensson E, Uronen-Hansson H, Pabst O, et al. Small intestinal CD103+dendritic cells display unique functional properties that are conserved between mice and humans. *J Exp Med* 2008; 205(9):2139–2149.
65. Matteoli G, Mazzini E, Iliev ID, et al. Gut CD103+ dendritic cells express indoleamine 2,3-dioxygenase which influences T regulatory/T effector cell balance and oral tolerance induction. *Gut* 2010; 59(5):595–604.
66. Mora JR, Iwata M, Eksteen B, et al. Generation of gut-homing IgA-secreting B cells by intestinal dendritic cells. *Science* 2006; 314(5802):1157–1160.
67. Johansson-Lindbom B, Svensson M, Pabst O, et al. Functional specialization of gut CD103+ dendritic cells in the regulation of tissue-selective T cell homing.*J Exp Med* 2005; 202(8):1063–1073.
68. Jang MH, Sougawa N, Tanaka T, et al. CCR7 is critically important for migration of dendritic cells in intestinal lamina propria to mesenteric lymph nodes. *J Immunol* 2006; 176(2):803–810.
69. Worbs T, Forster R. A key role for CCR7 in establishing central and peripheral tolerance. *Trends Immunol* 2007; 28(6):274–280.
70. Prescott SL, Macaubas C, Smallacombe T, Holt BJ, Sly PD, Holt PG. Development of allergen-specific T-cell memory in atopic and normal children. *Lancet* 1999; 353(9148):196–200.
71. Sigurs N, Hattevig G, Kjellman B, Kjellman NI, Nilsson L, Bjorksten B. Appearance of atopic disease in relation to serum IgE antibodies in children followed up from birth for 4 to 15 years. *J Allergy Clin Immunol* 1994; 94(4):757–763.
72. Holt PG. Prenatal versus postnatal priming of allergen specific immunologic memory: the debate continues. *J Allergy-Clin Immunol* 2008; 122(4):717–718.
73. Poole JA, Barriga K, Leung DY, et al. Timing of initial exposure to cereal grains and the risk of wheat allergy. *Pediatrics* 2006; 117(6):2175–2182.
74. Du Toit G, Katz Y, Sasieni P, et al. Early consumption of peanuts in infancy is associated with a low prevalence of peanut allergy. *J Allergy Clin Immunol* 2008; 122(5):984–991.
75. Strobel S, Ferguson A. Immune responses to fed protein antigens in mice. 3. Systemic tolerance or priming is related to age at which antigen is first encountered. *Pediatr Res* 1984; 18(7):588–594.
76. Hanson DG. Ontogeny of orally induced tolerance to soluble proteins in mice. I. Priming and tolerance in newborns. *J Immunol* 1981; 127(4):1518–1524.
77. Haverson K, Corfield G, Jones PH, et al. Effect of oral antigen and antibody exposure at birth on subsequent immune status. A study in neonatal pigs. *Int Arch Allergy Immunol* 2009; 150(2):192–204.
78. Alves AC, Ramaldes GA, Oliveira MC, et al. Ovalbumin encapsulation into liposomes results in distinct degrees of oral immunization in mice. *Cell Immunol* 2008; 254(1):63–73.
79. Untersmayr E, Jensen-Jarolim E. The role of protein digestibility and antacids on food allergy outcomes.*J Allergy Clin Immunol* 2008; 121(6):1301–1308; quiz 9–10.
80. Scholl I, Untersmayr E, Bakos N, et al. Antiulcer drugs promote oral sensitization and hypersensitivity to hazelnut allergens in BALB/c mice and humans. *AmJClin Nutr* 2005; 81(1):154–160.
81. Untersmayr E, Scholl I, Swoboda I, et al. Antacid medication inhibits digestion of dietary proteins and causes food allergy: a fish allergy model in BALB/c mice. *J Allergy Clin Immunol* 2003; 112(3):616–623.
82. Brunner R, Wallmann J, Szalai K, et al. Aluminium per se and in the anti-acid drug sucralfate promotes sensitization via the oral route. *Allergy* 2009; 64(6):890–897.
83. Untersmayr E, Bakos N, Scholl I, et al. Anti-ulcer drugs promote IgE formation toward dietary antigens in adult patients. *FASEB J* 2005; 19(6):656–658.
84. Janzi M, Kull I, Sjoberg R, et al. Selective IgA deficiency in early life: association to infections and allergic diseases during childhood. *Clin Immunol* 2009; 133(1):78–85.
85. Cunningham-Rundles C, Brandeis WE, Good RA, Day NK. Milk precipitins, circulating immune complexes, and IgA deficiency. *Proc Natl Acad Sci USA* 1978; 75(7):3387–3389.
86. Husby S, Oxelius VA, Svehag SE. IgG subclass antibodies to dietary antigens in IgA deficiency quantification and correlation with serum IgG subclass levels. *Clin Immunol Immunopathol* 1992; 62(1 Pt. 1):85–90.
87. DePaolo RW, Abadie V, Tang F, et al. Co-adjuvant effects of retinoic acid and IL-15 induce inflammatory immunity to dietary antigens. *Nature* 2011; 471(7337):220–224.
88. Atarashi K, Honda K. Microbiota in autoimmunity and tolerance. *Curr Opin Immunol* 2011; 23(6):761–768.
89. MacDonald TT, Carter PB. Isolation and functional characteristics of adherent phagocytic cells from mouse Peyer's patches. *Immunology* 1982; 45(4):769–774.
90. McClelland DB. Peyer's-patch-associated synthesis of immunoglobulin in germ-free, specific-pathogen-free, and conventional mice. *Scand J Immunol* 1976; 5(8):909–915.
91. Ishikawa H, Tanaka K, Maeda Y, et al. Effect of intestinal microbiota on the induction of regulatory CD25+ CD4+ T cells. *Clin Exp Immunol* 2008; 153(1):127–135.
92. Walton KL, Galanko JA, Balfour Sartor R, Fisher NC. T cell-mediated oral tolerance is intact in germ-free mice. *Clin Exp Immunol* 2006; 143(3):503–512.
93. Hooper LV, Wong MH, Thelin A, Hansson L, Falk PG, Gordon JI. Molecular analysis of commensal host-microbial relationships in the intestine. *Science* 2001; 291(5505):881–884.
94. Hall JA, Bouladoux N, Sun CM, et al. Commensal DNA limits regulatory T cell conversion and is a natural adjuvant of intestinal immune responses. *Immunity* 2008; 29(4):637–649.

95. Ivanov, II, Atarashi K, Manel N, et al. Induction of intestinal Th17 cells by segmented filamentous bacteria. *Cell* 2009; 139(3):485–498.
96. Gaboriau-Routhiau V, Rakotobe S, Lecuyer E, et al. The key role of segmented filamentous bacteria in the coordinated maturation of gut helper T cell responses. *Immunity* 2009; 31(4):677–689.
97. Round JL, Mazmanian SK. Inducible Foxp3+ regulatory T-cell development by a commensal bacterium of the intestinal microbiota. *Proc Natl Acad Sci USA* 2010; 107(27):12204–12209.
98. Bjorksten B, Sepp E, Julge K, Voor T, Mikelsaar M. Allergy development and the intestinal microflora during the first year of life. *J Allergy Clin Immunol* 2001; 108(4):516–520.
99. Thompson-Chagoyan OC, Fallani M, Maldonado J, et al. Faecal microbiota and short-chain fatty acid levels in faeces from infants with cow's milk protein allergy. *Int Arch Allergy Immunol* 2011; 156(3):325–332.
100. Rodriguez B, Prioult G, Hacini-Rachinel F, et al. Infant gut microbiota is protective against cow's milk allergy in mice despite immature ileal T-cell response. *FEMS Microbiol Ecol* 2012; 79(1):192–202.
101. Okamoto Y, Freihorst J, Ogra PL. Maternal determinants of neonatal immune response to ovalbumin: effect of breast feeding on development of anti-ovalbumin antibody in the neonate. *Int Arch Allergy Appl Immunol* 1989; 89(1):83–89.
102. Polte T, Hansen G. Maternal tolerance achieved during pregnancy is transferred to the offspring via breast milk and persistently protects the offspring from allergic asthma. *Clin ExpAllergy* 2008; 38(12):1950–1958.
103. Matson AP, Thrall RS, Rafti E, Puddington L. Breastmilk from allergic mothers can protect offspring from allergic airway inflammation. *Breastfeed Med* 2009; 4(3):167–174.
104. Fusaro AE, de Brito CA, Taniguchi EF, et al. Balance between early life tolerance and sensitization in allergy: dependence on the timing and intensity of prenatal and postnatal allergen exposure of the mother. *Immunology* 2009; 128(1 Suppl.):e541–e550.
105. Ando T, Hatsushika K, Wako M, et al. Orally administered TGF-beta is biologically active in the intestinal mucosa and enhances oral tolerance. *J Allergy Clin Immunology* 2007; 120(4):916–923.
106. Verhasselt V, Milcent V, Cazareth J, et al. Breast milk-mediated transfer of an antigen induces tolerance and protection from allergic asthma. *Nat Med* 2008; 14(2):170–175.
107. Matson AP, Zhu L, Lingenheld EG, et al. Maternal transmission of resistance to development of allergic airway disease. *J Immunol* 2007; 179(2):1282–1291.
108. Matson AP, Thrall RS, Rafti E, Lingenheld EG, Puddington L. IgG transmitted from allergic mothers decreases allergic sensitization in breastfed offspring. *Clin Mol Allergy* 2010; 8:9.
109. Baker K, Qiao SW, Kuo T, et al. Immune and non-immune functions of the (not so) neonatal Fc receptor, FcRn. *Semin Immunopathol* 2009; 31(2):223–236.
110. Jarvinen KM, Laine ST, Jarvenpaa AL, Suomalainen HK. Does low IgA in human milk predispose the infant to development of cow's milk allergy? *Pediatr Res* 2000; 48(4):457–462.
111. Labbok MH, Clark D, Goldman AS. Breastfeeding: maintaining an irreplaceable immunological resource. *Nat Rev Immunol* 2004; 4(7):565–572.
112. Bottcher MF, Jenmalm MC, Garofalo RP, Bjorksten B. Cytokines in breast milk from allergic and nonallergic mothers. *Pediatr Res* 2000; 47(1):157–162.
113. Hawkes JS, Bryan DL, James MJ, Gibson RA. Cytokines (IL-1beta, IL-6, TNF-alpha, TGF-beta1, and TGF-beta2) and prostaglandin E2 in human milk during the first three months postpartum. *Pediatr Res* 1999; 46(2):194–199.
114. Fox AT, Sasieni P, du Toit G, Syed H, Lack G. Household peanut consumption as a risk factor for the development of peanut allergy. *J Allergy Clin Immunol* 2009; 123(2):417–423.
115. Sicherer SH, Wood RA, Stablein D, et al. Maternal consumption of peanut during pregnancy is associated with peanut sensitization in atopic infants. *J Allergy ClinImmunol* 2010; 126(6):1191–1197.

8 *In Vitro* Diagnostic Methods in the Evaluation of Food Hypersensitivity

Robert G. Hamilton
Division of Allergy and Clinical Immunology, Departments of Medicine and Pathology, Johns Hopkins University School of Medicine, Baltimore, MA, USA

Key Concepts

- Positive serological measurements of food-specific IgE antibodies confirm sensitization in support of a clinical history-driven diagnosis of food allergy.
- Three IgE antibody autoanalyzers employed worldwide display comparable analytical sensitivity (0.1 kU_A/L) and excellent intra-assay precision and inter-assay reproducibility, but they detect different quantitative levels of IgE antibody for any given food specificity.
- Low quantitative levels of food-specific IgE antibody (<0.35 kU_A/L) have unknown clinical significance.
- A quantitative (kU_A/L) food-specific IgE level can be judiciously used as a risk factor for select food specificities to facilitate a decision about the need for an oral food challenge.
- Allergenic component-specific IgE serology can facilitate diagnosis by identifying pollen–food cross-reactivities and, in select cases (e.g., peanut), identifying a risk for severe food-induced allergic reactions.
- Food-specific IgG or IgG4 antibody measurements should not be performed in the diagnostic workup of a food-allergic patient as no objective evidence exists for their role in inducing immediate-type hypersensitivity reactions.
- Wheat, gliadin, endomysium, and tissue transglutaminase-specific IgG/IgA antibodies can be useful in the evaluation of patients for celiac disease.

Introduction

The clinical laboratory plays a seminal role in the diagnosis and management of an estimated 6% of children and 3.7% of adults who manifest allergic symptoms following the consumption of foods [1]. The detection of food-specific antibodies aids the clinician in distinguishing between immunologically mediated reactions (food allergy and celiac disease) and nonimmunologically mediated intolerance induced by food consumption. The diagnostic process begins with a thorough clinical history and physical examination, in which one or several allergic symptoms are associated with consumption of a food. These reactions can involve the skin (pruritus, urticaria, angioedema, flushing), GI tract (oral pruritus, nausea, vomiting, diarrhea), nasal/respiratory tract (nasal congestion, rhinorrhea, ocular pruritus, sneezing, nasal pruritus, laryngeal edema, wheezing, shortness of breath), and/or the cardiovascular system (light-headedness, syncope, hypotension).

Hypersensitivity as used in this chapter is a term to indicate an objectively defined and reproducible symptom (acute reactions, urticaria, oral allergy syndrome) that occurs following the consumption of or exposure to a food substance. Once the clinician develops a high degree of suspicion that a food exposure is inducing a hypersensitivity reaction, a second level in the diagnostic algorithm involves confirmation of sensitization by evaluation of the patient for food-specific antibody. This involves either an *in vivo* analysis for IgE antibody (e.g., skin testing, see Chapter 21) or an *in vitro* analysis for food-specific IgE, IgG, or IgA antibody that is performed in a clinical laboratory. The latter topic is addressed in this chapter. If the antibody result is discordant with the clinical history, then a third-level evaluation may involve an *in vivo* provocation analysis (e.g., oral food challenge, see Chapter 21). Laboratory testing is then able to help classify immunologically mediated food-induced symptoms into allergic hypersensitivity, which involves food-specific IgE antibody or a non-IgE-mediated hypersensitivity (e.g., celiac disease) that involves gliadin-specific IgG and IgA antibodies and immune cells.

Food Allergy: Adverse Reactions to Foods and Food Additives, Fifth Edition. Edited by Dean D Metcalfe, Hugh A Sampson, Ronald A Simon and Gideon Lack.

Food-specific antibody assays

IgE was identified as a unique immunoglobulin isotype and the mediator of immediate-type hypersensitivity reactions in 1967 [2]. That same year, the radioallergosorbent test was reported as a method of detecting allergen-specific IgE antibody in human serum [3]. The original test involved the covalent binding of a mixture of extracted components from a single allergen source (e.g., peanut) or a mixture of allergen extracts (e.g., peanut, chicken egg, cow's milk, soybean, wheat, cod fish) onto a single activated cellulose matrix (paper disc). When incubated with the patient's serum, antibodies specific for any of these components would bind. A buffer wash removed unbound serum proteins and bound IgE antibody was detected with an I^{125}-labeled anti-human IgE Fc reagent. The assay was initially calibrated using a birch pollen-specific IgE antibody (heterologous) serum that was incubated at multiple dilutions using birch pollen allergen discs. Relative levels of IgE antibody detected were reported relative to an arbitrarily defined unit and graded into class groups.

Over the years, extensive improvements have been made in the assay reagents even though the current IgE antibody assays employ the same basic chemistry [4]. New solid phase matrices are used that have a higher binding capacity. The assays generate a chemiluminescent or fluorescent response instead of the need for detection of radioactivity. The use of nonisotopic enzymatic labels as opposed to radioisotopes has lengthened the shelf-life (stability) of the reagents. Moreover, safety concerns related to the use of radioisotopes have been eliminated. The principal assay systems available widely throughout the world are autoanalyzers. The automation and random access capability provided by these computer-driven autoanalyzers have enhanced their intra-assay precision and inter-assay reproducibility [5]. Reduced misclassification and transcription errors are a result of eliminated reagent mix-up errors. A higher quality IgE antibody results with a shorter turnaround time. The assays today are calibrated using a generic heterologous calibration system that involves a total IgE two-site (capture and detection antibody) chemistry. Clinical assays available today employ an IgE standard that is traceable to the WHO's total serum IgE reference preparation (WHO 75/502). This has allowed closer agreement of results between assays and a common analytical sensitivity among the assays of 0.1 kIU/L (where 1 IU = 2.4 ng of IgE). Despite the enhanced lower limit of assay detection, IgE antibody results that are reported between 0.1 and 0.35 kU/L have an unknown clinical significance. These need to be interpreted by an experienced clinician who knows the patient's history and reported allergenic exposures. As IgE antibody levels increase above 0.35 kU/L, their relative level becomes increasingly predictive in food-allergic individuals of an immediate-type allergic process as judged by oral food provocation endpoints [6].

Despite extensive efforts to establish a common calibration system based on the WHO IgE reference preparation, the three principal assays (Table 8.1) that are used widely in most countries report slightly different results for any given food allergen specificity [5, 7, 8]. This is especially true when extracts of foods are used as reagents. Food allergen extraction is a variable process that results in different amounts of allergens being incorporated into the various assays' reagents. This results in excellent agreement among the three autoanalyzer systems in terms of qualitative detection (presence or absence) of IgE antibody in any given serum. However, quantitatively, the IgE antibody levels reported from these three assays do not precisely agree with each other [5, 7, 8]. It remains unclear whether the observed inter-assay variability can be resolved if the three assay systems that have different coupling chemistries use the identical extract or recombinant and native allergenic components as reagents.

One novel immunochromatographic IgE antibody assay has been developed for rapid detection of a limited number of aeroallergen and food allergen specificities [9]. The handheld cassette has been designed as a lateral flow point-of-care IgE antibody assay (e.g., ImmunoCAP Rapid, Thermo Fisher Scientific). Ten thin lines of allergen extracts are bound to an activated paper surface and a drop of blood is administered to the device. Following minutes, buffer is added to a conjugate well that migrates colloidal gold-anti-IgE up the paper. If IgE has bound to the allergen line, anti–IgE-gold binds, producing a red line that is

Table 8.1 Currently available allergen-specific IgE assays from clinical laboratories in North America.

Manufacturer[a]	Assay name	Instrument type	Data units
Hycor Biomedical	HYTEC 288	Autoanalyzer	kU_A/L—quantitative
Siemens Healthcare	Immulite System	Autoanalyzer	kU_A/L—quantitative
Thermo Fisher Scientific	ImmunoCAP System	Autoanalyzer	kU_A/L—quantitative
Thermo Fisher Scientific	ISAC System[a]	Chip microarray	ISU—semiquantitative
Thermo Fisher Scientific	ImmunoCAP Rapid	Lateral flow point-of-care test	Positive/negative—visual class 1–3. reader

[a]The ISAC is not FDA cleared for clinical patient testing.

visible by eye or an optical scanner. While this device has been configured with 10 food specificities, the US FDA has restricted its sale as a point-of-care test in the United States for the detection of food-specific IgE. Since the presence of IgE antibody is not synonymous with the presence of allergic disease, the FDA's decision resulted from a concern over anticipated misinterpretation of food-specific IgE antibody results by primary care physicians or patients that could lead to inappropriate avoidance of foods.

The most recent addition to the allergen-specific IgE testing methodology is the chip-based immuno-solid phase allergen chip or ISAC assay (Thermo Fisher Scientific). The ISAC is an activated chip which is imprinted with purified native or recombinant allergenic components (Tables 8.1 and 8.2) from more than 100 specificities in triplicate dots in a defined matrix pattern [10, 11]. A sample of human serum (30 μL) is layered over the allergen-coated chip area and specific antibodies of any isotype bind. Following a buffer wash, fluorescent-labeled anti-IgE is layered over the same surface to detect bound IgE. After a final buffer wash, bound fluorescence is quantified in a chip scanner. Antibody cross-reactivity, especially between pollen and food allergens is effectively assessed with the ISAC. Its analytical sensitivity approaches that of the singleplex assays and it reports results as ISU, which are semiquantitative. The fact that a fixed repertoire of allergen specificities must be analyzed is considered a constraining limitation of overtesting if only limited IgE antibody specificities are desired by the clinician. Moreover, a second concern is the potential for interference by non-IgE antibodies as a result of the use of allergen-limiting microdots.

An analogous chip-based microarray for IgE antibody detection has been reported that uses allergen extracts instead of allergenic components [12]. Its performance, however, against established predicate devices will require further documentation. Neither chip device is FDA cleared for clinical use. Thus, their data are currently used in supplemental support of diagnostic autoanalyzer-based singleplex IgE antibody results.

Table 8.2 Mainly species specific allergenic food components in serological IgE antibody assays.

Chicken egg (*Gallus domesticus*)	
Egg white	Gal d 1—ovomucoid
	Gal d 2—ovalbumin
	Gal d 3—conalbumin
Egg yolk	Gal d 5—albumin
Cow's milk (*Bos domesticus*)	Bos d 4-alpha lactalbumin
	Bos d 5-beta lactoglobulin
	Bos d 8-casein
	Bos d lactoferrin
Fish (Cod) (*Gadus morhua*)	Gad c 1-Parvalbumin—calcium binding protein
Shrimp (*Penaeus monodon*)	Pen m 2—arginine kinase
	Pen m 4
Nuts and seeds	
Cashewnut (*Anacardium occidentale*)	Ana o 2—legumin-like protein
Brazil nut (*Bertholletia exelsa*)	Ber e 1—2S albumin
Hazelnut (*Corylus avellana*)	Cor a 9—11S globulin
Walnut (*Juglans* spp.)	Jug r 1—2S albumin
	Jug r 2—7S vicilin-like globulin
Sesame (*Sesamum indicum*)	Ses i 1—2S albumin
Legumes	
Peanut (*Arachis hypogaea*)	Ara h 1—glycinin—seed storage
	Ara h 2—conglutin—trypsin inhibitor
	Ara h 3—glycinin—seed storage
	Ara h 6—conglutin—2S albumin
Soy (*Glycine max*)	Gly m 5
	Gly m 6—2S albumin
Cereals	
Buckwheat (*Fagopyrum esculentum*)	Fag e 2
Wheat (*Triticum aestivum*)	Tri a 14
	Tri a 19.010 (gliadin, gluten)
Fruit	
Kiwi (*Actinidia deliciosa*)	Act d 1—actinidin—cysteine protease
	Act d 5

Indications for allergen-specific IgE testing

According to NIAID Consensus Guidelines [1, 13], individuals who present with anaphylaxis or cutaneous, ocular, upper or lower respiratory tract, gastrointestinal, or cardiovascular symptoms within minutes to hours after ingesting a food are candidates for evaluation. In addition, children with eosinophilic, esophagitis, enterocolitis, enteropathy, and atopic dermatitis should be considered for evaluation. Detection of food-specific IgE in serum from individuals experiencing these conditions identifies the individual as sensitized and at a risk for a clinical reaction if reexposed subsequently to the same food. Multiple studies have identified hen's egg, cow's milk, peanuts, soybean products, wheat, tree nuts, and fish as accounting for 90% of food reactions in children [1, 13–16]. In contrast, adults experience allergic reactions most commonly to peanuts, tree nuts, fish, and shellfish. Importantly, the presence of food-specific IgE alone is not sufficient to consider an individual as having a food allergy without a linkage to an objectively collected history of a reaction following exposure to the food in question.

IgG and IgA antibody detection in celiac disease

Celiac disease is an autoimmune enteropathy in which the lining of the small intestine is damaged and absorption of nutrients is compromised. This leads to gastrointestinal symptoms which include abdominal pain, bloating, diarrhea, nausea, and vomiting and that overlap with food-specific IgE-mediated allergic symptoms. It is triggered by the ingestion of gluten found in wheat, barley, rye, and possibly oats that elicit an antibody response [17]. Historically, the only means of diagnosing celiac disease was through invasive biopsies. With the availability of IgG and IgA anti-gliadin analyses, the need for a diagnostic biopsy has been reduced. Elimination of gluten from the diet tends to restore intestinal villi and resume food adsorption. Some of the same assays in Table 8.1 and less automated ELISAs are used to detect IgG and IgA antibodies specifically for gliadin in wheat, and endomysium and tissue transglutaminase in the serum of patients suspected of having celiac disease [17–19]. The presence of serum tissue transglutaminase and endomysial IgA autoantibodies is predictive of small bowel abnormalities and thus indicative of celiac disease.

Food allergens

While there are several hundred foods that are known to contain allergens, only a small number (chicken egg, cow's milk, peanut, soybean, wheat, tree nuts, and fish) elicit the majority of food-induced allergic reactions [20]. Historically, allergenic molecules have been extracted from complex animal- and plant-based foodstuffs using different processing protocols. This leads to mixtures of both immunogenic (including allergenic) molecules that elicit antibodies and those which are not immunogenic. Ideally, a physiological extract of a food is prepared in such a manner that it preserves and contains all the allergenic molecules present in that food [21]. These food allergen extracts are then immobilized on a solid phase using one of several chemistries. Use of these food allergen-containing reagents should theoretically permit a comprehensive detection of IgE antibody against all the clinically relevant allergens in that particular food.

Occasionally, an important allergenic component is shown to be labile during the manufacturing process and it may be supplemented with native or recombinant allergen. This practice, however, can lead to unintended consequences due to structural similarity with molecules in other allergenic groups. One high-profile illustration of this involved the PR-10/Bet v 1 homologue cross-reactive family in which hazelnut was supplemented with labile Cor a 1 [22]. Due to a well-documented cross-reactivity between birch pollen-derived Bet v 1 and hazelnut Cor a 1, serum from birch pollen-allergic individuals containing IgE anti-Bet v 1 began being strongly detected and reported as high IgE anti-hazelnut levels using this reagent. Whether the reported hazelnut-specific IgE as measured in this assay results from cross-reactive IgE anti-Bet v 1 or a true Cor a 1 specificity is not easily determined by the clinician receiving the serological report. In contrast to cross-reactive Cora1 specific IgE, the presence of IgE anti-Cor a 9 and 14 (hazelnut storage proteins) provides evidence for direct hazelnut sensitization [23]. It is possible that cross-reactive IgE anti-Bet v 1 detection may be useful to some clinicians evaluating a suspected hazelnut-allergic individual. However, this has remained unclear and the clinical significance of cross-reactive IgE antibody is currently being further studied.

Allergenic food components

An added level of complexity occurs with foods since they are consumed either as raw foodstuffs or processed by boiling and roasting, or as dried or fermented foods. As such, it has been difficult for the manufacturers of IgE antibody assays to recreate the ideal presentation of food antigens in their reagents. Variations in the number and structure of antigenic epitopes also change or are destroyed during digestion in the gastrointestinal tract following natural exposure. Antigenic epitopes can also be created as neoantigens or destroyed during the manufacturer's processing (extraction, chemical coupling). Some food extracts, for example, those prepared from apples, can even show differences among the varieties. Others such as celery, hazelnut, and peanut appear to have more consistency in their composition among the different varieties [20]. Heat treatment is particularly a concern during the extraction step as it can often alter the allergenic potency of a diagnostically used food extract, especially for apples, hazelnut, and celery.

Increasingly the principal allergenic molecules in complex food extracts are being identified, isolated, cloned, sequenced, and reproduced as recombinant allergenic components [24]. Those recombinant allergens that do not maintain their antigenic epitopes as assessed empirically in IgE antibody-based diagnostic assays can be replaced with native molecules that are isolated directly from food extracts. Proteins with analogous structures and biological functions in different species of plants can be recognized by the same IgE antibody, even though there has been no known exposure to that allergen specificity. These interactions represent cross-reactivity of IgE antibodies across structurally similar molecules. Of the component allergens that have been identified and produced as recombinant proteins, there are a number of food proteins that reflect species specificity. A different set of food components can be used to identify IgE antibody that can cross-react among structurally similar families of allergenic proteins that are found in both foods and aeroallergens [25–27]. The food component specificities that are available for the assessment of IgE antibody in patient's sera on the microarray

Table 8.3 Cross-reactive food–aeroallergen components in serological IgE antibody assays.

Tropomyosin: actin-binding muscle protein that regulates actin mechanics in muscle contraction	
Anisakis-Herring worm (*Anisakis simplex*)	Ani s 3
German cockroach (*Blattella germanica*)	Bla g 7
Dust mite (*Dermatophagoides pteronyssinus*)	Der p 10
Shrimp (*Penaeus monodon*)	Pen m 1
Serum albumin: protein in blood that functions to transport fats and fatty acids to muscle tissue	
Cow (*Bos domesticus*)	Bos d 6
Dog (*Canis familaris*)	Can f 3
Horse (*Equus caballus*)	Equ c 3
Cat (*Felis domesticus*)	Fel d 2
Nonspecific lipid transfer proteins: conserved plant proteins that function to shuttle phospholipids and other fatty acids between cell membranes	
Peanut (*Arachis hypogaea*)	Ara h 9
Hazelnut (*Corylus avellana*)	Cor a 8
Walnut (*Juglans* spp.)	Jug r 3
Peach (*Prunus persica*)	Pru p 3
Mugwort	
Olive pollen	
Plane tree	
Pathogenesis related proteins: PR10 family (Bet v 1 homologues)	
Birch (*Betula verrucosa*)	Bet v 1
Hazel pollen (*Corylus avellana*)	Cor a 1.010
Hazelnut (*Corylus avellana*)	Cor a 1.040
Apple (*Malus domesticus*)	Mal d 1
Peach (*Prunus persica*)	Pru p 1
Soybean (*Glycine max*)	Gly m 4
Peanut (*Arachis hypogaea*)	Ara h 8
Kiwi (*Actinidia deliciosa*)	Act d 8
Celery	
Profilin: an actin-binding protein involved in the dynamic turnover and restructuring of the actin cytoskeleton	
Birch (*Betula verrucosa*)	Bet v 2
Natural rubber latex (*Hevea brasiliensis*)	Hev b 8
Mercury	
Timothy grass	
Carbohydrate cross-reactive determinants:	
Bromelain (pineapple)	MUXF3

chip-based ISAC (Thermo Fisher Scientific) are summarized in Table 8.2 (species specific) and Table 8.3 (food–aeroallergen cross-reactive). The latter group which shares extensive homology includes the PR-10/Bet v 1 homologue, lipid transfer protein, tropomysin, and profilin families that can promote pollen–food-allergic syndrome and allergens with carbohydrate cross-reactive determinants (CCDs) that exhibit extensive cross-reactivity among the foods.

Peanut is the one food specificity where component-specific IgE testing has been identified as adding diagnostically useful information in the quest to minimize oral food challenges. In an initial population-based birth cohort, component-resolved diagnostics using microarray analysis was used to differentiate 8-year-old children who were IgE anti-peanut positive and failed food challenge from those who passed the challenge and were thus deemed to be peanut tolerant [28]. This study reported that approximately one quarter (22.4%) of IgE anti-peanut extract-positive (sensitized) children actually failed an oral peanut challenge. Moreover, they identified Ara h 2 as the most important IgE anti-peanut component specificity that best predicted clinical allergy as evidenced by a failed oral peanut challenge. Subsequent studies [29, 30] have reproduced this observation that Ara h 2-specific IgE antibody can effectively differentiate between peanut-allergic and peanut-tolerant children. Using a 0.35 kU_A/L criterion for positivity, IgE anti-Ara h 2 by ImmunoCAP displayed a diagnostic sensitivity and specificity of 88% and 84%, respectively. Other investigators have stressed that not only IgE anti-Ara h 2 positivity, but also Ara h 1 and 3 positivity should be considered in the identification of individuals at risk for reactions to peanuts [31]. IgE anti-Ara h 1, Ara h 2, and Ara h 3 positivity were identified in 60.0%, 72.7%, and 43.6%, respectively, of peanut-allergic children. This contrasted with 7.4%, 1.5%, and 7.4% in the group of children who were peanut tolerant [31]. Quantitative levels of IgE anti-Ara h 1, 2, and 3 were also significantly higher in the peanut-allergic group. Finally, Ara h 8 is structurally similar to Bet v 1 in birch pollen. IgE anti-Ara h 8 positivity in the absence of IgE anti-Ara h 1, 2, and 3 tended to display tolerance to peanuts in most individuals [32]. Where reactions did occur in individuals with an exclusive IgE anti-Ara h 8 response, they tended to be mild and were restricted to the oral cavity. Thus, at present, peanut appears to be the principal food where component-resolved IgE antibody testing clearly provides enhanced diagnostic information over the peanut extract-based food-specific IgE measurement.

Food allergen epitopes

Currently available IgE antibody assays (Table 8.1) only provide a measure of the presence and concentration of IgE antibody to intact allergens extracted from foods. However, the specificity or diversity of the IgE antibody together with its concentration, affinity, and the IgE-specific activity (specific IgE/total IgE ratio) contributes to whether a state of sensitization (IgE positivity) will translate into the manifestation of an allergic symptom following a repeated allergen exposure [33, 34]. By identifying the patient's pattern of specific IgE-binding epitopes, the hope was that this additional information would provide insight into the patient's risk for a mild or severe reaction and the degree of persistence of their sensitivity from childhood into adulthood.

To this end, the specificity of specific IgE antibodies has been mapped to sequential (linear) and conformational IgE-binding epitopes on some food allergens [35]. Sequential epitopes that are formed by contiguous amino acids survive heat denaturation during cooking and gastrointestinal tract digestion, while conformation epitopes that depend on the tertiary structure of the allergen often do not survive denaturation. Protease-digested or chemically cleaved allergenic proteins were historically probed by Western blot analysis with IgE antibody-containing sera. The IgE-binding allergen fragments were then subsequently amino acid sequenced [36]. More recently, overlapping peptides that span the primary amino acid sequences of characterized food allergens are coupled to membranes or microarray chips and probed with IgE-containing sera [37, 38]. Sequential IgE-binding epitopes have been shown to span five to eight amino acids or longer. The number of amino acids and actual sequences in the linear epitopes recognized by milk-, egg-, and peanut-specific IgE tend to vary among patients. In contrast, studies of conformational epitopes have been more limited due to the difficulty in preserving the three-dimensional structure. They are, however, known to be important in oral allergy syndrome and respiratory allergy and they vary in their ability to withstand gastric digestion [39]. The greater the diversity of IgE-binding epitopes (or specificity of the IgE response), the more at risk the individual is for severe allergic reactions to peanut, egg, and milk [38–40], based on historical data. However, because the epitope-binding patterns for any given food are heterogeneous among patients with comparable food allergy histories, application of epitope mapping in the diagnosis and prognosis of food allergy is considered limited [41]. Moreover, since the detection of food-specific IgE antibody simply signifies sensitization to a peptide or protein, it is best viewed as a risk factor and not as a proof that allergen will cross-link IgE on effector cells and trigger mediator release.

Predictive quantitative allergen-specific IgE levels

The definitive test for the diagnosis of food allergy is an oral food challenge. However, since the controlled administration of food to a person who is possibly sensitized to that food is a time-consuming and potentially risky procedure, there has been great interest in developing an alternative method that could identify individuals who do not need food challenges. Using retrospectively and prospectively collected sera from a group of children with atopic dermatitis, specific IgE levels were identified that provided a 95% probability of failing a food challenge to milk, egg, peanut, and fish [42, 43]. These were landmark studies, because for the first time the allergy community considered a quantitative level of specific IgE antibody for select foods as defining a clinical decision point above which there was a high probability of failing an oral food challenge. This has had the consequence of reducing the number of oral food challenges in individuals.

Subsequent studies attempting to replicate these seminal initial findings have shown large differences in the observed IgE anti-food concentration that predicts a given probability of a failed food challenge. These differences in the reported predictive clinical decision levels among studies may be attributed to differences in the study subjects' diet, specific food, demographics (especially age), disease state (e.g., presence or absence of atopic dermatitis), and the challenge protocol and data analysis methods. Due to the wide range of reported food-specific IgE antibody concentrations associated with a 95% probability of failing an oral food challenge (e.g., Table 8.4), one must exercise judicious care when extrapolating a clinical significance of any quantitative measure of IgE antibody based on population-derived predictive probability values to an individual. While some clinicians have elected to use a specific IgE level that provides a reported 95% probability of an oral food challenge failure rate, others employ an antibody concentration decision criterion that represents a 50% likelihood of passing or failing a food challenge [50]. Limited data suggest that a correlation between the magnitude of specific IgE and severity of clinical reaction in egg-allergic children may exist [51]. However, in general, the magnitude of a food-specific IgE level does not predict the severity of the clinical reaction [52]. Additionally, there is a suggestion that a direct relationship exists between the IgE-specific activity (e.g., peanut-specific IgE to total IgE ratio) and the severity of a challenge reaction [53]. However, other investigators have found the specific to total IgE ratio to be no more helpful than the specific IgE level alone in predicting the severity outcome of a food challenge [54].

The allergen-specific IgE antibody level may also aid in predicting the natural history of an allergy to peanuts [55], tree nuts [56], cow's milk [57], and hen's egg [58]. These studies provide target levels of food-specific IgE antibody above which it is less likely that an individual will develop tolerance to a particular food as they mature into adulthood. Moreover, the more rapid the rate of decline of a food-specific IgE level, the more likely a subject is to develop tolerance to the food consumption over time [59].

Finally, the published food-specific IgE antibody data discussed in this overview that relate to predictive values for failing a food challenge and developing tolerance with age have been obtained using the ImmunoCAP System (Table 8.1). Since other autoanalyzers are known to report different results for any allergen specificity with the same serum, the question has arisen whether one can make decisions about the need for a food challenge using IgE antibody as measured in a non-ImmunoCAP assay. One

Table 8.4 Review of clinical studies reporting positive predictive values of food-specific IgE testing.

Study	No. subjects	% Atopic dermatitis	Average age (years)	Study design	Food	Total IgE median (kU/L) (range)	PPV value (%)/specific IgE level (kU/L)	Sens. for IgE level (%)	Spec. for IgE level (%)
Sampson and Ho [42]	196	100	5.2	Retrospective DBPCFC in 64%	Cow's milk	3000 (100–40 000)	95/32	51	98
Sampson [43]	62	61	3.8	Prospective DBPCFC in 34%	Cow's milk	[a]	95/15	57	94
Garcia-Ara et al. [44]	170	23	0.4	Prospective open controlled challenge in 95%	Cow'smilk	[a]	95/5	30	99
Celik-Bilgili et al. [45]	398	88	1.1	Prospective DBPCFC or open challenge in all	Cow'smilk	[a]	90/88.8	[a]	[a]
Sampson and Ho [42]	196	100	5.2	Retrospective DBPCFC in 64%	Hen's egg	3000 (100–40 000)	95/6	72	90
Sampson [43]	75	61	3.8	Prospective DBPCFC in 33%	Hen's egg	[a]	98/7	61	95
Celik-Bilgili et al. [45]	227	88	1.1	Prospective DBPCFC or open challenge in all	Hen's egg	[a]	95/12.6	[a]	[a]
Boyano Martinez et al. [46]	81	43	1.3	Prospective, Open controlled challenge in all	Egg white	40 (3–597)	94/0.35	91	77
Osterballe et al. [47]	56	100	2.2	Prospective, open challenge in all	Egg white	[a]	100/1.5	60	100
Sampson and Ho [42]	196	100	5.2	Retrospective DBPCFC in 64%	Peanut	3000 (100–40 000)	95/15	73	92
Sampson [43]	68	61	3.8	Prospective DBPCFC in 2%	Peanut	[a]	100/14	57	100
Maloney et al. [48]	234	57	6.1	Prospective; clinical history, no challenges	Peanut	[a]	99/13	60	96

Source: Modified from data in Reference 49.
[a]Not provided.

study has directly examined this question by analyzing sera in the ImmunoCAP and Immulite from patients with IgE positivity (>0.1 kUA/L) to chicken egg white, cow's milk, and/or peanut [60]. The IgE antibody levels from both assays for each of the three food specificities were highly correlated. However, more importantly, empirically determined Immulite/ImmunoCAP ratios (mean $\pm$ 1 SD) were 4.85 $\pm$ 1.79 kUA/L (egg), 2.33 $\pm$ 1.0 kUA/L (milk), and 1.86 $\pm$ 0.98 kUA/L (peanut). Since reported predictive values for the ImmunoCAP alone can vary among studies by up to 10-fold (Table 8.4), they are possibly best used in decision making as a relative and not an absolute benchmark for the need for an oral challenge. Thus, these inter-assay data that vary by less than fivefold [60] suggest that IgE anti-egg, milk, and peanut results as measured in the Immulite may also be useful as a relative benchmark for decision making about the need for a subsequent oral food challenge.

Analytes and assays with little or no confirmed value in the diagnosis of food allergy

There are a number of analytes that are measured by the clinical immunology laboratory that are limited in their diagnostic value during the workup of a patient suspected of having a food allergy.

Total serum IgE

The clinical laboratory performs a quantitative measurement of total serum IgE that in select circumstances can be of value in the diagnostic workup of a food allergy patient. In general, total serum IgE provides a rough indication of the atopic disposition of a patient. However, since the nonatopic population range is broad and varies with age, it remains limited in its predictive value for diagnosing allergic disease. The few applications where total serum IgE serves the clinician productively include (a) the determination of the suitability of the patient to receive anti-IgE treatment (Omalizumab/Xolair; 30 to 700 kU/L target range); (b) defining the dose of anti-IgE that needs to be administered, which is partially based on the patient's baseline total IgE level; (c) adjudicating the clinical significance with very low specific IgE antibody levels when the IgE-specific activity (specific IgE/total IgE ratio) [61] is high; and (d) part of the diagnostic workup for allergic bronchopulmonary aspergillosis where an elevated total serum IgE is a diagnostic criterion along with a positive IgE anti-*Aspergillus fumigatus* analysis.

Tryptase

The laboratory quantifies mast cell tryptase by immunoassay as a marker of mast cell degranulation during systemic anaphylaxis. Tryptase is a serine esterase with four subunits, each having an enzymatically active site. At rest, the mast cell contains 10–35 pg of tryptase. Upon activation of the mast cell, tryptase is dissociated from heparin and rapidly degrades into its monomers as a mature form which loses enzymatic activity. Total tryptase levels in the serum of healthy (nondiseased) adults average 5 μg/L (range 1–10 μg/L). During systemic anaphylaxis with hypotension, elevated levels of tryptase (>10 μg/L) can be detected in serum from 1 to 4 hours after the event [62]. A diagnosis of systemic mastocytosis is supported by a baseline total tryptase level >20 μg/L. Mature tryptase levels <1 μg/L are observed in nondiseased individuals and >1 μg/L of mature tryptase in serum indicates mast cell activation. Tryptase is thus used principally to verify mast cell degranulation following a suspected anaphylactic event and not as a routine diagnostic allergy test. There is recent indication that elevated baseline levels of mast cell tryptase may serve as a risk marker for severe insect venom anaphylaxis [63]. Whether baseline tryptase measurements may also serve equally well as a risk factor in severe reactions in the diagnostic workup of suspected food-allergic patients is yet to be determined.

Food antigen-specific IgG antibody

In 1982, one study showed that monoclonal antibodies specific for human IgG4 could induce histamine release from basophils [64]. This led to the suggestion that antigen-specific IgG4 antibodies are reaginic and to the present-day quest of disgruntled patients with negative IgE antibody serologies to seek IgG4 anti-food measurements to prove their "food allergy." This *in vitro* phenomenon was later shown to be a result of IgG4 anti-IgE autoantibodies bound to IgE (IgG–IgE complexes) on the surface of basophils which were activated to release histamine following the addition of human IgG4-specific monoclonal antibodies [65, 66]. Thus, based on all the objective data that are available, serological testing of IgG or IgG4 antibodies specific for food antigens is considered irrelevant in the laboratory workup of food allergy or intolerance [67]. In fact, food allergen-specific IgG and IgG4 antibodies can be viewed as markers of exposure to food components that are recognized by the human immune system as foreign. Since there is no objective evidence that IgG antibodies induce immediate-type hypersensitivity reactions, food-specific IgG or IgG4 antibody analyses should not be performed in the diagnostic workup of a patient with suspected allergic disease.

Basophil histamine release test

The BHR test assesses the release of histamine from peripheral blood basophils that occurs following the cross-linking of IgE antibodies that are bound to basophil surface receptors [68]. In general, there is a good correlation between the results of the BHR test and puncture skin test and serological measures of specific IgE antibody [69]. However, limitations associated with identifying the optimal concentration of the challenging food allergen and logistics of shipping whole blood in a timely manner to the laboratory have relegated the BHR test to a research assay rather than a routine diagnostic test. Finally, there are concerns about high spontaneous histamine release with specimens from food-allergic individuals [70], a problem with nonresponsive basophils in 10% of individuals [71], and the induction of histamine release by complement activation and direct activation by idiosyncratic reactions to aspirin which reduce the BHR test's overall diagnostic specificity.

Other analytes

Leukotrienes and prostaglandins have been used in research studies to monitor allergic inflammation. The CAST or CAST-ELISA has been designed to measure leukotrienes that are released from basophils following exposure to food allergens [72]. Concerns about allergen-extract contamination with endotoxin that can lead to false-positive CAST-ELISA results and the same concerns as the BHR test with logistics and optimization have limited the routine utility of this test in the diagnosis of food allergy.

A number of cytokines including IL-4, IL-5, IL-13, and interferon gamma have been extensively measured in research studies of food-induced allergic inflammation [73]. However, the levels of these cytokines in serum have never been shown to be diagnostically useful in the workup of an allergic patient.

Eosinophil cationic protein (ECP) is a research analyte that is used to follow the levels of eosinophils following food challenges in allergic individuals. While increased levels of ECP have been reported after positive oral food challenges [74], the results indicate that ECP measurements have limited value in the diagnostic workup of an allergic patient.

Laboratory considerations

Because the three primary IgE antibody autoanalyzers (Table 8.1) in use today have similar chemistries and total IgE heterologous calibration schemes and they all report to the same analytical sensitivity (0.1 kU_A/L), it is not possible to determine from the data in a laboratory report which method was used in the analysis. However, since the three assays are known to report different levels of IgE antibody [4–8], it is important to know what method was used to perform a particular IgE antibody analysis. It is therefore critical that the assay method be listed on the patient's final report. Moreover, the measurements need to be performed in a licensed clinical immunology laboratory that successfully participates in a peer-reviewed external proficiency survey, such as that conducted by the College of American Pathologists [5]. It is ultimately the responsibility of the clinician to require that these criteria are met before the IgE antibody data are used to support a clinical history and physical examination-based diagnosis of allergic disease [75].

Summary

Diagnosis of IgE-mediated food allergy remains based on the clinical history, and sensitization is confirmed with laboratory-based food allergen-specific IgE measurements. IgE antibody assay technology has improved with the development of reproducible autoanalyzers, highly quality controlled reagents, lateral flow point-of-care assays, and chip-based microarrays. While the latter two technologies can sometimes facilitate the diagnosis, the food allergen extract-based singleplex IgE antibody assay on autoanalyzers remains the principal diagnostic test for the workup of a suspected food-allergic individual. Three IgE antibody autoanalyzers are employed worldwide which display comparable analytical sensitivity (0.1 kU_A/L) and excellent intra-assay precision and inter-assay reproducibility. However, they detect different quantitative levels of IgE antibody for any given food specificity. Low quantitative levels of food-specific IgE antibody ($<0.35\ kU_A/L$) have unknown clinical significance. Quantitative (kU_A/L) food-specific IgE levels can be judiciously employed as risk factors for select food specificities to facilitate the clinician's decision about the need for an oral food challenge and to better assess the natural history of a patient's allergic reactions to select foods. Allergenic component-resolved diagnosis can identify pollen–food cross-reactivity and for select foods (e.g., peanut) it can identify a risk for severe food-induced allergic reactions. Food-specific IgG or IgG4 antibody measurements should not be performed in the diagnostic workup of a food-allergic patient as no objective evidence exists for their role in inducing immediate-type hypersensitivity reactions. Tests that have minimal or no diagnostic utility in the workup of a food-allergic patient include total serum IgE, tryptase, ECP, mediators (histamine, leukotrienes) and cytokines, and the basophil-based histamine and leukotriene release tests.

References

1. NIAID-Sponsored Expert Panel; Boyce JA, Assa'ad A, Burks AW, et al. Guidelines for the diagnosis and management of food allergy in the United States: report of the NIAID-sponsored expert panel. *J Allergy Clin Immunol* 2010; 126(Suppl. 6):1–58.
2. Hamilton RG. The science behind the discovery of IgE (invited, Allergy Archives). *J Allergy Clin Immunol* 2005; 115:648–652.
3. Wide L, Bennich H, Johansson SGO. Diagnosis of allergy by an in vitro test for allergen antibodies. *Lancet* 1967; 2:1105–1107.
4. Matsson P, Hamilton RG, Homburger HA, et al. *Analytical Performance Characteristics and Clinical Utility of Immunological Assays for Human Immunoglobulin E (IgE) Antibody of Defined Allergen Specificities*, 2nd edn. Clinical Laboratory Standards Institute 1/LA20-A, 2009.
5. Hamilton RG. Proficiency survey-based evaluation of clinical total and allergen-specific IgE assay performance. *Arch Pathol Lab Med* 2010; 134:975–982.
6. Sampson HA. Utility of food-specific IgE concentrations in predicting symptomatic food allergy. *J Allergy Clin Immunol* 2001; 107:891–896.
7. Wood RA, Segall N, Ahlstedt S, Williams PB. Accuracy of IgE antibody laboratory results. *Ann Allergy Asthma Immunol* 2007; 99:34–41.
8. Wang J, Godbold JH, Sampson HA. Correlation of serum allergy (IgE) tests performed by different assay systems. *J Allergy Clin Immunol* 2008; 121:1219–1224.
9. Sarratud T, Donnanno S, Terracciano L, et al. Accuracy of a point-of-care testing device in children with suspected respiratory allergy. *Allergy Asthma Proc* 2010; 31:11–17.
10. Jahn-Schmid B, Harwanegg C, Hiller R, et al. Allergen microarray: comparison to microarray using recombinant allergens with conventional diagnostic methods to detect allergen-specific serum immunoglobulin E. *Clin Exp Allergy* 2003; 33:1443–1449.
11. Scala E, Alessandri C, Palazzo P, et al. IgE recognition patterns of profilin, PR-10, and tropomyosin panallergens tested in 3,113 allergic patients by allergen microarray-based technology. *PLoS One* 2011; 6(9):e24912.
12. Dottorini T, Sole G, Nunziangeli L, et al. Serum IgE reactivity profiling in an asthma affected cohort. *PLoS One* 2011; 6(8):e22319.
13. Burks AW, Jones SM, Boyce JA, et al. NIAID-sponsored 2010 guidelines for managing food allergy: applications in the pediatric population. *Pediatrics* 2011; 128:955–965.
14. Sampson HA, McCaskin CC. Food hypersensitivity and atopic dermatitis: evaluation of 113 patients. *J Pediatr* 1985; 107:669–675.
15. Burks AW James JM, Hiegel A, et al. Atopic dermatitis and food hypersensitivity reactions. *J Pediatr* 1998; 132:132–136.
16. Bock SA, Atkins FM. Patterns of food hypersensitivity during sixteen years of double-blind, placebo-controlled food challenges. *J Pediatr* 1990; 117:561–567.

17. Riddle MS, Murray JA, Porter CK. The incidence and risk of celiac disease in a healthy US adult population. *Am J Gastroenterol* 2012; 107:1248–1255.
18. Dieterich W, Ehnis T, Baur M, et al. Identification of tissue transglutaminase as the autoantigen of celiac disease. *Nat Med* 1997; 3:797–801.
19. Wolters V, Vooijs-Moulaert AF, Burger H, et al. Human tissue transglutaminase enzyme-linked immunosorbent assay outperforms both the guinea pig based tissue transglutaminase assay and anti-endomysium antibodies when screening for celiac disease. *Eur J Pediatr* 2002; 161:284–287.
20. Vieths S, Hoffman A, Holzhauser T, et al. Factors influencing the quality of food extracts for in vitro and in vivo diagnosis. *Allergy* 1998; 53:65–71.
21. Vieths S, Scheurer S, Reidl J, et al. Optimized allergen extracts and recombinant allergens in diagnostic applications. *Allergy* 2001; 56:78–82.
22. Sicherer SH, Dhillon G, Laughery KA, et al. Caution: the Phadia hazelnut ImmunoCAP (f17) has been supplemented with recombinant Cor a 1 and now detects Bet v 1-specific IgE, which leads to elevated values for persons with birch pollen allergy. *J Allergy Clin Immunol* 2008; 122:413–414.
23. Masthoff LJN, Mattsson L, Zuidmeer-Jongejan L, et al. Sensitization to Cor a 9 and Cor a 14 is highly specific for hazelnut allergy with objective symptoms in Dutch children and adults. *J Allergy Clin Immunol* 2013; In press.
24. Breiteneder H, Ebner C. Molecular and biochemical classification of plant-derived food allergens. *J Allergy Clin Immunol* 2000; 106:27–36.
25. Sicherer SH. Clinical implications of cross-reactive food allergens. *J Allergy Clin Immunol* 2001; 108:881–890.
26. Soeria-Atmadja D, Onell A, Kober A, et al. Multivariate statistical analysis of large-scale IgE antibody measurements reveals allergen extract relationships in sensitized individuals. *J Allergy Clin Immunol* 2007; 120:1433–1440.
27. Jones SM, Magnolfi CF, Cooke SK, Sampson HA. Immunologic cross-reactivity among cereal grains and grasses in children with food hypersensitivity. *J Allergy Clin Immunol* 1995; 96:341–351.
28. Nicolaou N, Poorafshar M, Murray C, et al. Allergy or tolerance in children sensitized to peanut: prevalence and differentiation using component-resolved diagnostics. *J Allergy Clin Immunol* 2010; 125:191–197.
29. Dang TD, Tang M, Choo S, et al. Increasing the accuracy of peanut allergy diagnosis by using Ara h 2. *J Allergy Clin Immunol* 2012; 129:1056–1063.
30. Pedrosa M, Boyano-Martínez T, García-Ara MC, Caballero T, Quirce S. Peanut seed storage proteins are responsible for clinical reactivity in Spanish peanut-allergic children. *Pediatr Allergy Immunol* 2012; 23:654–659.
31. Ebisawa M, Movérare R, Sato S, et al. Measurement of Ara h 1-, 2-, and 3-specific IgE antibodies is useful in diagnosis of peanut allergy in Japanese children. *Pediatr Allergy Immunol* 2012; 23:573–581.
32. Asarnoj A, Nilsson C, Lidholm J, et al. Peanut component Ara h 8 sensitization and tolerance to peanut. *J Allergy Clin Immunol* 2012; 130:468–472.
33. Lund G, Willumsen N, Holm J, Christensen LH, Würtzen PA, Lund K. Antibody repertoire complexity and effector cell biology determined by assays for IgE-mediated basophil and T-cell activation. *J Immunol Methods* 2012; 383:4–20.
34. Christensen LH, Holm J, Lund G, et al. Several distinct properties of the IgE repertoire determine effector cell degranulation in response to allergen challenge. *J Allergy Clin Immunol* 2008; 122:298–304.
35. Lin J, Sampson HA. The role of immunoglobulin E-binding epitopes in the characterization of food allergy. *Curr Opin Allergy Clin Immunol* 2009; 9:357–363.
36. Elsayed S, Apold J, Aas K, Bennich H. The allergenic structure of allergen M from cod. I. Tryptic peptides of fragment TM1. *Int Arch Allergy Appl Immunol* 1976; 52:59–63.
37. Frank R. The SPOT synthesis technique: synthetic peptide arrays on membrane supports—principles and applications. *J Immunol methods* 2002; 267:13–26.
38. Shreffler WG, Beyer K, Chu THT, et al. Microarray immunoassay: association of clinical history, in vitro IgE function and heterogeneity of allergenic peanut epitopes. *J Allergy Clin Immunol* 2004; 113:776–782.
39. Shreffler WG, Lencer DA, Bardina L, Sampson HA. IgE and IgG4 epitope mapping by microarray immunoassay reveals the diversity of immune response to the peanut allergen. *J Allergy Clin Immunol* 2005; 116:511–517.
40. Chatchatee P, Jaarvinen KM, Bardina L, et al. Identification of IgE and IgG binding epitopes on beta and kappa casein in cow's milk allergic patients. *Clin Exp Allergy* 2001; 31:1256–1262.
41. Jarvinen KM, Beyer K, Vila L, et al. Specificity of IgE antibodies to sequential epitopes of hen's egg ovomucoid as a marker for persistence of egg allergy. *Allergy* 2007; 62:758–765.
42. Sampson HA, Ho DG. Relationship between food-specific IgE concentrations and the risk of positive food challenges in children and adolescents. *J Allergy Clin Immunol* 1997; 100:444–451.
43. Sampson HA. Utility of food-specific IgE concentrations in predicting symptomatic food allergy. *J Allergy Clin Immunol* 2001; 107:891–896.
44. Perry TT, Matsui EC, Kay Conover-Walker M, Wood RA. The relationship of allergen-specific IgE levels and oral food challenge outcome. *J Allergy Clin Immunol* 2004; 114:144–149.
45. Benhamou AH, Zamora SA, Eigenmann PA. Correlation between specific immunoglobulin E levels and the severity of reactions in egg allergic patients. *Pediatr Allergy Immunol* 2008; 19:173–179.
46. Sicherer SH, Morrow EH, Sampson HA. Dose-response in double-blind, placebo-controlled oral food challenges in children with atopic dermatitis. *J Allergy Clin Immunol* 2000; 105:582–586.
47. El-Khouly F, Lewis SA, Pons L, et al. IgG and IgE avidity characteristics of peanut allergic individuals. *Pediatr Allergy Immunol* 2007; 18:607–613.
48. Mehl A, Verstege A, Staden U, et al. Utility of the ratio of food-specific IgE/total IgE in predicting symptomatic food allergy in children. *Allergy* 2005; 60:1034–1039.

49. Fleischer DM, Conover-Walker MK, Christie L, Burks AW, Wood RA. The natural progression of peanut allergy: resolution and the possibility of recurrence. *J Allergy Clin Immunol* 2003; 112:183–189.
50. Fleischer DM, Conover-Walker MK, Matsui EC, Wood RA. The natural history of tree nut allergy. *J Allergy Clin Immunol* 2005; 116:1087–1093.
51. Skripak JM, Matsui EC, Mudd K, Wood RA. The natural history of IgE-mediated cow's milk allergy. *J Allergy Clin Immunol* 2007; 120:1172–1177.
52. Savage JH, Matsui EC, Skripak JM, Wood RA. The natural history of egg allergy. *J Allergy Clin Immunol* 2007; 120:1413–1417.
53. Shek LP, Soderstrom L, Ahlstedt S, Beyer K, Sampson HA. Determination of food specific IgE levels over time can predict the development of tolerance in cow's milk and hen's egg allergy. *J Allergy Clin Immunol* 2004; 114: 387–391.
54. Hamilton RG, Mudd K, White MA, Wood RA. Extension of food allergen specific IgE ranges from the ImmunoCAP to the IMMULITE systems. *Ann Allergy Asthma Immunol* 2011; 107:139–144.
55. Hamilton RG, MacGlashan DW Jr, Saini SS. IgE antibody-specific activity in human allergic disease. *Immunol Res* 2010; 47:273–284.
56. Van der Linden PW, Hack CE, Poortman J, et al. Insect sting challenge in 138 patients: relation between clinical severity of anaphylaxis and mast cell activation. *J Allergy Clin Immunol* 1992; 90:110–118.
57. Heine RG, Freeman T. Elevated baseline mast cell tryptase: a marker of severe insect venom anaphylaxis. *Curr Opin Allergy Clin Immunol* 2010; 10(4):309–311.
58. Fagan DL, Slaughter CA, Capra JD, Sullivan TJ. Monoclonal antibodies to immunoglobulin G4 induce histamine release from human basophils in vitro. *J Allergy Clin Immunol* 1982; 70:399–404.
59. Lichtenstein LM, Kagey-Sobotka A, White JM, Hamilton RG. Anti-human IgG causes basophil histamine release by acting on IgG–IgE complexes bound to IgE receptors. *J Immunol* 1992; 15:3929–3936.
60. Hamilton RG. Relevance of [IgG anti-IgE]-IgE complexes, IgG subclass and modern IgG antibody autoanalyzers in the dying IgG reagin story. *Allergy* 2009; 64:317–318.
61. Stapel SG, Asero R, Ballmer-Weber BK, et al. Testing for IgG4 against foods is not recommended as a diagnostic tool: EAACI Task Force report. *Allergy* 2008; 63:793–796.
62. James IM, Burks Jr AW. Food allergy: current diagnostic methods and interpretation of results. *Clin Allergy Immunol* 2000; 15:199–215.
63. Nolte H, Schiltz PO, Kruse A, Skov S. Comparison of intestinal mast cell and basophil histamine release in children with food allergic reactions. *Allergy* 1989; 44:554–565.
64. May CD, Remigo L. Observations of high spontaneous release of histamine from leukocytes in vitro. *Clin Allergy* 1982; 12:229–241.
65. Kleine-Tebbe J, Erdmann S, Knol EF, et al. Diagnostic tests based on human basophils: potentials, pitfalls and perspectives. *Int Arch Allergy Immunol* 2006; 141:79–90.
66. Van Rooyen C, Anderson R. Assessment of determinants of optimum performance of the CAST-2000 ELISA procedure. *J Immunol Methods* 2004; 288:1–7.
67. Scott-Taylor TH, Hourihane JB, Harper J, Strobel S. Patterns of food allergen-specific cytokine production by T lymphocytes of children with multiple allergies. *Clin Exp Allergy* 2005; 35:1473–1480.
68. Niggemann B, Beyer K, Wahn U. The role of eosinophils and eosinophil cationic protein in monitoring oral challenge tests in children with food sensitive atopic dermatitis. *J Allergy Clin Immunol* 1994; 94:963–971.
69. Hamilton RG. Responsibility for quality IgE antibody results rests ultimately with the referring physician [Invited Editorial]. *Ann Allergy Asthma Immunol* 2001; 86:353–354.
70. Garcia-Ara C, Boyano-Martinez T, Diaz-Pena JM, et al. Specific IgE levels in the diagnosis of immediate hypersensitivity to cow's milk protein in the infant. *J Allergy Clin Immunol* 2001; 107:185–190.
71. Celik-Bilgili S, Mehl A, Verstege A, et al. The predictive value of specific immunoglobulin E levels in serum for the outcome of oral food challenges. *Clin Exp Allergy* 2005; 35:268–273.
72. Boyano Martinez T, Garcia-Ara C, Diaz-Pena JM, et al. Validity of specific IgE antibodies in children with egg allergy. *Clin Exp Allergy* 2001; 31:1464–1469.
73. Osterballe M, Bindslev-Jensen C. Threshold levels in food challenge and specific IgE in patients with egg allergy: is there a relationship? *J Allergy Clin Immunol* 2003; 112:196–201.
74. Maloney JM, Rudengren M, Ahlstedt S, et al. The use of serum-specific IgE measurements for the diagnosis of peanut, tree nut, and seed allergy. *J Allergy Clin Immunol* 2008; 122:145–151.
75. Eckman J, Saini SS, Hamilton RG. Diagnostic evaluation of food-related allergic diseases. *Allergy Asthma Clin Immunol* 2009; 5:2.

2 Adverse Reactions to Food Antigens: Clinical Science

9 Theories on the Increasing Prevalence of Food Allergy

Katrina J. Allen[1,2,3] & Jennifer J. Koplin[1]

[1]Murdoch Children's Research Institute, Royal Children's Hospital, Melbourne, VIC, Australia
[2]The University of Melbourne Department of Paediatrics, Royal Children's Hospital, Melbourne, VIC, Australia
[3]Department of Allergy and Immunology, Royal Children's Hospital, Melbourne, VIC, Australia

Key Concepts

- Food allergy and adverse food reactions, including anaphylaxis, appear to be becoming more common.
- A family history of allergy is associated with an increased risk of food allergy; however, specific genetic risk factors for the development of food allergy remain poorly understood.
- Key theories to explain the rise in food allergy prevalence include changing microbial diversity, infant feeding practices, and changes in sun exposure (through vitamin D).
- Future studies will need to consider environmental factors in the context of genetic background.

Introduction

Is food allergy on the rise?

The prevalence of IgE-mediated food allergies appears to be increasing in industrialized countries [1] following the rapid rise in other allergic conditions such as asthma, eczema, and allergic rhinitis [2] although reliable, population-based data are limited. The key reason for the lack of evidence for changes in food allergy prevalence is that methodological issues such as selection bias related to sampling methodology and response rates, varying definitions of food allergy, and differences in the age group and foods being studied, make it difficult to compare existing studies. As food allergy is relatively uncommon compared to other allergic conditions such as asthma, studies need large sample sizes in order to detect even relatively large changes in prevalence.

Few large studies have attempted to measure the prevalence of food allergy in the same population at two time points using the same definition of food allergy. Those that do exist have primarily focused on peanut allergy. In a UK study, Venter et al. found that peanut sensitization varied from 1.3% to 3.3% to 2.0% in three sequential early childhood cohorts from the same geographic area, each surveyed 6 years apart, while reported peanut allergy increased from 0.5% to 1.4% then 1.2% [3]. While there was evidence that both peanut sensitization and allergy were significantly more common in the second cohort (born between 1994 and 1996) compared with the initial cohort (born in 1989), there was no evidence of a further increase in prevalence in the third cohort (born between 2001 and 2002). This study was limited by the small sample size ($n = 891$) in the final survey, as well as by low response rates in the second survey (43%), which may have led to inflated prevalence estimates if those at higher risk of allergic disease were more likely to participate in an allergy study. There were also differences in ages between the three studies, with the first conducted at 4 years of age, the second at 3–4 years, and the third at 3 years of age.

Between three US-wide phone surveys conducted in 1997, 2002, and 2007, the prevalence of self-reported peanut and/or tree nut allergy increased from 0.6% to 1.2% to 2.1% among children, although no change was observed for adults [4]. However, this increase in reported allergy was paralleled by a decreasing response rate across surveys (42% response rate in 2007), raising questions about whether these prevalence figures can be generalized to the wider population.

Enteropathy resulting from cow's milk is one of the better-understood, non-IgE-mediated food allergies. One prospective cohort study of newborns in Denmark found that the incidence of cow's milk enteropathy was 2.2% over the first year of life, with a high rate of resolution (97%) by 15 years of age [5]. Similarly, reports suggest a

Food Allergy: Adverse Reactions to Foods and Food Additives, Fifth Edition. Edited by Dean D Metcalfe, Hugh A Sampson, Ronald A Simon and Gideon Lack.

rapid rise in eosinophilic esophagitis—a condition that was first linked to food allergy in 1995 [6]. Coeliac disease is also reported to be rising in prevalence [7] although there are some suggestions that improved serological screening studies have increased the case finding for this disease, which has a reported prevalence of 0.5–1.0% of the community [8, 9].

There have been reports that hospitalizations for food-allergy-related anaphylaxis—the most serious and life-threatening manifestation—have increased markedly since 1990 in the United Kingdom, the United States, and Australia. The data from Australia were the most dramatic, with a fivefold increase, in 0- to 4-year olds over a 10-year time frame [10]. Poulos and colleagues found a continuous increase in the rates of hospital admission for angioedema (3.0% per year), urticaria (5.7% per year), and, importantly, anaphylaxis (8.8% per year), over a 10-year period from 1993 [11]. These findings certainly support the hypothesis for the rise in food allergy prevalence since anaphylaxis is a clearly objective clinical presentation. However, the possibility remains that the rise is in part due to increased ascertainment of cases or alternatively that more severe presentations of food allergy are on the rise.

Why do not we have better data?

Results of population studies examining food allergy prevalence have been hampered by small sample sizes, selection bias related to sampling methodology and response rates, and use of parental or self-report of allergy or a skin prick test result as a proxy for food allergy diagnosis. Even studies that have used the diagnostic gold standard of oral food challenge, where the allergen of interest is fed to the child, have been limited by a lack of predetermined objective criteria to define the outcome.

Oral food challenges are the gold standard for diagnosis of food allergy, however, these can be difficult to implement in large population-based studies as they are expensive and often have low uptake by participants. The HealthNuts study has demonstrated that it is possible to perform a large-scale study using oral food challenges to confirm food allergy in infants irrespective of skin prick test wheal size. However, until recently food challenge methodologies have not been standardized. Studies tend to rely on challenge protocols from local units, which can vary by challenge material used (e.g., peanut butter vs. peanut flour for peanut challenges), dosing regimens, and time intervals between administration. Most problematical, internationally standardized challenge stopping criteria have not been developed, although we were recently the first to publish predetermined stopping criteria used in the HealthNuts study [12].

Recruitment of a population-based sample poses difficulties that need to be overcome with respect to participation bias, with those at higher risk of allergy often more likely to participate in allergy studies. This can be overcome either by achieving high response rates or at least by measuring participation bias and taking this into account when analyzing data and reporting results.

Accurate baseline data will be vital to measure future changes in food allergy prevalence, including monitoring the effectiveness of guideline changes as understanding of environmental exposures linked to food allergy increases. We recently undertook the HealthNuts study to investigate the prevalence of food allergy in 1-year-old infants in Melbourne, using a sampling frame designed to recruit a representative population sample and predetermined criteria to assess food allergy outcomes at oral food challenge [13]. Recruitment occurred at childhood vaccination sessions. Participants' parents completed a questionnaire, and the infants received skin prick testing for commonly allergenic foods. Among 2848 participants (73% participation rate), those with any sensitization to one of the four foods (egg, peanut, sesame, and cow's milk) were invited to attend an allergy research clinic for formal oral food challenge. Using this method, the study found population-based prevalence of 2.9% (95% CI, 2.3–3.6%) for peanut allergy, 8.9% (95% CI, 7.8–10.0%) for egg allergy, 2.7% for cow's milk, and 0.8% (95% CI, 0.5–1.1%) for sesame allergy in 1-year-old infants [14].

Certainly, the rates reported in the HealthNuts study are the highest yet reported in the Western world, with up to 10% of 1-year-old infants in this study population exhibiting signs of IgE-mediated food allergy in a challenge setting. Although it is anticipated that many of those with egg or cow's milk allergy will develop tolerance to these foods in the first 3–4 years of life, the high prevalence of peanut allergy remains concerning, as only 20% of the children are expected to achieve resolution of this allergy by 5 years of age [15]. Furthermore, there is now evolving evidence that food allergy, including cow's milk and egg allergy, may represent the first step on the allergic pathway referred to as the "atopic march" [16]. Also recent evidence suggests a change in the natural history of food allergy with resolution occurring later among egg-allergic infants than previous reports [17]. As such, the question remains as to whether this reported high prevalence of food allergy may reflect a second and evolving epidemic of allergic disease, with an early onset in the form of food allergy that will translate into increased rates of asthma and other chronic allergic disease later in life [18].

The EuroPrevall birth cohort study, which includes over 12 000 infants from nine European countries, has been designed to examine between-country variations in food allergy, confirmed using the gold standard of double-blind placebo-controlled food challenge, in European children in the first 2–3 years of life. The advantages of this study design are that it allows assessment of regional differences in factors that might be related to food allergy risk and comparison of food allergy prevalence by region. The study has already reported large differences between countries in possible risk factors such as tobacco smoking during pregnancy and caesarean section delivery [19]. However, it poses analytical challenges related to identifying major contributing factors where there are multiple between-country differences including environmental, racial, genetic, and cultural differences.

What are the main theories for the rise in food allergy?

The rise in incidence in food allergy is likely to be driven by potentially modifiable environmental factors, since the rise is more rapid than genetic deviation would allow. At the most general level, it appears that these factors are linked to the "modern lifestyle," since food allergy is more common in developed than developing countries, and migrants appear to acquire the incident risk of allergy of their adopted country [20]. A whole host of factors have been examined with regards to general allergic disease but to date very few studies have investigated factors that might increase the risk of food allergy, and more importantly very few have used challenge-proven food allergy as an outcome when looking for causative factors. Since the majority of cases of food allergy occur early in an infant's life (most often when allergenic foods are first introduced into the infants diet), causative factors are likely to be prenatal, perinatal, or postnatal (Figure 9.1). The main hypotheses include the hygiene hypothesis (and fecal microbial diversity), the "Old Friends hypothesis," infant feeding factors (e.g., timing of introduction of solids including allergenic solids and breastfeeding), and other lifestyle factors that might impact on the infant's immunomodulatory status such as vitamin D, long-chain polyunsaturated fatty acids, folate, and exposure to tobacco smoke. Importantly, these factors may act singly or in concert and there is likely to be at least some component of gene–environment interaction. That is to say, lifestyle factors may have a differential effect depending on genetic status of the individual [21].

Associations have been found between several environmental factors and the development of eczema and atopy,

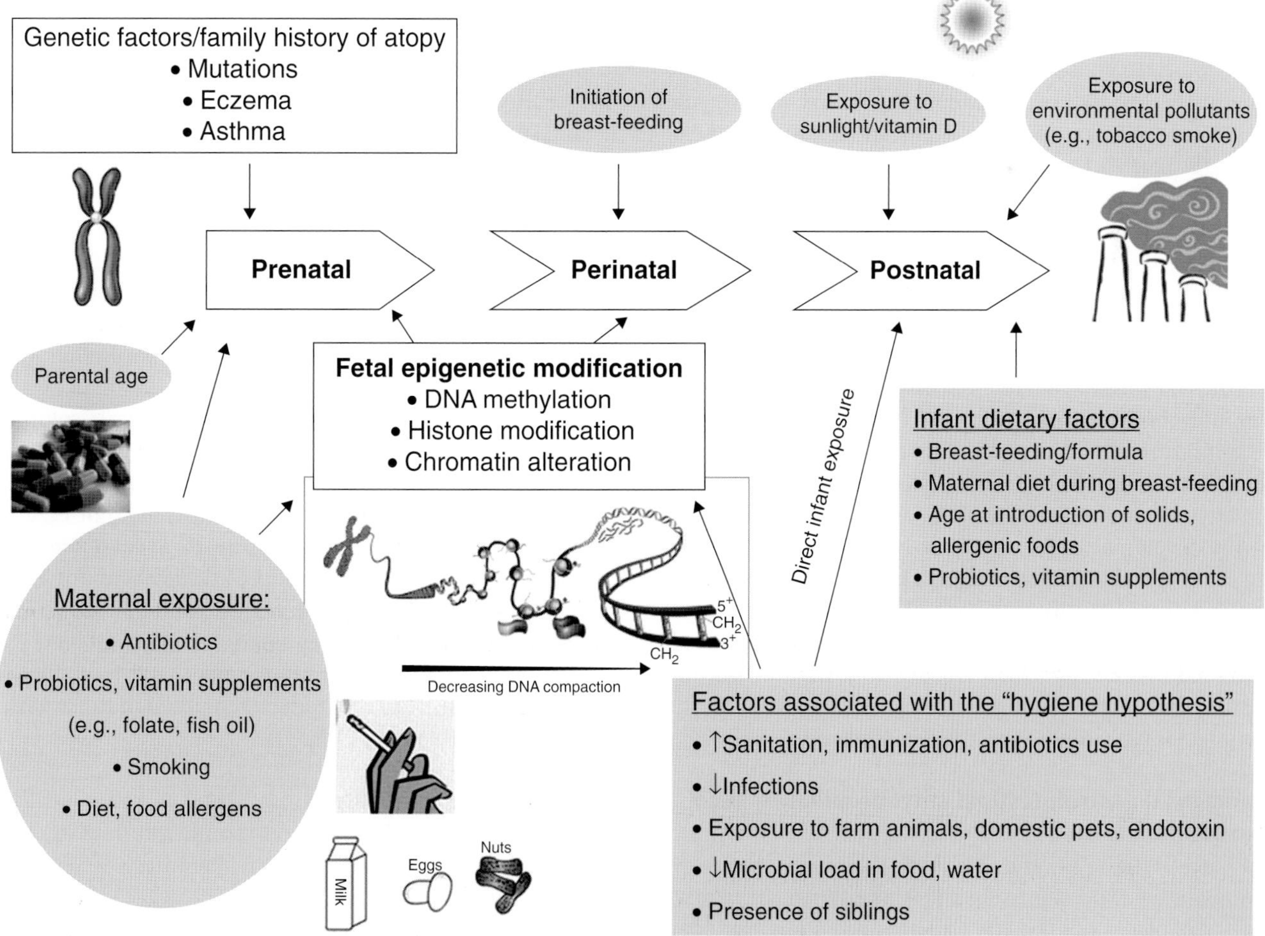

Figure 9.1 Potential genetic, epigenetic, and environmental factors contributing to an increase in IgE-mediated food allergy. Reproduced from Reference 21 with permission.

but these factors have not been formally examined in association with food allergy, despite the strong association between eczema and food allergy [22, 23]. Environmental factors associated with the hygiene hypothesis (i.e., the hypothesis that early exposure to microbial antigens promote healthy immune development and reduces the risk of developing allergies) and linked to allergic outcomes such as asthma or allergic sensitization include companion animal ownership [24], number of siblings [25], and exposure to farm animals [26]. Timing of introduction of solids [27] and breastfeeding regimes [28] have also been examined, but results have been conflicting, possibly contaminated by reverse causation [29].

Factors associated with a "modern lifestyle" include a myriad of changes to our level of public health including improved sanitation, secure water supplies (with associated decreased prevalence of *Helicobacter pylori* infection), widespread use of antibiotics and increasing rates of immunization, improved nutrition, decreased helminthic infestation, improved food quality (and presumably less microbial load in the food chain) as well as generally improved nutrition and associated obesity. These factors might work individually or in concert to affect a failure in the development of oral immune tolerance in the first year of life when development of IgE-mediated food allergy is most likely to occur. These factors have all come in to play some time in the last half of the twentieth century and yet the rise in food allergy prevalence appears in the context of the early part of the twenty-first century. If the hygiene hypothesis is found to be central to the rise of both atopy in general and food allergy more specifically, this effect might be expressed through a delayed generational effect and the impact of maternal epigenetic modification on fetal priming of the immune system.

Countries with a Westernized lifestyle appear to have the highest rates of allergic disease, and allergies are less common in developing countries. To date there has been little information on these differences or why they might be occurring. Emerging evidence suggests that changes in the environment related to a Western lifestyle and to economic development are the most important factors causing the rise in allergic disease [18]. In particular, improved hygiene, less exposure to microbial organisms, changes in diet (eating less fish and vegetables), less exposure to sunlight (reduced UV and therefore reduced vitamin D), and possibly increased use of antibiotics are thought to be the main factors contributing to the rise in allergy.

Commensal gastrointestinal microbe milieu—"fecal microbial diversity"

The maturation of the mucosal immune system is prompted by exposure to microbes after birth. In searching for explanations for food allergy, attention has been turned to the composition of and timing of exposure to gut microflora and their possible role in disease development or prevention. Recent research suggests that toll-like, receptor-dependent signals provided by intestinal bacteria may inhibit the development of allergic responses to food antigens via stimulation of regulatory T cells, a key player in the induction of oral tolerance [30]. One hypothesis to explain the increased incidence of sensitization to food allergens is that the reduction in early childhood infections or in exposure to microbial products (e.g., endotoxin) may impede the development of early immunoregulatory responses. This leaves the immune system more susceptible to inappropriate reactivity to innocuous antigens, resulting in an "allergic" reaction [31].

Postnatal development of mucosal immune homoeostasis is influenced by the type of commensal microbiota present in the neonatal period. It has been hypothesized that the predominance of bifidobacteria in breastfed infants may be protective against food allergy. The differences in the neonatal gut microbiota precede the development of atopy, suggesting a role for commensal intestinal bacteria in the prevention of allergy [32]. This has led to the hypothesis that probiotics may promote oral tolerance. Perinatal administration of *Lactobacillus casei* GG has been reported to reduce the incidence of atopic dermatitis, but not food allergy, in at-risk children during the first 4 years of life. However, the topic has remained controversial, with some studies finding consistent results [33], others failing to find evidence of a protective effect [34], and yet another finding a protective effect in the context of a caesarian-section birth [35].

After sampling microflora multiple times from 324 infants starting shortly after birth, Adlerberth and colleagues found no association with the lack of any particular flora and the development of food-specific IgE at 18 months of age [36]. It was found that caesarean section delivery was associated with *Clostridium difficile* colonization, as was a lack of older siblings; both factors that have been found to carry a risk of atopic disease in other studies. Another study did find an increased risk of eczema, recurrent wheeze, and sensitization to at least one food or aeroallergen and colonization of *C. difficile* at any number [37]. A recent systematic review found an association of caesarean section and increased risk of developing sensitization to food (and presumed associated food allergy) although this risk appears to be augmented in those with a family history of atopy [38].

The "Hygiene" hypothesis

The consideration of the composition of gut flora in childhood is part of a broader theory of allergic disease etiology, namely the "hygiene hypothesis." Avenues of investigation have included occurrence of viral, bacterial, and parasitic infections, exposure to endotoxin in particular, exposure to potential sources of infection and, true to the name, exposure to hand washing and general cleanliness.

Several epidemiological studies have semi-quantified exposure to pathogens via environmental circumstances, such as number of siblings, pet ownership, and child care attendance. A review of the literature in 2000 found that a sibling effect—higher numbers of siblings conveying a protective effect—existed for eczema, hay fever, atopic sensitization, and asthma and wheeze [25]. The weighted average odds ratio of being atopic by skin prick test or serum IgE, to food or aeroallergens or both, was 0.62 for three or more siblings. The authors concluded, however, that the hygiene hypothesis was not able to explain the association alone, hence there are questions raised as to how much *in utero* influences change susceptibility to allergy. There is a need to examine the sibling effect in confirmed food allergy as well as associated atopic disorders. No association was found between dog or cat exposure during the first year of life and confirmed food allergy in one study, although the number of allergic children considered was small ($N = 15$) [39]. A systematic review found a protective effect of cat or dog exposure on eczema at all ages, which in childhood is closely linked to food allergy, but it was found to be statistically insignificant when animal avoidance behavior was taken into account [40]. Day care attendance was found to be protective against wheeze in later childhood (0.8, 95% CI 0.6–1.0) [41], although this has recently been disputed [42]. Early day care attendance was found to be a risk factor for nonatopic eczema but not atopic eczema, raising the possibility that day care may be protective against persistence or development of sensitization [43].

Our own data are the first to look at these factors in relation to egg allergy in a population cohort of infants. Those who were sensitized at the population level underwent formal food challenge. Children with older siblings and those with a pet dog at home were less likely to develop egg allergy by 1 year of age (adjusted OR [aOR] 0.72, 95% CI 0.62, 0.83 per sibling and aOR 0.64, 95% CI 0.47, 0.89, respectively). Caesarean section delivery, antibiotic use in infancy, child care attendance, and maternal age were not associated with egg allergy. History of allergic disease in an immediate family member and having parents born in East Asia were strong risk factors for infantile egg allergy (aOR 1.90, 95% CI 1.44, 2.50 and aOR 3.24, 95% CI 2.39, 4.41, respectively) [44].

Specific infections that are acquired in childhood have been queried as causes of food allergy. *Helicobacter pylori* infection, the prevalence of which has decreased contemporaneously with the perceived increase in food allergy, has been implicated as a protector against food allergy. *Helicobacter pylori* seropositivity rates explained 32% of the difference between Finland and a geographically similar location in Russia, where infection was inversely related to atopy [45]. A study conducted in the United Kingdom found that *H. pylori* infection was associated with a reduced risk of asthma, eczema, or allergic rhinitis, but no statistically significant association was found with them individually [46], highlighting the need for sufficient sample size within similar studies. To consider whether rotavirus infection may contribute to the development of allergy, Firer et al. [47] examined anti-rotavirus antibody titers in children with cow's milk allergy. A higher proportion of non-IgE-mediated milk allergy cases had evidence of previous infection (76%) compared with IgE-mediated milk allergy (33%, $p = 0.01$). The KOALA study found that there was no association between rotavirus and norovirus seropositivity and eczema or atopy in the first 2 years of life [48].

The "Old Friends" hypothesis

Surprisingly, given the presumed teleological development of IgE immune mechanisms for the control of helminthic infections, until recently few investigators have examined whether decreased helminthic infestation (the "Old Friends" hypothesis) in Westernized countries could be linked to the rise in food allergy [49], even though there is an evolving interest in this area as a form of therapy as for inflammatory bowel disease [50]. There is a possibility that our findings above showing a protective role of dog ownership for egg allergy could be mediated through this mechanism.

Infant feeding practices

Early studies suggested that the delayed introduction of solids combined with maternal avoidance during pregnancy and lactation may protect against allergic disease through the prevention of sensitization. However, later follow-up of these cohorts showed that the protective effect was not maintained, suggesting the associations may have been contaminated by confounding. There is now emerging evidence that avoidance strategies are likely to be ineffective and may even be harmful with a new concept of an optimal "window of opportunity" for the development of gastrointestinal tolerance [51].

Until very recently, expert guidelines for infants with a family history of allergy typically recommended delaying introduction of allergenic foods (including avoiding eggs until 2 years and nuts until 3 years of age), as well as delaying solid foods until after 6 months and breastfeeding for at least 12 months with the aim of reducing the risk of food allergy. Until our own recent publication, no population study had directly examined the relationship between infant feeding in the first year of life and risk of confirmed infant food allergy, although data from Du Toit et al. suggested that early introduction of peanut in Israel may protect against peanut allergy [52]. In the HealthNuts study, compared with introduction at 4–6 months, introducing egg into the diet later was associated with higher rates of egg allergy (aOR 3.4 [1.8 to 6.5] for introduction after 12 months). Most interestingly, introduction of cooked egg such as scrambled, baked, or fried was more protective than simply introducing egg in baked goods, with those introducing cooked egg at 4–6 months being five times less likely to develop egg allergy than those waiting to the normally recommended time of 10–12 months of age, even after adjusting for confounding factors. There was no protective effect among infants who first introduced baked egg into their diet between 4 and 6 months presumably because a lower dose exposure does not provide protection. No other factors, such as maternal avoidance or prolonged breastfeeding, were associated with altered risk of food allergy after adjusting for confounders [53]. These results are the first evidence-based findings to inform the recently revised international feeding guidelines in Australia as well as in Europe and the United States that avoidance of allergenic foods in the first year of an infant's life is no longer recommended [54, 55].

Infant feeding data collected as part of birth cohort studies have been analyzed to investigate the relationship between solid food introduction and the later development of atopy. No study found any benefit on allergic outcome by delaying the introduction of solids and two found an association between the delayed introduction of milk [56] and egg [57, 58] and increased incidence of eczema and atopic sensitization. More recently, it has been suggested that children exposed to cereal grains before 6 months of age (as opposed to after 6 months of age) are protected from the development of wheat-specific IgE [59]. However, all studies collected feeding data retrospectively which makes the findings vulnerable to both recall bias and reverse causality. Nevertheless, these studies have raised the possibility that delaying the introduction of foods into an infant's diet (particularly of allergenic foods) is not beneficial.

Other aspects of infantile development are likely to be important in development of oral tolerance. The initial timing and dosage of dietary antigens has a profound effect on the change to bowel flora around the time of solid food introduction [60]. Exclusive breastfeeding appears to have a protective effect on the early development of asthma and atopic dermatitis up to 2 years of age, but the evidence for prevention of food allergies is less clear [28]. If exclusive breastfeeding is not possible, a hydrolyzed formula is recommended for the first 4 months of life in infants at high risk of food allergy (i.e., those with an atopic first-degree relative) [61]. However, this is likely to be revised in light of the recent publication of the largest randomized controlled trial of partially hydrolyzed formula to date, which showed no effect on the prevention of any allergic disease including food allergy to the age of 7 years [62]. Currently, there is no evidence for the protective role of maternal elimination diets during pregnancy [63].

Although all authorities agree that breast milk is the food of choice for infants, the evidence that it prevents allergic outcomes is contradictory, with different studies showing protection, no effect, and even increased risk [28]. This may be due to variations in breast milk composition or differences in maternal diet, but no studies have shown long-term benefits with regard to allergic outcomes. These conclusions also apply to the effect on the prevention of food allergy in particular. Given the current recommendations in many countries to delay the introduction of all complementary foods until 6 months and for much longer delays for specific allergenic foods, it is surprising that the evidence of the effects of delaying the introduction of allergenic foods into the infant diet is extremely limited. Obviously it would be unethical to mount a randomized trial of breastfeeding versus formula feeding from birth.

Vitamin D

Recent hypotheses that low vitamin D may increase the risk of food allergy [64] are supported by two lines of ecological enquiry. First, there is a strong latitudinal prevalence gradient, with those countries further from the equator (and thus lower ambient ultraviolet radiation) recording more admissions to hospital for food allergy-related events [65], and more prescriptions for adrenaline autoinjectors for the treatment of anaphylaxis [66]. These findings appear to be independent of longitude, physician density, or socioeconomic status. Second, season of birth may play a role with children attending emergency departments in Boston with a food-related acute allergic reaction more likely to be born in autumn/winter, when vitamin D levels reach their nadir, than in spring/summer [67] and similar links to birth seasonality in the Southern hemisphere [68].

We have recently confirmed that Melbourne, the most southern major city in Australia, has the highest reported prevalence of documented infantile food allergy in the world, with more than 10% of a population sample of 1-year-old infants having challenge-proven IgE-mediated food allergy [14]. In a separate study, we have shown that compared with the northern states, children residing in the southern states of Australia are six times more likely to have peanut allergy at age 6 years and twice as likely to have egg allergy than those in the northern states [69]. We have also shown that the delayed introduction of egg, one of breastfed infants' richest sources of vitamin D, increases the risk of developing egg allergy by age 12 months by at least fivefold [53]. Finally, increasing vitamin D insufficiency over the last 20 years [70], paralleling the rise in food allergy, is supported by data showing that up to 30% of pregnant women in Melbourne are vitamin D insufficient [71]. Vitamin D could influence the onset and resolution of food allergy via several plausible mechanisms. The vitamin D receptor is widely expressed in the immune system including T cells, in particular promoting the expression of interleukin (IL)-10-secreting T regulatory cells crucial to maintaining immune tolerance, [72] and potentially playing a key role in the induction of tolerance in food-allergic individuals [73]. Vitamin D metabolites also contribute to innate epithelial defenses by stimulating production of antimicrobial proteins such as cathelicidins [74, 75] and defensins [76]. Taken together, these findings increasingly point to a possible causal role for vitamin D deficiency in the epidemic of food allergy.

Genetic risk

Food allergy development is highly likely to be influenced by both genetic and environmental factors. The significant role that genetics plays in the disorders is reflected in a 64.3% concordance rate of peanut allergy between child monozygotic twins, compared with 6.8% ($p < 0.0001$) for dizygotic twins [77]. The heritability is estimated at 81.6% for peanut allergy (95% CI 41, 6–99.7%) and found to range from 15% to 35% for other specific foods in a separate study [78]. The heritability of non-IgE-mediated food allergy is not known, although with the characterization of the related syndromes, twin studies to deduce the genetic contribution to the syndromes should be possible. Coeliac disease, a specific example of food-triggered enteropathy, has shown a very high concordance rate for a multifactorial disease: 75% pairwise concordance (95% CI 62.0–94.0) was found among monozygotic twins compared with 11% concordance (95% CI 9.9–23.0%) among dizygotic twins [79].

A number of candidate gene association studies have been performed in an effort to elucidate genetic risk factors for food allergy but so far there has been little success. Candidate genes for food allergy might encompass genes known to be associated with asthma and eczema, which are closely related atopic disorders. Studies have investigated polymorphism(s) in genes including the major histocompatibility complex (MHC), human leukocyte antigen (HLA) class II gene family including HLA-DRB1, HLA-DQB1, and HLA-DPB1, cluster of differentiation 14 (CD14), forkhead box P3 (FOXP3), signal transducer and activator of transcription 6 (STAT6), serine protease inhibitor Karzal type 5 (SPINK5), IL-10, and IL-13. Each of these genes was found to be associated with the incidence or the severity of food allergy in single studies [21]. However, most of these associations have yet to be replicated in independent populations and thus a specific, confirmed locus for food allergy risk has not been identified.

A number of recent studies have linked null mutations (R501X and 2282del4) in the filaggrin gene (FLG) with an increased susceptibility to eczema [80], a condition that commonly occurs in infants with IgE-mediated food sensitivities. Individuals with two null alleles in FLG have been shown to be four to seven times more likely to have eczema than those without [81]. The filaggrin protein appears to play an essential role in epithelial integrity: a severe breakdown in the function of the protein produced can result in ichthyosis vulgaris. The association between eczema and IgE-mediated food allergy has been hypothesized to be mechanistic; it is possible that the route of sensitization is through damaged epithelia. We have recently demonstrated support for this concept. Again in the HealthNuts study, we assessed the association of FLG mutations with risk of both food sensitization and food allergy over and above the association with eczema association. After adjusting for eczema, FLG mutations were significantly associated with food sensitization (aOR 3.0; 95% CI 1.0–8.7; $p = 0.043$) but only showed a trend for association with food allergy (aOR 2.9; 95% CI 1.0–8.6; $p = 0.055$). Food-specific analyses showed that FLG mutations increased the risk of egg sensitization (aOR 4.4; 95% CI 1.1–17.2; $p = 0.034$), egg allergy (aOR 3.0; 95% CI 1.0–9.1; $p = 0.046$), and peanut sensitization (aOR 4.9; 95% CI 1.4–17.0; $p = 0.011$) but not peanut allergy (aOR 1.8; 95% CI 0.5–7.0; $p = 0.383$) [82]. Our findings extend those of Brown et al. [83] who in a multisite study of peanut allergy found that the FLG mutations were associated with a significantly increased risk of peanut allergy although history of eczema and sensitization status was not available, so assessment of the impact of FLG on these outcomes could not be assessed independently of food allergy.

A better understanding of the existing genetic predispositions to food allergy will lead to the determination of whether a rise in food allergy is occurring asymmetrically between high-risk and low-risk groups. Researchers found that the increasing incidence in type 1 diabetes was explained by an increased disease incidence among lower-risk HLA DR4-X and HLA DR3-X genotypes between 1950 and 2005, while the incidence of disease among the higher-risk HLA DR3-DR4 genotype remained constant [84], indicating a major role for recent environmental changes. Such research of immune disorders, including food allergy, may be pivotal in directing research toward plausible modifiable risk factors for disease.

Gene–environment interactions

Despite evidence that genetic predisposition plays a role in the development of food allergy, existing studies that have examined environmental risk factors for food allergy have done so without regard for the influence of genetic factors. There is growing awareness that the expression of diseases which appear to have a complex etiology, such as allergic disease in general and food allergy specifically, is likely to be dependent on a combination of both genes and the environment [21]. The continuous dialog between the genome and the environment (gene–environment interactions, G × E) is important for the pathogenesis of complex diseases, which exhibit a heritable component but do not follow Mendel's laws. Food allergy, like other complex diseases, is presumed to be caused by a combination of subtle genetic and environmental factors. G × E reflects how environmental exposures (including lifestyle and diet) interact with genetic predisposition to modify disease risk and/or outcome. An interaction is indicated when the simultaneous influence of two or more factors on a phenotype is not additive [85]. Thus, the presence of one factor affects the influence (manifestation of risk) associated with a second. For example, the effect of air pollution on allergic sensitization to inhalant and/or food allergens appears to be modified by the GSTP1 Ile105Val polymorphisms [86]. Additionally, the influence of the C-159T polymorphism on the CD14 gene could depend on the microbial stimulation from the environment, with individuals carrying the TT genotype appearing to have increased protection from eczema with dog exposure [39].

Epigenetics—the interface of genetics and environment

While emerging evidence exists for a role of both genetic and environmental factors in specifying the risk of allergy, it is becoming clear that epigenetic modification represents a major mechanism through which these factors interact. Epigenetics refers to the "structural adaptations of chromosomal regions so as to register, signal, or perpetuate altered activity states" [87]. This definition encompasses changes to gene expression that are mitotically and/or meiotically heritable independently of changes in DNA sequence. Epigenetic mechanisms regulate gene expression changes accompanying cell differentiation and represent a major mechanism underpinning the majority of environmentally mediated changes to gene expression. The epigenome can change and adapt to environmental stimuli over a relatively short timescale and is also subject to epigenetic "drift" over the life course in response to both environmental and stochastic factors [85]. These changes may possibly be transmitted to subsequent generations.

Epigenetic marks include changes to nucleotides and DNA-associated proteins through a number of mechanisms including methylation and histone deacetylation. Modifications of DNA and histone proteins can influence chromatin structure and expression by several mechanisms including through changes in electrostatic interactions between histones and DNA, causing particular regions to be more or less accessible to transcription factors and therefore gene expression. Mounting evidence suggests that early development (*in utero*, termed "fetal programming" and early postnatal) represents an especially sensitive time for epigenetic disruption, however, evidence suggests they can also occur during later periods and can influence gene expression differentially throughout the life span [87].

The "fetal origins" hypothesis (as it is now known) is supported by a large number of studies in animals and fewer, largely epidemiological studies in humans. The altered susceptibility to disease is believed to be "programmed" *in utero* by the maternal environment, for example, maternal nutrition, maternal body composition, levels of stress hormones. It has been proposed that fetal exposure to an inadequate intrauterine environment can result in a permanent adaptation of the developing fetus including the immune system [88]. The molecular mechanism(s) underlying this phenomenon are largely speculative but are now thought to be, at least in part, specified epigenetically. This has led to the "neo-Lamarckian" concept of environmental adaptation whereby an environmental exposure in one generation can produce epigenetic changes inherited by the next. The most studied maternal environments in this regard are diet, age, infection, stress, assisted reproductive technologies, alcohol, smoking, exposure to endocrine disruptors, toxins, and drugs. All have been shown to induce epigenetic change in offspring, and, in some cases, subsequent generations. To date no study has investigated the role of epigenetics in food allergy but given the emerging impact of this field and the evidence that environmental factors are likely to be critical factors in the rise of food allergy, the role of epigenetics to help determine disease mechanism or act as biomarkers of either food allergy development or subsequent tolerance is likely to be a fruitful field of enquiry.

Conclusion

Although the timing and magnitude of changes in food allergy prevalence remain poorly understood because high-quality data from the last 40–50 years are not available, existing evidence generally supports an increase in the prevalence of both IgE-mediated food allergy and severe food reactions including anaphylaxis. What is known about the epidemiology of food allergy indicates that the rise in food allergy is likely to be linked to factors associated with the modern lifestyle. To date insufficient evidence is available to allow firm conclusions about which aspect or aspects of the modern lifestyle are most important and whether these may be modifiable to prevent food allergy. Future studies that take into account genetic background when investigating environmental risk factors for food allergy will help to elucidate the important factors.

References

1. Allen KJ. Food allergy: is there a rising prevalence and if so why? *Med J Aust* 2011; 195:5–7.
2. Bjorksten B, Clayton T, Ellwood P, Stewart A, Strachan D, Phase III Study Group. Worldwide time trends for symptoms

of rhinitis and conjunctivitis: phase III of the International Study of Asthma and Allergies in Childhood. *Pediatr Allergy Immunol* 2008; 19:110–124.

3. Venter C, Hasan Arshad S, Grundy J, et al. Time trends in the prevalence of peanut allergy: three cohorts of children from the same geographical location in the UK. *Allergy* 2010; 65:103–108.
4. Sicherer SH, Munoz-Furlong A, Godbold JH, Sampson HA. US prevalence of self-reported peanut, tree nut, and sesame allergy: 11-year follow-up. *J Allergy Clin Immunol* 2010; 125:1322–1326.
5. Host A, Halken S, Jacobsen HP, Christensen AE, Herskind AM, Plesner K. Clinical course of cow's milk protein allergy/intolerance and atopic diseases in childhood. *Pediatr Allergy Immunol* 2002; 13:23–28.
6. Kelly KJ, Lazenby AJ, Rowe PC, Yardley JH, Perman JA, Sampson HA. Eosinophilic esophagitis attributed to gastroesophageal reflux: improvement with an amino acid-based formula. *Gastroenterology* 1995; 109:1503–1512.
7. Lohi S, Mustalahti K, Kaukinen K, et al. Increasing prevalence of coeliac disease over time. *Aliment Pharmacol Ther* 2007; 26:1217–1225.
8. West J, Logan RF, Hill PG, et al. Seroprevalence, correlates, and characteristics of undetected coeliac disease in England. *Gut* 2003; 52:960–965.
9. Fasano A, Berti I, Gerarduzzi T, et al. Prevalence of celiac disease in at-risk and not-at-risk groups in the United States: a large multicenter study. *Arch Intern Med* 2003; 163:286–292.
10. Liew WK, Williamson E, Tang MLK. Anaphylaxis fatalities and admissions in Australia. *J Allergy Clin Immunol* 2009; 123:434–442.
11. Poulos LM, Waters A-M, Correll PK, Loblay RH, Marks GB. Trends in hospitalizations for anaphylaxis, angioedema, and urticaria in Australia, 1993–1994 to 2004–2005. *J Allergy Clin Immunol* 2007; 120:878–884.
12. Koplin JJ, Tang ML, Martin PE, et al. Predetermined challenge eligibility and cessation criteria for oral food challenges in the HealthNuts population-based study of infants. *J Allergy Clin Immunol* 2012; 129:1145–1147.
13. Osborne NJ, Koplin JJ, Martin PE, et al. The HealthNuts population-based study of paediatric food allergy: validity, safety and acceptability. *Clin Exp Allergy* 2010; 40:1516–1522.
14. Osborne NJ, Koplin JJ, Martin PE, et al. Prevalence of challenge-proven IgE-mediated food allergy using population-based sampling and predetermined challenge criteria in infants. *J Allergy Clin Immunol* 2011; 127:668–676.
15. Ho MH, Wong WH, Heine RG, Hosking CS, Hill DJ, Allen KJ. Early clinical predictors of remission of peanut allergy in children. *J Allergy Clin Immunol* 2008; 121:731–736.
16. Allen KJ, Dharmage SC. The role of food allergy in the atopic march. *Clin Exp Allergy* 2010; 40:1439–1441.
17. Savage JH, Matsui EC, Skripak JM, Wood RA. The natural history of egg allergy. *J Allergy Clin Immunol* 2007; 120:1413–1417.
18. Prescott S, Allen KJ. Food allergy: riding the second wave of the allergy epidemic. *Pediatr Allergy Immunol* 2011; 22:155–160.
19. McBride D, Keil T, Grabenhenrich L, et al. The EuroPrevall birth cohort study on food allergy: baseline characteristics of 12,000 newborns and their families from nine European countries. *Pediatr Allergy Immunol* 2012; 23:230–239.
20. Cataldo F, Accomando S, Fragapane ML, Montaperto D. Are food intolerances and allergies increasing in immigrant children coming from developing countries? *Pediatr Allergy Immunol* 2006; 17:364–369.
21. Tan TH, Ellis JA, Saffery R, Allen KJ. The role of genetics and environment in the rise of childhood food allergy. *Clin Exp Allergy* 2012; 42:20–29.
22. Hill D, Heine R, Hosking C, et al. IgE food sensitization in infants with eczema attending a dermatology department. *J Pediatr* 2007; 151:359–363.
23. Hill DJ, Hosking CS. Food allergy and atopic dermatitis in infancy: an epidemiologic study. *Pediatr Allergy Immunol* 2004; 15:421–427.
24. Bisgaard H, Simpson A, Palmer C, et al. Gene-environment interaction in the onset of eczema in infancy: filaggrin loss-of-function mutations enhanced by neonatal cat exposure. *PLoS Med* 2008; 5:e131.
25. Karmaus W, Botezan C. Does a higher number of siblings protect against the development of allergy and asthma? A review. *J Epidemiol Community Health* 2002; 56:209–217.
26. Ege MJ, Bieli C, Frei R, et al. Prenatal farm exposure is related to the expression of receptors of the innate immunity and to atopic sensitization in school-age children. *J Allergy Clin Immunol* 2006; 117:817–823.
27. Zutavern A, Brockow I, Schaaf B, et al. Timing of solid food introduction in relation to atopic dermatitis and atopic sensitization: results from a prospective birth cohort study. *Pediatrics* 2006; 117:401–411.
28. Matheson MC, Allen KJ, Tang ML. Understanding the evidence for and against the role of breastfeeding in allergy prevention. *Clin Exp Allergy* 2012; 42:827–851.
29. Lowe AJ, Carlin JB, Bennett CM, et al. Atopic disease and breast-feeding—cause or consequence? *J Allergy Clin Immunol* 2006; 117:682–687.
30. Bashir MEH, Louie S, Shi HN, Nagler-Anderson C. Toll-like receptor 4 signaling by intestinal microbes influences susceptibility to food allergy. *J Immunol* 2004; 172:6978–6987.
31. Bailey M, Haverson K, Inman C, et al. The development of the mucosal immune system pre- and post-weaning: balancing regulatory and effector function. *Proc Nutr Soc* 2005; 64:451–457.
32. Kalliomaki M, Kirjavainen P, Eerola E, Kero P, Salminen S, Isolauri E. Distinct patterns of neonatal gut microflora in infants in whom atopy was and was not developing. *J Allergy Clin Immunol* 2001; 107:129–134.
33. Wickens K, Black PN, Stanley TV, et al. A differential effect of 2 probiotics in the prevention of eczema and atopy: a double-blind, randomized, placebo-controlled trial. *J Allergy Clin Immunol* 2008; 122:788–794.
34. Kopp MV, Hennemuth I, Heinzmann A, Urbanek R. Randomized, double-blind, placebo-controlled trial of probiotics for primary prevention: no clinical effects of *Lactobacillus GG* supplementation. *Pediatrics* 2008; 121:e850–e856.

35. Kuitunen M, Kukkonen K, Juntunen-Backman K, et al. Probiotics prevent IgE-associated allergy until age 5 years in cesarean-delivered children but not in the total cohort. *J Allergy Clin Immunol* 2009; 123:335–341.
36. Adlerberth I, Strachan DP, Matricardi PM, et al. Gut microbiota and development of atopic eczema in 3 European birth cohorts. *J Allergy Clin Immunol* 2007; 120:343–350.
37. Penders J, Thijs C, van den Brandt PA, et al. Gut microbiota composition and development of atopic manifestations in infancy: the KOALA Birth Cohort Study. *Gut* 2007; 56:661–667.
38. Koplin J, Allen K, Gurrin L, Osborne N, Tang MLK, Dharmage S. Is caesarean delivery associated with sensitization to food allergens and IgE-mediated food allergy: a systematic review. *Pediatr Allergy Immunol* 2008; 19:682–687.
39. Gern JE, Reardon CL, Hoffjan S, et al. Effects of dog ownership and genotype on immune development and atopy in infancy. *J Allergy Clin Immunol* 2004; 113:307–314.
40. Langan SM, Flohr C, Williams HC. The role of furry pets in eczema: a systematic review. *Arch Dermatol* 2007; 143:1570–1577.
41. Ball TM, Castro-Rodriguez JA, Griffith KA, Holberg CJ, Martinez FD, Wright AL. Siblings, day-care attendance, and the risk of asthma and wheezing during childhood. *N Engl J Med* 2000; 343:538–543.
42. Caudri D, Wijga A, Scholtens S, et al. Early daycare is associated with an increase in airway symptoms in early childhood but is no protection against asthma or atopy at 8 years. *Am J Respir Crit Care Med* 2009; 180:491–498.
43. Kusel MM, Holt PG, de Klerk N, Sly PD. Support for 2 variants of eczema. *J Allergy Clin Immunol* 2005; 116:1067–1072.
44. Koplin JJ, Dharmage SC, Ponsonby AL, et al. Environmental and demographic risk factors for egg allergy in a population-based study of infants. *Allergy* 2012; 67:1415–1422.
45. von Hertzen LC, Laatikainen T, Makela MJ, et al. Infectious burden as a determinant of atopy—a comparison between adults in Finnish and Russian Karelia. *Int Arch Allergy Immunol* 2006; 140:89–95.
46. McCune A, Lane A, Murray L, et al. Reduced risk of atopic disorders in adults with Helicobacter pylori infection. *Eur J Gastroenterol Hepatol* 2003; 15:637–640.
47. Firer MA, Hosking CS, Hill DJ. Possible role for rotavirus in the development of cows' milk enteropathy in infants. *Clin Allergy* 1988; 18:53–61.
48. Reimerink J, Stelma F, Rockx B, et al. Early-life rotavirus and norovirus infections in relation to development of atopic manifestation in infants. *Clin Exp Allergy* 2009; 39:254–260.
49. Levin ME, Le Souef PN, Motala C. Total IgE in urban Black South African teenagers: the influence of atopy and helminth infection. *Pediatr Allergy Immunol* 2008; 19:449–454.
50. Hamelmann E, Beyer K, Gruber C, et al. Primary prevention of allergy: avoiding risk or providing protection? *Clin Exp Allergy* 2008; 38:233–245.
51. Prescott SL, Smith P, Tang M, et al. The importance of early complementary feeding in the development of oral tolerance: concerns and controversies. *Pediatr Allergy Immunol* 2008; 19:375–380.
52. Du Toit G, Katz Y, Sasieni P, et al. Early consumption of peanuts in infancy is associated with a low prevalence of peanut allergy. *J Allergy Clin Immunol* 2008; 122:984–991.
53. Koplin JJ, Osborne NJ, Wake M, et al. Can early introduction of egg prevent egg allergy in infants? A population-based study. *J Allergy Clin Immunol* 2010; 126:807–813.
54. ASCIA. Infant feeding advice. *Australasian Society of Clinical Immunology and Allergy (ASCIA)* 2011; http://www.allergy.org.au/health-professionals/papers/ascia-infant-feeding-advice.
55. Greer FR, Sicherer SH, Burks AW. Effects of early nutritional interventions on the development of atopic disease in infants and children: the role of maternal dietary restriction, breast-feeding, timing of introduction of complementary foods, and hydrolyzed formulas. *Pediatrics* 2008; 121:183–191.
56. Snijders BE, Thijs C, van Ree R, van den Brandt PA. Age at first introduction of cow milk products and other food products in relation to infant atopic manifestations in the first 2 years of life: the KOALA Birth Cohort Study. *Pediatrics* 2008; 122:e115–e122.
57. Zutavern A, Brockow I, Schaaf B, et al. Timing of solid food introduction in relation to eczema, asthma, allergic rhinitis, and food and inhalant sensitization at the age of 6 years: results from the prospective birth cohort study LISA. *Pediatrics* 2008; 121:e44–e52.
58. Filipiak B, Zutavern A, Koletzko S, et al. Solid food introduction in relation to eczema: results from a four-year prospective birth cohort study. *J Pediatr* 2007; 151:352–358.
59. Poole JA, Barriga K, Leung DY, et al. Timing of initial exposure to cereal grains and the risk of wheat allergy. *Pediatrics* 2006; 117:2175–2182.
60. Stark PL, Lee A. The microbial ecology of the large bowel of breast-fed and formula-fed infants during the first year of life. *J Med Microbiol* 1982; 15:189–203.
61. Halken S, Host A. Prevention. *Curr Opin Allergy Clin Immunol* 2001; 1:229–236.
62. Lowe AJ, Hosking CS, Bennett CM, et al. Effect of a partially hydrolyzed whey infant formula at weaning on risk of allergic disease in high-risk children: a randomized controlled trial. *J Allergy Clin Immunol* 2011; 128:360–365.
63. Prescott SL, Tang ML. The Australasian Society of Clinical Immunology and Allergy position statement: summary of allergy prevention in children. *Med J Aust* 2005; 182:464–467.
64. Vuillermin PJ, Ponsonby AL, Kemp AS, Allen KJ. Potential links between the emerging risk factors for food allergy and vitamin D status. *Clin Exp Allergy;* 2013;43(6):599–607.
65. Rudders SA, Espinola JA, Camargo CA Jr. North–south differences in US emergency department visits for acute allergic reactions. *Ann Allergy Asthma Immunol* 2010; 104:413–416.
66. Camargo CA Jr, Clark S, Kaplan MS, Lieberman P, Wood RA. Regional differences in EpiPen prescriptions in the United States: the potential role of vitamin D. *J Allergy Clin Immunol* 2007; 120:131–136.
67. Vassallo MF, Banerji A, Rudders SA, Clark S, Camargo CA Jr. Season of birth and food-induced anaphylaxis in Boston. *Allergy* 2010; 65:1492–1493.
68. Mullins RJ, Clark S, Katelaris C, Smith V, Solley G, Camargo CA Jr. Season of birth and childhood food allergy in Australia. *Pediatr Allergy Immunol* 2011; 22:583–589.

69. Osborne NJ, Ukoumunne OC, Wake M, Allen KJ. Prevalence of eczema and food allergy is associated with latitude in Australia. *J Allergy Clin Immunol* 2012; 129:865–867.
70. Holick MF. Vitamin D deficiency. *N Engl J Med* 2007; 357:266–281.
71. Morley R, Carlin JB, Pasco JA, Wark JD, Ponsonby AL. Maternal 25-hydroxyvitamin D concentration and offspring birth size: effect modification by infant VDR genotype. *Eur J Clin Nutr* 2009; 63:802–804.
72. Cantorna MT, Mahon BD. D-hormone and the immune system. *J Rheumatol Suppl* 2005; 76:11–20.
73. Shreffler WG, Wanich N, Moloney M, Nowak-Wegrzyn A, Sampson HA. Association of allergen-specific regulatory T cells with the onset of clinical tolerance to milk protein. *J Allergy Clin Immunol* 2009; 123:43–52.
74. Liu PT, Stenger S, Li H, et al. Toll-like receptor triggering of a vitamin D-mediated human antimicrobial response. *Science* 2006; 311:1770–1773.
75. Yim S, Dhawan P, Ragunath C, Christakos S, Diamond G. Induction of cathelicidin in normal and CF bronchial epithelial cells by 1,25-dihydroxyvitamin D(3). *J Cyst Fibros* 2007; 6:403–410.
76. Wang TT, Dabbas B, Laperriere D, et al. Direct and indirect induction by 1,25-dihydroxyvitamin D3 of the NOD2/CARD15-defensin beta2 innate immune pathway defective in Crohn disease. *J Biol Chem* 2010; 285:2227–2231.
77. Sicherer SH, Furlong TJ, Maes HH, Desnick RJ, Sampson HA, Gelb BD. Genetics of peanut allergy: a twin study. *J Allergy Clin Immunol* 2000; 106:53–56.
78. Tsai H-J, Kumar R, Pongracicwz J, et al. Familial aggregation of food allergy and sensitization to food allergens: a family-based study. *Clin Exp Allergy* 2009; 39:101–109.
79. Greco L, Romino R, Coto I, et al. The first large population based twin study of coeliac disease. *Gut* 2002; 50:624–628.
80. Palmer CN, Irvine AD, Terron-Kwiatkowski A, et al. Common loss-of-function variants of the epidermal barrier protein filaggrin are a major predisposing factor for atopic dermatitis. *Nat Genet* 2006; 38:441–446.
81. Marenholz I, Nickel R, Rüschendorf F, et al. Filaggrin loss-of-function mutations predispose to phenotypes involved in the atopic march. *J Allergy Clin Immunol* 2006; 118:866–871.
82. Tan T, Ellis J, Koplin J, et al. Filaggrin loss-of-function mutations predict food sensitization but do not increase the risk of food allergy amongst sensitized infants. *J Allergy Clin Immunol* 2012; 130:1211–1213.
83. Brown SJ, Asai Y, Cordell HJ, et al. Loss-of-function variants in the filaggrin gene are a significant risk factor for peanut allergy. *J Allergy Clin Immunol* 2011; 127:661–667.
84. Fourlanos S, Varney MD, Tait BD, et al. The rising incidence of type 1 diabetes is accounted for by cases with lower-risk human leukocyte antigen genotypes. *Diabetes Care* 2008; 31:1546–1549.
85. Jirtle RL, Skinner MK. Environmental epigenomics and disease susceptibility. *Nat Rev Genet* 2007; 8:253–262.
86. Klose RJ, Bird AP. Genomic DNA methylation: the mark and its mediators. *Trends Biochem Sci* 2006; 31:89–97.
87. Bird A. Perceptions of epigenetics. *Nature* 2007; 447:396–398.
88. Barker DJ. In utero programming of chronic disease. *Clin Sci (Lond)* 1998; 95:115–128.

10 The Spectrum of Allergic Reactions to Foods

Stacie M. Jones[1] & A. Wesley Burks[2]

[1]Division of Allergy and Immunology, University of Arkansas for Medical Sciences and Arkansas Children's Hospital, Little Rock, AR, USA

[2]Department of Pediatrics, University of North Carolina, Chapel Hill, NC, USA

Key Concepts

- Immunoglobulin E-mediated food allergy is the most common and well-recognized form of food hypersensitivity.
- Allergic reactions to food range from mild to life-threatening.
- Risk factors for life-threatening anaphylaxis are important to recognize.
- Atopic dermatitis and asthma are allergic conditions in which hypersensitivity to food(s) may play a role in disease activity.
- Food allergy is often associated with eosinophilic gastrointestinal disorders and may induce clinical symptoms.

Introduction

An *adverse food reaction* is a general term that can be applied to a clinically abnormal response to an ingested food or food additive. The ingestion of food represents the greatest foreign antigenic load confronting the human immune system. In the vast majority of individuals, oral tolerance of food proteins is the norm. However, when oral tolerance fails, the immune system is primed to develop aberrant immune responses characteristic of food-allergic reactions [1]. Adverse food reactions are common and often assumed by patients to be allergic in nature. Interestingly, up to 35% of patients surveyed perceive that they or a family member have a food allergy; however, far fewer have confirmed food-allergic disease [2]. Food allergies are most prevalent in childhood with ~4% of US children <18 years of age reporting food allergy [3]. Additionally, food allergy prevalence increased from 1997 to 2007 by 18% [3]. Food allergy affects approximately 6–8% of children less than 3 years of age and has been described in recent publications as affecting more than 1–2% but less than 10% of the population [4–7]. The most common food allergens in children include milk, egg, soy, wheat, peanuts, tree nuts, fish, and shellfish, while peanuts, tree nuts, fish, and shellfish are the most common food allergens affecting adults [6]. About 2.5% of infants have hypersensitivity reactions to cow milk in the first year of life, with about 80% "outgrowing" the allergy by their fifth birthday [6, 8]. IgE-mediated reactions account for about 60% of milk-allergic reactions; about 25% of these infants retain their sensitivity into the second decade of life, and 35% go on to acquire other food allergies. About 1.5% of young children are allergic to eggs and 0.5% to peanuts [6, 9]. Some evidence suggests that the prevalence of peanut allergy has been increasing during the past two decades [10–12]. Children with atopic disorders tend to have a higher prevalence of food allergy; about 35% of children with moderate to severe atopic dermatitis (AD) have IgE-mediated food allergy [13], and about 6% of children with asthma have food-induced wheezing [14]. Adverse reactions to food additives have also been demonstrated to affect 0.5–1% of children [6, 15, 16]. Food allergy appears to be less common in adults, although adequate epidemiologic studies are lacking. A survey in the United States indicated that peanut and tree nut allergies together affect 1.1% of American adults [9, 17]. Overall, it is estimated that about 2% of adults in the United States are affected by food allergies [2, 7, 18]. Adverse reactions to foods are classified as either *food allergy (hypersensitivity)* or *food intolerance* [6].

Food allergy

Food allergy is defined as an adverse health effect arising from a specific immune response that occurs reproducibly

Food Allergy: Adverse Reactions to Foods and Food Additives, Fifth Edition. Edited by Dean D Metcalfe, Hugh A Sampson, Ronald A Simon and Gideon Lack.

on exposure to a given food [6]. This reaction occurs only in some patients, may occur after only a small amount of the substance is ingested, and is unrelated to any physiologic effect of the food or food additive. Food allergy occurs due to an immune response that typically involves the immunoglobulin E (IgE) mechanism, of which anaphylaxis is the best example [6]. Several other food hypersensitivity disorders involve cell-mediated immune responses that are associated with IgE production or may be entirely unrelated to IgE-mediated responses.

Food intolerance

Food intolerance is a general term describing an abnormal physiologic response to an ingested food or food additive [6]. This reaction has not been proven to be immunologic in nature, which distinguishes these reactions from those occurring as a result of food allergy. Food intolerance may be caused by many factors including toxic contaminants (e.g., histamine in scombroid fish poisoning, toxins secreted by infectious agents such as *Salmonella, Shigella,* and *Campylobacter*), pharmacologic properties of the food (e.g., caffeine in coffee, tyramine in aged cheeses, sulfites in red wine, monosodium glutamate in Asian food), characteristics of the host such as metabolic disorders (e.g., lactase deficiency), and idiosyncratic responses.

Spectrum of food-allergic responses

The spectrum of food-allergic responses can best be understood by categorizing reactions based on the types of primary immune mechanisms responsible for these adverse reactions. The spectrum of food-induced reactions ranges from benign manifestations of disease, such as flushing or rhinorrhea, to life-threatening symptoms such as anaphylaxis or enterocolitis syndrome. In this chapter, we will examine adverse food reactions that are based on the following immune-mediated mechanisms: (1) IgE mediated, (2) non-IgE mediated, (3) eosinophilic disorders, and (4) allergic responses due to combinations of immune mechanisms (Tables 10.1 and 10.2).

Table 10.1 Food allergy disorders mediated by IgE and mixed IgE and cellular mechanisms.

Immune mechanism	Disorders
IgE mediated	
Cutaneous	Flushing/pruritus
	Urticaria/angioedema
	Contact urticaria
	Morbilliform rashes
Respiratory	Rhinoconjunctivitis
	Laryngospasm
	Wheezing/bronchospasm
Gastrointestinal	Oral allergy syndrome
	Gastrointestinal anaphylaxis
Multisystem	Generalized anaphylaxis
	Food and exercise-induced anaphylaxis
Mixed IgE and cell mediated	
Cutaneous	Atopic dermatitis
Respiratory	Asthma
Gastrointestinal	Eosinophilic esophagitis
	Eosinophilic gastroenteritis

IgE-mediated reactions

IgE-mediated food-allergic reactions are typically rapid in onset (usually within minutes to 2 hours) and are the most widely known reactions associated with foods. Symptoms are believed to be caused by preformed mediator release from tissue mast cells and circulating basophils that have been previously sensitized to a specific food antigen [19]. Specific manifestations of IgE-mediated food hypersensitivity reactions can involve any system within the human body. These reactions frequently involve the skin, respiratory tract, gastrointestinal tract, and cardiovascular system. More severe symptoms and those involving multiple systems are defined by the term "generalized anaphylaxis" and are often life-threatening. Two additional distinct presentations of IgE-mediated food-allergic reactions are the oral allergy syndrome and food-dependent, exercise-induced anaphylaxis.

Cutaneous responses

The *skin* is the most common target organ in IgE-mediated food hypersensitivity reactions, and cutaneous symptoms occur in >80% of allergic reactions to foods [19]. The ingestion of food allergens can either lead to immediate cutaneous symptoms or exacerbate chronic conditions such as AD. Acute *urticaria* and *angioedema* are the most common cutaneous manifestations of food hypersensitivity reactions, generally appearing within minutes of ingestion of the food allergen. Food allergy may account for 20% of cases of acute urticaria [19, 20]. By comparison, food allergies underlying chronic urticaria and angioedema (defined as symptoms greater than 6-week duration) are uncommon. In adult patients with chronic urticaria evaluated by placebo-controlled food challenge, less than 10%

Table 10.2 Food allergies mediated by cellular (non-IgE) mechanisms.

Cutaneous	Allergic contact dermatitis
	Dermatitis herpetiformis
Respiratory	Food protein-induced pulmonary hemosiderosis (Heiner syndrome)
Gastrointestinal	Celiac disease
	Food protein-induced enterocolitis
	Food protein-induced enteropathy
	Food protein-induced proctocolitis

of symptoms were associated with food allergy despite the perception of food involvement in as many as 50% of patients [21].

Flushing, pruritus, and morbilliform rash are other acute cutaneous manifestations that commonly occur during allergic reactions to foods. These early symptoms often precede the development of urticaria, angioedema, or more serious adverse symptoms. Food can also cause allergic contact dermatitis (ACD) and contact urticaria. ACD is a form of eczema caused by cell-mediated allergic reactions to chemical haptens that may occur naturally in foods or are additives to foods [22]. Contact urticaria to foods may be either immunologic (IgE mediated) or nonimmunologic (direct histamine release). In this condition, urticarial lesions develop only on the area of skin that is in direct contact with the food. Occupational exposure to raw meats, seafood, raw vegetables, and fruits are among the foods that have been most commonly implicated in this form of food allergy [23–25].

Respiratory and ocular responses

Upper respiratory symptoms such as rhinorrhea, sneezing, nasal congestion, and pruritus are frequently experienced during allergic reactions to foods. Nasal symptoms typically occur in conjunction with other organ system involvement [5, 19]. *Ocular* symptoms commonly occur concurrently with respiratory manifestations of IgE-mediated reactions to foods [19]. Symptoms may include periocular erythema, pruritus, conjunctival erythema, and tearing. Isolated symptoms of rhinitis and/or conjunctivitis in response to food allergen ingestion are rare.

Lower respiratory symptoms are potentially life-threatening manifestations of IgE-mediated reactions to foods [14, 19]. Symptoms can include laryngospasm, cough, and wheezing and require prompt medical intervention. In a retrospective chart review of 253 failed oral food challenges, Perry et al. found that 26% of participants experienced lower respiratory symptoms, and each of the tested foods carried a similar risk for eliciting lower respiratory symptoms [26]. Although lower respiratory symptoms can occur in any person experiencing anaphylaxis to foods, patients with underlying asthma are at increased risk of severe symptoms. Lower respiratory symptoms due to food allergy are temporally related to ingestion and are typically accompanied by other organ system involvement. It is rare that chronic lower respiratory symptoms or poorly controlled asthma are sole manifestations of food allergy [14].

These points are illustrated by a large study of 480 patients with a history of an adverse food reaction undergoing double-blind placebo-controlled oral food challenges (DBPCFC). Positive reactions were observed in 185 patients, 39% of whom had respiratory and ocular symptoms [5]. Symptoms included combinations of periocular erythema, pruritus, and tearing; nasal congestion, pruritus, sneezing, and rhinorrhea; and coughing, voice changes, and wheezing. Isolated respiratory symptoms occurred in only 5%. One area of exception involves occupational exposure to potential food allergens. Adults working in the food processing and packing industries may develop occupational food allergies and present with rhinoconjunctivitis, with or without asthma [27–30].

Gastrointestinal responses

The signs and symptoms of food-induced IgE-mediated gastrointestinal allergy are most commonly seen as immediate gastrointestinal hypersensitivity but can also be manifested as oral allergy syndrome [31].

Immediate gastrointestinal hypersensitivity is a form of IgE-mediated food allergy, which may accompany allergic manifestations in other target organs [19, 32, 33]. The symptoms vary and may include nausea, abdominal pain or cramping, vomiting, and/or diarrhea. The onset of upper gastrointestinal symptoms (nausea, vomiting, pain) is generally minutes to 2 hours after ingestion of the offending food but lower gastrointestinal symptoms, such as diarrhea, may begin immediately or may be delayed for 2–6 hours after ingestion. Symptoms may be severe and protracted resulting in the need for fluid or electrolyte replacement.

The *oral allergy syndrome or pollen-food-related syndrome* is considered to be a form of contact urticaria that is confined almost exclusively to the oropharynx and rarely involves the lower respiratory tract or other target organs [33, 34]. Oral allergy syndrome is manifested by the rapid onset of pruritus and angioedema of the lips, tongue, palate, and throat. This syndrome has been reported in up to 50% of patients with pollen-induced rhinoconjunctivitis and is most commonly associated with the ingestion of fresh fruits and vegetables. For example, patients with ragweed allergy may experience symptoms following contact with melons (e.g., watermelons, cantaloupe, honeydew) and bananas. Birch pollen-sensitive patients often have symptoms following the ingestion of raw potatoes, carrots, celery, apples, pears, cherries, and hazelnuts. Mugwort-allergic patients may react to celery or mustard. Symptoms typically resolve spontaneously within minutes after ingestion ceases. Although symptoms rarely progress to involve other organ systems, progression to systemic involvement has been noted in ~10% of patients with anaphylaxis reported in not more than one to two. Tree nuts and peanuts causing oral symptoms are best avoided because of the frequency with which these foods cause more severe reactions. Peanut- and tree nut-associated oral symptoms are not usually defined as part of the oral allergy syndrome, but rather serve as a precursor "warning sign" for more advanced symptoms to follow [35–37]. In certain countries, such as in northern Europe, hazelnut allergy associated with IgE antibodies to Cor a and peanut allergy associated with antibodies with Ara h8 are more common causes of the oral allergy syndrome due to their cross-reactivity to tree pollens.

Generalized anaphylaxis

Anaphylaxis is defined as a "severe, potentially fatal, systemic allergic reaction that occurs suddenly after contact with an allergy-causing substance" [6, 19]. Food-induced generalized anaphylaxis involves multiple organ systems and has been estimated to account for 30–50% of all anaphylaxis treated in emergency department settings [38–41]. Peanuts, tree nuts, fish, and shellfish account for more anaphylactic reactions than any other foods. In generalized anaphylaxis, the onset of symptoms is abrupt, often occurring within minutes of ingestion. Symptoms are due to the effects of potent intracellular mediators such as histamine and tryptase that are released from mast cells and basophils during an allergic reaction and can involve any organ system [19]. Severe or life-threatening anaphylactic reactions involving the respiratory and cardiovascular systems can culminate in respiratory failure, hypotension, cardiac dysrhythmias, shock, and death if left untreated. A biphasic reaction may be seen in up to 20% of patients, noted as a recurrence of symptoms hours after the initial onset. This second phase may follow a quiescent, asymptomatic interval [6, 37, 42].

Recently, symptoms of "delayed" anaphylaxis have been described in patients (typically adolescents and adults) following ingestion of mammalian meats, such as beef, pork, and lamb [43, 44]. Symptoms are typical of anaphylaxis but begin 3–6 hours after meat ingestion rather than within the first 2 hours of exposure. This form of delayed anaphylaxis has been attributed to IgE antibodies to galactose-α-1,3-galactose (α-gal), a newly defined mammalian cross-reactive carbohydrate determinant. To date, patients have been described from a geographic region in the mid-south to Virginia with links to tick bite exposure.

Fatal and near-fatal reactions to foods have been described [35–37, 45]. Peanuts and tree nuts are the most common allergens reported in such cases. Risk factors associated with fatal food-induced anaphylaxis include adolescent or young adult age group, coexistent asthma, history of previous serious reaction, delayed administration of epinephrine, and absence of skin symptoms. In a series of 13 children with fatal or near-fatal anaphylactic reactions to food, all were known to have food allergies and had accidentally ingested peanuts (four patients), nuts (six patients), eggs (one patient), or milk (two patients) [37]. Twelve of the 13 had asthma that was well controlled. Six patients died, with only two of those receiving epinephrine within the first hour. By comparison, six of the seven survivors received epinephrine within 30 minutes. The correlation between absence of skin findings and fatal anaphylaxis has not been systematically studied, although it is postulated to result from the rapid development of hypotension, resulting in poor skin perfusion and minimal skin symptoms. An alternative explanation may be that patients lacking skin symptoms are not recognized as having anaphylaxis as quickly, leading to a delay in treatment and consequent poor outcome.

Food-associated, exercise-induced anaphylaxis

There have been increasingly more reports of patients with anaphylaxis that occurs only when the ingestion of food is coupled with exercise within a 2- to 4-hour time interval. This syndrome is known as food-associated, exercise-induced anaphylaxis [6, 46–49]. It appears to be most prevalent in adolescents and young adults, although there have been reports in middle-aged patients as well. Most patients react to one or two specific foods. Common causative foods include wheat, celery, and seafood [46–49]. Classically, the food can be ingested in the absence of exercise without development of symptoms. Alternatively, patients may exercise without eating the specific food without induction of symptoms. The coupling of specific food ingestion and exercise, however, produces a potentially life-threatening anaphylaxis.

Non-IgE-mediated reactions

Non-IgE-mediated food allergies typically present with more subacute or chronic symptoms isolated to the gastrointestinal tract that present within hours or days of food ingestion. Affected patients commonly present with a classic constellation of features that are consistent with well-described clinical disorders (Table 10.2). These disorders include food protein-induced enterocolitis, food protein-induced proctocolitis, food protein-induced gastroenteropathy, food-induced contact dermatitis, celiac disease with or without dermatitis herpetiformis (DH), allergic skin reactions, and food-induced pulmonary hemosiderosis. Although the precise immune mechanisms have not been described, evidence suggests a cell-mediated hypersensitivity response associated with all of these disorders.

Cutaneous responses

Food-induced ACD has been reported in individuals without IgE antibodies to the causal food [22, 50]. This reaction typically occurs in food handlers and can be confirmed by patch testing, thus indicating a cell-mediated immune response. Implicated foods frequently include fish, shellfish, meats, and eggs [23–25].

DH is a skin manifestation of celiac disease (gluten-sensitive enteropathy). DH is a chronic blistering skin rash characterized by chronic, pruritic papulovesicular lesions that are symmetrically distributed over the extensor surfaces of the extremities and on the buttocks [51–53]. Gastrointestinal symptoms and histopathologic findings within the gut mucosa are generally milder than those seen in patients presenting with primary gastrointestinal disease. Elimination of gluten from the diet typically results in resolution of skin and gastrointestinal lesions.

Gastrointestinal responses

Food protein-induced enterocolitis syndrome (FPIES) is a disorder which presents most commonly in early infancy [6, 54–56]. Acute symptoms are typically isolated to the gastrointestinal tract and consist of profuse, repetitive vomiting and sometimes diarrhea. Symptoms are often severe and may cause dehydration, hypotension, and shock, often leading to an erroneous diagnosis of sepsis. Cow's milk and/or soy protein in infant formulas or maternal breast milk are most often responsible for induction of symptoms, although FPIES due to solid food (e.g., cereal grains and meats) is often seen [55–57]. Objective findings on stool examination consist of gross or occult blood, polymorphonuclear neutrophils, eosinophils, Charcot–Leyden crystals, and positive reducing substances. IgE testing for food proteins is characteristically negative. Jejunal biopsies often reveal flattened villi, edema, and increased numbers of lymphocytes, eosinophils, and mast cells. A food challenge with the responsible protein generally results in vomiting and occasionally diarrhea within minutes to several hours, and occasionally leads to shock [31, 55].

Infants and children with FPIES are often allergic to both cow's milk and soy protein. Approximately 50% of children with cow's milk allergy will have concomitant soy allergy; therefore, it is recommended that infants with FPIES due to cow's milk also avoid soy products [31, 53, 55–57]. Elimination of the offending allergen generally results in resolution of the symptoms within 72 hours although secondary disaccharidase deficiency may persist longer. This disorder tends to subside by 18–24 months of age, but may last longer in a subset of children.

Food protein-induced enteropathy is characterized by diarrhea, vomiting, malabsorption, and poor weight gain [6, 58, 59]. It is clinically distinguishable from FPIES due to the presence of nonbloody stools. Vomiting is often less prominent, and reexposure does not elicit acute symptoms after a period of avoidance. Onset of symptoms is typically delayed for days to weeks and may require continual feeding of the culprit food protein. Other clinical features include abdominal pain and distension, as well as hypoproteinemia leading to peripheral edema. Patients typically present in the first year of life. The most common causal food is cow's milk although other foods such as soy, egg, and grains have been associated with food protein-induced enteropathy. Histologic examination reveals patchy villous atrophy mononuclear cell infiltrates and few eosinophils. Symptoms typically resolve within 72 hours after dietary elimination and it is usually outgrown within 12–24 months of dietary allergen avoidance.

Food protein-induced proctocolitis generally presents in the first few months of life and, like FPIES, is most often secondary to cow's milk and/or soy protein hypersensitivity [6, 31, 32]. Infants with this disorder often do not appear ill and generally present with bloody stools. Other distinguishing features include normal growth and absence of vomiting. Gastrointestinal lesions are usually confined to the rectum but can involve the entire large bowel and consist of eosinophilic infiltrates or abscesses in the epithelium and lamina propria. If lesions are severe with crypt destruction, PMNs are also prominent in this disorder. Food protein-induced proctocolitis typically resolves after 6–12 months of dietary allergen avoidance. Elimination of the offending food allergen leads to resolution of hematochezia within 72 hours, but the mucosal lesions may take up to 1 month to disappear and range from patchy mucosal injection to severe friability with small aphthoid ulcerations and bleeding.

Celiac disease (or gluten-sensitive enteropathy) is an extensive enteropathy leading to malabsorption [60, 61]. Total villous atrophy and an extensive cellular infiltrate are associated with sensitivity to gliadin, the alcohol-soluble portion of gluten found in wheat, rye, and barley. Celiac disease is almost exclusively limited to genetically predisposed individuals who express the HLA-DQ2 and/or HLA-DQ8 heterodimers [61–63]. Patients often have presenting symptoms of diarrhea or frank steatorrhea, abdominal distention and flatulence, failure to thrive, and occasionally nausea and vomiting. Oral ulcers and other extraintestinal symptoms secondary to malabsorption are sometimes associated. Serologic testing aids in the diagnosis and includes measurement of anti-IgA antibodies to human tissue transglutaminase (TTG) and anti-endomysial antibody (EMA) [60, 61]. Serologic testing to rule out low total serum IgA (IgA deficiency) is essential for the diagnosis of celiac disease. Confirmation with endoscopic biopsies is necessary for the diagnosis and reveals total villous atrophy and inflammatory infiltrates. Clinical symptoms and endoscopic findings resolve with strict dietary elimination of gluten that must be maintained for life.

Respiratory responses

Food-induced pulmonary hemosiderosis (Heiner syndrome) is a rare syndrome in infants characterized by recurrent pneumonia with pulmonary infiltrates, hemosiderosis, gastrointestinal blood loss, iron deficiency anemia, and failure to thrive [64, 65]. Symptoms are associated with non-IgE-mediated hypersensitivity to cow's milk with evidence of peripheral eosinophilia and the presence of cow's milk precipitins on diagnostic testing. Deposits of immunoglobulins and C3 may also be found on lung biopsy. Strict dietary elimination of milk results in reversal of symptoms.

Adverse food reactions associated with eosinophilic disease

Allergic eosinophilic gastrointestinal disorders are a group of disorders characterized by symptoms of postprandial gastrointestinal dysfunction associated with eosinophilic infiltration of at least one layer of the gastrointestinal tract, absence of vasculitis, and peripheral eosinophilia in about 50% of cases [4, 31, 58, 66]. These disorders are defined by the site(s) of involvement and include eosinophilic esophagitis (EoE) and eosinophilic gastroenteritis. Symptoms for each of these syndromes are related to the specific anatomical site of involvement. The pathogenesis of these disorders likely involves both IgE-mediated and cellular immune mechanisms.

Eosinophilic esophagitis

EoE is defined as a chronic immune/antigen-mediated esophageal disease characterized clinically by symptoms related to esophageal dysfunction and histologically by eosinophil-predominant inflammation [66]. Symptoms are typically severe or refractory gastrointestinal symptoms and include dysphagia, epigastric pain, and postprandial nausea and vomiting [66–68]. This disorder should be considered in patients of any age presenting with esophageal symptoms, especially when recalcitrant to symptomatic treatment, such as proton-pump inhibitors (PPIs) or other antireflux medications. Very young children may present with feeding disorders, whereas older children and adults present with dysphagia, vomiting, and abdominal pain. A history of food impaction is common.

Many patients with EoE have other atopic diseases. In a series of 103 children with EoE, rhinoconjunctivitis was present in 57% and wheezing was noted in 37%, while possible food allergy was cited in 46% [66, 69, 70]. In a retrospective review of 381 children with EoE, the most commonly implicated foods were cow's milk, egg, soy, corn, wheat, and beef. Implementation of an empiric 6-food elimination diet (e.g., milk, egg, soy, wheat, peanut/tree nuts, fish/shellfish) has been associated with reductions in eosinophilic inflammation and improved clinical symptoms, thus indicating that common food allergens play a role in EoE in a significant number of patients [53, 67, 70]. Most patients with evidence of food sensitivity tested positive for multiple foods, and children have evidence for more food allergy than adults [66, 68]. Elimination of these foods or the use of elemental diets typically results in clinical and histologic improvement. However, the pathophysiologic relationship between EoE and allergens, such as foods or aeroallergens, remains unclear.

Eosinophils are not normally found in the esophageal mucosa and symptoms are likely due to the release of eosinophilic mediators. EoE is clinically distinguishable from gastroesophageal reflux disease (GERD) due to its feature of being refractory to aggressive management with antacids, PPIs and promotility medications that are typically effective in the treatment of GERD. Other distinguishing characteristics include normal pH probe results, the presence of patient or family history of atopy, and peripheral eosinophilia. On endoscopy, EoE patients may have visually normal-appearing esophageal mucosa although esophageal furrowing and rings have been reported [66, 67, 71]. On histologic examination, esophageal biopsies in patients with EoE typically contain >15 eosinophils per HPF as compared with <5 eosinophils per HPF in patients with GERD [66]. Proximal and mid-esophageal lesions are common in EoE whereas reactive eosinophilic infiltrates due to GERD are often limited to the distal esophagus [66, 67, 72].

Eosinophilic gastroenteritis

Eosinophilic gastroenteritis can present at any age with abdominal pain, nausea, diarrhea, malabsorption, and weight loss [58, 73, 74]. In infants, it may present as outlet obstruction with postprandial projectile vomiting. In adolescents and adults, it can mimic irritable bowel syndrome [75]. Approximately one-half of patients have allergic disease, such as defined food allergies, asthma, eczema, or rhinitis [73]. However, in contrast to EoE, avoidance of implicated foods may have limited value [73, 74]. Eosinophilic gastroenteritis is characterized by eosinophilic infiltration of the stomach, small intestine, or both with variable involvement of the large intestine [76]. Symptoms may include vomiting, abdominal pain, diarrhea, malabsorption, and failure to thrive. Severe symptoms can mimic pyloric stenosis or other forms of gastric outlet obstruction when duodenal involvement is present. Since eosinophils may normally be found in the stomach and intestine, endoscopic findings are more difficult to interpret as compared to EoE. In addition, multiple sites may need to be biopsied to effectively exclude eosinophilic gastroenteritis due to the patchy nature of eosinophilic infiltration. Biopsies in eosinophilic gastroenteritis will typically show 20–40 eosinophils per HPF. Treatment may involve elimination of the potential offending food(s) or institution of an elemental diet with slow addition of foods. Similar to EoE, eosinophilic gastroenteritis usually follows a prolonged course requiring protracted therapy and dietary intervention for months to years. After dietary restriction, foods can be reintroduced slowly after avoidance and based on endoscopic and clinical evidence of disease resolution.

Food aversion

Food aversion may be an adverse manifestation of food allergy, especially in young infants and children. Food aversion is typically manifested as overt food refusal or avoidance of foods or food groups that are generally "safe" foods and not part of the medically indicated food restriction diet. This can occur among patients with any form of immune-based food allergy as a behavioral response to diet restriction and food allergy management. Nutritional outcomes can be poor if food aversion is not addressed. Behavioral management and counseling with a trained specialist (e.g., child psychologist) is necessary in most cases to resolve food aversion behavior and to resume normal dietary intake of safe foods.

Conditions associated with multiple immune mechanisms

Asthma

Asthma alone is an infrequent manifestation of food allergy. Although ingestion of food allergens is rarely the main aggravating factor in chronic asthma, there is some evidence to suggest that food antigens can provoke bronchial hyperreactivity [14, 77]. An exception is occupational asthma (often with accompanying rhinitis) in food-industry workers. "Baker's asthma," caused by IgE-mediated allergy to inhaled wheat proteins, is an example [78]. Patients with these conditions may not react to the food upon ingestion, rather only with inhalation exposure. More typically, asthma is seen as a component of more generalized, IgE-mediated reactions. Asthmatic reactions secondary to airborne food allergens have been reported in cases where susceptible individuals are exposed to vapors or steam emitted from cooking food, for example, fish, mollusks, crustacea, eggs, and garbanzo beans (chick pea) [27–30].

Another relationship between food allergy and asthma is that coexisting asthma is a significant risk factor for death from food-induced anaphylaxis. Conversely, substantially higher rates of food allergy are noted among children requiring intubation for asthma compared to a control group of asthmatic children [6, 35, 36, 79, 80].

Atopic dermatitis

AD is a chronic skin disorder that generally begins in early infancy and is characterized by typical distribution, extreme pruritus, chronically relapsing course, and association with asthma and allergic rhinitis [13]. Food allergy has been correlated with the development and persistence of AD, especially during infancy and early childhood. In children <5 years old, 35–40% will be allergic to at least one food [6, 13, 81–83]. These patients typically fail to respond to conventional medical therapy or may have frequent exacerbations of underlying skin disease if causal foods are not strictly avoided. The most common foods associated with AD include cow's milk, egg, peanut, soy, wheat, fish, and tree nuts. Due to the chronicity of symptoms, a trial of dietary elimination of the suspected food allergen and the use of diagnostic food challenges may be warranted to aid in the accurate diagnosis of food allergy in these children. Dietary elimination of relevant food allergens may result in clearing of the skin. However, some patients continue to have ongoing skin disease due to concomitant sensitization to aeroallergens or due to nonallergic triggers.

In one well-designed report, 113 patients with marked AD underwent DBPCFC [82]. Among the 101 positive food challenges observed in 63 children skin, gastrointestinal, and respiratory symptoms were observed in 84%, 52%, and 32% oral food challenges, respectively. Some patients were subsequently placed on elimination diets based upon these findings, with most exhibiting significant clinical improvement in skin symptoms. Although egg, peanut, and milk were responsible for most reactions, it was difficult to predict the patients with food allergy based upon history and laboratory information alone.

In a single center's experience evaluating over 2000 food challenges in 600 children with AD, ~40% of the DBPCFCs were positive [83]. Nearly 75% of the positive tests included cutaneous manifestations, principally consisting of macular, morbilliform, and/or pruritic rashes located in areas commonly affected by AD. Approximately 30% of positive tests consisted of skin rashes alone.

Summary

Inadvertent ingestion of food allergens in sensitized, allergic individuals may provoke a variety of cutaneous, respiratory, gastrointestinal symptoms, and/or systemic anaphylaxis with shock. Additionally, other non-IgE-mediated adverse food reactions can significantly alter quality of life and health outcomes and can pose serious, life-threatening reactions. A better understanding of the immunopathologic mechanisms associated with oral tolerance and food allergy development is critical to advancing our ability to better recognize the spectrum of adverse food reactions and to provide effective immunologic targets for therapeutic intervention.

References

1. Vickery BP, Scurlock AM, Jones SM, et al. Mechanisms of immune tolerance relevant to food allergy. *J Allergy Clin Immunol* 2011; 127(3):576–584.

2. Rona RJ, Keil T, Summers C, et al. The prevalence of food allergy: a meta-analysis. *J Allergy Clin Immunol* 2007; 120(3):638–646.
3. Branum AM, Lukacs SL. Food allergy among children in the United States. *Pediatrics* 2009; 124(6):1549–1555.
4. Bock SA. Prospective appraisal of complaints of adverse reactions to foods in children during the first 3 years of life. *Pediatrics* 1987; 79(5):683–688.
5. Bock SA, Atkins FM. Patterns of food hypersensitivity during sixteen years of double-blind, placebo-controlled food challenges. *J Pediatr* 1990; 117(4):561–567.
6. Boyce JA, Assa'ad A, Burks AW, et al. Guidelines for the diagnosis and management of food allergy in the United States: report of the NIAID-sponsored expert panel. *J Allergy Clin Immunol* 2010; 126(6 Suppl):S1–S58.
7. Chafen JJ, Newberry SJ, Riedl MA, et al. Diagnosing and managing common food allergies: a systematic review. *J Am Med Assoc* 2010; 303(18):1848–1856.
8. Sicherer SH, Leung DY. Advances in allergic skin disease, anaphylaxis, and hypersensitivity reactions to foods, drugs, and insects in 2010. *J Allergy Clin Immunol* 2011; 127(2):326–335.
9. Sicherer SH, Munoz-Furlong A, Godbold JH, et al. US prevalence of self-reported peanut, tree nut, and sesame allergy: 11-year follow-up. *J Allergy Clin Immunol* 2010; 125(6):1322–1326.
10. Grundy J, Matthews S, Bateman B, et al. Rising prevalence of allergy to peanut in children: data from 2 sequential cohorts. *J Allergy Clin Immunol* 2002; 110(5):784–789.
11. Sicherer SH, Munoz-Furlong A, Burks AW, et al. Prevalence of peanut and tree nut allergy in the US determined by a random digit dial telephone survey. *J Allergy Clin Immunol* 1999; 103(4):559–562.
12. Sicherer SH, Munoz-Furlong A, Sampson HA. Prevalence of peanut and tree nut allergy in the United States determined by means of a random digit dial telephone survey: a 5-year follow-up study. *J Allergy Clin Immunol* 2003; 112(6):1203–1207.
13. Eigenmann PA, Sicherer SH, Borkowski TA, et al. Prevalence of IgE-mediated food allergy among children with atopic dermatitis. *Pediatrics* 1998; 101(3):E8.
14. James JM. Respiratory manifestations of food allergy. *Pediatrics* 2003; 111(6 Pt 3):1625–1630.
15. Fuglsang G, Madsen G, Halken S, et al. Adverse reactions to food additives in children with atopic symptoms. *Allergy* 1994; 49(1):31–37.
16. Simon RA. Adverse reactions to food additives. *Curr Allergy Asthma Rep* 2003; 3(1):62–66.
17. Ben-Shoshan M, Harrington DW, Soller L, et al. A population-based study on peanut, tree nut, fish, shellfish, and sesame allergy prevalence in Canada. *J Allergy Clin Immunol* 2010;125(6):1327–1335.
18. Sloan AE, Powers ME. A perspective on popular perceptions of adverse reactions to foods. *J Allergy Clin Immunol* 1986; 78(1 Pt. 2):127–133.
19. Sicherer SH, Sampson HA. Food allergy: recent advances in pathophysiology and treatment. *Annu Rev Med* 2009; 60:261–277.
20. Sehgal VN, Rege VL. An interrogative study of 158 urticaria patients. *Ann Allergy* 1973; 31(6):279–283.
21. Kobza BA, Greaves MW, Champion RH, et al. The urticarias 1990. *Br J Dermatol* 1991; 124(1):100–108.
22. Warshaw EM, Belsito DV, Deleo VA, et al. North American Contact Dermatitis Group patch-test results, 2003–2004 study period. *Dermatitis* 2008; 19(3):129–136.
23. Jovanovic M, Oliwiecki S, Beck MH. Occupational contact urticaria from beef associated with hand eczema. *Contact Dermatitis* 1992; 27(3):188–189.
24. Delgado J, Castillo R, Quiralte J, et al. Contact urticaria in a child from raw potato. *Contact Dermatitis* 1996; 35(3):179–180.
25. Fisher AA. Contact urticaria from handling meats and fowl. *Cutis* 1982; 30(6):726, 729.
26. Perry TT, Matsui EC, Conover-Walker MK, et al. Risk of oral food challenges. *J Allergy Clin Immunol* 2004; 114(5):1164–1168.
27. Toskala E, Piipari R, Aalto-Korte K, et al. Occupational asthma and rhinitis caused by milk proteins. *J Occup Environ Med* 2004; 46(11):1100–1101.
28. Sherson D, Hansen I, Sigsgaard T. Occupationally related respiratory symptoms in trout-processing workers. *Allergy* 1989; 44(5):336–341.
29. Hudson P, Cartier A, Pineau L, et al. Follow-up of occupational asthma caused by crab and various agents. *J Allergy Clin Immunol* 1985; 76(5):682–688.
30. Storaas T, Steinsvag SK, Florvaag E, et al. Occupational rhinitis: diagnostic criteria, relation to lower airway symptoms and IgE sensitization in bakery workers. *Acta Otolaryngol* 2005; 125(11):1211–1217.
31. Sampson HA, Anderson JA. Summary and recommendations: classification of gastrointestinal manifestations due to immunologic reactions to foods in infants and young children. *J Pediatr Gastroenterol Nutr* 2000; 30(Suppl):S87–S94.
32. Crowe SE, Perdue MH. Gastrointestinal food hypersensitivity: basic mechanisms of pathophysiology. *Gastroenterology* 1992; 103(3):1075–1095.
33. Garcia-Careaga M Jr, Kerner JA Jr. Gastrointestinal manifestations of food allergies in pediatric patients. *Nutr Clin Pract* 2005; 20(5):526–535.
34. Egger M, Mutschlechner S, Wopfner N, et al. Pollen-food syndromes associated with weed pollinosis: an update from the molecular point of view. *Allergy* 2006; 61(4):461–476.
35. Bock SA, Munoz-Furlong A, Sampson HA. Fatalities due to anaphylactic reactions to foods. *J Allergy Clin Immunol* 2001; 107(1):191–193.
36. Bock SA, Munoz-Furlong A, Sampson HA. Further fatalities caused by anaphylactic reactions to food, 2001–2006. *J Allergy Clin Immunol* 2007; 119(4):1016–1018.
37. Sampson HA, Mendelson L, Rosen JP. Fatal and near-fatal anaphylactic reactions to food in children and adolescents. *N Engl J Med* 1992; 327(6):380–384.
38. Yocum MW, Butterfield JH, Klein JS, et al. Epidemiology of anaphylaxis in Olmsted County: a population-based study. *J Allergy Clin Immunol* 1999; 104(2 Pt. 1):452–456.
39. Clark S, Bock SA, Gaeta TJ, et al. Multicenter study of emergency department visits for food allergies. *J Allergy Clin Immunol* 2004; 113(2):347–352.

40. Sampson HA. Adverse reactions to foods. In: Adkinson N, Bochner BS, Yunginger JW, et al. (eds), *Middleton's Allergy Principles and Practice*. Mosby, 2003; pp. 1619–1643.
41. Clark S, Espinola J, Rudders SA, et al. Frequency of US emergency department visits for food-related acute allergic reactions. *J Allergy Clin Immunol* 2011; 127(3):682–683.
42. Lieberman P. Biphasic anaphylactic reactions. *Ann Allergy Asthma Immunol* 2005; 95(3):217–226.
43. Commins SP, Satinover SM, Hosen J, et al. Delayed anaphylaxis, angioedema, or urticaria after consumption of red meat in patients with IgE antibodies specific for galactose-alpha-1,3-galactose. *J Allergy Clin Immunol* 2009; 123(2):426–433.
44. Commins SP, Platts-Mills TA. Anaphylaxis syndromes related to a new mammalian cross-reactive carbohydrate determinant. *J Allergy Clin Immunol* 2009; 124(4):652–657.
45. Yunginger JW, Nelson DR, Squillace DL, et al. Laboratory investigation of deaths due to anaphylaxis. *J Forensic Sci* 1991; 36(3):857–865.
46. Du Toit G. Food-dependent exercise-induced anaphylaxis in childhood. *Pediatr Allergy Immunol* 2007; 18(5):455–463.
47. Beaudouin E, Renaudin JM, Morisset M, Codreanu F, Kanny G, Moneret-Vautrin DA. Food-dependent exercise-induced anaphylaxis—update and current data. *Eur Ann Allergy Clinical Immunol* 2006; 38(2):45–51.
48. Morita E, Kunie K, Matsuo H. Food-dependent exercise-induced anaphylaxis. *J Dermatol Sci* 2007; 47(2):109–117.
49. Romano A, Di Fonso M, Giuffreda F, et al. Diagnostic work-up for food-dependent, exercise-induced anaphylaxis. *Allergy* 1995; 50(10):817–824.
50. Hjorth N, Roed-Petersen J. Occupational protein contact dermatitis in food handlers. *Contact Dermatitis* 1976; 2(1):28–42.
51. Zone JJ. Skin manifestations of celiac disease. *Gastroenterology* 2005; 128(4 Suppl 1):S87–S91.
52. Fasano MB. Dermatologic food allergy *Pediatr Ann* 2006; 35(10):727–731.
53. Chehade M, Aceves SS. Food allergy and eosinophilic esophagitis. *Curr Opin Allergy Clin Immunol* 2010; 10(3):231–237.
54. Mehr S, Kakakios A, Frith K, et al. Food protein-induced enterocolitis syndrome: 16-year experience. *Pediatrics* 2009; 123(3):e459–e464.
55. Nowak-Wegrzyn A, Muraro A. Food protein-induced enterocolitis syndrome. *Curr Opin Allergy Clin Immunol* 2009; 9(4):371–377.
56. Sicherer SH. Food protein-induced enterocolitis syndrome: case presentations and management lessons. *J Allergy Clin Immunol* 2005; 115(1):149–156.
57. Nowak-Wegrzyn A, Sampson HA, Wood RA, et al. Food protein-induced enterocolitis syndrome caused by solid food proteins. *Pediatrics* 2003; 111(4 Pt 1):829–835.
58. Chehade M, Magid MS, Mofidi S, et al. Allergic eosinophilic gastroenteritis with protein-losing enteropathy: intestinal pathology, clinical course, and long-term follow-up. *J Pediatr Gastroenterol Nutr* 2006; 42(5):516–521.
59. Lake A. Food protein-induced gastroenteropathy in infants and children. In: Metcalfe DD, Sampson HA, Simon R (eds), *Food Allergy Adverse Reactions to Foods and Food Additives*. St. Louis, MO: Mosby, 1991; pp. 173–185.
60. Hill ID, Dirks MH, Liptak GS, et al. Guideline for the diagnosis and treatment of celiac disease in children: recommendations of the North American Society for Pediatric Gastroenterology, Hepatology and Nutrition. *J Pediatr Gastroenterol Nutr* 2005; 40(1):1–19.
61. Fasano A, Araya M, Bhatnagar S, et al. Federation of International Societies of Pediatric Gastroenterology, Hepatology, and Nutrition consensus report on celiac disease. *J Pediatr Gastroenterol Nutr* 2008; 47(2):214–219.
62. Papadopoulos GK, Wijmenga C, Koning F. Interplay between genetics and the environment in the development of celiac disease: perspectives for a healthy life. *J Clin Invest* 2001; 108(9):1261–1266.
63. Sollid LM, Thorsby E. HLA susceptibility genes in celiac disease: genetic mapping and role in pathogenesis. *Gastroenterology* 1993; 105(3):910–922.
64. Heiner DC, Sears JW, Kniker WT. Multiple precipitins to cow's milk in chronic respiratory disease. A syndrome including poor growth, gastrointestinal symptoms, evidence of allergy, iron deficiency anemia, and pulmonary hemosiderosis. *Am J Dis Child* 1962; 103:634–654.
65. Lee SK, Kniker WT, Cook CD, et al. Cow's milk-induced pulmonary disease in children. *Adv Pediatr* 1978; 25:39–57.
66. Liacouras CA, Furuta GT, Hirano I, et al. Eosinophilic esophagitis: updated consensus recommendations for children and adults. *J Allergy Clin Immunol* 2011; 128(1):3–20.
67. Aceves SS, Newbury RO, Dohil R, et al. Distinguishing eosinophilic esophagitis in pediatric patients: clinical, endoscopic, and histologic features of an emerging disorder. *J Clin Gastroenterol* 2007; 41(3):252–256.
68. Liacouras CA, Spergel JM, Ruchelli E, et al. Eosinophilic esophagitis: a 10-year experience in 381 children. *Clin Gastroenterol Hepatol* 2005; 3(12):1198–1206.
69. Noel RJ, Putnam PE, Rothenberg ME. Eosinophilic esophagitis. *N Engl J Med* 2004; 351(9):940–941.
70. Spergel JM, Andrews T, Brown-Whitehorn TF, et al. Treatment of eosinophilic esophagitis with specific food elimination diet directed by a combination of skin prick and patch tests. *Ann Allergy Asthma Immunol* 2005; 95(4):336–343.
71. Liacouras CA, Ruchelli E. Eosinophilic esophagitis. *Curr Opin Pediatr* 2004; 16(5):560–566.
72. Rothenberg ME. Biology and treatment of eosinophilic esophagitis. *Gastroenterology* 2009; 137(4):1238–1249.
73. Masterson JC, Furuta GT, Lee JJ. Update on clinical and immunological features of eosinophilic gastrointestinal diseases. *Curr Opin Gastroenterol* 2011; 27(6):515–522.
74. Oh HE, Chetty R. Eosinophilic gastroenteritis: a review. *J Gastroenterol* 2008; 43(10):741–750.
75. Talley NJ, Shorter RG, Phillips SF, et al. Eosinophilic gastroenteritis: a clinicopathological study of patients with disease of the mucosa, muscle layer, and subserosal tissues. *Gut* 1990; 31(1):54–58.
76. Rothenberg ME. Eosinophilic gastrointestinal disorders (EGID). *J Allergy Clin Immunol* 2004; 113(1):11–28.
77. James JM. Food allergy, respiratory disease, and anaphylaxis. In: Leung DY, Sampson HA, Geha RS, Szefler SJ (eds), *Pediatric Allergy: Principles and Practice*. St. Louis, MO: Mosby, 2003; pp. 529–537.

78. Roberts G, Lack G. Relevance of inhalational exposure to food allergens. *Curr Opin Allergy Clin Immunol* 2003; 3(3):211–215.
79. Roberts G, Patel N, Levi-Schaffer F, et al. Food allergy as a risk factor for life-threatening asthma in childhood: a case-controlled study. *J Allergy Clin Immunol* 2003; 112(1):168–174.
80. Sampson HA, Munoz-Furlong A, Campbell RL, et al. Second symposium on the definition and management of anaphylaxis: summary report—Second National Institute of Allergy and Infectious Disease/Food Allergy and Anaphylaxis Network symposium. *J Allergy Clin Immunol* 2006; 117(2):391–397.
81. Burks AW, James JM, Hiegel A, et al. Atopic dermatitis and food hypersensitivity reactions. *J Pediatr* 1998; 132(1):132–136.
82. Sampson HA, McCaskill CC. Food hypersensitivity and atopic dermatitis: evaluation of 113 patients. *J Pediatr* 1985; 107(5):669–675.
83. Sicherer SH, Sampson HA. Food hypersensitivity and atopic dermatitis: pathophysiology, epidemiology, diagnosis, and management. *J Allergy Clin Immunol* 1999; 104(3 Pt. 2):S114–S122.

11 Cutaneous Reactions: Atopic Dermatitis and Other IgE- and Non-IgE-Mediated Skin Reactions

David M. Fleischer & Donald Y.M. Leung

University of Colorado Denver School of Medicine, Division of Pediatric Allergy and Immunology, National Jewish Health, Denver, CO, USA

Key Concepts

- Food allergy plays a role in the pathogenesis of atopic dermatitis (AD) in a subset of patients.
- Approximately one-third of children with moderate to severe AD are affected by food allergy.
- Eighty percent of food allergy diagnosed by food challenge in children with AD is caused by milk, egg, and peanut. The most common food allergens in adults are peanut, tree nuts, fish, and shellfish.
- Eliminating the offending food allergen(s) can improve skin lesions in patients with food allergy.

Introduction

Atopic dermatitis (AD) usually begins in early infancy and is typified by extreme pruritus, a chronic relapsing course, and a distinctive pattern of skin distribution. The prevalence of AD varies according to geographic location, ranging from 1% to 20%, with the highest prevalence in northern Europe [1, 2]. The onset of AD occurs during the first 6 months of life in 45% of children, during the first year of life in 60%, and before the age of 5 years in 85% of affected individuals [3]. AD is often the first step in the atopic march, with more than 50% of affected children developing asthma and allergic rhinitis [4, 5]. Triggers for AD include food allergens, inhalant respiratory allergens, irritant substances, and infectious organisms such as *Staphylococcus aureus* [6, 7] (Table 11.1). In this chapter, we will review how the ingestion of certain foods can trigger AD. Mechanistic investigations demonstrate that cutaneous reactions triggered by foods involve both IgE- and non-IgE-mediated skin reactions.

Immunopathophysiology of AD

The pathophysiology of AD involves an interaction between defects in skin barrier function, environmental allergens, infectious agents, various host susceptibility genes, and immunologic responses. It also involves multiple cell types including T-lymphocytes, dendritic cells (DCs), macrophages, keratinocytes, mast cells, and infiltrating inflammatory cells. While a full understanding is not yet complete, some important insights into the allergic mechanisms involved in the initiation and maintenance of skin inflammation in AD have been elucidated [10–12].

Skin barrier dysfunction resulting from gene mutations in the epidermal differentiation complex and defects in keratinocyte differentiation has emerged as a major cause of AD. Loss-of-function mutations in filaggrin (FLG), a protein involved in aggregation of keratin in the upper epidermis, can result in AD [13]. Furthermore, FLG null mutation leads to enhanced allergen penetration through the skin and systemic IgE sensitization to environmental allergens. Relevant to the subject of this textbook, FLG mutations have been reported to be a significant risk factor for peanut allergy [14–16].

The most common cause of reduced skin barrier function in AD is likely due to abnormalities in keratinocyte differentiation [17]. Cytokines secreted during the AD skin immune response, including IL-4, IL-13, and IL-22, have been found to reduce epidermal differentiation [18]. AD results from not only loss of skin barrier proteins but also

Food Allergy: Adverse Reactions to Foods and Food Additives, Fifth Edition. Edited by Dean D Metcalfe, Hugh A Sampson, Ronald A Simon and Gideon Lack.

Table 11.1 Triggers of AD.

Food allergens (most common)	Aeroallergens	Microorganisms
Cow's milk	Pollen	Bacteria *Staphylococcus aureus* *Streptococcus* species
Egg	Mold	
Soy	Dust mite	
Wheat	Animal dander	Fungi/yeasts *Trichophyton* species *Malassezia* (formerly known as *Pityrosporum ovale/orbiculare*) species *Candida* species
Peanut	Cockroach	
Tree nuts		
Fish		
Shellfish		

Source: Reproduced from Reference 8.

Table 11.2 Association between AD and food allergy.

Clinical studies
- Appropriate dietary elimination leads to improvement in AD
- Double-blind, placebo-controlled food challenges reproduce skin symptoms
- The use of a hydrolyzed formula compared to a cow's milk formula in high-risk infants reduces infant and childhood allergy and infant cow's milk allergy

Laboratory studies
- Presence of elevated food-specific IgE antibodies
- LCs bear high-affinity IgE receptors and can present allergen to T-cells
- Plasma histamine elevation during positive OFCs
- Elevated histamine-releasing factors in children when consuming diet with allergenic food
- Increased spontaneous basophil histamine release while ingesting causal food
- Eosinophils are activated during positive food challenge
- T-cells, cloned from active lesions of AD, can react with food allergen
- Children allergic to milk with AD have CLA+, milk-reactive T-cells.

Source: Modified from Reference 25.

lipid abnormalities, increased protease activity, as well as reduced expression of antimicrobial genes, required for the innate immune response to microbial invasion [19, 20]. Acute AD skin lesions are associated with increased expression of Th2 cytokines, notably IL-4 and IL-13. IL-4 and IL-13 mediate antibody isotype switching to IgE synthesis and IgE receptor upregulation and induce expression of adhesion molecules required for infiltration of inflammatory cells into the skin. Epidermal keratinocytes in AD express increased thymic stromal lymphopoietin (TSLP) [21], a cytokine that enhances DC-driven Th2 cell differentiation. Mechanical injury, allergen exposure, and microbial infection increase TSLP release from keratinocytes and may thereby increase IgE responses [22]. The maintenance of chronic AD involves increased production of IL-22, which induces keratinocyte proliferation and downregulation of FLG expression [23].

Serum IgE levels are elevated in ~85% of patients with AD and often contain food allergen-specific and aeroallergen-specific IgE antibodies. The role of allergen-specific IgE in the pathogenesis of AD involves a number of cell types. Langerhans cells (LCs) in AD lesions have allergen-specific IgE antibodies on their surface [24], and this makes them 100- to 1000-fold more efficient at presenting allergen to T-cells than LCs, which do not express the high-affinity IgE receptor (FcεRI) [25]. Th2 cytokines upregulate FcεRI on LCs and other antigen-presenting cells. IgE-bearing FcεRI inflammatory dendritic epidermal cells (IDECs) are prominent in chronic AD skin lesions. It is believed not only that IDECs are involved in cell recruitment and IgE-mediated antigen presentation to T-cells, but that they also release IL-12 and IL-18 and promote Th1 cytokine production by priming naive T-cells into IFN-γ-producing T-cells, which together may lead to the switch from an initial Th2-type immune response to a Th1-type immune response.

Role of food allergy in AD

A large and growing body of evidence supports the pathogenic role of food allergy in skin reactions particularly in children (Table 11.2). Three patterns of cutaneous reactions to food may occur in AD: (1) immediate-type allergic reactions, such as urticaria and angioedema, which occur within 2 hours after food ingestion, and suggest an IgE-mediated mechanism; (2) pruritus within 2 hours soon after food ingestion, which also suggests an IgE-mediated mechanism, with subsequent scratching leading to an AD exacerbation; and (3) delayed reactions with AD exacerbations that occur after 6–48 hours, either with or without a previous immediate-type response, suggestive of a non-IgE-mediated reaction or a cutaneous late-phase reaction of IgE-mediated hypersensitivity [27].

Clinical evidence

The clinical evidence supporting the role of food allergy in AD is based on three areas of clinical investigation: elimination diet studies; double-blind, placebo-controlled food challenge (DBPCFC) studies; and preventive studies of AD. Multiple clinical studies have shown that elimination of pertinent food allergens can lead to improvement in AD symptoms, that repeat oral challenge with the offending food(s) can lead to redevelopment of skin symptoms, and that AD and food hypersensitivity can be partially prevented by prophylactic elimination of highly allergic foods from infant diets and possibly from diets of breast-feeding mothers.

Elimination diet studies

Numerous studies have addressed the therapeutic effect of dietary elimination on the treatment of AD. Atherton et al. [28] showed that 14 of 20 subjects (70%) with AD between the ages of 2 and 8 years showed significant improvement after completing a 12-week, double-blind, controlled, cross-over trial of an egg and cow's milk (CM) exclusion diet. Neild et al. [29] found only 10 of 40 AD subjects benefited from an egg and CM exclusion diet, yielding a response rate to the diet that was not statistically significant. Juto et al. [30] reported on 20 AD infants treated with a strict elimination diet for up to 6 weeks. Seven infants had complete resolution of their rash, 12 had some skin improvement while on the diet, and the remaining infant had no change in skin condition. While the cumulative results of the above studies provide support for the role of food allergy in AD, most of the trials failed to control confounding factors such as other potential AD triggers, placebo effect, or observer bias.

In one of the original prospective follow-up studies of the natural history of food hypersensitivity in children with AD, Sampson and Scanlon [31] studied 34 subjects with AD, of whom 17 had food allergy diagnosed by DBPCFCs. These 17 subjects were placed on appropriate elimination diets and experienced significant improvement in their clinical symptoms. Comparisons made at 1–2-year and 3–4-year follow-ups with 12 control subjects who did not have food allergy and 5 subjects with food allergy who were noncompliant with their diet showed that the 17 food-allergic subjects with appropriate dietary restriction demonstrated highly significant improvement in their AD compared with the control groups.

Lever et al. [32] performed a randomized, controlled trial of an egg exclusion diet in 55 children who presented to a dermatology clinic with AD and possible egg sensitivity identified by IgE testing before randomization. True egg sensitivity was confirmed by DBPCFC after the trial. The 55 children were randomized either to a 4-week regimen, in which mothers received general advice on the care of AD and additional specific advice from a dietician about an egg elimination diet (diet group), or to a control group in which only general advice was provided. There was a significantly greater mean reduction in surface area affected by AD in the diet group than in the control group. There was also significant improvement in symptom severity scores for the diet group, compared to the control group.

Oral food challenge studies

Almost 35 years ago, researchers used the DBPCFC to demonstrate that food allergens can cause symptoms of rash and pruritus in children with food allergy-associated AD [33]. Twenty years later, in two studies, Burks et al. [34, 35] also used the DBPCFC to study 165 children with mild to severe AD. Sixty percent of the subjects with AD had a positive skin prick test (SPT) to at least one of the following foods: milk, egg, soy, wheat, peanut, cashew, and codfish. They performed 266 DBPCFCs, and 64 subjects, 38.7% of the total group with AD, were found to have food allergy.

Sampson and colleagues [31, 36–38] published a number of articles using DBPCFCs to identify foods that are trigger factors of AD. In the initial evaluation of 470 subjects with a median age of 4.1 years (range 3 months to 24 years), serum total IgE concentration was elevated in 376 subjects (80%), with a median of 3410 IU/mL and range of 1.5–45,000 IU/mL. Foods used in the DBPCFCs were selected based on skin and IgE testing results and/or a clinical history suggestive of food allergy, and these foods were eliminated from the subject's diet for at least 7–10 days prior to admission. A total of 1776 DBPCFCs were performed during the studies and 714 (40%) were positive and 1062 were negative. Cutaneous reactions during challenges developed in the vast majority of subjects (529 (74%) of the 714 DBPCFC-positive cases). The cutaneous reactions comprised a pruritic, erythematous, macular, or morbilliform rash that occurred primarily in previously affected AD sites. The development of skin symptoms occurred only in 214 (30%) of the positive reactions, and typical urticaria was rarely seen, and if present, consisted of only a few lesions. However, intense pruritus and scratching often led to superficial excoriations and occasionally bleeding.

Almost all symptoms during the DBPCFCs began between 5 minutes and 2 hours after starting the challenge. Immediate-type response symptoms generally occurred abruptly and lasted 1–2 hours. A few patients had a delayed second episode of pruritus including pruritus and urticaria, scratching, and transient morbilliform rash 6–10 hours after the initial challenge. This morbilliform rash may represent the acute phase of AD, and it is induced in the oral food challenges (OFCs) by acute consumption of a food that previously caused symptoms on a chronic basis [39]. Clinical reactions to milk, egg, soy, and wheat accounted for nearly 75% of the reactions in the studies. Some subjects had repeated reactions during a series of daily OFCs and subsequently had an increasingly severe AD exacerbation. These data provide further evidence that ingestion of a causal food can trigger itching, scratching, and the reappearance of typical AD lesions.

Prevention of food hypersensitivity and AD through diet

In addition to the above-mentioned studies that have shown that AD can improve through elimination diets of offending foods and that reintroduction of these foods during DBPCFCs can elicit symptoms, many studies have been performed in an attempt to prevent food allergy and AD through dietary means during pregnancy, lactation, and early infant feeding. Studies attempting to prevent CM and egg allergies by maternal CM and egg avoidance during late pregnancy have failed to show a reduction in food allergy, any other atopic disorder, or sensitization from birth through age 5 years. Additionally, maternal weight gain during pregnancy was negatively affected by these dietary restrictions. A Cochrane meta-analysis [40] confirmed the above findings, and the authors concluded that the prescription of an antigen avoidance diet to a high-risk woman during pregnancy is unlikely to substantially reduce the child's risk of atopic diseases, and such a diet may adversely affect maternal or fetal nutrition, or both. Another review of this issue by Muraro et al. [41] stated that there is no conclusive evidence for a protective effect of a maternal exclusion diet during pregnancy.

It has been suggested that the presence of food antigens in breast milk might sensitize an infant if the mother does not avoid these foods in her diet during lactation. However, results of studies during the 1980s and 1990s examining this hypothesis have been contradictory. These contradictory studies, along with consideration of many others, led both a Cochrane analysis [40] and a recent meta-analysis [41] to conclude that while the prescription of an antigen avoidance diet to high-risk women during lactation may reduce the child's risk of developing AD, there is inconclusive evidence to show a preventative effect of maternal diet during lactation on atopic disease in childhood. Furthermore, one cannot state for certain whether food antigens in breast milk will induce allergy or be immunoprotective in any given recipient [42].

Of the many studies regarding the association between breast-feeding and AD, some have shown a protective effect [43, 44], whereas others have shown a lack of association [45], and some have even shown a positive association [46, 47]. To assist in sorting out the discrepancies in the above studies, Yang et al. [48] performed a systematic review and meta-analysis of 21 prospective cohort studies in developed countries that compared breast-feeding with CM formula feeding on the development of AD. Statistical analysis revealed that exclusive breast-feeding for at least 3 months was not significantly protective against the development of AD compared with CM formula (OR 0.89, 95% CI 0.76–1.04). Although exclusive breast-feeding compared to use of conventional formula was associated with a decreased risk of AD (OR 0.7, 95% CI 0.5–0.99) when only cohorts with a positive family history of atopy were examined, this effect was lost when a controversial study was excluded from the analysis (OR 0.94, 95% CI 0.81–1.08). This led the authors to conclude that overall there was no strong evidence of a protective effect of exclusive breast-feeding for at least 3 months against AD onset in childhood.

The effect of breast-feeding on the development of food allergy is difficult to determine, as both AD and asthma are closely associated with the development of food allergy. There are a limited number of studies that have examined breast-feeding's role on the outcomes of specific food allergies, and the results may be affected by other dietary variables such as the length and extent of exclusivity of breast-feeding. After reviewing the existing studies, Muraro et al. [41] determined that exclusive breast-feeding for at least 4 months is related to a lower cumulative incidence of CM allergy until 18 months of age. However, no firm conclusions about the role of breast-feeding in either the primary prevention of or delay in onset of other specific food allergies can be made at this time.

Many studies have been performed exploring the use of various infant formulas, including conventional CM formula, partial whey hydrolysate formula (pHF), extensive casein hydrolysate formulas (eHFs), and soy protein-based formulas in the prevention of allergy. A 2006 systematic review [49] determined that there is no evidence to support prolonged feeding with a hydrolyzed formula to prevent allergy in preference to exclusive breast-feeding. In high-risk infants who are not able to be completely breast-fed, there is evidence that the use of a hydrolyzed formula compared to a CM formula reduces infant and childhood allergy and infant CM allergy. A more recent meta-analysis of formula consumption and risk of AD found that infants who were fed pHF had a lower risk of AD than those fed CM formula (summary relative risk estimate (SRRE) 0.45, 95% CI 0.40–0.70) [50]. Although some studies show a slight benefit of eHFs compared with pHFs, there is inconclusive evidence at this time to determine whether feeding with an eHF has any advantage over a pHF [51, 52]. There is convincing evidence that feeding with a soy formula is not recommended in high-risk infants for the prevention of allergy [53].

Early studies regarding the timing of solid food introduction demonstrated some benefit in delaying early solid food introduction [54, 55], but more recent studies have shown a lack of protective effect [56]. The conflicting data from the studies taken as a whole do not currently allow an authoritative statement regarding the relation between the introduction of solids and the development of allergy to be made. Therefore, the advantage of delaying highly allergic solid food introduction beyond 4–6 months is unconfirmed. Delaying solid food introduction may even increase the risk of allergy (e.g., milk, egg, and wheat allergy) [57–59].

IgE- and non-IgE-mediated mechanisms

Several lines of laboratory evidence also provide support for the role of food-specific IgE in AD. To show that food ingestion led to IgE-mediated reactions, Sampson and Jolie [60] sought markers of mast cell activation in 33 subjects with AD who underwent DBPCFCs to evaluate the role of histamine in food hypersensitivity by monitoring changes in circulating plasma histamine. Only the group of subjects with positive DBPCFCs demonstrated a significant rise in plasma histamine; subjects who consumed placebo or had negative DBPCFCs showed no demonstrable rise in plasma histamine. The rise in plasma histamine that was observed implicated the role of mast cell or basophil mediators in the pathogenesis of food allergy in AD.

Mechanisms that involve IgE antibody, other than direct IgE-mediated activation of cutaneous mast cells, may also play a role in the inflammatory process in AD. Sampson et al. [61] studied 63 subjects with AD and food hypersensitivity documented by DBPCFCs, 20 subjects with AD but no food allergy based on negative DBPCFCs, and 18 normal controls. Subjects with AD and food allergy had higher rates of mean spontaneous histamine release than the other two subject groups. The high rate of histamine release appeared to depend on continued ingestion of the offending food, because once a subject was placed on the appropriate elimination diet for 9–12 months, the spontaneous histamine release returned to normal levels. Another important finding was the identification of spontaneously produced cytokines called histamine-releasing factors (HRFs) from peripheral blood mononuclear cells (PBMCs) of food-allergic subjects with high spontaneous histamine release. HRF *in vitro* could activate basophils from other food-allergic subjects, but not from nonfood-allergic subjects. Normal controls did not produce HRFs, and subjects with food allergy who adhered to an elimination diet had a decrease in the rate of spontaneous HRF production. The HRF was found to activate basophils through surface-bound IgE. Several different forms of IgE have been identified [62], and it has been proposed that HRFs may interact with certain of these IgE isoforms.

Basophil histamine release (BHR) had been proposed as an *in vitro* correlate to *in vivo* allergic responses [63]. BHR as a method of diagnosing food allergy was reported by Nolte [64] to correlate well with SPTs, RASTs, and open OFCs, but not with histamine release from intestinal mast cells obtained by duodenal biopsy in children. Another study comparing BHR, SPTs, and DBPCFCs, however, showed that the BHR assay was no more effective in predicting clinical sensitivity than SPTs [65]. The clinical application of BHR is further complicated by several factors: it is not a widely available test, blood needs to be processed within a certain amount of time for cells to be viable, and there are no standardized methods for performing BHR. BHR assays are now primarily used in research settings.

A relatively new technique used to study the mediator effects of basophils, the basophil activation test (BAT), has the potential to overcome the pitfalls of BHR. The emerging ability to measure basophil activation as an assay for immediate hypersensitivity has the potential to provide diagnostic or prognostic utility in food allergy [66]. Allergen desensitization in studies has been shown to induce basophil hyporesponsiveness to allergen-induced degranulation [67, 68], and *in vivo* constitutive activation of basophils correlates with CD203c expression measured directly *ex vivo* by flow cytometry [66]. Some have found that CD203c is expressed at very high levels in patients with AD and food allergy [66]. The assessment of BAT as a clinical diagnostic tool for food allergy in AD remains in its early stages, however. Monitoring the BAT for patients with food allergy on various elimination diets or following OFCs with subjective or late-phase reactions may also prove to be an important clinical tool, but further studies are needed. Whether the BAT also becomes a diagnostic tool for food allergy or an additional piece of information to help decide when to perform an OFC on a patient who may have outgrown a particular food allergy remains to be seen.

Other data support a key role of eosinophils in the pathogenesis of food-sensitive AD, particularly in the late-phase IgE response. Studies of the late-phase reactions after the initial mast cell activation have shown that the terminal stages of IgE-mediated allergic reactions are characterized by infiltration of inflammatory cells, including eosinophils [69, 70]. Although blood eosinophilia is common in AD patients, increased numbers of activated eosinophils have not always been found in biopsies of AD lesions. However, eosinophil degranulation and release of potent mediators clearly occurs. Leiferman et al. [71] found extensive dermal deposition of eosinophil-derived MBP in lesional biopsies of 18 subjects with AD but not in normal-appearing skin in affected subjects, suggesting that the assessment of eosinophil involvement cannot be based simply on the eosinophil numbers in tissue. Suomalainen et al. [72] studied 28 challenge-proven CM-allergic subjects and showed increased levels of eosinophil cationic protein (ECP) in the subjects with cutaneous symptoms only, which indicated that ingestion of an offending food in an allergic patient can lead to activation of circulating eosinophils that may then infiltrate the skin of AD patients. Another study confirmed the finding of significantly elevated plasma ECP levels in subjects with AD [73].

Several important studies have helped clarify the role of food allergen-specific T-cells in the underlying inflammatory process in AD, showing that cell-mediated immunity also occurs in patients with food-sensitive AD in addition to IgE-mediated hypersensitivity. Food antigen-specific T-cells have been isolated and cloned from active AD lesions [74–76]. Researchers have also been able to routinely identify food antigen-specific T-cells from peripheral blood in subjects with food allergy-associated AD [75–77]. There has been disagreement in the literature, though, about the validity of *in vitro* T-lymphocyte proliferation responses to specific foods in AD. Kondo, Agata, and colleagues [78, 79] demonstrated that proliferative responses of PBMCs to the offending food antigen in subjects with nonimmediate types of food allergy (rash developing at least 2 hours after OFC) were significantly higher than those of healthy controls and subjects with immediate types of food allergy, respectively, indicating that the proliferative response of PBMCs to food antigens is specific to each offending food antigen in nonimmediate types of food allergy-related AD. On the other hand, others have found increased lymphocyte proliferative responses to relevant foods also in subjects with immediate reactions [76]. Overall, the clinical utility of lymphocyte proliferation assays in food-allergic patients is considered marginal due to considerable overlap in individual responses to the test, as Hoffman et al. [80] found them to be neither diagnostic nor predictive of clinical reactivity in individual subjects with milk allergy because lymphocytes of many control patients were highly responsive to milk antigens, and lymphocytes of many subjects with milk allergy were not.

Further evidence of T-lymphocyte involvement in the development of AD in food-allergic patients relates to the homing of allergen-specific T-cells to the skin [75]. The extravasation of T-cells at sites of inflammation is critically dependent on the activity of homing receptors that are involved in endothelial cell recognition and binding. Two such homing receptors, cutaneous lymphocyte-associated antigen (CLA) and L-selectin, have been shown to be selectively involved in T-cell migration to the skin and peripheral lymph nodes, respectively. Significantly higher expression of CLA occurred in casein-reactive T-cells from children with milk-induced AD than *Candida albicans*-reactive T-cells from the same subjects, and from either casein- or *C. albicans*-reactive T-cells from the control groups. In contrast, the percentage of L-selectin-expressing T-cells did not significantly differ among the three groups.

The role of non-IgE-mediated food-induced hypersensitivity in AD remains unclear [81], likely in part due to the raging debate for several decades whether food can act as a provocation factor for late eczematous reactions. Atopy patch tests (APTs) have been proposed as a mode of diagnosis of non-IgE-mediated food allergy and in identifying allergens in delayed-onset clinical reactions. The patch test reaction seems to be specific for sensitized patients with AD, as it does not occur in healthy volunteers or in patients suffering from asthma or rhinitis [82]. The outcome of APTs in different studies shows large variations due to differences in patient selection and, more importantly, differences in methodology. These facts make interpretation of studies somewhat difficult due to reliability issues, but a number of investigators, as discussed in the diagnostic section below, have examined the use of the APTs in addition to SPTs for the diagnosis of non-IgE-mediated food allergy, primarily in patients with AD.

Epidemiology of food allergy in AD

The prevalence of food allergy in patients with AD differs depending on the age of the patient and the severity of AD. Burks et al. [34], using DBPCFCs, diagnosed food allergy in 15 of 46 children (33%) with AD ranging from mild to severe that were referred to allergy or dermatology clinics. In a larger study published 10 years later of 165 children with AD referred to the allergy clinic, Burks et al. [35] diagnosed food allergy in 64 children (38.7%) utilizing DBPCFCs. Ascertainment bias could have affected the results of these two studies since many of the patients were referred to an allergist, so Eigenmann et al. [38] addressed this potential bias by evaluating 63 unselected children referred to a university-based dermatologist for assessment of moderate to severe AD. Again OFCs were used as part of the evaluation, and ultimately 23 of 63 (37%, 95% CI 25–50%) were found to have clinically significant IgE-mediated food hypersensitivity. In an epidemiologic study of IgE-mediated food allergy in 74 Swiss children with AD referred to an allergist or dermatologist, Eigenmann and Calza [83] found that 25 of the 74 children (33.8%) were food allergic using OFCs and other tests. While the above studies did not stratify children by the severity of AD [34, 38, 82] or demonstrate a direct relationship between severity of AD and presence of food allergy [35], Guillet and Guillet [84] attempted this in a study of 250 children with AD. They found that increased severity of AD and younger age of children directly correlated with the presence of food allergy. Finally, two more studies, neither of which performed OFCs, looked at the prevalence of food allergy in two prospective birth cohorts in Australia. In the first, Hill et al. [85] found a cumulative prevalence of AD of 24%. The contribution of IgE food sensitization to the burden of AD was calculated as an attributable risk percent; this calculation estimated that IgE food sensitization was responsible for 65% and 64% of AD in the at-risk cohort at 6 and 12 months, respectively. In the second study, Hill and Hosking [86] discovered a cumulative prevalence of AD of 28.9%. The association between IgE-mediated food allergy and AD was assessed using only SPT cutoffs and was stratified by groups of AD severity. As the severity of AD increased, so did the frequency of IgE-mediated food allergy and reported adverse food reactions, from 12% in the least severe AD group, up to 69% in the most severe AD group.

Epidemiologic studies of food allergy in adults with severe AD are comparatively limited, which may in part be due to the fact that most food allergy is outgrown in children, with the notable exceptions of peanut, tree nuts, fish, and shellfish. In a double-blind, controlled study using an antigen-free formula (Vivasorb) compared with placebo diet in 33 severe AD adults, Munkvad et al. [87] found that food allergy played little role in the etiology of AD in adults because the antigen-free diet did not significantly reduce symptoms. de Maat-Bleeke and Bruijnzeel-Koomen [88] also failed to discover a significant role of food allergy in adult AD. However, one study from Japan found that 44% of the 195 adults with AD had positive challenges to foods, although the causative foods listed were uncommon allergens, including chocolate, coffee, and rice [89]. Finally, a recent German study [90] found that certain adult subjects were sensitized to pollen allergens, and according to those pollen allergens, also sensitized to pollen-associated food allergens.

Diagnosis of food hypersensitivity in patients with AD

General approach

The diagnosis of food allergy (Fig. 11.1) must first begin with a careful medical history since the information gathered will be used to guide the best mode of diagnosis. It is well documented in several studies where DBPCFCs were used to diagnose food allergy that only about 40% of patient histories of suspected food-induced allergic reactions could be verified [91]. The history should focus on the food(s) and quantity of food suspected of provoking the reaction, the type of symptoms attributed to food ingestion (acute vs. chronic), the timing between ingestion and onset of symptoms, patterns of reactivity, the most recent reaction, and whether other associated activities play a role in inducing symptoms (e.g., exercise, alcohol ingestion). When gathering the history, one must also be aware of other foods eaten at the same time, potentially contaminated foods that may have been packaged on nondedicated lines, and hidden sources of ingredients.

Once a symptom history is established, the search for a food-related etiology needs to be put in context with the prevalence that food allergy is implicated as the causative factor. The prevalence of food hypersensitivities is greatest in the first few years of life, affecting about 6% of children less than 3 years of age, then decreasing to a steady prevalence of 3.7% by late childhood through adulthood [92]. Furthermore, although any food could theoretically cause an allergic reaction, a small number of foods account for about 90% of verified food reactions: milk, egg, soy,

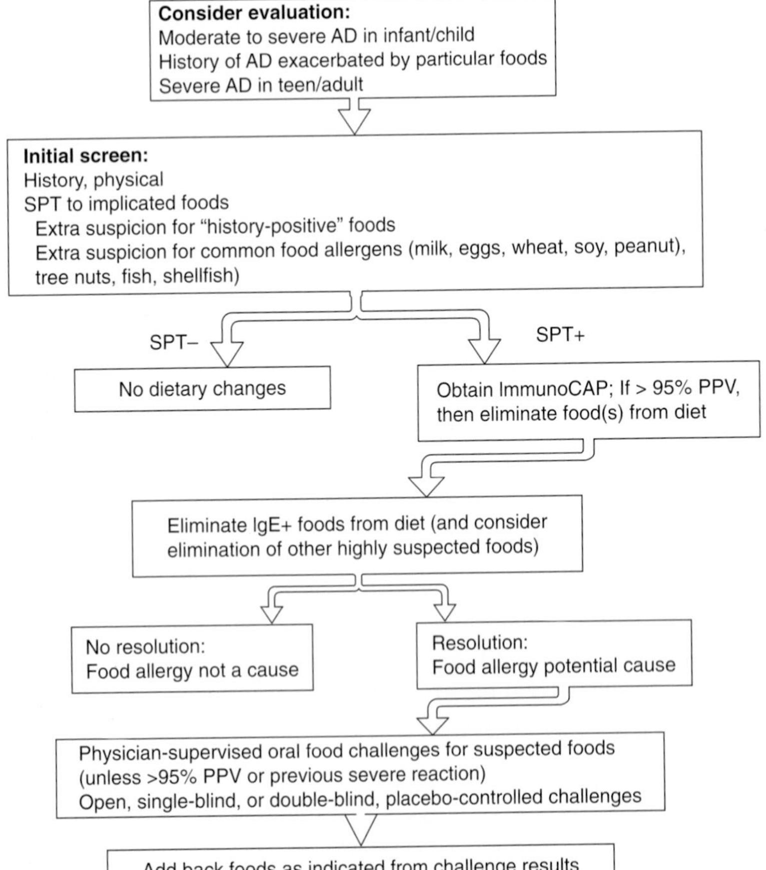

Figure 11.1 General approach to the evaluation of food allergy in atopic dermatitis. Adapted from Reference 8.

wheat, peanut, tree nuts, and fish in children; and peanuts, tree nuts, fish, and shellfish in adults.

Once a thorough history has been obtained, the physical examination should focus on detecting other atopic features, which are more commonly found in patients with IgE-mediated allergic reactions. After completing the history and physical, the physician should determine whether the patient's findings implicate a food-induced disorder and whether an IgE-mediated or non-IgE-mediated mechanism is most likely responsible. When food allergy has been identified as the likely cause of symptoms, confirmation of the diagnosis and identification of the implicated food(s) can begin. A number of tools exist that aid in the diagnosis of food allergy. In general, laboratory tests are more useful in delineating the specific foods responsible for IgE-mediated reactions, whereas they are of limited or no value in non-IgE-mediated disorders. Available studies include *in vivo* tests such as SPT, OFCs, elimination diets, and APTs and *in vitro* tests such as quantification of food-specific IgE and the BAT. The utility of these test modalities will be briefly discussed.

In vivo and *in vitro* laboratory testing

SPTs are commonly used to screen patients with suspected IgE-mediated food reactions. When an SPT is positive, it indicates the possible association between the food tested and the patient's reactivity to that food because the positive predictive accuracies of SPTs are less than 50% compared to DBPCFCs. However, a positive SPT may be considered diagnostic in patients who have experienced a systemic anaphylactic reaction to an isolated food. On the other hand, negative responses virtually exclude the possibility of an IgE-mediated reaction because their negative predictive value (NPV) exceeds 95% [93]. The accuracy of SPTs varies depending on which food antigen is being studied, the quality of the food extract, and the technical skills of the tester. As a result of a study by Bock et al. [94], intradermal skin tests (ISTs) to food extracts were found to have no positive advantage over SPTs, and it was concluded that the increased sensitivity of ISTs would lead to even more false-positive tests than seen with the prick technique [95]. Fresh food skin prick tests (FFSPTs) are often required. Commercially prepared extracts frequently lack the labile proteins that are responsible for IgE-mediated sensitivity to many fruits and vegetables because they are degraded or lose allergenicity during extract preparation [96]. Negative SPTs with commercially available extracts that contradict a convincing history of a food-induced allergic reaction should be repeated with the fresh food before concluding that food-specific IgE is absent [97].

Another way to identify food-specific IgE that is more widely available to the general practitioner is the CAP-System fluorescent-enzyme immunoassay (FEIA), although the sensitivity is slightly less than SPTs. The development of the CAP-System FEIA allowed better quantification of food-specific IgE antibodies, which have been shown in key studies to be more predictive of symptomatic IgE-mediated food hypersensitivity. In a retrospective study on 196 children and adolescents (mean age 5.2 years) with AD, Sampson and Ho [65] compared the food-specific IgE levels with the results of DBPCFCs and found that concentrations of 6 kU_A/L or greater for egg, 32 kU_A/L or greater for CM, 15 kU_A/L or greater for peanut, and 20 kU_A/L or greater for codfish were 95% predictive of an allergic reaction. Therefore, a patient with a food-specific IgE level greater than the 95% positive predictive value (PPV) could be considered reactive and an OFC would not be warranted. If, however, the food-specific IgE level was less than the 95% PPV, a patient may be reactive but would need an OFC to confirm the diagnosis. There are several caveats with this study that affect its use in the general population: first, all patients had AD, and these patients tend to have higher IgE levels; and second, this group of patients had a much higher prevalence of food allergy than is seen in most populations. Because of these factors, Sampson performed a prospective study of 100 children (median age 3.8 years) not selected for AD (only 61% had this disorder) with similar results except the 95% PPV cut-off was lower for milk at 15 kU_A/L [95].

APTs have been proposed as a mode of diagnosis of non-IgE-mediated food allergy and in identifying allergens in delayed-onset IgE-mediated clinical reactions. A number of investigators have examined the use of the APTs in addition to SPTs and food-specific IgE levels by CAP-System FEIA for the diagnosis of non-IgE-mediated food allergy, primarily in patients with AD. Roehr et al. [98] performed 173 challenges in 98 patients with AD and used APTs, SPTs, and food-specific IgE levels to CM, egg, soy, and wheat to see if the combination of a positive APT result plus a positive food-specific IgE level, a positive SPT, or both would make DBPCFCs unnecessary. Positive APT results alone correlated with high PPVs for CM (95%), hen's egg (94%), and wheat (94%), but with only a 50% PPV for soy (only four children reacted to soy). Combining the APT with proof of specific IgE for CM (0.35 kU_A/L) and for egg (17.5 kU_A/L) increased the PPVs to 100%, thus making DBPCFCs superfluous. Adding SPTs to the other two tests did not further improve results. More recent studies [99, 100], however, have not been able to duplicate the results from Roehr and colleagues, finding that APTs had poor reliability, added only minimal predictive value, and were inferior to DBPCFCs in evaluation of food allergy. In a recent review of literature on APT since 2004, Turjanmaa [101] stated there is accumulating evidence that a small subset of patients with AD shows positive APTs when specific IgE to the same allergen is negative, but that because the APT lacks standardization and until the methodology improves, the specificity, sensitivity, and PPVs and NPVs cannot be calculated properly.

One must be extremely careful in interpreting tests for food-specific IgE antibodies as clinical errors occur when the above tests are overinterpreted or various limitations are not fully appreciated, such as not considering the medical history, epidemiology of food allergy (causal foods, cross-reactivity, and age), and specific test limitations (sensitivity, specificity, technique, and reagents). One must also appreciate that the results from studies like Sampson's [65, 95] and others may not be applicable beyond the specific food, the test studied, and the characteristics of the study population (e.g., children). Another common pitfall is the assumption that a negative test result indicates a lack of allergy, but this has been shown not to be the case [102].

Elimination diets and oral food challenges

The purpose of an elimination diet is to determine if a patient's symptoms will resolve when foods are restricted from the diet. If a patient's symptoms persist despite a very strict avoidance diet, it is unlikely that the food accounts for the patient's complaints [103]. The type of diet chosen will depend on the clinical presentation being evaluated and the results of IgE antibody tests. Elimination of one or more foods may be the obvious course of action and therapeutic in the case of an acute reaction to a food and the presence of a positive test for IgE to that food. It may also be especially helpful in evaluating infants who are on a very limited diet. In an oligoantigenic diet, a large number of foods suspected to cause chronic problems are removed, and the patient is given a list of allowed foods. This type of diet is useful for evaluation of chronic disorders such as AD. In the most extreme diet, the elemental diet, a hydrolyzed formula provides all the nutrition. This diet may be necessary when the other diets mentioned above have failed, but the suspicion for food-related illness remains high. If a patient's symptoms do not disappear on an elemental diet, then it is very unlikely that ingested substances are the problem [103, 104].

If symptoms resolve on an elimination diet, some form of OFC is generally warranted. OFCs are performed by feeding suspected foods in gradually increasing amounts over hours or days under the supervision of a physician. OFCs can be done openly, single-blind, or double-blind and placebo-controlled. The DBPCFC is considered to be the "gold standard" for the diagnosis of food allergy, and it is the least prone to bias and confounding factors [65, 104]. OFCs can be used to assess any kind of adverse response to foods. If an elimination diet did not alleviate symptoms and suspicion is still high for a food-related cause, then the OFC may be needed to resolve the issue. For non-IgE-mediated reactions, OFCs are often the only means of diagnosis [105].

The decision to perform OFCs should not be taken lightly as severe anaphylactic reactions can occur, and they are time consuming, cost intensive, and stressful to the patient and families. In the patient with a convincing history of anaphylaxis and a positive test for specific IgE to the causal food, an OFC is generally not needed as it places patients at risk for severe reactions [105]. Given the risk of anaphylaxis during an OFC, the physician must be prepared to treat it with emergency medications and equipment. OFCs are usually done in a graded fashion with dose increases every 15–60 minutes and a period of observation once the OFC is finished. If a patient has tolerated all the food in the challenge, then clinical reactivity has generally been ruled out in that a negative OFC has a high NPV [106]. However, for blinded challenges, all negative challenges should be confirmed by an open feeding of the suspected food made in its commonly prepared state and served in normal meal-size quantities under medical supervision to exclude the rare false-negative challenge response [103].

Fleischer et al. in a recently published paper demonstrated the importance of a careful and guided approach with respect to the diagnosis of food allergy in AD patients because of the higher likelihood of false-positive tests with higher IgE levels in AD patients. In 125 patients referred to an outpatient treatment program for AD and food allergy, 96% had AD, and all were on an elimination diet. A total of 364 OFCs were performed on foods that had been avoided at the time of admission, and 325 (89%) were negative. Many of the patients had excluded foods that they had never eaten or foods they had once tolerated without known reaction, and many of the foods that could now be introduced back into the diet after negative OFCs had been eliminated solely on the basis of serum IgE testing. The importance of a detailed clinical history followed by careful use of SPTs, IgE testing when indicated, and the need for OFCs to confirm or refute true reactivity in the accurate diagnosis of food allergy is demonstrated here.

Management

In addition to the medical management of AD using hydration therapy, topical corticosteroids, topical calcineurin inhibitors, antibiotics for secondary bacterial infections, and environmental avoidance of triggers, the only currently available treatments for food allergy are strict dietary elimination of the causative food(s) and being prepared to treat a potential reaction after accidental ingestion. The complete elimination of food proteins, though, is not an easy task, and lack of complete elimination can lead to puzzling results. Therefore, with any of these diets, specific information needs to be reviewed carefully to ensure adherence, as it is common for patients to make errors. For example, eliminating egg from someone's diet means reading labels for key words such as ovalbumin, lysozyme, and globulin. However, reading labels on US food products has become an easier task since the implementation in January 2006 of the Food Allergen Labeling and Consumer Protection Act of 2004, which requires clear labels for the major food allergens (milk, egg, soy, wheat, peanut, tree nuts, fish, and shellfish). Contamination of the food being eliminated and hidden ingredients in nonlabeled products such as in restaurants can still be issues that hinder strict avoidance. Organizations such as Food Allergy Research and Education (http://www.foodallergy.org) may provide assistance for patients. When multiple foods are eliminated from the diet, it may also be necessary to consult the aid of a nutritionist to maintain a balanced diet.

Unfortunately, accidental ingestions of known allergenic foods are relatively common. Therefore, patients, family members, and other caregivers must have an emergency action plan in place for such occasions. This plan includes readily available injectable epinephrine, oral antihistamines, bronchodilators, and knowledge of when to seek urgent medical attention. Patients that have had prior severe reactions, those with underlying asthma, and patients allergic to peanut, tree nuts, fish, and shellfish may be more at risk for acute, severe, or even fatal food-induced anaphylactic reactions [107]. Prompt administration of epinephrine at the initial signs of a severe reaction needs to be emphasized because reports of fatal and near-fatal reactions have been associated with delayed epinephrine use [107]. Routine follow-up to assess growth and nutrition and to retest for progression or possible resolution of food allergy is crucial as well.

Natural history of food hypersensitivity

Fortunately most children with food-induced eczema will lose or "outgrow" their allergies to milk, egg, soy, and wheat [108], and this usually corresponds to the resolution or improvement of their AD [26]. However, patients allergic to peanut, tree nuts, fish, or shellfish are much less likely to lose their clinical reactivity; only ~20% of children who have had a reaction to peanut early as a child may outgrow their peanut sensitivity [109, 110], while only ~10% may outgrow tree nut allergy [111]. From the Sampson and Scanlon study on the natural history of food allergy in AD [31], about one-third of children outgrew their clinical reactivity over 1–3 years with strict compliance to the elimination diet, which was believed to have helped in speedier resolution. Three factors emerged to be most important in determining the likelihood of patients losing clinical reactivity: (1) the specific food(s) to which the patient was allergic, meaning that patients allergic to milk, egg, soy, or wheat were much more likely to outgrow these allergies than those with peanut, tree nut, fish, or shellfish allergies; (2) the food-specific IgE level, that is, the higher the level of food-specific IgE, the less likely clinical tolerance will develop in subsequent years; and (3) the degree of strict adherence to the diet, that is, patients who continued to ingest small amounts of food allergen or had frequent accidental ingestions were less likely to develop clinical tolerance. New studies, however, are challenging this concept of strict avoidance of foods to speed the resolution of food allergy for certain foods, in that some patients with egg and milk allergies are able to tolerate baked products that contain extensively heated egg and milk protein, respectively [112–114]. Regular consumption of these baked products can accelerate the resolution of egg and milk allergies, but should only be done under the supervision of an allergist after a food challenge to ensure it is safe to consume such foods, and that their regular consumption will not secondarily affect the patient's AD.

Clinical tolerance is acquired more quickly than the loss of food-specific IgE measured by SPT or *in vitro* allergen-specific IgE testing [31, 115], as these tests can remain positive for many years after the food has been reintroduced into the diet. Therefore, it is important to follow patients with food allergy regularly with intermittent OFCs when appropriate to determine if food allergy persists. Although food allergy and AD may resolve, many of these infants and children often go on to develop allergic rhinitis and/or asthma [10, 11]. In one study, ~90% of children with egg-specific IgE and AD developed respiratory allergies and asthma [8].

Conclusions

Both IgE-mediated and non-IgE-mediated mechanisms have been observed in AD and other food-induced skin diseases including urticaria and dermatitis herpetiformis (Chapter 17). Early in life, the role of allergens, especially food allergens, is clearly important particularly in AD and urticaria. A careful history with appropriate diagnostic testing coupled with a comprehensive treatment program can alter the disease and life for patients with AD and food hypersensitivity.

References

1. The International Study of Asthma and Allergies in Childhood (ISAAC) Steering Committee. Worldwide variation in prevalence of symptoms of asthma, allergic rhinoconjunctivitis, and atopic eczema: ISAAC. *Lancet* 1998; 351:1225–1232.

2. Shaw TE, Currie GP, Koudelka CW, et al. Eczema prevalence in the United States: data from the 2003 National Survey of Children's Health. *J Invest Dermatol* 2011; 131(1): 67–73.
3. Kay J, Gawkrodger DJ, Mortimer MJ, et al. The prevalence of childhood atopic eczema in a general population. *J Am Acad Dermatol* 1994; 30:35–39.
4. Lau S, Nickel R, Niggeman B, et al. The development of childhood asthma: lessons from the German Multicentre Allergy Study (MAS). *Paediatr Respir Rev* 2002; 3:265–272.
5. Spergel JM, Paller JS. Atopic dermatitis and the atopic march. *J Allergy Clin Immunol* 2003; 112:S118–S127.
6. Novak N, Allam JP, Bieber T. Allergic hyperactivity to microbial components: a trigger factor of "intrinsic" atopic dermatitis?. *J Allergy Clin Immunol* 2003; 112:215–216.
7. Scheynius A, Johansson C, Buentke E, et al. Atopic eczema/dermatitis syndrome and Malassezia. *Int Arch Allergy Immunol* 2002; 127:161–169.
8. Leung D. *Pediatric Allergy: Principles and Practice*. St. Louis, MO: Mosby, 2003.
9. Barnes KC. An update on the genetics of atopic dermatitis: scratching the surface in 2009. *J Allergy Clin Immunol* 2010; 125(1):16–29.e1–11; quiz 30–31.
10. Boguniewicz M, Leung DY. Recent insights into atopic dermatitis and implications for management of infectious complications. *J Allergy Clin Immunol* 2010; 125(1):4–13; quiz 4–5.
11. Guttman-Yassky E, Nograles KE, Krueger JG. Contrasting pathogenesis of atopic dermatitis and psoriasis. Part II: Immune cell subsets and therapeutic concepts. *J Allergy Clin Immunol* 2011; 127(6):1420–1432.
12. Irvine AD, McLean WH, Leung DY. Filaggrin mutations associated with skin and allergic diseases. *N Engl J Med* 2011; 365(14):1315–1327.
13. Brown SJ, Asai Y, Cordell HJ, et al. Loss-of-function variants in the filaggrin gene are a significant risk factor for peanut allergy. *J Allergy Clin Immunol* 2011; 127(3):661–667.
14. O'Regan GM, Kemperman PM, Sandilands A, et al. Raman profiles of the stratum corneum define 3 filaggrin genotype-determined atopic dermatitis endophenotypes. *J Allergy Clin Immunol* 2010; 126(3):574–580.e1.
15. Miajlovic H, Fallon PG, Irvine AD, et al. Effect of filaggrin breakdown products on growth of and protein expression by *Staphylococcus aureus*. *J Allergy Clin Immunol* 2010; 126(6):1184–1190.e3.
16. Suarez-Farinas M, Tintle SJ, Shemer A, et al. Nonlesional atopic dermatitis skin is characterized by broad terminal differentiation defects and variable immune abnormalities. *J Allergy Clin Immunol* 2011; 127(4):954–964.e1–4.
17. Howell MD, Kim BE, Gao P, et al. Cytokine modulation of atopic dermatitis filaggrin skin expression. *J Allergy Clin Immunol* 2007; 120(1):150–155.
18. Broccardo CJ, Mahaffey S, Schwarz J, et al. Comparative proteomic profiling of patients with atopic dermatitis based on history of eczema herpeticum infection and *Staphylococcus aureus* colonization. *J Allergy Clin Immunol* 2011; 127(1):186–193.e1–11.
19. De Benedetto A, Kubo A, Beck LA. Skin barrier disruption: a requirement for allergen sensitization? *J Invest Dermatol* 2012; 132(3 Pt 2):949–963.
20. Ziegler SF, Artis D. Sensing the outside world: TSLP regulates barrier immunity. *Nat Immunol* 2010; 11(4):289–293.
21. Oyoshi MK, Larson RP, Ziegler SF, et al. Mechanical injury polarizes skin dendritic cells to elicit a T(H)2 response by inducing cutaneous thymic stromal lymphopoietin expression. *J Allergy Clin Immunol* 2010; 126(5):976–984.e1–5.
22. Gutowska-Owsiak D, Schaupp AL, Salimi M, et al. Interleukin-22 downregulates filaggrin expression and affects expression of profilaggrin processing enzymes. *Br J Dermatol* 2011; 165(3):492–498.
23. Bruynzeel-Koomen C, van Wichen DF, Toonstra J, et al. The presence of IgE molecules on epidermal Langerhans cells in patients with atopic dermatitis. *Arch Dermatol Res* 1986; 278(3):199–205.
24. Mudde GC, Bheekha R, Bruijnzeel-Koomen CA. Consequences of IgE/CD23-mediated antigen presentation in allergy. *Immunol Today* 1995; 16(8):380–383.
25. Sicherer SH, Sampson HA. Food hypersensitivity and atopic dermatitis: pathophysiology, epidemiology, diagnosis, and management. *J Allergy Clin Immunol* 1999; 104:S114–S122.
26. Wuthrich B. Food-induced cutaneous adverse reactions. *Allergy* 1998; 53:S56–S60.
27. Atherton DJ, Sewell M, Soothill JF, et al. A double-blind controlled crossover trial of an antigen-avoidance diet in atopic eczema. *Lancet* 1978; 1:401–403.
28. Neild VS, Marsden RA, Bailes JA, et al. Egg and milk exclusion diets in atopic eczema. *Br J Dermatol* 1986; 114:117–123.
29. Juto P, Engberg S, Winberg J. Treatment of infantile atopic dermatitis with a strict elimination diet. *Clin Allergy* 1978; 8:493–500.
30. Sampson HA, Scanlon SM. Natural history of food hypersensitivity in children with atopic dermatitis. *J Pediatr* 1989; 115:23–27.
31. Lever R, MacDonald C, Waugh P, et al. Randomised controlled trial of advice on an egg exclusion diet in young children with atopic eczema and sensitivity to eggs. *Pediatr Allergy Immunol* 1998; 9:13–19.
32. Bock S, Lee W, Remigio L, et al. Studies of hypersensitivity reactions to food in infants and children. *J Allergy Clin Immunol* 1978; 62:3327–3334.
33. Burks AW, Mallory SB, Williams LW, et al. Atopic dermatitis: clinical relevance of food hypersensitivity reactions. *J Pediatr* 1988; 113:447–451.
34. Burks AW, James JM, Hiegel A, et al. Atopic dermatitis and food hypersensitivity reactions. *J Pediatr* 1998; 132:132–136.
35. Sampson HA, McCaskill CC. Food hypersensitivity and atopic dermatitis: evaluation of 113 patients. *J Pediatr* 1985; 107:669–675.
36. Sampson HA, Metcalfe DD. Food allergies [Review]. *J Am Med Assoc* 1992; 268:2840–2844.
37. Eigenmann PA, Sicherer SH, Borkowski TA, et al. Prevalence of IgE-mediated food allergy among children with atopic dermatitis. *Pediatrics* 1998; 101:E8.

38. Sicherer SH, Sampson HA. Role of food allergens. In: Leung DY, Greaves MW (eds.) *Allergic Skin Disease: A Multidisciplinary Approach*, 1st edn. Philadelphia, PA: Marcel Dekker, 2000; pp. 403–422.
39. Kramer MS, Kakuma R. Maternal dietary antigen avoidance during pregnancy or lactation, or both, for preventing or treating atopic disease in the child. *Cochrane Database Syst Rev* 2003;4:CD0001333.
40. Muraro A, Dreborg S, Halken S, et al. Dietary prevention of allergic diseases in infants and small children. Part III. Critical review of published peer-reviewed observational and interventional studies and final recommendations. *Pediatr Allergy Immunol* 2004;15:291–307.
41. Friedman NJ, Zeiger RS. The role of breast-feeding in the development of allergies and asthma. *J Allergy Clin Immunol* 2005;115:1238–1248.
42. Kull I, Bohme M, Wahlgren C-F, et al. Breast-feeding decreases the risk for childhood eczema. *J Allergy Clin Immunol* 2005;116:657–661.
43. Laubereau B, Brockow I, Zirngibl A, et al. Effect of breast-feeding on the development of atopic dermatitis during the first 3 years of life—results from the GINI-birth cohort study. *J Pediatr* 2004;144:602–607.
44. Ludvigsson JF, Mostrom M, Ludvigsson J, et al. Exclusive breastfeeding and the risk of atopic dermatitis in some 8300 infants. *Pediatr Allergy Immunol* 2005;16:201–208.
45. Pesonen M, Kallio MJ, Ranki A, et al. Prolonged exclusive breastfeeding is associated with increased atopic dermatitis: a prospective follow-up study of unselected healthy new-borns from birth to age 20 years. *Clin Exp Allergy* 2006;36:1011–1018.
46. Flohr C, Nagel G, Weinmayr G, et al. Lack of evidence for a protective effect of prolonged breastfeeding on childhood eczema: lessons from the International Study of Asthma and Allergies in Childhood (ISAAC) Phase Two. *Br J Dermatol* 2011; 165(6):1280–1289.
47. Yang YW, Tsai CL, Lu CY. Exclusive breastfeeding and incident atopic dermatitis in childhood: a systematic review and meta-analysis of prospective cohort studies. *Br J Dermatol* 2009; 161(2):373–383.
48. Osborn DA, Sinn J. Formulas containing hydrolyzed protein for prevention of allergy and food intolerance in infants. *Cochrane Database Syst Rev* 2006; 4:CD003664.
49. Alexander DD, Cabana MD. Partially hydrolyzed 100% whey protein infant formula and reduced risk of atopic dermatitis: a meta-analysis. *J Pediatr Gastroenterol Nutr* 2010; 50(4):422–430.
50. von Berg A, Koletzko S, Filipiak-Pittroff B, et al. Certain hydrolyzed formulas reduce the incidence of atopic dermatitis but not that of asthma: three-year results of the German Infant Nutritional Intervention Study. *J Allergy Clin Immunol* 2007; 119:718–725.
51. von Berg A, Filipiak-Pittroff B, Kramer U, et al. Preventive effect of hydrolyzed infant formulas persists until age 6 years: long-term results from the German Infant Nutritional Intervention Study (GINI). *J Allergy Clin Immunol* 2008; 121(6):1442–1447.
52. Osborn DA, Sinn J. Soy formula for the prevention of allergy and food intolerance in infants. *Cochrane Database Syst Rev* 2006; 3:CD003741.
53. Fergusson DM, Horwood LJ, Shannon FT. Early solid feeding and recurrent childhood eczema: a 10-year longitudinal study. *Pediatrics* 1990; 86:541–546.
54. Kajosaari M. Atopy prophylaxis in high-risk infants: prospective 5-year follow-up study of children with six months exclusive breastfeeding and solid food elimination. *Adv Exp Med Biol* 1991; 310:453–458.
55. Zutavern A, Brockow I, Schaaf B, et al. Timing of solid food introduction in relation to atopic dermatitis and atopic sensitization: results from a prospective birth cohort study. *Pediatrics* 2006; 117:401–411.
56. Katz Y, Rajuan N, Goldberg MR, et al. Early exposure to cow's milk protein is protective against IgE-mediated cow's milk protein allergy. *J Allergy Clin Immunol* 2010; 126(1):77–82.e1.
57. Koplin JJ, Osborne NJ, Wake M, et al. Can early introduction of egg prevent egg allergy in infants? A population-based study. *J Allergy Clin Immunol* 2010; 126(4):807–813.
58. Poole JA, Barriga K, Leung DY, et al. Timing of initial exposure to cereal grains and the risk of wheat allergy. *Pediatrics* 2006; 117:2175–2182.
59. Sampson HA, Jolie PL. Increased plasma histamine concentrations after food challenges in children with atopic dermatitis. *N Engl J Med* 1984; 311:372–376.
60. Sampson HA, Broadbent KR, Bernhisel-Broadbent J. Spontaneous release of histamine from basophils and histamine-releasing factor in patients with atopic dermatitis and food hypersensitivity. *N Engl J Med* 1989; 321:228–232.
61. Lyczak JB, Zhang K, Saxon A, et al. Expression of novel secreted isoforms of human immunoglobulin E proteins. *J Biol Chem* 1996; 271:3428–3436.
62. Du Buske LM. Introduction: basophil histamine release and the diagnosis of food allergy. *Allergy Proc* 1993; 14:243–249.
63. Nolte H. The clinical utility of basophil histamine release. *Allergy Proc* 1993; 14:251–254.
64. Sampson HA, Ho DG. Relationship between food-specific IgE concentrations and the risk of positive food challenges in children and adolescents. *J Allergy Clin Immunol* 1997; 100:444–451.
65. Shreffler WG. Evaluation of basophil activation in food allergy: present and future applications. *Curr Opin Allergy Clin Immunol* 2006; 6:226–233.
66. Sobotka AK, Dembo M, Goldstein B, et al. Antigen-specific desensitization of human basophils. *J Immunol* 1979; 122:511–517.
67. Satti MZ, Cahen P, Skov PS, et al. Changes in IgE- and antigen-dependent histamine-release in peripheral blood of Schistosoma mansoni-infected Ugandan fishermen after treatment with praziquantel. *BMC Immunol* 2004; 5:6.
68. Demoly P, Piette V, Bousquet J. In vivo methods for study of allergy. In: Adkinson NF, Yunginger JW, Busse WW, et al. (eds), *Middleton's Allergy: Principles and Practice*, 6th edn. Philadelphia, PA: Mosby, 2003; pp. 631–632.

69. Abramovits W. Atopic dermatitis. *J Am Acad Dermatol* 2005; 53:S86–S93.
70. Leiferman KM, Ackerman SJ, Sampson HA, et al. Dermal deposition of eosinophil-granule major basic protein in atopic dermatitis. Comparison with onchocerciasis. *N Engl J Med* 1985; 313:282–285.
71. Suomalainen H, Soppi E, Isolauri E. Evidence for eosinophil activation in cow's milk allergy. *Pediatr Allergy Immunol* 1994; 5:27–31.
72. Magnarin M, Knowles A, Ventura A, et al. A role for eosinophils in the pathogenesis of skin lesions in patients with food-sensitive atopic dermatitis. *J Allergy Clin Immunol* 1995; 96:200–208.
73. van Reijsen FC, Felius A, Wauters EA. T-cell reactivity for a peanut-derived epitope in the skin of a young infant with atopic dermatitis. *J Allergy Clin Immunol* 1998; 101:207–209.
74. Abernathy-Carver KJ, Sampson HA, Parker LJ, et al. Milk-induced eczema is associated with the expansion of T cells expressing cutaneous lymphocyte antigen. *J Clin Invest* 1995; 95:913–918.
75. Reekers R, Beyer K, Niggemann B, et al. The role of circulating food antigen-specific lymphocytes in food allergic children with atopic dermatitis. *Br J Dermatol* 1996; 135:935–941.
76. Werfel T, Ahlers G, Schmidt P, et al. Detection of kappa-casein-specific lymphocyte response in milk-responsive atopic dermatitis. *Clin Exp Allergy* 1996; 26:1380–1386.
77. Kondo N, Fukutomi O, Agata H, et al. Proliferative responses of lymphocytes to food antigens are useful for detection of allergens in nonimmediate types of food allergy. *J Invest Allergol Clin Immunol* 1997; 7:122–126.
78. Agata H, Kondo N, Fukutomi O, et al. Effect of elimination diets in food-specific IgE antibodies and lymphocyte proliferative responses to food antigens in atopic dermatitis patients exhibiting sensitivity to food allergens. *J Allergy Clin Immunol* 1993; 91:668–679.
79. Hoffman KM, Ho DG, Sampson HA. Evaluation of the usefulness of lymphocyte proliferation assays in the diagnosis of allergy to cow's milk. *J Allergy Clin Immunol* 1997; 99:360–366.
80. Sampson HA. Eczema and food hypersensitivity. In: Metcalfe DD, Sampson HA, Simon RA (eds), *Food Allergy: Adverse Reactions to Foods and Food Additives*, 3rd edn. Malden: Blackwell Publishing, 2003; pp. 144–159.
81. De Bruin-Weller MS, Knol EF, Bruijnzeel-Koomen C. Atopy patch testing—a diagnostic tool? *Allergy* 1999; 54:784–791.
82. Eigenmann PA, Calza AM. Diagnosis of IgE-mediated food allergy among Swiss children with atopic dermatitis. *Pediatr Allergy Immunol* 2000; 11:95–100.
83. Guillet G, Guillet MH. Natural history of sensitizations in atopic dermatitis. A 3-year follow-up in 250 children: food allergy and high risk of respiratory symptoms. *Arch Dermatol* 1992; 128:187–192.
84. Hill DJ, Sporik R, Thorburn J, et al. The association of atopic dermatitis in infancy with immunoglobulin E food sensitization. *J Pediatr* 2000; 137:475–479.
85. Hill DJ, Hosking CS. Food allergy and atopic dermatitis in infancy: an epidemiologic study. *Pediatr Allergy Immunol* 2004; 15:421–427.
86. Munkvad M, Danielsen L, Hoj L, et al. Antigen-free diet in adult patients with atopic dermatitis. A double-blind controlled study. *Acta Derm Venereol* 1984; 64:524–528.
87. de Maat-Bleeker F, Bruijnzeel-Koomen C. Food allergy in adults with atopic dermatitis. *Monogr Allergy Basel Karger* 1996; 32:157–163.
88. Uenishi T, Sugiura H, Uehara M. Role of foods in irregular aggravation of atopic dermatitis. *J Dermatol* 2003; 30:91–97.
89. Worm M, Forschner K, Lee HH, et al. Frequency of atopic dermatitis and relevance of food allergy in adults in Germany. *Acta Derm Venereol* 2006; 86:119–122.
90. Bock SA, Atkins FM. Patterns of food hypersensitivity during sixteen years of double-blind, placebo-controlled food challenges. *J Pediatr* 1990; 117:561–567.
91. Sicherer SH, Sampson HA. Food allergy. *J Allergy Clin Immunol* 2006; 117:S470–S475.
92. Sampson HA. Food allergy. Part 2. Diagnosis and management. *J Allergy Clin Immunol* 1999; 103:981–989.
93. Bock SA, Lee WY, Remigio L, et al. Appraisal of skin tests with food extracts for diagnosis of food hypersensitivity. *Clin Allergy* 1978; 8:559–564.
94. Sampson HA. Utility of food-specific IgE concentrations in predicting symptomatic food allergy. *J Allergy Clin Immunol* 2001; 107:891–896.
95. Ortolani C, Ispano M, Pastorello EA, et al. Comparison of results of skin prick tests (with fresh foods and commercial food extracts) and RAST in 100 patients with oral allergy syndrome. *J Allergy Clin Immunol* 1989; 83:683–690.
96. Eigenmann PA, Sampson HA. Interpreting skin prick tests in the evaluation of food allergy in children. *Pediatr Allergy Immunol* 1998; 9:186–191.
97. Roehr CC, Reibel S, Ziegert M, et al. Atopy patch tests, together with determination of specific IgE levels, reduce the need for oral food challenges in children with atopic dermatitis. *J Allergy Clin Immunol* 2001; 107:548–553.
98. Breuer K, Heratizadeh A, Wulf A, et al. Late eczematous reactions to food in children with atopic dermatitis. *Clin Exp Allergy* 2004; 34:817–824.
99. Mehl A, Rolinck-Werninhaus C, Staden U, et al. The atopy patch test in the diagnostic workup of suspected food-related symptoms in children. *J Allergy Clin Immunol* 2006; 118:923–929.
100. Turjanmaa K. The role of atopy patch tests in the diagnosis of allergy in atopic dermatitis. *Curr Opin Allergy Clin Immunol* 2005; 5:425–428.
101. Sicherer SH, Bock SA. An expanding evidence base provides food for thought to avoid indigestion in managing difficult dilemmas in food allergy. *J Allergy Clin Immunol* 2006; 117:1419–1422.
102. Bock SA, Sampson HA, Atkins FA, et al. Double-blind, placebo-controlled food challenge (DBPCFC) as an office procedure: a manual. *J Allergy Clin Immunol* 1988; 82:986–997.
103. Sicherer SH. Food allergy: when and how to perform oral food challenges. *Pediatr Allergy Immunol* 1999; 10:226–234.
104. Sicherer SH. Food allergy. *Lancet* 2002; 360:701–710.
105. Sampson HA. Use of food-challenge tests in children. *Lancet* 2001; 358:1832–1833.

106. Sampson HA, Mendelson LM, Rosen JP. Fatal and near-fatal anaphylactic reactions to foods in children and adolescents. *N Engl J Med* 1992; 327:380–384.
107. Bock SA. The natural history of food sensitivity. *J Allergy Clin Immunol* 1982; 69:173–177.
108. Skolnick HS, Conover-Walker MK, Sampson HA, et al. The natural history of peanut allergy. *J Allergy Clin Immunol* 2002; 107:367–374.
109. Fleischer DM, Conover-Walker MK, Christie L, et al. The natural progression of peanut allergy: resolution and the possibility of recurrence. *J Allergy Clin Immunol* 2003; 112:183–189.
110. Fleischer DM, Conover-Walker MK, Matsui EC, et al. The natural history of tree nut allergy. *J Allergy Clin Immunol* 2005; 116:1087–1093.
111. Lemon-Mule H, Sampson HA, Sicherer SH, et al. Immunologic changes in children with egg allergy ingesting extensively heated egg. *J Allergy Clin Immunol* 2008; 122(5):977–983.e1.
112. Kim JS, Nowak-Wegrzyn A, Sicherer SH, et al. Dietary baked milk accelerates the resolution of cow's milk allergy in children. *J Allergy Clin Immunol* 2011; 128(1):125–131.e2.
113. Konstantinou GN, Kim JS. Paradigm shift in the management of milk and egg allergy: baked milk and egg diet. *Immunol Allergy Clin North Am* 2012; 32(1):151–164.
114. Fleischer DM, Conover-Walker MK, Christie L, et al. Peanut allergy: recurrence and its management. *J Allergy Clin Immunol* 2004; 114:1195–1201.
115. Nickel R, Kulig M, Forster G, et al. Sensitization to hen's egg at the age of 12 months is predictive for allergen sensitization to common indoor and outdoor allergens at the age of 3 years. *J Allergy Clin Immunol* 1997; 99:613–617.

12 Oral Allergy Syndrome

Julie Wang
Division of Allergy and Immunology, Department of Pediatrics, Elliot and Roslyn Jaffe Food Allergy Institute, Icahn School of Medicine at Mount Sinai, New York, NY, USA

Key Concepts

- Oral allergy syndrome (OAS) explains the relationship between allergic rhinitis and certain food allergies through homologous proteins in the plant kingdom.
- Wide regional variability exists for OAS.
- It is a contact allergy that primarily results in mild symptoms limited to the oropharyngeal area.
- The diagnosis of OAS is currently suboptimal, as *in vivo* and *in vitro* tests are poor predictors of clinical reactivity.
- The management of OAS relies on food avoidance, but may evolve to include immunotherapy in the future.

Introduction

The first report of hypersensitivity to fruits and vegetables in patients with pollen allergy occurred 70 years ago when Tuft et al. described four individuals with hay fever who experienced localized symptoms with fresh fruits and vegetables [1]. In 1970, the observation that ragweed allergy was commonly associated with allergy to melon and banana was described [2]. Ragweed-allergic patients experienced immediate oral symptoms after eating melons or bananas. No one had anaphylaxis, and none of the nonpollen-allergic patients reported symptoms with these fruits. Soon after, similar associations were reported for birch pollen and apple allergy [3] as well as for mugwort and celery allergy [4]. These pollen–fruit–vegetable associations had similar characteristics of localized symptoms after ingestion of fresh plant-derived products.

The term oral allergy syndrome (OAS) has been used to describe such symptoms with ingestion of fresh fruits and vegetables in pollen-allergic patients. This is an IgE-mediated allergy that is due to cross-reacting, homologous proteins between pollens and food proteins [5]. Since conserved proteins are widely expressed throughout the plant kingdom, it is not surprising that homologous proteins are being identified in a growing number of plant-derived foods. In fact, cross-reactivities between pollens and fruits and vegetables have been increasingly reported in recent years, coincident with the increased prevalence of allergic rhinitis. There has been tremendous progress in the last few decades leading to a better understanding of these cross-reacting allergens.

Epidemiology

OAS is the most common food allergy in adults, with more than half of food-allergic individuals reporting oropharyngeal symptoms after ingestion of fresh fruits and vegetables [6, 7]. Unlike classic IgE-mediated food allergy, it can develop after years of tolerance to the food. A study of an unselected adult population in Denmark revealed that 10% of adults have both allergic rhinitis and OAS [8]. Among individuals with allergic rhinitis, the prevalence of OAS ranged from 30% to 70% depending on location, likely due to differences in pollen distribution and dietary habits [8–11]. Osterballe et al. [8] found that a higher probability of clinical allergy to plant-derived foods occurred in individuals who had sensitization to multiple pollens (birch, grass, and/or mugwort). Fewer studies have reported the prevalence of OAS in children. An Italian study found that 29% of children with allergic rhinitis to grass reported food allergy symptoms [12].

In addition to regional variations in prevalence, different foods are responsible for OAS in different locations. In a

Food Allergy: Adverse Reactions to Foods and Food Additives, Fifth Edition. Edited by Dean D Metcalfe, Hugh A Sampson, Ronald A Simon and Gideon Lack.

study of 274 English adults who were allergic to at least one pollen (birch, grass, and/or mugwort), 34% had OAS to apple, 25% to potato, 23% to carrot, 23% to celery, 22% to peach, and 16% to melon [9]. In contrast, OAS was most commonly due to hazelnut, kiwi, apple, and celery root in Italy [8]. Pollen-allergic adults in Sweden most often reported symptoms with hazelnut, apple, tomato, carrot, and peanut [13], whereas in Spain, peach was the most common fruit allergy [14].

Regional differences also exist in the patterns of associations. Patients with allergy to apple, but not birch pollen have not been reported in northern and middle Europe, but are commonly seen in Spain [15]. In Spain, apple allergy is, instead, associated with grass pollen allergy [16]. Different patterns of kiwi allergen recognition are evident in various parts of Europe as well [17]. Kiwi is associated with grass pollen allergy in Italy, but with birch pollen allergy in Spain [12]. New sensitizations have also been reported when people are exposed to new environments. Two patients who tolerated jackfruit in the Philippines, a birch-free environment, reportedly reacted to jackfruit when they developed sensitization to birch pollen while in Switzerland [18]. These highlight the role of regional exposures on the development of cross-sensitization.

Clinical features

OAS is an IgE-mediated allergy that is generally mild. It is a contact allergy resulting in local symptoms such as lip/mouth itching, swelling, hoarseness, papulae, and in rare cases, blisters [15]. The onset of symptoms is rapid, with most symptoms appearing within 5 minutes of exposure to the triggering food [19]. However, symptoms may be delayed, appearing after 30 minutes in 7% of cases [19]. The degree of clinical reactivity can have seasonal variations. In one study, 44% of birch pollen-allergic individuals reported worsening of symptoms during the birch pollen season [11], which has been postulated to be due to upregulation of birch pollen allergens (Bet v 1 and 2) in pollen during maturation [20]. However, symptoms are still present outside of the birch pollen season for the majority of patients (86.8%) [11]. Symptoms can occur outside the oropharynx as well. In a study of 706 patients with OAS, 13.6% had extra-oral gastrointestinal symptoms, 13.9% reported laryngeal edema, and 2.1% of individuals experienced anaphylaxis (Table 12.1) [21].

Table 12.1 Symptoms of oral allergy syndrome.

Symptoms
Localized symptoms
Lip/mouth swelling
Lip/mouth itching
Hoarseness
Papulae
Laryngeal edema
Systemic symptoms
Cutaneous—urticaria/angioedema, atopic dermatitis flare
Rhinitis
Conjunctivitis
Wheezing
Gastrointestinal symptoms—abdominal pain/cramps, nausea, vomiting, diarrhea
Anaphylaxis

Molecular basis/pathogenesis

IgE-mediated food allergies can be classified according to the route of sensitization [22]. Class I allergy is due to sensitization via the gastrointestinal tract, whereas class II allergy indicates that the primary allergic sensitization is to inhalant allergens. Class I allergy often presents in childhood, while class II allergy is more commonly observed in adults. Complete food allergens, which have the ability to both sensitize and elicit symptoms, induce class I allergy. In contrast, class II allergy is triggered by incomplete food allergens, which do not typically cause sensitization, but can elicit symptoms because of cross-reactivity to the homologous sensitizer [23]. OAS is classified as a class II allergy since the pollen allergens are the sensitizers and homologous proteins in plant-derived foods elicit symptoms. These food allergens are generally heat-labile and susceptible to gastric digestion, thus inducing symptoms primarily in the oropharynx.

There are several hypotheses explaining the localization of symptoms present in OAS. Amlot et al. proposed that oral symptoms are predominant because there is a high concentration of mast cells in oropharyngeal mucosa [5]. Local symptoms may also be due to a high concentration of allergens on the oral mucosa that are rapidly released when in contact with saliva [15]. Alternatively, high concentrations of T cells in the oropharyngeal lymphoid tissue can have food-specific T-cell responses since cross-reactivity has been found at the T-cell level [24, 25].

Allergens

A variety of plant proteins have been identified to play a role in OAS. These include pathogenesis-related (PR) proteins, proteinase and α-amylase inhibitors, peroxidases, profilins, seed storage proteins, thiol proteases, and lectins [26]. Many of these are distributed throughout the plant kingdom, accounting for the extensive IgE cross-reactivity between taxonomically unrelated plant foods.

PR proteins are plant-defense proteins that are expressed in response to stress from the environment, chemicals, or infection [27]. Most PR proteins causing OAS belong to the PR-10 family. IgE antibodies to the major birch pollen

(Bet v 1) cross-react with homologous plant food allergens belonging to the PR-10 protein family. Symptoms are often mild, since these Bet v 1-related proteins are unstable to heat and digestion [28, 29]. The most common fruits causing symptoms in Bet v 1-allergic individuals include members of the order Rosaceae, such as apple, pear, cherry, and apricot (Table 12.2). Homologous proteins are also found in celery, carrot, hazelnut, soy, and peanut.

Lipid transfer proteins (LTPs) belong to the PR-14 family [30] and have been identified as major allergens involved in nonpollen plant food allergies; the term LTP syndrome has since been used to describe these patients. LTPs comprise a family of polypeptides that have the ability to transfer phospholipids from liposomes to mitochondria and are found throughout the plant kingdom [22]. They are defense proteins upregulated by some plants in response to fungal infection [31]. First identified as the major allergen in peach as well as an allergen for apple in 1999 [32, 33], LTPs have since been discovered in other related foods, including apricot [34], plum [35], and cherry [36] (Table 12.2). LTPs have also been identified in various unrelated plant products such as peanut, corn, asparagus, grape, lettuce, sunflower seeds, latex, and mugwort [18, 37, 38].

A larger, non-PR-related protein family that is implicated in OAS includes the profilins (Table 12.2) [22]. These are small (12–15 kDa) proteins that bind actin and have an important role regulating the cytoskeleton. Profilins are also sensitive to heat and gastric digestion [39]. The first profilin identified was a minor birch pollen protein, Bet v 2 [40]. Patients with pollen allergy and plant food allergy have a high frequency of IgE reactivity to Bet v 2. Patients sensitized to Bet v 2 also have reactivity to latex, grass, olive tree, and mugwort pollens, suggesting that reactivity to Bet v 2 may be a marker for broad aeroallergen sensitization [41]. Wensing et al. [42] similarly reported that profilin is responsible for a broader spectrum of cross-reactivity than Bet v 1. The authors found that those sensitized to both Bet v 1 and profilin had significantly more specific IgE to foods than those sensitized only to Bet v 1. However, this broad sensitization was not always correlated with clinical reactivity. Therefore, the clinical role for profilin remains unclear, since sensitization to profilin is rarely associated with clinical symptoms [43].

A group of high molecular weight allergens (45–60 kDa) has been identified in various pollen and foods [44]. These are highly cross-reactive IgE-binding structures and have been named cross-reactive carbohydrate determinants (CCDs) [35]. They are ubiquitous in pollen and plant-derived foods and have also been identified in hymenoptera venom [44]. Thirty to forty percent of pollen-allergic individuals have evidence of IgE against CCDs, which exhibit broad *in vitro* cross-reactivity [45] and heat stability [46]. Their immunological activity was demonstrated by Foetisch et al. [47] who showed that the tomato glycoprotein, β-fructofuranosidase, could induce histamine release when basophils were sensitized by serum from tomato-allergic patients. However, the role of CCDs in OAS remains uncertain as the *in vivo* relevance has not been demonstrated.

Table 12.2 List of allergens mentioned in this chapter (scientific names in parenthesis).

Allergen
Bet v 1 homologs (PR-10)
Apple (Mal d 1)
Apricot (Pru ar 1)
Carrot (Dau c 1)
Celery (Api g 1)
Cherry (Pru av 1)
Hazelnut (Cor a 1.04)
Jackfruit (Art i)
Peanut (Ara h 8)
Pear (Pyr c 1)
Soy (Gly m 4) (starvation-associated message 22)
Strawberry (Fra a 1)
Lipid transfer proteins (LTPs)
Asparagus (Aspa o 1)
Apple (Mal d 3)
Apricot (Pru ar 3)
Cherry (Pru av 3)
Grape (Vit v 1)
Hazelnut (Cor a 8)
Lettuce (Lac s 1)
Maize, corn (Zea m 14)
Mugwort (Art v 3)
Parietaria (Par j 1 and 2)
Peach (Pru p 3)
Peanut (Ara h 9)
Strawberry (Fra a 3)
Tomato (Lyc e 3)
Walnut (Jug r 3)
Profilin
Almond (Pru du 4)
Apple (Mal d 4)
Banana (Mus xp 1)
Bell pepper (Cap a 2)
Birch (Bet v 2)
Carrot (Dau c 4)
Celery (Api g 4)
Hazelnut (Cor a 2)
Latex (Hev b 8)
Melon (Cuc m 2)
Mugwort (Art v 4)
Peach (Pru p 4)
Ragweed (Amb a 8)
Soy (Gly m 3)
Strawberry (Fra a 4)
TIMOTHY grass (Phl p 12)
Tomato (Lyc e 1)

Source: Adapted from the International Union of Immunological Societies (IUIS) List of Allergens. A complete list can be found at www.allergen.org

Pollen-food syndromes

Birch–fruit–vegetable syndrome

Foods belonging to the order Rosaceae, which include apple, pear, peach, and almond, most commonly cause symptoms in birch-allergic patients. Bet v 1, the major birch tree allergen, accounts for most of this cross-reactivity [48]. The prevalence of birch–fruit syndrome is variable depending on geographic location. A US study reported that 75.9% of birch pollen-allergic patients had clinical symptoms with apple [49]. Lower rates have been reported in Europe, with 34% of birch pollen patients in Denmark reporting symptoms with apple [3], and 9% of birch pollen patients in Italy having symptoms with apple [8].

The primary sensitization in birch–fruit syndrome is to birch pollen, and the symptoms elicited by foods are a secondary phenomenon [20]. A Bet v 1 homolog was identified in apple in 1991 (Mal d 1) [49]. There is a high degree of homology between Bet v 1 and the plant food allergens. Bet v 1 and Mal d 1 share 64.5% sequence homology [15], and Cor a 1 (hazelnut) is 72% homologous with Bet v 1 [28]. Bet v 1-related proteins have also been identified in peanut [29] and soy [50].

Celery–birch–mugwort–spice syndrome

Celery has been found to have cross-reactivity with both birch and mugwort pollens. In areas where birch trees are prevalent, celery allergy is due to Bet v 1 homologues. However, celery allergy does exist in birch-free areas; in these cases, mugwort pollen allergens may be the primary sensitizer [22]. Wuthrich et al. [51] reported that patients with celery–birch allergy had undetectable or low specific IgE to cooked and uncooked celery. In contrast, patients with celery–mugwort association had positive IgE to cooked and uncooked celery, suggesting different allergens are involved in these two associations. Similarly, Hoffmann-Sommergruber et al. [52] examined two groups of celery-allergic individuals from two different geographic locations, one from Switzerland (birch trees present) and one from southern France (birch-free). The authors found that in Switzerland, all the patients had positive skin testing to birch and commercial celery extract. In contrast, only 25% of patients in southern France had positive skin testing to birch pollen and commercial celery extract, but all had sensitization to mugwort pollen. Immunoblots from these patients revealed IgE against high molecular weight proteins in the range of 28–69 kDa and two had IgE reactivity to a 12–13 kDa protein, suggesting that CCDs and profilin may be playing a role, rather than Bet v 1 homologues.

Bet v 1 and profilins have also been identified in various spices, including anise (Pim a 1 and 2), coriander (Cor s 1 and 2), cumin (Cum c 1 and 2), fennel (Foe v 1 and 2), and parsley (Pet c 1 and 2) [53]. Cross-reactivity between mugwort and mustard has been demonstrated [54]. Thus, the term celery-birch-mugwort-spice syndrome has been used to describe these cross-reactivities.

Ragweed–melon–banana association

Up to 50% of ragweed-allergic patients have specific IgE to at least one member of the gourd family Cucurbitaceae (e.g., watermelon, cantaloupe, honeydew, zucchini, cucumber) [55]. In fact, this association was the first report linking pollen and fruit allergy [2]. Melon allergy occurs mainly in association with pollen allergy, even in ragweed-free locations [56].

Profilin has been identified in both melon [22] and banana [57]. Melon profilin is highly susceptible to pepsin digestion [58]; therefore, melon allergy usually causes symptoms limited to the oropharynx. However, one study reported that nearly 20% of melon-allergic individuals experienced symptoms outside the mouth [59] and in another study, 11% had anaphylaxis [60], suggesting that other more stable allergens such as LTPs may be involved as well. It has also been reported that pollen-allergic patients with melon allergy have higher rates of asthma than pollen-allergic individuals without melon allergy, suggesting a more severe phenotype [59].

Lipid transfer protein syndrome

In a group of mugwort-allergic patients in southern Spain who had IgE to LTP in both mugwort (Art v 3) and peach (Pru p 3), the authors found that the pollen protein was the primary allergen, indicating that LTPs can act as class II allergens [61]. More commonly, however, LTPs appear to act as the primary sensitizer (class I allergen), which likely occurs in 15–20% of patients with allergies to fruits and/or vegetables who have no reported symptoms of allergic rhinitis and negative skin tests to pollens [19, 62]. Individuals with allergies to plant-derived foods without associated pollen allergy have several features distinguishing them from those with OAS-associated pollen allergy [16]. Individuals without pollen allergy had significantly more systemic reactions (82% vs. 45%), including anaphylaxis (73% vs. 18%), and had less oral symptoms (64% vs. 91%) when compared to those with pollen allergy. Individuals without pollen allergy were older at the onset of symptoms to fruits and vegetables (19 years of age vs. ~12 years). In addition, those without pollen allergy mainly reacted to fruits in the order Rosaceae whereas those with pollen allergy had more diverse sensitizations to different families of fruits and had reactions to a greater number of foods in general. Although the nonpollen-allergic group was more likely to have systemic reactions, those with pollen allergy appeared to have a higher risk of asthma [22].

Apple allergy in Spain (birch-free area) tends to be more severe (>35% systemic reactions) than apple allergy in other locations, and the major allergen in these cases has been identified as Mal d 3, an LTP [63]. The authors proposed that apple allergy in Spain is a result of cross-reactivity with peach proteins rather than with birch pollen proteins because peach is introduced in early childhood in that country and consumed in large quantities. Peach allergy develops at a younger age than apple allergy, and therefore the primary sensitization is believed to be to peach LTP, Pru p 3.

The systemic reactions that occur with LTP syndrome are likely due to the stability of LTPs in acidic and proteolytic conditions of the gastrointestinal tract [63] as well as their resistance to heating [28, 46]. For example, celery-allergic patients have been shown to have positive food challenges to cooked celery under double-blind, placebo-controlled conditions [46]. The heat resistance of LTP has also been demonstrated for hazelnut, maize, and cherry [28, 30, 64]. Thus, commercial foods that have been thermally processed may still cause symptoms in some sensitized individuals.

Latex–fruit syndrome

The first report of an allergic reaction to banana in a latex-allergic patient was published in 1991 [65]. Soon thereafter, cross-reactivity between latex and various fruits were demonstrated, and this was termed latex–fruit syndrome [66]. Significant cross-reactivity between latex and fruit allergens was demonstrated by Blanco et al. [66] who reported that 13 of 25 patients (52%) with latex allergy had specific IgE to fruits. Similar studies have reported that up to 88% of latex-allergic adults have evidence of specific IgE to plant-derived foods [67, 68]. Although there is a high degree of immunologic cross-reactivity between the latex and fruit allergens, the clinical significance appears to be much lower. A study from Germany of 136 latex-allergic patients showed that although 69% had specific IgE to fruits, only 32% had clinical symptoms [69]. Similarly, among melon-allergic patients, 68% had detectable latex-specific IgE, but only 26% were clinically reactive [60].

The primary sensitization is believed to be to latex, generally via inhalation. In a study of children with atopic dermatitis, all of the children who had latex-specific IgE also had IgE to various foods, mostly potato, tomato, sweet pepper, and avocado [70]. However, none of the children with elevated IgE to avocado, chestnut, and kiwi had ever had exposure to these foods.

Several latex allergens have been implicated in the latex–fruit syndrome. Class I chitinases (Hev b 11) belonging to the PR-3 protein family have been identified in chestnut, avocado, and banana [71]. The N-terminal region of Hev b 11 is related to hevein (Hev b 6.02), which is an important latex allergen that has several cross-reactive epitopes. Low-level inhibition of IgE binding to hevein, a major latex allergen, can be demonstrated with class I chitinases from several fruits [72], suggesting that these two allergens share some IgE-binding epitopes. In fact, Hev b 11 and hevein share 58% sequence identity at the chitin-binding domain [72]. Another major latex allergen Hev b 2 (β-1,3-glucanase, PR-2 protein family) is also involved in the latex–fruit syndrome and has been identified in bell peppers [73]. Furthermore, Hev b 8 (profilin), a minor latex allergen, has been demonstrated to have cross-reactivity with some fruits [74]. Thus, many latex allergens may contribute to food allergies in latex-sensitive individuals.

While some individuals with latex–fruit syndrome experience only oral symptoms, others can have systemic reactions [75]. These more severe symptoms may be due to the stability of some latex allergens. Hevein has been demonstrated to be stable in simulated gastric fluid [23]. In addition, although class I chitinase in avocado is extensively degraded in simulated gastric fluid, the peptides have been shown to retain their IgE-binding epitopes and can induce positive skin test results [76].

Differences have been observed between patients allergic to latex (without fruit allergy) and those with allergy to both latex and fruit. Blanco et al. [71] showed that chestnut and avocado class I chitinases were able to induce positive skin prick test (SPT) responses in more than 60% of patients with latex–fruit allergy, but did not result in positive tests in control subjects who were latex allergic, but not fruit allergic. Pooled serum from latex-allergic and not fruit-allergic individuals also does not detect class I chitinases in several fruit extracts [71]. In addition, different HLA associations have been identified for those with latex–fruit syndrome as compared to those with only latex allergy, suggesting a genetic basis for the latex–fruit syndrome [77].

Diagnosis

History remains the most important component in the diagnosis of any food allergy. Since some plant foods, including peanut and hazelnut, are known to cause both class I and class II food allergy, documentation of the onset and type of symptoms can guide proper characterization and management of the allergy.

SPTs and serum-specific IgE levels (sIgE) are the main diagnostic tools available for food allergy diagnosis. However, these tests are not very reliable for the diagnosis of OAS. The results may be variable depending on which food is being tested since there can be significant cross-reactivity between allergens that have common epitopes. Furthermore, SPT and sIgE are poor predictors of clinical reactivity. SPTs rely on commercial extracts that may not contain all of the relevant allergens. Some plant food allergens are heat labile [28, 29] and lose potency and sensitivity during processing of the extracts. In addition, proteases from the fruits themselves can affect potency. As an example, the pineapple protease bromelain destroys pineapple profilin in extracts prepared without protease inhibitor [74]. For some exotic fruits, low yield of protein for extracts has been problematic [74].

SPT with fresh fruits and vegetables generally correlates better with clinical reactivity when compared to commercial extracts, but this type of testing is not standardized [78, 79]. A study by Anhoej et al. [80] showed that the negative predictive value for SPT with fresh hazelnut, apple, and melon was greater than 90%. The positive predictive value was more variable, ranging from 50% to 85%. Sensitivity was high for all three (89–97%) and the specificities were greater than 70%. Freezing does not alter the antigenic properties of fresh fruits; therefore, SPT with frozen fruits is an acceptable alternative if fresh fruits are not available [81]. Of note, ripeness of the plant food can affect the sensitivity of SPT, since allergenicity has been demonstrated to increase with ripening in banana [82] and peach [83]. Differences in storage conditions and different cultivars can lead to variations in allergenicity as well [84–86]. Apples in prolonged cold storage under controlled atmosphere conditions are less allergenic than apples stored at 2°C in normal air, and Golden delicious apples are generally more allergenic than Santana apples [84].

A study comparing SPT with fresh foods and sIgE (ImmunoCAP®, Thermo Fisher Scientific, Waltham, MA, USA) in patients with OAS to melons demonstrated comparable positive predictive values (42% for SPT vs. 44% for sIgE) [87]. The negative predictive value was slightly higher for SPT with fresh food (77% SPT vs. 70% sIgE).

While SPT and sIgE results indicate allergic sensitization, positive results do not always correlate with clinical reactivity. Therefore, double-blind, placebo-controlled food challenge remains the gold standard for the diagnosis of food allergy. With respect to OAS, however, there are no standardized protocols for food challenges, and issues relating to adequate blinding of fresh foods remain a major concern.

Management

There are currently no consensus guidelines for the management of OAS. A survey of allergists revealed a tremendous variation in management strategies used [88]. The authors suggested that this may be due, in part, to the imprecise definition of OAS and lack of accurate and standardized diagnostic tests. Recommendations range from avoidance of only the offending fruits or vegetables to eliminating the entire botanical family. Allergy to one food, however, does not necessarily indicate allergy to all members of the botanical family. For example, 63% of peach-allergic individuals react to more than one Prunoideae fruit [89], and 46% have clinical cross-reactivity with other Rosaceae fruits [90]. A study of 65 adults in Madrid with OAS revealed that only 8% of the positive *in vivo* and *in vitro* tests for cross-reacting foods resulted in positive food challenges [91]. This supports the recommendation not to eliminate entire families of cross-reactive foods, which would be unnecessarily restrictive. However, the authors noted that in this series of patients, there were an additional 18 clinically relevant allergens, previously unknown to the patients, which were detected on further testing and food challenges. Therefore, they suggested that oral challenges be performed to related foods that the patients had not yet eaten subsequent to the most recent allergic reaction.

Table 12.3 Allergenicity of different apple cultivars.

Golden Delicious,	High allergenic
Jonagold, Gala	Moderate allergenic
Elstar, Fuji, Granny Smith	Low allergenic
Santana, Elize, Braeburn	

Ranking from nine Dutch patients (northern Europe) based on SPT with fresh apple and double-blind, placebo-controlled food challenges [84].

As previously stated, allergenicity can vary between different cultivars of fruits (Table 12.3) [84]. Therefore, some individuals may tolerate lower allergenic cultivars. In addition, this information may be useful in breeding novel, lower allergenic cultivars. Some report symptoms only when eating certain parts of the fruit, indicating that allergen distribution is not uniform. In fact, Mal d 1 (Bet v 1 homolog) is present in both the peel and pulp of apples, whereas, Mal d 3 (LTP) is most abundant in peel.

For individuals with OAS due to heat-labile proteins, heating the fruits and vegetables can denature the relevant proteins, thus allowing symptom-free consumption. Anecdotal evidence has suggested that briefly heating apples (e.g., by microwaving) may be sufficient to denature Mal d 1 allergens, without compromising the integrity of the fruit; however, this has not been confirmed by controlled studies.

It is important to note that there is a potential for systemic reactions with OAS. In fact, ~2% of patients experience anaphylaxis [21]. Risk factors for systemic reactions include prior history of a systemic reaction to the food, reaction to cooked forms of the food [30, 46], positive SPT to the food extract [92], lack of pollen sensitization [16], and sensitization to LTP [32] (Table 12.4). Thus, self-injectable epinephrine should

Table 12.4 Risk factors for severe symptoms of oral allergy syndrome.

- History of systemic reaction to the food
- Reaction to cooked forms of the food [30, 46]
- Positive skin test result to the food extract [92]
- Lack of pollen sensitization [16]
- Sensitization to LTP [32]

be prescribed, and education on the management of severe reactions provided.

In addition, the presence of other atopic conditions and concurrent medication use should be considered. Chronic use of antihistamines may mask mild OAS symptoms, prompting increased consumption of the triggering foods, which may increase the risk of systemic symptoms. This is a particular concern for patients who are already taking allergy medications for their allergic rhinitis symptoms [93].

Future directions

Advancements in the understanding of relevant allergens for OAS have led to the development of improved diagnostic tools as well as exploration into possible treatment strategies.

Component-resolved diagnosis

Improved diagnostic tools can facilitate diagnosis and management of OAS since it is often difficult to distinguish between class I allergy and class II allergy because a single food can be the trigger for both types of reactions. Peanut and hazelnut are two examples. For peanut, the major allergens involved in class I peanut allergy are Ara h 1, 2, 3 whereas the primary allergen responsible for pollen-related allergy is Ara h 8 (Bet v 1 homolog) [94]. The ability to measure specific IgE to these individual proteins has been shown to facilitate the characterization of peanut allergy. Nicolaou et al. detected significant differences in the pattern of recognition to these various peanut proteins using a microarray assay among peanut-allergic and peanut-tolerant children. The results suggested that IgE response to Ara h 2 was an important predictor of clinical allergy [95]. Furthermore, geographic variations in these different types of peanut allergy were reported by Vereda et al. [94]. When comparing clinical and immunologic features of peanut-allergic patients from the United States, Spain, and Sweden, Americans most frequently had IgE to the major peanut allergens (Ara h 1–3), whereas Spanish subjects were more often sensitized to LTP (Ara h 9), and Swedish patients had the highest sensitization rate to the Bet v 1 homolog (Ara h 8). These immunologic variations were associated with differing clinical features of peanut allergy. Similarly for hazelnut, Cor a 8 (LTP) and Cor a 9 (11S globulin) are involved in the more severe type of allergy, and Cor a 9 shares structural homology with other allergenic tree nuts [96]. In contrast, the pollen-related allergy to hazelnut is due to Cor a 1 (Bet v 1 homolog). With increased knowledge of the responsible allergens and the ability to identify these relevant allergens using component-resolved diagnosis, we may improve our ability to standardize the diagnosis of OAS, better assess risk of severe reactions, and allow more informed management of our patients.

Immunotherapy

Since immunotherapy is an effective treatment for allergic rhinitis and OAS is due to cross-reactivity with pollens, pollen immunotherapy would seem to be a logical treatment for OAS. Several studies have examined the efficacy of pollen immunotherapy with varying results. A study of birch immunotherapy for apple allergy in adults found a reduction in oral symptoms in 79% and decreased skin test sizes in 86%, but an increase in apple-specific IgE was observed in 43% [97]. This study was limited by lack of objective outcomes and placebo controls. Another study of birch subcutaneous immunotherapy (SCIT) found decreased symptoms (based on double-blind, placebo-controlled food challenges) and SPT in the treated group, but there was no placebo SCIT group for comparison [98]. Instead, the comparison was made with a group who used medication for symptomatic treatment. Researchers in Spain examined the effect of SCIT on plane tree pollen-associated allergy to plant foods (i.e., hazelnut, walnut, lettuce, peach, and cherry) [99]. In this open label study, 16 patients underwent 1 year of plane tree pollen SCIT, and open food challenges were performed before and after SCIT. Treatment with SCIT resulted in significant improvements in 55%, accompanied by a decrease in sIgE and increase in food-specific IgG_4.

In contrast, a pediatric study from Sweden indicated no beneficial effect of birch SCIT or oral immunotherapy for food-allergic symptoms [100]. A study of birch pollen sublingual immunotherapy found that although significant improvements in nasal provocation scores were seen in some subjects, apple-induced OAS was not significantly reduced [101]. A more recent study comparing SCIT and sublingual immunotherapy (SLIT) for birch-related apple allergy also noted minimal effects with SLIT [102].

Immunotherapy with recombinant allergens is another approach that has been explored. In one study, 44 patients received one preseasonal treatment of SCIT using a mixture of Bet v 1 fragments, a hypoallergenic Bet v 1-trimer, or aluminum hydroxide alone (placebo) [103]. Symptom improvement was seen in 28% of subjects on active treatment compared to only 5% of placebo-treated subjects.

Immunotherapy with specific food allergens has also been explored. In a study using apple oral immunotherapy, 63% of subjects on active treatment were able to tolerate at least 128 g of apple after 8 months of treatment as compared to 0/13 controls [104]. This effect was due to short-term desensitization rather than induction of oral tolerance as relapse of the allergy occurred in two subjects after their apple consumption was discontinued.

While immunotherapy is sparking tremendous interest for the treatment of food allergy, results to date are inconsistent for OAS, likely owing to study design variations regarding allergens, dosing, and duration of treatment. Furthermore, difficulties in objective evaluations for improvement in symptoms of OAS as well as seasonal and geographic variations in symptom severity and occurrence complicate comparisons between studies. Thus, immunotherapy remains an unproven therapeutic approach for OAS.

T-cell cross-reactivity

PR-10 proteins have been shown to have cross-reactivity at the T-cell level [24, 25]. Reekers et al. [105] reported that some patients with hypersensitivity to birch pollen and atopic dermatitis developed worsening of their skin symptoms after oral challenge with birch pollen-related foods. The authors also found birch pollen-specific T-cell responses in the skin lesions of these patients. The carboxy-terminal end of Bet v 1 (142–156) has been identified as an immunodominant T-cell epitope in many patients with birch–fruit–vegetable syndrome [106]. Bet v 1 (142–156)-specific T-cell clones cross-reacted with Rosaceae fruit allergens in apple and cherry, but less cross-reactivity occurred with vegetables of the Apiaceae family, celery and carrot. Interestingly, celery and carrot allergens were more potent activators of the T-cell clones than apple and peach allergens.

A recent study showed that in patients who have birch pollen allergy and atopic dermatitis, worsening of skin lesions without oral symptoms can be observed when eating cooked fruits and vegetables (i.e., apple, carrot, and celery) [107]. These authors suggest that eating birch-related fruits and vegetables outside the birch season can lead to pollen-specific T-cell activation (high IL-4 and thus elevated IgE) and maintenance of the allergic immune response perennially. This raises the question of whether patients should continue to consume the related plant food products outside of the pollen season despite lack of immediate symptoms.

Conclusions

OAS is a continually expanding entity as more allergens and cross-reactivities are identified and characterized, thus making diagnosis and management more challenging. The common unifier to these cross-reactivity syndromes is the presence of a plant-derived food allergy, which can often be attributed to homologous plant proteins. With increased knowledge of relevant allergens, improved diagnostic tools and effective treatments may be possible.

References

1. Tuft L, Blumstein GI. Studies in food allergy. II. Sensitization in fresh fruits: clinical and experimental observations. *J Allergy* 1942; 13:574–581.
2. Anderson LB Jr, Dreyfuss EM, Logan J, et al. Melon and banana sensitivity coincident with ragweed pollinosis. *J Allergy* 1970; 45:310–319.
3. Hannuksela M, Lahti A. Immediate reactions to fruits and vegetables. *Contact Dermatitis* 1977; 3:79–84.
4. Wuthrich B, Hofer T. Food allergy: the celery-mugwort-spice syndrome. Association with mango allergy? *Dtsch Med Wochenschr* 1984; 109:981–986.
5. Amlot PL, Kemeny DM, Zachary C, et al. Oral allergy syndrome (OAS): symptoms of IgE-mediated hypersensitivity to foods. *Clin Allergy* 1987; 17:33–42.
6. Castillo R, Delgado J, Quiralte J, et al. Food hypersensitivity among adult patients: epidemiological and clinical aspects. *Allergol Immunopathol (Madr)* 1996; 24:93–97.
7. Mattila L, Kilpelainen M, Terho EO, et al. Food hypersensitivity among Finnish university students: association with atopic diseases. *Clin Exp Allergy* 2003; 33:600–606.
8. Osterballe M, Hansen TK, Mortz CG, et al. The clinical relevance of sensitization to pollen-related fruits and vegetables in unselected pollen-sensitized adults. *Allergy* 2005; 60:218–225.
9. Bircher AJ, Van Melle G, Haller E, et al. IgE to food allergens are highly prevalent in patients allergic to pollens, with and without symptoms of food allergy. *Clin Exp Allergy* 1994; 24:367–374.
10. Eriksson NE, Formgren H, Svenonius E. Food hypersensitivity in patients with pollen allergy. *Allergy* 1982; 37:437–443.
11. Geroldinger-Simic M, Zelniker T, Aberer W, et al. Birch pollen-related food allergy: clinical aspects and the role of allergen-specific IgE and IgG_4 antibodies. *J Allergy Clin Immunol* 2011; 127:616–622.
12. Ricci G, Righetti F, Menna G, et al. Relationship between bet v 1 and bet v 2 specific IgE and food allergy in children with grass pollen respiratory allergy. *Mol Immunol* 2005; 42:1251–1257.
13. Ghunaim N, Gronlund H, Kronqvist M, et al. Antibody profiles and self-reported symptoms to pollen-related food allergens in grass pollen-allergic patients from northern Europe. *Allergy* 2005; 60:185–191.
14. Cuesta-Herranz J, Lazaro M, Martinez A, et al. Pollen allergy in peach-allergic patients: sensitization and cross-reactivity to taxonomically unrelated pollens. *J Allergy Clin Immunol* 1999; 104:688–694.
15. Pastorello EA, Ortolani C. Oral allergy syndrome. In: Metcalfe DD, Sampson HA, Simon RA (eds), *Food Allergy: Adverse*

Reactions to Foods and Food Additives, 3rd edn. Massachusetts: Blackwell Publishing, 2003; pp. 169–182.

16. Fernandez-Rivas M, van Ree R, Cuevas M. Allergy to Rosaceae fruits without related pollinosis. *J Allergy Clin Immunol* 1997; 100:728–733.
17. Bublin M, Mari A, Ebner C, et al. IgE sensitization profiles toward green and gold kiwifruits differ among patients allergic to kiwifruit from 3 European countries. *J Allergy Clin Immunol* 2004; 114:1169–1175.
18. van Ree R. Clinical importance of cross-reactivity in food allergy. *Curr Opin Allergy Clin Immunol* 2004; 4:235–240.
19. Ortolani C, Ispano M, Pastorello E, et al. The oral allergy syndrome. *Ann Allergy* 1988; 61:47–52.
20. Valenta R, Kraft D. Type 1 allergic reactions to plant-derived food: a consequence of primary sensitization to pollen allergens. *J Allergy Clin Immunol* 1996; 97:893–895.
21. Ortolani C, Pastorello EA, Farioli L, et al. IgE-mediated allergy from vegetable allergens. *Ann Allergy* 1993; 71(5):470–476.
22. Egger M, Mutschlechner S, Wopfner N, et al. Pollen-food syndromes associated with weed pollinosis: an update from the molecular point of view. *Allergy* 2006; 61:461–476.
23. Yagami T, Haishima Y, Nakamura A, et al. Digestibility of allergens extracted from natural rubber latex and vegetable foods. *J Allergy Clin Immunol* 2000; 106:752–762.
24. Bohle B, Radakovics A, Jahn-Schmid B, et al. Bet v 1, the major birch pollen allergen, initiates sensitization to api g 1, the major allergen in celery: evidence at the T cell level. *Eur J Immunol.* 2003;33:3303–3310.
25. Fritsch R, Bohle B, Vollmann U, et al. Bet v 1, the major birch pollen allergen, and mal d 1, the major apple allergen, cross-react at the level of allergen-specific T helper cells. *J Allergy Clin Immunol* 1998; 102:679–686.
26. Breiteneder H, Ebner C. Molecular and biochemical classification of plant-derived food allergens. *J Allergy Clin Immunol* 2000; 106:27–36.
27. Hoffmann-Sommergruber K. Plant allergens and pathogenesis-related proteins. What do they have in common? *Int Arch Allergy Immunol* 2000; 122:155–166.
28. Pastorello EA, Vieths S, Pravettoni V, et al. Identification of hazelnut major allergens in sensitive patients with positive double-blind, placebo-controlled food challenge results. *J Allergy Clin Immunol* 2002; 109:563–570.
29. Mittag D, Akkerdaas J, Ballmer-Weber BK, et al. Ara h 8, a bet v 1-homologous allergen from peanut, is a major allergen in patients with combined birch pollen and peanut allergy. *J Allergy Clin Immunol* 2004; 114:1410–1417.
30. Pastorello EA, Pompei C, Pravettoni V, et al. Lipid-transfer protein is the major maize allergen maintaining IgE-binding activity after cooking at 100 degrees C, as demonstrated in anaphylactic patients and patients with positive double-blind, placebo-controlled food challenge results. *J Allergy Clin Immunol* 2003; 112:775–783.
31. Molina A, Segura A, Garcia-Olmedo F. Lipid transfer proteins (nsLTPs) from barley and maize leaves are potent inhibitors of bacterial and fungal plant pathogens. *FEBS Lett* 1993; 316:119–122.
32. Pastorello EA, Farioli L, Pravettoni V, et al. The major allergen of peach (*Prunus persica*) is a lipid transfer protein. *J Allergy Clin Immunol* 1999; 103:520–526.
33. Sanchez-Monge R, Lombardero M, Garcia-Selles FJ, et al. Lipid-transfer proteins are relevant allergens in fruit allergy. *J Allergy Clin Immunol* 1999; 103:514–519.
34. Pastorello EA, D'Ambrosio FP, Pravettoni V, et al. Evidence for a lipid transfer protein as the major allergen of apricot. *J Allergy Clin Immunol* 2000; 105:371–377.
35. Pastorello EA, Farioli L, Pravettoni V, et al. Characterization of the major allergen of plum as a lipid transfer protein. *J Chromatogr B Biomed Sci Appl* 2001; 756:95–103.
36. Scheurer S, Pastorello EA, Wangorsch A, et al. Recombinant allergens Pru av 1 and Pru av 4 and a newly identified lipid transfer protein in the in vitro diagnosis of cherry allergy. *J Allergy Clin Immunol* 2001; 107:724–731.
37. Krause S, Reese G, Randow S, et al. Lipid transfer protein (Ara h 9) as a new peanut allergen relevant for a Mediterranean allergic population. *J Allergy Clin Immunol* 2009; 124:771–778.
38. Pastorello EA, Farioli L, Pravettoni V, et al. The maize major allergen, which is responsible for food-induced allergic reactions, is a lipid transfer protein. *J Allergy Clin Immunol* 2000; 106:744–751.
39. Breiteneder H, Radauer C. A classification of plant food allergens. *J Allergy Clin Immunol* 2004; 113:821–830.
40. Valenta R, Duchene M, Pettenburger K, et al. Identification of profilin as a novel pollen allergen; IgE autoreactivity in sensitized individuals. *Science* 1991; 253:557–560.
41. Diez-Gomez ML, Quirce S, Cuevas M, et al. Fruit-pollen-latex cross-reactivity: implication of profilin (bet v 2). *Allergy* 1999; 54:951–961.
42. Wensing M, Akkerdaas JH, van Leeuwen WA, et al. IgE to bet v 1 and profilin: cross-reactivity patterns and clinical relevance. *J Allergy Clin Immunol* 2002; 110:435–442.
43. Pauli G, Oster JP, Deviller P, et al. Skin testing with recombinant allergens rBet v 1 and birch profilin, rBet v 2: diagnostic value for birch pollen and associated allergies. *J Allergy Clin Immunol* 1996; 97:1100–1109.
44. Ebo DG, Hagendorens MM, Bridts CH, et al. Sensitization to cross-reactive carbohydrate determinants and the ubiquitous protein profilin: mimickers of allergy. *Clin Exp Allergy* 2004; 34:137–144.
45. Mari A. Multiple pollen sensitization: a molecular approach to the diagnosis. *Int Arch Allergy Immunol* 2001; 125: 57–65.
46. Ballmer-Weber BK, Hoffmann A, Wuthrich B, et al. Influence of food processing on the allergenicity of celery: DBPCFC with celery spice and cooked celery in patients with celery allergy. *Allergy* 2002; 57:228–235.
47. Foetisch K, Westphal S, Lauer I, et al. Biological activity of IgE specific for cross-reactive carbohydrate determinants. *J Allergy Clin Immunol* 2003; 111:889–896.
48. Breiteneder H, Pettenburger K, Bito A, et al. The gene coding for the major birch pollen allergen Betv1, is highly homologous to a pea disease resistance response gene. *EMBO J* 1989; 8:1935–1938.

49. Ebner C, Birkner T, Valenta R, et al. Common epitopes of birch pollen and apples—studies by western and northern blot. *J Allergy Clin Immunol* 1991; 88:588–594.
50. Mittag D, Vieths S, Vogel L, et al. Soybean allergy in patients allergic to birch pollen: clinical investigation and molecular characterization of allergens. *J Allergy Clin Immunol* 2004; 113:148–154.
51. Wuthrich B, Stager J, Johansson SG. Celery allergy associated with birch and mugwort pollinosis. *Allergy* 1990; 45:566–571.
52. Hoffmann-Sommergruber K, Demoly P, Crameri R, et al. IgE reactivity to api g 1, a major celery allergen, in a central European population is based on primary sensitization by Bet v 1. *J Allergy Clin Immunol* 1999; 104:478–484.
53. Scholl I, Jensen-Jarolim E. Allergenic potency of spices: hot, medium hot, or very hot. *Int Arch Allergy Immunol* 2004; 135:247–261.
54. Figueroa J, Blanco C, Dumpierrez AG, et al. Mustard allergy confirmed by double-blind placebo-controlled food challenges: clinical features and cross-reactivity with mugwort pollen and plant-derived foods. *Allergy* 2005; 60:48–55.
55. Enberg RN, Leickly FE, McCullough J, et al. Watermelon and ragweed share allergens. *J Allergy Clin Immunol* 1987; 79:867–875.
56. Cuesta-Herranz J, Lazaro M, Figueredo E, et al. Allergy to plant-derived fresh foods in a birch- and ragweed-free area. *Clin Exp Allergy* 2000; 30:1411–1416.
57. Grob M, Reindl J, Vieths S, et al. Heterogeneity of banana allergy: characterization of allergens in banana-allergic patients. *Ann Allergy Asthma Immunol* 2002; 89: 513–516.
58. Rodriguez-Perez R, Crespo JF, Rodriguez J, et al. Profilin is a relevant melon allergen susceptible to pepsin digestion in patients with oral allergy syndrome. *J Allergy Clin Immunol* 2003; 111:634–639.
59. Figueredo E, Cuesta-Herranz J, De-Miguel J, et al. Clinical characteristics of melon (*Cucumis melo*) allergy. *Ann Allergy Asthma Immunol* 2003; 91:303–308.
60. Rodriguez J, Crespo JF, Burks W, et al. Randomized, double-blind, crossover challenge study in 53 subjects reporting adverse reactions to melon (*Cucumis melo*). *J Allergy Clin Immunol* 2000; 106:968–972.
61. Lombardero M, Garcia-Selles FJ, Polo F, et al. Prevalence of sensitization to artemisia allergens art v 1, art v 3 and art v 60 kDa. Cross-reactivity among art v 3 and other relevant lipid-transfer protein allergens. *Clin Exp Allergy* 2004; 34:1415–1421.
62. Hernandez J, Garcia Selles FJ, Pagan JA, et al. Immediate hypersensitivity to fruits and vegetables and pollenosis. *Allergol Immunopathol (Madr)* 1985; 13:197–211.
63. Fernandez-Rivas M, Bolhaar S, Gonzalez-Mancebo E, et al. Apple allergy across Europe: how allergen sensitization profiles determine the clinical expression of allergies to plant foods. *J Allergy Clin Immunol* 2006; 118:481–488.
64. Scheurer S, Lauer I, Foetisch K, et al. Strong allergenicity of pru av 3, the lipid transfer protein from cherry, is related to high stability against thermal processing and digestion. *J Allergy Clin Immunol* 2004; 114:900–907.
65. M'Raihi L, Charpin D, Pons A, et al. Cross-reactivity between latex and banana. *J Allergy Clin Immunol* 1991; 87:129–130.
66. Blanco C, Carrillo T, Castillo R, et al. Latex allergy: clinical features and cross-reactivity with fruits. *Ann Allergy* 1994; 73:309–314.
67. Beezhold DH, Sussman GL, Liss GM, et al. Latex allergy can induce clinical reactions to specific foods. *Clin Exp Allergy* 1996; 26:416–422.
68. Ebo DG, Bridts CH, Hagendorens MM, et al. The prevalence and diagnostic value of specific IgE antibodies to inhalant, animal and plant food, and ficus allergens in patients with natural rubber latex allergy. *Acta Clin Belg* 2003; 58: 183–189.
69. Brehler R, Theissen U, Mohr C, et al. "Latex-fruit syndrome": frequency of cross-reacting IgE antibodies. *Allergy* 1997; 52:404–410.
70. Tucke J, Posch A, Baur X, et al. Latex type I sensitization and allergy in children with atopic dermatitis. Evaluation of cross-reactivity to some foods. *Pediatr Allergy Immunol* 1999; 10:160–167.
71. Blanco C, Diaz-Perales A, Collada C, et al. Class I chitinases as potential panallergens involved in the latex-fruit syndrome. *J Allergy Clin Immunol* 1999; 103:507–513.
72. Wagner S, Breiteneder H. The latex-fruit syndrome. *Biochem Soc Trans* 2002; 30:935–940.
73. Wagner S, Radauer C, Hafner C, et al. Characterization of cross-reactive bell pepper allergens involved in the latex-fruit syndrome. *Clin Exp Allergy* 2004; 34:1739–1746.
74. Reindl J, Rihs HP, Scheurer S, et al. IgE reactivity to profilin in pollen-sensitized subjects with adverse reactions to banana and pineapple. *Int Arch Allergy Immunol* 2002; 128:105–114.
75. Yagami T. Allergies to cross-reactive plant proteins. Latex-fruit syndrome is comparable with pollen-food allergy syndrome. *Int Arch Allergy Immunol* 2002; 128:271–279.
76. Diaz-Perales A, Blanco C, Sanchez-Monge R, et al. Analysis of avocado allergen (Prs a 1) IgE-binding peptides generated by simulated gastric fluid digestion. *J Allergy Clin Immunol* 2003; 112:1002–1007.
77. Blanco C, Sanchez-Garcia F, Torres-Galvan MJ, et al. Genetic basis of the latex-fruit syndrome: association with HLA class II alleles in a Spanish population. *J Allergy Clin Immunol* 2004; 114:1070–1076.
78. Ortolani C, Ispano M, Pastorello EA, et al. Comparison of results of skin prick tests (with fresh foods and commercial food extracts) and RAST in 100 patients with oral allergy syndrome. *J Allergy Clin Immunol* 1989; 83:683–690.
79. Osterballe M, Scheller R, Stahl Skov P, et al. Diagnostic value of scratch-chamber test, skin prick test, histamine release and specific IgE in birch-allergic patients with oral allergy syndrome to apple. *Allergy* 2003; 58:950–953.
80. Anhoej C, Backer V, Nolte H. Diagnostic evaluation of grass- and birch-allergic patients with oral allergy syndrome. *Allergy* 2001; 56:548–552.
81. Begin P, Des Roches A, Nguyen M, et al. Freezing does not alter antigenic properties of fresh fruits for skin testing in patients with birch tree pollen-induced oral allergy syndrome. *J Allergy Clin Immunol* 2011; 127:1624–1626.

82. Clendennen SK, May GD. Differential gene expression in ripening banana fruit. *Plant Physiol* 1997; 115:463–469.
83. Brenna OV, Pastorello EA, Farioli L, et al. Presence of allergenic proteins in different peach (*Prunus persica*) cultivars and dependence of their content on fruit ripening. *J Agric Food Chem* 2004; 52:7997–8000.
84. Bolhaar ST, van de Weg WE, van Ree R, et al. In vivo assessment with prick-to-prick testing and double-blind, placebo-controlled food challenge of allergenicity of apple cultivars. *J Allergy Clin Immunol* 2005; 116:1080–1086.
85. Carnes J, Ferrer A, Fernandez-Caldas E. Allergenicity of 10 different apple varieties. *Ann Allergy Asthma Immunol* 2006; 96:564–570.
86. Vlieg-Boerstra BJ, van de Weg WE, van der Heide S, et al. Identification of low allergenic apple cultivars using skin prick tests and oral food challenges. *Allergy* 2010; 66:491–498.
87. Rodriguez J, Crespo JF, Burks W, et al. Randomized, double-blind, crossover challenge study in 53 subjects reporting adverse reactions to melon (*Cucumis melo*). *J Allergy Clin Immunol* 2000; 106:968–972.
88. Ma S, Sicherer SH, Nowak-Wegrzyn A. A survey on the management of pollen-food allergy syndrome in allergy practices. *J Allergy Clin Immunol* 2003; 112:784–788.
89. Pastorello EA, Ortolani C, Farioli L, et al. Allergenic cross-reactivity among peach, apricot, plum, and cherry in patients with oral allergy syndrome: an in vivo and in vitro study. *J Allergy Clin Immunol* 1994; 94:699–707.
90. Rodriguez J, Crespo JF, Lopez-Rubio A, et al. Clinical cross-reactivity among foods of the Rosaceae family. *J Allergy Clin Immunol* 2000; 106:183–189.
91. Crespo JF, Rodriguez J, James JM, et al. Reactivity to potential cross-reactive foods in fruit-allergic patients: implications for prescribing food avoidance. *Allergy* 2002; 57: 946–949.
92. Asero R. Detection and clinical characterization of patients with oral allergy syndrome caused by stable allergens in Rosaceae and nuts. *Ann Allergy Asthma Immunol* 1999; 83:377–383.
93. Mari A, Ballmer-Weber BK, Vieths S. The oral allergy syndrome: improved diagnostic and treatment methods. *Curr Opin Allergy Clin Immunol* 2005; 5:267–273.
94. Vereda A, van Hage M, Ahlstedt S, et al. Peanut allergy: clinical and immunologic differences among patients from 3 different geographic regions. *J Allergy Clin Immunol* 2011; 127:603–607.
95. Nicolaou N, Poorafshar M, Murray C, et al. Allergy or tolerance in children sensitized to peanut: prevalence and differentiation using component-resolved diagnostics. *J Allergy Clin Immunol* 2010; 125:191–197.
96. Flinterman AE, Akkerdaas JH, Knulst AC, et al. Hazelnut allergy: from pollen-associated mild allergy to severe anaphylactic reactions. *Curr Opin Allergy Clin Immunol* 2008; 8:261–265.
97. Asero R. Effects of birch pollen-specific immunotherapy on apple allergy in birch pollen-hypersensitive patients. *Clin Exp Allergy* 1998; 28:1368–1373.
98. Bolhaar ST, Tiemessen MM, Zuidmeer L, et al. Efficacy of birch-pollen immunotherapy on cross-reactive food allergy confirmed by skin tests and double-blind food challenges. *Clin Exp Allergy* 2004; 34:761–769.
99. Alonso R, Enrique E, Pineda F, et al. An observational study on outgrowing food allergy during non-birch pollen-specific, subcutaneous immunotherapy. *Int Arch Allergy Immunol* 2007; 143:185–189.
100. Moller C. Effect of pollen immunotherapy on food hypersensitivity in children with birch pollinosis. *Ann Allergy* 1989; 62:343–345.
101. Kinaciyan T, Jahn-Schmid B, Radakovics A, et al. Successful sublingual immunotherapy with birch pollen has limited effects on concomitant food allergy to apple and the immune response to the Bet v 1 homolog Mal d 1. *J Allergy Clin Immunol* 2007; 119:937–943.
102. Mauro M, Russello M, Incorvaia C, et al. Birch-apple syndrome treated with birch pollen immunotherapy. *Int Arch Allergy Immunol* 2011; 156:416–422.
103. Niederberger V, Reisinger J, Valent P, et al. Vaccination with genetically modified birch pollen allergens: immune and clinical effects on oral allergy syndrome. *J Allergy Clin Immunol* 2007; 119:1013–1016.
104. Kopac P, Rudin M, Gentinetta T, et al. Continuous apple consumption induces oral tolerance in birch-pollen-associated apple allergy. *Allergy* 2012; 67:280–285.
105. Reekers R, Busche M, Wittmann M, et al. Birch pollen-related foods trigger atopic dermatitis in patients with specific cutaneous T-cell responses to birch pollen antigens. *J Allergy Clin Immunol* 1999; 104:466–472.
106. Jahn-Schmid B, Radakovics A, Luttkopf D, et al. Bet v 1142-156 is the dominant T-cell epitope of the major birch pollen allergen and important for cross-reactivity with bet v 1-related food allergens. *J Allergy Clin Immunol* 2005; 116:213–219.
107. Bohle B, Zwolfer B, Heratizadeh A, et al. Cooking birch pollen-related food: divergent consequences for IgE- and T cell-mediated reactivity in vitro and in vivo. *J Allergy Clin Immunol* 2006; 118:242–249.

13 The Respiratory Tract and Food Hypersensitivity

Graham Roberts

Department of Paediatric Allergy and Respiratory Medicine, University Hospital Southampton NHS Foundation Trust, Southampton, UK

Key Concepts

- Food hypersensitivity in early life is a known risk factor for the development of later asthma.
- Food hypersensitivity and asthma frequently coexist.
- Chronic aerosolized exposure can lead to the development of asthma, as in Baker's asthma.
- Coexistent asthma is associated with anaphylaxis.
- Coexistent food hypersensitivity increases the risk of life-threatening exacerbation of asthma.

Introduction

The coassociation of food hypersensitivity and respiratory tract problems has become much more appreciated in the last decade [1, 2]. Food hypersensitivity and asthma are both allergic diseases and therefore frequently coexist. Respiratory tract symptoms and signs are frequently part of food hypersensitivity reactions and it is now recognized that foods can, particularly in the aerosolized form, precipitate exacerbations of asthma. Additionally, the presence of asthma is associated with a greater risk of morbidity and mortality from food hypersensitivity, while there are also data suggesting that the presence of food hypersensitivity increases the chances of life-threatening exacerbation of asthma. Finally, food hypersensitivity in early life is a known risk factor to the development of later asthma, although it is unclear whether there is a causal link or they are associated because of shared genetic and environmental predispositions. The currently available asthma guidelines say very little about food allergy [3–6]. It is important that clinicians are aware of the link between food hypersensitivity and respiratory tract problems and it is this that this chapter will focus on.

Epidemiology

Asthma

Asthma is defined as reversible airway obstruction due to airway inflammation and bronchial hyperresponsiveness [6]. Symptoms of wheeze, chest tightness, and shortness of breath are elicited by stereotypic precipitants such as exercise, cold air, and specific allergens or irritants. Typically symptoms are reversed within minutes of the use of a bronchodilator. While the prevalence of asthma was increasing, it has been relatively stable over the last decade at around one in seven of the population in developed countries [7]. While most children, teenagers, and adults have mild to moderate asthma that is readily controllable with appropriate treatment, a minority have problematic asthma leading to more morbidity and mortality [8]. It is being increasingly recognized that there is more than one phenotype of asthma. Preschool children tend to have a phenotype that is associated with viral-induced exacerbations; they are often nonatopic and under these circumstances frequently outgrow their symptoms by the time they get to school. Atopic children with asthma tend to develop symptoms early on in life which are much more persistent. There are several more adult-related phenotypes, in particular, one associated with obesity. Although the literature is not clear, it would seem that food allergy is associated with early-onset atopic asthma.

Food Allergy: Adverse Reactions to Foods and Food Additives, Fifth Edition. Edited by Dean D Metcalfe, Hugh A Sampson, Ronald A Simon and Gideon Lack.

Food hypersensitivity

It is thought that food hypersensitivity has increased in prevalence over the last couple of decades [9] and now affects 1 in 20 young children and approximately 1 in 50 adults [10]. There is a perception that food allergy is much more frequent, but many symptoms that people associate with food allergy do not have an immunological basis. Food hypersensitivity can be divided into two broad groups of immune reactions, those that are IgE mediated and those that are non-IgE mediated [11]. The IgE-mediated reactions are characterized by symptoms that start within 1–2 hours of contact with the allergen, some patients may also experience late phase reaction 4–8 hours later. Non-IgE-mediated reactions are characterized by delayed onset with symptoms starting 4–48 hours after contact, often involving the gastrointestinal tract or the skin.

Respiratory presentations of food allergy

Upper respiratory tract

Recurrent or chronic rhinitis

Symptoms of rhinitis are an underrecognized but common manifestation of food hypersensitivity reactions. For example, in one series of children undergoing double-blind, placebo-controlled food challenges, two-thirds developed rhinitis during the challenge [12]. Usually rhinitis occurs in association with other clinical manifestations, such as urticaria, angioedema, nausea, vomiting, or abdominal pain. Generally, the connection between the food and the symptoms is obvious and so food hypersensitivity seems not to be a frequent cause of chronic rhinitis symptoms. Many parents connect their child's symptoms of blocked nasal passages and nasal discharge to food, particularly cow's milk, but this link has never been proven.

Recurrent or chronic otitis media

Serious otitis media has a number of etiologies of which the most usual is a recurrent viral upper respiratory tract infection often in association with eustachian tube dysfunction. Allergic airway inflammation may cause additional eustachian tube dysfunction increasing the risk and severity of otitis media effusion. The potential role of food allergy in inducing recurrent otitis media has been examined, but the data are currently not conclusive [13].

Lower respiratory tract

Lower respiratory tract symptoms and signs occur less frequently than cutaneous upper respiratory tract or gastrointestinal problems in food challenges. In one series of double-blind, placebo-controlled food challenges, one in six of the positive challenges was characterized by lower respiratory tract symptoms [12]. Usually, these lower respiratory tract symptoms are associated with other manifestations of acute allergic reactions, such as urticaria, angioedema, rhinoconjunctivitis, nausea, and vomiting.

Any lower respiratory tract symptoms related to food hypersensitivity would satisfy the criteria for anaphylaxis [14]. Where the symptoms and signs are more localized to the respiratory tract, there may be some debate as to whether a presentation is one of acute asthma or anaphylaxis. This has the potential to lead to confusion and suboptimal therapy. Such a presentation ought to be labeled anaphylaxis and managed using an anaphylaxis protocol with the use of intra-muscular adrenaline with inhaled bronchodilators as an adjunct.

The development of lower respiratory tract symptoms at food challenge may actually underrepresent the number of patients who have respiratory reactions to a food allergen. In one series with adolescents and young adults with asthma and food allergy, about half developed lower respiratory tract symptoms of cough, laryngeal reactions, or wheeze. Only half developed a reduced FEV_1, although all had increased bronchial hyperresponsiveness several hours after the challenge [15]. It, therefore, seems that food allergens can induce significant bronchial hyperresponsiveness without any impaired pulmonary function; this though may lead patients to be at risk of an exacerbation of their asthma over the subsequent weeks if they come into contact with another trigger for their asthma.

Allergens

Any food can theoretically precipitate a hypersensitivity reaction, although some do this more commonly than others. Typical food allergens are peanuts, tree nuts, milk, egg, fish, and shellfish (Box 13.1). These have been demonstrated to cause food hypersensitivity reactions within double-blind, placebo-controlled, food challenge testing [16, 17]. Some food allergens seem to be more prone to precipitating respiratory tract symptoms. For example, respiratory reactions were reported in half of those responding to one survey if they had a peanut or tree nut allergy [18] and the presence of asthma was a risk factor for these patients to have a more severe reaction. Some foods become readily aerosolized and these have been documented to cause reactions by inhalation route. These include poppy seeds [19], carrot [20], sunflower seeds [21], lupin [22], and soya bean [23].

Box 13.1 Common food allergens implicated in respiratory reactions

All respiratory reactions	Severe reactions (anaphylaxis)
Hens' egg	Peanuts
Cows' milk	Tree nuts
Peanuts	Shellfish
Tree nuts	
Fish	
Shellfish	

Many patients with asthma report that food additives worsen their respiratory symptoms, including monosodium glutamate, sulfites, and aspartame [24]. But double-blind, placebo-controlled trials with additives have failed to demonstrate a reaction in more than 1 in 20 patients [25–27]. About a third of subjects do experience adverse reactions with monosodium glutamate, but these seem to be restricted to headaches, muscle tightening, numbness, weakness, and flushing.

Routes of exposure

Oral ingestion

Oral ingestion is the route of exposure that one normally associates with food allergens. A number of authors have published data looking at hypersensitivity reactions within a controlled trial setting. For example, in a series of more than 700 patients with food hypersensitivity, bronchospasm developed in around 10% of children [17]. These studies involve a series of increasing doses of the potential allergy and a protocol that stops the challenge at the first objective symptom. As the initial signs are usually cutaneous, such as urticaria and edema, they are likely to underreport respiratory involvement. James et al. monitored 88 children with atopic dermatitis undergoing double-blind, placebo-controlled food challenges with spirometry [12]. Approximately 15% of them developed lower respiratory tract symptoms including wheeze, with half of them experiencing a 20% drop in their FEV_1.

Inhalation food allergens

The ability of aerosolized food to cause food hypersensitivity reactions is less appreciated. There are though many examples in the literature of respiratory reactions associated with aerosolized food proteins. Fish protein seems to be readily aerosolizable even without cooking and reactions are reported by patients within this context [28, 29]. Fish protein can be detected from air samples within, for example, a fish market [30]. The factors that determine how readily different foods become aerosolized have not been studied, although in general, boiling or steaming might be more likely to generate appreciable quantities of aerosolized protein. There have also been self-reports of allergic reactions to peanuts on commercial airlines [31]. In one report 0.4% of individuals reported a reaction to a peanut or tree nut by the inhalational exposure on a commercial airliner, although direct contact could not be ruled out. Peanut allergen has been detected in the filter system of commercial airlines [32]. Some commercial airlines now control what snacks are available in-flight. A number of other foods have additionally been implicated in causing allergic reactions by inhalational route; they include milk [33], green bean [34], lentils [35], buckwheat [36], egg [37], and seafood [38].

Occupational exposure to aerosolized foods is known to lead to the development of asthma in adult life. Perhaps 10% of adult asthma is related to occupational exposure [39]; an example is Baker's asthma [40]. Baker's asthma results from an occupational exposure to airborne cereal grain or amylase. Patients develop cough and wheeze with the likelihood of development of symptoms being related to the level of exposure [41, 42]. Affected workers have positive skin prick test to specific allergy to wheat proteins. Occupational exposure to aerosolized egg protein can give rise to similar symptoms in confectionery workers and egg processors [43, 44]. Other examples include soya, cocoa, garlic, and buckwheat [39]. It is intriguing that the majority of adults affected by food-induced occupational asthma can ingest the allergen without symptoms [40]. This may be due to the localized production of specific IgE in the respiratory mucosa [45]. Alternatively, food allergens may have become denatured before they reach the gastrointestinal tract [46].

Foods have also been found to behave as more general environmental aeroallergens beyond the work environment. A prime example is the epidemic of asthma seen in the 1970s and 1980s in Barcelona. Cases were clustered around the port area, with exacerbations sudden in onset and often causing very severe symptoms with fatalities being reported. A case–control approach was taken to investigate the cause, epidemics were found to be associated with days when soya was being unloaded at the port, and three quarters of cases had specific IgE to soya compared to less than half the controls [47]. Similar asthma epidemics have been related to aerosolized soya at Cartagena [48].

Control challenge data exploring the relationship between inhalational exposure and symptoms in children are very limited. There is one small series of 12 children who presented to allergy clinic with reported symptoms on inhalation exposure [49]. All had evidence of specific IgE to the suspected food allergen and had coexistent asthma. Implicated foods were fish, milk, chickpeas, buckwheat, or eggs. Nine of the children consented to a bronchial challenge and five developed objective signs of wheeze, plus lung function changes on bronchial food challenge. Two children also developed a late phase reaction. For these children, dietary avoidance alone was not sufficient and their asthma symptoms only improved when the families stopped cooking the foods in the house.

Given that the prevalence of asthma is around 1 in 15, and for food hypersensitivity is lower at 1–2%, the coexistence of asthma and food hypersensitivity in affected individuals, be they children or adults, is unexpectedly high. There are a number of possible reasons for this observation. It may result from common genetic or environmental risk factors, or the presence of one of these two diagnoses may make it more likely for a patient to go on to present with the other.

What is the link between the respiratory tract and food hypersensitivity?

Epidemiological associations

Many investigators have looked for evidence of food hypersensitivity in groups of patients who have asthma. For example, in a group of 500 children from a US inner city asthma cohort, nearly a half had evidence of IgE sensitization to at least one food with a fifth having levels at or above 50% of the positive predictive value for clinical reactivity for at least one food [50]. Sensitization though does not equate always with food hypersensitivity and there is a potential that this cohort was not representative of the general population of patients with asthma. In a Hong Kong study, investigators examined more than 200 children with asthma and a smaller group of match controls. Again, about half of the patients with asthma had positive specific IgE to food, compared to only a quarter of the controls, confirming the results of the US study [51] where investigators have used a population approach. In the United States, 8000 adult participants in the National Health and Nutrition Examination Survey had specific IgE measured to the common food allergens assessed [52]. Using age-specific IgE criteria to define food hypersensitivity, 2.5% were defined as having clinical food allergy. In the participants with reported asthma, probable food allergy was found to be 6.6% (odds ratio 2.8, 95% CI, 1.7–4.5). Figures for likely food hypersensitivity were 1.9% in those with asthma and 0.9% in those without asthma. Additionally, participants with likely allergy were far more likely to have required an emergency department visit because of their asthma in the past year (8.5% vs. 1.3%). In France, more than 6000 schoolchildren have been assessed for a range of atopic disease [53]. Around 2% reported symptoms of food hypersensitivity and most were sensitized. Around two-thirds of children with food allergy had current asthma compared to only 1 in 15 of the others. In a cross-sectional epidemiological adult study, more than 100 randomly selected young adults underwent skin prick testing to common food allergens. Around 1% had probable IgE-mediated food allergy. They were much more likely than others to have current asthma [54].

Food allergy as a risk factor for asthma

In childhood the expression of atopy progresses with age [55]. This so-called "allergic march" usually starts initially with eczema, and food allergies with allergic asthma and rhinitis appearing later in childhood. This clinical picture is mirrored in terms of sensitization, with infants being predominately sensitized to foods whereas school age children are predominately sensitized to aeroallergen [56]. Interestingly sensitization to foods, particularly egg, is predictive of development of asthma in childhood [57, 56] and adult life [58]. For example, in the German MAS birth cohort of more than 500 participants, children with long-lasting sensitization to food allergens, by serum-specific IgE, had a 5.5 times higher risk of developing asthma than children who were only transiently sensitized [56]. Within the Isle of Wight birth cohort, an association has been seen between infant egg allergy and later asthma with the association being even more apparent when the coexisting infant eczema was included [57]. There are two potential explanations for this temporal association: food allergy and asthma may both be manifestations of the same process seen at different points in the maturation of the child; alternatively sensitization or allergy to food allergens itself may have a causal role in the development of asthma. So sensitization and allergy to food allergens in early life seem to be predictive of the later development of asthma.

There is an intriguing association between filaggrin mutations, food hypersensitivity, and asthma which might shed further light on this area. Filaggrin is important in maintaining the skin barrier and there are several loss-of-function mutations in the gene encoding filaggrin which are strong genetic risk factors for eczema and coexisting asthma, although the protein is not expressed in the airway [59, 60]. In more than 800 individuals from the German MAS cohort, the association between three filaggrin mutations and asthma was examined. In infants with eczema and coexisting sensitization to food allergens, the filaggrin mutations perfectly predicted childhood asthma; filaggrin and early sensitization to food allergens interacted synergistically in this relationship [61]. This adds to the evidence that sensitization to food allergens is involved in the pathogenesis of childhood asthma.

Table 13.1 Studies assessing the relationship between coexisting asthma and allergic reactions to food.

References	Design	Association of allergic reactions to food with asthma
Uguz et al. [73]	Prospective questionnaire, allergy support group	Severe reactions: 26/30 (86%), $p < 0.008$
Jarvinen et al. [74]	Retrospective questionnaire, tertiary allergy clinic	Single versus multiple adrenaline: 43 (56%) versus 17 (94%), $p = 0.005$
Manivannan et al. [75]	Medical record review, population based	Single versus multiple adrenaline: none, $p = 0.17$
Simon et al. [76]	Retrospective questionnaire, allergy support group	Autoinjector used versus not: 214/428 (50%) versus 560/1377 (41%), $p = 0.001$
Rudders et al. [77]	Medical record review, emergency department based	Anaphylaxis versus not: 48 versus 31, $p = 0.008$

The pathogenesis of childhood asthma is still unclear although we are now recognizing that the airway epithelium and innate response to pathogens are likely to be key factors in the process [62]. The importance of allergen exposure was recognized much earlier [63]. Using animal models, the process can be examined. For example, aerosolized ovalbumin, without an adjuvant, results in IgE sensitization and increased methacholine airway responsiveness but no airway inflammation [64]. In mice sensitized to ovalbumin by intraperitoneal injection, chronic low dose-inhaled exposure to ovalbumin resulted in both bronchial hyperresponsiveness and airway inflammation [65]. More recent mouse models have also managed to mimic the airway remodeling seen in asthma with chronic exposure [66]. So it seems that, in a sensitized animal, exposure-aerosolized food allergen can lead to the development of asthma. This mirrors the experience with occupational asthma, for example, Baker's asthma. Interestingly, young infants with food allergen sensitization have altered airway function [67].

Asthma as a risk factor for anaphylaxis

Asthma is a common factor in fatal or near fatal anaphylaxis. In the published series, about 90% of cases had coexisting asthma [68–71, 72]. Uncontrolled asthma seemed to be a common factor in these cases. A similar association is seen with less severe anaphylactic reactions (Table 13.1). For example, of 1094 clinic patients with peanut or tree nut allergy, a third had had lower respiratory symptoms with reactions, with the odds ratio for these being 2.7 (95% CI 1.7–4.2) and 6.8 (4.1–11.3) for mild and moderate-to-severe asthma, respectively [78]. Using data from a UK general practice database, it has been found that mild-to-moderate asthma is associated with an increased risk of anaphylaxis (relative risk 2.07, 95% CI, 1.65–2.60) with severe asthma being associated with an even greater risk (3.29, 2.47–3.47) [79]. Patients with coexisting allergic rhinitis or atopic dermatitis and those using antihistamines, oral steroids, or antibiotics were particularly at risk of experiencing anaphylaxis. This leads to the question of why coexisting asthma is a risk factor for anaphylaxis; is it merely identifying patients with severe food hypersensitivity, or do the pathological features of the asthmatic airway mean that a patient experiencing an allergic reaction is more likely to develop lower airway problems?

Food hypersensitivity as a risk factor for severe exacerbations of asthma

While most children with asthma have relatively mild disease, a minority have severe disease with life-threatening exacerbations despite modern pharmacotherapy [80, 81]. A number of risk factors have been identified for severe exacerbations of asthma [82], including coexisting food hypersensitivity [1, 83, 84]. For example, in a case–control study on life-threatening asthma in children, 10 out of 19 children with life-threatening asthma (53%) had food hypersensitivity compared to 4 out of 38 (11%) of controls (adjusted odds ratio 5.9, 95% CI 1.1–33) [85]. Food hypersensitivity has also been found to be a risk factor for any hospitalization with asthma in children and adults [86, 87]. This has important implications for asthma management as 4–8% of patients with asthma have coexisting food hypersensitivity [85].

Managing a patient presenting with food-induced respiratory symptom

Medical history

A comprehensive medical history should be obtained in patients suspected of having food hypersensitivity-induced respiratory symptoms [1, 88]. The history should include questions about the timing of the reaction in relation to food ingestion, the minimum quantity of food required to cause symptoms, the reproducibility of the symptoms, and current or past clinical history suggestive of a specific food hypersensitivity. With a history of an unexplained sudden exacerbation of asthma, the preceding food ingestion should be explored.

Physical examination

Signs of allergic disease such as atopic dermatitis will help to establish that the patient is atopic. The examination may reveal signs of chronic severe asthma, such as a Harrison's sulcus.

Skin testing for food allergy

Skin prick testing can rapidly provide reliable diagnostic information to support or refute the diagnosis of a food allergy. Testing should preferably be directed by the history as there is always the possibility of false-positive responses, particularly in the face of severe eczema. The diameter of the wheal response is predictive of the risk of clinical food allergy. Results though need to be interpreted in the light of the clinical history [89]. Where a result is inconclusive, laboratory testing or a challenge should be arranged.

Laboratory testing for food allergy

Laboratory assessment of food allergy involved the measurement of food-specific IgE in the serum. As the assay system is highly sensitive, this approach has a higher sensitivity to skin prick tests. The magnitude of the result is related to the risk of clinical allergy, with again the result needing to be interpreted in relation to the clinical history [90].

Oral food challenges

If there is a clinical suspicion of a food-induced respiratory symptoms that is supported by skin prick testing or specific IgE results, an elimination diet should be implemented under the supervision of a dietician. Resolution of symptoms would provide support to the diagnosis although with infrequent, intermittent reactions, this may be difficult. Oral food challenges can be very useful in confirming or refuting a diagnosis of food-induced symptoms. Challenges should be conducted in a hospital setting with available personnel and equipment to manage systemic anaphylaxis and severe bronchospasm. Patients should be well on the day of challenge with a FEV_1 of at least 80% predicted. Double-blind, placebo-controlled food challenges are the gold standard and are essential when the symptoms are subjective. With a history of objective symptoms or when a food hypersensitivity needs to be formally ruled out, an open challenge will suffice. Increasing doses of the food allergy are given at 20- to 30-minute intervals until objective symptoms develop or the top dose (equivalent to an age-appropriate portion) is consumed. Where a patient experiences a reaction, the possibility of a late-phase respiratory reaction must be considered.

Intervention

Once a food hypersensitivity has been confirmed as a cause for respiratory symptoms, strict avoidance of the allergen should be instigated. This may need to include both ingestion and contact with the allergen in an aerosolized form. The assistance of a dietician should be sought to avoid nutritional deficiencies, such as calcium deficiency. Growth parameters should be closely monitored in children on elimination diets. Patients with food hypersensitivity should have an individualized written emergency plan to help them manage their clinical symptoms in the case of an accidental exposure to the food allergen. Self-injectable adrenaline should be immediately available particularly as it is an effective bronchodilator. In the case of coexisting asthma, prioritization should be given to asthma management to minimize chronic airway inflammation.

Summary and conclusions

The coassociation of food hypersensitivity and respiratory tract problems are now being recognized not only because they are both allergic diseases but also, food hypersensitivity reactions frequently manifested in the respiratory tract, particularly in the face of aerosolized allergen. Chronic aerosolized exposure can lead to the development of asthma, as in Baker's asthma. Additionally, the presence of asthma is associated with a higher risk of morbidity and mortality from food hypersensitivity while food hypersensitivity increases the risk of life-threatening exacerbation of asthma. Lastly, food hypersensitivity in early life is a known risk factor to the development of later asthma although it is unclear whether there is a causal link, since asthma-like pathology develops in animal models with chronic aerosolized food allergy exposure. It is important that clinicians are aware that patients with coexisting food hypersensitivity and asthma are at increased risk and require careful management.

References

1. Roberts G, Lack G. Relevance of inhalational exposure to food allergens. *Curr Opin Allergy Clin Immunol* 2003; 3:211–215.
2. Roberts G, Lack G. Food allergy and asthma. *Paediatr Respir Rev* 2003; 4:205–212.
3. Bacharier LB, Boner A, Carlsen KH, et al. Diagnosis and treatment of asthma in childhood: a PRACTALL consensus report. *Allergy* 2008; 63(1):5–34.
4. British Thoracic Society Scottish Intercollegiate Guidelines Network. British guideline on the management of asthma. *Thorax* 2008; 63(Suppl. 4): iv1–iv121.
5. Global Initiative for Asthma [GINA]. (2009) *Global Strategy for the Diagnosis and Management of Asthma in Children 5 Years*

and Younger. Available at www.ginasthma.org/; last accessed August 2013.

6. Papadopoulos NG, Arakawa H, Carlsen K-H, et al. International Consensus on [ICON] Pediatric Asthma. *Allergy* 2012; 67:976–997.
7. Anderson HR, Gupta R, Strachan DP, Limb ES. 50 years of asthma: UK trends from 1955 to 2004. *Thorax* 2007; 62(1):85–90.
8. Bush A, Hedlin G, Carlsen KH, de Benedictis F, Lodrup-Carlsen K, Wilson N. Severe childhood asthma: a common international approach? *Lancet* 2008; 372(9643):1019–1021.
9. Grundy J, Matthews S, Bateman B, Dean T, Arshad SH. Rising prevalence of allergy to peanut in children: data from 2 sequential cohorts. *J Allergy Clin Immunol* 2002; 110(5):784–789.
10. Rona RJ, Keil T, Summers C, et al. The prevalence of food allergy: a meta-analysis. *J Allergy Clin Immunol* 2007; 120(3):638–646.
11. Johansson SG, Bieber T, Dahl R, et al. Revised nomenclature for allergy for global use: report of the Nomenclature Review Committee of the World Allergy Organization, October 2003. *J Allergy Clin Immunol* 2004; 113(5):832–836.
12. James JM, Bernhisel-Broadbent J, Sampson HA. Respiratory reactions provoked by double-blind food challenges in children. *Am J Respir Crit Care Med* 1994; 149(1):59–64.
13. Skoner AR, Skoner KR, Skoner DP. Allergic rhinitis, histamine, and otitis media. *Allergy Asthma Proc* 2009; 30(5):470–481.
14. Sampson HA, Muñoz-Furlong A, Campbell RL, et al. Second symposium on the definition and management of anaphylaxis: summary report—Second National Institute of Allergy and Infectious Disease/Food Allergy and Anaphylaxis Network Symposium. *J Allergy Clin Immunol* 2006; 117(2):391–397.
15. James JM, Eigenmann PA, Eggleston PA, Sampson HA. Airway reactivity changes in asthmatic patients undergoing blinded food challenges. *Am J Respi Crit Care Med* 1996; 153(2):597–603.
16. Eigenmann PA, Zamora SA. An internet-based survey on the circumstances of food-induced reactions following the diagnosis of IgE-mediated food allergy. *Allergy* 2002; 57:449–453.
17. Rancé F, Kanny G, Dutau G, Moneret-Vautrin DA. Food hypersensitivity in children: clinical aspects and distribution of allergens. *Pediatr Allergy Immunol* 1999; 10(1):33–38.
18. Sicherer SH, Furlong TJ, Munoz-Furlong A, Burks AW, Sampson HA. A voluntary registry for peanut and tree nut allergy: characteristics of the first 5149 registrants. *J Allergy Clin Immunol* 2001; 108(1):128–132.
19. Keskin O, Sekerel BE. Poppy seed allergy: a case report and review of the literature. *Allergy Asthma Proc* 2006; 27:396–398.
20. Moreno-Ancillo A, Gil-Adrados AC, Cosmes PM, Penide CF. Role of Dau c 1 in three different patterns of carrot-induced asthma. *Allergol Immunopathol (Madr)* 2006; 34:116–120.
21. Palma-Carlos AG, Palma-Carlos ML, Tengarrinha F. Allergy to sunflower seeds. *Eur Ann Allergy Clin Immunol* 2005; 37(5):183–186.
22. Moreno-Ancillo A, Gil-Adrados AC, Dominguez-Noche C, Cosmes PM. Lupine inhalation induced asthma in a child. *Pediatr Allergy Immunol* 2005; 16(6):542–544.
23. Rodrigo M-J, Cruz M-J, García M-D-M, Antó J-M, Genover T, Morell F. Epidemic asthma in Barcelona: an evaluation of new strategies for the control of soybean dust emission. *Int Arch Allergy Immunol* 2004; 134(2):158–164.
24. Zhou Y, Yang M, Dong BR. Monosodium glutamate avoidance for chronic asthma in adults and children. *Cochrane Database Syst Rev* 2012; (6):CD004357. doi:10.1002/14651858.CD004357.pub4
25. Onorato J, Merland N, Terral C, et al. Placebo-controlled double-blind food challenge in asthma. *J Allergy Clin Immunol* 1986; 78:1139–1146.
26. Bock SA, Atkins FM. Patterns of food hypersensitivity during sixteen years of double-blind, placebo-controlled food challenges. *J Pediatr* 1990; 117:561–567.
27. Yang WH, Drouin MA, Herbert M, Mao Y, Karsh J. The monosodium glutamate symptom complex: assessment in a double-blind, placebo-controlled, randomized study. *J Allergy Clin Immunol* 1997; 99:757–762.
28. Crespo JF, Pascual C, Dominguez C, et al. Allergic reactions associated with airborne fish particles in IgE-mediated fish hypersensitive patients. *Allergy* 1995; 50:257–261.
29. Rodriguez J, Reano M, Vives R, et al. Occupational asthma caused by fish inhalation. *Allergy* 1997; 52:866–869.
30. Taylor AV, Swanson MC, Jones RT, et al. Detection and quantitation of raw fish aeroallergens from an open-air fish market. *J Allergy Clin Immunol* 2000; 105:166–169.
31. Sicherer SH, Furlong TJ, DeSimone J, Sampson HA. Self-reported allergic reactions to peanut on commercial airliners. *J Allergy Clin Immunol* 1999; 104:186–189.
32. Jones RT, Stark D, Sussman G, Yunginger JW. Recovery of peanut allergen from ventilation filters of commercial airliners. *J Allergy Clin Immunol* 1996; 97:423.
33. Rossi GL, Corsico A, Moscato G. Occupational asthma caused by milk proteins: report on a case. *J Allergy Clin Immunol* 1994; 93:799–801.
34. Daroca P, Crespo JF, Reano M, et al. Asthma and rhinitis induced by exposure to raw green beans and chards. *Ann Allergy Asthma Immunol* 2000; 85:215–218.
35. Kalogeromitros D, Armenaka M, Galatas I, et al. Anaphylaxis induced by lentils. *Ann Allergy Asthma Immunol* 1996; 77:480–482.
36. Gohte CJ, Wieslander G, Ancker K, Forsbeck M. Buckwheat allergy: health food, an inhalation health risk. *Allergy* 1983; 38:155–159.
37. Kemp AS, Van Asperen PP, Douglas J. Anaphylaxis caused by inhaled pavlova mix in egg-sensitive children. *Med J Aust* 1988; 149(11–12):712–713.
38. Desjardins A, Malo JL, L'Archeveque J, et al. Occupational IgE-mediated sensitization and asthma caused by clam and shrimp. *J Allergy Clin Immunol* 1995; 96:608–617.
39. Bernstein DI, Bernstein IL. Occupational asthma. In: Middleton E, Reed CE, Ellis EF, et al. (eds), *Allergy Principles and Practice*, 3rd edn. MO: Mosby, 1988.
40. Brisman J. Baker's asthma. *Occup Environ Med* 2002; 59:498–502.

41. Cullinan P, Cook A, Nieuwenhuijsen MJ, et al. Allergen and dust exposure as determinants of work-related symptoms and sensitization in a cohort of flour exposed workers: a case-control analysis. *Ann Occup Hyg* 2001; 45:97–103.
42. Brisman J, Jarvholm B, Lillienberg L. Exposure–response relations for self reported asthma and rhinitis in bakers. *Occup Environ Med* 2000; 57:335–340.
43. Bernstein DI, Smith AB, Moller DR, et al. Clinical and immunologic studies among egg-processing workers with occupational asthma. *J Allergy Clin Immunol* 1987; 80:791–797.
44. Boeniger MF, Lummus ZL, Biagini RE, et al. Exposure to protein aeroallergens in egg processing facilities. *Appl Occup Environ Hyg* 2001; 16:660–670.
45. Huggins KG, Brostoff J. Local production of specific IgE antibodies in allergic rhinitis patients with negative skin tests. *Lancet* 1975; 2:148–150.
46. Taylor SL, Lehrer SB. Principles and characteristics of food allergens. *Crit Rev Food Sci Nutr* 1996; 36(Suppl.):S91–S118.
47. Anto JM, Sunyer J, Rodriguez-Roisin R, et al. Community outbreaks of asthma associated with inhalation of soybean dust. Toxicoepidemiological Committee. *N Engl J Med* 1989; 320:1097–1102.
48. Hernando L, Navarro C, Marquez M, et al. Asthma epidemics and soybean in Cartagena (Spain). *Lancet* 1989; 1:502.
49. Roberts G, Golder N, Lack G. Bronchial challenges with aerosolized food in asthmatic children with food allergy. *Allergy* 2002; 57:713–717.
50. Wang J, Visness CM, Sampson HA. Food allergen sensitization in inner-city children with asthma. *J Allergy Clin Immunol* 2005; 115:1076–1080.
51. Leung TF, Lam CW, Chan IH, Li AM, Tang NL. Sensitization to common food allergens is a risk factor for asthma in young Chinese children in Hong Kong. *J Asthma* 2002; 39(6):523–529.
52. Liu AH, Jaramillo R, Sicherer SH, et al. National prevalence and risk factors for food allergy and relationship to asthma: results from the National Health and Nutrition Examination Survey 2005–2006. *J Allergy Clin Immunol* 2010; 126(4):798–806.
53. Penard-Morand C, Raherison C, Kopferschmitt C, et al. Prevalence of food allergy and its relationship to asthma and allergic rhinitis in schoolchildren. *Allergy* 2005; 60(9):1165–1171.
54. Woods RK, Thien F, Raven J, Walters EH, Abramson M. Prevalence of food allergies in young adults and their relationship to asthma, nasal allergies, and eczema. *Ann Allergy Asthma Immunol* 2002; 88(2):183–189.
55. Wahn U. What drives the allergic march? *Allergy* 2000; 55:591–599.
56. Kulig M, Bergmann R, Tacke U, et al. Long-lasting sensitization to food during the first two years precedes allergic airway disease. The MAS Study Group, Germany. *Pediatr Allergy Immunol* 1998; 9:61–67.
57. Tariq SM, Matthews SM, Hakim EA, Arshad SH. Egg allergy in infancy predicts respiratory allergic disease by 4 years of age. *Pediatr Allergy Immunol* 2000; 11:162–167.
58. Rhodes HL, Thomas P, Sporik R, et al. A birth cohort study of subjects at risk of atopy. *Am Rev Resp Crit Care Med* 2002; 165:176–180.
59. van den Oord RA, Sheikh A. Filaggrin gene defects and risk of developing allergic sensitisation and allergic disorders: systematic review and meta-analysis. *BMJ* 2009; 339: b2433.
60. Irvine AD, McLean WH, Leung DY. Filaggrin mutations associated with skin and allergic diseases. *N Engl J Med* 2011; 365(14):1315–1327.
61. Marenholz I, Kerscher T, Bauerfeind A, et al. An interaction between filaggrin mutations and early food sensitization improves the prediction of childhood asthma. *J Allergy Clin Immunol* 2009; 123(4):911–916.
62. Holgate ST, Arshad SH, Roberts GC, Howarth PH, Thurner P, Davies DE. A new look at the pathogenesis of asthma. *Clin Sci* 2010; 118:439–450.
63. Sporik R, Holgate ST, Platts-Mills TAE, Cogswell JJ. Exposure to house dust mite allergen and the development of astshma in childhood. A prospective study. *N Engl J Med* 1990; 323:502–507.
64. Renz H, Smith HR, Henson JE, Ray BS, Irvin CG, Gelfand EW. Aerosolized antigen exposure without adjuvant causes increased IgE production and increased airway responsiveness in the mouse. *J Allergy Clin Immunol* 1992; 89(6):1127–1138.
65. Temelkovski J, Hogan SP, Shepherd DP, Foster PS, Kumar RK. An improved murine model of asthma: selective airway inflammation, epithelial lesions and increased methacholine responsiveness following chronic exposure to aerosolised allergen. *Thorax* 1998; 53(10):849–856.
66. McMillan SJ, Lloyd CM. Prolonged allergen challenge in mice leads to persistent airway remodelling. *Clin Exp Allergy* 2004 ; 34(3):497–507.
67. Teague WG. Food allergen sensitization as a determinant of disturbed airway function in young infants: first step on the path to persistent asthma? *J Allergy Clin Immunol* 2008; 122(4):766–767.
68. Sampson HA, Mendelson L, Rosen JP. Fatal and near-fatal anaphylactic reactions to food in children and adolescents. *N Engl J Med* 1992; 327(6):380–384.
69. Bock SA, Munoz-Furlong A, Sampson HA. Fatalities due to anaphylactic reactions to foods. *J Allergy Clin Immunol* 2001; 107(1):191–193.
70. Bock SA, Munoz-Furlong A, Sampson HA. Further fatalities caused by anaphylactic reactions to food, 2001–2006. *J Allergy Clin Immunol* 2007; 119: 2016–2018.
71. Pumphrey RS, Gowland MH. Further fatal allergic reactions to food in the United Kingdom, 1999–2006. *J Allergy Clin Immunol* 2007; 119(4):1018–1019.
72. Macdougall CF, Cant AJ, Colver AF. How dangerous is food allergy in childhood? The incidence of severe and fatal allergic reactions across the UK and Ireland. *Arch Dis Child* 2002; 86:236–239.
73. Uguz A, Lack G, Pumphrey R, et al. Allergic reactions in the community: a questionnaire survey of members of the anaphylaxis campaign. *Clin Exp Allergy* 2005; 35(6):746–750.

74. Jarvinen KM, Sicherer SH, Sampson HA, Nowak-Wegrzyn A. Use of multiple doses of epinephrine in food-induced anaphylaxis in children. *J Allergy Clin Immunol* 2008; 122(1):133–138.
75. Manivannan V, Campbell RL, Bellolio MF, Stead LG, Li JT, Decker WW. Factors associated with repeated use of epinephrine for the treatment of anaphylaxis. *Ann Allergy Asthma Immunol* 2009; 103(5):395–400.
76. Simons FE, Clark S, Camargo CA Jr. Anaphylaxis in the community: learning from the survivors. *J Allergy Clin Immunol* 2009; 124(2):301–306.
77. Rudders SA, Banerji A, Corel B, Clark S, Camargo Jr CA. Multicenter study of repeat epinephrine treatments for food-related anaphylaxis. *Pediatrics* 2010; 125(4):e711–e718.
78. Summers CW, Pumphrey RS, Woods CN, McDowell G, Pemberton PW, Arkwright PD. Factors predicting anaphylaxis to peanuts and tree nuts in patients referred to a specialist center. *J Allergy Clin Immunol* 2008; 121:632–638.
79. Gonzalez-Perez A, Aponte Z, Vidaurre CF, Rodriguez LA. Anaphylaxis epidemiology in patients with and patients without asthma: a United Kingdom database review. *J Allergy Clin Immunol* 2010; 125(5):1098–1104.
80. Bush A, Saglani S. Management of severe asthma in children [Review]. *Lancet* 2010; 376(9743):814–825.
81. Hedlin G, Bush A, Lodrup CK, et al. Problematic severe asthma in children, not one problem but many: a GA2LEN initiative. [Review]. *Eur Respir J* 2010; 36(1):196–201.
82. Alvarez GG, Schulzer M, Jung D, Fitzgerald JM. A systematic review of risk factors associated with near-fatal and fatal asthma. *Can Respir J* 2005; 12(5):265–270.
83. Vogel NM, Katz HT, Lopez R, Lang DM. Food allergy is associated with potentially fatal childhood asthma. *J Asthma* 2008; 45(10):862–866.
84. Bergstrom SE, Boman G, Eriksson L, et al. Asthma mortality among Swedish children and young adults, a 10-year study. *Respir Med* 2008; 102(9):1335–1341.
85. Roberts G, Patel N, Levi-Schaffer F, Habibi P, Lack G. Food allergy as a risk factor for life-threatening asthma in childhood: a case-controlled study. *J Allergy Clin Immunol* 2003; 112(1):168–174.
86. Berns SH, Halm EA, Sampson HA, Sicherer SH, Busse PJ, Wisnivesky JP. Food allergy as a risk factor for asthma morbidity in adults. *J Asthma* 2007; 44(5):377–381.
87. Simpson AB, Glutting J, Yousef E. Food allergy and asthma morbidity in children. *Pediatr Pulmonol* 2007; 42(6):489–495.
88. Bird JA, Burks AW. Food allergy and asthma. *Prim Care Respir J* 2009; 18(4):258–265.
89. Du Toit G, Santos A, Roberts G, Fox AT, Smith P, Lack G. The diagnosis of IgE-mediated food allergy in childhood. *Pediatr Allergy Immunol* 2009; 20(4):309–319.
90. Stiefel, Roberts G. How to use serum specific IgE measurements in diagnosing and monitoring food allergy. *Arch Dis Child Educ Pract Ed*.2012; 97:29–36.

14 Anaphylaxis and Food Allergy

Hugh A. Sampson
Translational Biomedical Sciences, Jaffe Food Allergy Institute Department of Pediatrics, Icahn School of Medicine at Mount Sinai, New York, NY, USA

Key Concepts

- Food allergy is the leading single cause of anaphylaxis treated in emergency departments in the United States.
- Any food may cause an anaphylactic reaction, but peanut, tree nuts, milk, fish, and shellfish are most often implicated in severe and fatal reactions.
- A careful clinical history is critical for the accurate diagnosis of food-induced anaphylaxis; an algorithm of clinical symptoms has been proposed, which provides a universal standard for accurately diagnosing anaphylaxis.
- Laboratory studies are not diagnostic of anaphylaxis, simply supportive.
- All patients at risk for a food-induced anaphylactic reaction should be provided with an emergency plan and appropriate medications, for example, epinephrine autoinjector, to initiate therapy in case of an accidental allergen ingestion.

Introduction

Although fatal allergic reactions have been recognized for over 4500 years [1], it was not until the last century that the syndrome of anaphylaxis was fully characterized. In their classic studies, Portier and Richet (1902) described the rapid death of several dogs that they were attempting to immunize against the toxic sting of the sea anemone [2]. Since this reaction represented the opposite of their intended "prophylaxis," they coined the term "anaphylaxis," or "without or against protection." From these studies, they concluded that anaphylaxis required a latent period for sensitization and reexposure to the sensitizing material. Shortly thereafter Schlossman (1905) reported a patient who developed acute shock after the ingestion of cow's milk [3]. The first modern-day series of food anaphylaxis in man was published in 1969 by Golbert and colleagues [4]. They described 10 cases of anaphylaxis following the ingestion of various foods, including different legumes, fish, and milk. The reports by Yunginger [5] and then Sampson [6] and Bock [7–9] further characterized the natural course of near-fatal and fatal food-induced anaphylactic reactions. Similar findings were reported more recently from Australia [10].

Definitions

The term "food-induced anaphylaxis" refers to a serious allergic reaction following the ingestion of a food, typically IgE-mediated, which is generally rapid in onset and may progress to death [11]. Typically, the term ***anaphylaxis*** connotes an immunologically mediated event that occurs after exposure to certain foreign substances, whereas the term ***anaphylactoid*** indicates a clinically indistinguishable reaction that is not believed to be IgE-mediated but probably involves many of the same mediators, for example, histamine. The syndrome results from the generation and release of a variety of potent biologically active mediators and their concerted effects on various target organs. "Biphasic anaphylaxis" is defined as a recurrence of symptoms that develops following the apparent resolution of the initial anaphylactic event. Biphasic reactions have been reported to develop in 1–20% of anaphylactic reactions and typically occur within 1–4 hours following the resolution of the initial symptoms, although some cases have been reported up to 72 hours later [12]. "Protracted anaphylaxis" is defined as an anaphylactic reaction that

Food Allergy: Adverse Reactions to Foods and Food Additives, Fifth Edition. Edited by Dean D Metcalfe, Hugh A Sampson, Ronald A Simon and Gideon Lack.

lasts for hours or in extreme cases, days [6–13]. "Food-associated, exercise-induced anaphylaxis" refers to a food-induced anaphylactic reaction that occurs only when the patient exercises within several hours of ingesting a food; when the food is consumed without subsequent exercise or when exercise occurs without the ingestion of the food allergen, the patient will not experience allergic symptoms [14–16].

Anaphylaxis is recognized by a constellation of cutaneous, respiratory, cardiovascular, and gastrointestinal signs and symptoms occurring singly or in combination. To facilitate and standardize the diagnosis of anaphylaxis, the National Institute of Allergy and Infectious Diseases (NIAID) and the Food Allergy & Anaphylaxis Network (FAAN) convened an international panel of experts from various medical specialties that deal with anaphylactic cases. An algorithm was proposed, as depicted in Table 14.1 [17], and later shown to be a sensitive indicator of anaphylaxis in the emergency department (ED) setting [18]. Since anaphylactic reactions may present with varied degrees of severity, which may influence the form of treatment rendered, Table 14.2 presents a simplified scoring system based upon the diagnostic algorithm of anaphylaxis proposed by the NIAID-FAAN working group. This chapter focuses on allergic reactions to foods that manifest as signs and symptoms fulfilling the proposed definition of anaphylaxis.

Table 14.1 Diagnostic criteria for anaphylaxis [17].

Anaphylaxis is highly likely when any one of the following three criteria is fulfilled:

1. Acute onset of an illness (minutes to several hours) with involvement of the skin, mucosal tissue, or both (e.g., generalized hives, pruritus, or flushing, swollen lips–tongue–uvula) **AND AT LEAST ONE OF THE FOLLOWING**
- **a.** Respiratory compromise (e.g., dyspnea, wheeze–bronchospasm, stridor, reduced peak expiratory flow, hypoxemia)
- **b.** Reduced blood pressure or associated symptoms of end-organ dysfunction (e.g., hypotonia (collapse), syncope, incontinence)

2. Two or more of the following that occur rapidly after exposure *to a **likely** allergen for that patient* (minutes to several hours):
- **a.** Involvement of the skin–mucosal tissue (e.g., generalized hives, itch-flush, swollen lips–tongue–uvula)
- **b.** Respiratory compromise (e.g., dyspnea, wheeze–bronchospasm, stridor, reduced peak expiratory flow, hypoxemia)
- **c.** Reduced blood pressure or associated symptoms of end-organ dysfunction (e.g., hypotonia (collapse), syncope, incontinence)
- **d.** Persistent gastrointestinal symptoms (e.g., crampy abdominal pain, vomiting)

3. Reduced BP after exposure *to **known** allergen for that patient* (minutes to several hours):
- **a.** Infants and children: low systolic blood pressure (age-specific) or greater than 30% decrease in systolic blood pressure[a]
- **b.** Adults: systolic blood pressure <90 mm Hg or greater than 30% decrease from that patient's baseline

PEF, peak expiratory flow; BP, blood pressure.
[a]Low systolic BP for children: 1 month–1 year <70 mm Hg; 1–10 years < [70 mm Hg + (2 × age)]; 11–17 years <90 mm Hg.

Table 14.2 Grading severity of anaphylaxis.

Grade	Defined by
(1) ***Mild*** (skin and subcutaneous tissues, GI, and/or mild respiratory)	Flushing, urticaria, periorbital erythema or angioedema, mild dyspnea, wheezing and upper respiratory symptoms, mild abdominal pain, and/or emesis
(2) ***Moderate*** (mild symptoms + features suggesting moderate respiratory, cardiovascular, or GI symptoms)	Marked dysphagia, hoarseness, and/or stridor, SOB, wheezing and retractions, crampy abdominal pain, recurrent vomiting and/or diarrhea, and/or mild dizziness
(3) ***Severe*** (hypoxia, hypotension, or neurological compromise)	Cyanosis or $SpO_2 \leq 92\%$ at any stage, hypotension, confusion, collapse, loss of consciousness, or incontinence

Prevalence

The prevalence of anaphylaxis is uncertain since unlike many disorders, there is no requirement to report such reactions to a national registry. In addition, it is likely that many cases are misdiagnosed [19, 20]. Also contributing to this lack of scientific data is the fact that many patients who experience a mild anaphylactic reaction recognize the causative relationship to a specific food, self-medicate and simply attempt to avoid that food rather than consult a physician.

In a retrospective survey, Yocum and Khan [21] reviewed all cases of anaphylaxis treated in the Mayo Clinic Emergency Department (United States) over a 3.5-year period. Records were reviewed on all patients experiencing respiratory obstructive symptoms and/or cardiovascular symptoms plus evidence of allergic mediator release, for example, urticaria. Overall, 179 patients were identified; 66% were female, 49% were atopic, and 37% had experienced an immediate reaction to the responsible allergen in the past. A probable cause was identified in 142 cases (Table 14.3). Allergic reactions to food were found to be the most common single cause of anaphylactic reactions outside of the hospital, more frequent than reactions to bee sting and drugs combined. A follow-up study looking at the incidence of anaphylaxis in Olmstead County revealed a 26% increase in cases of anaphylaxis between 1990 and 2000, with about one-third of reactions due to food allergy [22]. Food-induced anaphylactic reactions account for over one-half of the anaphylactic reactions in children treated in EDs and are most often due to peanut, tree nuts, milk, fish, or shellfish. Pumphrey [23] and Moneret-Vautrin [24] reported similar findings in the

Table 14.3 Three-year retrospective survey of anaphylaxis occurring outside of the hospital treated by the Mayo Clinic Emergency Department [7].

Presumed etiology of anaphylaxis	Number	Percentage (%)
Food	59	33
Idiopathic	34	19
Hymenoptera	25	14
Medications	23	13
Exercise	12	7
Other	8	4
False diagnosis	18	10
Foods implicated in 18 patients who were skin tested:		
Peanut	4	
Cereals	6	
Egg	2	
Nuts	9	
Milk	2	

United Kingdom and France, respectively. In Italy, Novembre reported that food allergy was responsible for about one-half of severe anaphylactic episodes in children treated in EDs [25], and a survey of South Australian preschool and school-age children revealed a parent-reported food-induced anaphylaxis rate of 0.43 per 100 school children, which accounted for over one-half of all cases of anaphylaxis in this age group [26]. Similarly, the Canadian Pediatric Surveillance Program reported that 81% of anaphylaxis cases in children were due to food [27]. In a more recent survey from Australia, 526 children with generalized allergic reactions were seen in a local ED, 57 were diagnosed with anaphylaxis. This represented an incidence of 9.3 in 1000 ED visits for generalized allergic reactions and an anaphylaxis incidence of 1 in 1000 [28]. Liew and coworkers reported an incidence of hospital admissions for food-induced anaphylaxis of about 6/100 000 population in 2005, a 350% increase over the previous 11 years [10]. In a similar series of 304 adults attending an ED in the same city over a 1-year period, 162 were diagnosed with acute allergic reactions and 142 with anaphylaxis, including 60 whose anaphylaxis was severe and one of whom died, for an anaphylaxis presentation incidence of 1 in 439 [29].

The first of several reports on fatal food-induced anaphylaxis was in 1988 by Yunginger and colleagues who reported seven cases of fatal anaphylaxis evaluated during a 16-month period [5]. In all but possibly one case, the victims unknowingly ingested a food which had provoked a previous allergic reaction. Similarly, six fatal and seven near-fatal food-induced anaphylactic reactions in children (ages 2–17 years) were accumulated from three metropolitan areas over a 14-month period [6]. Common risk factors were noted in these cases: all patients had asthma (although generally well controlled); all patients were unaware that they were ingesting the food allergen; all patients had experienced previous allergic reactions to the incriminated food, although in most cases symptoms had been much milder; and all patients had immediate symptoms with about half experiencing a quiescent period prior to a major respiratory collapse. In both these early series, no patient who died received adrenaline immediately, however, three patients with near-fatal reactions did receive adrenaline within 15 minutes of developing symptoms but still went on to develop respiratory collapse and hypotension requiring mechanical ventilation and vasopressor support for 12 hours to 3 weeks. None of these patients investigated had a significant increase in serum tryptase.

In two reports by Bock and coworkers [7, 8], 63 cases of fatal food-induced anaphylaxis were evaluated. As in earlier series, peanuts and tree nuts accounted for more than 90% of the fatalities, but in the second report, milk accounted for 4 of 31 deaths. In these series, all but two of the patients were known to have asthma and most of the individuals did not have epinephrine available at the time of their fatal reaction. Of the cumulative 63 fatal food anaphylaxis cases reported, however, six individuals (~10%) had received epinephrine in a timely manner but failed to respond. In an earlier series of 48 fatal cases reviewed by Pumphrey, three patients (~6%) died despite receiving epinephrine from a self-administration kit appropriately at the onset of their reaction [23].

The incidence of food-dependent exercise-induced anaphylaxis appears to be increasing, possibly due to the increased popularity of exercising over the past decade. Two forms of food-dependent exercise-induced anaphylaxis have been described; reactions following the ingestion of specific foods (e.g., egg, celery, shellfish, wheat) [16, 17, 30–35, 32, 33, 36–38] and rarely reactions following the ingestion of any food [39, 40]. Anaphylaxis will occur when a patient exercises within 2–4 hours of ingesting a food, but otherwise the patient can ingest the food without any apparent reaction and can exercise without any apparent reaction as long as the specific food (or any food in the case of nonspecific reactors) has not been ingested within the past several hours. This disorder is twice as common in females and greater than 60% of cases occur in individuals younger than 30 years of age. In a survey of 199 individuals experiencing exercise-induced anaphylaxis, ingestion of food within 2 hours of exercise was felt to be a factor in the development of attacks in 54% of the cases [31]. More recently, several cases of food- and aspirin-dependent exercise-induced anaphylaxis have been reported [41–43]. Symptoms generally start with a sensation of generalized pruritus that progresses to urticaria and erythema, respiratory obstruction, and cardiovascular collapse. Patients with specific food-dependent exercise-induced anaphylaxis generally have positive prick skin tests to the food and occasionally these patients will have a history of "outgrowing" an allergy to the causative food when they were younger. As discussed below, specific management of this disorder involves identifying the food(s) that cause the reaction (i.e., double-blind placebo-controlled food challenge (DBPCFC) with exercise).

Several factors appear to predispose an individual to food-induced anaphylaxis including a personal history of atopy, family history of atopy, age, and dietary exposure. Atopic patients with asthma are at increased risk of developing more severe food-allergic reactions [6–9, 44–46]. In the reports of Yunginger et al. [5], Sampson et al. [6], and Bock et al. [7, 8], the majority of individuals were highly atopic, and all had histories of asthma. Although atopy reportedly does not predispose individuals to an increased risk of anaphylaxis, it does tend to predispose to more severe reactions. In general, it has been thought that individuals inherit the ability to produce antigen-specific IgE to food proteins and that hypersensitivity to a specific food is not inherited. However, in a report evaluating twins with peanut allergy, there was a significant concordance rate of peanut allergy among monozygotic twins compared with dizygotic twins, suggesting strongly that there is a major genetic influence on the inheritence of peanut allergy [47].

Age may play a factor in predisposing an individual to food-induced anaphylaxis. The prevalence of food allergy appears greatest in the first 2 years of life and decreases with age [48]. Consequently, exposure to foods during the first year (e.g., cow milk, egg, soy, wheat, and peanut (as peanut butter in the United States)) is more apt to induce hypersensitization. Allergic reactions to milk, egg, soybean, and wheat are generally "outgrown" with age [48], [49]. The age of onset of milk allergy is usually in the first year of life, with the majority of infants "outgrowing" their sensitivity by 7–8 years of age [50–52]. While most food hypersensitivities are outgrown during childhood, food sensitivity to peanuts, tree nuts, sesame, fish, and shellfish often persist into adulthood [48, 53]. Only about 20% of children diagnosed with peanut allergy early in life outgrow their peanut allergy [54, 55] and about 10% outgrow their tree nut allergy [56].

Dietary exposure can influence the occurrence of food-induced anaphylaxis in several ways. Different populations and nationalities may consume more of certain foods, and the increased exposure may result in an increased prevalence of that specific food allergy. In the United States, peanut is one of the most common food allergies [57, 58], Americans ingest several tons of peanuts daily (FDA, 1986). By contrast, in Scandinavia, where fish consumption is high, the incidence of allergic reactions to codfish is increased (FDA, 1986). Rice and buckwheat allergy are quite rare in the United States but not uncommon in Japan where these foods are frequently ingested [59].

Table 14.4 Foods most frequently implicated in food-induced anaphylaxis.

Peanut	
Tree nuts	Hazel nuts (filberts), walnuts, cashews, pistachios, Brazil nuts
Fish	Less often tuna
Shellfish	Shrimp, crab, lobster, oyster, scallop
Cow milk	Goat milk
Hens egg	
Seeds	Cotton seed, sesame seed, pine nuts, sunflower seed
Beans	Soybeans, green peas, pinto beans, garbanzo beans, green beans
Fruit	Banana, kiwi
Cereal grains	Wheat, barley, oat, buckwheat
Potato	

Etiology

Foods

A large variety of foods have been reported to precipitate an anaphylactic reaction. The list of foods that may induce an anaphylactic reaction is unlimited, and in theory, any food protein is capable of causing an anaphylactic reaction. As indicated in Table 14.4, certain foods tend to be cited most frequently as the cause of anaphylaxis, although any food may be the cause. Foods most often responsible for anaphylactic reactions include peanuts (and to a much lesser extent other legumes such as soybeans, lupine, lentils, peas, garbanzo beans), fish (e.g., codfish, whitefish, salmon), shellfish (shrimp, lobster, crab, scallops, oyster), tree nuts (hazelnuts, cashews, pistachio, walnuts, pecans, Brazil nuts, almonds), cow milk, egg, fruits (banana, kiwi), seeds (sesame seed, mustard), and cereals or grains (wheat, rice, rye, millet, buckwheat) [15]. The potency of particular foods to induce an anaphylactic reaction appears to vary and is also dependent upon the sensitivity of the individual. In general, it appears that for some foods such as peanuts, microgram quantities may be sufficient to induce a reaction.

Prior exposure and sensitization to food allergens theoretically must precede the initial anaphylactic reaction. However, there have been numerous reports of an anaphylactic reaction occurring after the first known exposure to a food substance. In one series of children allergic to peanuts and tree nuts, a significant number of these patients reacted on their first known exposure to the food [60, 61]. Several possibilities may account for this apparent paradox: infants may be sensitized to foods passed in maternal breast milk during lactation; sensitization may occur following allergen contact on the skin in infants with atopic dermatitis [62, 63]; sensitization may develop following an unknown exposure to a food antigen (e.g., milk formula given during the night in the newborn nursery, food given by another caregiver (e.g., baby sitter or grandparent), or food contained in another product that was not suspected of containing the antigen in question); and sensitization may occur because of cross-sensitization to a similar allergen (e.g., kiwi or banana allergy in a latex-sensitive individual) [64]. Some data suggest that sensitization may occur *in utero* [65].

Food additives

Although food additives are often suspected of provoking anaphylactic reactions, very few food additives have been proven to provoke an anaphylactic reaction. One of the initial reports detailed an atopic, nonasthmatic patient who experienced an anaphylactic reaction after consuming a restaurant meal, which contained significant sodium bisulfite [66]. Specific IgE to sodium bisulfite was demonstrated by skin testing and transfer of passive cutaneous anaphylaxis, and an oral food challenge produced itching of the ears and eyes, nausea, warmness, cough, tightness in the throat, and erythema of the shoulders. These symptoms resolved following treatment with epinephrine. There have been other scattered case reports in the literature confirming sulfite-induced anaphylaxis [67, 68]. A number of natural additives have been implicated in anaphylactic reactions, including annatto, psyllium and guar gum [67–71].

Clinical features

The hallmark of a food-induced anaphylactic reaction is the onset of symptoms within seconds to minutes following the ingestion of the food allergen. The time course of the appearance and perception of symptoms and signs will differ among individuals. Almost invariably, at least some symptoms will begin within the first hour after the exposure. Generally, the later the onset of anaphylactic signs and symptoms, the less severe the reaction. About 10–30% of patients will experience a biphasic reaction [6, 72–74], where patients typically develop classical symptoms initially, appear to be recovering (and may become asymptomatic), and then experience the recurrence of significant, often catastrophic symptoms, which may be more refractory to standard therapy. The intervening quiescent period may last up to 1–3 hours. In the report by Sampson and colleagues, three of seven patients with near-fatal anaphylaxis experienced protracted anaphylaxis, with symptoms lasting from 1 to 21 days [6]. Most reports suggest that the earlier epinephrine is administered in the course of anaphylaxis the better the chance of a favorable prognosis [75], but there are no data to indicate that the timing of epinephrine affects the prevalence of biphasic or protracted symptoms [72]. In addition, it should be noted that in about 5–10% of cases in which patients have received an initial injection of epinephrine in a timely manner, they still progressed to fatal anaphylaxis [7, 8]. Even with appropriate treatment in a medical facility, it rarely may be impossible to reverse an anaphylactic reaction once it has begun.

The symptoms of anaphylaxis are generally related to the gastrointestinal, respiratory, cutaneous, and cardiovascular systems [11]. Other organ systems may be affected but much less commonly. The sequence of symptom presentation and severity will vary from one individual to the next. Additionally, one patient who experiences anaphylaxis to more than one type of food may experience a different sequence of symptoms with each food. While many patients will develop similar allergic symptoms on subsequent occasions following the ingestion of a food allergen, patients with asthma and peanut and/or nut allergy seem to be less predictable. There are many cases of peanut-allergic children who reacted with minimal cutaneous and gastrointestinal symptoms as a young child who later developed asthma and then experienced a catastrophic anaphylactic event after ingesting peanut in their teenage years.

The first symptoms experienced often involve the oropharynx. Symptoms may include edema and pruritus of the lips, oral mucosa, palate, and pharynx [11, 76, 77]. Young children may be seen scratching at their tongue, palate, anterior neck, or external auditory canals (presumably from referred pruritus of the posterior pharynx). Evidence of laryngeal edema includes a "dry staccato" or croupy cough and/or dysphonia and dysphagia. Gastrointestinal symptoms include nausea, vomiting, crampy abdominal pain, and diarrhea. Emesis generally contains large amounts of "stringy" mucus. Respiratory symptoms may consist of a deep repetitive cough, stridor, dyspnea, and/or wheezing. Cutaneous symptoms of anaphylaxis may include flushing, urticaria, angioedema, and/or an erythematous macular rash. The development of cardiovascular symptoms, along with airway obstruction, is of greatest concern in anaphylactic reactions. Although cardiovascular symptoms occur less frequently in food-induced anaphylactic reactions compared to insect sting or medication-induced anaphylaxis, it is important to recognize the symptoms early and the potential complications. Symptoms associated with hypotension can include nausea, vomiting, diaphoresis, dyspnea, hypoxia, dizziness, seizures, and collapse [78]. Extravasation of fluid and vasodilatation can lead to a decrease in circulating blood volume of up to 35% within 10 minutes [79]. In addition, cardiac dysfunction associated with nonspecific electrocardiographic changes and normal coronary arteries have been reported [80]. Therefore, placing the patient in a supine position (as tolerated) and elevating the legs to prevent pooling of blood in the lower extremities and aggressive fluid resuscitation is recommended. In fact, upright posture has been found to lead to fatalities in cases of food-induced anaphylactic shock [81].

Other signs and symptoms reported frequently in anaphylaxis include periocular and nasal pruritus, sneezing, diaphoresis, disorientation, fecal or urinary urgency or incontinence, and uterine cramping (manifested as lower back pain similar to "labor" pains). Patients often report an impending "sense of doom." In some instances, the initial manifestation of anaphylaxis may be the loss of consciousness. Death may ensue in minutes but has been reported to occur days to weeks after anaphylaxis [7, 8, 23], with late deaths generally resulting from organ damage experienced early in the course of anaphylaxis.

Several factors appear to increase the risk of more severe anaphylactic reactions. Patients taking β-adrenergic antagonists or calcium channel blockers may be resistant to standard therapeutic regimens and therefore at increased risk for severe anaphylaxis [11, 40, 77–82]. Patients with asthma appear to be at increased risk for severe symptoms as noted in a number of reports concerning fatal and near-fatal food anaphylactic reactions [6, 7]. Similar findings have been reported in patients with insect-sting allergy [83] and from patients experiencing anaphylaxis as a result of immunotherapy [84, 85]. In these patients, acute bronchospasm developed along with other symptoms of anaphylaxis.

The skin is the most commonly affected organ in anaphylaxis, appearing in more than 80% of cases [11, 73]. However, up to 20% of cases do not present with skin findings, particularly in children reacting to foods [6, 28]. In these cases, a history of allergy and possible exposure, along with symptoms consistent with criteria 2 listed on Table 14.1 would establish the diagnosis. In rare cases, hypotension has been reported to be the primary symptom of anaphylaxis. These situations would satisfy the third criteria if the patient had exposure to a known allergen. The annual incidence of anaphylaxis with cardiovascular compromise is 8–10 per 100 000 inhabitants [86, 87]. In six cases of fatal food-induced anaphylaxis [6], initial symptoms developed within 3–30 minutes and severe respiratory symptoms within 20–150 minutes. Symptoms involved the lower respiratory tract in 6 of 6 children, the gastrointestinal tract in 5 of 6 patients, and the skin in only 1 of 6 children. Anaphylaxis should never be considered ruled out on the basis of absent skin symptoms.

Diagnosis

Using the algorithm presented in Table 14.1, the diagnosis of anaphylaxis should be readily apparent [17, 18]. Young children presenting with anaphylaxis most often present with cutaneous and gastrointestinal symptoms [28], whereas adults will often have cutaneous, respiratory, and cardiovascular symptoms [80]. In many cases where a food is implicated, the inciting food is obvious from the temporal relationship between the ingestion and the onset of symptoms. The initial step in determining the cause of an episode of anaphylaxis is a very careful history, especially when the cause of the episode is not straightforward [88, 89]. Specific questions to address include the type and quantity of food eaten, the last time the food was ingested, the time frame between ingestion and the development of symptoms, the nature of the food (cooked or uncooked), other times when similar symptoms occurred (and if the food in question was eaten on those occasions), and whether any other precipitating factors appear to be involved, for example, exercise, alcohol, NSAIDs.

Basically, any food may precipitate an anaphylactic reaction, but there are a few specific foods which appear to be most often implicated in the etiology of food-induced anaphylactic reactions: peanuts, tree nuts, milk, fish, and shellfish. In cases where the etiology of the anaphylactic reaction is not apparent, a dietary history should review all ingredients of the suspected meal including any possible concealed ingredients or food additives. The food provoking the reaction may be merely a contaminant (knowingly or unknowingly) in the meal. For example, peanuts or peanut butter are frequently added to cookies, candies, pastries, or sauces such as chili, spaghetti, and barbecue sauces. Chinese restaurants frequently use peanut butter to "glue" the overlapping ends of an egg roll, pressed or "extruded" peanut oil in their cooking, and the same wok to cook a variety of different meals resulting in residual contaminant carryover. Another infrequent (but not rare) cause of food contamination occurs during the manufacturing process. This contamination may happen with scraps of candy or dough that are "reworked" into the next batch of candy or cookies, or in processing plants where there is a production change from one product to the next. As an example, a reaction to almond butter by a peanut-allergic patient started an investigation that determined that 10% of the almond butter produced in that plant was contaminated with peanut butter (FDA, 1986). This occurred after a production change in the manufacturing process from peanut butter to almond butter. Other examples include popsicles run on the same line as creamsicles (milk), fruit juices packaged in individual cartons where milk products have been packaged, milk-free desserts packaged in dairy plants [90], and so on. Food items with "natural flavoring" designated on the label may contain an unsuspected allergen, for example, casein in canned tuna fish, hot dogs or bologna, soy in a variety of baked goods, and so on. However, the *Food Allergen Labeling and Consumer Protection Act (FALCPA)* enacted in January, 2006, in the United States mandated that foods containing any amount of milk, egg, peanut, tree nuts, fish, shellfish, soy, or wheat must declare the food in plain language on the ingredient label, that is, "milk" and not "sodium caseinate." FALCPA has made label reading to ascertain ingredients much easier for millions of Americans. In the European Common Market countries, similar legislation has been enacted, and sesame is included in the list of foods that must be declared.

Food allergy can develop at any age, although it appears more commonly in the first 3 years of life. Not uncommonly, a patient will present who has tolerated a food (i.e., shrimp) for his or her entire life and then at some point in mid-adulthood experiences a major allergic reaction after ingestion of the food. These patients may experience no forewarning of their impending episode, but on detailed questioning will not infrequently describe some minor symptoms previously, such as oral pruritus or nausea and cramping. It is also possible that cooking or processing of some foods may remove, diminish, or even enhance their allergenicity.

Some conditions may be confused with food anaphylaxis. Among these clinical problems are scromboid poisoning, factitious allergic emergency, and vasovagal collapse. In the absence of urticaria and angioedema, one must consider arrhythmia, myocardial infarction, hereditary angioedema, aspiration of a bolus of food, pulmonary embolism, and seizure disorders. Following the algorithm in Table 14.1 should enable physicians to accurately identify individuals with anaphylaxis.

With the presence of laryngeal edema, especially when accompanied by abdominal pain, the diagnosis of hereditary angioedema must be considered. In general, this disorder is slower in onset, does not include urticaria, and often there is a family history of similar reactions [91, 92]. Systemic mastocytosis results in flushing, tachycardia, pruritus, headache, abdominal pain, diarrhea, and syncope. A factitious allergic emergency may occur when patients knowingly and secretively ingest a food substance to which they are known to be allergic.

In vasovagal syncope, the patient may collapse after an injection or a painful or disturbing situation. The patient typically looks pale and complains of nausea prior to the syncopal episode, but does not complain of pruritus or become cyanotic. Respiratory difficulty does not occur and symptoms are almost immediately relieved by recumbency. Profuse diaphoresis, slow pulse, and maintenance of blood pressure generally complete the syndrome [93], but asystole and bradycardia have been reportedly associated with blood drawing [94]. Hyperventilation may cause breathlessness and collapse. It is usually not associated with other signs and symptoms of anaphylaxis, except peripheral and perioral tingling sensations.

Laboratory evaluation

The laboratory evaluation of patients with an anaphylactic reaction should be directed at identifying specific IgE antibodies to the food in question. IgE antibody can be recognized *in vivo* by prick or puncture skin testing. Although not absolute, a negative prick/puncture skin test is an excellent predictor for a negative IgE-mediated food reaction to the suspected food. In contrast, a positive prick skin test does not necessarily mean that the food is the inciting agent, but in a patient with a classic history of anaphylaxis to ingestion of an isolated food and a positive prick/puncture skin test to that food, this laboratory test appears to be a good positive predictor of allergic reactivity. In cases of food-associated or aspirin-associated exercise-induced anaphylaxis, prick skin tests performed following exercise/ingestion of aspirin are enhanced compared with tests done prior to exercise/aspirin ingestion in many patients [42].

There are some limitations to skin testing which need to be recognized. There is speculation that skin testing shortly following the anaphylactic event may fail to yield a positive response owing to temporary anergy. Although not demonstrated in food allergy, this phenomenon has been demonstrated in Hymenoptera sensitivity following an insect sting [95]. Possible causes of false-negative prick skin tests include improper skin test technique, concomitant use of antihistamines, or the use of food extracts with reduced or inadequate allergenic potential. With some foods, the processing of the food for commercial extracts may diminish antigenicity [96]. This is especially true for some fruits and vegetables, and occasionally shellfish. However, if there is a high index of suspicion that a food may have precipitated an anaphylactic reaction even though the prick skin test is negative, the patient should be tested with the natural food utilizing the "prick-plus-prick" method to ensure an absence of detectable IgE antibody [97]. Some caution should be exercised in doing this procedure since the amount of antigen on the prick device will not be controlled, and appropriate negative controls also should be performed.

Appropriate skin testing is indicated in each patient, although *in vitro* measurement of food-specific IgE may be evaluated initially. In many patients with anaphylaxis, limited prick skin testing is necessary to confirm the etiology of the anaphylactic reaction. In cases of idiopathic anaphylaxis, more extensive prick testing may occasionally prove helpful in making the diagnosis [98]. The clinician must decide how many skin tests are practical and justified, taking into account the anticipated low yield of positive results in idiopathic anaphylaxis and the value of discovering an etiology in this serious disorder.

Intradermal skin tests are sometimes performed following negative prick/puncture skin tests in other allergic diseases, but the diagnostic significance of a positive intradermal test to food following a negative prick/puncture test is of no clinical benefit [99], except in cases of delayed anaphylaxis due to galactose-α-1,3-galactose in red meat [100, 101]. Fatal anaphylactic reactions have been documented following intradermal skin tests to foods

[84, 102], so extra caution should be exercised if intradermal tests are performed (if done at all). **Under no circumstances should an intradermal skin test be performed prior to performing a prick/puncture test.** In cases where extreme hypersensitivity is suspected, alternative approaches may be warranted including the further dilution of the food extract prior to prick skin testing or the use of a food-specific IgE *in vitro* tests, for example, UniCAP®; Thermo Fisher Scientific, Uppsala, Sweden. The UniCAP System appears to be slightly more sensitive than the older standard RAST. In a number of studies, predictive curves and diagnostic decision points have been established using the UniCAP System for predicting a positive food challenge for at least milk, egg, and peanuts [103–105]. At the present, there is no laboratory test that will predict the potential severity of an allergic reaction. A study investigating peanut-allergic patients' IgE binding to allergenic peanut epitopes demonstrated that individuals with binding to large numbers of epitopes (epitope diversity) tended to have more severe reactions than those binding fewer epitopes [106].

Massive activation of mast cells during anaphylaxis results in a dramatic rise in plasma histamine and somewhat later a rise in plasma serum tryptase [107, 108]. Plasma histamine rises over the first several minutes of a reaction, generally remains elevated for only several minutes, requires special collection techniques, and will breakdown unless the plasma sample is frozen immediately. Consequently, measurement of plasma histamine to document anaphylaxis is often impractical except in research situations. Whether measurement of urinary methylhistamine will be useful in the documentation of anaphylaxis remains to be demonstrated. Serum tryptase rises over the first hour and may remain elevated for many hours. It is fairly stable at room temperature and can be obtained from postmortem specimens [108]. Total tryptase has been shown to be markedly elevated in some cases of bee sting or drug-induced anaphylaxis [108], but several recent studies have found it less often elevated than plasma histamine [88, 109, 110, 107]. Unfortunately, total tryptase is rarely elevated in food-induced anaphylaxis [6, 40]. Mature β-tryptase is a better indicator of mast cell activation, and if the assay for β-tryptase becomes more available, it may prove to be a better indicator of anaphylaxis than total tryptase [88]. Other mediators being evaluated for potential use as a laboratory marker of anaphylaxis include carboxypeptidase and platelet-activating factor (PAF) [88, 111, 112]. A recent study found that PAF levels were elevated in 20%, 66.7%, and 100% of patients with mild, moderate, and severe anaphylactic reactions, respectively, whereas histamine values were increased from 40% to 57% to 70% and tryptase from 0% to 60% across the three grades of anaphylaxis [112].

DBPCFCs are the "gold standard" for diagnosing food allergy, but are contraindicated in patients with an unequivocal history of anaphylaxis following the isolated ingestion of a food to which they have evidence of significant IgE antibodies [40, 111]. However, if several foods were ingested and the patient has positive skin tests to several foods, it is essential that the responsible food be identified. Patients have been reported who experienced repeated anaphylactic reactions because physicians incorrectly assumed that they had identified the responsible food [6]. Young children who experience anaphylactic reactions to foods other than peanuts, tree nuts, fish, and shellfish may eventually outgrow their clinical reactivity, so an oral food challenge may be warranted following an extended period of food elimination with no history of reactions to accidental ingestions.

Treatment

Treatment of food-induced anaphylaxis may be subdivided into acute and long-term management. While management of an acute attack is something physicians spend hours preparing for, it is the long-term measures that provide the best quality of life for the food-allergic patient.

Acute management

Fatalities may occur if treatment of a food-induced anaphylactic reaction is not immediate [5–8], [6] (Table 14.5). Data from the review of fatal bee sting-induced anaphylactic reactions indicate that the longer the initial therapy is delayed, the greater the incidence of complications and fatalities [113]. Although epinephrine is clearly the medicine of first choice for the treatment of anaphylaxis, a multicenter study of United States emergency room visits for food allergies revealed that only 16% of 678 patients presenting to the emergency room with acute allergic reactions to foods received epinephrine. Even in the group determined to have anaphylaxis (51%), only 22% received epinephrine [114]. Initial treatment must be preceded by a rapid assessment to determine the extent and severity of the reaction, the adequacy of oxygenation, cardiac output and tissue perfusion, any potential confounding medications (e.g., β-blockers), and the suspected cause of the reaction [40, 111]. The patient should be placed in the supine position with the legs elevated, if tolerated, to help maintain adequate perfusion and blood pressure [81]. Initial therapy should be directed at the maintenance of an effective airway and circulatory system. The first step in the acute management of anaphylaxis is the intramuscular injection of 0.01 ml/kg of aqueous epinephrine 1:1000 (maximal dose 0.3–0.5 ml, or 0.3–0.5 mg). Intravenous administration of epinephrine may cause fatal arrhythmias or myocardial infarction, particularly in adults, and

Table 14.5 Acute management of anaphylaxis.

Rapid assessment of	extent and severity of symptoms adequacy of oxygenation, cardiac output, and tissue perfusion potential confounding medications suspected cause of the reaction
Initial therapy	**Epinephrine**—0.01 mg/kg/dose up to 0.3–0.5 mg i.m. up to 3 times every 15–20 min (EpiPen®, Twinject®, Auvi-Q®, and epinephrine ampule—1:1000) oxygen—40–100% by mask lie patient in supine position with legs elevated, if tolerated intravenous fluids—30 ml/kg of crystalloid up to 2 l (or more depending upon blood pressure and response to meds)
Secondary medications	nebulized albuterol—may be continous antihistamines: H_1 antagonist (diphenhydramine—1 mg/kg up to 75 mg; cetirizine—0.25 mg/kg up to 10 mg) H_2 antagonist (cimetidine—4 mg/kg up to 300 mg; ranitidine—1–2 mg/kg up to 150 mg) corticosteroids: solumedrol—1–2 mg/kg/dose dopamine—for hypotension refractory to epinephrine (2—20 μg/kg/min) norepinephrine—for hypotension refractory to epinephrine glucagon—(5–15 μg/min) for hypotension refractory to epinephrine and norepinephrine; especially patients on β-blockers
Discharge	Emergency plan and medications Appointment for evaluation of cause if not known

should be reserved for refractory hypotension requiring cardiopulmonary resuscitation [115]. In patients with pulmonary symptoms, supplemental oxygen should be administered.

In order to ensure that patients receive epinephrine as early as possible, it is important that they, their family members, and other care providers are instructed in the self-administration of epinephrine. Preloaded syringes with epinephrine are available and should be given to any patients at risk for food-induced anaphylaxis, that is, patients with a history of a previous anaphylactic reaction and patients with asthma and food allergy, especially if they are allergic to peanuts, nuts, fish, or shellfish. A number of epinephrine autoinjectors are available in the United States, Europe, and Asia, and are mostly intended for a single intramuscular injection. All are obtained in two doses: 0.3 mg for those weighing over 28 kg and 0.15 mg for those weighing less than 28 kg. Children are generally advanced to the 0.3 mg dose when they reach 23 kg–28 kg [40], depending upon the severity of previous reactions. Since parent or caregivers attempting to measure and administer epinephrine from a vial is so inaccurate [116], the 0.15 mg epinephrine dose is often used in small children weighing 8 kg or more. Those individuals who experienced previous severe symptoms should be advanced to the 0.3 mg dose earlier than those with a history of milder reactions. Since most autoinjectors can deliver only a single dose, two autoinjectors may be prescribed for patients who have experienced a previous anaphylactic reaction or who are at high risk and do not have ready access to a medical center. It is imperative that the patient and/or family members practice with appropriate training devices to ensure their ability to use the device proficiently in case of an emergency. Also, it should be made clear to the patients that these preloaded devices carry a 1-year shelf life and therefore should be renewed each year.

Sustained-release preparations of epinephrine are not an appropriate treatment for acute anaphylaxis. While inhaled epinephrine (either nebulized or via metered-dose inhaler) was recommended in the past [117], a study by Simon and coworkers demonstrated that most children and adolescents are unable to inhale sufficient epinephrine to produce adequate systemic levels [118, 119]. Lesser doses may be beneficial to reverse laryngeal edema or persistent bronchospasm.

Once epinephrine has been administered, other therapeutic modalities may be of benefit. Studies have suggested that the combination of an H_1 antihistamine (i.e., diphenhydramine—1 mg/kg up to 75 mg) either intramuscularly or intravenously and an H_2 antihistamine (i.e., 4 mg/kg up to 300 mg of cimetidine) administered intravenously may be more effective than either administered alone [77, 120]. Both histamine antagonists should be infused slowly if given intravenously since rapid infusion of diphenhydramine is associated with arrhythmias and cimetidine with falls in blood pressure. The role of corticosteroids in the treatment of anaphylaxis remains to be established [40, 121]. However, most authorities recommend giving prednisone (1 mg/kg orally) for mild to moderate episodes of anaphylaxis and solumedrol (1–2 mg/kg intravenously) for severe anaphylaxis in an attempt to modulate the late-phase response [11]. Patients who have been receiving glucocorticosteroid therapy for other reasons should be assumed to have hypothalamic–pituitary–adrenal axis suppression and should be administered stress doses of hydrocortisone intravenously during resuscitation. If wheezing is prominent, an aerosolized β-adrenergic agent (e.g., albuterol) is recommended intermittently or continuously, depending upon the patient's symptoms and the availability of cardiac monitoring. Intravenous aminopylline may also be useful for recalcitrant respiratory symptoms. Aerosolized epinephrine may be useful for preventing life-threatening upper airway edema; however, in about 10%, a tracheotomy may be required to prevent fatal laryngeal obstruction [122]. Hypotension, due to a shift in fluid from the intravascular to extravascular space, may be severe and refractory to epinephrine and antihistamines. Laying the patient in the recumbent position (if tolerated) and raising the legs immediately improves cardiovascular return [123]. Depending upon the blood pressure, large volumes of crystalloid (e.g., lactated Ringer's solution or normal saline) infused rapidly are frequently required to reverse the hypotensive state [124]. An alternative to crystalloid solution is the colloid, hydroxyethal starch. Children may need up to 30 ml/kg of crystalloid over the first hour [125] and adults up to 2 l [80] over the first hour to control hypotension. Patients taking β-blockers may require much larger volumes (e.g., 5–7 l) of fluid before pressure is stabilized [126].

Although epinephrine and fluids are the mainstay of treatment for hypotension, the use of other vasopressor drugs may be necessary [40, 77]. Dopamine administered at a rate of 2–20 μg/kg/min while carefully monitoring the blood pressure may be lifesaving. In addition, 1–5 mg of glucagon given as a bolus followed by an infusion of 5–15 μg/min titrated against clinical response may be helpful in refractory cases or in patients taking β-blockers. The best approach to treating patients experiencing anaphylaxis while taking β-adrenergic blocking drugs remains uncertain. If combined β_1 and β_2 receptor blockers (e.g., propranolol) are used, it may be possible to administer epinephrine for its α-adrenergic activity and isoproterenol in an attempt to overcome the β-blockade. Since patients may experience a biphasic response, all patients should be monitored for a minimum of 4 hours, longer in cases of more severe anaphylaxis [40].

Although controversial, some authorities have suggested the use of activated charcoal in an attempt to prevent further absorption of food allergens from the gut [127]. However, the volume required and the disagreeable taste often precludes patients from taking adequate quantities and the consequences of aspiration are grave. Others have suggested that some attempts should be made to evacuate the stomach, if vomiting has not already occurred such as gastric lavage when large amounts of the allergen have been ingested. Whether or not these measures are beneficial in ameliorating food-induced anaphylaxis remain to be demonstrated.

Patients who are at risk for food-induced anaphylaxis should have medical information concerning their condition available on them at all times, for example, MedicAlert™ bracelet or necklace. This information may be lifesaving since it will expedite the diagnosis and appropriate treatment of a patient experiencing an anaphylactic reaction.

Long-term management

The life-threatening nature of anaphylaxis makes prevention the cornerstone of therapy (Table 14.6). If the causative food allergen is not clearly delineated, an evaluation to determine the etiology should be promptly initiated so that a lethal reoccurrence can be prevented, as discussed above. The central focus of prevention of food-induced anaphylaxis requires the appropriate identification and complete dietary avoidance of the specific food allergen [11, 40], especially those at higher risk for anaphylaxis, as discussed previously. An educational process is imperative to ensure the patient and family understand how to avoid all forms of the food allergen and the potential severity of a reaction if the food is inadvertently ingested. *Food Allergy Research and Education* is a nonprofit organization in the United States. (http://www.foodallergy.org) that can assist in providing patients information about food allergen avoidance and which has several programs for schools and parents of children with food allergies and anaphylaxis. Self-injectable epinephrine should be prescribed and patients or parents should be thoroughly educated in the use of the device.

Table 14.6 Long-term management of food-induced anaphylaxis.

Identify positively, food which provoked anaphylactic reaction
Educate patient, family, and/or care providers how to avoid all exposure to food allergen
Provide patient at risk with self-injectable epinephrine and thoroughly teach them when and how to use this medication (i.e., practice with Epi-Pen[R] trainer)
Provide patient with liquid antihistamine (diphenhydramine or hydroxyzine) and teach them when and how to use this medication
Establish a formal ***Emergency Plan*** in case of a reaction: proper use of "emergency medications" transportation to nearest emergency facility (capable of resuscitation and endotracheal tube placement)

It is not uncommon for patients experiencing a previous food-allergic reaction to subsequently demonstrate some instinctive avoidance measure. This may be typified by extreme dislike for the taste or even smell of the offending food. A very proactive role is required for the sensitized person to completely avoid a food that has caused a previous anaphylactic reaction. For many this may even require total removal of the food from the household. Educational measures must be directed at the patient, his or her family, and school personnel, and other caretakers, or fellow workers so that they understand the potential severity and scope of the problem. If a patient ingests a food prepared outside the home, they must always be very cautious and not hesitate to ask very specific and detailed questions concerning ingredients of foods they are planning to eat. Unfortunately, it is not uncommon for patients dining in restaurants to ingest a food that they were assured did not exist in the meal they were eating.

Although changes in food labeling laws in the United States and Europe have simplified somewhat the reading of labels for food-allergic individuals, several problems still remain. These problems fall into one of four categories: (1) misleading labels, for example, "non-dairy" creamers usually contain some milk proteins; (2) ingredient switches, for example, a name brand food may alter the ingredients with no significant change on the label; (3) "natural flavoring" designation often allows a product to contain a small amount of other food proteins for purposes of flavoring without having to identify that protein, for example, casein in canned tuna fish; and (4) inadvertent contamination which may occur when more than one product is run on a line and residual protein from the previous run adulterates the subsequent run, for example, non-dairy ice cream desserts. It is still imperative that patients and their families scrupulously read all labels of products because certain food allergens may unexpectedly occur.

Prognosis

For many young children diagnosed with anaphylaxis to foods such as milk, egg, wheat, and soybeans, there is good possibility that the clinical sensitivity may be outgrown after several years. Children who develop their food sensitivity after 3 years of age are less likely to lose their food reactions over a several year period. Approximately 20% of children who develop peanut allergy early in life [54, 55] will outgrow this sensitivity. There are rare reports of children who appear to outgrow their peanut allergy only to have allergic reactivity recur at a later date [128, 129]. Allergies to foods such as tree nuts, fish, and seafood are generally not outgrown and these individuals appear likely to retain their allergic sensitivity for a lifetime [48]. With better characterization of allergens and understanding of the immunologic mechanism involved in this reaction, investigators have developed several therapeutic modalities potentially applicable to the treatment and eventual prevention of food allergy. Among the therapeutic options currently under investigation, there is peptide immunotherapy, mutated allergen protein immunotherapy, DNA immunization, immunization with immunostimulatory sequences, a Chinese herbal formulation, and anti-IgE therapy [130, 131]. These novel forms of treatment for allergic disease hold promise for the safe and effective treatment of food-allergic individuals and the prevention of food allergy in the future.

References

1. Sheffer A. Anaphylaxis. *J Allergy Clin Immunol* 1985; 75(2):227–233.
2. Portier P, Richet C. De l'action anaphylactique de certains venins. *C R Soc Biol (Paris)* 1902; 54:170–172.
3. Anderson J, Sogn DD. (eds) *Adverse Reactions to Foods*, National Institute of Allergy & Infectious Disease, NIH Publication No 84-2442, Bethesda, MD, 1984.
4. Golbert TM, Patterson R, Pruzansky JJ. Systemic allergic reactions to ingested antigens. *J Allergy* 1969; 44(2):96–107.
5. Yunginger JW, Sweeney KG, Sturner WQ, et al. Fatal food-induced anaphylaxis. *J Am Med Assoc* 1988; 260:1450–1452.
6. Sampson HA, Mendelson LM, Rosen JP. Fatal and near-fatal anaphylactic reactions to food in children and adolescents. *N Engl J Med* 1992; 327:380–384.
7. Bock SA, Munoz-Furlong A, Sampson HA. Fatalities due to anaphylactic reactions to foods. *J Allergy Clin Immunol* 2001; 107(1):191–193.
8. Bock SA, Munoz-Furlong A, Sampson HA. Further fatalities caused by anaphylactic reactions to food, 2001–2006. *J Allergy Clin Immunol* 2007; 119(4):1016–1018.
9. Gonzalez-Perez A, Aponte Z, Vidaurre CF, et al. Anaphylaxis epidemiology in patients with and patients without asthma: a United Kingdom database review. *J Allergy Clin Immunol* 2010; 125(5):1098–1104.
10. Liew WK, Williamson E, Tang ML. Anaphylaxis fatalities and admissions in Australia. *J Allergy Clin Immunol* 2009; 123(2):434–442.
11. Sampson HA, Munoz-Furlong A, Bock A, et al. Symposium on the definition and management of anaphylaxis: summary report. *J Allergy Clin Immunol* 2005; 115(3):584–591.
12. Lieberman P. Biphasic anaphylactic reactions. *Ann Allergy Asthma Immunol* 2005; 95(3):217–226.
13. Lieberman P. Anaphylaxis. *Med Clin North Am* 2006; 90(1):77–95.
14. Sampson HA. Anaphylaxis and emergency treatment. *Pediatrics* 2003; 111(6 Pt 3):1601–1608.
15. Sicherer SH, Sampson HA. Food allergy. *J Allergy Clin Immunol* 2006; 117(2):S470–S475.
16. Du TG. Food-dependent exercise-induced anaphylaxis in childhood. *Pediatr Allergy Immunol* 2007; 18(5):455–463.
17. Sampson HA, Munoz-Furlong A, Campbell RL, et al. Second symposium on the definition and management of anaphylaxis: summary report–Second National Institute of Allergy and Infectious Disease/Food Allergy and Anaphylaxis Network Symposium. *J Allergy Clin Immunol* 2006; 117(2):391–397.
18. Campbell RL, Hagan JB, Manivannan V, et al. Evaluation of national institute of allergy and infectious diseases/food allergy and anaphylaxis network criteria for the diagnosis of anaphylaxis in emergency department patients. *J Allergy Clin Immunol* 2012; 129(3):748–752.
19. Klein JS, Yocum MW. Underreporting of anaphylaxis in a community emergency room. *J Allergy Clin Immunol* 1995; 95(2):637–638.
20. Sorensen H, Nielsen B, Nielsen J. Anaphylactic shock occurring outside hospitals. *Allergy* 1989; 44:288–290.
21. Yocum MW, Khan DA. Assessment of patients who have experienced anaphylaxis: a 3-year survey. *Mayo Clin Proc* 1994; 69:16–23.
22. Decker WW, Campbell RL, Manivannan V, et al. The etiology and incidence of anaphylaxis in Rochester, Minnesota: a report from the Rochester Epidemiology Project. *J Allergy Clin Immunol* 2008; 122(6):1161–1165.
23. Pumphrey RSH, Stanworth SJ. The clinical spectrum of anaphylaxis in north-west England. *Clin Exper Allergy* 1996; 26:1364–1370.

24. Moneret-Vautrin DA, Kanny G. Food-induced anaphylaxis. A new French multicenter survey. *Ann Gastroenterol Hepatol (Paris)* 1995; 31(4):256–263.
25. Novembre E, Cianferoni A, Bernardini R, et al. Anaphylaxis in children: clinical and allergologic features. *Pediatrics* 1998; 101(4):E8.
26. Boros CA, Kay D, Gold MS. Parent reported allergy and anaphylaxis in 4173 south Australian children. *J Paediatr Child Health* 2000; 36(1):36–40.
27. Simons FER, Chad Z, Gold MS. Anaphylaxis in children: realtime reporting from a national network. *Allergy Clin Immunol Int-J World Allergy Org* 2004; (Suppl):242–244.
28. Braganza SC, Acworth JP, Mckinnon DRL, et al. Paediatric emergency department anaphylaxis: different patterns from adults. *Arch Dis Child* 2006; 91(2):159–163.
29. Brown AF, McKinnon D, Chu K. Emergency department anaphylaxis: a review of 142 patients in a single year. *J Allergy Clin Immunol* 2001; 108(5):861–866.
30. Dohi M, Suko M, Sugiyama H, et al. Food-dependent, exercise-induced anaphylaxis: a study on 11 Japanese cases. *J Allergy Clin Immunol* 1991; 87(1 Pt 1):34–40.
31. Horan R, Sheffer A. Food-dependent, exercise-induced anaphylaxis. *Immunol Allergy Clin North Am* 1991; 11:757–766.
32. Romano M, di Fonso M, Guiffreda F, et al. Food-dependent exercise-induced anaphylaxis: clinical and laboratory findings in 54 subjects. *Int Arch Allergy Appl Immunol* 2001; 125(3):264–272.
33. Morita E, Kunie K, Matsuo H. Food-dependent exercise-induced anaphylaxis. *J Dermatol Sci* 2007; 47(2):109–117.
34. Aihara Y, Takahashi Y, Kotoyori T, et al. Frequency of food-dependent, exercise-induced anaphylaxis in Japanese junior-high-school students. *J Allergy Clin Immunol* 2001; 108(6):1035–1039.
35. Teo SL, Gerez IF, Ang EY, et al. Food-dependent exercise-induced anaphylaxis—a review of 5 cases. *Ann Acad Med Singapore* 2009; 38(10):905–909.
36. Maulitz R, Pratt D, Schocket A. Exercise-induced anaphylactic reaction to shellfish. *J Allergy Clin Immunol* 1979; 63(6):433–434.
37. Kushimito H, Aoki T. Masked type I wheat allergy.Relation to exercise-induced anaphylaxis. *Arch Dermatol* 1985; 121(3):355–360.
38. Asero R, Mistrello G, Roncarolo D, et al. Lipid transfer protein: a pan-allergen in plant-derived foods that is highly resistant to pepsin digestion. *Int Arch Allergy Immunol* 2000; 122(1):20–32.
39. Novey HS, Fairshter RD, Sainess K, et al. Postprandial exercise-induced anaphylaxis. *J Allergy Clin Immunol* 1983; 71(5):498–504.
40. Boyce JA, Assa'ad A, Burks AW, et al. Guidelines for the diagnosis and management of food allergy in the United States: report of the NIAID-sponsored expert panel. *J Allergy Clin Immunol* 2010; 126(6 Suppl):S1–S58.
41. Harada S, Horikawa T, Ashida M, et al. Aspirin enhances the induction of type I allergic symptoms when combined with food and exercise in patients with food-dependent exercise-induced anaphylaxis. *Br J Dermatol* 2001; 145(2):336–339.
42. Aihara M, Miyazawa M, Osuna H, et al. Food-dependent exercise-induced anaphylaxis: influence of concurrent aspirin administration on skin testing and provocation. *Br J Dermatol* 2002; 146(3):466–472.
43. Matsuo H, Morimoto K, Akaki T, et al. Exercise and aspirin increase levels of circulating gliadin peptides in patients with wheat-dependent exercise-induced anaphylaxis. *Clin Exp Allergy* 2005; 35(4):461–466.
44. Iribarren C, Tolstykh IV, Miller MK, et al. Asthma and the prospective risk of anaphylactic shock and other allergy diagnoses in a large integrated health care delivery system. *Ann Allergy Asthma Immunol* 2010; 104(5):371–377.
45. Atkins FM, Steinberg SS, Metcalfe DD. Evaluation of immediate adverse reactions to foods in adult patients. II. A detailed analysis of reaction patterns during oral food challenge. *J Allergy Clin Immunol* 1985; 75:356–363.
46. de Martino M, Novembre E, Cozza G, et al. Sensitivity to tomato and peanut allergens in children monosensitized to grass pollen. *Allergy* 1988; 43(3):206–213.
47. Sicherer SH, Furlong TJ, Maes HH, et al. Genetics of peanut allergy: a twin study. *J Allergy Clin Immunol* 2000; 106(1 Pt 1):53–56.
48. Sicherer SH, Sampson HA. Food allergy. *J Allergy Clin Immunol* 2010; 125(Suppl 2):S116–S125.
49. Sampson HA, Scanlon SM. Natural history of food hypersensitivity in children with atopic dermatitis. *J Pediatr* 1989; 115:23–27.
50. Wood RA. The natural history of food allergy. *Pediatrics* 2003; 111(6 Pt 3):1631–1637.
51. Cantani A, Micera M. Natural history of cow's milk allergy. An eight-year follow-up study in 115 atopic children. *Eur Rev Med Pharmacol Sci* 2004; 8(4):153–164.
52. Host A. Cow's milk protein allergy and intolerance in infancy. *Pediatr Allergy Immunol* 1994; 5(Suppl 5):5–36.
53. Bock SA, Atkins FM. The natural history of peanut allergy. *J Allergy Clin Immunol* 1989; 83:900–904.
54. Hourihane JO, Roberts SA, Warner JO. Resolution of peanut allergy: case-control study. *BMJ* 1998; 316(7140):1271–1275.
55. Skolnick HS, Conover-Walker MK, Koerner CB, et al. The natural history of peanut allergy. *J Allergy Clin Immunol* 2001; 107(2):367–374.
56. Fleischer DM, Conover-Walker MK, Matsui EC, et al. The natural history of tree nut allergy. *J Allergy Clin Immunol* 2005; 116(5):1087–1093.
57. Sampson HA. Clinical practice. Peanut allergy. *N Engl J Med* 2002; 346(17):1294–1299.
58. Settipane G. Anaphylactic deaths in asthmatic patients. *Allergy Proc* 1989; 10:271–274.
59. Sampson HA. Update of food allergy. *J Allergy Clin Immun* 2004; 113(5):805–819.
60. Sicherer SH, Burks AW, Sampson HA. Clinical features of acute allergic reactions to peanut and tree nuts in children. *Pediatrics* 1998; 102(1):e6.
61. Sicherer SH, Munoz-Furlong A, Burks AW, et al. Prevalence of peanut and tree nut allergy in the United States of America. *J Allergy Clin Immun* 1999; 103(4):559–562.
62. Lack G, Fox D, Northstone K, et al. Factors associated with the development of peanut allergy in childhood. *N Engl J Med* 2003; 348(11):977–985.

63. Fox AT, Sasieni P, Du TG, et al. Household peanut consumption as a risk factor for the development of peanut allergy. *J Allergy Clin Immunol* 2009; 123(2):417–423.
64. Moneret-Vautrin D, Beaudouin E, Widmer S, et al. Prospective study of risk factors in natural rubber latex hypersensitivity. *J Allergy Clin Immunol* 1993; 92(5):668–677.
65. Warner JA, Miles EA, Jones AC, et al. Is deficiency of interferon gamma production by allergen triggered cord blood cells a predictor of atopic eczema? *Clin Exp Allergy* 1994; 24(5):423–430.
66. Prenner BM, Stevens JJ. Anaphylaxis after ingestion of sodium bisulfite. *Ann Allergy* 1976; 37(3): 180–182.
67. Twarog FJ, Leung DY. Anaphylaxis to a component of isoetharine (sodium bisulfite). *J Am Med Assoc* 1982; 248(16):2030–2031.
68. Clayton D, Busse W. Anaphylaxis to wine. *Clin Allergy* 1980; 10(3):341–343.
69. Ebo DG, Ingelbrecht S, Bridts CH, et al. Allergy for cheese: evidence for an IgE-mediated reaction from the natural dye annatto. *Allergy* 2009; 64(10):1558–1560.
70. James JM, Cooke SK, Barnett A, et al. Anaphylactic reactions to a psyllium-containing cereal. *J Allergy Clin Immunol* 1991; 88:402–408.
71. Papanikolaou I, Stenger R, Bessot JC, et al. Anaphylactic shock to guar gum (food additive E412) contained in a meal substitute. *Allergy* 2007; 62(7):822.
72. Lee JM, Greenes DS. Biphasic anaphylactic reactions in pediatrics. *Pediatrics* 2000; 106(4):762–766.
73. Webb LM, Lieberman P. Anaphylaxis: a review of 601 cases. *Ann Allergy Asthma Immunol* 2006; 97(1):39–43.
74. Tole JW, Lieberman P. Biphasic anaphylaxis: review of incidence, clinical predictors, and observation recommendations. *Immunol Allergy Clin North Am* 2007; 27(2):309–326.
75. Gold MS, Sainsbury R. First aid anaphylaxis management in children who were prescribed an epinephrine autoinjector device (EpiPen). *J Allergy Clin Immunol* 2000; 106(1 Pt 1):171–176.
76. Sampson HA. Anaphylaxis and emergency treatment. *Pediatrics* 2004; 111(6):1601–1608.
77. Lieberman P, Nicklas RA, Oppenheimer J, et al. The diagnosis and management of anaphylaxis practice parameter: 2010 update. *J Allergy Clin Immunol* 2010; 126(3):477–480.
78. Brown SGA. Clinical features and severity grading of anaphylaxis. *J Allergy Clin Immunol* 2004; 114(2):371–376.
79. Fisher MM. Clinical observations on the pathophysiology and treatment of anaphylactic cardiovascular collapse. *Anaesth Intensive Care* 1986; 14(1):17–21.
80. Brown SGA. Cardiovascular aspects of anaphylaxis: implications for treatment and diagnosis. *Curr Opin Allergy Clin Immunol* 2005; 5(4):359–364.
81. Pumphrey RSH. Fatal posture in anaphylactic shock. *J Allergy Clin Immunol* 2003; 112(2):451–452.
82. Kivity S, Yarchovsky J. Relapsing anaphylaxis to bee sting in a patient treated with B-blocker and Ca blocker. *J Allergy Clin Immunol* 1990; 85(3):669–670.
83. Settipane G, Chafee R, Klein DE, et al. Anaphylactic reactions to Hymenoptera stings in asthmatic patients. *Clin Allergy* 1980; 10(6):659–665.
84. Lockey R, Benedict L, Turkeltaub P, et al. Fatalities form immunotherapy and skin testing. *J Allergy Clin Immunol* 1987; 79:660–667.
85. Reid MJ, Lockey RF, Turkeltaub PC, et al. Survey of fatalities from skin testing and immunotherapy 1985–1989. *J Allergy Clin Immunol* 1993; 92(1 Pt 1):6–15.
86. Yocum MW, Butterfield JH, Klein JS, et al. Epidemiology of anaphylaxis in Olmsted County: a population-based study. *J Allergy Clin Immunol* 1999; 104:452–456.
87. Helbling A, Hurni T, Mueller UR, et al. Incidence of anaphylaxis with circulatory symptoms: a study over a 3-year period comprising 940,000 inhabitants of the Swiss Canton Bern. *Clin Exp Allergy* 2004; 34(2):285–290.
88. Simons FE, Frew AJ, Ansotegui IJ, et al. Risk assessment in anaphylaxis: current and future approaches. *J Allergy Clin Immunol* 2007; 120 1(Suppl):S2–S24.
89. Simons FE. Anaphylaxis: recent advances in assessment and treatment. *J Allergy Clin Immunol* 2009; 124(4):625–636.
90. Gern J, Yang E, Evrard H, et al. Allergic reactions to milk-contaminated "nondairy" products. *N Engl J Med* 1991; 324:976–979.
91. Tricker ND, Malone KM, Ellis MM. Hereditary angioedema: a case report and literature review. *Gen Dent* 2002; 50(6):540–543.
92. Frank MM. Hereditary angioedema: the clinical syndrome and its management in the United States. *Immunol Allergy Clin North Am* 2006; 26(4):653–668.
93. Alboni P, Brignole M, Degli Uberti EC. Is vasovagal syncope a disease? *Europace* 2007; 9(2):83–87.
94. Wakita R, Ohno Y, Yamazaki S, et al. Vasovagal syncope with asystole associated with intravenous access. *Oral Surg Oral Med Oral Pathol Oral Radiol Endod* 2006; 102(6):e28–e32.
95. Settipane G, Chafee F. Natural history of allergy of Hymenoptera. *Clin Allergy* 1979; 9:385–390.
96. Ortolani C, Ispano M, Pastorello EA, et al. Comparison of results of skin prick tests (with fresh foods and commercial food extracts) and RAST in 100 patients with oral allergy syndrome. *J Allergy Clin Immunol* 1989; 83(3):683–690.
97. Rosen JP, Selcow JE, Mendelson LM, et al. Skin testing with natural foods in patients suspected of having food allergies: is it a necessity? *J Allergy Clin Immunol* 1994; 93:1068–1070.
98. Stricker WE, Anorve-Lopez E, Reed CE. Food skin testing in patients with idiopathic anaphylaxis. *J Allergy Clin Immunol* 1986; 77(3):516–519.
99. Bock S, Buckley J, Holst A, et al. Proper use of skin tests with food extracts in diagnosis of food hypersensitivity. *Clin Allergy* 1978;8:559–564.
100. Gronlund H, Adedoyin J, Commins SP, et al. The carbohydrate galactose-alpha-1,3-galactose is a major IgE-binding epitope on cat IgA. *J Allergy Clin Immunol* 2009; 123(5):1189–1191.
101. Commins SP, Satinover SM, Hosen J, et al. Delayed anaphylaxis, angioedema, or urticaria after consumption of red meat in patients with IgE antibodies specific for galactose-alpha-1,3-galactose. *J Allergy Clin Immunol* 2009; 123(2):426–433.
102. Lockey RF. Adverse reactions associated with skin testing and immunotherapy. *Allergy Proc* 1995; 16(6):293–296.

103. Sampson HA. Utility of food-specific IgE concentrations in predicting symptomatic food allergy. *J Allergy Clin Immunol* 2001; 107(5):891–896.
104. Yunginger JW, Ahlstedt S, Eggleston PA, et al. Quantitative IgE antibody assays in allergic diseases. *J Allergy Clin Immunol* 2000; 105(6 Pt 1):1077–1084.
105. Komata T, Soderstrom L, Borres MP, et al. The predictive relationship of food-specific serum IgE concentrations to challenge outcomes for egg and milk varies by patient age. *J Allergy Clin Immunol* 2007; 119(5):1272–1274.
106. Shreffler WG, Beyer K,Chu TH, et al. Microarray immunoassay: association of clinical history, in vitro IgE function, and heterogeneity of allergenic peanut epitopes. *J Allergy Clin Immun* 2004; 113(4):776–782.
107. Schwartz L, Metcalfe DD, Miller J, et al. Tryptase levels as an indicator of mast-cell activation in systemic anaphylaxis and mastocytosis. *N Engl J Med* 1987; 316(26):1622–1626.
108. Schwartz LB, Yunginger JW, Miller J, et al. Time course of appearance and disappearance of human mast cell tryptase in the circulation after anaphylaxis. *J Clin Invest* 1989; 83(5):1551–1555.
109. Lin RY, Schwartz LB, Curry A, et al. Histamine and tryptase levels in patients with acute allergic reactions: an emergency department-based study. *J Allergy Clin Immunol* 2000; 106(1 Pt 1):65–71.
110. Brown SG, Blackmean KE, Heddle RJ. Can serum mast cell tryptase help diagnose anaphylaxis? *Emerg Med Australas* 2004; 16(2):120–124.
111. Simons FE, Ardusso LR, Bilo MB, et al. 2012 Update: World Allergy Organization Guidelines for the assessment and management of anaphylaxis. *Curr Opin Allergy Clin Immunol* 2012; 12(4):389–399.
112. Vadas P, Perelman B, Liss G. Platelet-activating factor, histamine, and tryptase levels in human anaphylaxis. *J Allergy Clin Immunol* 2013; 131(1):144–149.
113. Barnard J. Studies of 400 Hymentoptera sting deaths in the United States. *J Allergy Clin Immunol* 1973; 52:259–264.
114. Clark S, Bock SA, Gaeta TJ, et al. Multicenter study of emergency department visits for food allergies. *J Allergy Clin Immun* 2004; 113(2):347–352.
115. Brown SG, Blackmean KE, Stenlake V, et al. Insect sting anaphylaxis; prospective evaluation of treatment with intravenous adrenaline and volume resuscitation. *Emerg Med J* 2004; 21:149–154.
116. Simons FE, Chan ES, Gu X, et al. Epinephrine for the out-of-hospital (first-aid) treatment of anaphylaxis in infants: is the ampule/syringe/needle method practical? *J Allergy Clin Immunol* 2001; 108(6):1040–1044.
117. Muller U, Mosbech H, Aberer W, et al. EAACI position statement: adrenaline for emergency kits. *Allergy* 1995; 50:783–787.
118. Simons FE, Gu X, Johnston LM, et al. Can epinephrine inhalations be substituted for epinephrine injection in children at risk for systemic anaphylaxis? *Pediatrics* 2000; 106(5):1040–1044.
119. Warren JB, Doble N, Dalton N, et al. Systemic absorption of inhaled epinephrine. *Clin Pharmacol Ther* 1986; 40(6):673–678.
120. Simons FE. Anaphylaxis. *J Allergy Clin Immunol* 2010; 125(Suppl 2):S161–S181.
121. Choo KJ, Simons FE, Sheikh A. Glucocorticoids for the treatment of anaphylaxis. *Cochrane Database Syst Rev* 2012; 4:CD007596.
122. Delage C, Irey NS. Anaphylactic deaths: a clinicopathologic study of 43 cases. *J Forensic Sci* 1972; 17(4):525–540.
123. Simons FE. Anaphylaxis pathogenesis and treatment. *Allergy* 2011; 66(Suppl 95):31–34.
124. Brown AF. Anaphylactic shock:mechanisms and treatment. *J Accid Emerg Med* 1995; 12(2):89–100.
125. Saryan J, O'Loughlin J. Anaphylaxis in children. *Pediatr Ann* 1992; 21:590–598.
126. Eon B, Papazian L, Gouin F. Management of anaphylactic and anaphylactoid reactions during anesthesia. *Clin Rev Allergy* 1991; 9(3–4):415–429.
127. Vadas P, Perelman B. Activated charcoal forms non-IgE binding complexes with peanut proteins. *J Allergy Clin Immunol* 2003; 112(1):175–179.
128. Busse PJ, Nowak-Wegrzyn A, Noone SA, et al. Recurrent peanut allergy. *N Engl J Med* 2002; 347(19):1535–1538.
129. Fleischer DM, Connover-Walker MK, Christie L, et al. Peanut allergy: recurrence and its management. *J Allergy Clin Immunol* 2004; 114(5):1195–1202.
130. Nowak-Wegrzyn A, Sampson HA. Future therapies for food allergies. *J Allergy Clin Immunol* 2011; 127(3):558–573.
131. Wang J, Sampson HA. Treatments for food allergy: how close are we? *Immunol Res* 2012; 54(1–3):83–94.

15 Infantile Colic and Food Allergy

Ralf G. Heine[1,2,3] & David J. Hill[2]

[1]Department of Allergy & Immunology, Royal Children's Hospital, Melbourne, Australia
[2]Murdoch Childrens Research Institute, Melbourne, Australia
[3]Department of Paediatrics, The University of Melbourne, Melbourne, Australia

Key Concepts

- The term "infantile colic" describes episodes of paroxysmal unexplained crying and fussing (for more than 3 hours per day) in otherwise healthy young infants.
- Colic symptoms typically start in the first weeks of life and gradually resolve around 4–5 months of age.
- Although the etiology of colic is multifactorial, there is increasing evidence linking this condition to gastrointestinal food protein allergies (non-IgE-mediated).
- In breast-fed infants, hypersensitivity reactions may be caused by ingestion of intact food proteins contained in breast milk.
- In formula-fed infants, extensively hydrolyzed (casein- or whey-predominant) or amino acid-based formulas have been shown to improve colic symptoms, whereas soy, partially hydrolyzed or lactose-free cow's milk formulas offered no therapeutic benefit.
- Maternal elimination diets have been shown to significantly reduce the crying duration in breast-fed infants with colic.
- Several recent randomized trials on the effect of probiotic supplementation in young infants with colic have demonstrated a significant reduction in crying duration.

Introduction

Persistent crying is a common pediatric problem that affects more than 20% of young infants [1]. In the majority, the distressed behavior commences at 2 weeks of age, peaks at about 6 weeks, and gradually resolves around 4–5 months of age [2, 3]. A Canadian study showed that 6.4% of infants still had colic at 3 months of age [4]. Although the etiology of infantile colic is multifactorial, there is increasing evidence linking persistent crying and distress in the young infant to food allergy [5, 6]. Interactive factors and behavior patterning also influence the clinical course of infantile colic [7].

Crying and fussing, especially in the evening, are normal developmental phenomena in the first months of life [2]. Unexplained paroxysms of irritability, fussing, or crying that persist for more than 3 hours per day, for more than 3 days per week, and for at least 3 weeks are considered a separate clinical condition termed "colic" [3, 8]. During such episodes, the legs may be drawn up to the abdomen and the infant may become flushed. Abdominal distension and increased passage of flatus are often noted. Parents may attribute these episodes to pain. However, the infant appears generally well, and it has been estimated that in about 5% of infants an underlying medical etiology can be identified [7, 9].

Epidemiology of colic

Prevalence figures for infantile colic vary greatly, depending on the definition of colic and recruitment method used in epidemiological studies [1]. No population-based prevalence study, using generally accepted diagnostic criteria for colic, has to date been performed. Many studies are biased toward severe colic or families presenting in crisis [1]. For example, mothers with depressive symptoms may be more likely to seek help for their crying infant [10, 11]. In addition, parents perceive persistent crying as more worrisome if there are associated symptoms such as regurgitation [12] or feeding difficulties [13] which may lead to an

Food Allergy: Adverse Reactions to Foods and Food Additives, Fifth Edition. Edited by Dean D Metcalfe, Hugh A Sampson, Ronald A Simon and Gideon Lack.

Table 15.1 Prevalence of infantile colic.

Author	Country	Year	Prevalence (%)
Hide and Guyer [14]	England	1982	16
Rubin and Prendergast [15]	England	1984	26
Carey [16]	United States	1984	10
Michelsson et al. [17]	Finland	1990	14
Hogdall et al. [18]	Denmark	1991	19
Rautava et al. [11]	Finland	1993	28
Lehtonen and Korvenranta [19]	Finland	1995	13
Canivet et al. [20]	Sweden	1996	11
Canivet et al. [21]	Sweden	2002	9.4
Clifford et al. [22]	Canada	2002	24
Wake et al. [23]	Australia	2006	19.1

overestimate of underlying medical conditions. Table 15.1 shows the prevalence of colic reported from several Western countries.

Clinical classification of crying syndromes

The etiology of infantile colic is multifactorial, and our understanding of the mechanisms leading to distressed behavior in early infancy is incomplete. The term "colic" implies that the infants' distress is related to visceral pain or spasm, although this mechanism has never been conclusively demonstrated. Therefore, alternative terms such as "persistent crying" or "distressed behavior" have been used.

In the following discussion, the term "colic" will be used interchangeably with each of these terms while not implying a particular pathological mechanism.

Barr has suggested four main crying syndromes in infancy [7]. These syndromes may overlap clinically:

- Infantile colic
- Persistent mother–infant-distress syndrome
- The temperamentally "difficult" infant
- The dysregulated infant

According to this model, infantile colic is considered part of normal emotional development, in which an infant displays diminished capacity to regulate crying duration [7]. If colic is unresolved for several weeks, this may lead to disturbances in the mother–infant relationship that is the persistent mother–infant-distress syndrome; this group often presents with associated organic manifestations, including feeding difficulties [13, 24], gastroesophageal reflux (GER) [24–27], esophagitis [28], lactose malabsorption [29, 30], or gastrointestinal motility disturbance [31]. Many of these manifestations have been linked to food protein allergy [25, 31]. The temperamentally "difficult" infant may be predisposed to negative affect and have an increased tendency for persistent crying. The last category, the "dysregulated" infant, is thought to have a central dysregulation leading to poor self-calming, poor tolerance to change, and hyperalert arousal [7].

Infantile and parental factors associated with infantile colic

Infantile factors

Brazelton [2] used parental recording on cry charts to document the natural history of distressed behavior in infancy [2, 8]. Barr et al. [32] developed 24-hour cry charts which they validated against voice-activated audiotape recordings of crying infants. Using these validated cry charts, Hunziker and Barr [33] confirmed Brazelton's [2] findings.

There are significant differences in the pattern and duration of distressed behavior of colicky and non-colicky infants [34]. Figure 15.1 shows the higher levels of distressed behavior in the colicky infants compared to non-colicky infants. The evaluation of distressed behavior on an hour-by-hour basis found a predominance of nocturnal symptoms, but prolonged episodes of crying also occurred during other periods of the day. These prolonged and inconsolable episodes of crying appear to be features that are specific for infantile colic in the first weeks of life [35]. It is important to distinguish colic symptoms from sleep-waking problems which are also a common concern in young infants. Evidence from longitudinal studies suggests that infants with colic symptoms around 5–6 weeks of age generally do not have a sleep problem at 12 weeks of age, suggesting different etiologies for colic and persistent sleep-waking problems in early infancy [36].

Children with a past history of colic are at increased risk of experiencing negative emotions, negative moods during meals and more likely to report abdominal pain in early childhood, suggesting that infant temperament may be a factor contributing to infantile colic [37]. However,

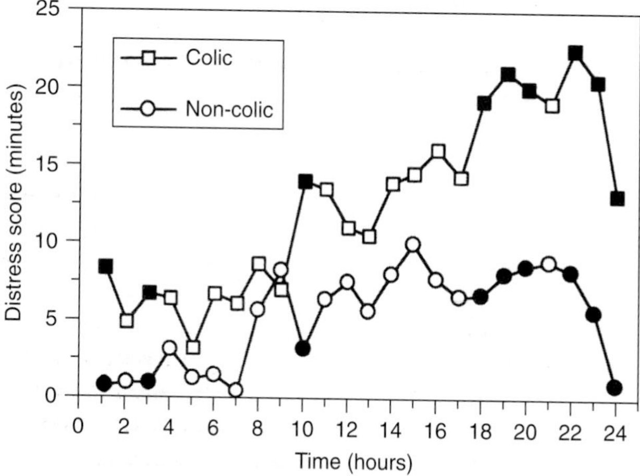

Figure 15.1 Comparison of diurnal variation in distress scores for infants with and without colic; hourly mean duration of crying and fussing time, recorded over 24 hours. Filled symbols mark periods with a significant difference in crying and fussing between groups ($p < 0.05$). From Reference 34.

the majority of colicky infants will develop normal parent–child relationships. Only a small number will progress to a more generalized "persistent mother–infant-distress syndrome" [38]. An Australian study of distressed infants found that persistent crying and sleep problems in the first 2 years of life are usually transient [23]. A 10-year follow-up study of 96 infants with a history of infantile colic found a high prevalence of recurrent abdominal pain, allergic disorders, and psychological abnormalities [39]. Another follow-up study of 75 school-age children with a history of hospitalization for severe colic reported a significantly higher prevalence of mental health problems and mental disorders, compared to community controls [40]. Unremitting, severe persistent crying beyond 3 months of age may also be a marker of cognitive deficits in later childhood [41].

Maternal factors

The unpredictable, prolonged, and unexplained nature of crying in colicky infants is a source of great concern and anxiety for parents [42, 43]. Maternal anxiety during late pregnancy has been shown to be a risk factor for infantile colic [44]. Studies by Rautava et al. in Finnish infants suggested an association between colic and maternal distress during pregnancy and childbirth or unsatisfactory sexual relationships, but not between colic and sociodemographic factors [11, 45]. Mothers who report excessive infant crying are also more likely to perceive a lack of positive reinforcement from their infant [46].

Maternal report of a sleep problem in their infant was significantly associated with depressive symptoms [10, 47]. This may indicate that maternal depressive symptoms during the early infant period are caused by, or compounded by, sleep deprivation [47]. A recent study reported that persistent, rather than transient, infant distress was associated with maternal depression and parent stress [23].

Behavior interventions and parental support

Several studies have assessed the importance of behavioral and interactive factors in infantile colic. Taubman [48] compared parental counseling and dietary interventions in a study of 21 colicky infants. He found that increasing parental responsiveness had a similar effect on persistent crying as the introduction of a cow's milk-free diet. Interestingly, the distressed behavior of diet-responsive colicky infants decreased further with parental counseling.

Barr et al. [49] studied the effect of supplemental carrying in 66 colicky infants. In 6-week-old colicky infants, a significant treatment benefit of supplemental carrying could not be demonstrated, whereas non-colicky crying improved. Wolke et al. [50] examined the effect of different supportive strategies in 92 mothers of infants with colic. After 3 months, infant distress had improved in all patients. Infants of mothers who had received advice on behavior modification improved their distress by 51%, compared with 37% in infants of mothers who were receiving empathic support, and 35% in the control group.

Colic as a manifestation of food protein allergy

Cow's milk is one of the first food allergens that is introduced into the diet of infants. Cow's milk allergy (CMA) therefore represents one of the first allergic manifestations in early infancy which affects about 2% of infants. Early studies have demonstrated a high prevalence of colic in infants with CMA. In a sequential cohort of 100 patients with challenge-proven CMA, 44% of infants displayed irritable and colicky behavior during the cow's milk challenge [51]. Several trials have since demonstrated a treatment benefit for soy and extensively hydrolyzed formulae in infants with colic, even when no other symptoms of food protein allergy were evident [52–58].

Differences between breast- and formula-fed infants

In contrast to breast-fed infants, formula-fed infants often develop infantile colic before 6 weeks of age [2, 59]. There are significant differences in the diurnal variation of distressed behavior between breast- and formula-fed infants. While total distress levels were similar over a 24-hour period, formula-fed infants showed significantly more distress in the morning hours than breast-fed infants, whereas breast-fed infants were more distressed in the afternoon (Fig. 15.2) [34, 60]. Axelsson et al. [61] noted that about 4 hours after maternal cow's milk ingestion, beta-lactoglobulin appeared in breast milk, and the highest concentrations were found in breast milk 8–12 hours after ingestion. Paganelli et al. [62] demonstrated that cow's

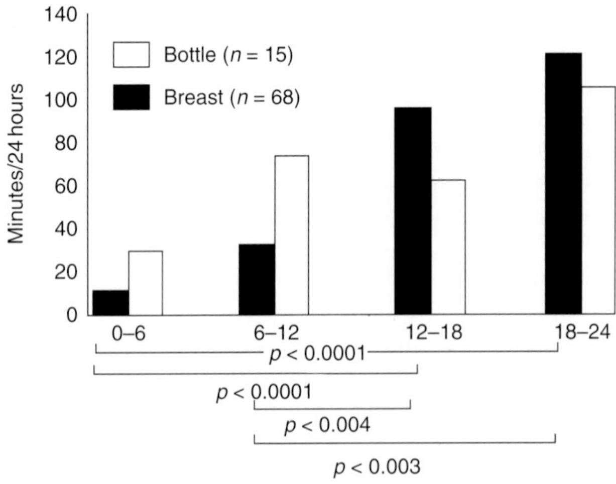

Figure 15.2 Bottle-fed infants show more distress before midday, whereas breast-fed infants have significantly more distress in the afternoon and evening. From Reference 60.

milk antigen appeared in serum within 1 hour of ingestion. Thus, formula feeding with a large dose of ingested antigens may elicit a more rapid distress response than prolonged low-dose antigen exposure through breast milk. A recent study in 94 mother–infant dyads suggests that breast-fed infants have a significantly lower incidence of colic, lower severity of colic symptoms, and longer nocturnal sleep duration, compared to formula-fed infants [63]. The authors of that study speculated that melatonin in breast milk may ameliorate colic symptoms in young infants.

Food allergy in breast-fed infants

Breast milk contains a range of intact food proteins (e.g., cow's milk, egg, peanut, or wheat) that may elicit immune responses via the neonatal gut-associated lymphatic tissue (GALT) [64–68]. Food allergic reactions via breast milk have been demonstrated after maternal cow's milk challenge [69]. Infants with multiple food protein allergy (MFPA), a rare form of non-IgE-mediated food allergy and impaired tolerance development, present with severe persistent crying [70–73]. These infants develop severe irritability after ingestion of breast milk or formula, that is, cow's milk, soy, or extensively hydrolyzed formula. Associated clinical features of MFPA include regurgitation/vomiting, persistent diarrhea, and poor weight gain. The absence of eczema in the majority of infants with persistent crying suggests non-IgE-mediated mechanisms. The association of MFPA with severe infantile colic led to the hypothesis that persistent crying in early infancy may be a manifestation of non-IgE-mediated food allergy.

Development of food allergy in children with previous infantile colic

The absence of atopic manifestations in the majority of infants with colic suggests that non-IgE-mediated mechanisms predominate in the pathogenesis of infantile colic. However, a study from Finland found that infants with a history of colic are at increased risk of atopy, as compared to non-colicky infants [74]. In that study, of 116 infants with atopy at 2 years of age, 44 (38%) had presented with infantile colic. By contrast, a prospective study of 983 infants found no evidence of an increased risk for asthma and other atopic manifestations in infants with colic [75].

Intestinal microbiota in infants with colic

There are significant differences in the composition of intestinal microbiota in infants with and without colic. Typically, bifidobacteria and lactobacilli are the predominant gut bacteria in breast-fed infants [76]. Savino et al. [77] found that breast-fed infants with colic were less frequently colonized with lactobacilli and carried more gram-negative gut bacteria. Also the type of lactobacilli appeared to vary between infants with and without colic [78]. While *Lactobacillus lactis* and *L. brevis* were only found in infants with colic, *L. acidophilus* was only found in healthy infants. These findings are in keeping with a more recent study which analyzed fecal microbial composition of infants with colic, using molecular techniques [79]. It remains unclear how these different bacterial microbiota are involved in the pathogenesis of infantile colic.

A higher degree of fecal microbial biodiversity is associated with a decreased risk of allergic disorders and asthma [80, 81]. Infants with colic have a lower degree of fecal microbial biodiversity and increased levels of fecal calprotectin. Calprotectin is a marker of neutrophilic intestinal inflammation, and the elevated levels suggest that intestinal inflammation is part of the pathophysiology of infantile colic [82]. In that study, *Klebsiella spp.* was more commonly found in infants with colic, compared to control infants, suggesting a possible role of this organism in its etiology. Specific lactobacilli may suppress colonization of the neonatal gut with gas-producing coliform bacteria and confer a protective effect against colic [83]. Several randomized clinical trials have examined the effect of the probiotic strain, *L. reuteri* DSM 17938 on colic symptoms [84–86]. Studies from Italy [84] and Poland [85] showed a dramatic reduction in crying duration after 3–4 weeks of treatment with *L. reuteri* in breast-fed infants with colic, compared to the placebo response. Infants were treated with a daily dose of 10^8 colony-forming units (5 drops). The Italian study by Savino et al. [84] found a significant reduction in crying duration by at least 50% in 20 of 25 infants (80%), compared to 8 of 21 (38%) infants, after 7 days of treatment ($p = 0.006$). The group differences remained significant at 14 days and 21 days. The Polish study by Szajewska et al. [85] was performed in 80 exclusively, or predominantly breast-fed infants and found similar response rates at 7, 14, 21, and 28 days of probiotic treatment [85]. Data from an Australian study are still unpublished [86]. While both currently available studies [84,85] suggest a strong treatment benefit for the probiotic supplementation with *L. reuteri*, subject numbers were relatively small. Further trials are awaiting completion which will provide additional data to inform therapeutic recommendations, including data on formula-fed infants [86].

Infantile colic and gastrointestinal disorders

Gastroesophageal reflux, esophagitis, and infantile colic

Persistent distress and feeding refusal in the early infant period are frequently attributed to GER [25, 26, 87]. This is based on the assumption that acid reflux, even in the absence of esophagitis, may be associated with pain and feeding resistance. Crying itself does not appear to increase

GER [88]. Distressed infants are often treated with antireflux medications on an empirical basis [24, 89]. However, a causal relationship between GER and distress has never been conclusively demonstrated [28].

GER is considered pathological if it is associated with acid-peptic complications (esophagitis, esophageal strictures, etc.), failure to thrive, or respiratory complications (aspiration, persistent wheeze, stridor, apneic episodes). In three retrospective series of infants with severe persistent distress, abnormally frequent acid reflux was demonstrated by esophageal 24-hour pH monitoring in 15–25% of infants studied [24, 28, 89]. This exceeds the expected prevalence of 5–10% in young infants [90] and may in part be explained by selection bias in infants referred for gastroenterological investigation. Infants with abnormally frequent or prolonged GER on pH monitoring usually presented with overt regurgitation and non-regurgitant "silent" GER was uncommon [24, 28]. The duration of crying and fussing per day did not correlate with the severity of GER [24]. In a randomized clinical trial of infants with colic or persistent crying, treatment with ranitidine and cisapride was no better than placebo [91]. In a similar subsequent randomized trial, omeprazole, a proton pump inhibitor, was not effective in treating crying infants [92]. In that study, effective acid suppression was achieved in the infants on active medication, but not on placebo. Both studies make a direct causal relationship between GER and colic unlikely [91, 92].

Esophageal 24-hour pH monitoring is the definitive diagnostic test for the quantification of acid reflux. In a study of 125 distressed infants with symptoms of GER, one quarter of infants had an abnormal pH study, and one quarter had histological esophagitis. However, there was poor diagnostic agreement between abnormal pH monitoring and histological esophagitis [28]. This may indicate a non-acid-peptic etiology of the esophagitis in these infants. Esophagitis was frequently associated with gastritis or duodenitis, suggesting the presence of a more generalized upper gastrointestinal inflammatory process in infants with persistent distress [93].

There is evidence supporting the hypothesis that GER and esophagitis in infancy may be caused by CMA [31]. Previous studies have provided clinical evidence of gastric dysrhythmias in infants with CMA, presenting with vomiting and GER [94]. Iacono et al. demonstrated that in more than 42% of infants with histological esophagitis, reflux symptoms improved after treatment with extensively hydrolyzed formula and relapsed on subsequent blinded formula challenges [95]. Other authors have also found evidence of food protein-induced GER [25].

The differential diagnosis of GERD in infancy includes eosinophilic esophagitis (EOE). EOE is an immunologically mediated pan-esophagitis with an increase in mucosal eosinophils in T-helper 2-type allergic inflammatory response [96, 97]. Symptoms in infancy include unsettled behavior, regurgitation, as well as feeding difficulties or refusal [98]. The diagnosis relies on the demonstration of more than 15–20 eosinophils per high power field on esophageal biopsy [99]. While infants with EOE respond poorly to treatment with proton pump inhibitors, most will remit after empirical or targeted elimination diets, including amino acid-based formulas (AAFs) [96, 100]. EOE is discussed in detail in Chapter 16.

Colic and intestinal spasm

In a systematic review of treatments for infantile colic, dicyclomine, an anticholinergic agent, was found to be effective [53]. It is no longer used in the treatment of colic because of its potentially serious side effects in infancy [101]. The therapeutic effect in colicky infants was poorly understood but may have been due to antispasmodic properties on intestinal smooth muscle. Another anticholinergic agent, cimetropium bromide, has been shown to significantly shorten the duration of crying episodes in infants with infantile colic [102]. This drug, a synthetic scopolamine derivative, appears to have fewer serious side effects than dicyclomine. About three quarters of infants responded to treatment with cimetropium bromide. The mean duration of crying episodes was 17.3 minutes for active medication and 47.5 minutes for placebo ($p < 0.005$). Although not conclusive, these findings may add further weight to the hypothesis that infantile colic is associated with visceral pain that is relieved by these medications.

Animal models of food hypersensitivity have provided direct evidence of gastrointestinal spasm and motility disturbance in response to dietary antigen challenge [103]. In sensitized rats, mucosal exposure to food protein antigens resulted in gastric [104] or intestinal smooth muscle contraction [105, 106]. The potential importance of disturbed gut motility in colic is further supported by the finding of increased levels of the hormone motilin, a prokinetic gastrointestinal hormone, both postnatally and at the age of onset of persistent crying [107, 108]. Maternal smoking during pregnancy and lactation has been linked to an increased risk of infantile colic and elevated serum motilin levels [109]. Among infants with colic, formula-fed infants have higher motilin levels than breast-fed infants [110]. Another gastrointestinal hormone, ghrelin, was also found to be significantly increased in infantile colic, as compared to healthy control infants [110]. These findings may provide further insights into the etiology of distress in young infants and should stimulate further research into the role of abnormal gut motility in infants with colic.

Lactose malabsorption

Infants with lactose malabsorption often experience abdominal pain and may present with unsettled behavior or prolonged crying. Despite this, lactose malabsorption is generally not considered to be a significant factor in infants with persistent crying [5, 6]. Several studies have assessed the effect of lactose-free formula on persistent crying. Moore et al. [29] examined the effects of lactose on breath hydrogen production in infants with and without colic. That study found that breath hydrogen concentrations, after intake of human milk or lactose-containing formula, were higher in infants with colic, compared to controls. However, two subsequent randomized controlled trials found no significant clinical benefit for lactose restriction in breast-fed or formula-fed infants with colic [30, 111]. A more recent double-blind, placebo-controlled study in 53 infants found a minor improvement of colic symptoms after preincubation of milk with lactase [112]. However, the response appeared to be variable, and the trial remained inconclusive. Low-lactose formula or pretreatment of breast milk with lactase are therefore not recommended in the treatment of infantile colic or persistent crying [53].

Dietary treatment of colic

The self-limiting course of infantile colic makes the assessment of therapeutic interventions difficult, and no firm conclusions can be drawn unless proper double-blind placebo-controlled randomized trials are performed. Only few well-designed randomized trials on the treatment of colic have been conducted, and many previous studies had some shortfalls in methodology or study design. This review will focus predominantly on the role of hypoallergenic diets in the treatment of infantile colic.

Hypoallergenic formulas

Several clinical trials have assessed the effects of formula on colic and demonstrated a significant treatment benefit of hypoallergenic formulae [53]. In a study of 70 infants with severe colic, 50 (71%) improved after a change to soy formula, and relapsed within 24 hours after cow's milk challenge [113]. Other studies have shown an improvement in colic symptoms in response to extensively hydrolyzed formula [114–116]. A meta-analysis of these studies found a significant beneficial treatment effect for extensively hydrolyzed formulae in infants with colic [5, 53]. Non-response after treatment with hypoallergenic formulae may in some infants be due to the residual allergenicity of extensively hydrolyzed whey or casein formula [73, 117]. In infants who are intolerant to extensively hydrolyzed formula, AAF has been shown to be effective and safe [118, 119]. Several groups have assessed the effect of AAF on persistent crying [70, 93, 120, 121]. These uncontrolled studies provided preliminary evidence that AAF may be effective in reducing persistent crying. However, further prospective trials are required to assess the efficacy and cost-effectiveness of this approach in the community.

Maternal elimination diets

Maternal elimination diets reduce the secretion of food proteins into breast milk and may provide a treatment for a proportion of breast-fed infants with colic [122]. Jakobsson and Lindberg [123] noted that one-third of breast-fed infants with colic improved after maternal dietary cow's milk elimination, and relapsed on reintroduction of cow's milk into the mother's diet. Evans et al. [54], however, were unable to confirm these findings. A more recent clinical trial examined the role of a broad-based hypoallergenic maternal elimination diet in 91 exclusively breast-fed infants under 6 weeks of age with colic [52]. Mothers were randomly allocated to a low-allergen diet (avoiding cow's milk, soy, wheat, egg, peanut, nuts, fish, and shellfish) or an unrestricted control diet. Clinical response after 1 week was defined as a reduction in cry/fuss duration by at least 25%, as assessed by validated 48-hour cry charts. Significantly more infants responded to the maternal low-allergen diet compared with the control diet, although symptomatic improvement occurred in both treatment arms. After 1 week, the clinical response rate in the low-allergen group was 74%, compared to 37% in the control group—a risk reduction of 37% in favor of the maternal elimination diet. This corresponded with a reduction in crying duration by 274 minutes/48 hours in the low-allergen group versus 102 minutes/48 hours in the control group; $p = 0.028$ (Fig. 15.3). Despite these reductions

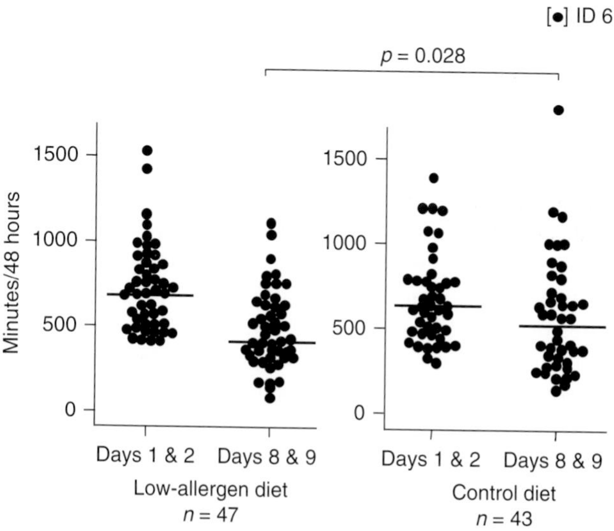

Figure 15.3 Effect of a maternal elimination diet in 90 breast-fed infants less than 6 weeks of age. There was a significantly greater reduction in cry/fuss duration for infants on the low-allergen diet, compared to infants of mothers on the unrestricted control diet. With permission from Reference 52.

in crying, the maternal overall assessment of treatment response ("better," "same," or "worse") did not significantly differ between the two interventions. That study suggested that maternally ingested food proteins are transferred into breast milk and may contribute to colic symptoms in breast-fed infants. However, the exact mechanisms remain to be defined. The relative contribution of a multiple food elimination diet, as compared to cow's milk elimination alone, could not be differentiated.

Investigation and management of infants with colic and suspected food allergy

Due to a lack of clear diagnostic markers for non-IgE-mediated CMA in infancy, the clinical management of colic is often empirical rather than evidence based. While CMA appears to be increased in infants with persistent crying, the majority of infants with colic does not appear to suffer from underlying food allergies. Most treatments initiated at the peak of crying around 6 weeks of age are no better than placebo, as spontaneous improvement of colic symptoms usually occurs toward 3–4 months of age [124]. In recent years, elimination of cow's milk protein from the maternal diet or use of hypoallergenic formula have become common strategies in the treatment of infantile colic [125]. Studies supporting this practice, however, had some methodological limitations and are mostly not population based.

The diagnostic evaluation of underlying food allergies in infants with colic is limited as reactions are generally non-IgE-mediated CMA [126]. Skin prick testing or measurement of cow's milk-specific serum IgE antibodies is therefore not clinically useful in these infants. The diagnosis of non-IgE-mediated CMA relies on demonstration of a reduction in crying duration after cow's milk elimination, and a relapse of symptoms after cow's milk challenge. A positive challenge may also be associated with other symptoms, such as increased vomiting/regurgitation, diarrhea, or eczema [127].

As infantile colic generally improves toward 3–4 months of age, the persistence of symptoms beyond 4 months may indicate a higher risk of underlying pathologies, including CMA. In infants with severe or unremitting colic symptoms beyond 4 months and those with other clinical features of CMA (persistent diarrhea, vomiting, or eczema), a limited trial of a cow's milk protein-free diet should be considered [128]. In younger infants with colic, the clinical response to a dairy-free diet is more variable. Formula-fed infants with colic and suspected CMA should be commenced on an extensively hydrolyzed formula [53]. Lactose-free formula is not recommended. In breast-fed infants, a maternal elimination diet may be effective, and continuation of breast feeding should be encouraged [52].

In infants who improved within 2–4 weeks of commencing a hypoallergenic formula or cow's milk-free diet, the diagnosis of CMA should be confirmed by subsequent cow's milk challenge—either with cow's milk-based formula or via the maternal diet. However, as food elimination and challenge sequences are cumbersome, parents are often not motivated to perform formal food challenges after clinical remission has been achieved. This may lead to unnecessary elimination diets and may predispose to poor nutritional outcomes. Elimination diets should be closely supervised by an experienced dietician in order to prevent insufficient macro- or micronutrient intakes for both mother and infant, and growth parameters of the infant should be monitored [129]. Many infants with colic and CMA will tolerate cow's milk protein from 9 to 12 months of age. However, some infants will remain allergic to cow's milk until 2–3 years of age [128]. It is therefore important that infants are reviewed at regular intervals until tolerance to cow's milk protein has been demonstrated.

Conclusion

Infantile colic is a common pediatric problem in the first months of life. No general consensus has emerged about its most likely multifactorial etiology. Behavioral and interactional factors strongly influence the natural history of infantile colic. Infants with colic appear generally well and in only 5% of distressed infants, a medical explanation for the distress can be found. GER, esophagitis, or lactose intolerance, although sometimes present in infants with colic, are not likely to be the cause of the persistent distress, and empirical treatment with gastric acid-suppressing medications or lactose-free formula is ineffective.

In formula-fed infants with moderate to severe unremitting colic beyond 3–4 months of age, a trial of a hypoallergenic formula should be attempted. Breast-fed infants may respond to a maternal cow's milk protein-free diet. After remission of symptoms, the diet can be gradually normalized and food proteins introduced into the diet, as tolerated. Elimination diets should be closely supervised by an experienced dietician, and growth parameters be monitored. In addition to any dietary interventions, successful management of infants with colic and their families should address the adverse effects of prolonged parental stress and maternal depression.

References

1. Lucassen PL, Assendelft WJ, van Eijk JT, et al. Systematic review of the occurrence of infantile colic in the community. *Arch Dis Child* 2001; 84:398–403.
2. Brazelton TB. Crying in infancy. *Pediatrics* 1962; 29:579–588.
3. Illingworth RS. Three-months' colic. *Arch Dis Child* 1954; 29:165–174.

4. Clifford TJ, Campbell MK, Speechley KN, et al. Sequelae of infant colic: evidence of transient infant distress and absence of lasting effects on maternal mental health. *Arch Pediatr Adolesc Med* 2002; 156:1183–1188.
5. Lucassen PL, Assendelft WJ. Systematic review of treatments for infant colic. *Pediatrics* 2001; 108:1047–1048.
6. Garrison MM, Christakis DA. A systematic review of treatments for infant colic. *Pediatrics* 2000; 106:184–190.
7. Barr RG. Colic and crying syndromes in infants. *Pediatrics* 1998; 102:1282–1286.
8. Wessel MA, Cobb JC, Jackson EB, et al. Paroxysmal fussing in infancy, sometimes called colic. *Pediatrics* 1954; 14:421–435.
9. Freedman SB, Al-Harthy N, Thull-Freedman J. The crying infant: diagnostic testing and frequency of serious underlying disease. *Pediatrics* 2009; 123:841–848.
10. Hiscock H, Wake M. Infant sleep problems and postnatal depression: a community-based study. *Pediatrics* 2001; 107:1317–1322.
11. Rautava P, Helenius H, Lehtonen L. Psychosocial predisposing factors for infantile colic. *BMJ* 1993; 307:600–604.
12. Nelson SP, Chen EH, Syniar GM, et al. Prevalence of symptoms of gastroesophageal reflux during infancy. A pediatric practice-based survey. Pediatric Practice Research Group. *Arch Pediatr Adolesc Med* 1997; 151:569–572.
13. Hillervik-Lindquist C. Studies on perceived breast milk insufficiency. A prospective study in a group of Swedish women. *Acta Paediatr Scand Suppl* 1991; 376:1–27.
14. Hide DW, Guyer BM. Prevalence of infant colic. *Arch Dis Child* 1982; 57:559–560.
15. Rubin SP, Prendergast M. Infantile colic: incidence and treatment in a Norfolk community. *Child Care Health Dev* 1984; 10:219–226.
16. Carey WB. "Colic"—primary excessive crying as an infant-environment interaction. *Pediatr Clin North Am* 1984; 31:993–1005.
17. Michelsson K, Rinne A, Paajanen S. Crying, feeding and sleeping patterns in 1 to 12-month-old infants. *Child Care Health Dev* 1990; 16:99–111.
18. Hogdall CK, Vestermark V, Birch M, et al. The significance of pregnancy, delivery and postpartum factors for the development of infantile colic. *J Perinat Med* 1991; 19:251–257.
19. Lehtonen L, Korvenranta H. Infantile colic. Seasonal incidence and crying profiles. *Arch Pediatr Adolesc Med* 1995; 149:533–536.
20. Canivet C, Hagander B, Jakobsson I, et al. Infantile colic–less common than previously estimated? *Acta Paediatr* 1996; 85:454–458.
21. Canivet C, Jakobsson I, Hagander B. Colicky infants according to maternal reports in telephone interviews and diaries: a large Scandinavian study. *J Dev Behav Pediatr* 2002; 23:1–8.
22. Clifford TJ, Campbell MK, Speechley KN, et al. Infant colic: empirical evidence of the absence of an association with source of early infant nutrition. *Arch Pediatr Adolesc Med* 2002; 156:1123–1128.
23. Wake M, Morton-Allen E, Poulakis Z, et al. Prevalence, stability, and outcomes of cry-fuss and sleep problems in the first 2 years of life: prospective community-based study. *Pediatrics* 2006; 117:836–842.
24. Heine RG, Jordan B, Lubitz L, et al. Clinical predictors of pathological gastro-oesophageal reflux in infants with persistent distress. *J Paediatr Child Health* 2006; 42:134–139.
25. Heine RG. Gastroesophageal reflux disease, colic and constipation in infants with food allergy. *Curr Opin Allergy Clin Immunol* 2006; 6:220–225.
26. Putnam PE. GERD and crying: cause and effect or unhappy coexistence? *J Pediatr* 2002; 140:3–4.
27. Feranchak AP, Orenstein SR, Cohn JF. Behaviors associated with onset of gastroesophageal reflux episodes in infants. Prospective study using split-screen video and pH probe. *Clin Pediatr* 1994; 33:654–662.
28. Heine RG, Cameron DJ, Chow CW, et al. Esophagitis in distressed infants: poor diagnostic agreement between esophageal pH monitoring and histopathologic findings. *J Pediatr* 2002; 140:14–19.
29. Moore DJ, Robb TA, Davidson GP. Breath hydrogen response to milk containing lactose in colicky and noncolicky infants. *J Pediatr* 1988; 113:979–984.
30. Ståhlberg MR, Savilahti E. Infantile colic and feeding. *Arch Dis Child* 1986; 61:1232–1233.
31. Heine RG. Allergic gastrointestinal motility disorders in infancy and early childhood. *Pediatr Allergy Immunol* 2008; 19:383–391.
32. Barr RG, Kramer MS, Boisjoly C, et al. Parental diary of infant cry and fuss behaviour. *Arch Dis Child* 1988; 63:380–387.
33. Hunziker UA, Barr RG. Increased carrying reduces infant crying: a randomized controlled trial. *Pediatrics* 1986; 77:641–648.
34. Hill DJ, Menahem S, Hudson I, et al. Charting infant distress: an aid to defining colic. *J Pediatr* 1992; 121:755–758.
35. Barr RG, Paterson JA, MacMartin LM, et al. Prolonged and unsoothable crying bouts in infants with and without colic. *J Dev Behav Pediatr* 2005; 26:14–23.
36. St James-Roberts I, Peachey E. Distinguishing infant prolonged crying from sleep-waking problems. *Arch Dis Child* 2011; 96:340–344.
37. Canivet C, Jakobsson I, Hagander B. Infantile colic. Follow-up at four years of age: still more "emotional." *Acta Paediatr* 2000; 89:13–17.
38. Barr RG. Crying in the first year of life: good news in the midst of distress. *Child Care Health Dev* 1998; 24:425–439.
39. Savino F, Castagno E, Bretto R, et al. A prospective 10-year study on children who had severe infantile colic. *Acta Paediatr Suppl* 2005; 94:129–132.
40. Brown M, Heine RG, Jordan B. Health and well-being in school-age children following persistent crying in infancy. *J Paediatr Child Health* 2009; 45:254–262.
41. Rao MR, Brenner RA, Schisterman EF, et al. Long term cognitive development in children with prolonged crying. *Arch Dis Child* 2004; 89:989–992.
42. St James-Roberts IS, Conroy S, Wilsher K. Bases for maternal perceptions of infant crying and colic behaviour. *Arch Dis Child* 1996; 75:375–384.
43. Forsyth BW, Leventhal JM, McCarthy PL. Mothers' perceptions of problems of feeding and crying behaviors. A prospective study. *Am J Dis Child* 1985; 139:269–272.

44. Canivet CA, Östergren PO, Rosen AS, et al. Infantile colic and the role of trait anxiety during pregnancy in relation to psychosocial and socioeconomic factors. *Scand J Public Health* 2005; 33:26–34.
45. Rautava P, Lehtonen L, Helenius H, et al. Infantile colic: child and family three years later. *Pediatrics* 1995; 96:43–47.
46. Beebe SA, Casey R, Pinto-Martin J. Association of reported infant crying and maternal parenting stress. *Clin Pediatr* 1993; 32:15–19.
47. Vik T, Grote V, Escribano J, et al. Infantile colic, prolonged crying and maternal postnatal depression. *Acta Paediatr* 2009; 98:1344–1348.
48. Taubman B. Parental counseling compared with elimination of cow's milk or soy milk protein for the treatment of infant colic syndrome: a randomized trial. *Pediatrics* 1988; 81:756–761.
49. Barr RG, McMullan SJ, Spiess H, et al. Carrying as colic "therapy": a randomized controlled trial. *Pediatrics* 1991; 87:623–630.
50. Wolke D, Gray P, Meyer R. Excessive infant crying: a controlled study of mothers helping mothers. *Pediatrics* 1994; 94:322–332.
51. Bishop JM, Hill DJ, Hosking CS. Natural history of cow milk allergy: clinical outcome. *J Pediatr* 1990; 116:862–867.
52. Hill DJ, Roy N, Heine RG, et al. Effect of a low-allergen maternal diet on colic among breastfed infants: a randomized, controlled trial. *Pediatrics* 2005; 116:e709–715.
53. Lucassen PL, Assendelft WJ, Gubbels JW, et al. Effectiveness of treatments for infantile colic: systematic review. *BMJ* 1998; 316:1563–1569.
54. Evans RW, Fergusson DM, Allardyce RA, et al. Maternal diet and infantile colic in breast-fed infants. *Lancet* 1981; 1:1340–1342.
55. Campbell JP. Dietary treatment of infant colic: a double-blind study. *J R Coll Gen Pract* 1989; 39:11–14.
56. Lothe L, Lindberg T, Jakobsson I. Cow's milk formula as a cause of infantile colic: a double-blind study. *Pediatrics* 1982; 70:7–10.
57. Hill DJ, Hudson IL, Sheffield LJ, et al. A low allergen diet is a significant intervention in infantile colic: results of a community-based study. *J Allergy Clin Immunol* 1995; 96:886–892.
58. Forsyth BW. Colic and the effect of changing formulas: a double-blind, multiple-crossover study. *J Pediatr* 1989; 115:521–526.
59. Lucas A, St James-Roberts I. Crying, fussing and colic behaviour in breast- and bottle-fed infants. *Early Hum Dev* 1998; 53:9–18.
60. Hill DJ, Hosking CS. Infantile colic and food hypersensitivity. *J Pediatr Gastroenterol Nutr* 2000; 30(Suppl):S67–76.
61. Axelsson I, Jakobsson I, Lindberg T, et al. Bovine beta-lactoglobulin in the human milk. A longitudinal study during the whole lactation period. *Acta Paediatr Scand* 1986; 75:702–707.
62. Paganelli R, Atherton DJ, Levinsky RJ. Differences between normal and milk allergic subjects in their immune responses after milk ingestion. *Arch Dis Child* 1983; 58:201–206.
63. Cohen Engler A, Hadash A, Shehadeh N, et al. Breastfeeding may improve nocturnal sleep and reduce infantile colic: potential role of breast milk melatonin. *Eur J Pediatr* 2012; 171:729–732.
64. Brandtzaeg P. The gut as communicator between environment and host: immunological consequences. *Eur J Pharmacol* 2011; 668(Suppl 1):S16–32.
65. Sorva R, Mäkinen-Kiljunen S, Juntunen-Backman K. Beta-lactoglobulin secretion in human milk varies widely after cow's milk ingestion in mothers of infants with cow's milk allergy. *J Allergy Clin Immunol* 1994; 93:787–792.
66. Palmer DJ, Gold MS, Makrides M. Effect of maternal egg consumption on breast milk ovalbumin concentration. *Clin Exp Allergy* 2008; 38:1186–1191.
67. Vadas P, Wai Y, Burks W, et al. Detection of peanut allergens in breast milk of lactating women. *J Am Med Assoc* 2001; 285:1746–1748.
68. Chirdo FG, Rumbo M, Anon MC, et al. Presence of high levels of non-degraded gliadin in breast milk from healthy mothers. *Scand J Gastroenterol* 1998; 33:1186–1192.
69. Järvinen KM, Mäkinen-Kiljunen S, Suomalainen H. Cow's milk challenge through human milk evokes immune responses in infants with cow's milk allergy. *J Pediatr* 1999; 135:506–512.
70. Hill DJ, Cameron DJ, Francis DE, et al. Challenge confirmation of late-onset reactions to extensively hydrolyzed formulas in infants with multiple food protein intolerance. *J Allergy Clin Immunol* 1995; 96:386–394.
71. Hill DJ, Heine RG, Cameron DJ, et al. The natural history of intolerance to soy and extensively hydrolyzed formula in infants with multiple food protein intolerance. *J Pediatr* 1999; 135:118–121.
72. de Boissieu D, Matarazzo P, Rocchiccioli F, et al. Multiple food allergy: a possible diagnosis in breastfed infants. *Acta Paediatr* 1997; 86:1042–1046.
73. de Boissieu D, Dupont C. Allergy to extensively hydrolyzed cow's milk proteins in infants: safety and duration of amino acid-based formula. *J Pediatr* 2002; 141:271–273.
74. Kalliomäki M, Laippala P, Korvenranta H, et al. Extent of fussing and colic type crying preceding atopic disease. *Arch Dis Child* 2001; 84:349–350.
75. Castro-Rodriguez JA, Stern DA, Halonen M, et al. Relation between infantile colic and asthma/atopy: a prospective study in an unselected population. *Pediatrics* 2001; 108:878–882.
76. Johnson CL, Versalovic J. The human microbiome and its potential importance to pediatrics. *Pediatrics* 2012; 129:950–960.
77. Savino F, Cresi F, Pautasso S, et al. Intestinal microflora in breastfed colicky and non-colicky infants. *Acta Paediatr* 2004; 93:825–829.
78. Savino F, Bailo E, Oggero R, et al. Bacterial counts of intestinal *Lactobacillus* species in infants with colic. *Pediatr Allergy Immunol* 2005; 16:72–75.
79. Pärtty A, Kalliomäki M, Endo A, Salminen S, Isolauri E. Compositional development of *Bifidobacterium* and *Lactobacillus microbiota* is linked with crying and fussing in early infancy. *PLoS One* 2012; 7:e32495.

80. van Nimwegen FA, Penders J, Stobberingh EE, et al. Mode and place of delivery, gastrointestinal microbiota, and their influence on asthma and atopy. *J Allergy Clin Immunol* 2011; 128:948–955 e1-3.
81. Ege MJ. Intestinal microbial diversity in infancy and allergy risk at school age. *J Allergy Clin Immunol* 2011; 128:653–654.
82. Rhoads JM, Fatheree NY, Norori J, et al. Altered fecal microflora and increased fecal calprotectin in infants with colic. *J Pediatr* 2009; 155:823–828.
83. Savino F, Cordisco L, Tarasco V, et al. Antagonistic effect of Lactobacillus strains against gas-producing coliforms isolated from colicky infants. *BMC Microbiol* 2011; 11:157.
84. Savino F, Cordisco L, Tarasco V, et al. *Lactobacillus reuteri* DSM 17938 in infantile colic: a randomized, double-blind, placebo-controlled trial. *Pediatrics* 2010; 126:e526–533.
85. Szajewska H, Gyrczuk E, Horvath A. *Lactobacillus reuteri* DSM 17938 for the management of infantile colic in breastfed infants: a randomized, double-blind, placebo-controlled trial. *J Pediatr* 2013; 162:257–262.
86. Sung V, Hiscock H, Tang M, et al. Probiotics to improve outcomes of colic in the community: Protocol for the Baby Biotics randomised controlled trial. *BMC Pediatr* 2012; 12:135.
87. Hyman PE. Gastroesophageal reflux: one reason why baby won't eat. *J Pediatr* 1994; 125:S103–109.
88. Orenstein SR. Crying does not exacerbate gastroesophageal reflux in infants. *J Pediatr Gastroenterol Nutr* 1992; 14: 34–37.
89. Heine RG, Jaquiery A, Lubitz L, et al. Role of gastro-oesophageal reflux in infant irritability. *Arch Dis Child* 1995; 73:121–125.
90. Vandenplas Y, Goyvaerts H, Helven R, et al. Gastroesophageal reflux, as measured by 24-hour pH monitoring, in 509 healthy infants screened for risk of sudden infant death syndrome. *Pediatrics* 1991; 88:834–840.
91. Jordan B, Heine RG, Meehan M, et al. Effect of antireflux medication, placebo and infant mental health intervention on persistent crying: a randomized clinical trial. *J Paediatr Child Health* 2006; 42:49–58.
92. Moore DJ, Tao BS, Lines DR, et al. Double-blind placebo-controlled trial of omeprazole in irritable infants with gastroesophageal reflux. *J Pediatr* 2003; 143:219–223.
93. Hill DJ, Heine RG, Cameron DJ, et al. Role of food protein intolerance in infants with persistent distress attributed to reflux esophagitis. *J Pediatr* 2000; 136:641–647.
94. Ravelli AM, Tobanelli P, Volpi S, et al. Vomiting and gastric motility in infants with cow's milk allergy. *J Pediatr Gastroenterol Nutr* 2001; 32:59–64.
95. Iacono G, Carroccio A, Cavataio F, et al. Gastroesophageal reflux and cow's milk allergy in infants: a prospective study. *J Allergy Clin Immunol* 1996; 97:822–827.
96. Liacouras CA, Furuta GT, Hirano I, et al. Eosinophilic esophagitis: updated consensus recommendations for children and adults. *J Allergy Clin Immunol* 2011; 128:3–20.
97. Straumann A, Bauer M, Fischer B, et al. Idiopathic eosinophilic esophagitis is associated with a T(H)2-type allergic inflammatory response. *J Allergy Clin Immunol* 2001; 108:954–961.
98. Noel RJ, Putnam PE, Rothenberg ME. Eosinophilic esophagitis. *N Engl J Med* 2004; 351:940–941.
99. Liacouras CA. Clinical presentation and treatment of pediatric patients with eosinophilic esophagitis. *Gastroenterol Hepatol* 2011; 7:264–267.
100. Heine RG, Nethercote M, Rosenbaum J, et al. Emerging management concepts for eosinophilic esophagitis in children. *J Gastroenterol Hepatol* 2011; 26:1106–1113.
101. Williams J, Watkins-Jones R. Dicyclomine: worrying symptoms associated with its use in some small babies. *Br Med J (Clin Res Ed)* 1984; 288:901.
102. Savino F, Brondello C, Cresi F, Oggero R, Silvestro L. Cimetropium bromide in the treatment of crisis in infantile colic. *J Pediatr Gastroenterol Nutr* 2002; 34:417–419.
103. Catto-Smith AG, Tan D, Gall DG, et al. Rat gastric motor response to food protein-induced anaphylaxis. *Gastroenterology* 1994; 106:1505–1513.
104. Catto-Smith AG, Patrick MK, Scott RB, et al. Gastric response to mucosal IgE-mediated reactions. *Am J Physiol* 1989; 257:G704–708.
105. Scott RB, Tan DT, Miampamba M, et al. Anaphylaxis-induced alterations in intestinal motility: role of extrinsic neural pathways. *Am J Physiol* 1998; 275:G812–821.
106. Oliver MR, Tan DT, Kirk DR, et al. Colonic and jejunal motor disturbances after colonic antigen challenge of sensitized rat. *Gastroenterology* 1997; 112:1996–2005.
107. Lothe L, Ivarsson SA, Lindberg T. Motilin, vasoactive intestinal peptide and gastrin in infantile colic. *Acta Paediatr Scand* 1987; 76:316–320.
108. Lothe L, Ivarsson SA, Ekman R, et al. Motilin and infantile colic. A prospective study. *Acta Paediatr Scand* 1990; 79:410–416.
109. Shenassa ED, Brown MJ. Maternal smoking and infantile gastrointestinal dysregulation: the case of colic. *Pediatrics* 2004; 114:e497–505.
110. Savino F, Grassino EC, Guidi C, et al. Ghrelin and motilin concentration in colicky infants. *Acta Paediatr* 2006; 95:738–741.
111. Miller JJ, McVeagh P, Fleet GH, et al. Effect of yeast lactase enzyme on "colic" in infants fed human milk. *J Pediatr* 1990; 117:261–263.
112. Kanabar D, Randhawa M, Clayton P. Improvement of symptoms in infant colic following reduction of lactose load with lactase. *J Hum Nutr Diet* 2001; 14:359–363.
113. Iacono G, Carroccio A, Montalto G, et al. Severe infantile colic and food intolerance: a long-term prospective study. *J Pediatr Gastroenterol Nutr* 1991; 12:332–335.
114. Lucassen PL, Assendelft WJ, Gubbels JW, et al. Infantile colic: crying time reduction with a whey hydrolysate: a double-blind, randomized, placebo-controlled trial. *Pediatrics* 2000; 106:1349–1354.
115. Lothe L, Lindberg T. Cow's milk whey protein elicits symptoms of infantile colic in colicky formula-fed infants: a double-blind crossover study. *Pediatrics* 1989; 83:262–266.
116. Jakobsson I, Lothe L, Ley D, et al. Effectiveness of casein hydrolysate feedings in infants with colic. *Acta Paediatr* 2000; 89:18–21.
117. Vanderhoof JA, Murray ND, Kaufman SS, et al. Intolerance to protein hydrolysate infant formulas: an underrecognized

cause of gastrointestinal symptoms in infants. *J Pediatr* 1997; 131:741–744.

118. Isolauri E, Sutas Y, Makinen-Kiljunen S, et al. Efficacy and safety of hydrolyzed cow milk and amino acid-derived formulas in infants with cow milk allergy. *J Pediatr* 1995; 127:550–557.
119. Niggemann B, Binder C, Dupont C, et al. Prospective, controlled, multi-center study on the effect of an amino-acid-based formula in infants with cow's milk allergy/intolerance and atopic dermatitis. *Pediatr Allergy Immunol* 2001; 12:78–82.
120. Estep DC, Kulczycki A, Jr. Colic in breast-milk-fed infants: treatment by temporary substitution of neocate infant formula. *Acta Paediatr* 2000; 89:795–802.
121. Estep DC, Kulczycki A, Jr. Treatment of infant colic with amino acid-based infant formula: a preliminary study. *Acta Paediatr* 2000; 89:22–27.
122. Palmer DJ, Makrides M. Diet of lactating women and allergic reactions in their infants. *Curr Opin Clin Nutr Metab Care* 2006; 9:284–288.
123. Jakobsson I, Lindberg T. Cow's milk proteins cause infantile colic in breast-fed infants: a double-blind crossover study. *Pediatrics* 1983; 71:268–271.
124. Hall B, Chesters J, Robinson A. Infantile colic: a systematic review of medical and conventional therapies. *J Paediatr Child Health* 2012; 48:128–137.
125. Iacovou M, Ralston RA, Muir J, et al. Dietary management of infantile colic: a systematic review. *Matern Child Health J* 2012; 16:1319–1331.
126. Moravej H, Imanieh MH, Kashef S, et al. Predictive value of the cow's milk skin prick test in infantile colic. *Ann Saudi Med* 2010; 30:468–470.
127. Heine RG, Elsayed S, Hosking CS, et al. Cow's milk allergy in infancy. *Curr Opin Allergy Clin Immunol* 2002; 2:217–225.
128. Allen KJ, Davidson GP, Day AS, et al. Management of cow's milk protein allergy in infants and young children: an expert panel perspective. *J Paediatr Child Health* 2009; 45:481–486.
129. Arvola T, Holmberg-Marttila D. Benefits and risks of elimination diets. *Ann Med* 1999; 31:293–298.

16 Eosinophilic Esophagitis, Gastroenteritis, and Colitis

Amanda Muir & Chris A. Liacouras

Pediatric Gastroenterology, Division of Gastroenterology and Nutrition, The Children's Hospital of Philadelphia, Philadelphia, PA, USA

Key Concepts

- Food allergens play a strong role in the pathogenesis of eosinophilic esophagitis (EoE).
- Elimination or elemental diets are highly effective treatments for EoE.
- EoE is distinct from eosinophilic gastroenteritis (EoG).
- It is essential to distinguish EoG from inflammatory bowel disease.

Primary disorders involving an accumulation of eosinophils in the gastrointestinal (GI) tract include EoE, EoG, and eosinophilic colitis. The goal of this chapter is to provide an overview of these conditions.

Eosinophilic esophagitis

Introduction

Our understanding of eosinophilic esophagitis (EoE) has evolved over the past 30 years from isolated case reports of patients with prominent esophageal eosinophilia (often misclassified as gastroesophageal reflux) to a well-defined clinical disorder. This disease has been given several names including EoE, allergic esophagitis, primary EoE, and idiopathic EoE.

Definition

EoE is a distinct disease defined by a clinicopathologic diagnosis involving a localized eosinophilic inflammation of the esophagus. Since symptoms are similar to gastroesophageal reflux, esophageal endoscopic biopsies are required to establish the diagnosis. EoE is defined as the presence of 15 or more eosinophils in the most severely involved high-powered field (HPF) (4003) isolated to the esophagus and associated with characteristic clinical symptoms, which do not respond to adequate proton-pump inhibitor (PPI) therapy. Other recognized causes of esophageal eosinophilia should be excluded before making the diagnosis (Table 16.1).

Incidence and prevalence

In 2003, the incidence and prevalence of EoE in children 0–19 years of age were reported to be 1 and 4.3 per 10,000 children, respectively [1]. Studies have suggested a rising prevalence of EoE in the last 10 years [2]. In adults, the prevalence of esophageal eosinophilia has been reported to be as high as 0.2–2.4% in a large nation-wide endoscopic database analysis [3]. The male to female ratio in both children and adults is approximately 3:1 [3, 4].

Etiology

The exact etiology of EoE is unknown; however, EoE is believed to be a mixed IgE and non-IgE-mediated allergic response to food antigens, with non-IgE cell-mediated responses predominating [5]. The identified esophageal eosinophilia is thought to represent only part of a complex cellular and molecular cascade of interactions between Th2 cells, mast cells, cytokines such as IL-5 and IL-13, endogenous chemokines such as eotaxin-1 and eotaxin-3, and eosinophils [6].

While several studies have documented resolution of EoE with the strict avoidance of food antigens, in 1995, Kelly et al. published a sentinel paper on EoE [7]. Kelly studied 10 patients with symptoms of chronic gastroesophageal reflux who failed medical and surgical therapy (six patients had ongoing symptoms and esophageal eosinophilia despite undergoing a fundoplication). Because the suspected etiology was an abnormal immunologic response to specific unidentifiable food antigens, patients

Food Allergy: Adverse Reactions to Foods and Food Additives, Fifth Edition. Edited by Dean D Metcalfe, Hugh A Sampson, Ronald A Simon and Gideon Lack.

Table 16.1 Differential diagnosis of esophageal eosinophilia.

- Gastroesophageal reflux
- Inflammatory bowel disease
- Food allergy
- Eosinophilic gastroenteritis
- Celiac disease
- Parasitic infection
- Connective tissue disease
- Drug allergy
- Hypereosinophilic syndrome
- Autoimmune enteropathy
- Candida esophagitis
- Viral esophagitis (herpes or cytomegalovirus (CMV))
- Churg–Strauss syndrome

were placed on a strict diet consisting of an amino acid-based formula for a median of 17 weeks. Symptomatic improvement was seen within an average of 3 weeks after the introduction of the elemental diet (resolution in eight patients, improvement in two). All 10 patients demonstrated a significant histologic improvement in their esophageal eosinophilia. Subsequently, all patients reverted to previous symptoms upon reintroduction of foods. Open food challenges were then conducted with a return of symptoms with challenges to milk (seven patients), soy (four patients), wheat (two patients), peanut (two patients), and egg (one patient) [7].

Rothenberg et al. recently described the first EoE susceptibility locus at 5q22. One of the genes at this locus, thymic stromal lymphopoietin (TSLP) was found to be overexpressed in esophageal biopsy samples of patients with EoE compared to normal controls [8]. TSLP is a Th2 type cytokine expressed by epithelial cells of the airway, gastrointestinal (GI) tract, and skin. The cytokine TSLP has been previously linked to asthma [9], allergic rhinitis [10], and eczema [11] making it a likely gene of interest in the pathogenesis of EoE.

Several authors have suggested that aeroallergens may play a role in the development of EoE. Mishra and Rothenberg used a mouse model to show that the inhalation of Aspergillus may cause EoE [12]. They found that the allergen-challenged mice developed elevated levels of esophageal eosinophils and features of epithelial cell hyperplasia that mimic EoE. In addition, Spergel reported a case of a 21-year-old female with EoE, asthma, and allergic rhinoconjunctivitis who became symptomatic from her EoE during pollen seasons followed by resolution during winter months [13]. Further epidemiology studies have shown that rates of EoE diagnosis increase in the summer and fall and decrease in the winter suggesting seasonality possibly linked to the prominent aeroallergens at these time periods [14].

Table 16.2 Clinical symptoms of eosinophilic esophagitis.

- Vomiting
- Regurgitation
- Dysphagia
- Nausea
- Epigastric pain
- Chest pain
- Esophageal food impaction
- Irritability/feeding difficulties
- Nighttime cough

Clinical features

Although the current reports suggest that patients with EoE are predominantly young Caucasian males, EoE can occur at any age or race and in either sex. Those affected typically present with one or more of the following symptoms: vomiting, regurgitation, nausea, epigastric, or chest pain, dysphagia, water brash, globus, or decreased appetite [15]. Others will drink large quantities of water after each bite or over-chew their food in an attempt to compensate for these symptoms. Less common symptoms include growth failure, hematemesis, and esophageal dysmotility. Symptoms can be frequent and severe in some patients while extremely intermittent and mild in others (Table 16.2). The majority of children experience vomiting, chronic nausea, or regurgitation while older children and adolescents develop heartburn, epigastric pain, or episodes of dysphagia. Up to 50% of patients manifest additional allergy-related symptoms such as asthma, eczema, or rhinitis. Furthermore, up to 50% of patients have one or more parents with history of allergy. EoE should be strongly considered in those patients who have severe or refractory symptoms of gastroesophageal reflux, especially those who are refractory to medication.

Other complications that can occur with EoE include failure to thrive, malnutrition, feeding intolerance, esophageal strictures, hiatal hernia, small caliber esophagus, and esophageal perforation. Esophageal fungal or viral superinfection may also occur. Any patient who is being considered for surgical correction of gastroesophageal reflux (fundoplication) should first be evaluated endoscopically for EoE to prevent unnecessary surgery [16].

Diagnosis

Children with chronic refractory symptoms of gastroesophageal reflux disease (GERD) or dysphagia should undergo evaluation for EoE. While laboratory and radiological assessment may be appropriate in most cases, all patients should undergo an upper endoscopy with biopsy. The diagnosis of EoE is made when there is an isolated severe histologic esophagitis, unresponsive to aggressive acid blockade, associated with symptoms similar to those seen in GERD or dysphagia.

Upper endoscopy should be performed to directly visualize the esophagus and to obtain tissue samples for pathologic investigation. EoE is best defined as the presence of at least 15 eosinophils per HPF isolated strictly to the esophagus. In 1999, Ruchelli evaluated 102 patients presenting with GERD symptoms who also were found to have at least one esophageal eosinophil without any other GI abnormalities [17]. Patients were subsequently treated with acid blockade. It was demonstrated that the treatment response could be classified into three categories. Patients who improved and had a lasting response had on average 1.1 eosinophils per HPF, patients who relapsed upon completion of therapy had 6.4 eosinophils per HPF, and patients who remained symptomatic despite therapy had on average 24.5 eosinophils per HPF. Other histologic abnormalities often found in conjunction with eosinophilia include microabcesses, extracellular eosinophilic granules, basal cell hyperplasia, dilated intercellular spaces, and lamina propria fibrosis [18, 19].

Since EoE has been described as a patchy disease, multiple esophageal biopsies should be obtained from the proximal and distal esophagus [19]. In the past, early reports suggested that EoE patients developed proximal or mid-esophageal eosinophilia; however, recent information demonstrates that severe mucosal eosinophilia can occur in any portion (proximal, mid, distal) of the esophagus [20–22]. To make an accurate diagnosis, the remainder of the GI tract must be normal; thus, biopsies should be obtained from the gastric antrum and duodenum to rule out other diseases.

EoE has been associated with visual findings on endoscopy in 68% of patients: concentric ring formation (called "trachealization" or a "feline esophagus"), longitudinal linear furrows, and patches of small, white papules on the esophageal mucosal surface [23]. Most investigators believe that the esophageal rings and furrows are a response to full-thickness esophageal tissue inflammation. The white papules appear to represent the formation of eosinophilic abscesses. However, the esophagus may be visually normal on endoscopy in over 30% of patients. Therefore, whenever the diagnosis of EoE is suspected, esophageal biopsies must be performed.

In 2000, Fox utilized high-resolution probe endosonography in patients with EoE in order to determine the extent of tissue involvement [24]. He compared eight patients with EoE to four control patients without esophagitis. He discovered that the esophageal tissue layers were thicker in EoE patients compared to controls (total wall thickness 2.8 vs. 2.2 mm, *p*, 0.01; combined mucosal and submucosal thickness 1.6 versus 1.1 mm, *p*, 0.01; muscularis propria thickness 1.3 vs. 1.0 mm, *p*, 0.05). These findings suggested that EoE patients had more than just surface involvement of eosinophils.

While other noninvasive tests have been used in an attempt to diagnose EoE, upper endoscopy with biopsy is the only test that can precisely determine the diagnosis of EoE. The other noninvasive GI diagnostic tests include radiographic upper GI (UGI) series, pH probe, and manometry. Although radiographs demonstrate anatomic abnormalities, they do not identify tissue eosinophilia. However, in patients suspected of having esophageal strictures, a UGI can provide important information. Patients with EoE usually have normal or borderline normal pH probes. Patients may have mild GERD secondary to abnormalities in esophageal motility due to tissue eosinophilic infiltration; however, there have been no specific manometric findings of EoE to date.

Allergy testing

Once EoE is suspected, patients should be encouraged to seek an allergy consultation. Serum peripheral eosinophilia or elevated IgE levels are not present in the majority of patients. Furthermore, these tests have been found to be unreliable due to the fact that they usually respond to environmental allergens as well as ingested or inhaled allergens. Serum allergen-specific testing for food-specific IgE antibodies has a very limited role in EoE due to its low sensitivity. Use of a combination of peripheral blood absolute eosinophil count (AEC), levels of eosinophil-derived neurotoxin (EDN), and eotaxin-3 as noninvasive biomarkers are under investigation; however, these tests do not currently appear to have the sensitivity or negative predictive value needed for widespread clinical practice [25].

A combination of skin prick testing (SPT) and atopy patch testing (APT) attempts to identify IgE and non-IgE-based causative food allergens, respectively. Furthermore, SPT for aeroallergen sensitivity is warranted given the possible causality between these antigens and EoE [18]. In a study population of 146 pediatric patients, elimination diet based on foods identified by a combination of SPT and APT led to resolution of esophageal eosinophilia in 67% of patients, and histologic improvement in 82% of patients [5, 26]. In EoE patients, SPT most frequently identifies positive reactions to egg, milk, and soy. Given the non-IgE-mediated mechanism of most of the food reactions in EoE patients, APT may play an important role in the successful identification of causative food antigens. Presently, the lack of standardization of APT methodologies in addition to variability in technique and interpretation are likely explanations for the nonuniform results of APT. Interpretation is based on a no reaction, or 1, 2, 3 scale depending on the degree of erythema, papules, and/or vesicles. The most common foods identified by APT are corn, soy, and wheat [26].

Treatment

Acute management

Several treatment options are available to patients diagnosed with EoE. Currently, most investigators do not believe that esophageal acid exposure is the etiology of EoE; however, because of the severity of mucosal and submucosal diseases seen in EoE, secondary acid reflux often occurs. Additionally, because there may be some histologic overlap between patients with EoE and those with GERD, it is important to exclude acid reflux as a cause of esophageal inflammation. Acid reflux may cause significant esophageal eosinophilia. Therefore, patients suspected of having EoE should be prescribed a PPI so that GERD can be excluded. A case series by Ngo and colleagues have identified several patients with significant esophageal eosinophilia that resolved 1 month after taking a PPI medication [27]. Patients should be treated with 8–12 weeks of therapy with a PPI prior to histologic diagnosis to eliminate GERD as a potential diagnosis. The adult dosage is 20–40 mg up to twice daily and the pediatric dosing is 1 mg/kg twice daily [18].

Adult gastroenterologists have reported the use of esophageal dilation for their patients who present acutely with esophageal strictures secondary to EoE. While esophageal dilation may relieve dysphagia and improve an esophageal stricture, many physicians describe esophageal tearing during endoscopy and dilation [28–31]. Previously, high rates of esophageal perforation (up to 5%) after attempted esophageal endoscopic dilation in EoE had been described [31, 32]. More recently, the rate of esophageal perforation in EoE has been reevaluated and it was found to be more consistent with 1% [33]. While esophageal dilation can provide up to 23 months of symptom relief, it does not provide any degree of mucosal healing unless used concurrently with other therapeutic options [34]. Thus while the risk associated with dilation is much lower than previously thought, it is important to consider medical or dietary therapy prior to the dilation and perform dilation on a case by case basis [18].

Systemic corticosteroids were the first medical treatment shown to be effective in improving both symptoms and esophageal histology in patients with EoE [35]. Patients were treated with oral solumedrol (average dose 1.5 mg/kg/day; maximum dose 48 mg/day) for 1 month. Symptoms were significantly improved in 19 of 20 patients by an average of 8 days. A repeat endoscopy with biopsy (4 weeks after the initiation of therapy) demonstrated almost complete normalization of esophageal histology. However, upon discontinuation of corticosteroids, 90% had recurrence of symptoms. Oral corticosteroids should be used whenever patients have severe dysphagia (with or without strictures) or other clinical symptoms that may be contributing to possible hospitalization because of a feeding disorder, poor weight gain, or dehydration. While systemic steroids work rapidly, their disadvantages include the fact that they cannot be used chronically, that they do not cure the disease, and that they often have serious side effects with a prolonged use (bone, growth, and mood abnormalities).

Instead of prescribing systemic steroids, topical corticosteroids can be utilized [36–39]. Medications, such as fluticasone propionate, can be sprayed into the pharynx and swallowed. Within a few weeks, both clinical symptoms and esophageal histology dramatically improve. In a study by Konikoff, the authors conducted a randomized, double-blind, placebo-controlled trial of swallowed fluticasone in patients with active EoE [40]. Thirty-six patients were randomly assigned to receive either 880 mg of fluticasone daily or placebo. Of these, 50% of the fluticasone-treated patients achieved complete histologic remission compared with 9% of patients who received placebo. In addition, resolution of clinical symptoms occurred more frequently with fluticasone than with placebo. The authors concluded that swallowed fluticasone was effective in inducing histologic remission and clinical symptoms in EoE in a significant number of patients.

The advantage of using topical steroids is that their side effects are less than that seen with systemic steroids. The disadvantages include not treating the disease fully (the disease generally recurs when the treatment is discontinued) and the development of possible side effects such as epistaxis, dry mouth, and esophageal candidiasis. When using topical, swallowed corticosteroids, the initial dose varies from 110 to 880 mg, twice daily, depending on the patient's age and size. Patients do not eat, drink, or rinse their mouth for 20–30 minutes after using this medication. Other atopic diseases should be controlled as rhinitis and environmental allergies may be linked to EoE. The patient should undergo endoscopy after 2–3 months of therapy. If improved, fluticasone can be weaned empirically. The medication can be discontinued as tolerated; however, in many patients the disease recurs. Recently, the use of a swallowed viscous budesonide solution has been reported with some effectiveness [41].

Several other medications have also been utilized. Cromolyn sodium has been used as a therapy for EoE in a small number of patients. However, cromolyn sodium did not demonstrate any histologic or clinical improvement in a series of 14 patients [42]. Leukotriene receptor antagonists have also been utilized to treat EoE [43]. Doses of 10 mg/day were prescribed to patients in remission while on topical steroids, however, after 3 months of treatment, there was little change in symptoms or histology. While the advantage of using a leukotriene receptor antagonist is that it has minimal side effects and it may alleviate the patient's clinical symptoms, there have been no reports documenting improvement in the patient's histology. Additionally, the patient's clinical symptoms recur when the medication is discontinued.

Dietary therapy has been reported to be extremely effective for pediatric patients with EoE [7, 12]. While there has been no definitive evidence that EoE is a food allergy, the removal of food antigens has been clearly demonstrated to successfully treat both the clinical symptoms and the underlying histopathology in well over 95% of patients with EoE. The elimination of causative foods can follow several therapeutic regimens. First, specific food elimination can be based on allergy testing and clinical history [26, 44]. Second, the most likely causative foods can be removed regardless of history. Recently, a study utilized the removal of six foods (milk, eggs, wheat, soy, nuts, shellfish), without the aid of allergy testing, and demonstrated resolution of symptoms in over two-thirds of patients [13]. When comparing these studies, similar outcomes occur. In both studies, food elimination successfully improved symptoms in approximately 75% of patients. Moreover, although esophageal histology also significantly improved, in most patients it did not normalize.

While every attempt should be made to identify and eliminate potential food allergens through food elimination, a significant number of patients remain symptomatic and continue to have abnormal esophageal histology. In these cases, the administration of a strict diet utilizing an amino acid-based formula is often necessary. As established by Kelly and Liacouras, the use of an elemental diet in children is greater than 95% successful in resolving both the clinical symptoms and histologic abnormalities of EoE [7, 12]. Although the strict use of an amino acid-based formula (typically provided by nasogastric tube feeding) may be difficult for patients (and parents) to comprehend, its benefits outweigh the risks of other treatments. Once the esophagus is healed, foods are reintroduced systematically. Since the clinical symptoms are often erratic, endoscopy with biopsy should be performed in order to determine the improvement in esophageal histology.

In our experience of over 164 compliant patients, who were treated with an amino acid-based diet, 97% of patients had a clinical and histologic improvement in their EoE [42]. In those that required an elemental diet, over 84% had specific food antigens identified and were able to discontinue the elemental diet after approximately 6 months using a graded food reintroduction protocol (Table 16.3). Dietary restriction using a combination of patch and SPT alone without the need for an elemental diet was successful in over 50% of 130 children [44]. Elimination of the responsible foods usually does not lead to immediate

Table 16.3 EoE food introduction following an elemental diet.

A	B	C	D
Vegetables (Non-legume) Carrots, squash Sweet potato Spinach, broccoli Lettuce Fruit Grapes, pear Peaches, plum Apricot, cherries Orange, grapefruit, lemon, Lime, cherries, Strawberries, Blueberries Other fruits	Apple, banana, Kiwi, pineapple, Mango, watermelon, honeydew, Cantaloupe, papaya, guava, avocado Legumes Lima beans, Chickpeas, white/black/red beans, string beans Peas White potato	Grains Rice, oat, barley, rye Meat[a] Lamb, chicken, turkey, pork Fish/shellfish Tree nuts Almond, walnut, hazelnut, brazil nut, pecan	Milk Corn Peanut Wheat Beef Soy Egg

[a]Progress from well cooked to rarer.

resolution of symptoms. Rather, improvement of symptoms occurs approximately 1–3 weeks after the removal of the causative antigen. Also, in patients with EoE, symptoms do not always occur immediately after food reintroduction and may return after several days to weeks. In some cases, the responsible food antigens must be identified using a systematic approach: foods are eliminated for 6–8 weeks and repeat endoscopy is performed. New foods are typically introduced every 7 days and repeat biopsies are performed based on clinical symptoms or after five to eight new foods are introduced. Nutritional support is also an important component in the management of EoE patients. Foods considered to be the most antigenic for EoE include milk, eggs, soy, corn, wheat, and beef.

Finally, other medications are being developed that target specific chemokines and other inflammatory mediators involved in eosinophil proliferation, recruitment, and activation. Medications such as anti-interleukin-5 (anti-IL-5), very late activating antigen, and monoclonal eotaxin antibody may benefit those patients who have severe EoE. A small study of four patients identified with severe long-standing EoE showed that treatment with anti-IL-5 improved peripheral blood and esophageal eosinophilia as well as clinical symptoms and dysphagia [45]. Further studies, however, showed more mixed results. Spergel et al. performed a double-blind, randomized placebo control trial in 2012. They enrolled 226 children and adolescents with EoE. After 12 weeks of treatment, they found that while the eosinophil counts had decreased significantly in the treatment groups, there was no significant improvement in patient-reported symptoms or physician global assessment [46].

Long-term management

The focus of long-term management of EoE should be to provide symptom relief along with histologic healing. At this point, topical corticosteroids and dietary restriction have both been shown to be successful in the long-term treatment of EoE. Several reports have demonstrated esophageal healing and symptom resolution with dietary therapy ranging from the removal of a few foods to the use of a total elemental diet strictly using an amino acid-based formula.

Unlike infantile milk protein allergy, the majority of patients with EoE require long-term, indefinite food antigen removal. In our series of 231 patients, only a few patients appeared to "outgrow" their food allergy; however, recent evidence suggests that an increasing number of patients may develop "tolerance" if the food antigens are removed for a prolonged period of time (years) [47].

With regard to medical therapy, because of the possibility of secondary gastroesophageal reflux due to chronic esophageal inflammation, acid blockade is effective in improving the patient's symptoms. Recent adult literature suggests that PPI therapy may be associated with a significantly increased risk of hip fractures if used for more than 1 year [48]. Further research into the safety of long-term PPI therapy in adults and children is needed, and the risk–benefit ratio of any medication should always be evaluated in the individual patient clinical context. Topical, swallowed fluticasone has been shown to be an effective treatment for EoE [23, 40]. Unfortunately, when therapy is discontinued, EoE almost always recurs. While the long-term use of topical steroids appears reasonably safe, several side effects have been reported which include esophageal candidiasis, epistaxis, and dry mouth. In addition, long-term effects on growth, bone health, and esophageal fibrosis are currently not known.

Eosinophilic gastroenteritis (gastroenterocolitis)

Introduction

Eosinophilic gastroenteritis or gastroenterocolitis (EoG) is a general term that describes a constellation of symptoms and a pathologic infiltration of the GI tract by eosinophils. EoG was originally described by Kaijser in 1937 [49]. It is a disorder characterized by tissue eosinophilia that can affect different layers of the bowel wall, anywhere from the mouth to the anus. In 1970, Klein classified EoG into three categories: mucosal, muscular, and serosal [50].

Definition

There are no strict diagnostic criteria for EoG, and its definition has been largely shaped by multiple case reports and case series. A combination of GI complaints with supportive histologic findings is sufficient to make the diagnosis of EoG and investigate the differential diagnosis (Table 16.4).

Prevalence

Currently, the prevalence of EoG is not known. Our clinical experience is that EoG occurs less frequently than inflammatory bowel disease in children (7 per 100 000 children) [53].

Etiology

The exact etiology of EoG remains unknown, although it is now recognized to occur as a result of both IgE- and non-IgE-mediated sensitivity [54]. The association between IgE-mediated inflammatory response (typical allergy) and EoG is supported by the increased likelihood of other allergic disorders such as atopic disease, food allergies, and seasonal allergies [55, 56]. Specific foods have been

Table 16.4 Differential diagnosis of eosinophilic gastroenteritis.

Celiac disease	
Chronic granulomatous disease	Infectious
	Ancylostoma caninium (hookworm)
Connective tissue	*Anisakis*
Diseases/vasculitis	*Ascaris*
Systemic lupus erythematosus	EBV
Scleroderma	*Enterobius vermicularis* (pinworm)
Dermatomyositis	*Eustoma rotundatum*
Polymyositis	*Giardia lamblia*
Churg–Strauss syndrome	*Helicobacter pylori*
Polyarteritis nodosa	*Schistosomiasis trichus*
Others	
	Strongyloides
Food allergies	*Toxocara canis*
	Trichinella spiralis
Hypereosinophilic syndrome	Others
Inflammatory bowel disease[a]	
Inflammatory fibroid polyp	
Malignancy	
Medications	
Azathioprine	
Carbamazepine	
Clofazimine	
Enalapril	
Gemfibrozil	
Gold	
Others [51, 52]	

Note this list is not exhaustive—case reports of other etiologies have been reported.

[a]In our experience, inflammatory bowel disease (often in young children) can initially manifest histologically as eosinophilia.

implicated in the cause of EoG [57, 58]. In contrast, the role of non-IgE-mediated immune dysfunction, in particular the interplay between lymphocyte-produced cytokines and eosinophils, has also received attention. IL-5 is a chemoattractant responsible for tissue eosinophilia [59]. Desreumaux et al. found that among patients with EoG, the levels of IL-3, IL-5, and granulocyte–macrophage colony-stimulating factor (GM-CSF) were significantly increased as compared to control patients [60]. Once recruited to the tissue, eosinophils may further recruit similar cells through their own production of IL-3 and IL-5, as well as production of leukotrienes [61]. This mixed type of immune dysregulation in EoG has implications in the way this disorder is diagnosed, as well as in the way it is treated [62].

Clinical features

EoG affects patients of all ages, with a slight male predominance. Most commonly, eosinophils infiltrate only the mucosa, leading to symptoms associated with malabsorption, such as growth failure, weight loss, diarrhea, and hypoalbuminemia. Additional symptoms of EoG include colicky abdominal pain, bloating, dysphagia, and vomiting [62–64]. Other features of severe disease include GI bleeding, iron deficiency anemia, protein losing enteropathy (hypoalbuminemia), and growth failure [63]. Approximately 75% of affected patients have elevated blood eosinophil levels [63]. Rarely, ascites can occur [65, 66]. In addition, up to 50% of patients have a past or family history of atopy [67].

In an infant, EoG may present in a manner similar to hypertrophic pyloric stenosis, with progressive vomiting, dehydration, electrolyte abnormalities, and thickening of the gastric outlet [68, 69]. When an infant presents with this constellation of symptoms, in addition to atopic symptoms such as eczema and reactive airway disease, an elevated eosinophil count, or a strong family history of atopic disease, then EoG should be considered before surgical intervention.

Uncommon presentations of EoG include an acute abdomen (even mimicking acute appendicitis), isolated ulceration, obstruction, or mass lesions [70–74]. There also have been reports of serosal infiltration with eosinophils, with associated abdominal distention, eosinophilic ascites, and bowel perforation [66, 72, 75–78].

Diagnosis

EoG should be considered in any patient with a history of chronic symptoms including vomiting, abdominal pain, diarrhea, anemia, hypoalbuminemia, or poor weight gain in combination with the presence of eosinophils in the GI tract. The number of eosinophils that are defined as abnormal depends on the location in the GI tract, and has geographic variability [79, 80].

A number of tests may aid in the diagnosis of EoG; however, no single test is pathognomonic and there are no standards for diagnosis. Eosinophils in the GI tract must be documented before EoG can be truly entertained as a diagnosis. This is most readily done with biopsies of the upper GI tract through esophagogastroduodenoscopy and the lower tract through colonoscopy with terminal ileal intubation. In our experience, inflammatory bowel disease is an important entity in the differential diagnosis, and eosinophilia can be the initial presentation especially in young children. Mucosal EoG may affect any portion of the GI tract. A review of the biopsy findings in 38 children with EoG revealed that all patients examined had mucosal eosinophilia of the gastric antrum [67]. Seventy-nine percent of the patients also demonstrated eosinophilia of the proximal small intestine, with 60% having esophageal involvement, and 52% having involvement of the gastric corpus. Those with colonic involvement tended to be under 6 months of age and were ultimately classified as having allergic colitis.

Radiographic contrast studies may demonstrate mucosal irregularities or edema, wall thickening, ulceration, or luminal narrowing. A lacy mucosal pattern of the gastric antrum known as *areae gastricae* is a unique finding that may be present in patients with EoG [81].

Evaluation of other causes of eosinophilia should be undertaken that include parasitic infection, inflammatory bowel disease, neoplasm, chronic granulomatous disease, collagen vascular disease, and the hypereosinophilic syndrome [82–86] (Table 16.4). Specifically, consultations with an allergist, gastroenterologist, infectious disease specialist, and rheumatologist should be obtained. Signs of intestinal obstruction warrant abdominal imaging and surgical consultation.

Laboratory evaluation

In contrast to EoE, peripheral eosinophilia or an elevated IgE level occurs in approximately 70% of affected individuals [87]. Allergic investigation is the same as for patients with EoE; however, it is less often revealing. Infectious workup should include stool ova and parasite testing on three separate stool samples, serum (and possibly tissue) Epstein–Barr virus (EBV) PCR, giardia antigen, and *Helicobacter pylori* testing [88–93]. Rheumatologic testing should be considered in the appropriate clinical context [94, 95]. Measures of absorptive activity such as the D-xylose absorption test and lactose hydrogen breath testing may reveal evidence of malabsorption, reflecting small intestinal damage. Inflammatory bowel disease serologies may also be considered, but with the recognition that they have limited sensitivity especially in younger children [95, 96]. Negative anti-*Saccharomyces cerevisiae* (ASCA) and perinuclear antineutrophil cytoplasmic antibodies (pANCA) do not exclude the diagnosis of inflammatory bowel disease.

Treatment

Acute management

Since EoG is a rare and difficult disease to diagnose, randomized trials for its treatment are lacking and there is considerable debate as to which treatment is best.

Food allergy is considered one of the underlying causes of EoG, and its management is the same as described previously for EoE. In some cases, the administration of a strict diet, utilizing an elemental formula, has been shown to be successful [56, 97, 98]. Unfortunately, unlike EoE, elemental diets are not uniformly successful for patients with EoG.

When the use of a restricted diet fails, corticosteroids are often employed due to their high likelihood of success in attaining remission [64]. However, when weaned, the duration of remission is variable and can be short lived, leading to the need for repeated courses or continuous low doses of steroids [99]. In addition, the chronic use of corticosteroids carries an increased likelihood of undesirable side effects, including cosmetic problems (cushingoid facies, hirsutism, and acne), decreased bone density, impaired growth, and personality changes. A response to these side effects has been to look for substitutes that may act as steroid-sparing agents, while still allowing for control of symptoms. Budesonide (Entocort®) is a steroid formulation with less systemic toxicity that has been successful for some patients with EoG [100, 101].

Orally administered cromolyn sodium has been used with some success [63, 101–104], and recent reports have detailed the efficacy of other oral anti-inflammatory medications. Montelukast, a selective leukotriene receptor antagonist used to treat asthma, has been reported to be successful in the treatment of two patients with EoG, both alone and in combination with corticosteroids [105–109]. Treatment of EoG with inhibition of leukotriene D4, a potent chemotactic factor for eosinophils, relies on the theory that the inflammatory response in EoG is perpetuated by the presence of eosinophils already present in the mucosa. Suplatast tosilate and ketotifen have also been reported as treatments for EoG [104, 105]. Anti-IL-5 therapy for EoG is also being investigated.

Long-term management

As with EoE, every attempt should be made to identify and restrict potential food allergens in a stepwise approach. Given the limited possibilities for treatment of EoG, the combination of therapies incorporating the best chance of success with the smallest likelihood of side effects should be employed.

When other treatments fail, corticosteroids remain a reliable treatment for EoG, with attempts at limiting the total dose, or the number of treatment courses where possible. Due to the diffuse and inconsistent nature of symptoms in this disease, serial endoscopy with biopsy is a useful and important modality for monitoring disease progression. Particularly in younger children, protean manifestations of inflammatory bowel disease should be considered with every endoscopy.

Eosinophilic proctocolitis

Introduction

Eosinophilic proctocolitis (EoP), also known as allergic proctocolitis or milk protein proctocolitis, has been recognized as one of the most common etiologies of rectal bleeding in infants [67, 106, 107]. This disorder is characterized by the onset of rectal bleeding, generally in children less than 2 months of age.

Definition

EoP is strictly defined as an abnormal number of eosinophils confined to the colon. However, in clinical practice, endoscopy is usually not performed. The diagnosis is established when infants present with rectal bleeding that resolves when placed on a protein hydrolysate formula.

Prevalence

It is felt that up to 7.5% of the population in developed countries exhibit cow's milk allergy, although there is wide variation in the reported data [108–110]. Soy protein allergy is felt to be less common than cow's milk allergy, with a reported prevalence of approximately 0.5% [111]. However, soy-protein intolerance becomes more prominent in individuals who have developed milk-protein-induced proctocolitis, with a prevalence from 15% to 50% or more in milk-protein-sensitized individuals [112].

Etiology

The GI tract plays a major role in the development of oral tolerance to foods. Through the process of endocytosis by the enterocytes, food antigens are generally degraded into non-antigenic proteins [113, 114]. Although the GI tract serves as an efficient barrier to ingested food antigens, this barrier may not be mature for the first few months of life [115]. As a result, ingested antigens may have an increased propensity for being presented intact to the immune system. These intact antigens have the potential for stimulating the immune system, and driving an inappropriate response directed at the GI tract. Because the major component of the young infant's diet is milk or formula, it stands to reason that the inciting antigens in EoP are derived from the proteins found in them. Cow milk and soy proteins are the foods most frequently implicated in EoP.

Commercially available infant formulas most commonly utilize cow's milk as the protein source. There are at least 25 known immunogenic proteins within cow milk, with the caseins and β-lactoglobulin serving as the most antigenic [111]. For this reason, substitution of a soy-protein-based formula for a milk-protein-based formula in patients with suspected milk protein proctocolitis is often unsuccessful. However, because of the expense of protein hydrolysate formulas, practitioners may attempt to use soy formulas initially.

Maternal breast milk represents a different challenge to the immune system. Up to 50% of the cases of EoP occur in breast-fed infants; but, rather than developing an allergy to human milk protein, it is felt that the infants are manifesting allergy to antigens ingested by the mother and transferred via the breast milk. The transfer of maternal dietary protein via breast milk was first demonstrated in 1921 [116]. More recently, the presence of cow milk antigens in breast milk has been established [117–119].

When a problem with antigen handling occurs, whether secondary to increased absorption through an immature GI tract or through a damaged epithelium secondary to gastroenteritis, sensitization of the immune system results. Once sensitized, the inflammatory response is perpetuated with continued exposure to the inciting antigen. This may explain the reported relationship between early exposures to cow's milk protein or viral gastroenteritis and the development of allergy [120–122].

Clinical manifestations

Diarrhea, rectal bleeding, and increased mucus production are the typical symptoms seen in patients who present with EoP [67, 123]. There is a bimodal age distribution with the majority of patients presenting in infancy (mean age at diagnosis of 60 days) and the other group presenting in adolescence and early adulthood [124].

The typical infant with EoP is well appearing with no constitutional symptoms. Rectal bleeding begins gradually, initially appearing as small flecks of blood. Usually, increased stool frequency occurs accompanied by water loss or mucus streaks. The development of irritability or straining with stools is also common and can falsely lead to the initial diagnosis of anal fissuring. Atopic symptoms such as eczema and reactive airway disease may be associated. Continued exposure to the inciting antigen causes increased bleeding and may, on rare occasions, cause anemia or poor weight gain. Despite the progression of symptoms, the infants are generally well appearing. Other manifestations of GI tract inflammation such as vomiting, abdominal distention, or weight loss almost never occur (Table 16.5).

Table 16.5 Characteristics of eosinophilic proctocolitis.

- Clinical symptoms
  - Blood-streaked stools
  - Diarrhea
  - Mild abdominal pain
  - 3 months of age
  - Usually normal weight gain
  - Well appearing
  - Eczema, atopy
- Laboratory features
  - Fecal leukocytes, eosinophils
  - Mild peripheral eosinophilia
  - Rarely
    - Hypoalbuminemia
    - Anemia
  - Skin prick test, food-specific serum IgE testing negative (usually not needed)

Diagnosis

EoP is primarily a clinical diagnosis, although several laboratory parameters and diagnostic procedures may be useful. Initial assessment should be directed at the overall health of the child. A toxic appearing infant is not consistent with the diagnosis of EoP and should prompt evaluation for other causes of GI bleeding.

Stool studies for bacterial pathogens, such as *Salmonella* and *Shigella*, should be performed in the setting of rectal bleeding. In particular, an assay for *Clostridium difficile* toxins A and B should also be considered. While *C. difficile* may cause colitis, infants may be asymptomatically colonized with this organism [125, 126]. A stool specimen may be analyzed for the presence of white blood cells, and specifically for eosinophils. The sensitivity of these tests is not well documented, and the absence of a positive finding on these tests does not exclude the diagnosis [127]. Eosinophils can also accumulate in the colon in other conditions such as pin and hookworm infections, drug reactions, vasculitis, and inflammatory bowel disease. Depending on the clinical situation, it may be important to exclude these diagnoses especially in older children.

Although not always necessary, flexible sigmoidoscopy may be useful to demonstrate the presence of colitis. Visually, one may find erythema, friability, or frank ulceration of the colonic mucosa. Alternatively, the mucosa may appear normal or show evidence of lymphoid hyperplasia [128, 129]. Histological findings typically include increased eosinophils in focal aggregates within the lamina propria, with generally preserved crypt architecture. Findings may be patchy, so that care should be taken to examine many levels of each specimen if necessary [130, 131].

Laboratory evaluation

A complete blood count is useful, as the majority of infants with EoP have a normal or borderline low hemoglobin level. An elevated serum eosinophil count may be present. A stool smear for eosinophils (Wright stain) may also support the diagnosis. Stool cultures for ova and parasites, bacteria, and *C. difficile* toxins should be obtained in the appropriate clinical setting.

Treatment

Acute management

In a well-appearing patient with a history consistent with EoP, it is acceptable to make an empiric formula change. Given the high degree of reactivity to both milk and soy protein in sensitized individuals, a protein hydrolysate formula is often the best choice [121]. However, in mild cases, soy formulas may be attempted initially given the expense of protein hydrolysate formulas. Resolution of symptoms begins almost immediately after the elimination of the problematic food. Although symptoms may linger for several days to weeks, continued improvement is the rule. If symptoms do not quickly improve or persist beyond 4–6 weeks, other antigens should be considered, as well as other potential causes of rectal bleeding. In breast-fed infants, dietary restriction of milk and soy-containing products for the mother may result in improvement; however, care should be taken to ensure that the mother maintains adequate protein and calcium intake from other sources.

Long-term management

EoP in infancy is generally benign and withdrawing the milk protein trigger resolves the condition. Though gross blood in the stool usually disappears within 72 hours, occult blood loss may persist for longer [124]. The prognosis is excellent and the majority of patients are able to tolerate the introduction of the responsible milk protein by 1–3 years of age. Given the unlikely possibility of an allergic reaction following milk reintroduction, milk challenges should be performed in a physician's office at 1 year of age. If a reaction does occur, infants are typically rechallenged at 15 months of age and then referred to an allergist. The prognosis for older onset EoP is less favorable than the infant presentation and is typically chronic and relapsing.

References

1. Noel RJ, Putnam PE, Rothenberg ME. Eosinophilic esophagitis. *N Engl J Med* 2004; 351:940–941.
2. Cherian S, Smith NM, Forbes DA. Rapidly increasing prevalence of eosinophilic oesophagitis in Western Australia. *Arch Dis Child* 2006; 91:1000–1004.
3. Kapel RC, Miller JK, Torres C, et al. Eosinophilic esophagitis: a prevalent disease in the United States that affects all age groups. *Gastroenterology* 2008; 134(5):1316–1321.
4. Franciosi JP, Tam V, Liacouras CA, et al. A case-control study of sociodemographic and geographic characteristics of 335 children with eosinophilic esophagitis. *Clin Gastroenterol Hepatol* 2009; 7(4):415–419.
5. Spergel JM, Beausoleil JL, Mascarenhas M, et al. The use of skin prick tests and patch tests to identify causative foods in eosinophilic esophagitis. *J Allergy Clin Immunol* 2002; 109:363–368.
6. Mishra A, Rothenberg ME. Intratracheal IL-13 induces eosinophilic esophagitis by an IL-5, eotaxin-1, and STAT6-dependent mechanism. *Gastroenterology* 2003; 125:1419–1427.
7. Kelly KJ, Lazenby AJ, Rowe PC, et al. Eosinophilic esophagitis attributed to gastroesophageal reflux: improvement with an amino acid-based formula. *Gastroenterology* 1995; 109:1503–1512.
8. Rothenberg ME, Spergel JM, Sherrill JD, et al. Common variants at 5q22 associate with pediatric eosinophilic esophagitis. *Nat Genet* 2010; 42(4):289–291.
9. Ying S, O'Connor B, Ratoff J, et al. Thymic stromal lymphopoietin expression is increased in asthmatic airways and correlates with expression of th2-attracting chemokines and disease severity. *J Immunol* 2005; 174(12):8183–8190.
10. Bunyavanich S, Melen E, Wilk JB, et al. Thymic stromal lymphopoietin (TSLP) is associated with allergic rhinitis in children with asthma. *Clin Mol Allergy* 2011; 9:1.
11. Soumelis V, Reche PA, Kanzler H, et al. Human epithelial cells trigger dendritic cell-mediated allergic inflammation by producing TSLP. *Nat Immunol* 2002; 3(7):673–680.
12. Mishra A, Hogan SP, Brandt EB, et al. An etiological role for aeroallergens and eosinophils in experimental esophagitis. *J Clin Invest* 2001; 107:83–90.
13. Fogg MI, Ruchelli E, Spergel JM. Pollen and eosinophilic esophagitis. *J Allergy Clin Immunol* 2003; 112:796–797.
14. Prasad GA, Alexander JA, Schleck CD, et al. Talley NJ epidemiology of eosinophilic esophagitis over three decades in Olmsted County, Minnesota. *Clin Gastroenterol Hepatol* 2009; 7(10):1055–1061.
15. Liacouras CA, Markowitz JE. Eosinophilic esophagitis: a subset of eosinophilic gastroenteritis. *Curr Gastroenterol Rep* 1999; 1:253–258.
16. Liacouras CA. Failed Nissen fundoplication in two patients who had persistent vomiting and eosinophilic esophagitis. *J Pediatr Surg* 1997; 32:1504–1506.
17. Ruchelli E, Wenner W, Voytek T, et al. Severity of esophageal eosinophilia predicts response to conventional gastroesophageal reflux therapy. *Pediatr Dev Pathol* 1999; 2:15–18.
18. Liacouras CA, Furuta GT, Hirano I, et al. Eosinophilic esophagitis: updated consensus recommendations for children and adults. *J Allergy Clin Immunol* 2011; 128(1): 3–20.
19. Aceves SS, Newbury RO, Dohil R, et al. Esophageal remodeling in pediatric eosinophilic esophagitis. *J Allergy Clin Immunol* 2007; 119(1):206–212.
20. Steiner SJ, Gupta SK, Croffie JM, et al. Correlation between number of eosinophils and reflux index on same day

esophageal biopsy and 24 hour esophageal pH monitoring. *Am J Gastroenterol* 2004; 99:801–805.

21. Straumann A, Spichtin HP, Grize L, et al. Natural history of primary eosinophilic esophagitis: a follow-up of 30 adult patients for up to 11.5 years. *Gastroenterology* 2003; 125:1660–1609.
22. Katzka DA. Eosinophilic esophagitis. *Curr Treat Options Gastroenterol* 2003;6:49–54.
23. Orenstein SR, Shalaby TM, Di Lorenzo C, et al. The spectrum of pediatric eosinophilic esophagitis beyond infancy: a clinical series of 30 children. *Am J Gastroenterol* 2000; 95:1422–1430.
24. Fox VL, Nurko S, Teitelbaum JE, et al. High-resolution EUS in children with eosinophilic "allergic" esophagitis. *Gastrointest Endosc* 2003; 57:30–36.
25. Konikoff MR, Blanchard C, Kirby C, et al. Potential of blood eosinophils, eosinophil-derived neurotoxin, and eotaxin-3 as biomarkers of eosinophilic esophagitis. *Clin Gastroenterol Hepatol* 2006; 4:1328–1336.
26. Spergel JM, Brown-Whitehorn T, Beausoleil JL, et al. Predictive values for skin prick test and atopy patch test for eosinophilic esophagitis. *J Allergy Clin Immunol* 2007; 119:509–511.
27. Ngo P, Furuta GT, Antonioli DA, et al. Eosinophils in the esophagus–peptic or allergic eosinophilic esophagitis? Case series of three patients with esophageal eosinophilia. *Am J Gastroenterol* 2006; 101:1666–1670.
28. Straumann A, Rossi L, Simon HU, et al. Fragility of the esophageal mucosa: a pathognomonic endoscopic sign of primary eosinophilic esophagitis? *Gastrointest Endosc* 2003; 57:407–412.
29. Kaplan M, Mutlu EA, Jakate S, et al. Endoscopy in eosinophilic esophagitis: "feline" esophagus and perforation risk. *Clin Gastroenterol Hepatol* 2003; 1:433–437.
30. Croese J, Fairley SK, Masson JW, et al. Clinical and endoscopic features of eosinophilic esophagitis in adults. *Gastrointest Endosc* 2003; 58:516–522.
31. Lucendo AJ, De Rezende L. Endoscopic dilation in eosinophilic esophagitis: a treatment strategy associated with a high risk of perforation. *Endoscopy* 2007; 39:376.
32. Eisenbach C, Merle U, Schirmacher P, et al. Perforation of the esophagus after dilation treatment for dysphagia in a patient with eosinophilic esophagitis. *Endoscopy* 2006; 38:E43–E44.
33. Jung KW, Gundersen N, Kopacova J, et al. Occurrence of and risk factors for complications after endoscopic dilation in eosinophilic esophagitis. *Gastrointest Endosc* 2011; 73(1):15–21.
34. Schoepfer AM, Gonsalves N, Bussmann C, et al. Esophageal dilation in eosinophilic esophagitis: effectiveness, safety, and impact on the underlying inflammation. *Am J Gastroenterol* 2010; 105(5):1062–1070.
35. Liacouras CA, Wenner WJ, Brown K, et al. Primary eosinophilic esophagitis in children: successful treatment with oral corticosteroids. *J Pediatr Gastroenterol Nutr* 1998; 26:380–385.
36. Faubion Jr WA, Perrault J, Burgart LJ, et al. Treatment of eosinophilic esophagitis with inhaled corticosteroids. *J Pediatr Gastroenterol Nutr* 1998; 27:90–93.
37. Arora AS, Perrault J, Smyrk TC. Topical corticosteroid treatment of dysphagia due to eosinophilic esophagitis in adults. *Mayo Clin Proc* 2003; 78:830–835.
38. Noel RJ, Putnam PE, Collins MH, et al. Clinical and immunopathologic effects of swallowed fluticasone for eosinophilic esophagitis. *Clin Gastroenterol Hepatol* 2004; 2:568–575.
39. Remedios M, Campbell C, Jones DM, et al. Eosinophilic esophagitis in adults: clinical, endoscopic, histologic findings, and response to treatment with fluticasone propionate. *Gastrointest Endosc* 2006; 63:3–12.
40. Konikoff MR, Noel RJ, Blanchard C, et al. A randomized, double-blind, placebo-controlled trial of fluticasone propionate for pediatric eosinophilic esophagitis. *Gastroenterology* 2006; 131:1381–1391.
41. Aceves SS, Dohil R, Newbury RO, et al. Topical viscous budesonide suspension for treatment of eosinophilic esophagitis. *J Allergy Clin Immunol* 2005; 116:705–706.
42. Liacouras CA, Spergel JM, Ruchelli E, et al. Eosinophilic esophagitis: a 10-year experience in 381 children. *Clin Gastroenterol Hepatol* 2005; 3:1198–1206.
43. Lucendo AJ, De Rezende LC, Jiménez-Contreras S, et al. Montelukast was inefficient in maintaining steroid-induced remission in adult eosinophilic esophagitis. *Dig Dis Sci* 2011; 56(12):3551–3558.
44. Spergel JM, Andrews T, Brown-Whitehorn TF, et al. Treatment of eosinophilic esophagitis with specific food elimination diet directed by a combination of skin prick and patch tests. *Ann Allergy Asthma Immunol* 2005; 95:336–343.
45. Stein ML, Collins MH, Villanueva JM, et al. Anti-IL-5 (mepolizumab) therapy for eosinophilic esophagitis. *J Allergy Clin Immunol* 2006; 118:1312–1319.
46. Spergel JM, Rothenberg ME, Collins MH, et al. Reslizumab in children and adolescents with eosinophilic esophagitis: results of a double-blind, randomized, placebo-controlled trial. *J Allergy Clin Immunol* 2012; 129(2):456–463.
47. Liacouras CA. Eosinophilic esophagitis: treatment in 2005. *Curr Opin Gastroenterol* 2006; 22:147–152.
48. Yang YX, Lewis JD, Epstein S, et al. Long-term proton pump inhibitor therapy and risk of hip fracture. *J Am Med Assoc* 2006; 296:2947–2953.
49. Kaijser R. Zur Kenntnis der allergischen Affektioner desima Verdeanungaskanal von Standpunkt desmia Chirurgen aus. *Arch Klin Chir* 1937; 188:36–64.
50. Klein NC, Hargrove RL, Sleisenger MH, et al. Eosinophilic gastroenteritis. *Medicine (Baltimore)* 1970; 49:299–319.
51. Barak N, Hart J, Sitrin MD. Enalapril-induced eosinophilic gastroenteritis. *J Clin Gastroenterol* 2001; 33:157–158.
52. Kakumitsu S, Shijo H, Akiyoshi N, et al. Eosinophilic enteritis observed during alpha-interferon therapy for chronic hepatitis C. *J Gastroenterol* 2000; 35:548–551.
53. Kugathasan S, Judd RH, Hoffmann RG, et al. Epidemiologic and clinical characteristics of children with newly diagnosed inflammatory bowel disease in Wisconsin: a statewide population-based study. *J Pediatr* 2003; 143:525–531.
54. Spergel JM, Pawlowski NA. Food allergy. Mechanisms, diagnosis, and management in children. *Pediatr Clin North Am* 2002; 49:73–96, vi.

55. Park HS, Kim HS, Jang HJ. Eosinophilic gastroenteritis associated with food allergy and bronchial asthma. *J Korean Med Sci* 1995; 10:216–219.
56. Justinich C, Katz A, Gurbindo C, et al. Elemental diet improves steroid-dependent eosinophilic gastroenteritis and reverses growth failure. *J Pediatr Gastroenterol Nutr* 1996; 23:81–85.
57. Leinbach GE, Rubin CE. Eosinophilic gastroenteritis: a simple reaction to food allergens? *Gastroenterology* 1970; 59:874–889.
58. Caldwell JH, Sharma HM, Hurtubise PE, et al. Eosinophilic gastroenteritis in extreme allergy. Immunopathological comparison with nonallergic gastrointestinal disease. *Gastroenterology* 1979; 77:560–564.
59. Kelso A. Cytokines: structure, function and synthesis. *Curr Opin Immunol* 1989; 2:215–225.
60. Desreumaux P, Bloget F, Seguy D, et al. Interleukin 3, granulocyte-macrophage colony-stimulating factor, and interleukin 5 in eosinophilic gastroenteritis. *Gastroenterology* 1996; 110:768–774.
61. Takafuji S, Bischoff SC, De Weck AL, et al. IL-3 and IL-5 prime normal human eosinophils to produce leukotriene C4 in response to soluble agonists. *J Immunol* 1991; 147:3855–3861.
62. Kweon MN, Kiyono H. Eosinophilic gastroenteritis: a problem of the mucosal immune system? *Curr Allergy Asthma Rep* 2003; 3:79–85.
63. Kelly KJ. Eosinophilic gastroenteritis. *J Pediatr Gastroenterol Nutr* 2000; 30:S28–S35.
64. Whitington PF, Whitington GL. Eosinophilic gastroenteropathy in childhood. *J Pediatr Gastroenterol Nutr* 1988; 7:379–385.
65. Talley NJ, Shorter RG, Phillips SF, et al. Eosinophilic gastroenteritis: a clinicopathological study of patients with disease of the mucosa, muscle layer, and subserosal tissues. *Gut* 1990; 31:54–58.
66. Santos J, Junquera F, de Torres I, et al. Eosinophilic gastroenteritis presenting as ascites and splenomegaly. *Eur J Gastroenterol Hepatol* 1995; 7:675–678.
67. Goldman H, Proujansky R. Allergic proctitis and gastroenteritis in children. Clinical and mucosal biopsy features in 53 cases. *Am J Surg Pathol* 1986; 10:75–86.
68. Aquino A, Domini M, Rossi C, et al. Pyloric stenosis due to eosinophilic gastroenteritis: presentation of two cases in mono-ovular twins. *Eur J Pediatr* 1999; 158:172–173.
69. Khan S, Orenstein SR. Eosinophilic gastroenteritis masquerading as pyloric stenosis. *Clin Pediatr (Phila)* 2000; 39:55–57.
70. Redondo-Cerezo E, Cabello MJ, Gonzalez Y, et al. Eosinophilic gastroenteritis: our recent experience: one-year experience of atypical onset of an uncommon disease. *Scand J Gastroenterol* 2001; 36:1358–1360.
71. Shweiki E, West JC, Klena JW, et al. Eosinophilic gastroenteritis presenting as an obstructing cecal mass—a case report and review of the literature. *Am J Gastroenterol* 1999; 94:3644–3645.
72. Huang FC, Ko SF, Huang SC, et al. Eosinophilic gastroenteritis with perforation mimicking intussusception. *J Pediatr Gastroenterol Nutr* 2001; 33:613–615.
73. Siahanidou T, Mandyla H, Dimitriadis D, et al. Eosinophilic gastroenteritis complicated with perforation and intussusception in a neonate. *J Pediatr Gastroenterol Nutr* 2001; 32:335–337.
74. Markowitz JE, Russo P, Liacouras CA. Solitary duodenal ulcer: a new presentation of eosinophilic gastroenteritis. *Gastrointest Endosc* 2000; 52:673–676.
75. Deslandres C, Russo P, Gould P, et al. Perforated duodenal ulcer in a pediatric patient with eosinophilic gastroenteritis. *Can J Gastroenterol* 1997; 11:208–212.
76. Wang CS, Hsueh S, Shih LY, et al. Repeated bowel resections for eosinophilic gastroenteritis with obstruction and perforation. Case report. *Acta Chir Scand* 1990; 156:333–336.
77. Hoefer RA, Ziegler MM, Koop CE, et al. Surgical manifestations of eosinophilic gastroenteritis in the pediatric patient. *J Pediatr Surg* 1977; 12:955–962.
78. Lerza P. A further case of eosinophilic gastroenteritis with ascites. *Eur J Gastroenterol Hepatol* 1996; 8:407.
79. Lowichik A, Weinberg AG. A quantitative evaluation of mucosal eosinophils in the pediatric gastrointestinal tract. *Mod Pathol* 1996; 9:110–114.
80. Pascal RR, Gramlich TL, Parker KM, et al. Geographic variations in eosinophil concentration in normal colonic mucosa. *Mod Pathol* 1997; 10:363–365.
81. Teele RL, Katz AJ, Goldman H, et al. Radiographic features of eosinophilic gastroenteritis (allergic gastroenteropathy) of childhood. *Am J Roentgenol* 1979; 132:575–580.
82. DeSchryver-Kecskemeti K, Clouse RE. A previously unrecognized subgroup of "eosinophilic gastroenteritis". Association with connective tissue diseases. *Am J Surg Pathol* 1984; 8:171–180.
83. Dubucquoi S, Janin A, Klein O, et al. Activated eosinophils and interleukin 5 expression in early recurrence of Crohn's disease. *Gut* 1995; 37:242–246.
84. Levy AM, Yamazaki K, Van Keulen VP, et al. Increased eosinophil infiltration and degranulation in colonic tissue from patients with collagenous colitis. *Am J Gastroenterol* 2001; 96:1522–1528.
85. Griscom NT, Kirkpatrick Jr JA, Girdany BR, et al. Gastric antral narrowing in chronic granulomatous disease of childhood. *Pediatrics* 1974; 54:456–460.
86. Harris BH, Boles Jr ET. Intestinal lesions in chronic granulomatous disease of childhood. *J Pediatr Surg* 1973; 8:955–956.
87. Caldwell JH, Tennenbaum JI, Bronstein HA. Serum IgE in eosinophilic gastroenteritis. Response to intestinal challenge in two cases. *N Engl J Med* 1975; 292:1388–1390.
88. Tsibouris P, Galeas T, Moussia M, et al. Two cases of eosinophilic gastroenteritis and malabsorption due to *Enterobious vermicularis*. *Dig Dis Sci* 2005; 50:2389–2392.
89. Chira O, Badea R, Dumitrascu D, et al. Eosinophilic ascites in a patient with toxocara canis infection. A case report. *Rom J Gastroenterol* 2005; 14:397–400.
90. Van Laethem JL, Jacobs F, Braude P, et al. *Toxocara canis* infection presenting as eosinophilic ascites and gastroenteritis. *Dig Dis Sci* 1994; 39:1370–1372.
91. Papadopoulos AA, Tzathas C, Polymeros D, et al. Symptomatic eosinophilic gastritis cured with *Helicobacter pylori* eradication. *Gut* 2005; 54:1822.

92. Montalto M, Miele L, Marcheggiano A, et al. Anisakis infestation: a case of acute abdomen mimicking Crohn's disease and eosinophilic gastroenteritis. *Dig Liver Dis* 2005; 37: 62–64.
93. Koga M, Fujiwara M, Hotta N, et al. Eosinophilic gastroenteritis associated with Epstein–Barr virus infection in a young boy. *J Pediatr Gastroenterol Nutr* 2001; 33:610–612.
94. Sunkureddi PR, Baethge BA. Eosinophilic gastroenteritis associated with systemic lupus erythematosus. *J Clin Gastroenterol* 2005; 39:838–839.
95. Schwake L, Stremmel W, Sergi C. Eosinophilic enterocolitis in a patient with rheumatoid arthritis. *J Clin Gastroenterol* 2002; 34:487–488.
96. Reese GE, Constantinides VA, Simillis C, et al. Diagnostic precision of anti-Saccharomyces cerevisiae antibodies and perinuclear antineutrophil cytoplasmic antibodies in inflammatory bowel disease. *Am J Gastroenterol* 2006; 101:2410–2422.
97. Vandenplas Y, Quenon M, Renders F, et al. Milk-sensitive eosinophilic gastroenteritis in a 10-day-old boy. *Eur J Pediatr* 1990; 149:244–245.
98. Chehade M, Magid MS, Mofidi S, et al. Allergic eosinophilic gastroenteritis with protein-losing enteropathy: intestinal pathology, clinical course, and long-term follow-up. *J Pediatr Gastroenterol Nutr* 2006; 42:516–521.
99. Chen MJ, Chu CH, Lin SC, et al. Eosinophilic gastroenteritis: clinical experience with 15 patients. *World J Gastroenterol* 2003; 9:2813–2816.
100. Siewert E, Lammert F, Koppitz P, et al. Eosinophilic gastroenteritis with severe protein-losing enteropathy: successful treatment with budesonide. *Dig Liver Dis* 2006; 38: 55–59.
101. Tan AC, Kruimel JW, Naber TH. Eosinophilic gastroenteritis treated with non-enteric-coated budesonide tablets. *Eur J Gastroenterol Hepatol* 2001; 13:425–427.
102. Van Dellen RG, Lewis JC. Oral administration of cromolyn in a patient with protein-losing enteropathy, food allergy, and eosinophilic gastroenteritis. *Mayo Clin Proc* 1994; 69:441–444.
103. Moots RJ, Prouse P, Gumpel JM. Near fatal eosinophilic gastroenteritis responding to oral sodium chromoglycate. *Gut* 1988; 29:1282–1285.
104. Di Gioacchino M, Pizzicannella G, Fini N, et al. Sodium cromoglycate in the treatment of eosinophilic gastroenteritis. *Allergy* 1990; 45:161–166.
105. Tien FM, Wu JF, Jeng YM, et al. Clinical features and treatment responses of children with eosinophilic gastroenteritis. *Pediatr Neonatol* 2011; 52(5):272–278.
106. Jenkins HR, Pincott JR, Soothill JF, et al. Food allergy: the major cause of infantile colitis. *Arch Dis Child* 1984; 59:326–329.
107. Troncone R, Discepolo V. Colon in food allergy. *J Pediatr Gastroenterol Nutr* 2009; 48(Suppl 2):S89–S91.
108. Gerrard JW, MacKenzie JW, Goluboff N, et al. Cow's milk allergy: prevalence and manifestations in an unselected series of newborns. *Acta Paediatr Scand Suppl* 1973; 234: 1–21.
109. Host A, Halken S. A prospective study of cow milk allergy in Danish infants during the first 3 years of life. Clinical course in relation to clinical and immunological type of hypersensitivity reaction. *Allergy* 1990; 45:587–596.
110. Strobel S. Epidemiology of food sensitivity in childhood—with special reference to cow's milk allergy in infancy. *Monogr Allergy* 1993; 31:119–130.
111. Simpser E. Gastrointestinal allergy. In: Altschuler SM, Liacouras CA (eds), *Clinical Pediatric Gastroenterology.* Philadelphia, PA: Churchill Livingstone, 1998; pp. 113–118.
112. Eastham EJ. Soy protein allergy. In: Hamburger RN (ed.), *Allergology, Immunology, and Gastroenterology.* New York: Raven Press, 1989; pp. 223–236.
113. Heyman M, Grasset E, Ducroc R, et al. Antigen absorption by the jejunal epithelium of children with cow's milk allergy. *Pediatr Res* 1988; 24:197–202.
114. Husby S, Host A, Teisner B, et al. Infants and children with cow milk allergy/intolerance. Investigation of the uptake of cow milk protein and activation of the complement system. *Allergy* 1990; 45:547–551.
115. Kerner Jr JA. Formula allergy and intolerance. *Gastroenterol Clin North Am* 1995; 24:1–25.
116. Shannon WR. Demonstration of food proteins in human breast milk by anaphylactic experiments in guinea pig. *Am J Dis Child* 1921; 22:223–225.
117. Makinen-Kiljunen S, Palosuo T. A sensitive enzyme-linked immunosorbent assay for determination of bovine beta- lactoglobulin in infant feeding formulas and in human milk. *Allergy* 1992; 47:347–352.
118. Axelsson I, Jakobsson I, Lindberg T, et al. Bovine beta-lactoglobulin in the human milk. A longitudinal study during the whole lactation period. *Acta Paediatr Scand* 1986; 75:702–707.
119. Pittschieler K. Cow's milk protein-induced colitis in the breast-fed infant. *J Pediatr Gastroenterol Nutr.* 1990;10:548–549.
120. Vandenplas Y, Hauser B, Van den Borre C, et al. Effect of a whey hydrolysate prophylaxis of atopic disease. *Ann Allergy* 1992; 68:419–424.
121. Juvonen P, Mansson M, Jakobsson I. Does early diet have an effect on subsequent macromolecular absorption and serum IgE? *J Pediatr Gastroenterol Nutr* 1994; 18:344–349.
122. Kaczmarski M, Kurzatkowska B. The contribution of some environmental factors to the development of cow's milk and gluten intolerance in children. *Rocz Akad Med Bialymst* 1988; 33–34:151–165.
123. Katz AJ, Twarog FJ, Zeiger RS, et al. Milk-sensitive and eosinophilic gastroenteropathy: similar clinical features with contrasting mechanisms and clinical course. *J Allergy Clin Immunol* 1984; 74:72–78.
124. Hill SM, Milla PJ. Colitis caused by food allergy in infants. *Arch Dis Child* 1990; 65:132–133.
125. Donta ST, Myers MG. Clostridium difficile toxin in asymptomatic neonates. *J Pediatr* 1982; 100:431–434.
126. Cooperstock MS, Steffen E, Yolken R, et al. *Clostridium difficile* in normal infants and sudden infant death syndrome: an association with infant formula feeding. *Pediatrics* 1982; 70:91–95.
127. Hirano K, Shimojo N, Katsuki T, et al. Eosinophils in stool smear in normal and milk-allergic infants. *Arerugi* 1997; 46:594–601.

128. Anveden-Hertzberg L, Finkel Y, Sandstedt B, et al. Proctocolitis in exclusively breast-fed infants. *Eur J Pediatr* 1996; 155:464–467.

129. Odze RD, Bines J, Leichtner AM, et al. Allergic proctocolitis in infants: a prospective clinicopathologic biopsy study. *Hum Pathol* 1993; 24:668–674.

130. Machida HM, Catto Smith AG, Gall DG, et al. Allergic colitis in infancy: clinical and pathologic aspects. *J Pediatr Gastroenterol Nutr* 1994; 19:22–26.

131. Goldman H. Allergic disorders. In: Ming S-C, Goldman H (eds), *Pathology of the Gastrointestinal Tract*. Philadelphia, PA: WB Saunders, 1992; pp. 171–187.

17 Gluten-Sensitive Enteropathy

Alberto Rubio-Tapia[1] & Joseph A. Murray[1,2]

[1]Division of Gastroenterology and Hepatology, Mayo Clinic, Rochester, MN, USA
[2]Department of Immunology, Mayo Clinic, Rochester, MN, USA

Key Concepts

- Celiac disease is a permanent intolerance to ingested gluten with damage to the small intestine that resolves with the removal of gluten from the diet.
- Celiac disease affects 1 in 141 residents of the United States.
- Celiac disease is strongly associated with the HLA class II genes that encode the molecules DQ2 and DQ8.
- Celiac disease can present with a wide range of multisystem symptoms.
- The mainstay of treatment of celiac disease is lifelong adherence to a diet that excludes foods containing gluten (wheat, barley, and rye).

Introduction

Celiac disease (CD), also known as gluten-sensitive enteropathy, is the end result of collision between the human immune system and the widespread cultivation of wheat (the major food source that fueled Western civilization). The point of contact is the lining of the small intestine. The collision results in inflammation and architectural changes of the absorptive mucosa in those susceptible to CD. The inflammation leads to destruction and eventual loss of absorptive surface (villi), increased net secretion, and potentially a multitude of consequences of malabsorption (Figure 17.1).

CD is defined as a permanent intolerance to ingested gluten that damages the small intestine in genetically predisposed individuals and that resolves with the removal of gluten from the diet [1].

Classically, CD causes increased loss of ingested fat and fatty acids in the stool, malnutrition, and deficiency of micronutrients (iron, folate, and the fat-soluble vitamins) that may result in a syndrome of severe malabsorption. However, the disorder frequently presents with only the vaguest symptoms or may remain entirely silent for many years despite much damage to the intestine [2]. The disease is a global health problem, and cases have been described in Western and Eastern populations [3]. The disorder usually completely resolves with the exclusion of gluten from the diet, but reoccurs when gluten is reintroduced. Although it was once thought to be a rare disease, it is now recognized as a common chronic disorder affecting as much as 1% the general population in Western countries [4].

Other forms of intolerance to wheat/gluten

Although CD is the best-recognized pathologic consequence of gluten ingestion, wheat and gluten may be implicated in other syndromes that partly resemble CD.

Clinical syndromes of chronic diarrhea that respond to gluten exclusion have been described in people who lack the architectural changes of CD in the small intestine. The term non-celiac gluten sensitivity is used for conditions in which gluten ingestion leads to morphological or symptomatic manifestations despite the absence of CD [5]. A double-blind randomized placebo-controlled trial demonstrated that ingestion of gluten causes symptoms in patients with non-celiac gluten sensitivity [6].

Wheat may induce a more classic allergic response that is characterized by IgE or eosinophil-mediated responses; its diagnosis is made by eliciting a history of an immediate reaction to wheat including urticaria, wheezing, and angioedema. While skin prick testing would support suspect food items, ultimately double-blind food challenge may be needed as proof [7].

Food Allergy: Adverse Reactions to Foods and Food Additives, Fifth Edition. Edited by Dean D Metcalfe, Hugh A Sampson, Ronald A Simon and Gideon Lack.

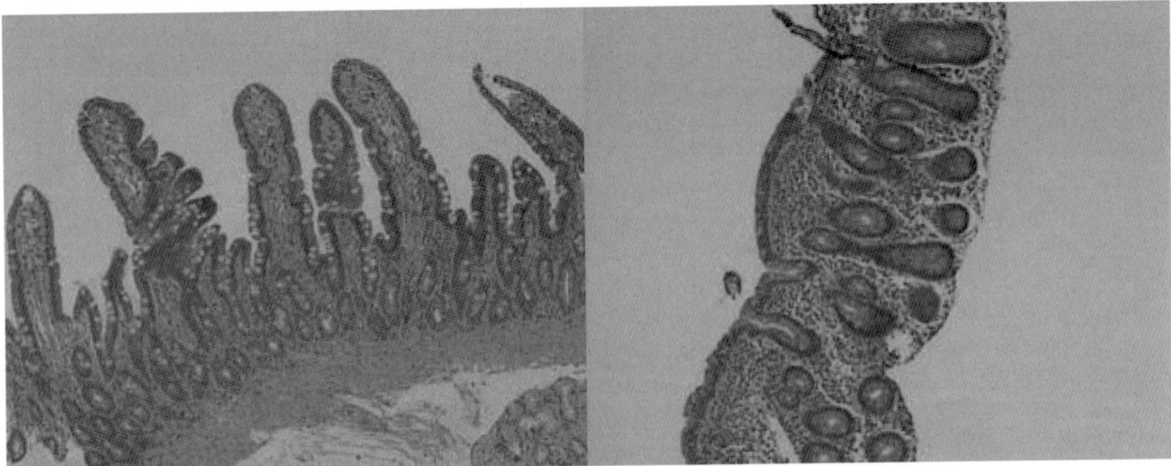

Figure 17.1 Histologic findings in celiac disease. A normal mucosa on the left in contrast with the typical changes of the mucosal lesion of CD on the right. There is loss of the villous structures and hyperplasia of the crypts. Lymphocytes and plasma cells predominate in the inflamed lamina propria. Intraepithelial lymphocytes increase in density (magnification 200×).

Etiology

The intestinal lesion in CD is characterized by architectural and inflammatory changes in the mucosa of the small intestine. The inflammatory response consists of increased numbers of lymphocytes, plasma cells, and macrophages in the lamina propria, and increased lymphocytes in the surface layer of the epithelium (intraepithelial lymphocytes). The normally tall thin villi are shortened and flattened, and crypt layer is increased in depth. These changes may be patchy or continuous, and may affect a variable length of the small intestine [8]. All these changes may result in substantial loss of the absorptive function of the small intestine.

The combination of genetic predisposition, environmental insults, and the intestinal immune system culminates in the intestinal mucosal damage of CD.

Genetics

The genetic basis of the disease comes of the recognition that CD occurs more commonly in families or relatives of probands (Table 17.1).

Table 17.1 Risk of celiac disease in relatives of known celiacs.

Likelihood of a second case	50%
Sibling	10–20%
Parent	5–10%
Sibling sharing at-risk HLA	40%
Child	5–10%
Niece/nephew	5% or less
Grandchild	5%

CD is a complex trait with several genes involved in disease susceptibility. CD is strongly associated with the human leukocyte antigen (HLA) class II genes located in chromosome 6 that encode the molecules DQ2 and DQ8. The majority (95%) of patients carry genes that encode the haplotype DQ2 (DQA1*05/DQB1*01), and the remaining patients express DQ8 (DQA1*03/DQB1*0302) [9]. Such is the strength of the association that the carriage of one of these HLA haplotypes is virtually essential for the disease to occur (high negative predictive value). However, HLA DQ2 is present in 30% individuals from the general population and consequently the positive predictive value is low. Even more, there is a gene dosage effect in which homozygosity increases the risk of the disease, and may influence in severity or age of onset.

There are several possible reasons that these HLA genotypes increase the risk of CD. First, these HLA haplotypes are associated with an increased risk of autoimmune diseases in general due to the escape of autoreactive T cells from thymic selection. People with these HLA genotypes develop a larger repertoire of T cells that are potentially self-reactive. Second, a unique binding affinity exists between DQ2 or DQ8 and certain peptide fragments of wheat (especially if they have undergone modification) that may occur in the gut.

HLA haplotypes confer at least 40–50% of genetic predisposition [10]. There are other genes involved in the susceptibility for CD both within and outside the HLA region [11]. Genome-wide linkage analyses have identified a number of putative "celiac loci." A locus on the 5q31-33q (CELIAC2) [12] region contains a number of cytokine genes and has been implicated in other autoimmune diseases. A loci on chromosome 2q33 (CELIAC3) encompassing the CTLA4 gene has been associated in several studies but is considered to confer only a very modest risk for CD [13]. A locus on chromosome 19 (CELIAC4) has been demonstrated to confer risk for CD in certain populations [14]. A locus on chromosome 7q was reported recently in a large set of North American families (ethnically homogeneous sample) with a minimum of two cases of CD [15].

Non-HLA risk factors for CD may help to improve identification of high-risk individuals but the diagnostic gain of combining non-HLA genes compared to using HLA only is small [16]. Further refinement of non-HLA gene-based diagnostic and prognostic models is necessary to be helpful in clinical practice.

Environmental factors

It has long been known that CD is triggered by the cereal proteins, collectively known as "gluten," that are derived from wheat, barley, and rye. These cultivated grain plants (plant tribe Triticeae) are closely related grasses from the family Poaceae. The storage proteins of these grains are needed for seed germination. The proteins most harmful to those susceptible to CD are gliadins and glutenins in wheat, hordeins in barley, and secalins in rye [17]. The avidins in oats, although long suspected as harmful, are not toxic to the vast majority of celiacs [18, 19].

These toxic proteins are large and complex, and they contain many separate amino acid sequences (epitopes) that can elicit vigorous responses in CD. These proteins consist of remarkably large proportions of glutamine (35%) and proline (20%) residues [20]. Proline residues are especially important because they confer to proteins a high resistance to proteolysis in the intestine. This incomplete digestion favors the persistence of immunogenic peptide epitopes [21]. Additionally, proline residues favor immunological reaction to gluten by (1) enhancing recognition and presentation of peptides by HLA-DQ2-containing cells and (2) selective deamidation of glutamine by tissue transglutaminase (tTG) that enhances the immunogenic proprieties of the gluten.

Past history of infectious gastroenteritis [22], rotavirus infection [23], and infant feeding practices (abrupt introduction of gluten without breast-feeding) [24] have been associated with an increased risk of CD. It is possible that other disease triggers may be identified in the future.

Intestinal permeability modulation

Gluten-induced increased intestinal permeability is an early phenomenon in CD pathogenesis [25]. Increased intestinal permeability allows the entry of gliadin peptides and enhances the immune response in the lamina propria [26]. The responsible mechanisms are complex and include tight-junction (intercellular) dysfunction, transepithelial translocation, and epithelial apoptosis [27, 28]. The molecular details of these processes are beyond the scope of this chapter, but are potential targets for non-dietary therapies for CD.

Immunologic factors

The intestinal mucosa responds constantly to myriad foreign antigens in the gut lumen including food, bacteria, viruses, and toxins. It must do so in a way that protects the host from pathogens and toxins but allows the controlled entry of nutrients. The gut immune system is a delicately balanced milieu in which both the innate and adaptive arms of the immune system are in a controlled state of chronic inflammation. In CD, the consumption of gluten disturbs this homeostasis, resulting in unchecked inflammation in the intestinal mucosa (Figure 17.2).

Adaptive immune response

Cellular immunity seems to play the major role in the intestinal damage of CD [29]. The pathogenic sequence of events has been elucidated primarily through *in vivo* challenge studies in treated patients with CD and *in vitro* challenge studies on biopsies from treated and untreated patients [30]. The accumulation and activation of gluten-reactive memory T cells in the duodenal mucosa play a crucial role in the immunopathogenesis of CD. Activated T cells increase in the small intestine, and many of them respond specifically to gluten [31]. The response is dominated by an HLA-restricted Th1 type cytokine response characterized by IFN-γ, tumor necrosis factor (TNF), and other pro-inflammatory cytokines. These cytokines induce a migration of lymphocytes into the surface epithelium, subsequent recruitment of activated lymphocytes, macrophages, and plasma cells into the lamina propria, and deposition of complement in the subepithelial layer [32].

The surface epithelial layer is infiltrated with an increased number of predominantly CD8 T lymphocytes [33]. Most of these cells express the $\alpha\beta$ receptor, but an increased proportion of cells express the $\gamma\delta$ receptor. The intraepithelial cells in the surface layer also express the natural killer (NK) cell surface marker CD94 [34]. These cells migrate into the intraepithelial compartment in response to gliadin, an effect that may be mediated by interleukin (IL)-15, expressed on the surface of enterocytes [1]. These cells may be affected by innate response to gluten or other noxious stimuli. The innate response provides the costimulatory signals needed to expand the initial adaptive response [35]. Enterocytes, monocytes, and dendritic cells (DCs) may also play a crucial role in amplifying the initial adaptive response. Indeed, CD11c$^+$ cells (a unique subset of DCs) are responsible for antigen presentation of gluten to T cells in the celiac lesion. Even more, a DC-T-cell interaction at the mucosal site is an early event in the inflammatory response to gluten exposure [36].

The complex interrelationship between the surface enterocytes and the supporting fibroblasts is disrupted, leading

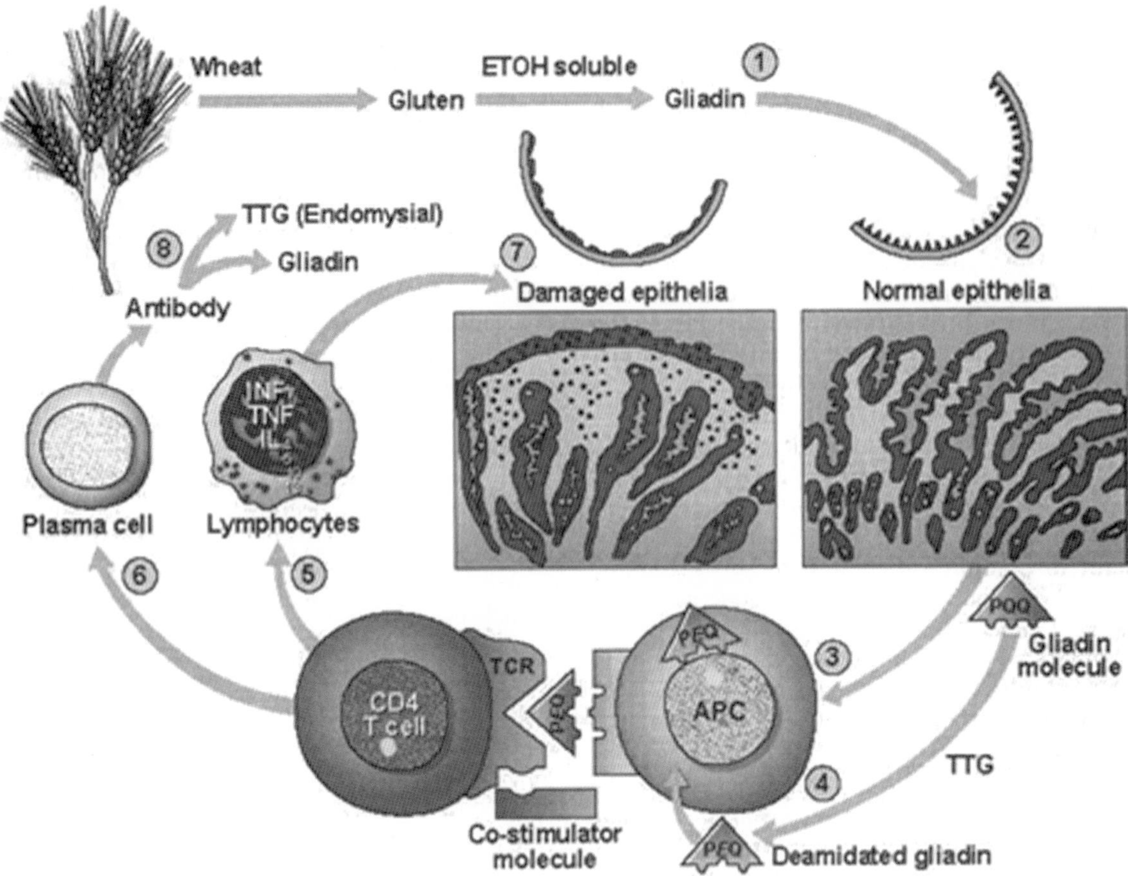

Figure 17.2 Pathogenesis of celiac disease. The steps that lead to CD are shown in this illustration. (1) Gliadin, the alcohol-soluble fraction of wheat, and similar proteins from rye and barley, undergo partial digestion in the gut. (2) The resulting peptides cross the gut epithelial barrier. (3) Native gliadin molecules are taken up by APCs as is, or (4) they undergo deamidation (glutamine [Q] is changed to glutamic acid [E]), after which they are presented to activated T cells. These activated T cells in turn activate the (5) cellular and (6) humoral pathways. (7) The T cells cause production of more cytokines and recruitment of other inflammatory markers that lead to epithelial damage. (8) The plasma cells produce antibodies directed against both gliadin and autoantibodies. It is not clear how these antibodies cause disease in the gut, but cross-reactive antibodies may cause dermatitis herpetiformis. Both environmental (predominantly gluten) and genetic factors give rise to the inflammation that leads to the destruction of the absorptive surface of the intestine. Adapted from Encyclopedia of Gastroenterology, copyright The Mayo Foundation with permission of Mayo Foundation for Medical Education and Research. All rights reserved.

to loss of the orderly migration and differentiation of the villous surface. The thickening of the crypt is not so much a response to loss of surface enterocytes as it is the result of inflammation and remodeling of the mucosa. The inflammatory response likely also damages the structural support and the microcirculation of the villi, causing villous atrophy. This damage is the most intense in the proximal small intestine, and it decreases distally as demonstrated by wireless capsule endoscopy [37, 38]. Surface lymphocytic infiltration of the stomach and colon may also be seen. The rectal mucosa of untreated CD responds to rectal exposure to gluten [39].

Humoral response

A potent humoral response occurs in untreated CD. The intestinal mucosa in CD contains increased numbers of plasma cells secreting IgA, IgG, and IgM directed against gluten peptides, and antibodies against connective tissue autoantigens. Rapid accumulation of $DC11c^{+}CD14^{+}$ occurs after gluten challenge in treated CD and precedes architectural changes [40]. The duodenal plasma cell compartment in CD is enriched with transglutaminase 2-specific IgA autoantibodies secreting cells [41]. Those antibodies are found in the intestinal juice and the serum. The dynamics of the humoral response seem to parallel those of cellular injury, although antibodies may arise before mucosal relapse and disappear before healing. Secreted IgA against gliadin may be a vain attempt to exclude a harmful antigen, while anti-connective tissue antibodies may target host antigen(s) in the connective tissue of the jejunum, umbilical cord, and endomysium. The main autoantigen target is the enzyme tTG [42].

Gliadin antibodies can be seen in other intestinal conditions, but the connective tissue antibodies are highly specific to CD. The humoral response may have a role in some of the extraintestinal manifestations seen in CD, including dermatitis herpetiformis (DH), hyposplenism, IgA nephropathy, liver disease, and hypoparathyroidism [43].

Host modification of gluten by tTG

An intriguing feature of tTG is that its substrate is glutamine, which constitutes 35% of α-gliadin amino acids. tTG itself may complex with gliadin thereby providing gliadin-responsive T cells to help tTG-responsive but inactive B cells to generate a potent self-directed antibody response [44]. It seems likely that tTG modifies the gliadin peptides, increasing the binding affinity for the antigen-presenting site of the two HLA molecules [45]. Interestingly, the deamidated peptides are not recognized in the context of DQ types that are not involved in CD [46]. This host modification of the external antigen may be a crucial step in expanding the immune response to the exogenous gliadin molecule once tTG has been released.

Epidemiology

CD has raised considerable interest in the past few years with the demonstration of its high prevalence (up to 1% in almost every studied country). This new insight in prevalence has been possible, in part, due to the use and availability of celiac serological tests.

CD has been described in all the continents of the world, in developed and developing countries, and in a diversity of racial groups [3]. Thus, the old concept of CD as a "rare and predominantly European disease" is completely incorrect.

A recent study using a nationally representative sample estimated the prevalence of CD in the United States of 0.71% (1 in 141) with a marked predominance among non-Hispanic whites [47].

However, CD remains an underdiagnosed disorder with less than 1:10 affected being diagnosed. The increasing number of cases detected by serology from the Denver studies, in which a birth cohort of subjects that share the HLA haplotypes for CD has been followed up serologically on an annual basis, supports the concept of delayed detection [48]. However, CD may develop at any time in people with confirmed absence of CD autoimmunity in the past [3, 49].

The incidence of CD varies internationally but there appears to be a trend to increasing incidence in many countries [50, 51]. The prevalence of CD in the United States increased four times in the last 50 years [52].

The reasons for the increasing incidence and prevalence are not clear but are likely related to environmental factors. There has been an increase in wheat consumption globally, but especially in North America over the last 20 years, with a 70% increase in per capita wheat consumption, largely reflecting an increase in convenience for prepackaged convenience foods. The increased exposure to gluten can result in a major number of symptomatic subjects explaining increasing incidence. This explanation is not enough to explain increasing trends of CD because a high percentage of the newly detected cases has mild symptoms or are completely asymptomatic and most cases with CD remain undiagnosed.

Modification of wheat to enhance production cannot be ruled out as a possible contributory factor for the increasing incidence of CD, but it is not proven to date. Even more, the use of new technologies to improve agriculture has increased the production and distribution of wheat worldwide.

Natural history of celiac disease

CD is a chronic disease and one that will persist unless treated. It may be asymptomatic despite being otherwise fully evolved in terms of villous atrophy and positive serology. The conditions required for CD to start exist from early life with a combination of genetic predisposition and the consumption of the inciting grains.

There are four possible outcomes to CD once it develops. Some patients will be symptomatic and obtain diagnosis and treatment. Others will be symptomatic but will not receive the diagnosis and leave untreated. Yet more patients will remain asymptomatic and never be diagnosed, and a few patients who would have remained asymptomatic are diagnosed by some type of screening detection.

Many patients may remain untreated and the ultimate outcome of untreated CD is really unknown. Emerging evidence suggests that undiagnosed (hence untreated) CD may increase the risk of death over time (decades) [52].

Clinical presentation

The classic constellation of symptoms and signs characterizing the malabsorptive syndrome of CD includes diarrhea, steatorrhea, weight loss or failure to thrive, bloating, and flatulence with multiple deficiency states [53] (Table 17.2). More common and difficult to recognize are the other ways in which CD presents, the so-called "nonclassical" presentations [54]. It can mimic many common clinical entities

Table 17.2 Presentations of celiac disease (partial list).

Gastrointestinal	Nongastrointestinal
Steatorrhea	Dermatitis herpetiformis
Chronic diarrhea	Infertility
Weight loss	Anemia
Elevated transaminases	Dementia
Recurrent pancreatitis	Osteoporosis
Bloating, abdominal pain	Neuropathy
Failure to thrive	Dental enamel defects
Enteropathy-associated T cell lymphoma	Ataxia
Vomiting	Osteomalacia
Duodenal obstruction	Tetany

(CD is considered the "modern impostor") including irritable bowel syndrome, deficiencies of single micronutrients, especially iron, folate, B12, and the fat-soluble vitamins. Other "nonclassical" presentations are secondary osteoporosis, osteomalacia, ataxia, dementia, fatigue, neuropathy, and chorea.

The presentation of CD in children similarly can result in stunting of growth and intellectual development, epilepsy, and dental abnormalities as single symptoms without the more classic malabsorption symptoms of malnourished pot-bellied infant with steatorrhea [55].

CD is defined according to the clinical presentation and has been likened to an iceberg, "the celiac iceberg." The tip of the iceberg represents the most obvious part of the clinical spectra (classic malabsorption). If the patient's symptoms are characteristic of the malabsorption syndrome (diarrhea, steatorrhea, weight loss, and fatigue), then the adjective "classical" is used. Then there is the "nonclassical" CD, an adjective applied when patients have nonspecific symptoms such as abdominal discomfort, bloating, indigestion, or nongastrointestinal symptoms (microcytic anemia). Thus, this group of patients had minimal symptoms but can be detected clinically if there is a high suspicion for the diagnosis. Paradoxically, the "nonclassical" is now the most frequent presentation of CD in the United States. Finally, there is the submerged part of the iceberg where patients have histological evidence of CD but remain undetected. Some of that portion consists of identifiable at-risk groups such as families of people with CD and subjects with CD-associated diseases. In "silent" CD, intestinal biopsies show the characteristic morphologic changes in an asymptomatic patient. Autoantibodies may or may not be present. "Latent" disease refers to genetically susceptible persons, without symptoms or histologic evidence of CD who will ultimately go on to develop CD. These cases are found by following up persistently positive autoantibodies such as endomysial or tTG antibodies, in patients with DH who initially have an apparently normal small intestine who then develop CD while on a gluten-containing diet, or occasionally in asymptomatic family members of an index case.

Celiac crisis

A life-threatening presentation of CD has been reported in children and less frequently in adults [56, 57]. Profuse acute diarrhea, dehydration, hypokalemia, and severe metabolic acidosis; the so-called "celiac crisis" needs emergent life-saving therapy [58]. This dramatic clinical scenario can be a spontaneous clinical presentation or precipitated by the gluten challenge in patients very sensitive to the gluten.

Dermatitis herpetiformis

DH is characterized by chronic, intensely pruritic, polymorphic rash that causes vesicles–bullae on extensor surfaces of the elbows, knees, buttocks, and scalp [59]. There is a slight male preponderance of DH [60]. It is a skin manifestation of the intestinal immune response to ingested gluten that is characterized by the deposition of IgA granules at the dermo-epidermal junction. The source of these IgA deposits in the skin is unknown, but they may be produced in the intestinal mucosa and are likely cross-reactive with the closely related skin-based autoantigen epidermal transglutaminase, which is similar to tTG (the primary autoantigen in the gut) [61]. The intestinal damage may be asymptomatic at the time of presentation of the skin rash, but it is indistinguishable from that seen in CD. A positive serological test strengthens the certainly of the skin diagnosis, and would also mandate examination of the patient for consequences of malabsorption. However, it is not necessary to perform these antibody tests or even an intestinal biopsy to establish the etiologic role of intestinal gluten exposure in DH. That can be reliably inferred by the demonstration of the granular IgA deposits in the skin. The serology test may be useful in cases in which there remains some doubt, for example, in distinguishing it from bullous linear IgA disease, which is not a gluten-sensitive disorder. Gliadin antibodies may be seen in other bullous skin disorders and are not particularly helpful in this setting [62].

Many patients in the United States with DH have not been treated with a gluten-free diet (GFD), but rather with dapsone, which suppresses only the skin rash. The usual starting dose is 100 mg/day; however, dapsone does not prevent intestinal damage, but its benefit on the rash may delay or divert the patient from taking the appropriate dietary measures. Many of these patients may present years later with gastrointestinal (GI) symptoms, anemia, and severe metabolic bone disease or even malignancies. Additionally, dapsone side effects include methemoglobinemia, hemolytic anemia, and a severe idiosyncratic reaction called dapsone hypersensitivity syndrome [63]. Thus, a lifelong GFD must be recommended as the mainstay of the long-term treatment of DH.

Diagnostic tests for celiac disease

An important consideration is whether the patient has been on a GFD prior the testing. All of the tests, including the intestinal biopsies may have returned to normal, making confirmation difficult without reintroducing gluten into the diet.

The pre-modern diagnosis of CD was based on the constellation of features, especially steatorrhea and weight loss or failure to thrive, that are hallmarks of frank malabsorption. Almost simultaneously in the 1950s, advances in understanding of the specific pathologic lesion in the small intestinal mucosa and its gluten-induced etiology enhanced the precision with which the disease could be diagnosed; diagnosis included the response to therapy. Current guidelines require histological evidence of enteropathy and a positive response of symptoms or signs to a GFD. The earlier requirement for three sets of biopsies (one at diagnosis, after treatment with GFD, and after gluten challenge) was both cumbersome and, in most cases, unnecessary to establish and confirm a diagnosis of CD.

Serological testing has greatly facilitated the identification of CD in people with clinical presentations too mild to justify the invasiveness of a biopsy as the initial diagnostic test. The ready availability of serology has made detection accessible to primary care doctors and their patients in primary care. Not only are more people being diagnosed, but many other issues have arisen about the accuracy of the diagnosis and how to incorporate serologic testing into the diagnostic approach (Figure 17.3). Indeed, the new guidelines from the European Society for Pediatric Gastroenterology, Hepatology, and Nutrition proposed the option for the diagnosis of CD without intestinal biopsy in children with symptoms and high titers of tTG antibodies (>10 times the upper limit of normal). If the patient accepts this option, testing for HLA is necessary and endomysial antibodies should be investigated in a different blood sample [65].

Serology

A summary of diagnostic performance of the serological tests available for CD diagnosis is shown in Table 17.3. Conventional anti-gliadin antibodies are no longer

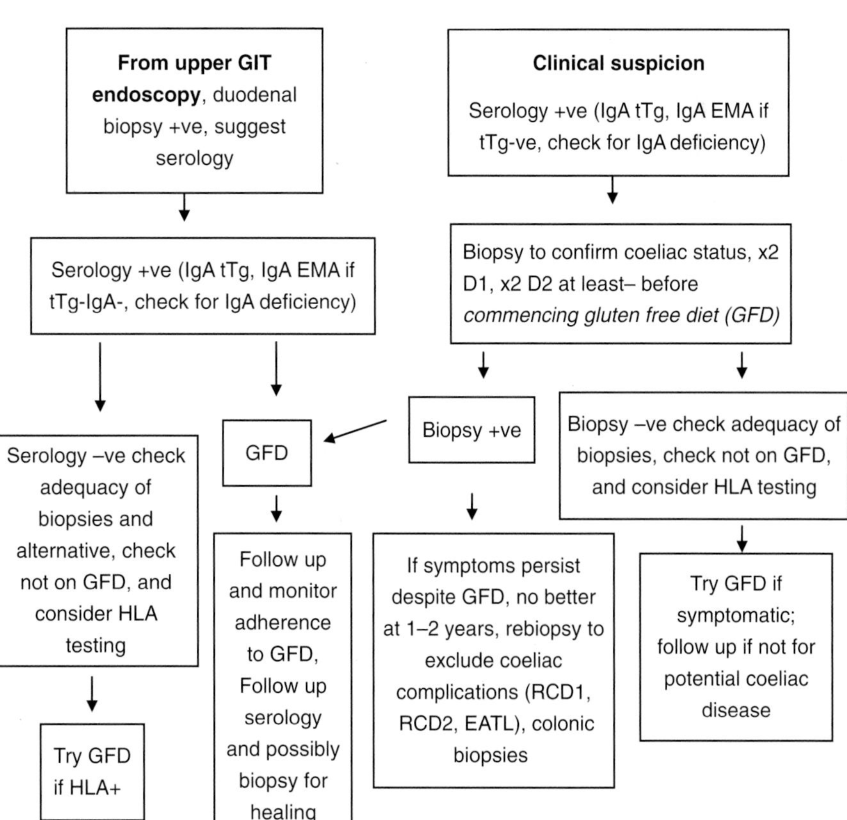

Figure 17.3 Approach to the diagnosis of celiac disease by using combined serology and histology. Reprinted from Reference 64.

Table 17.3 Serological tests for celiac disease.

Substrate/antigen	Antibody isotype	Sensitivity (%)	Specificity (%)
Gliadin	IgA	31–100	85–100
Gliadin	IgG	46–100	67–100
Endomysium	IgA[a]	57–100	95–100
Tissue transglutaminase	IgA[a]	92–98	98
Deamidated gliadin peptides	IgA[a]	88	95

[a]IgG is available but not recommended in patients without IgA deficiency.

recommended. The serologic test of choice for CD diagnosis is IgA tTG antibody [66].

Intestinal biopsies

Multiple biopsies from the duodenum are necessary because the celiac lesion could be patchy. A biopsy of the bulb in addition to four biopsies of distal duodenum may improve diagnostic yield for CD [67, 68]. A duodenal bulb biopsy from either 9- or 12-o'clock position may be the ideal site within the bulb [69]. Unfortunately, adherence to submitting multiple biopsies (≥4 specimens) is low (about 35%) in the United States [70]. The biopsy must be interpreted by an expert pathologist with recognition of the whole spectrum of the histological lesion in CD. The most used histological classification is that described by Marsh [38]. Briefly, Marsh type 0 is a normal mucosa. Marsh type 1, or "infiltrative" lesion, is characterized by intraepithelial lymphocytosis in the absence of another abnormality but is not specific for CD. Marsh type 2, or "hyperplastic" lesion, is characterized by intraepithelial lymphocytosis with crypt hyperplasia. Marsh type 3, or "atrophic" lesion, is characterized by partial atrophy (3a), subtotal atrophy (3b), and total atrophy (3c) [71]. Marsh type 4 refers to the most severe "hypoplastic" lesion. Corraza et al. proposed a simplified classification with just three histological groups for celiac patients with increased intraepithelial lymphocytes (>25/100 enterocytes): A, non-atrophic; B1, atrophic, villous-crypt ratio <3:1; and B2, atrophic, without detectable villi [72]. The simplified classification has higher interobserver agreement than modified Marsh classification.

Gluten challenge

It is no longer necessary to re-challenge most patients who have a well-established diagnosis of CD. However, in patients first diagnosed under the age of 3 years or those who have already embarked on a GFD and are seeking a confirmation of the diagnosis, a formal gluten challenge may be desirable [73]. This is not usually needed if the patient had a biopsy while on gluten-containing diet. Review of the original histology slides, if available, may suffice to confirm the diagnosis. The absence of HLA DQ2 and DQ8 made CD highly unlikely and the challenge unnecessary.

The length of time it takes to relapse with gluten challenge is quite variable [74]. The gluten in three to four slices of whole wheat bread daily should be sufficient to produce damage in 2–4 weeks, although it can take longer for the full pattern of injury to occur. Some very sensitive patients may need a reduction of this dose to prevent severe symptoms. Most patients relapse within 6 months although, in rare cases, it may take years to relapse.

Treatment

Dietary therapy

The mainstay of treatment of CD is lifelong adherence to a diet that excludes foods containing gluten [75] (Table 17.4). Patients may have difficulty accepting that something as fundamental to their diet as wheat can injure them. The patient can be motivated with the expectation of what can often be a dramatic improvement in general well-being in addition to improvement of GI symptoms [76]. A GFD should result in a prompt and even dramatic improvement in symptoms [77]. The recovery is more rapid and complete in children than adults. Resolution of symptoms may take 3–6 months, and complete healing of the intestine may take longer, especially in adults [78].

Detailed instruction from an experienced, well-informed dietitian is invaluable for most patients. In the absence of dietary instruction, many patients unfortunately resort to books or the internet for information and may not fully understand important details. Inadvertent gluten intake or an overly restricted diet deficient in essential nutrients may be adopted. A CD support group can provide local information and emotional support to newly diagnosed patients.

Oats were once thought to be toxic for most CD patients, but recent controlled studies have shown that a moderate amount of a pure oat product did not impair healing of the intestine or cause a relapse. However, contamination of commercial oat products with other grains may occur. Vigilance is needed on the part of the patient and physician if a decision is made to incorporate oats in the diet.

Hidden sources of gluten are frequently present in what seem to be safe foods. Ingredient lists of gluten-free foods must be reviewed regularly for changes. It may be difficult to ascertain the exact grain source of ingredients because of production outsourcing. Even non-food items may be sources of trace gluten and can cause symptoms in more sensitive patients. Contamination of supposedly gluten-free products can also occur.

Lactose intolerance affects one half of celiacs at diagnosis but usually resolves with mucosal restoration. Temporarily limiting lactose ingestion or using lactase may be necessary.

Table 17.4 Sources of gluten in the diet.

Gluten-containing grains and flours
Wheat
Rye
Malt
Barley
Triticale (wheat–rye hybrid)
Couscous
Kamut
Spelt
Semolina
Gluten-containing foods
Bread
Breaded foods
Cakes
Cookies
Crackers
Croutons
Pasta
Pizza
Stuffing
Toast
Commonly overlooked sources of gluten
Beer
Broth
Brown rice syrup
Coating mixes
Caramel color
Cereal products
Catsup and mustard
Candy bars
Cheese spreads
Chip and dip mixes
"Cornflour" in Europe
Hot chocolate mixes or cocoa
Imitation bacon or seafood marinades
Instant coffee and tea, salad dressings
Modified food starch
Natural flavorings
Nondairy creamer
Non-fat processed food
Malt or malt flavoring
Processed meats and poultry
Some brands of ice cream
Sausage products
Sauces
Soup bases
Soy sauce
Stuffings
Thickeners
Tomato sauce
Unexpected sources of gluten
Medications (both prescription and OTC)
Tooth paste, denture fixatives
Glues, pastes, and dry wall filler
Airborne flour
Communion wafers
Cross contamination

Vitamin or mineral supplements are given to correct deficiencies of iron, folate, B12, calcium, and fat-soluble vitamins as needed. Marked osteopenia and osteoporosis are common in both men and women. Patients with decreased axial bone density should be advised to obtain at least 1200 mg of calcium and replacement doses of vitamin D. Secondary hyperparathyroidism may occur but tetany is rare. Pancreatic enzyme supplementation may be useful in very malnourished patients, and this may accelerate weight return.

All patients should be followed up to ensure compliance with, and a response to, the GFD [79]. Adolescents seem especially likely to be noncompliant with the dietary restrictions [80]. All antibody levels diminish with the institution of a GFD, often within weeks; by 6 months both tTG-IgA and EMA-IgA may be undetectable. The gliadin antibody titers, however, often persist for a year or more into the GFD. Repeat testing is used to monitor the diet. However, a negative test is not entirely reliable as an indicator of low-level gluten ingestion. Improved absorption may cause patients to gain excess weight, increase absorption of medications such as thyroid replacement, or develop increased cholesterol.

Non-dietary therapies

The better knowledge of CD pathogenesis may make possible the development of non-dietary therapies [81]. The current explored approaches include (1) enzymatic alteration of wheat, (2) oral enzyme supplements, (3) polymeric binders, (4) intestinal permeability modification, and (5) induction of immune tolerance.

Prevention

Breast feeding and gradual introduction of gluten

Protective factors, such as breast feeding and delayed introduction of large quantities of gluten into the infant diet, seem to reduce the likelihood of developing CD in early age. This practical knowledge derives of the experience and analysis of the "Swedish epidemic of CD" [82]. In Sweden, a high incidence of CD was observed after national infant-feeding polices were changed to favor the introduction of larger quantities of gluten at the age of 6 months, after weaning was complete.

The incidence of symptomatic CD (clinically detected) in children under 2 years of age returned to "pre-epidemic" values after a national change in infant feeding recommendations was proposed in 1996: a slow introduction to gluten during weaning was stressed, the recommendation being the introduction of smaller quantities of gluten at the age of 4 months with continued breast feeding, instead of larger quantities at the age of 6 months at the time of weaning [83]. However, no difference was found in undiagnosed CD between the screened children born before and those born after 1996. However, when screened, fully 3% of children born during the epidemic period were found to have a CD [24]. Thus, a slow introduction of gluten in infancy could protect some children from developing symptomatic CD, but it might not protect them from subclinical or silent forms of this disease in childhood.

Vaccines

Currently, there are no vaccines for CD. However, as the gluten is clearly identified as the most important environmental factor, and the auto-antigen (tTG) is known, the development of a vaccine is hypothetically possible. Prophylactic vaccination against pneumococcal infections may be appropriate in the context of CD-associated hyposplenism [84]. Patients with CD have a good immune response to the polyvalent pneumococcal vaccine [85]. On the other hand, a lack of response to hepatitis B vaccine has been reported in CD [86].

Persistent or recurring symptoms

Patients with previously diagnosed CD who have persistent or recurrent diarrhea despite apparent adherence to GFD should undergo a careful dietary review and a check of their serology [87, 88]. If both are negative and it is less than 6 months since diagnosis, treatment with lactose-restricted diet, pancreatic supplements (especially if there are features of malabsorption and low fecal-elastase 1) should be started. Colonic biopsies may identify microscopic colitis. If it has been longer than 6 months since diagnosis, it may be prudent to re-biopsy the small intestine to assess for improvement. Other causes of recurrent symptoms are small-intestinal bacterial overgrowth, irritable bowel syndrome, and refractory CD [89].

Refractory celiac disease

Refractory celiac disease (RCD) is a combination of continued or recurrent severe malabsorption, progressive malnutrition, intestinal villous atrophy on repeat biopsy, and increased mortality despite compliance with a GFD for more than 6 months [90]. This condition affects approximately 3% of CD patients. Usually tTG and EMA antibodies are negative. Patients may have extensive small-intestinal ulcerations extending beyond the distal duodenum (ulcerative jejunoileitis) with a high risk of perforation, obstruction, and transformation to lymphoma [91]. Other uncommon complications are mesenteric lymph node cavitation and collagenous sprue (subepithelial collagen band thicker than 10 μm). Enteric protein loss may be marked. The clinical presentation includes profound malnutrition, weight loss, abdominal pain, and fever.

Enteropathy-associated T-cell lymphoma should be carefully sought. CT scanning, small bowel radiography, capsule endoscopy, PET scan, and double-balloon enteroscopy have been used to establish the diagnosis.

The presence of aberrant intraepithelial lymphocytes ($CD3$-$CD3c^{+}$, $CD8^{-}$) by immunohistochemistry (>50%) or flow cytometry (>20%) and T cell clones on molecular analysis is the hallmark of RCD II [92, 93). The abnormal clone of intraepithelial lymphocyte expresses cytoplasmic CD3 but lose the surface CD8 marker (and other T-cell markers), and demonstrates clonal T-cell receptor (TCR) gamma gene rearrangement. The absence of a T cell clone (RCD I) has a much better prognosis, with good clinical response to steroids or immunosuppression likely. Older age at diagnosis and hypoalbuminemia may be associated with increased mortality risk [94, 95]. Parenteral nutrition support allows correction of the nutritional problems, but some patients require home total parenteral nutrition for survival. Prognosis of RCD II is poor, with 50% of patients suffering a fatal outcome most often after progression to overt lymphoma. Currently, there is no effective treatment for RCD II. Steroids and immunosuppressive drugs should be used with caution and frequently are ineffective. A third of the patients with RCD II were clinically and histologically improved with the use of 2-clorodeoxyadenosine, or cladribine; however, the T cell abnormal clone persisted in all the patients and in 40% the disease progressed to overt lymphoma [96]. The use of alemtuzumab (anti-CD52 monoclonal antibody) [97] or autologous hematopoietic stem cell transplantation has been reported as a successful treatment for overt T-cell lymphoma [98]. Interleukin 15 blockade represent one promising option for the future treatment of RS type II [99].

Mortality in celiac disease

Patients with CD have a modestly increased mortality risk, with the most common cause of death being cardiovascular disorders [100]. Malignancies are also a common cause of death in patients with CD [101]. The risk of malignancy is highest during the first 3 years after diagnosis, and remains higher if CD is left untreated [102].

The development of hypoalbuminemia, anemia, recurrent steatorrhea, weight loss, lymphadenopathy, fevers, and malaise in a previously stable patient should prompt a search for neoplasm.

Patients with untreated CD have a particularly high risk of enteropathy-associated T-cell lymphoma [103], an otherwise rare form of high grade and frequently lethal lymphoma. Adenocarcinoma of the small intestine, nasopharyngeal, melanoma, and esophageal cancer are also more common in CD [104]. On the other hand, a lower incidence of breast cancer has been reported in women with CD.

Nonmalignant complications also play a role in mortality in CD. Cardiovascular disease was the most frequent cause of death among patients with CD from a large population-based study [100].

References

1. Di Sabatino A, Ciccocioppo R, Cupelli F, et al. Epithelium derived interleukin 15 regulates intraepithelial lymphocyte Th1 cytokine production, cytotoxicity, and survival in coeliac disease. *Gut* 2006; 55(4):469–477.
2. Lee SK, Green PH. Celiac sprue (the great modern-day imposter). *Curr Opin Rheumatol* 2006; 18(1):101–107.
3. Catassi C. The world map of celiac disease. *Acta Gastroenterol Latinoam* 2005; 35(1):37–55.
4. Fasano A, Berti I, Gerarduzzi T, et al. Prevalence of celiac disease in at-risk and not-at-risk groups in the United States: a large multicenter study. *Arch Intern Med* 2003; 163(3):286–292.
5. Ludvigsson JF, Leffler DA, Bai JC, et al. The Oslo definitions for coeliac disease and related terms. *Gut* 2013; 62:43–52.
6. Biesiekierski JR, Newnham ED, Irving PM, et al. Gluten causes gastrointestinal symptoms in subjects without celiac disease: a double-blind randomized placebo-controlled trial. *Am J Gastroenterol* 2011; 106(3):508–514.
7. Palosuo K. Update on wheat hypersensitivity. *Curr Opin Allergy Clin Immunol* 2003; 3(3):205–209.
8. Marsh MN. Gluten, major histocompatibility complex, and the small intestine. A molecular and immunobiologic approach to the spectrum of gluten sensitivity ('celiac sprue'). *Gastroenterology* 1992; 102(1):330–354.
9. Tollefsen S, Arentz-Hansen H, Fleckenstein B, et al. HLA-DQ2 and -DQ8 signatures of gluten T cell epitopes in celiac disease. *J Clin Invest* 2006; 116(8):2226–2236.
10. van Heel DA, Hunt K, Greco L, et al. Genetics in coeliac disease. *Best Pract Res Clin Gastroenterol* 2005; 19(3):323–339.
11. Ahn R, Ding YC, Murray J, et al. Association analysis of the extended MHC region in celiac disease implicates multiple independent susceptibility loci. *PLoS One* 2012; 7(5):e36926.
12. Greco L, Corazza G, Babron MC, et al. Genome search in celiac disease. *Am J Hum Genet* 1998; 62(3):669–675.
13. Holopainen P, Naluai AT, Moodie S, et al. Candidate gene region 2q33 in European families with coeliac disease. *Tissue Antigens* 2004; 63(3):212–222.
14. Van Belzen MJ, Meijer JW, Sandkuijl LA, et al. A major non-HLA locus in celiac disease maps to chromosome 19. *Gastroenterology* 2003; 125(4):1032–1041.
15. Garner CP, Ding YC, Steele L, et al. Genome-wide linkage analysis of 160 North American families with celiac disease. *Genes Immun* 2007; 8(2):108–114.
16. Romanos J, van Diemen CC, Nolte IM, et al. Analysis of HLA and non-HLA alleles can identify individuals at high risk for celiac disease. *Gastroenterology* 2009; 137(3):834–840.
17. Molberg O, Uhlen AK, Jensen T, et al. Mapping of gluten T-cell epitopes in the bread wheat ancestors: implications for celiac disease. *Gastroenterology* 2005; 128(2):393–401.
18. Holm K, Maki M, Vuolteenaho N, et al. Oats in the treatment of childhood coeliac disease: a 2-year controlled trial and a long-term clinical follow-up study. *Aliment Pharmacol Ther* 2006; 23(10):1463–1472.
19. Haboubi NY, Taylor S, Jones S. Coeliac disease and oats: a systematic review. *Postgrad Med J* 2006; 82(972):672–678.
20. Vader LW, Stepniak DT, Bunnik EM, et al. Characterization of cereal toxicity for celiac disease patients based on protein homology in grains. *Gastroenterology* 2003; 125(4):1105–1113.
21. Qiao SW, Bergseng E, Molberg O, et al. Antigen presentation to celiac lesion-derived T cells of a 33-mer gliadin peptide naturally formed by gastrointestinal digestion. *J Immunol* 2004; 173(3):1757–1762.
22. Riddle MS, Murray JA, Porter CK. The incidence and risk of celiac disease in a healthy US adult population. *Am J Gastroenterol* 2012; 107(8):1248–1255.
23. Stene LC, Honeyman MC, Hoffenberg EJ, et al. Rotavirus infection frequency and risk of celiac disease autoimmunity in early childhood: a longitudinal study. *Am J Gastroenterol* 2006; 101(10):2333–2340.
24. Myleus A, Ivarsson A, Webb C, et al. Celiac disease revealed in 3% of Swedish 12-year-olds born during an epidemic. *J Pediatr Gastroenterol Nutr* 2009; 49(2):170–176.
25. Clemente MG, De Virgiliis S, Kang JS, et al. Early effects of gliadin on enterocyte intracellular signalling involved in intestinal barrier function. *Gut* 2003; 52(2):218–223.
26. Drago S, El Asmar R, Di Pierro M, et al. Gliadin, zonulin and gut permeability: effects on celiac and non-celiac intestinal mucosa and intestinal cell lines. *Scand J Gastroenterol* 2006; 41(4):408–419.
27. Macdonald TT, Monteleone G. Immunity, inflammation, and allergy in the gut. *Science* 2005; 307(5717):1920–1925.
28. Duerksen DR, Wilhelm-Boyles C, Parry DM. Intestinal permeability in long-term follow-up of patients with celiac disease on a gluten-free diet. *Dig Dis Sci* 2005; 50(4):785–790.
29. Jabri B, Kasarda DD, Green PH. Innate and adaptive immunity: the yin and yang of celiac disease. *Immunol Rev* 2005; 206:219–231.
30. Jabri B, Sollid LM. Mechanisms of disease: immunopathogenesis of celiac disease. *Nat Clin Pract Gastroenterol Hepatol.* 2006;3(9):516–525.
31. Molberg O, Solheim Flaete N, Jensen T, et al. Intestinal T-cell responses to high-molecular-weight glutenins in celiac disease. *Gastroenterology* 2003; 125(2):337–344.
32. Sollid LM. Celiac disease as a model of gastrointestinal inflammation. *J Pediatr Gastroenterol Nutr* 2005; 40(Suppl 1):S41–S42.
33. Kakar S, Nehra V, Murray JA, et al. Significance of intraepithelial lymphocytosis in small bowel biopsy samples with normal mucosal architecture. *Am J Gastroenterol* 2003; 98(9):2027–2033.
34. Collin P, Wahab PJ, Murray JA. Intraepithelial lymphocytes and coeliac disease. *Best Pract Res Clin Gastroenterol* 2005; 19(3):341–350.

35. Stepniak D, Koning F. Celiac disease–sandwiched between innate and adaptive immunity. *Hum Immunol* 2006; 67(6):460–468.
36. Raki M, Tollefsen S, Molberg O, et al. A unique dendritic cell subset accumulates in the celiac lesion and efficiently activates gluten-reactive T cells. *Gastroenterology* 2006; 131(2):428–438.
37. Murray JA, Rubio-Tapia A, Van Dyke CT, et al. Mucosal atrophy in celiac disease: extent of involvement, correlation with clinical presentation, and response to treatment. *Clin Gastroenterol Hepatol* 2008; 6(2):186–193.
38. Marsh MN, Crowe PT. Morphology of the mucosal lesion in gluten sensitivity. *Baillieres Clin Gastroenterol* 1995; 9(2):273–293.
39. Ensari A, Marsh MN, Morgan S, *et al.* Diagnosing coeliac disease by rectal gluten challenge: a prospective study based on immunopathology, computerized image analysis and logistic regression analysis. *Clin Sci (Lond)* 2001; 101(2):199–207.
40. Beitnes AC, Raki M, Brottveit M, et al. Rapid accumulation of CD14+CD11c +dendritic cells in gut mucosa of celiac disease after in vivo gluten challenge. *PLoS One* 2012; 7(3):e33556.
41. Di Niro R, Mesin L, Zheng NY, et al. High abundance of plasma cells secreting transglutaminase 2-specific IgA autoantibodies with limited somatic hypermutation in celiac disease intestinal lesions. *Nat Med* 2012; 18(3):441–445.
42. Dieterich W, Ehnis T, Bauer M, *et al.* Identification of tissue transglutaminase as the autoantigen of celiac disease. *Nat Med* 1997; 3(7):797–801.
43. Hernandez L, Green PH. Extraintestinal manifestations of celiac disease. *Curr Gastroenterol Rep* 2006; 8(5):383–389.
44. Skovbjerg H, Noren O, Anthonsen D, et al. Gliadin is a good substrate of several transglutaminases: possible implication in the pathogenesis of coeliac disease. *Scand J Gastroenterol* 2002; 37(7):812–817.
45. Qiao SW, Raki M, Gunnarsen KS, *et al.* Posttranslational modification of gluten shapes TCR usage in celiac disease. *J Immunol* 2011; 187(6):3064–3071.
46. Kim CY, Quarsten H, Bergseng E, et al. Structural basis for HLA-DQ2-mediated presentation of gluten epitopes in celiac disease. *Proc Natl Acad Sci USA* 2004; 101(12):4175–4179.
47. Rubio-Tapia A, Ludvigsson JF, Brantner TL, et al. The prevalence of celiac disease in the United States. *Am J Gastroenterol* 2012; 107(10):1538–1544.
48. Hoffenberg EJ, MacKenzie T, Barriga KJ, et al. A prospective study of the incidence of childhood celiac disease. *J Pediatr* 2003; 143(3):308–314.
49. Vilppula A, Kaukinen K, Luostarinen L, et al. Increasing prevalence and high incidence of celiac disease in elderly people: a population-based study. *BMC Gastroenterol* 2009; 9:49.
50. Steens RF, Csizmadia CG, George EK, et al. A national prospective study on childhood celiac disease in the Netherlands 1993–2000: an increasing recognition and a changing clinical picture. *J Pediatr* 2005; 147(2):239–243.
51. Murray JA, Van Dyke C, Plevak MF, et al. Trends in the identification and clinical features of celiac disease in a North American community, 1950–2001 *Clin Gastroenterol Hepatol* 2003; 1(1):19–27.
52. Rubio-Tapia A, Kyle RA, Kaplan EL, et al. Increased prevalence and mortality in undiagnosed celiac disease. *Gastroenterology* 2009; 137(1):88–93.
53. Rostom A, Murray JA, Kagnoff MF. American Gastroenterological Association (AGA) Institute technical review on the diagnosis and management of celiac disease. *Gastroenterology* 2006; 131(6):1981–2002.
54. Rampertab SD, Pooran N, Brar P, et al. Trends in the presentation of celiac disease. *Am J Med* 2006; 119(4):355. e9–e14.
55. Fasano A. Clinical presentation of celiac disease in the pediatric population. *Gastroenterology* 2005; 128(4 Suppl 1):S68–S73.
56. Baranwal AK, Singhi SC, Thapa BR, et al. Celiac crisis. *Indian J Pediatr* 2003; 70(5):433–435.
57. Wolf I, Mouallem M, Farfel Z. Adult celiac disease presented with celiac crisis: severe diarrhea, hypokalemia, and acidosis. *J Clin Gastroenterol* 2000; 30(3):324–326.
58. Jamma S, Rubio-Tapia A, Kelly CP, et al. Celiac crisis is a rare but serious complication of celiac disease in adults. *Clin Gastroenterol Hepatol* 2010; 8(7):587–590.
59. Oxentenko AS, Murray JA. Celiac disease and dermatitis herpetiformis: the spectrum of gluten-sensitive enteropathy. *Int J Dermatol* 2003; 42(8):585–587.
60. Turchin I, Barankin B. Dermatitis herpetiformis and gluten-free diet. *Dermatol Online J* 2005; 11(1):6.
61. Sardy M, Karpati S, Merkl B. Epidermal transglutaminase (TGase 3) is the autoantigen of dermatitis herpetiformis. *J Exp Med* 2002; 195(6):747–757.
62. Karpati S. Dermatitis herpetiformis: close to unravelling a disease. *J Dermatol Sci* 2004; 34(2):83–90.
63. Sener O, Doganci L, Safali M, et al. Severe dapsone hypersensitivity syndrome. *J Investig Allergol Clin Immunol* 2006; 16(4):268–270.
64. Walker MM, Murray JA. An update in the diagnosis of coeliac disease. *Histopathology* 2011; 59:166–179.
65. Husby S, Koletzko S, Korponay-Szabo IR, et al. European Society for Pediatric Gastroenterology, Hepatology, and Nutrition guidelines for the diagnosis of coeliac disease. *J Pediatr Gastroenterol Nutr* 2012; 54(1):136–160.
66. Leffler DA, Schuppan D. Update on serologic testing in celiac disease. *Am J Gastroenterol* 2010; 105(12):2520–2524.
67. Bonamico M, Thanasi E, Mariani P, et al. Duodenal bulb biopsies in celiac disease: a multicenter study. *J Pediatr Gastroenterol Nutr* 2008; 47(5):618–622.
68. Hopper AD, Cross SS, Sanders DS. Patchy villous atrophy in adult patients with suspected gluten-sensitive enteropathy: is a multiple duodenal biopsy strategy appropriate? *Endoscopy* 2008; 40(3):219–224.
69. Kurien M, Evans KE, Hopper AD, et al. Duodenal bulb biopsies for diagnosing adult celiac disease: is there an optimal biopsy site? *Gastrointest Endosc* 2012; 75(6):1190–1196.
70. Lebwohl B, Kapel RC, Neugut AI, et al. Adherence to biopsy guidelines increases celiac disease diagnosis. *Gastrointest Endosc* 2011; 74(1):103–109.
71. Oberhuber G. Histopathology of celiac disease. *Biomed Pharmacother* 2000; 54(7):368–372.

72. Corazza GR, Villanacci V, Zambelli C, et al. Comparison of the interobserver reproducibility with different histologic criteria used in celiac disease. *Clin Gastroenterol Hepatol* 2007; 5(7):838–843.
73. National Institutes of Health Consensus Development Conference Statement on Celiac Disease, June 28–30, 2004. *Gastroenterology* 2005;128(4 Suppl 1):S1–S9.
74. Laurin P, Wolving M, Falth-Magnusson K. Even small amounts of gluten cause relapse in children with celiac disease. *J Pediatr Gastroenterol Nutr* 2002; 34(1):26–30.
75. See J, Murray JA. Gluten-free diet: the medical and nutrition management of celiac disease. *Nutr Clin Pract* 2006; 21(1):1–15.
76. Case S. The gluten-free diet: how to provide effective education and resources. *Gastroenterology* 2005;128(4 Suppl 1):S128–S134.
77. Murray JA, Watson T, Clearman B, et al. Effect of a gluten-free diet on gastrointestinal symptoms in celiac disease. *Am J Clin Nutr* 2004; 79(4):669–673.
78. Rubio-Tapia A, Rahim MW, See JA, et al. Mucosal recovery and mortality in adults with celiac disease after treatment with a gluten-free diet. *Am J Gastroenterol* 2010; 105(6):1412–1420.
79. Schuppan D, Dennis MD, Kelly CP. Celiac disease: epidemiology, pathogenesis, diagnosis, and nutritional management. *Nutr Clin Care* 2005; 8(2):54–69.
80. Pietzak MM. Follow-up of patients with celiac disease: achieving compliance with treatment. *Gastroenterology* 2005; 128(4 Suppl 1):S135–S141.
81. Stoven S, Murray JA, Marietta E. Celiac disease: advances in treatment via gluten modification. *Clin Gastroenterol Hepatol* 2012; 10(8):859–862.
82. Ivarsson A, Persson LA, Nystrom L, et al. Epidemic of coeliac disease in Swedish children. *Acta Paediatr* 2000; 89(2):165–171.
83. Ivarsson A, Hernell O, Stenlund H, et al. Breast-feeding protects against celiac disease. *Am J Clin Nutr* 2002; 75(5):914–921.
84. Johnston SD, Robinson J. Fatal pneumococcal septicaemia in a coeliac patient. *Eur J Gastroenterol Hepatol* 1998; 10(4):353–354.
85. McKinley M, Leibowitz S, Bronzo R, et al. Appropriate response to pneumococcal vaccine in celiac sprue. *J Clin Gastroenterol* 1995; 20(2):113–116.
86. Noh KW, Poland GA, Murray JA. Hepatitis B vaccine nonresponse and celiac disease. *Am J Gastroenterol* 2003; 98(10):2289–2292.
87. Rubio-Tapia A, Barton SH, Murray JA. Celiac disease and persistent symptoms. *Clin Gastroenterol Hepatol* 2011; 9(1):13–17.
88. Krauss N, Schuppan D. Monitoring nonresponsive patients who have celiac disease. *Gastrointest Endosc Clin N Am* 2006; 16(2):317–327.
89. Abdulkarim AS, Burgart LJ, See J, et al. Etiology of nonresponsive celiac disease: results of a systematic approach. *Am J Gastroenterol* 2002; 97(8):2016–2021.
90. Trier JS, Falchuk ZM, Carey MC, et al. Celiac sprue and refractory sprue. *Gastroenterology* 1978; 75(2):307–316.
91. Elsing C, Placke J, Gross-Weege W. Ulcerative jejunoileitis and enteropathy-associated T-cell lymphoma. *Eur J Gastroenterol Hepatol* 2005; 17(12):1401–1405.
92. Rubio-Tapia A, Murray JA. Classification and management of refractory coeliac disease. *Gut* 2010; 59(4):547–557.
93. Cellier C, Delabesse E, Helmer C, et al. Refractory sprue, coeliac disease, and enteropathy-associated T-cell lymphoma. French Coeliac Disease Study Group. *Lancet* 2000; 356(9225):203–208.
94. Rubio-Tapia A, Kelly DG, Lahr BD, et al. Clinical staging and survival in refractory celiac disease: a single center experience. *Gastroenterology* 2009; 136(1):99–107.
95. Malamut G, Afchain P, Verkarre V, et al. Presentation and long-term follow-up of refractory celiac disease: comparison of type I with type II. *Gastroenterology* 2009; 136(1):81–90.
96. Al-Toma A, Goerres MS, Meijer JW, et al. Cladribine therapy in refractory celiac disease with aberrant T cells. *Clin Gastroenterol Hepatol* 2006; 4(11):1322–1327.
97. Vivas S, Ruiz de Morales JM, Ramos F, et al. Alemtuzumab for refractory celiac disease in a patient at risk for enteropathy-associated T-cell lymphoma. *N Engl J Med* 2006; 354(23):2514–2515.
98. Rongey C, Micallef I, Smyrk T, et al. Successful treatment of enteropathy-associated T cell lymphoma with autologous stem cell transplant. *Dig Dis Sci* 2006; 51(6):1082–1086.
99. Cellier C, Cerf-Bensussan N. Treatment of clonal refractory celiac disease or cryptic intraepithelial lymphoma: A long road from bench to bedside. *Clin Gastroenterol Hepatol* 2006; 4(11):1320–1321.
100. Ludvigsson JF, Montgomery SM, Ekbom A, et al. Small-intestinal histopathology and mortality risk in celiac disease. *J Am Med Assoc* 2009; 302(11):1171–1178.
101. Viljamaa M, Kaukinen K, Pukkala E, et al. Malignancies and mortality in patients with coeliac disease and dermatitis herpetiformis: 30-year population-based study. *Dig Liver Dis* 2006; 38(6):374–380.
102. West J, Logan RF, Smith CJ, et al. Malignancy and mortality in people with coeliac disease: population based cohort study. *BMJ* 2004; 329(7468):716–719.
103. Halfdanarson TR, Litzow MR, Murray JA. Hematologic manifestations of celiac disease. *Blood* 2007; 109(2):412–421.
104. Green PH, Fleischauer AT, Bhagat G, et al. Risk of malignancy in patients with celiac disease. *Am J Med* 2003; 115(3):191–195.

18 Food Protein-Induced Enterocolitis and Enteropathies

Jay A. Lieberman & Anna Nowak-Węgrzyn

Division of Allergy and Immunology, Department of Pediatrics, Icahn School of Medicine at Mount Sinai, New York, NY, USA

Key Concepts

- Food protein-induced enterocolitis and enteropathies are non-IgE-mediated gastrointestinal food allergic disorders.
- Food protein-activated intestinal lymphocytes elaborate inflammatory cytokines that result in increased intestinal permeability, malabsorption, dysmotility, diarrhea, pain, and failure to thrive.
- Food protein-induced enterocolitis syndrome (FPIES) is typically caused by cow's milk and soy; rice is the most common solid food cause, but cereal grains (oat, barley), fish, poultry, and vegetables may also cause FPIES.
- Classic infantile food protein-induced enteropathy was caused by cow's milk, soy, and wheat; recent reports describe subtle enteropathy in older children and adults with delayed food allergy to cow's milk and cereal grains as well as in children with multiple IgE-mediated food allergies.
- The majority of FPIES and food protein-induced enteropathies resolve by age 3 years.

Introduction

Allergic reactions to foods affecting the gastrointestinal tract have been known since ancient times. Hippocrates observed that cow's milk caused gastrointestinal symptoms as well as urticaria, and that some infants fed cow's milk developed prolonged diarrhea, vomiting, and failure to thrive that resolved only after removal of cow's milk from their diet. At present, gastrointestinal immune reactions to cow's milk proteins that are mediated by T lymphocytes with or without the contribution of specific IgE antibody are estimated to account for up to 40% of cow's milk protein hypersensitivity in infants and young children [1–7].

Food protein-induced enterocolitis syndrome (FPIES) and enteropathies represent non-IgE-mediated gastrointestinal food hypersensitivities. Their prevalence is not well characterized but they are well established as distinct clinical entities. Their pathophysiology requires further characterization; current evidence indicates that T-lymphocyte-mediated responses play an important role, whereas IgE antibodies to the offending foods are of minimal or no significance in the pathophysiology of these disorders [8]. In the absence of definitive laboratory tests, diagnosis relies predominantly on clinical responses to elimination diets with resolution of symptoms, oral food challenges (OFCs) with reappearance of symptoms following ingestion of the offending food, and endoscopy and biopsy findings as well as exclusion of causes such as infections, inflammatory bowel disease, ischemia, metabolic disorders, and others.

Table 18.1 summarizes the most important features of the clinical conditions induced by dietary proteins in children that are reviewed in this chapter, including FPIES, enteropathy, and iron deficiency anemia caused by cow's milk. They were defined using the consensus criteria developed by a workshop jointly sponsored by European Society of Pediatric Gastroenterology, Hepatology and Nutrition and North American Society for Pediatric Gastroenterology and Nutrition in November 1998 and further commented on in the most recent guidelines for the diagnosis and management of food allergy in the United States [8, 9].

Food protein-induced enterocolitis syndrome

FPIES manifests as profuse vomiting and diarrhea in young infants and is most commonly caused by cow's milk, soy, and rice proteins. Other solid foods have been reported;

Food Allergy: Adverse Reactions to Foods and Food Additives, Fifth Edition. Edited by Dean D Metcalfe, Hugh A Sampson, Ronald A Simon and Gideon Lack.

Table 18.1 Comparison of FPIES, food protein-induced enteropathy, and iron deficiency anemia due to cow's milk.

	FPIES	Enteropathy	Iron deficiency anemia
Age at onset	1 day–1 year	Dependent on age of exposure to antigen; Cow's milk and soy up to 2 years	2–20 months
Food proteins implicated			
Most common	Cow's milk, soy	Cow's milk, soy	Cow's milk
Less common	Rice, oat, barley, chicken, turkey, fish, pea, sweet potato	Wheat, egg	
Multiple food hypersensitivities	Both cow's milk and soy in up to 60%	Rare	No
Feeding at the time of onset	Formula	Formula	Cow's milk, nonhumanized cow's milk-based formula
Atopic background			
Family history of atopy	40–70%	Unknown	Unknown
Personal history of atopy	30%	22%	Unknown
Symptoms			
Emesis	Prominent	Intermittent	No
Diarrhea	Severe	Moderate	Minimal
Bloody stools	Severe	Rare	No
Edema	Acute, severe	Moderate	Mild
Shock	Possible	No	No
Failure to thrive	Moderate	Moderate	Minimal
Laboratory Findings			
Anemia	Moderate	Moderate	Moderate
Hypoalbuminemia	Acute	Moderate	Mild
Methemoglobinemia	May be present	No	No
Acidemia	May be present	No	No
Allergy evaluation			
Food skin prick test	Negative[a]	Negative	Negative
Serum food-allergen IgE	Negative[a]	Negative	Negative
Total IgE	Normal	Normal	Normal
Peripheral blood eosinophilia	No	No	No
Biopsy findings	Patchy, variable	Variable, increased crypt length	Mild
Villous injury	Prominent	No	No
Colitis	Occasional	No	No
Mucosal erosions	No	No	No
Lymphoid nodular hyperplasia	Prominent	No	No
Eosinophils		Few	
Food challenge	Vomiting in 3–4 h; diarrhea in 5–8 h	Vomiting and/or diarrhea in 40–72 h	Usually not necessary
Treatment	Protein elimination, 80% respond to casein hydrolysate and symptoms clear in 3–10 days; Re-challenge in 1.5–2 years	Protein elimination, symptoms clear in 1–3 weeks, rechallenge and biopsy in 1–2 years	Whole cow's milk protein elimination, feeding with humanized cow's milk-based formulas
Natural History	Cow's milk: Most resolve by 2 years Soy: 25–100% resolved by 2 years	Most cases resolve in 2–3 years	Most cases resolve by 3 years
Reintroduction of the food into the diet	Inpatient food challenge	Home, gradually advancing	Home, gradually advancing

[a]If positive, may be a risk factor for persistent disease.

onset of symptoms at older ages may occur with shellfish [8].

Historical perspective

Rubin, in 1940, reported intestinal bleeding due to cow's milk allergy in newborns [10]. Gryboski et al. and Powell described infants presenting in the first 6 weeks of life with recurrent vomiting, bloody diarrhea, and abdominal distension while being fed with cow's milk-based formula [11–14]. Many appeared dehydrated and severely ill. Sepsis evaluations were negative but improvement was achieved with intravenous (IV) fluids or hydrolyzed casein-based formula, but not with soy-based formula. Reintroduction of cow's milk-based formula resulted in recurrence of severe emesis and elevation of the peripheral blood neutrophil count. Subsequently Powell characterized major features of the disorder, and established criteria for the diagnosis of cow's milk-induced enterocolitis and a standard challenge protocol [15]. Reports of a series of infants with food protein-induced enterocolitis by Sicherer et al. (16 patients) and Burks et al. (43 patients) further characterized clinical features and refined food challenge protocols [16, 17]. More recent reports have identified various solid foods as triggers for FPIES [18–28].

Prevalence

In a birth cohort of 13 019 infants under 12 months of age in Israel, 0.34% were diagnosed with cow's milk FPIES during physician-supervised OFCs [29]. In comparison, 0.5% infants were diagnosed as having IgE-mediated cow milk allergy. Although it is impossible to extrapolate results from Israel to other patient populations, this study suggests that FPIES may be a more common condition than previously assumed. Prevalence estimates for other countries have not been reported.

Clinical characteristics

Cow's milk/soy FPIES

FPIES is commonly caused by cow's milk or soy proteins in formula-fed infants, with many reacting to both foods; and onset of symptoms from first days to 12 months of life; later onset is associated with delayed introduction of milk or soy protein in breast-fed infants [13, 14]. FPIES is extremely rare in exclusively breast-fed infants, with very few reports of reactions to the offending foods in the breast milk, perhaps suggesting an important role of breast feeding in FPIES [22, 30, 31].

In the most severe cases, symptoms may manifest within the first days of life with severe, bloody diarrhea, lethargy, abdominal distension, hypoactive bowel sounds, weight loss, failure to thrive, dehydration, metabolic acidosis and electrolyte abnormalities, anemia, elevated white blood count with eosinophilia, and hypoalbuminemia [13, 32]. Intramural gas may be noted on abdominal radiographs, prompting a diagnosis of necrotizing enterocolitis, sepsis evaluation, and treatment with antibiotics [13, 32, 33]. Ileus resulting in laparoscopy was reported [34, 35]. Overall, 75% of infants with FPIES appear acutely ill including 15% who are hypotensive and require hospitalization as well as extensive evaluation before the diagnosis of FPIES is established. Methemoglobinemia has also been reported, and when present, is typically associated with severe reactions and profound acidemia [16, 36].

Young infants presenting with chronic symptoms while being continuously fed with cow's milk or soy formula improve promptly when placed on IV fluids or with casein hydrolysate-based formula. However, upon reintroduction of the offending food, they develop dramatic symptoms, including shock in 15–20% of cases. Based on Powell's experience with 14 positive follow-up challenges in 18 infants, repetitive emesis started within 1–2 hours following ingestion and diarrhea within 2–10 hours (mean onset, 5 hours) with blood, mucous, leukocytes, eosinophils, and increased carbohydrate content in the stool [14]. Peripheral blood neutrophil counts were elevated in all positive challenges, peaking at 6 hours following ingestion with a mean increase of 9900 cells/mm^3 and the range 5500–16 800 cells/mm^3.

Solid food FPIES

Rare case reports initially described infants with typical features of FPIES provoked by ingestion of solid foods such as rice, chicken, turkey, egg white, green pea, and peanut [16, 18, 19, 21, 37]. Subsequently, larger series of patients with solid food FPIES were published [22–24, 26, 28]. In adults, crustacean shellfish (shrimp, crab, and lobster) and fish hypersensitivity may provoke a similar syndrome with severe nausea, abdominal cramps, protracted vomiting, and diarrhea [8].

In one series of infants with solid food FPIES, 65% were previously diagnosed with cow's milk and/or soy FPIES and were fed with casein hydrolysate- or amino acid-based formula; 35% were breast-fed at the time of FPIES onset, again suggesting that breast milk may confer a protective effect against FPIES development [22]. The mean age at onset of solid food FPIES tends to be higher. Infants often present with a history of multiple reactions and have undergone extensive evaluations for alternative etiologies (infectious, toxic, and metabolic) before the diagnosis of FPIES is established [22, 24, 26, 28]. Delayed diagnosis may be explained by a common perception that grains, for example, rice, and vegetables have low allergenic potential and are not considered as a cause of severe food allergic reactions, as well as lack of definitive diagnostic tests and the unusual nature of symptoms.

Table 18.2 Differential diagnosis of food protein-induced enterocolitis syndrome.

Allergic	Nonallergic
Food protein-induced proctocolitis Food protein-induced enteropathy Eosinophilic gastroenteropathies Cow's milk-induced gastroesophageal reflux	Necrotizing enterocolitis Sepsis Gastrointestinal infection (*Salmonella, Shigella, Campylobacter, Yersinia* spp., parasites) Hirschprung's disease Intussusception Volvulus Metabolic disorder Congenital cardiac defect Neurologic disorder

Diagnosis and management of FPIES

Diagnosis of FPIES relies on history, clinical features, exclusion of other etiologies, and OFC; Table 18.2 lists the differential diagnoses. The vast majority (over 90%) of patients in large series have negative skin prick tests and undetectable allergen-specific IgE antibodies to the offending foods [16, 17, 28, 29]. Although OFC is the gold standard for diagnosing FPIES, the majority of infants do not need to undergo confirmatory challenges, especially if they have a classic history of severe reactions and become asymptomatic following elimination of the suspected food. However, OFCs are necessary to determine when a patient "outgrows" FPIES. In the infants with chronic diarrhea, stool samples test positive for occult blood and show the presence of intact polymorphonuclear neutrophils, eosinophils, and Charcot–Leyden crystals. Some patients develop carbohydrate malabsorption and show reducing substances in the stool.

The atopy patch test (APT) has been evaluated in 19 infants (ages 5–30 months) with FPIES confirmed by an OFC [38]. APT predicted the outcome of an OFC in 28 of 33 instances; all positive OFCs had a positive APT, but five patients with positive APT did not react to an OFC. These findings have not been confirmed by other investigators, so at this time, the role of APT in the diagnosis of FPIES requires further rigorous evaluation.

Given the description of the typical constellation of clinical symptoms and strict criteria for a positive OFC, endoscopic examination is not performed routinely in patients with suspected FPIES. However, prior to establishment of diagnostic criteria, endoscopic evaluations were done in ill infants with cow's milk and/or soy FPIES and rectal bleeding. They reported rectal ulceration and bleeding with friability of the mucosa in most patients; endoscopy was normal in a minority of children. Plain radiological imaging or with barium contrast in infants with ongoing chronic symptoms of diarrhea, rectal bleeding, and/or failure to thrive showed air fluid levels consistent with intestinal obstruction, nonspecific narrowing, and thumbprinting of the rectum and sigmoid, as well as thickening of the plicae circulares in the duodenum and jejunum with excess luminal fluid. Striking, ribbon-like jejunum with loss of valvulae and separation of bowel loops, suggesting thickening of the bowel wall was reported [34, 39]. In extreme cases of ileus, in which laparotomy was performed, distention of small bowel loops and marked thickening of the wall of jejunum distal to Treitz's ligament with diffuse subserosal bleeding was observed [34, 35]. However, the bowel may appear grossly normal in FPIES without the complication of ileus [40]. Follow-up studies performed on a restricted diet in asymptomatic patients documented the resolution of radiological abnormalities. Radiological findings are nonspecific and can also be seen in celiac disease, intestinal lymphangiectasia, immunodeficiency, or Crohn's disease. However, they may alert the physician to the possibility of allergic colitis in a child presenting with chronic symptoms of diarrhea, failure to thrive, anemia, and hypoalbuminemia.

Oral food challenge in FPIES

OFCs can be used to establish the diagnosis of FPIES or to evaluate the possibility that FPIES has been "outgrown" in a patient with known or suspected FPIES. Depending on the clinical severity, follow-up challenges should be performed every 18–24 months to determine tolerance in patients without accidental reactions [41]. Guidelines for preparation and interpretation of the OFC for FPIES are summarized in Table 18.3; Box 18.1 contains a practical

Table 18.3 Oral food challenge in FPIES.

Challenge protocol
High-risk procedure, requires immediate availability of fluid resuscitation, secure intravenous access
Baseline peripheral neutrophil count
Gradual (over 1 h) administration of food protein 0.06–0.6[a] g/kg body weight, generally not to exceed total 3 g protein or 10 g of total food for an initial feeding
If no reaction in 2–3 h, administer a regular age appropriate serving of the food followed by several hours of observation
Majority of positive challenges require treatment with intravenous fluids and steroids
Criteria for a positive challenge
Symptoms
Emesis (typically in 2–4 h)
Diarrhea (typically in 5–8 h)
Laboratory findings
Fecal leukocytes
Fecal eosinophils
Increase in peripheral neutrophil count >3500 cells/mm^3 peaking at 6 h
Interpretation of the challenge outcome
Positive challenge: three of five criteria positive
Equivocal: two of five criteria positive

Source: Based on data from References 15, 41, 42, and 43.
[a]Lower dose recommended in children with history of previous severe reaction.

Box 18.1 Food challenge preparation for food protein-induced enterocolitis syndrome.

1. Obtain current weight of the patient.
2. Calculate the amount of protein per kg body weight; range 0.06–0.6 g protein per kg body weight; typically 0.15–0.3 g protein per kg body weight.
3. Weigh the equivalent of the calculated protein dose; do not exceed 10 g of the food challenged.
4. Mix the amount calculated with a vehicle of choice, such as rice milk for a total weight of 200 mL.
5. Administer in three doses over 30–45 minutes.

The child's weight is 10 kg.

Total dose of milk protein: 0.15 g × 10 kg = 1.5 g = 42 mL of skim milk = 1.4 oz skim milk [8 oz = 236.5 mL contains 8.4 g milk protein]. Add 42 mL of skim milk to a safe[a] rice milk for a total volume 100[b] mL and administer in 3 doses over 30–45 minutes.

Source: Adapted from Reference 43, with permission.
[a]Vehicles used in the oral food challenges should be carefully selected to avoid contamination with food allergens to which the patient undergoing challenge is allergic.
[b]100 mL is used to simplify calculations. The total amount of food should be the smallest amount needed that will mask the challenge food and will be reasonable for the patient to consume at one sitting.

example for calculating the quantity of food to use in the challenge.

OFCs involve the administration of food protein, 0.06–0.6 g/kg body weight, with lower doses (0.06 g/kg) used in children with prior severe reactions [15, 16, 42]. Generally, the amount served initially during an OFC does not exceed 3 g of food protein or 10 g of total food by weight (usually less than 100 mL of liquid food such as cow's milk or infant formula). The calculated amount of food is divided in three equal portions and served over 45 minutes [44]. The patient is observed for 4 hours and if asymptomatic, a second feeding, typically an age-appropriate regular serving amount is given followed by observation for several hours [43]. OFCs in FPIES are a high-risk procedure and should be performed under physician supervision with secure IV access for fluid resuscitation [16]. IV hydration is the first-line therapy; however, corticosteroids are often used empirically for severe reactions, based on presumed pathophysiology that involves T-cell-mediated intestinal inflammation. Epinephrine should be available for severe cardiovascular reactions with hypotension/shock, however, rapid rehydration with IV fluids (up to 20 mL/kg) is the mainstay of therapy and the efficacy of epinephrine in FPIES has not been demonstrated.

Dietary management of FPIES

For patients with suspected or confirmed FPIES, strict dietary avoidance of the offending food protein(s) should be recommended and appropriate guidelines for avoidance provided. Given of the high risk of concomitant cow's milk and soy FPIES (up to 60% of cases), extensively hydrolyzed casein formulas are recommended for infants and young children that cannot be breast fed [14, 16, 41]. Eighty percent of patients with cow's milk and/or soy FPIES respond to extensively hydrolyzed casein formula with resolution of symptoms within 3–10 days. Up to 10–20% of patients require amino-acid-based formula or temporary IV therapy [45, 46].

Proposed guidelines for solid food introduction to infants with cow's milk- or soy-induced FPIES (especially those with atopic dermatitis) take into account that up to one-third of these children appear to develop a reaction to solid food and include (1) delayed introduction of solid foods and (2) suggested yellow fruits and vegetables instead of cereal grains as first foods [22, 43]. In some series, infants with solid food FPIES are at high risk to react to other foods, as 80% are reactive to more than one food protein, 65% react to cow's milk and/or soy, and those with a history of reactions to one grain have at least a 50% chance of reacting to other grains [22, 24]. Therefore, infants with solid food FPIES may benefit from empiric avoidance of grains, legumes, and poultry in the first year of life [43]. Introduction of cow's milk and soy in infants without a prior history of reactivity to these foods may be attempted after 1 year of age, preferably under physician supervision. Tolerance to one food from each "high-risk category" such as soy for legumes, chicken for poultry, or oat for grains might be considered as an indication of increased likelihood of tolerance to the remaining foods from the same category [43].

Natural history of FPIES

Rates for the development of tolerance vary by report, likely reflecting differences in geography, patient selection, and timing of challenges. A summary of reports from various countries is seen in Table 18.4. FPIES rarely develops to foods following first exposure beyond 1 year of age. For example, wheat allergy has not been reported in infants with oat- or rice-induced FPIES, but introduction of wheat was significantly delayed, presumably avoiding the "window of immunologic susceptibility" for FPIES development [22, 43]. Sicherer et al. noted three patients who initially presented with and two that developed positive skin prick tests to commercial extracts of cow's milk and detectable serum milk-specific IgE antibodies (1 and 3 years after the diagnosis) [16]. All five patients remained sensitive to the offending food and showed only symptoms consistent with FPIES. They had no IgE-mediated symptoms of

Table 18.4 Resolution of FPIES for common foods.

Study	Sicherer (1998)	Nowak (2003)	Hwang (2009)	Mehr (2009)	Katz (2011)
Country of origin	United States	United States	Republic of Korea	Australia	Israel
Food					
Milk	60% resolved by 30 months	60% resolved by 36 months	100% resolved by 20 months	N/A	94% tolerant by 30 months
Soy	25% resolved by 36 months	27% resolved by 36 months	100% tolerant by 14 months	83% tolerant by 36 months	N/A
Rice	N/A	40% resolved by 36 months	N/A	80% tolerant by 36 months	N/A
Oat	N/A	66% resolved by 36 months	N/A	N/A	N/A

urticaria, wheezing, or anaphylaxis when challenged. Similarly, persistence of oat and soy allergy 2–3 years after the initial reaction was observed in two patients with detectable serum IgE antibodies to these foods [22]. Therefore, initial presence or development of IgE to food protein may indicate a more protracted course. It may be prudent to include skin prick testing and/or measurement of serum food-specific IgE in the initial as well as follow-up evaluations to identify patients at risk for persistent FPIES.

Genetics

The genetics of FPIES and the role of heredity are unknown. FPIES appears to be slightly more frequent in males than females, with a ratio of 60:40. Family history of atopy is positive in 40–80% of patients reported but only rarely family history is positive for food allergy, in about 20% of the cases [16, 22, 41, 43]. In the authors' experience, FPIES is rarely seen in more than one family member.

Pathology

Because the diagnosis of FPIES is based on clinical criteria, endoscopy and biopsy are not routinely performed. However, previously, endoscopic evaluations and biopsies were obtained in infants with symptoms consistent with FPIES. These cases with available biopsy data highlight inflammatory responses in the colon. Endoscopic evaluation revealed diffuse colitis with variable degrees of ileal involvement; in the most severe cases, focal erosive gastritis and esophagitis is found with prominent eosinophilia and villus atrophy. Colon mucosa can appear mildly friable to demonstrating severe spontaneous hemorrhage, and minute ulcers similar to those seen in ulcerative colitis can be found [12, 41]. Crypt abscesses have been identified in some patients [47].

Jejunal biopsies reveal a mild to severe degree of villus atrophy, edema, and increased numbers of lymphocytes, IgM- and IgA-containing plasma cells, eosinophils, and mast cells [47, 48].

Pathophysiology

Based on clinical manifestations of severe emesis and dehydration, it is hypothesized that local intestinal inflammation induced upon food allergen ingestion leads to increased intestinal permeability and fluid shift. In asymptomatic children with suspected egg white FPIES, gastrointestinal absorption of ovalbumin as measured by serum levels of ovalbumin did not differ between children who subsequently had a positive oral challenge to egg white and those who had no symptoms on egg challenge, suggesting that baseline antigen absorption is normal and does not predispose to FPIES [49].

Cytokines secreted by food-allergen-stimulated T lymphocytes affect intestinal permeability. Interleukin-4 (IL-4), interferon-γ (IFN-γ), and tumor necrosis factor-α (TNF-α) synergistically increase intestinal permeability, whereas transforming growth factor-β1 (TGF-β1) protects the epithelial barrier of the gut from the penetration of foreign antigens by antagonizing the action of IFN-γ [50–53].

Several original studies investigated lymphocyte responses and cytokine release in the patients with FPIES. From these studies, it appears that peripheral blood mononuclear cells (PBMCs) from children with cow's milk- or soy-induced FPIES have increased proliferation in response to milk or soy proteins; however, this response does not appear to be different than response in patients with IgE-mediated milk or soy allergy [54–56]. Mori et al. showed that $CD3^+$ T cells isolated from PBMCs show increased IL-4 and decreased IFN-γ staining immediately after a positive OFC in a single FPIES patient. Follow-up OFC in the same patient once tolerance had been established showed a shift toward decreased IL-4 staining and increased IL-10 staining, suggesting that in patients with active FPIES, the offending food may deviate the immune response toward a T helper type II response, while tolerance is IL-10-mediated [57].

TNF-α is a potent proinflammatory cytokine that induces neutrophil activation and increases intestinal permeability *in vitro* by altering the tight junctions between epithelial cells [58]. Because of these known effects of

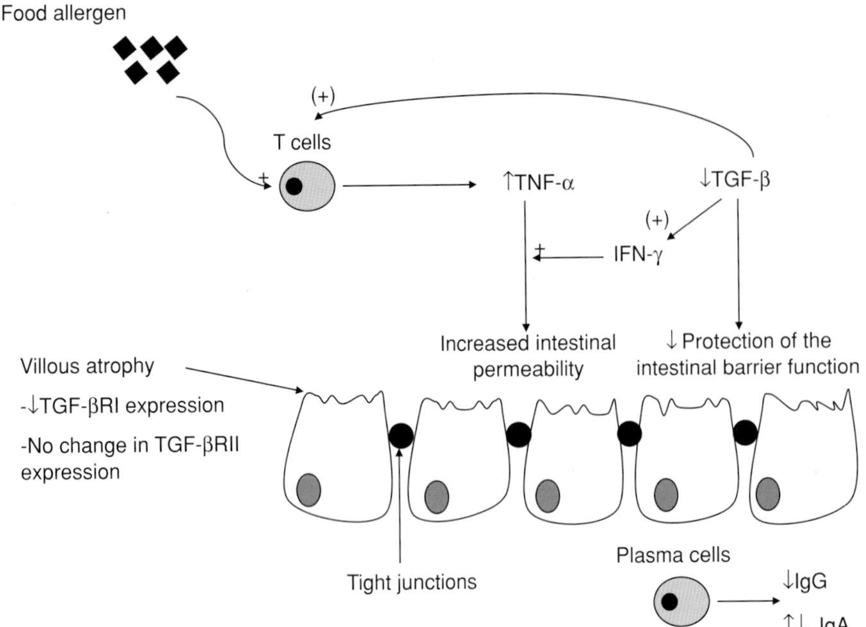

Figure 18.1 Summary of our current understanding of the immune mechanisms of food protein-induced enterocolitis syndrome (FPIES). Reprinted with permission from Caubet JC, Nowak-Węgrzyn A. Current understanding of the immune mechanisms of food protein-induced enterocolitis syndrome. *Expert Rev Clin Immunol* 2011; 7(3):317–327. doi: 10.1586/eci.11.13.

TNF-α, its role in this gastrointestinal cow's milk hypersensitivity has been investigated in a number of studies that included subsets of infants with cow's milk-induced FPIES. Heyman suggested that TNF-α secreted by circulating milk protein-specific T cells increased intestinal permeability, thus contributing to the influx of antigen into the submucosa with further activation of antigen-specific lymphocytes [59]. Lower quantities of intact cow's milk protein required to stimulate TNF-α secretion, and prolonged secretion of TNF-α by PBMCs were reported in patients with active intestinal cow's milk allergy, compared to patients with cutaneous symptoms and those who outgrew cow's milk allergy [60]. Cow's milk-stimulated fecal TNF-α was also found in increased concentrations following positive challenges in children with cow's milk allergy.

Investigating local mucosal characteristics, Chung found generally depressed TGF-β expression in duodenal biopsies from all 28 infants with challenge-proven cow's milk FPIES [61]. Expression of type 1 TGF-β receptors was significantly lower in the patients with villous atrophy compared with patients who did not have villous atrophy ($p < 0.001$). This was negatively correlated with the severity of villous atrophy ($r = -0.59$, $p < 0.001$). In contrast to depressed TGF-β, TNF-α expression on epithelial and lamina propria cells was significantly greater in the patients with villous atrophy ($p < 0.01$), suggesting that imbalance in TGF-β/TNF-α may be important in the pathophysiology of FPIES.

Humoral immune responses are generally not considered to be an important mechanism in FPIES. Interestingly, an increase in serum food antigen-specific IgA and IgG antibody levels has been noted in the FPIES patients [62]. Shek et al. found lower levels of serum cow's milk-specific IgG_4 antibody levels ($p < 0.05$) and a trend for higher IgA antibody levels in patients with cow's milk FPIES when compared to the control group [56]. The role of IgG and IgA antibodies in the pathogenesis of FPIES needs to be explored further. A working model of the inflammatory response in FPIES is shown in Figure 18.1.

Food protein-induced enteropathy

Food protein-induced enteropathy is a syndrome of small bowel injury with resulting malabsorption, similar to celiac disease although less severe [8].

Historical perspective

The first report of malabsorption syndrome with diarrhea, emesis, and impaired growth induced by cow's milk feedings in infants was published in 1905 [63]. Subsequent reports, including a large series of cow's milk protein-sensitive Finnish infants, defined clinical features of this disorder [64–70]. The reported incidence of food protein-induced enteropathy peaked in the 1960s in Finland, with virtual disappearance of severe jejunal damage caused by cow's milk protein in the past 20 years [71]. Infant feeding practices have been implicated as a cause of the changing prevalence of food protein-induced enteropathy, with the highest incidence of classic severe enteropathy attributed to feedings with nonhumanized, high-protein infant formulas and the lowest incidence in breast-fed infants

[72–74]. Recently, intestinal enteropathy was reported in older children with delayed-type allergic reactions to cow's milk as well as in children with multiple food allergies; however, it remains to be established whether these older children represent a milder phenotype of enteropathy or whether they have a different disease caused by cow's milk hypersensitivity [75–77].

Clinical features of food protein-induced enteropathy

Food protein-induced enteropathy presents with protracted diarrhea in the first 9 months of life, typically the first 1–2 months, within weeks following the introduction of cow's milk formula. Food proteins such as soybean, wheat, and egg have also been confirmed as causes of enteropathy, frequently in children with coexistent cow's milk protein-induced enteropathy [78–81].

More than 50% of the affected infants have vomiting and failure to thrive and some present with abdominal distension, early satiety, and malabsorption. In many infants, the onset of symptoms is gradual; in others, it mimics acute gastroenteritis with transient emesis and anorexia complicated by protracted diarrhea. It may be difficult to distinguish food protein-induced enteropathy from post-enteritis-induced lactose intolerance, especially since these two conditions may overlap [81]. Acute small bowel injury caused by viral enteritis has been postulated to predispose children to subsequent food protein-induced enteropathy, or alternatively to unmask underlying food protein hypersensitivity [69, 80, 82, 83]. Diarrhea generally resolves within 1 week following cow's milk protein elimination, although some infants require prolonged IV nutrition [70].

Moderate anemia (typically due to iron deficiency) is present in 20–69% of infants with cow's milk protein-induced enteropathy [70, 71]. Bloody stools are typically absent but occult blood can be found in 5% of patients [84]. Malabsorption is common, and evidence of hypoproteinemia, steatorrhea, sugar malabsorption, and deficiency of vitamin K-dependent factors can be seen [69, 85].

Diagnosis and management of food protein-induced enteropathy

Food protein-induced enteropathy is diagnosed by the confirmation of villous injury, crypt hyperplasia, and inflammation on small bowel biopsy obtained in a symptomatic patient who is being fed a diet containing the offending food allergen [47, 86–89]. Elimination of the food allergen should lead to resolution of clinical symptoms within 1–3 weeks [70]. Villous atrophy should improve within 4 weeks but complete resolution may take up to 1.5 years. Infants with severe initial manifestations may require prolonged bowel rest and parenteral nutrition for days or weeks. Diagnostic confirmatory challenges and measurement of specific serologies for celiac disease may be necessary to distinguish between food-protein enteropathy and celiac disease, or to identify multiple food allergens. In the clear-cut cases, OFCs are not absolutely required for confirmation of the diagnosis. The OFCs should be performed periodically to assess the development of oral tolerance.

Milk IgA and milk IgG precipitins may be elevated with active disease, but the diagnostic utility of these tests is unknown, particularly in view of the high prevalence of positive results in many other gastrointestinal inflammatory disorders in childhood [70]. Classically, food-specific IgE antibodies are undetectable and skin prick tests are negative [90]. Patch skin tests may be a useful screen for some gastrointestinal food hypersensitivity (cow's milk, wheat) [9]. However, biopsies were not obtained and the association of positive patch tests with gastrointestinal changes remains to be determined.

Studies have examined using serum concentrations of granzymes A (GrA) and B (GrB), soluble Fas, and CD30 (markers of activated cytotoxic lymphocytes) for the diagnosis of cow's milk-sensitive enteropathy [91]. GrB is present more often in patients with cow's milk-sensitive enteropathy as compared to controls, and serum levels of both granzymes were higher in untreated food-allergic patients; these markers should be confirmed in larger studies, however, prior to their routine clinical use.

Natural history of food protein-induced enteropathy

Food protein-induced enteropathy resolves clinically in the majority of children by age 1–2 years; however, the proximal jejunal mucosa may be persistently abnormal at that time [70]. Mucosal healing continues during feeding with the implicated food once clinical tolerance is achieved [87]. In children with less severe disease who were diagnosed at an older age, tolerance also developed at an older age, however, most became tolerant by 3 years [73]. Of note, 5 of 54 infants with challenge-confirmed cow's milk-induced enteropathy were ultimately diagnosed with celiac disease that persisted beyond infancy [70]. In contrast, transient wheat enteropathy with or without associated cow's milk protein-induced enteropathy has been reported in a number of studies, including transient wheat enteropathy following enteritis [82, 92, 93]. Strict criteria for the diagnosis of transient wheat-induced enteropathy were established and include evidence of small bowel villous injury, resolution with gluten avoidance and persistent normal small bowel mucosa for 2 or more years after re-introducing gluten to the diet [94]. The course of food protein-induced enteropathy in older children has not been characterized.

Pathologic features of food protein-induced enteropathy

The degree of villous injury is variable, ranging from severe to mild, with most biopsy specimens revealing patchy,

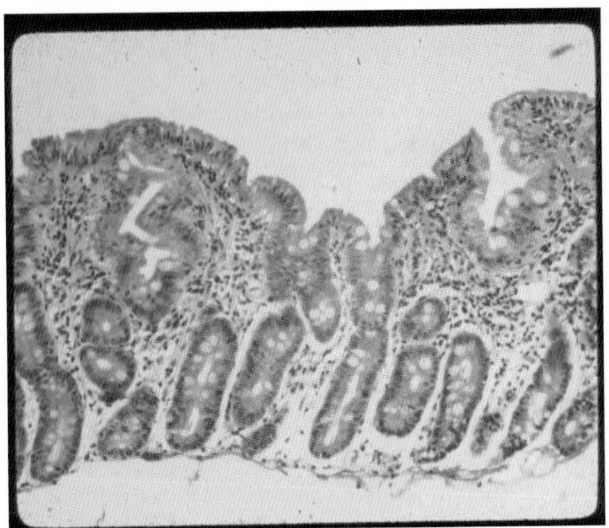

Figure 18.2 Biopsy of duodenal mucosa obtained from a 6-month-old infant with cow's milk protein-induced enteropathy. Hematoxylin and eosin stain, original magnification 200×. Villous blunting, elongated crypts, and numerous lymphocytes can be seen in the intestinal epithelium. Slide and description were generously provided by Dr Keith Benkov, Division of Pediatric Gastroenterology, Icahn School of Medicine at Mount Sinai, New York, NY, USA.

subtotal villous atrophy [47, 70, 87–89] (Figure 18.2). In more recent reports, patterns of enteropathy are more subtle, without obvious villous atrophy but with noticeable villous blunting and reduced crypt–villous ratio [76, 77, 86]. Intestinal mucosa is thin and crypts can be elongated [70, 73, 76, 95] (Figure 18.2). Intraepithelial lymphocytes are prominent, while infiltration with eosinophils is inconsistent [76, 86, 95–97]. Lymphocytes can also be found in the lamina propria. Increased apoptosis of duodenal intraepithelial lymphocytes can be found [98]. Noncaseating granulomas were also reported in one case [99].

Mucosal lipid content may be increased [100]. Columnar cells of the normal jejunum are replaced by crypt cells of a more cuboidal, immature type [66]. The epithelial cells bear short microvilli that contain large aggregates of lysozymes and abnormal nuclei [88]. The basement membrane is unevenly thickened. The epithelial cell renewal rate is markedly increased as a result of the increased mitotic rate [101, 102]. Immunohistochemical studies of the mucosal biopsies in untreated and challenge-positive infants demonstrate a nonspecific increase in mucosal IgA, IgG, and IgM, with inconsistent increase in IgE [103, 104]. The histological features of soybean- or cereal-induced enteropathy are similar to those noted for cow's milk [76, 78, 80, 105, 106].

Pathophysiology of food protein-induced enteropathy

T lymphocytes appear to play a central role in the pathophysiology of food protein-induced enteropathy. Activated T cells in the lamina propria of the fetal human small intestine can produce crypt hypertrophy and villous atrophy [107, 108]. Increased intraepithelial lymphocytes are predominantly $CD3^+$ α/β suppressor/cytotoxic $CD8^+$ T cells [109]. In some series, between 50% and 100% of patients with severe enteropathy have increased density of γ/δ T cells in the epithelium, similar to celiac disease and autoimmune enteropathy [110, 111]. Similar increases were also detected in older children with delayed gastrointestinal symptoms of cow's milk allergy [75, 76, 91, 112]. Many T cells express HLA-DR (human major histocompatibility complex, class II, human leukocyte antigens-DR), suggestive of an activated state. Following a cow's milk elimination diet, these cells diminish [76, 109, 112]. Increased numbers of cytotoxic intraepithelial lymphocytes expressing T-cell-restricted intracellular antigen (TIA1) are found in biopsies from infants as well as from school-age children [113–115]. Activation of cytotoxic duodenal intraepithelial lymphocytes (IELs) is also confirmed by analysis of expression of cytotoxic granule components such as perforin and granzyme A and B [91, 115]. These IELs correlate with serum-soluble Fas ligand concentration, suggesting a role for Fas-mediated apoptosis in the pathogenesis [116].

Mononuclear cells from biopsies of children with cow's milk enteropathy have significantly higher expression of VCAM-1 than that of control children [48]. The number of lymphocytes positive for gut homing receptor $\alpha 4/\beta 7$ is increased in the lamina propria in adults and untreated children with delayed food allergy [76, 117]. These patients also show higher numbers of ICAM-1^+ cells in the lamina propria.

In addition to lymphocytic infiltration, evidence of eosinophilic and mast cell infiltration and degranulation can be seen in biopsy specimens from patients with cow's milk enteropathy with increased levels of histamine and extracellular major basic protein (MBP), and the severity of villous atrophy was positively correlated with the deposition of MBP [89, 118].

As for humoral changes, the number of IgA- and IgM-bearing cells in the lamina propria increase significantly (average 2.4 times) following positive cow's milk challenge in these patients, a finding which is also seen in soy-induced enteropathy following an oral challenge with soy [105, 119]. The presence of IgE in the mucosal biopsies was reported by two groups but was not confirmed in large series of infants [120].

Cytokine patterns vary in patients with milk-induced enteropathy depending on the experimental system. Following stimulation with cow's milk protein *in vitro*, a higher proportion of cells isolated from jejunal biopsies of patients with enteropathy secreted IFN-γ and IL-4 than from control subjects, with IFN-γ-secreting cells being 10 times more numerous than IL-4-secreting cells [121]. IL-10-secreting cells were reduced, further implicating

Table 18.5 Summary of pathologic and immunologic features of food protein-induced enteropathy.

Characteristics	Infantile enteropathy
Offending foods	Cow's milk, soybean, wheat
Pathology	
Villous atrophy	Patchy, mild to severe
Intraepithelial and lamina propria lymphocytes	Increased
Eosinophilic infiltration	Variable
Mucosal lipid content	Increased
Crypt cells	Immature, cuboidal
Basement membrane	Unevenly thickened
Epithelial cell renewal rate	Increased
Mucosal IgA, IgG, IgM	Nonspecific increase
Mucosal IgE	Inconsistent increase
Pathophysiology	
Intraepithelial lymphocytes-cytotoxic $CD8^+$ phenotype	Predominantly α/β, fewer γ/δ
Increased markers of $CD8^+$ activation	HLA-DR T-cell-restricted intracellular antigen
High expression of lymphocyte adhesion molecules	VCAM-1, ICAM-1, $\alpha4/\beta7$
Mast cells activation	High mucosal histamine content
Eosinophil activation	Deposits of extracellular major basic protein
Cytokine patterns upon stimulation of cells isolated from jejunal biopsies with cow's milk *in vitro*	Increased IFN-γ $\gg$ increased IL-4
Spontaneous cytokine release in duodenal biopsy samples	Reduced IL-10

a predominance of the Th1-type responses involved. Table 18.5 summarizes the most important pathologic and immunologic features of food protein-induced enteropathy.

Iron deficiency anemia

Infants with cow's milk protein-induced occult rectal bleeding, anemia, hypoproteinemia, and respiratory signs were originally reported by Wilson, Heiner, and Lahey in 1962 [122]. Symptoms manifested between 2 and 20 months of age, frequently following the transition from breast feeding or formula to regular cow's milk. Hypoproteinemia was caused by increased intestinal protein leakage, but malabsorption and growth retardation were absent [123]. Subsequently, cow's milk-induced anemia and hypoproteinemia were reported in 1 in 7000 infants in a large prospective study from Scandinavia [124].

Pulmonary hemosiderosis has been reported in children with cow's milk-induced anemia and respiratory symptoms of chronic cough, hemoptysis, recurrent lung infiltrates, wheezing, and persistent rhinitis [124–131]. Recently, a single case of buckwheat-induced hemosiderosis and melena was described [132]. Respiratory symptoms and anemia resolved following elimination of the offending food and relapsed upon oral challenge. Iron-laden macrophages were recovered from bronchial or gastric washings or at lung biopsy. Skin prick tests and serum food-specific IgE levels were negative but high titers of serum milk and buckwheat precipitins were reported. Increased proliferation of PBMCs upon stimulation with buckwheat flour was observed in one patient with buckwheat-induced pulmonary hemosiderosis [133]. Biopsy specimens of the lung revealed deposits of IgG, IgA, and complement components, without evidence of IgE [128]. Pulmonary symptoms tend to be persistent, with relapses described in 6- and 8-year-olds but the natural history of food protein-induced pulmonary hemosiderosis is unknown. Considering the seriousness of pulmonary hemorrhage, diagnostic OFCs must be done with extreme caution under close physician supervision in the hospital setting and only when potential benefits outweigh the risks, such as identification of an offending food in a patient with ongoing symptoms or determination of tolerance after a long period of food avoidance without accidental reactions.

Whole cow's milk was associated with iron depletion in a large proportion (27%) of infants from 4 to 12 months of age, mostly attributable to reduced iron absorption [134]. Heat treatment of pasteurized cow's milk reduced the incidence of occult fecal blood loss from 40% to less than 10% in 6-month-old infants, whereas feeding with humanized cow's milk-based formula completely prevented fecal blood loss [135]. Pathophysiology of this disorder is unknown; the limited biopsy data reveal minimal lymphocytic infiltrates and cytotoxicity, and no significant increase in local antibody synthesis [136].

Conclusion

Food protein-induced enterocolitis, enteropathy, and anemia in infants and children have been reviewed. Invariably, they respond well to strict dietary elimination of the offending food protein. Most are outgrown within 3 years of life but subtle enteropathy in school-age children and adults with symptoms of delayed food allergy is being increasingly recognized. In addition, occasional cases of FPIES persisting into the teenage years are being seen. Considering the increasing prevalence of allergic disease in general, as well as food hypersensitivities specifically, one may anticipate increasing frequency of these disorders [137, 138]. As more insight into the pathophysiology of these disorders is gained, noninvasive diagnostic tests may become available. Heightened awareness and increased attention should lead to early, accurate diagnosis and management.

References

1. Host A, Halken S. A prospective study of cow milk allergy in Danish infants during the first 3 years of life. *Allergy* 1990; 45:587–596.
2. Host A. Cow's milk protein allergy and intolerance in infancy. Some clinical, epidemiological and immunological aspects. *Pediatr Allergy Immunol* 1994; 5(Suppl. 6):5–36.
3. Jakobsson I, Lindberg T. A prospective study of cow's milk protein intolerance in Swedish infants. *Acta Pediatr Scand* 1979; 68:853–859.
4. Schrander JJ, van den Bogart JP, Forget PP, Schrander-Stumpel CT, Kuijten RH, Kester Ad. Cow's milk protein intolerance in infants under 1 year of age: a prospective epidemiological study. *Eur J Pediatr* 1993; 152:640–644.
5. Sampson HA. Epidemiology of food allergy. *Pediatr Allergy Immunol* 1996; 7(Suppl. 9):42–50.
6. Eggesbo M, Botten G, Halvorsen R, Magnus P. The prevalence of CMA/CMPI in young children: the validity of parentally perceived reactions in a population-based study. *Allergy* 2001; 56:393–402.
7. Hill DJ, Firer MA, Shelton MJ, Hosking CS. Manifestations of milk allergy in infancy: clinical and immunologic findings. *J Pediatr* 1986; 109:270–276.
8. Sampson HA, Anderson JA. Summary and recommendations: classification of gastrointestinal manifestations due to immunologic reactions to foods in infants and young children. *J Pediatr Gastroenterol Nutr* 2000; 30:S87–S94.
9. Boyce JA, Assa'ad A, Burks AW, et al. Guidelines for the diagnosis and management of food allergy in the United States: report of the NIAID-sponsored expert panel. *J Allergy Clin Immunol* 2010; 126(6 Suppl.):S1–S58.
10. Rubin MI. Allergic intestinal bleeding in the newborn; a clinical syndrome. *Am J Med Sci* 1940; 200:385–390.
11. Gryboski J, Burkle F, Hillman R. Milk induced colitis in an infant. *Pediatrics* 1966; 38:299–302.
12. Gryboski J. Gastrointestinal milk allergy in infancy. *Pediatrics* 1967; 40:354–362.
13. Powell GK. Enterocolitis in low-birth-weight infants associated with milk and soy protein intolerance. *J Pediatr* 1976; 88(5):840–844.
14. Powell GK. Milk- and soy-induced enterocolitis of infancy. *J Pediatr* 1978; 93(4):553–560.
15. Powell GK. Food protein-induced enterocolitis of infancy: differential diagnosis and management. *Comp Ther* 1986; 12(2):28–37.
16. Sicherer SH, Eigenmann PA, Sampson HA. Clinical features of food-protein-induced entercolitis syndrome. *J Pediatr* 1998; 133(2):214–219.
17. Burks AW, Casteel HB, Fiedorek SC, Willaims LW, Pumphrey CL. Prospective oral food challenge study of two soybean protein isolates in patients with possible milk or soy protein enterocolitis. *Pediatr Allergy Immunol* 1994; 5:40–45.
18. Cavataio F, Carroccio A, Montalto G, Iacono G. Isolated rice intolerance: clinical and immunologic characteristics in four infants. *J Pediatr* 1996; 128:558–560.
19. Borchers SD, Li BUK, Friedman RA, McClung HJ. Rice-induced anaphylactoid reaction. *J Pediatr Gastroenterol Nutr* 1992; 15:321–324.
20. Vitoria JC, Camarero C, Sojo A, Ruiz A, Rodriguez-Soriano J. Enteropathy related to fish, rice, and chicken. *Arch Dis Child* 1982; 57:44–48.
21. Vandenplas Y, Edelman R, Sacré L. Chicken-induced anaphylactoid reaction and colitis. *J Pediatr Gastroenterol Nutr* 1994; 19:240–241.
22. Nowak-Wegrzyn A, Sampson HA, Wood RA, Sicherer SH. Food protein-induced enterocolitis syndrome caused by solid food proteins. *Pediatrics* 2003; 111(4 Pt. 1):829–835.
23. Zapatero RL, Alonso LE, Martin FE, Martinez Molero MI. Food-protein-induced enterocolitis syndrome caused by fish. *Allergol Immunopathol (Madr)* 2005; 33(6):312–316.
24. Hojsak I, Kljaic-Turkalj M, Misak Z, Kolacek S. Rice protein-induced enterocolitis syndrome. *Clin Nutr* 2006; 25(3):533–536.
25. Gray HC, Foy TM, Becker BA, Knutsen AP. Rice-induced enterocolitis in an infant: TH1/TH2 cellular hypersensitivity and absent IgE reactivity. *Ann Allergy Asthma Immunol* 2004; 93(6):601–605.
26. Levy Y, Danon YL. Food protein-induced enterocolitis syndrome—not only due to cow's milk and soy. *Pediatr Allergy Immunol* 2003; 14(4):325–329.
27. Bruni F, Peroni DG, Piacentini GL, De Luca G, Boner AL. Fruit proteins: another cause of food protein-induced enterocolitis syndrome. *Allergy* 2008; 63(12):1645–1646.
28. Mehr S, Kakakios A, Frith K, Kemp AS. Food protein-induced enterocolitis syndrome: 16-year experience. *Pediatrics* 2009; 123(3)459–464.
29. Katz Y, Goldberg MR, Rajuan N, Cohen A, Leshno M. The prevalence and natural course of food protein-induced enterocolitis syndrome to cow's milk; a large-scale, prospective population-based study. *J Allergy Clin Immunol* 2011; 127(3):647–643.
30. Monti G, Castagno E, Liguori SA, et al. Food protein-induced enterocolitis syndrome by cow's milk proteins passed through breast milk. *J Allergy Clin Immunol* 2011; 127(3):679–680.
31. Tan J, Campbell D, Mehr S. Food protein-induced enterocolitis syndrome in an exclusively breast-fed infant—an uncommon entity. *J Allergy Clin Immunol* 2012; 129(3):873.
32. Faber MR, Rieu P, Semmekrot BA, Van Krieken JH, Tolboom JJ, Draaisma JM. Allergic colitis presenting within the first hours of premature life. *Acta Paediatr* 2005; 94(10):1514–1515.
33. Eggertsen SC, Pereira PK. Necrotizing enterocolitis and milk protein intolerance. Causes of rectal bleeding in a term infant. *J Fam Pract* 1989; 28(2):219–223.
34. Masumoto K, Takahashi Y, Nakatsuji T, Arima T, Kukita J. Radiological findings in two patients with cow's milk allergic enterocolitis. *Asian J Surg* 2004; 27(3):238–240.
35. McIlhenny J, Sutphen JL, Block CA. Food allergy presenting as obstruction in an infant. *AJR Am J Roentgenol* 1988; 150(2):373–375.

36. Murray KF, Christie DL. Dietary protein intolerance in infants with transient methemoglobinemia and diarrhea. *J Pediatr* 1993; 122:90–92.
37. Muraro A, Dreborg S, Halken S, et al. Dietary prevention of allergic diseases in infants and small children. Part I: immunologic background and criteria for hypoallergenicity. *Pediatr Allergy Immunol* 2004; 15(2):103–111.
38. Fogg MI, Brown-Whitehorn TA, Pawlowski NA, Spergel JM. Atopy patch test for the diagnosis of food protein-induced enterocolitis syndrome. *Pediatr Allergy Immunol* 2006; 17(5):351–355.
39. Richards DG, Somers S, Issenman RM, Stevenson GW. Cow's milk protein/soy protein allergy: gastrointestinal imaging. *Radiology* 1988; 167:721–723.
40. Jayasooriya S, Fox AT, Murch SH. Do not laparotomize food-protein-induced enterocolitis syndrome. *Pediatr Emerg Care* 2007; 23(3):173–175.
41. Sicherer SH. Food protein-induced entercolitis syndrome: clinical perspectives. *J Pediatr Gastroenterol Nutr* 2000; 30(S):45–49.
42. Nowak-Wegrzyn A, Assa'ad A, Bahna SL, Bock SA, Sicherer SH, Teuber SS. Work group report: oral food challenge testing. *J Allergy Clin Immunol* 2009; 123(6 Suppl.):S365–S383.
43. Sicherer SH. Food protein-induced enterocolitis syndrome: case presentations and management lessons. *J Allergy Clin Immunol* 2005; 115(1):149–156.
44. Mofidi S, Bock SA. *A Health Professional's Guide to Food Challenges*. Fairfax, VA: The Food Allergy and Anaphylaxis Network, 2004.
45. Vanderhoof JA, Murray ND, Kaufman SS, et al. Intolerance to protein hydrolysate infant formulas: an underrecognized cause of gastrointestinal symptoms in infants. *J Pediatr* 1997; 131(5):741–744.
46. Kelso JM, Sampson HA. Food protein-induced enterocolitis to casein hydrolysate formulas. *J Allergy Clin Immunol* 1993; 92(6):909–910.
47. Fontaine JL, Navarro J. Small intestinal biopsy in cow's milk protein allergy in infancy. *Arch Dis Child* 1975; 50:357–362.
48. Chung HL, Hwang JB, Kwon YD, Park MH, Shin WJ, Park JB. Deposition of eosinophil-granule major basic protein and expression of intercellular adhesion molecule-1 and vascular cell adhesion molecule-1 in the mucosa of the small intestine in infants with cow's milk-sensitive enteropathy. *J Allergy Clin Immunol* 1999; 103:1195–1201.
49. Powell GK, McDonald PJ, VanSickle GJ, Goldblum RM. Absorption of food protein antigen in infants with food protein-induced enterocolitis. *Dig Dis Sci* 1989; 34(5):781–788.
50. Colgan SP, Resnick MB, Parkos CA, et al. Il-4 directly modulates function of a model human intestinal epithelium. *J Immunol* 1994; 153:2122–2129.
51. Madara JL, Stafford J. Interferon-gamma directly affects barrier function of cultured intestinal epithelial monolayers. *J Clin Invest* 1997; 100:204–215.
52. Adams RB, Planchon SM, Roche JK. IFN-gamma modulation of epithelial barrier function. Time course, reversibility, and site of cytokine binding. *J Immunol* 1993; 150:2356–2363.
53. Planchon SM, Martins CAP, Guerrant RL, Roche JK. Regulation of intestinal barrier function by TGF-beta 1. *J Immunol* 1994; 153:5730–5739.
54. VanSickle GJ, Powell GK, McDonald PJ, Goldblum RM. Milk and soy protein-induced entercolitis: evidence for lymphocyte sensitization to specific food proteins. *Gastroenterology* 1985; 88(6):1915–1921.
55. Hoffman KM, Ho DG, Sampson HA. Evaluation of the usefulness of lymphocyte proliferation assays in the diagnosis of cow's milk allergy. *J Allergy Clin Immunol* 1997; 99:360–366.
56. Shek LP, Soderstrom L, Ahlstedt S, Beyer K, Sampson HA. Determination of food specific IgE levels over time can predict the development of tolerance in cow's milk and hen's egg allergy. *J Allergy Clin Immunol* 2004; 114(2):387–391.
57. Mori F, Barni S, Cianferoni A, Pucci N, de Martino M, Novembre E. Cytokine expression in CD3+ cells in an infant with food protein-induced enterocolitis syndrome (FPIES): case report. *Clin Dev Immunol* 2009; 679381.
58. Rodriguez P, Heyman M, Candalh C, et al. Tumour necrosis factor-alpha induces morphological and functional alterations of intestinal HT29 cl.19A cell monolayers. *Cytokine* 1995; 7:441–448.
59. Heyman M, Darmon N, Dupont C, et al. Mononuclear cells from infants allergic to cow's milk secrete tumor necrosis factor alpha, altering intestinal function. *Gastroenterology* 1994; 106:1514–1523.
60. Benlounes N, Candalh C, Matarazzo P, Dupont C, Heyman M. The time-course of milk antigen-induced TNF-alpha secretion differs according to the clinical symptoms in children with cow's milk allergy. *J Allergy Clin Immunol* 1999; 104(4):863–869.
61. Chung HL, Hwang JB, Park JJ, Kim SG. Expression of transforming growth factor β1, transforming growth factor type I and II receptors, and TNF-α in the mucosa of the small intestine in infants with food protein-induced enterocolitis syndrome. *J Allergy Clin Immunol* 2002; 109(1):150–154.
62. McDonald PJ, Goldblum RM, VanSickle GJ, Powell GK. Food protein-induced enterocolitis: altered antibody response to ingested antigen. *Pediatr Res* 1984; 18:751–755.
63. Schlossmann NA. Uber die giftwirkung des artfremden eiweisses in der milch auf den organismus des sauglings. *Arch Kinderheilkunde* 1905; 41:99–103.
64. Lamy M, Nezelof C, Jos J, Frezal J, Rey J. Biopsy of intestinal mucosa in children: First results of study of malabsorption syndromes. *Presse Med* 1963; 71:1267–1270.
65. Davidson M, Burnstine MC, Kugler MM, Baure CH. Malabsorption defect induced by ingestion of lactoglobulin. *J Pediatr* 1965; 66:545–554.
66. Kuitunen P. Duodeno-jejunal histology in the malabsorption syndrome in infants. *Ann Paediatr Fenn* 1966; 12:101–132.
67. Visakorpi JK, Immonen P. Intolerance to cow's milk and wheat gluten in the primary malabsorption syndrome in infancy. *Acta Pediatr Scand* 1967; 56:49–56.
68. Liu HY, Tsao MU, Moore B, Giday Z. Bovine milk protein-induced intestinal malabsorption of lactose and fat in infants. *Gastroenterology* 1968; 54(1):27–34.

69. Harrison M, Kilby A, Walker-Smith JA, et al. Cow's milk protein intolerance: a possible association with gastroenteritis, lactose intolerance, and IgA deficiency. *BMJ* 1976; 1:1501–1504.
70. Kuitunen P, Visakorpi JK, Savilahti E, Pelkonem P. Malabsorption syndrome with cow's milk intolerance: Clinical findings and course in 54 cases. *Arch Dis Child* 1975; 50:251–256.
71. Savilahti E. Food-induced malabsorption syndromes. *J Pediatr Gastroenterol Nutr* 2000; 30:S61–S66.
72. Saarinen K, Juntunen-Backman K, Jarvenpaa A-L, et al. Supplementary feeding in maternity hospitals and the risk of cow's milk allergy: a prospective study of 6209 infants. *J Allergy Clin Immunol* 1999; 104:457–461.
73. Verkasalo M, Kuitunen P, Savilahti E. Changing pattern of cow's milk intolerance. *Acta Pediatr Scand* 1981; 70:289–295.
74. Vitoria JC, Sojo A, Rodriguez-Soriano J. Changing pattern of cow's milk protein intolerance. *Acta Pediatr Scand* 1990; 79:566–567.
75. Kokkonen J, Haapalahti M, Laurila K, Karttunemn TJ, Maki M. Cow's milk protein-sensitive enteropathy at school age. *J Pediatr* 2001; 139:797–803.
76. Veres G, Westerholm-Ormio M, Kokkonen J, Arato A, Savilahti E. Cytokines and adhesion molecules in duodenal mucosa of children with delayed-type food allergy. *J Pediatr Gastroenterol Nutr* 2003; 37(1):27–34.
77. Latcham F, Merino F, Lang A, et al. A consistent pattern of minor immunodeficiency and subtle enteropathy in children with multiple food allergy. *J Pediatr* 2003; 143(1):39–47.
78. Ament ME, Rubin CE. Soy protein—another cause of the flat intestinal lesion. *Gastroenterology* 1972; 62:227–234.
79. Iyngkaran N, Abdin Z, Davis K, et al. Acquired carbohydrate intolerance and cow milk protein-sensitive enteropathy in young infants. *J Pediatr* 1979; 95:373–378.
80. Iyngkaran N, Yadav M, Boey CG, Kamath KR, Lam KL. Causative effect of cow's milk protein and soy protein on progressive small bowel mucosal damage. *J Gastroenterol Hepatol* 1989; 4:127–136.
81. Walker-Smith JA. Cow's milk intolerance as a cause of postenteritis diarrhea. *J Pediatr Gastroenterol Nutr* 1982; 1:163–175.
82. Walker-Smith JA. Transient gluten intolerance. *Arch Dis Child* 1970; 45:523–526.
83. Iyngkaran N, Robinson NJ, Sumithran E, Lam SK, Putchucheary SD, Yadav M. Cow's milk protein-sensitive enteropathy. An important factor in prolonging diarrhoea in acute infective enteritis in early infancy. *Arch Dis Child* 1978; 53:150–153.
84. Lake AM. Food protein-induced colitis and gastroenteropathy in infants and children. In: Metcalfe DD, Sampson HA, Simon RA (eds), *Food Allergy: Adverse Reactions to Foods and Food Additives*. Cambridge, MA: Blackwell Scientific Publications, 1997; pp. 277–286.
85. Iyngkaran N, Abidin Z. One hour D-xylose in the diagnosis of cow's milk protein sensitive enteropathy. *Arch Dis Child* 1982; 57:40–43.
86. Paajanen L, Vaarala O, Karttunen R, Tuure T, Korpela R, Kokkonen J. Increased IFN-gamma secretion from duodenal biopsy samples in delayed-type cow's milk allergy. *Pediatr Allergy Immunol* 2005; 16(5):439–444.
87. Iyngkaran N, Yadav M, Boey CG, Lam KL. Effect of continued feeding of cow's milk on asymptomatic infants with milk protein sensitive enteropathy. *Arch Dis Child* 1988; 63:911–915.
88. Kuitunen P, Rapola J, Savilahti E, Visakorpi JK. Response of the mucosa to cow's milk in the malabsorption syndrome with cow's milk intolerance. *Acta Pediatr Scand* 1973; 62:585–595.
89. Shiner M, Ballard J, Brook CGD, Herman S. Intestinal biopsy in the diagnosis of cow's milk protein intolerance without acute symptoms. *Lancet* 1979; 29:1060–1063.
90. Baehler P, Chad Z, Gurbindo C, Bonin AP, Bouthillier L, Seidman EG. Distinct patterns of cow's milk allergy in infancy defined by prolonged, two stage double-blind, placebo-controlled food challenges. *Clin Exp Allergy* 1996; 26:254–261.
91. Augustin MT, Kokkonen J, Karttunen R, Karttunen TJ. Serum granzymes and CD30 are increased in children's milk protein sensitive enteropathy and celiac disease. *J Allergy Clin Immunol* 2005; 115(1):157–162.
92. Burgin-Wolff A, Gaze H, Hadziselimovic F, et al. Antigliadin and antiendomysium antibody determination for coeliac disease. *Arch Dis Child* 1991; 66(8):941–947.
93. Meuli R, Pichler WJ, Gaze H, Lentze MJ. Genetic difference in HLA-DR phenotypes between coeliac disease and transitory gluten intolerance. *Arch Dis Child* 1995; 72(1):29–32.
94. McNeish AS, Rolles CJ, Arthur LJ. Criteria for diagnosis of temporary gluten intolerance. *Arch Dis Child* 1976; 51(4):275–278.
95. Maluenda C, Philips AD, Briddon A, Walker-Smith JA. Quantitative analysis of small intestinal mucosa in cow's milk-sensitive enteropathy. *J Pediatr Gastroenterol Nutr* 1984; 3:349–356.
96. Kuitunen P, Kosnai I, Savilahti E. Morphometric study of the jejunal mucosa in various childhood enteropathies with special reference to intraepithelial lymphocytes. *J Pediatr Gastroenterol Nutr* 1982; 1:525–531.
97. Kosnai I, Kuitunen P, Savilahti E, Sipponen P. Mast cells and eosinophils in the jejunal mucosa of patients with intestinal cow's milk allergy and celiac disease. *J Pediatr Gastroenterol Nutr* 1984; 3:368–372.
98. Augustin MT, Kokkonen J, Karttunen TJ. Evidence for increased apoptosis of duodenal intraepithelial lymphocytes in cow's milk sensitive enteropathy. *J Pediatr Gastroenterol Nutr* 2005; 40(3):352–358.
99. Ozbek OY, Canan O, Ozcay F, Bilezikci B. Cows milk protein enteropathy and granulomatous duodenitis in a newborn. *J Paediatr Child Health* 2007; 43(6):494–496.
100. Variend S, Placzek M, Raafat F, Walker-Smith JA. Small intestinal mucosal fat in childhood enteropathies. *J Clin Pathol* 1984; 37:373–377.
101. Kosnai I, Kuitunen P, Savilahti E, Rapola J, Kohegyi J. Cell kinetics in the jejunal epithelium in malabsorption syndrome with cow's milk protein intolerance and coeliac disease of childhood. *Gut* 1980; 21(1041):1046.

102. Savidge TC, Shmakov AN, Walker-Smith JA, Phillips AD. Epithelial cell proliferation in childhood enteropathies. *Gut* 1996; 39:185–193.
103. Stern M, Dietrich R, Muller J. Small intestinal mucosa in coeliac disease and cow's milk protein intolerance: morphometric and immunofluorescent studies. *Eur J Pediatr* 1982; 139:101–105.
104. Rosekrans PC, Meijer CJ, Cornelise CJ, van der Wal AM, Lindeman J. Use of morphometry and immunohistochemistry of small intestinal biopsy specimens in the diagnosis of food allergy. *J Clin Pathol* 1980; 33:125–130.
105. Perkkio M, Savilahti E, Kuitunen P. Morphometric and immunohistochemical study of jejunal biopsies from children with intestinal soy allergy. *Eur J Pediatr* 1981; 137:63–69.
106. Poley JR, Klein AW. Scanning electron microscopy of soy protein-induced damage of small bowel mucosa in infants. *J Pediatr Gastroenterol Nutr* 1983; 2:271–287.
107. da Cunha Ferreira R, Forsyth LE, Richman PI, Wells C, Spencer J, MacDonald TT. Changes in the rate of crypt epithelial cell proliferation and mucosal morphology induced by a T-cell-mediated response in human small intestine. *Gastroenterology* 1990; 98:1255–1263.
108. MacDonald TT, Spencer J. Evidence that activated mucosal T cells play a role in the pathogenesis of enteropathy in human small intestine. *J Exp Med* 1988; 167:1341–1349.
109. Nagata S, Yamashiro Y, Ohtsuka Y, et al. Quantitative analysis and immunohistochemical studies on small intestinal mucosa of food-sensitive enteropathy. *J Pediatr Gastroenterol Nutr* 1995; 20:44–48.
110. Chan K, Phillips AD, Walker-Smith JA, Koskimies S, Spencer J. Density of gamma/delta T cells in small bowel mucosa related to HLA-DQ status without celiac disease. *Lancet* 1993; 342:492–493.
111. Pesce G, Pesce F, Fiorino N, et al. Intraepithelial gamma/delta-positive T lymphocytes and intestinal villous atrophy. *Int Arch Allergy Immunol* 1996; 110:233–237.
112. Kokkonen J, Holm K, Karttunen TJ, Maki M. Enhanced local immune response in children with prolonged gastrointestinal symptoms. *Acta Paediatr* 2004; 93(12):1601–1607.
113. Augustin M, Karttunen TJ, Kokkonen J. TIA1 and mast cell tryptase in food allergy of children: increase of intraepithelial lymphocytes expressing TIA1 associates with allergy. *J Pediatr Gastroenterol Nutr* 2001; 32(1):11–18.
114. Hankard GF, Matarazzo P, Duong JP, et al. Increased TIA1-expressing intraepithelial lymphocytes in cow's milk protein intolerance. *J Pediatr Gastroenterol Nutr* 1997; 25(1):79–83.
115. Augustin MT, Kokkonen J, Karttunen TJ. Duodenal cytotoxic lymphocytes in cow's milk protein sensitive enteropathy and coeliac disease. *Scand J Gastroenterol* 2005; 40(12):1398–1406.
116. Kokkonen TS, Augustin MT, Kokkonen J, Karttunen R, Karttunen TJ. Serum and tissue CD23, IL-15 and FAS-L in cow's milk protein-sensitive enteropathy and in celiac disease. *J Pediatr Gastroenterol Nutr* 2012; 54(4):525–531.
117. Veres G, Helin T, Arato A, et al. Increased expression of intercellular adhesion molecule-1 and mucosal adhesion molecule alpha4beta7 integrin in small intestinal mucosa of adult patients with food allergy. *Clin Immunol* 2001; 99(3):353–359.
118. Raithel M, Matek M, Baenkler HW, Jorde W, Hahn EG. Mucosal histamine content and histamine secretion in Crohn's disease, ulcerative colitis and allergic enteropathy. *Int Arch Allergy Immunol* 1995; 108:127–133.
119. Savilahti E. Immunochemical study of the malabsorption syndrome with cow's milk intolerance. *Gut* 1973; 14:491–501.
120. Van Spreeuwel JP, Lindenman J, Van Maanen J, Meyer CJLM. Increased numbers of IgE-containing cells in gastric and duodenal biopsies: an expression of food allergy secondary to chronic inflammation? *J Clin Pathol* 1984; 37:601–606.
121. Hauer AC, Breese EJ, Walker-Smith JA, MacDonald TT. The frequency of cells secreting interferon gamma and interleukin-4,-5, and -10 in the blood and duodenal mucosa of children with cow's milk hypersensitivity. *Pediatric Res* 1997; 42:629–638.
122. Wilson JF, Heiner DC, Lahey ME. Evidence of gastrointestinal dysfunction in infants with iron deficiency anemia: a preliminary report. *J Pediatr* 1962; 60:787–789.
123. Woodruff CW, Clark JL. The role of fresh cow's milk in iron deficiency. I. Albumin turnover in infants with iron deficiency anemia. *Am J Dis Child* 1972; 24:18–23.
124. Lundstrom U, Perkkio M, Savilahti E, Siimes M. Iron deficiency anemia with hypoproteinemia. *Am J Dis Child* 1983; 58:438–441.
125. Heiner DC, Sears JW. Chronic respiratory disease associated with multiple circulating precipitins to cow's milk. *Am J Dis Child* 1960; 100:500–502.
126. Boat TF, Polmar SH, Whitman V, et al. Hyperreactivity to cow milk in young children with pulmonary hemosiderosis and cor pulmonale secondary to nasopharyngeal obstruction. *J Pediatr* 1975; 87:23–29.
127. Lee SK, Kniker WT, Cook CD, Heiner DC. Cow's milk-induced pulmonary disease in children. *Adv Pediatr* 1978; 25:39–57.
128. Fossati G, Perri M, Careddu G, Mirra N, Carnelli V. Pulmonary hemosiderosis induced by cow's milk proteins: a discussion of a clinical case. *Pediatr Med Chir* 1992; 14(2):203–207.
129. Cohen GA, Hartman G, Hamburger RN, O'Connor RD. Severe anemia and chronic bronchitis associated with a markedly elevated specific IgG to cow's milk protein. *Ann Allergy* 1985; 55(1):38–40.
130. Moissidis I, Chaidaroon D, Vichyanond P, Bahna SL. Milk-induced pulmonary disease in infants (Heiner syndrome). *Pediatr Allergy Immunol* 2005; 16(6):545–552.
131. Cohen GA, Berman BA. Pulmonary hemosiderosis. *Cutis* 1985; 35(2):106, 108–109.
132. Agata H, Kondo N, Fukutomi O, et al. Pulmonary hemosiderosis with hypersensitivity to buckwheat. *Ann Allergy Asthma Immunol* 1997; 78:233–237.
133. Kondo N, Fukutomi O, Agata H, Yokoyama Y. Proliferative responses of lymphocytes to food antigens are useful for detection of allergens in nonimmediate types of food allergy. *J Investig Allergol Clin Immunol* 1997; 7(2):122–126.

134. Fuchs G, DeWeir M, Hutchinson S, Sundeen M, Schwartz S, Suskind R. Gastrointestinal blood loss in older infants: impact of cow milk versus formula. *J Pediatr Gastroenterology Nutrition* 1993; 16:4–9.

135. Fomon SJ, Ziegler EE, Nelson SE, Edwards BB. Cow milk feeding in infancy: gastrointestinal blood loss and iron nutritional status. *J Pediatr* 1981; 98:540–542.

136. Savilahti E, Verkasalo M. Intestinal cow's milk allergy: pathogenesis and clinical presentation. *Clin Rev Allergy* 1984; 2(1):7–23.

137. Holt PG, Macaubas C, Prescott SL, Sly PD. Primary sensitization to inhalant allergens. *Am J Respir Crit Care Med* 2000; 162:S91–S94.

138. Sicherer SH, Munoz-Furlong A, Sampson HA. Prevalence of peanut and tree nut allergy in the United States determined by means of a random digit dial telephone survey: a 5-year follow-up study. *J Allergy Clin Immunol* 2003; 112(6):1203–1207.

19 Occupational Reactions to Food Allergens

André Cartier[1], Sangeeta J. Jain[2], Laurianne G. Wild[2], Maxcie M. Sikora[3], Matthew Aresery[4], & Samuel B. Lehrer[5]

[1]Université de Montréal, Hôpital du Sacré-Coeur de Montréal, Montreal, QC, Canada
[2]Section of Clinical Immunology, Allergy and Rheumatology, Tulane University Health and Sciences Center, New Orleans, LA, USA
[3]Alabama Allergy and Asthma Center, Birmingham, AL, USA
[4]Maine General Medical Center, Augusta, ME, USA
[5]Tulane University, New Orleans, LA, USA

Key Concepts

- Occupational diseases have significant social and economic impact on workers and society as a whole.
- Workers in the food industry, an industry that employs over 16 million people in the United States, are exposed to a variety of food and nonfood materials that can cause a wide range of work-related diseases.
- Asthma, rhinitis, conjunctivitis, hypersensitivity pneumonitis, and dermatitis are common manifestations associated with occupational exposure to food allergens/antigens.
- Since symptoms can be poorly specific, the diagnosis of occupational asthma relies on objective evidence of work-related asthma as confirmed by either monitoring of peak expiratory flow and nonspecific bronchial responsiveness at and off work or by specific inhalation challenges. Similarly, occupational rhinitis, hypersensitivity pneumonitis, and occupational dermatitis should be confirmed objectively.
- Early diagnosis and removal from the exposure environment result in the best prognosis for occupational disease in the food industry.
- Since the removal from the exposure environment is not always possible, improvement of environmental conditions and use of protective devices is warranted.

Introduction

The United States Bureau of Labor Statistics reported that in 2010 there were 139 million employed civilian individuals, of which approximately 16.5 million work in some aspect of the food preparation and service industry. In addition, the USDA estimates there are up to 3 million Americans employed in the farming sector [1]. These workers can be exposed to a wide variety of substances that potentially may lead to hypersensitivity diseases. Most sensitizing materials are food-derived protein allergens, such as flour and shellfish. Nonfood agents may also induce allergic or immunologic disease (e.g., honey bees, grain storage mites, antibiotics, thermophilic actinomycetes, rubber boots, as well as chemicals like metabisulfites). It is well established that these materials can affect the skin, eyes, gastrointestinal tract, and respiratory system. With occupational exposure to food allergens/antigens, the routes of exposure are primarily through inhalation and skin contact, and vary depending on agents and industries. The ensuing diseases include occupational asthma (OA), occupational rhinitis (OR), conjunctivitis, hypersensitivity pneumonitis (HP) (or extrinsic allergic alveolitis), and occupational dermatitis (OD).

Making a diagnosis of one of these occupational diseases can have significant social and economic impact on both the individual and society as a whole. Diagnosing an occupational disease is often difficult, as it requires confirmation of a causal relationship between exposure at work and disease. Although most cases are new onset disease, this is not exclusive; for example, the history of previous asthma does not exclude OA. In the case of OD, the skin inflammation should improve while away from the workplace. In occupational lung diseases, unfortunately, the symptoms may be slow to resolve or still remain long after removal from the workplace. Each of these types of reactions will be discussed in greater detail. Several pertinent examples of each of the aforementioned diseases in occupational settings have been chosen to illustrate important points.

Food Allergy: Adverse Reactions to Foods and Food Additives, Fifth Edition. Edited by Dean D Metcalfe, Hugh A Sampson, Ronald A Simon and Gideon Lack.

Definitions/classifications

Occupational asthma refers to *de novo* asthma or the recurrence of previously quiescent asthma induced by sensitization to a specific substance, either high molecular weight (HMW) or low molecular weight (LMW) agents, which is termed sensitizer-induced OA, or by exposure to an inhaled irritant at work, which is termed irritant-induced OA [2]. The latter form encompasses reactive airways dysfunction syndrome (RADS) and irritant-induced asthma, which occur after acute high-level exposure to irritant gas, smoke, fumes, vapors [2, 3], or repeated lower level exposures to irritant compounds [2, 4], and does not require a period of latency. This form of OA will not be discussed further in the context of food-induced occupational reactions, although it may be seen in this industry due to accidental exposure, such as ammonia spills from refrigeration systems. Work-exacerbated asthma (not discussed in this chapter) is defined as preexisting or concurrent asthma that is worsened by work factors, for example, exercise or exposure to irritants such as cold air, dust, or fumes in excessive quantity.

Occupational rhinitis is defined as "an inflammatory condition of the nose, which is characterized by intermittent or persistent symptoms (e.g., nasal congestion, sneezing, rhinorrhea, itching) and/or variable nasal airflow limitation and/or hypersecretion, due to causes and conditions attributable to a particular work environment and not to stimuli encountered outside the workplace" [5]. Depending on the need for a latency period, OR is classified as either allergic or nonallergic. The allergic type encompasses both immunoglobulin E (IgE)-mediated (caused by a wide variety of HMW agents, particularly found in the food industry, and some LMW agents) or non-IgE-mediated OR (caused mainly by LMW agents acting as haptens). The nonallergic type of OR encompasses different types of rhinitis caused by the work environment through irritant, nonimmunologic mechanisms.

Hypersensitivity pneumonitis, or extrinsic allergic alveolitis, is an immunologically mediated inflammatory disease involving the terminal airways of the lung associated with intense or repeated exposure to various inhaled allergens. The result of this exposure is initially a lymphocytic alveolitis, followed by granuloma formation and eventually irreversible pulmonary fibrosis in the untreated patient [6, 7].

Occupational skin disorders include contact dermatitis and contact urticaria (OCU) [8]. Cutaneous manifestations of occupational exposure are generally divided into irritant contact dermatitis (ICD) and allergic contact dermatitis (ACD) or a combination of ICD and ACD. ICD is diagnosed based on history, clinical appearance, and distribution of skin lesions. It is a nonimmunologic form of dermatitis where agents have a direct toxic effect on the skin, for example, wet work, detergents, alkalis, solvents, and friction, and which is the most common type of occupational contact dermatitis. On the other hand, ACD represents an immunologically mediated disorder involving a delayed or type IV hypersensitivity reaction as the result of a T-cell-mediated immune response to skin sensitizers. Occupational contact urticaria can have either a nonimmunological or immunological mechanism involving an immediate or type I hypersensitivity reaction, associated with the presence of allergen-specific IgE. It is associated with proteins in food (particularly among cooks, bakers, caterers, and food handlers) and latex gloves and with some LMW agents.

Prevalence and incidence

Determining prevalence or incidence of occupational diseases with any certainty is difficult, particularly in the food industry. Both employees and physicians tend to under-report health problems and epidemiologic data on agricultural workers and food handlers remain scanty. However, as the importance of occupational lung disease has become better recognized, national databases have been established to monitor these data, including the SWORD [9] and SHIELD [10] in the United Kingdom, PROPULSE [11] in Canada, and SENSOR [12] in the United States. According to the World Health Organization, as many as 300 million people of all ages and ethnicities suffer from asthma worldwide [13]. In the United States, it is estimated that 18.7 million adults have asthma [14]. The exact prevalence of OA is unknown, but epidemiologic studies suggest that 9–15% of all cases of adult-onset asthma are attributable to occupational exposure [15, 16]. Its overall frequency has probably been stable during the last 10 years, although the causative agents have varied in frequency [17]. There is, however, some suggestion that its incidence has decreased in some countries [18–20]. In those food-related industries in which prevalence of OA is available, rates do not significantly differ from those found in nonfood industries. For example, OA occurs in 3–10% [21,22] of workers exposed to green coffee beans, 9% to as many as 50% of snow crab-processing workers [23], and 4–30% of bakers [24–27].

The prevalence of OR worldwide has been reported to be between 5% and 15% depending on the exposure environment [28]. OR occurs three times more frequently than asthma in the occupational setting. Its prevalence in subjects with OA is 76–92% [29, 30]. In healthcare workers exposed to latex gloves, sensitization has been reported as high as 20% with OR occurring in 9–12% [31, 32]. In seafood-processing workers, the prevalence of probable OR is as high as 15% [23] although rhinitis symptoms are reported by as many as 34.5% of workers. Similarly, nasal symptoms were reported by 24% of fish-food factory workers [33]. OR often coexists with OA and frequently precedes the development of asthma in the work environment [30]. In 59 workers with laboratory animal allergy, Gross et al. reported that OR preceded the development of OA in 45% of subjects and occurred at the same time in 55% [34].

The incidence of HP is more difficult to determine because of generally low occurrence of disease, problems with differential diagnosis, and the lack of prospective epidemiologic studies. Incidence also depends on exposure levels of the offending antigen and varies widely in different industries or even in areas of the same plant. For example, in one study, it was estimated that farmer's lung, one form of HP, affects less than 1–6% of farmers [35]. However, in a survey among 1054 farmers who grind moldy hay, the prevalence of farmer's lung was reported at 8.3–11.4% [36] while in others, it was estimated to be 4.2 per 1000 farmers [37] or less [38].

OD remains one of the most prevalent occupational diseases, with dermatitis of the hands being the most common [8]. However, most epidemiologic studies of dermatologic reactions in food industry workers have included only subjects already diagnosed with occupational skin disease. Consequently, although types of skin reactions can be distinguished and many of the important etiologic agents can be identified, the true prevalence of disease remains difficult to determine. In a study of 1052 workers in the Finnish food industry, 17% were identified as having a skin disease [39]. In that study, 8.5% of 541 female workers had OD, most commonly caused by fish, meat, and vegetables. Of the 196 workers handling food, hand dermatitis was present in 15%. In a 5-year retrospective study, 3662 consecutive patients, including 180 food handlers, were patch tested [40]. In 91 (50.5%) of 180 subjects, dermatitis resulted from an occupational exposure, of which 25 (13.8%) of 180 were from exposure to meats or vegetables. Patch tests were positive in 59 of 180 patients (32.7%). Another study involving 5285 patients in northern Bavaria found the incidence of OD was highest in pastry chefs (76%) and cooks (69%), followed closely by food-processing industry workers and butchers (63%) [41]. Hjorth and colleague evaluated 33 cases of OD occurring in restaurant kitchen workers [42]. Metals, onions, and garlic were implicated most frequently in contact dermatitis; fish and shellfish were the major agents responsible for provoking contact urticaria. The same food allergens were also identified as the most important in a study of caterers [43].

Using questionnaires, Smith estimated the mean annual incidence of skin conditions in the food manufacturing industry to be 2103 per million employees per year and 1414 per million employees per year in the retail/catering industry [44]. Other data on OD come from the EPIDERM and OPRA (Occupational Physicians Reporting Activity) surveillance plan which have been collecting data on occupational skin diseases in the United Kingdom since 1993. The dermatologists and occupational physicians that provided data for these studies report an annual incidence of occupational contact dermatitis of 12.9 per 100 000 [45]. The prevalence of OCU has also been increasing over the last 30 years; however, there is limited data on its epidemiology as it often coexists with other occupational skin diseases. A retrospective analysis in an Australian clinic found that OCU was diagnosed in 8.3% of occupational skin diseases with 151 cases in a 12-year period [46]. Among the non-latex contact urticaria, 47% of OCU were found in the food service industry. These results are comparable to those reported by the EPIDERM group in the United Kingdom [47]. These studies include non-food-related industries and there are limited data on the prevalence of OCU in the food industry alone.

Risk factors

Both industrial and individual factors are associated with an increased risk of developing occupational hypersensitivity. The best studies have been done in OA and OR. Physicochemical properties of occupational agents, as well as dose, duration, route of exposure, allergenic potency, and industrial hygiene and engineering practices influence the potential of occupational agents to induce allergic disease. The level of exposure in different settings is clearly a major determinant for many occupational agents [25, 48–50].

As only a small proportion of exposed workers develop occupational allergic reactions, host factors clearly play an important role in disease development. These factors may include atopy, genetic predisposition, cigarette smoking, and possibly preexisting increased nonspecific bronchial responsiveness (NSBR).

Atopy

Although OA is frequently associated with increased production of specific IgE antibodies, atopy *per se* is not always associated with an increased incidence of OA. In general, the association between atopy and OA is found consistently in OA caused by HMW agents. However, the association is not high and other factors are equally likely to be important in the ultimate development of disease such as the degree of exposure and concentration of the suspected agent. Atopy is associated with an increased risk of sensitization to snow crab, prawn, green coffee, castor bean, and bakery allergens. While atopy is associated with an increased risk of developing OA in workers exposed to bakery allergens [51], this has not been confirmed for workers exposed to salmon [52], with data on snow crab workers being inconsistent [23, 29]. Although an association between sensitization to HMW agents and atopy has been observed in many food-related work environments, atopy and the development of OR have not been linked. Unlike OA, there is no higher incidence of HP disease in atopic subjects.

The role of atopy has not been clearly defined in the pathophysiology of occupational dermatoses. Atopic dermatitis in particular may predispose workers to develop ICD; however, it does not appear to predispose to ACD. In a prospective follow-up study evaluating hand dermatitis in bakers, confectioners, and bakery shop assistants, Bauer et al. found that atopic individuals had a 3.9-fold relative risk of developing hand dermatitis. Total serum IgE levels did not correlate, however, with disease [53].

Genetics

There has been considerable interest in identifying markers of genetic susceptibility in OA. As reviewed by Bernstein [54], initial HLA studies found that workers with diisocyanate-associated asthma had a higher frequency of the alleles DQB1*0503 and DQB1*0201/0301 than asymptomatic controls, while DQA1*0101 and DQB1*0501 were reduced in diisocyanate-associated asthma. However, these results were not confirmed in other studies. Therefore, while specific HLA-DR, HLA-DQ, and HLA-DP alleles have been shown to confer either susceptibility or protection, these findings have not been consistently reproducible. There have been no genome-wide association studies done yet on OA to food allergens.

As with OA, no specific genetic basis has been clearly identified for HP. The nature of the antigen, the quantity of antigen inhaled and frequency of exposure, and finally host susceptibility are important. A study by Camarena et al. looked at polymorphisms of the major histocompatibility complex (MHC) class II alleles in 44 patients with pigeon breeders' disease, a form of HP. An increase of one HLA-DRB1 allele and one HLA-DQB1 allele were noted when MHC typing was performed by PCR-specific sequence oligonucleotide analysis. However, there was no specific association between the alleles in question and the development of HP [55].

Very little data exist for the genetic basis of OD. However, Holst studied ICD in monozygotic and dizygotic twins and found a high degree of concordance among monozygotic twins [56].

Smoking

The role of cigarette smoke, including exposure to second-hand smoke, is not clear in development, exacerbation, or pathogenesis of OA. Exposure to cigarette smoke increases bronchial epithelial permeability [57], which might potentially allow inhaled antigens increased access to immunocompetent cells and evoke an immune response. One study showed that smokers were more likely than nonsmokers to have a positive specific IgE test to workplace allergens, especially HMW allergens [58].

Smoking has been associated with an increased risk of developing sensitization to high molecular agents in the seafood industry, particularly to prawns [59], crab [23], and fish (pilchard, anchovy, and salmon) [60]. It is also associated with an increased risk of developing OA in snow crab- and salmon-processing workers [29, 52] and in workers exposed to green coffee dust and castor bean dust [61].

HP is uncommon in smokers, unlike other pulmonary diseases in which smoking increases frequency of disease. Several studies have shown an underrepresentation of smokers among patients with HP. The mechanism by which smoking seems to prevent the development of HP is not known. It may be through an impairment of immune cellular function induced by smoking [62–64]. However, Dangman et al. reported that smoking affects the laboratory and clinical findings used in the diagnosis of HP, making the confirmation of HP difficult, which may contribute to the apparent protective effect of smoking [65]. More studies are needed to confirm the role that smoking plays in the development of HP. Nevertheless, once HP has started, smoking does not appear to be protective [66].

Bronchial responsiveness

Although there has been no study in food-processing workers, there is no evidence that increased NSBR is a risk factor for the development of OA [2, 51, 67].

Agents associated with allergic occupational diseases of food workers

Hundreds of agents are known to cause OA and rhinoconjunctivitis. Most of these substances are chemicals, pharmaceuticals, wood dusts, and metals [68, 69]. In addition, more than 100 agents encountered in food or food-related industry are known to induce OA [70] and OR. In some industries, such as coffee factories, snow crab processing, and bakeries, OA is a well-recognized problem. In other types of workplaces, only individual case reports have been reported. Agents encountered in food industries that are known to cause OA and OR are listed in Tables 19.1 and 19.2. A more wide-ranging list of airway-sensitizing agents can be found in various reviews [78, 79]. Similarly,

Table 19.1 Food allergens responsible for occupational asthma and rhinitis.

Agent	Occupational exposure
Cereals	
Wheat, rye, barley	Baker, pastry maker
Gluten	Baker
Corn	Making stock feed
Rice	Rice miller
Plants, vegetables, fruits, and spices	
Spinach	Baker (handling spinach)
Asparagus	Harvesting asparagus
Broccoli, cauliflower	Plant breeder, restaurant worker
Artichoke	Warehouse (packaging artichokes)
Bell pepper	Greenhouse worker
Courgette (zucchini)	Warehouse (packaging courgette)
Carrot	Cook (handling and cutting raw carrots)
Tomatoes (flower)	Greenhouse grower
Raspberry	Chewing gum coating
Citrus fruit (limonene)	Fruit handler [71]
Peach	Farmer [72], factory worker handling peaches
Aniseed	Meat industry (handling spices)
Saffron (pollen)	Saffron worker
Hop	Baker, brewery chemist
Soybean	Dairy food product company, baker, animal food preparation
Chicory	Factory producing inulin from chicory roots, chicory grower
Coffee bean (raw and roasted)	Roasting green coffee beans
Green bean	Handling green beans
Lima bean	Food processing making dough [73]
Cacao	Confectionery
Anise	Anise liqueur factory
Almond	Almond-processing plant
Olive oil	Olive mill worker
Devil's tongue root (maiko)	Food processor
Garlic	Sausage makers, garlic harvesters, spice factory, packing and handling garlic
Aromatic herbs (rosemary, thyme, bay leaf, garlic)	Butcher (handling spices)
Paprika, coriander, mace	Butcher, greenhouse worker
Seeds	
Red onion (*Allium cepa*) seed	Seed-packing factory worker
Sesame seed	Miller (grounding waste bread for animal food), baker
Fennel seed	Sausage-manufacturing plant
Lupine seed	Agricultural research worker
Buckwheat flour	Health food products, noodle maker, cook
Seafood and fish	
Arthropods	
Snow crab, Alaskan king crab, dungeness crab, tanner crab, rock crab	Crab-processing worker
Prawn, shrimp, clam	Prawn processor, food processor (lyophilized powder), fishmonger, seafood delivery
Lobster	Cook, fishmonger
Mollusks	
Cuttlefish	Deep sea fisherman
Mussels	Mussels opener, cook
King and queen scallop	Processor
Abalone	Fisherman
Octopi	Processor
Fish	
Salmon, pilchard, anchovy, plaice, hake, tuna, trout	Fish processor, fishmonger
Herbal teas	
Tea	Green tea factory, tea packer
Cinnamon	Worker processing cinnamon
Chamomile	Tea-packing plant worker
Sarsaparilla root	Herbal tea worker
Ginger	Herbal tea worker [74]
Mushrooms	
Boletus edulis (porcino or king bolete)	Pasta factory
Saccharomyces cerevisiae	Mixing baker's yeast
Mushroom powder	Food manufacturer
Pleurotus cornucopiae	Mushroom grower
Farm products	
Pork (raw)	Meat-processing plant
Beef (raw)	Cook
Lamb (raw)	Cutting raw lamb meat
Hog	Pig farmer
Cow	Dairy farmer
Poultry (turkey, chicken)	Food-processing plant, poultry slaughterhouse
Egg	Confectionary worker, bakery, egg-processing plant
Pheasant, quail, dove	Breeder
Milk derivatives	
α-Lactalbumin	Candy maker, baker
Lactoserum	Cheese maker, baker [75, 76]
Casein	Delicatessen factory, milking sheep, candy maker
Rennet	Cheese maker
Bee, honey, pollen	Beekeeper, honey processor, cereal producer

Source: Adapted from References 70 and 77 with permission.

Siracusa et al. have compiled a comprehensive list of agents responsible for OR [80].

Organic dust derived from bacteria, fungi, protozoa, plant and animal products, and simple chemicals can induce HP. A list of agents encountered in food industries that are known to induce HP are given in Table 19.3. Many of these materials are of fungal origin. Coffee dust has been omitted from this list because the single case of "coffee worker's lung" was subsequently re-described as cryptogenic fibrosing alveolitis associated with rheumatoid arthritis [81].

Table 19.2 Food additives and contaminants responsible for occupational asthma and rhinitis.

Food additives	Occupational exposure
Colorants	
Carmine	Butcher (production of sausages)
Chinese red rice (derived from *Monascus ruber*)	Delicatessen manufacturing plant
Fungal enzymes (α-amylase, cellulase, xylanase)	Baker
Glucoamylase	Baker
Pectinase, glucanase	Fruit salad processing
Papain, bromelain	Meat tenderizer
Thickening agents	
Carob bean flour	Jam factory, ice cream maker
Pectin	Candy maker, preparation of jam
Konjac glucomannan	Food-manufacturing plant
Castor oil	Factory and dock workers
Vitamins (thiamine)	Manufacturing-enriched breakfast cereals
Gluten	Biscuit maker
Sodium metabisulfite	Producer spraying potatoes
Food contaminants	Occupational exposure
Insects	
Poultry mites (*Ornithonyssus sylviarum*)	Poultry worker
Grain storage mites (*Glycyphagus destructor*)	Grain worker
Ephestia kuehniella	Cereal stocker, baker
Champignon flies	Champignon cultivator
Cockroaches (*Blattella* spp.)	Baker
Granary weevils (*Sitophilus granarius*)	Baker
Rice flour beetles (*Tribolium confusum*)	Baker
Fungi	
Aspergillus niger	Brewer (contaminated malt)
Chrysonilia (Neurospora) sitophila	Service operator of coffee dispenser
Aspergillus, Alternaria spp.	Baker
Verticillium albo-atrum	Greenhouse tomato grower
Parasites	
Anisakis simplex	Fish-processing workers, frozen fish factory
Plants	
Hoya (sea squirts)	Oysters handlers
Others	
Soft red coral	Spiny lobster fisherman

Source: Adapted from References 70 and 77 with permission.

A wide variety of foods, additives, and flavorings, as well as materials used in food preparation, are known to induce several types of occupational skin disease. Table 19.4 lists etiologic agents, along with diagnoses. Some materials, such as seafood and garlic, commonly induce dermatitis, whereas others, including nonfood items such as betadine, are seldom reported to cause occupational skin disease.

Table 19.3 Etiology of hypersensitivity pneumonitis occurring in food and food-related industries.

Agent	Source/exposure	Disorders
Thermophilic actinomycetes		
Saccharopolyspora rectivirgula	Moldy hay Moldy compost	Farmer's lung Mushroom workers' lung
Thermoactinomyces sacchari	Moldy sugar cane	Bagassosis
T. vulgaris	Moldy compost	Mushroom workers' lung
Moldy hay	Farmer's lung	
T. viridis	Vineyards	Vineyard sprayers' lung
Fungi		
Aspergillus clavatus	Moldy barley/malt	Malt workers' lung
A. clavatus	Moldy cheese	Cheese workers' lung
A. flavus	Moldy corn	Farmer's lung
A. fumigatus	Vegetable compost	
A. oryzae	Soy sauce brewer	
Cladosporium	Moldy hay	Farmer's lung
Mucor stolonifer	Moldy paprika pods	Paprika slicers' disease
Penicillium sp.	Moldy hay	Farmer's lung
P. casei, P. roqueforti	Cheese	Cheese workers' lung
Botrytis cinerea	Moldy grapes	Wine growers' lung
Fusarium solani	Moldy onion and potatoes	Onion and potato sorter
Insects		
Grain weevil (*Sitophilus granarius*)	Infested wheat	Millers' lung
Cheese mites (*Acarus siro*)	Cheese	Cheese workers' lung
Animal products		
Duck proteins	Feathers	Duck fever
Chicken proteins	Chicken products Hen litter	Feather pluckers' disease
Turkey proteins	Turkey products	Turkey handlers' disease
Goose proteins	Feathers	
Bird proteins	Fishermen	
Fish meal	Fishmeal workers	
Plant products		
Miscellaneous		
Mushrooms	Spores	Mushroom workers' disease
Erwinia herbicola (Enterobacter agglomerans)	Contaminated grain	Grain workers' lung
Tea plants		Tea growers' lung
Oyster shells	Oyster shell dust	
Cork	Cork dust from wine bottles	
Prawn	Factory workers	Prawn-processing workers

Source: Adapted from Reference 77 with permission.

Table 19.4 Dermatitis in food processing and food service workers.

Industry	Exposure	Diagnosis
Moldy hay		
Milk controllers, milk recorders, milkers	Bronopol, Kathon CG	Contact dermatitis
Milk testers	Chrome, dichromate	Contact dermatitis
Milk analyzers	Dichromate	Allergic contact dermatitis
Ewe milker	Wool	Contact dermatitis
Celery harvesters	Celery fungus (*Sclerotinia sclerotiorum*)	Phototoxic dermatitis
Apple packers	Apples sprayed with ethoxyquin	Allergic contact dermatitis
Orange pickers	Omite-CR	Contact dermatitis
Greenhouse worker	Ginger (Zingiber mioga rosc.)	Contact dermatitis [82]
Grocery workers	Celery (furocoumarins)	
Mushroom harvesters	Shiitake mushrooms	Contact dermatitis
Food Preparation		
Fish factory workers	Fish, mustard	Dermatitis, contact urticaria
Cooks	Mustard, rape	Contact dermatitis
Cooks	Garlic/onions	Contact dermatitis
Cooks	Paprika, curry	Contact dermatitis
Salad makers	Mustard	Allergic contact dermatitis
Food workers	Cashew nuts (cardol)	Contact dermatitis
Sandwich makers	Codfish, plaice, chicken, onion, garlic	Contact dermatitis
Sandwich maker	Parmesan cheese	Contact urticaria [83]
Pizza maker	Olives	Contact urticaria [84]
Food worker (cannery)	Asparagus	Contact dermatitis [85]
Food workers	Lettuce	Contact dermatitis
Food workers	Lettuce, chicory, endive	Contact dermatitis
Bakers	Sodium metabisulfite	Contact dermatitis
	Persulfate	Contact dermatitis
	Cinnamon	Allergic Contact dermatitis [86, 87]
	Sorbic acid	Dermatitis
	Propyl gallate	Allergic contact dermatitis
	Dodecyl gallate	Dermatitis
	Chromium	Contact dermatitis
	Flour mite	Contact dermatitis
	Sugar mite	Dermatitis
	Karaya gum	Dermatitis
	Flour	Contact urticaria
Herb packer	Basil	Allergic contact dermatitis [88]
Butchers/Poultry Processors		
Butchers	Rubber boots	Allergic contact dermatitis
Butchers	Knife handle	Contact dermatitis

Table 19.4 *(Continued)*

Industry	Exposure	Diagnosis
Butchers	Povidone-iodine	Allergic contact dermatitis
Slaughter men	Blood (cow and pig), gut casings	Contact urticaria, Eczema
Butchers	Calf's liver, pig's gut, beef	Urticaria
Poultry workers	Various	Irritant allergic dermatitis, eczema
Chicken vaccinators	Antibiotics	Contact dermatitis
Delicatessen store	Salami	Allergic contact dermatitis [89]
Seafood		
Fish market workers	Shrimp	Allergic contact urticaria
Caterers	Shrimp	Contact urticaria
Seafood processors	Prawns	Dermatitis
Crabs processors	Crabs	Urticaria, dermatitis
Oyster shuckers	Oysters	Dermatitis
Mussel processors	Mussels	Dermatitis
Food handlers	Fish and shellfish	Contact dermatitis
Food handlers	Cuttlefish	Contact dermatitis
Fishermen	Fish	Contact dermatitis
Fish workers	Fish	Contact urticaria
Cooks	Fish	Contact urticaria
Caterers	Fish	Dermatitis
Trawlermen	Bryozoa	Contact dermatitis
Fishermen	Rubber boots	Contact dermatitis
Fishnet repairers	Fishnets	Contact dermatitis
Miscellaneous		
Snackbar meat prod	Penicillin residues	Contact dermatitis
Spice workers	Turmeric, cinnamon, cinnamic aldehyde	Allergic contact dermatitis
Margarine manufacturers, workers	Octyl gallate	Contact dermatitis
Peanut butter manufacturers	Octyl gallate	Contact dermatitis
Processing plant workers	Green coffee beans	Allergic contact dermatitis
Food workers	Sesame oil	Contact sensitivity
Food workers	Artichokes	Eczema
Confectioners	Cardamom	Allergic contact dermatitis
Cookie workers	"Thin mint" cookies	Eczema
Beekeepers	Propolis	Dermatitis
Beekeepers	Beeswax (poplar resin)	Dermatitis
Coconut climber	Coconut trees/coconuts	Dermatitis
Fruit handler (citrus)	Limonene	Allergic contact dermatitis [71]
Bartender	Citrus peel, geraniol citral	Allergic contact dermatitis

Source: Adapted from Reference 77 with permission.

Asthma in seafood workers

The seafood industry is an example of a sector of the food industry that has continued to grow to meet world demands and consequently has had greater exposures and corresponding disease. In 2005, the world's production of fish, crustaceans, and mollusks reached 140.5 million tons. Of this amount, 95 million tons were derived from capture fisheries and 45.5 million tons were from aquaculture [90]. This makes seafood one of the most highly traded commodities in the world market and the number of fishers and fish farmers has been growing steadily in response. With this increase in the production and consumption of seafood have come more allergic reactions in the occupational setting [91].

De Besche [92] published the first report of occupational allergy from seafood in a 1937 paper describing a fisherman with asthma, angioedema, and conjunctivitis. Since De Besche's time, seafood-processing plants have become technologically advanced with varying processing procedures. Crab, fish, mussel, and prawn processing cause an aerosolized protein exposure to which workers can become sensitized by inhalation [93, 94]. Table 19.5 lists sources of allergen exposures in the seafood industry [95]. One study suggested that higher concentration of the dust mite *Dermatophagoides pteronyssinus* may pose a risk to workers who spend significant amounts of time on fishing boats [96]. Non-seafood agents may also be implicated. These include various contaminants such as parasites, marine toxins, bacterial toxins, chemical additives, and spices. The reported prevalence of OA due to seafood alone varies from 4% to 36% [94].

Crab processing is associated with the highest prevalence of OA and occupational allergies among the seafood industry. Furthermore, OA is also more commonly associated with shellfish (4–36%) versus bony fish (2–8%) [95]. In the United States, a 1982 National Institute for Occupational Safety and Health (NIOSHA) investigation concluded that during the crab-processing season in

Table 19.5 Common processing techniques employed for seafood groups and sources of potential high-risk exposure to seafood products.

Seafood category	Processing techniques	Preservation techniques	Sources of occupational exposure to seafood products
Crustaceans			
Crabs, lobsters, crawfish	Cooking (boiling or steaming), "tailing" lobsters, "cracking," butchering, and degilling crabs, manual picking of meat, cutting, grinding, mincing, scrubbing and washing, cooling	Deep freezing, pasteurizing, sterilization, liquid freezing	Inhalation of wet aerosols from lobster "tailing," crab "cracking," butchering and degilling, boiling, scrubbing and washing, spraying, cutting, grinding, mincing, prawn "blowing," cleaning processing lines/tanks with pressurized water
Prawns	Heading, peeling, deveining, prawn "blowing" (water jets or compressed air)	Deep freezing, drying	Dermal contact from unprotected handling of prawn; hand immersion in water containing extruded gut material
Molluscs			
Oysters, mussels, clams, scallops, abalone	Washing, oyster "shucking," shellfish depuration, chopping, dicing, slicing	Deep freezing, freezing, sterilization, smoking, cooking	Inhalation of wet aerosols from oyster "shucking," washing Dermal contact from unprotected handling of molluscs
Finfish			
Various species	Heading, degutting, skinning, mincing, filleting, trimming, cooking (boiling or steaming), spice/batter application, frying, milling, bagging	Deep freezing, drying, smoking, sterilization, liquid freezing	Inhalation of wet aerosols from fish heading, degutting, boiling Inhalation of dry aerosols from fishmeal bagging Dermal contact from unprotected handling

Source: Modified from Reference 95 with permission.

Alaska, the monthly incidence of new cases of asthma was 80 times that reported for the general population, controlling for age [97]. Cartier et al. and Gautrin et al. reported a high prevalence of OA and occupational allergies to snow crab in processing workers of Quebec [29] or Newfoundland-Labrador [23]. Indeed, while work-related respiratory symptoms reached nearly a third of all workers, OA, either confirmed by monitoring of peak expiratory flows (PEFs) and NSBR [29] or based on history and evidence of specific sensitization to crab [23] was confirmed in about 16% of all workers. Sensitization to crab, as confirmed by positive skin prick tests or specific IgE ranged from 18.4% [23] to 31.6% [29]. Brushing and cleaning cooked crab is a process generating particularly high levels of allergens in the air [23]. Shrimp processing is also associated with a high prevalence of sensitization (±20%) [23, 98] but confirmed cases of OA are not frequent.

Rhinitis in bakers

Baker's rhinitis is a frequent cause of OR and often precedes the development of asthma. It was first described in the 1700s by Bernardo Ramazzini who reported in his treatise *De Morbis Artificum Diatriba* respiratory symptoms in bakers caused by exposure to flour dust. However, prior to this, there were anecdotal reports of Roman slaves who used facial cloths to protect their noses from inhaling flour. Allergen sources are found in flour and may include cereal proteins such as rye, wheat, barley, as well as grain mite, flour beetles, *Aspergillus fumigatus*, and microbial enzymes (alpha amylase, glucoamylase, and cellulase). A large, prospective study of apprentice bakers found that an increase in sensitization and work-related symptoms to allergens including bakers' dust, wheat, corn, rye, oatmeal, and barley increase with the duration of work exposure. The incidence of rhinitis was 6.5% after 1 year and 10.8% after 2 years. This study also showed that skin prick testing to occupational allergens was positive in 4.6% after 1 year and 8.2% after 2 years [99].

Mushroom worker's lung

During 2010–2011, 110 growers in the United States produced 845 million pounds of mushrooms valued at 952 million dollars [100]. HP among mushroom workers was first reported in 1959 [101] and the term "mushroom worker's lung" (MWL) was coined in 1967 [102]. After an outbreak of seven cases of MWL between April 1982 and April 1985, a cross-sectional respiratory morbidity survey was conducted at the mushroom farm where the outbreak occurred [103]. Other than the outbreak subjects, 20% of the more heavily exposed workers reported occasionally experiencing symptoms consistent with MWL. Serologic tests showed that almost all workers, from different work areas on the farm, had specific IgG against these mushrooms showing that they had been exposed to antigens that could potentially cause disease. However, there were no radiographic changes noted. In Japan, a study of mushroom workers reported that 71% of 69 previously healthy workers developed chronic cough within the first 3 months of working and at least two of these patients had HP [104].

Mushroom worker's lung is caused by a variety of antigens associated with cultivation of mushrooms, notably microorganisms and mushroom spores. The specific exposures depend on where an individual works in the operation, harvest conditions and which mushroom species are involved. Most cultivated mushrooms are grown in compost. During fermentation of compost, temperatures as high as 60°C are generated and thermophilic organisms flourish. Meanwhile, a growth medium is inoculated with mushroom spores; after growth begins, this material is transferred onto grain. The combination, called spawn, is mixed with fermented compost prior to seeding mushroom beds. High levels of thermophilic actinomycetes are liberated during the mixing process. Thermophilic organisms are the traditional source of MWL including *Thermomonospora* sp., *Streptomyces* sp., *Thermoactinomyces vulgaris*, and *Saccharopolyspora rectivirgula* (formerly known as *Micropolyspora faeni*, *Micropolyspora rectivirgula*, and/or *Faenia rectivirgula*) [105].

Mushroom spores *per se* can also cause HP in sensitive individuals and this is particularly true in more exotic mushrooms such as oyster [106] and shiitake [107], which spore continuously and have become more popular in recent years. Most commercial mushrooms (*Agaricus* sp.) are harvested prior to sporulation; however, workers can be exposed to high spore levels if picking occurs after this stage. OA and dermatitis have also been reported in mushroom growers [108, 109].

Dermatitis in bakers

Occupational dermatitis in the food handler can manifest as irritant contact dermatitis, allergic contact dermatitis or allergic contact urticaria. In addition to OA and OR, bakers are at risk for the development of occupational dermatitis [100]. Occupational dermatitis in the Baker is a good example of how one occupation can be associated with the various forms of occupational skin diseases. These forms of dermatitis are associated with exposure to dough, flour, additives (see Table 19.6), and flavorings. Most reactions are irritant (non-immunologic), rather than immunologic (allergic contact dermatitis and allergic contact urticaria) in nature, and result from continuous exposure to wet, sticky dough, sweetening agents, or flavorings. Irritant responses can be distinguished from immunologic (allergic contact urticaria and allergic contact dermatitis) reactions by patch testing with the putative agents. Flour itself can induce allergic contact urticaria and flour contaminants (i.e., mites) can induce occupational dermatoses in sensitized workers.

Table 19.6 Additives encountered by bakers that can cause skin disease.

Irritants	Allergens
Emulsifiers	Benzoyl peroxide
Acetic acid	Potassium bromate
Lactic acid	Cinnamon oil
Calcium acetate/sulfate	Limonene, oil of yeast
Potassium iodide/bromate	Balsam of Peru
Potassium bicarbonate	*p*-amino-azo-benzene
Bleaching agents	Eugenol
Ascorbic acid	Vanilla
	Sorbic acid
	Karaya gum
	Ammonium persulfate
	Sodium metabisulfite

Source: Reproduced from Reference 77 with permission.

Relationship of sensitization routes: inhalation at the workplace versus ingestion at home

The relationship between sensitization by inhalation and symptoms following inhalation or ingestion of the same or a related antigen is intriguing. Exposure to food allergens typically occurs only via ingestion. Having subjects sensitized to traditional food allergens by inhalation presents an opportunity to compare elements of the two exposure routes. Most food-related occupational allergens have not been shown to induce symptoms following ingestion by workers sensitized by inhalation. In some individuals, certain allergens can elicit symptoms following inhalation and ingestion: a spice factory worker who developed asthma following inhalation of garlic dust noted the immediate onset of wheezing after eating garlic-containing foods [111]. A provocative challenge with garlic aerosol produced an immediate 35% reduction in forced expiratory volume in 1 second (FEV1). An oral challenge with 1600 mg of garlic (in capsules) induced apprehension, flushing, and nausea within 10 minutes. Diarrhea, increased pulse rate, and a 21% reduction in FEV1 appeared within 2 hours. In contrast to the immediate response to inhalation challenge and natural ingestion of garlic-containing foods, maximal symptoms were noted 2 hours after laboratory challenge, suggesting that inhalation of garlic vapors or absorption through the oral mucosa was necessary to produce an immediate response. Buckwheat [112], pineapple protease [113], snow crab [29], and honey/pollen [114, 115] have also been shown to produce allergic reactions following inhalation and ingestion by sensitive subjects.

Some individuals sensitized by inhalation to one occupational agent report symptoms following ingestion of a related antigen. A bird breeder developed OA following exposure to birds concomitant with an extreme gastrointestinal sensitivity to ingested chicken eggs. The primary sensitization involved bird serum antigens, which cross-reacted with ingested egg yolk proteins [116]. Butcher and colleagues [117] described an individual who developed and lost sensitivity to toluene diisocyanate vapor and ingested radishes, which contain isothiocyanates.

Diagnosis

History and physical examination

Individuals with suspected OA usually experience episodic dyspnea, chest tightness, cough, and wheezing. Typically, symptoms are worse at work, improving over weekends or holidays. However, the relationship to work exposure may be masked by intermittent exposure or by symptoms being worse at home in the evening or not improving over short periods such as weekends. Any questionnaire should include not only information about the current job, but also previous jobs. The history should identify whether symptoms began a short time after a job or workplace changed, if new materials or processes were introduced into the workplace, if agents with known asthma-inducing potential are used in the workplace, and if other workers exhibit similar symptoms. Usually, a latent period occurs between first exposure and development of symptoms. The length of this latency can range from weeks to more than 30 years [118]. The occurrence of rhinitis, conjunctivitis, or skin rashes at work in a subject with asthma is surely suggestive of OA, although not enough to confirm the diagnosis [119]. As with all occupational diseases, a high index of suspicion is needed to make a diagnosis. However, a highly suggestive history of OA is not sufficient to confirm the diagnosis. Even in the hands of experts, the predictive value of a positive questionnaire is 67%; the expert is better at excluding the diagnosis with a negative predictive value of 83% [120]. Physical examination is nonspecific and does not confirm the diagnosis of asthma ("all that wheezes is not asthma") but may be helpful in excluding other conditions.

OR manifests as nasal congestion, itch, sneeze, and rhinorrhea with exposure to the work environment. Like other forms of occupational disease, symptoms typically improve with removal from the work environment. As in OA, the history of workplace exposure is extremely important. A medication history is equally important as symptoms may be masked with the use of certain medications. Symptoms initially felt to be related to the work environment may become prolonged or worsen after removal from the culprit environment with the overuse of certain medications. For example, rhinitis medicamentosa may develop as a result of chronic topical decongestant use for the treatment of OR. Physical findings in OR are nonspecific and similar to findings in rhinitis from nonoccupational causes.

The clinical presentation of HP is often classified as acute, subacute, or chronic. In the acute presentation, flu-like symptoms including fever, chills, and cough often result in its confusion with a bacterial or viral respiratory infection. The symptoms usually begin 4–12 hours after work exposure. The subacute form may have a more prolonged course of shortness of breath, weight loss, and fatigue. In chronic disease, the antigen exposure is not interrupted and the subject may go on to develop restrictive pulmonary disease that may not be reversible. In the acute form of HP, physical examination reveals fine bilateral crackles. Occasionally, rhonchi or wheezes can be detected, although asthma rarely constitutes a part of this disease syndrome. As with OA, history is important and disease must be temporally correlated with exposure.

In evaluating patients with occupational skin disease, physical examination is also important. The appearance helps to determine whether the dermatitis is endogenous (constitutional), contact, or a combination of the two. Secondary bacterial infections may also be involved, thus making morphology-based diagnosis more difficult. Distribution may suggest a probable cause. Approximately 90% of OD involves the hands, usually the backs and palmar surface of the wrist [121]. When occupational disease is suspected, matching the location of the dermatitis and the exposure source becomes necessary. Actual or simulated workplace practices may aid in accomplishing this task.

In the differential diagnosis, contact dermatitis caused by nonoccupational exposure and endogenous dermatitis needs consideration. Often OD is multifactorial, with irritants, allergens, endogenous factors, and secondary bacterial infection all causally involved. When taking the worker's history, it is important to ask about other work aside from their primary occupation, as well as hobbies, since they may have potential exposures at these sites. The worker should also be asked about treatments that have been attempted either by the worker or by the worker's physician, as some of these treatments may be the actual cause of the problem or may exacerbate the current skin condition.

Laboratory tests

Asthma/rhinitis

When a subject with suspected OA is evaluated, the diagnosis of asthma needs to be objectively confirmed by demonstrating either reversible airways obstruction or increased NSBR, as assessed by methacholine or histamine inhalation challenge. Confirming the diagnosis of asthma does not, however, confirm the diagnosis of OA. The relationship between work exposure and asthma needs to be confirmed by other means, such as monitoring of PEFs and NSBR at and away from work or by specific inhalation challenges. However, the absence of increased NSBR in a subject who has been off work for some time (usually weeks, although a few days may be enough) does not exclude the diagnosis of OA. Return to work or a specific challenge may then be associated with increased NSBR [122, 123]. Alternatively, normal NSBR in a symptomatic worker still at work makes the diagnosis unlikely [2, 51, 124].

Skin prick tests with common environmental antigens, including pollens, molds, and dusts, are used to identify atopic individuals. In addition, skin testing with specific occupational allergens may assist in establishing a diagnosis of OA or monitoring workplace populations; positive skin tests are not themselves diagnostic of disease as they are merely indicative of exposure and sensitization. The lack of standardized skin test reagents has made it difficult to do skin testing with predictive reliability. Further, with most LMW agents, skin test results are of little value. As with all skin testing, care must be exercised; particularly with allergens of extreme potency, such as bromelain and latex, which may induce systemic reactions [125].

Specific IgE levels can be assessed using several methods (RAST, ImmunoCap or ELISA). Like skin prick tests, specific IgE assays can be used to evaluate both individuals and populations. Although they are less sensitive than skin tests, such *in vitro* methods of IgE antibody detection are more convenient for the testing of industrial populations. Serum can be collected during the worker's regular plant physical, so that the employee does not have to be removed from the production line for testing, and a physician's presence is not required. These tests can also be used for retrospective studies as long as sera have been stored.

Finally, the results of skin testing and specific IgE tests must correlate with clinical symptoms. For example, in crab-processing workers, the positive predictive value of a positive skin test and positive specific IgE by RAST testing was 76% and 89%, respectively [126]. These figures will vary with the offending allergen, the sensitivity of HMW agents being usually higher with a lower specificity [127]. Therefore, negative skin tests or specific IgE do not exclude the diagnosis of asthma/rhinitis, while positive tests do not confirm it.

As a noninvasive assessment of respiratory inflammation, sputum analysis has been proposed in the diagnosis of OA. Lemière et al. have shown increased sputum eosinophils and sputum eosinophil cationic protein in subjects when at work compared with the periods away from work [128]. Comparison of induced sputum in HMW and LMW agents in exposed workers showed that eosinophil percentages were higher in nonoccupational asthmatics and in asthmatics with HMW-induced asthma than in normal subjects and in subjects with OA due to LMW agents [129]. The clinical utility of these analyses remains to be determined.

As in OA, in making the diagnosis of OR, allergen-specific IgE should be measured if the test is available. The presence of allergen-specific IgE helps support the diagnosis of OR when the history is suggestive.

Hypersensitivity pneumonitis

Peripheral blood leukocytosis, with or without eosinophilia, occurs in HP [130]. Chest radiographs (CXR) are usually consistent with a diffuse interstitial or alveolar filling process; occasionally findings suggest pulmonary edema in the acute phase. If episodes are infrequent, radiographs may be normal. Airspace consolidation, reticulonodular patterns, and interstitial fibrosis which may be described as a honeycombing pattern are seen in acute, subacute, and chronic disease, respectively. A high-resolution CT scan is more sensitive than CXR or traditional CT for evaluation of parenchymal abnormalities and may show abnormalities when the CXR is normal. An example of the radiographic changes seen in HP is shown in Figure 19.1. Unlike the characteristic reversible obstructive pattern seen in asthma patients, HP subjects classically have a restrictive pattern. However, spirometry, like CXR, may be normal between attacks or prior to developing chronic disease. When changes are noted, they are typically restrictive defects with decreased lung volumes and diffusion capacity. Oxygen desaturation particularly with exercise may also be seen. Finally, a mixed obstructive/restrictive pattern is also frequently seen.

Precipitating antibodies (or specific IgG) against the offending antigen can be helpful in making the diagnosis, but it should be noted that studies have shown that between 3% and 50% of asymptomatic subjects may also have precipitins. False negatives may also occur because of problems with sera concentration, use of nonstandardized commercial extracts, or because the test was done with the wrong antigen. Elevations in immunoglobulins, particularly IgG, are seen. Immunoglobulin M (IgM) and A (IgA) may also be elevated, but IgE is not usually elevated. Increases in erythrocyte sedimentation rate and C-reactive proteins are secondary to the active inflammatory process. Skin testing for immediate hypersensitivity is of no value in making a diagnosis of HP [132].

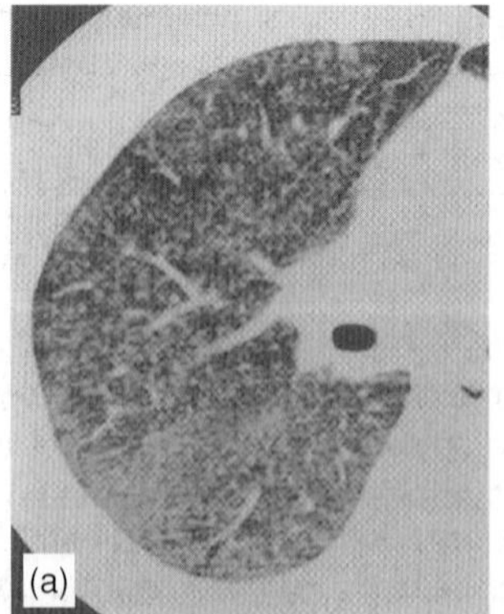

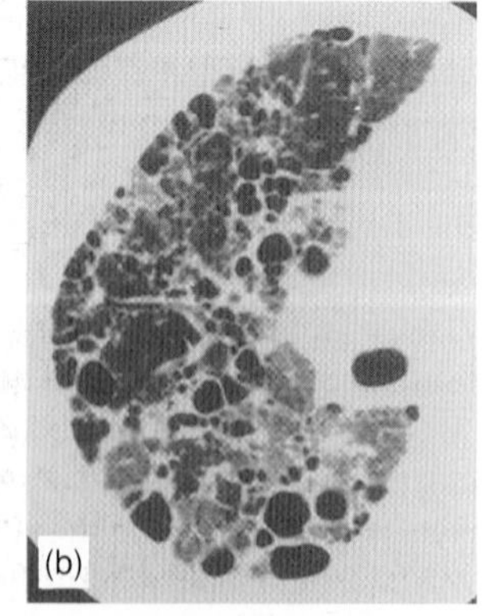

Figure 19.1 High-resolution CT scan in HP 39-year-old woman with HP presenting initially (a) with diffusely distributed centrilobular nodules and patchy ground-glass opacity on high-resolution CT scan. Follow-up study at 6 years (b) showed progression of parenchymal changes, forming honeycomb cysts, traction bronchiectasis, and bullae. Reproduced from Reference 131, with permission from Elsevier.

Bronchoalveolar lavage (BAL) shows variable cellular presentations. Classically, neutrophilia is seen within the first 48 hours after antigen challenge followed by lymphocytosis. The lymphocytosis may be of $CD4^+$ or $CD8^+$ T-lymphocytes. The CD4/CD8 ratio will depend on the specific time course in the disease during which the BAL is performed. BAL CD4/CD8 ratios have been variable in different studies and among specific causative allergens of HP [132–134]. Aside from the type of allergen, the dose of the allergen and stage of disease may also affect the ratio.

When clinical history and laboratory data are not sufficient to make a diagnosis, a lung biopsy may be needed. Lung biopsy may be performed by transbronchial or thoracoscopic/open biopsy, depending on the location and ability to obtain affected lung tissue. This also allows one to rule out infectious etiologies or other conditions [135].

Allergic contact dermatitis

In ACD, the patch test, which was first devised by Jadassohn in 1895, represents the only practical assay for diagnosis [136]. A common, commercially available patch test kit in the United States is the T.R.U.E. Test (GlaxoSmithKline, Research Triangle Park, NC). However, in the case of food allergens, ready-made patch testing is often not available. In these cases, one must prepare a personalized tray. If this is to be done, it is critical that the agents are prepared at proper concentrations so as not to give an irritant effect [137–139].

The Finn chamber is an example of an apparatus used to perform patch testing with a variety of agents that the clinician could select and/or prepare. It is a commonly used method of patch testing in which multiple 8-mm aluminum cups are filled with the test material and applied to the upper half of the back with an adhesive. The area that the chamber is to be applied to should be free of rash or large amounts of hair. The patch is affixed to the skin with tape. The patient is instructed not to shower during the period that the patch test is on. After 48–72 hours, the patch is removed and the underlying skin examined. The area should be examined on more than one occasion including at 72 hours, 96 hours, and 1 week. Using only one reading can decrease accuracy and may cause difficulty in differentiating irritant from allergic response. The interpretation of patch testing should be performed by individuals skilled in such procedures. As with all testing, false positives and false negatives are possible. False positives may

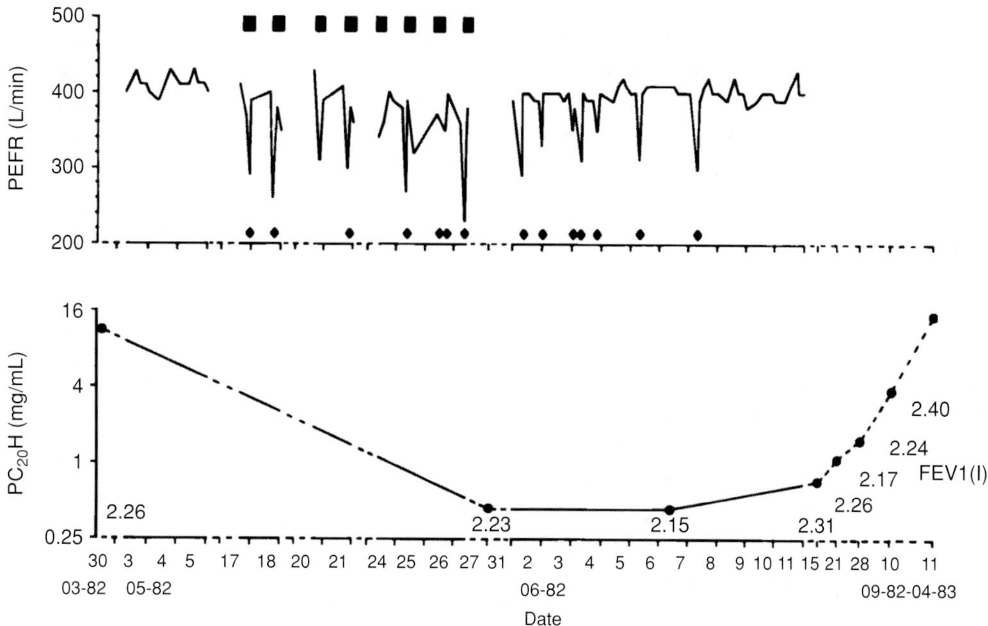

Figure 19.2 Monitoring of histamine bronchial responsiveness and peak expiratory flow (PEF) in a crab-processing worker. The upper panel illustrates the variation in PEF before and upon return to work in a crab-processing worker. Squares represent days at work. Upon return to work, there is a large variation in PEF associated with symptoms requiring two puffs of albuterol taken as needed (closed losanges). PEFs continued to fluctuate following work withdrawal for a few days. The lower panel illustrates the change in PC20 (provocative concentration of histamine inducing a 20% fall in FEV1), which decreased significantly upon return to work, while baseline FEV1 had not changed significantly when the subject was seen in the clinic. Return to baseline was only progressive and took almost 1 year. (Adapted from Reference 29, with permission from *Journal of Allergy and Clinical Immunology*.

occur because of the use of irritant substances or because of a pressure reaction over the applied site. False negatives may be because of material concentration, improper vehicles, or inappropriate reading times [140].

Monitoring pulmonary function

Pulmonary function testing (PFT) is used in helping to make the diagnosis of occupational lung disease, as well as for monitoring disease progression. In order to confirm OA, monitoring of PEF has proven to be very useful, with sensitivity of 81–100% and specificity of 74–89% compared to specific challenges [141–143]. Workers are asked to measure their PEF, the best of three reproducible (±20 l/min) being kept for analysis, ideally every 2 hours from awakening to bedtime or at least 4 times per day and when symptomatic. Peak flow meters offer the advantages of being cheap, portable, and readily available. However, PEF measurements are effort dependent, and compliance has been shown to be poor, especially when workers are seeking compensation [144, 145]. Although PEF is less reliable in assessing change in airway caliber, monitoring of FEV1 using portable devices has not proven more reliable [146]. When monitoring of PEF is done, it is important to keep medication at a minimum, using short-acting β-2 agonists on demand only and, if they are taken, keeping the dose of inhaled steroids or theophylline constant [147]. Monitoring of FEV1 before and after work shifts has not proven to be sensitive or specific enough [148, 149]. Finally, monitoring of NSBR coupled with monitoring of PEF may prove useful in certain cases as NSBR may increase upon return to work, improving (or decreasing) when taken off work. Figure 19.2 illustrates monitoring of PEF and histamine PC20 (i.e., the provocative concentration of histamine inducing a 20% fall in FEV1) in a snow crab-processing worker with OA [29]. When there is discrepancy between monitoring of PEF and NSBR, specific inhalation challenges, either in the laboratory or at work, may allow better accuracy of the diagnosis. While monitoring of PEF (and NSBR) can confirm the diagnosis of OA, it does not allow for the identification of the offending agents.

Specific inhalation challenge

Traditionally, challenges with food allergens are performed by ingestion. When dealing with asthma, to simulate industrial exposures, inhalation challenges must be performed. They are indicated if previous investigation with monitoring of PEF (and NSBR) was inconclusive or not possible to perform; for example, the subject was unable to return to work, or if the offending agent has not been identified. These tests can be done either in the laboratory or, occasionally, at work although the latter is less well controlled. They are safe when performed by trained personnel under the close supervision of an expert physician and offer the advantage of giving the diagnosis rapidly. Challenge testing in this manner should only be performed in a controlled setting that has the resources to handle medical emergencies.

Specific inhalation challenges done in the laboratory are considered by many as the reference standard for the diagnosis of OA and identification of the etiologic agent [2, 51, 150]. Nevertheless, false-positive (especially in unstable asthma) and false-negative reactions (due to loss of specific bronchial reactivity, using the wrong agent or taking medication prior to the challenge) may still occur. Although these tests are not well standardized, guidelines have been developed and should be followed [150, 151]. Subjects should be on minimum medication, stopping their medication according to standard recommendations, and the stability of the asthma should be assessed on a control day. The FEV1 is the most reliable index to monitor the bronchial response, PEF being less reliable, especially during the late asthmatic response [152, 153], and should be monitored for at least 7–8 hours after the end of exposure. In certain cases, challenge at work with similar monitoring of FEV1 may also confirm the diagnosis of OA, especially when the offending agent is unknown.

Respiratory response patterns seen in individuals with OA resulting from exposure to food antigens do not differ from those observed in subjects with allergic lung disease due to exposure to common environmental or other occupational antigens [154]. The most common types of asthmatic responses following exposure with HMW agents are immediate (65%), late, and dual (22%) [154]. Figure 19.3 illustrates these responses in sensitized snow crab-processing workers. In the immediate response, a decline in FEV1 occurs within minutes of exposure, reaches a peak within 20–30 minutes, and resolves within an hour or 2. In late reactions, the FEV1 decline starts 3–4 hours after exposure and is maximal between 6 and 10 hours. Dual responses are a combination of immediate and late responses. In some cases, a pattern of recurrent nocturnal asthma has been described, with falls in airway caliber occurring at approximately the same time on successive nights following a single exposure [155, 156]; the latter is probably due to increased NSBR. Atypical patterns have also been described but are less common with HMW agents.

Nasal challenge is necessary to secure the diagnosis of OR, but is not widely used. Furthermore, they are time consuming and not standardized. Although many methods of objective assessment of the nasal physiologic response to challenge are available, most are cumbersome and impractical. Acoustic rhinometry uses a piezoelectric spark to generate a three-dimensional image of the nasal passages, allowing measurement of nasal volume and cross-sectional area. This measurement can be used rapidly and repeatedly in nasal challenges [157, 158].

Specific inhalation challenges have limited value in most HP patients with the possible exception of some patients with acute disease. When it is performed, baseline PFTs are conducted, then exposure is done progressively and in a closed environment, using either nebulized extracts of suspected antigens or exposing the subject to the suspected agent in the same way as at work. The lack of standardized extracts is an additional complicating factor in being able to nebulize a standard amount of extract for challenge testing. The subject's symptoms and PFTs are followed serially, looking for clinical (fever) and spirometric changes described for acute disease which are more easily characterized than the symptoms in chronic disease [159]. Monitoring of the CBC is useful to track resolution of leukocytosis and eosinophilia [159]. Aside from a controlled chamber challenge, another potential consideration in subjects with acute disease is a re-exposure challenge to the suspected workplace.

Prognosis

While OA was considered a self-limited disease, most studies have shown that this is not the case. Thus, the majority of workers are still symptomatic or have abnormal pulmonary function after they have left the workplace [160, 161]. No study has been performed strictly in workers in the food industry, except follow-up studies on individuals with OA who are employed as snow crab workers, but it is likely that it is similar to other industries. In snow crab workers who were taken off work, improvement of FEV1 reaches a plateau after 1 year, while improvement of NSBR seems to plateau at 2 years. Similarly, there is a concurrent reduction in specific IgE antibodies, which does not seem to reach a plateau. The most relevant factors responsible for duration of symptoms after work withdrawal seem to be the duration of exposure after onset of symptoms, the total duration or exposure, and the degree of impairment in FEV1 as well as the degree of bronchial hyperresponsiveness at diagnosis [162, 163].

Similar patterns of improvement are seen with other causes of OA [160, 161]. Individuals who continue to work are thus at risk to develop irreversible disease, stressing the importance of early removal from exposure. Even reduction of exposure may expose workers to worsening of asthma [164]. While NSBR usually improves with work withdrawal, most workers will still exhibit persistent specific bronchial responsiveness if re-challenged with the agent responsible for their OA, after several years off work [165].

The socioeconomic consequences of OA are not negligible [166–168] and vary between countries according to the compensation systems and retraining programs. This stresses the importance of making a proper diagnosis.

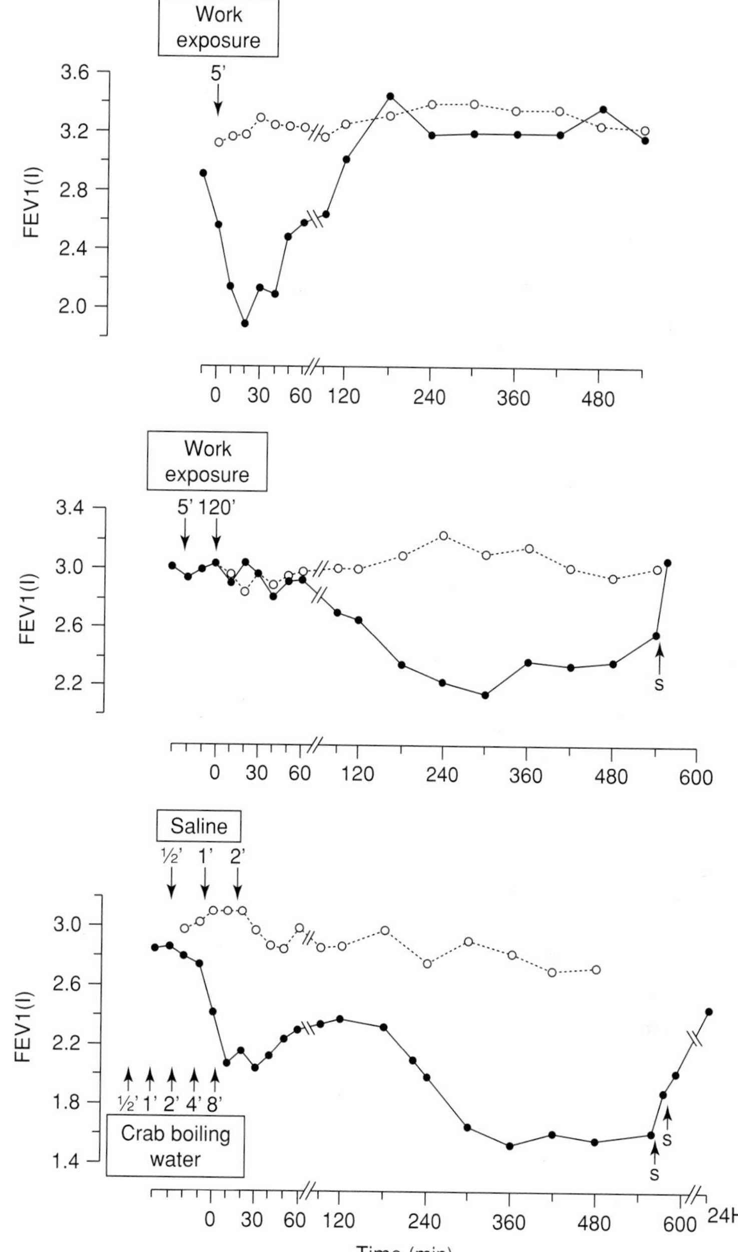

Figure 19.3 Specific inhalation challenges in crab-processing workers. The upper panel illustrates the change in FEV1 in a worker presenting an immediate type of asthmatic reaction, after a 5-minute exposure in the workplace. The middle panel illustrates a late asthmatic reaction occurring about 2 hours after 125 minutes of exposure in the workplace with full recovery at the end of the day post-albuterol (S). The lower panel illustrates a dual asthmatic response following the inhalation of crab boiling water in the laboratory. (Adapted from Reference 29, with permission from *Journal of Allergy and Clinical Immunology*.

In Quebec, where workers are no longer exposed to their offending agent once the diagnosis is made, about one-third of subjects find an adequate job with the same employer while one-third find a different job with another employer. Only 8% of subjects remain unemployed after 2 years of follow-up. Quality of life of subjects with OA in the same province is slightly though significantly less satisfactory than subjects with common asthma of comparable severity [169, 170]. In other countries, the situation is less favorable, with the number of subjects still unemployed varying between 25% and 69% [168, 171]. In many situations, workers have to stay in the same environment, which may be associated with deterioration in their asthma. Moscato et al. showed that subjects with OA who stayed at work needed more medication than those who ceased to be exposed [172]. Although much work has been put into the identification of prognostic indicators for OA, the prognosis of OR has not been as well studied. However, workers with OR have a lower quality of life [173].

The clinical prognosis for individuals with HP depends primarily on the amount of damage at the time of diagnosis and the ability of the individual to avoid contact with the etiologic agent, although this may not affect PFTs and CXRs [174, 175]. When HP is diagnosed early and ongoing exposure with the antigen is avoided, the outcomes are generally good and clinical, radiographic and pulmonary function return to baseline. Most of the recovery should occur within several months. If the patient still has changes after 6 months away from the exposure, the changes are likely to be permanent. With delays in diagnosis and treatment, subjects may progress to the chronic form of the disease, which may lead to irreversible changes as well. Patients may also go on to develop symptoms of asthma or emphysema. As with diagnosis, there are also no pathognomonic prognostic markers for HP. There have also been reports of continued decline in lung function despite removal from the inciting agent at the acute stage. In particular, there was continued decline in diffusing capacity of the lung for CO (DL,CO) and total lung capacity (TLC) over several years. If the subject does progress to the chronic fibrosis stage, they may go on to respiratory failure and death or right-sided heart failure.

The majority of individuals with contact dermatitis have an excellent prognosis, provided that exposure to the allergen is eliminated. If an employee cannot change jobs, dermatitis can become chronic. Chronic dermatitis can also occur in some subjects despite the apparent elimination of allergen exposure. This condition is particularly troublesome in industrial settings and may reflect complex exposures or mixed disease, endogenous, or irritant dermatitis.

Prevention and treatment

The best "treatment" of allergic occupational disease is prevention [176]. Reduction of exposure levels is the only way to reduce significantly the incidence of respiratory symptoms among workers, although some individuals may still be sensitized at very low levels. This may be achieved, for example, by enclosing the responsible process, improving ventilation and personal protection devices, and modifying the process by encapsulating the agent. While threshold limit values have been established to prevent exposure to irritant levels of various agents, threshold limit values to prevent sensitization are not known for most agents [49, 177]. However, once an individual has developed clinical evidence of OA, asthmatic responses will occur at minute exposure levels, usually less than any industrial plant can maintain. The specific treatment of OA, aside from removal of the inciting agent, is the same as non-OA.

Pre-employment screening and periodic health monitoring, with education of workers about risk of disease and means to reduce exposure, have been suggested as ways to prevent the development of allergic respiratory disease. Questions arise over which tests are appropriate. Skin prick testing with specific allergens may prove useful for monitoring, although positive responses do not necessarily correlate with disease and, as for atopy, do not predict adequately who will develop OA [51, 178]. Furthermore, human rights issues and laws protecting workers against discrimination would not allow using pre-screening to exclude subjects from being hired. However, monitoring of skin prick tests for specific allergens during work in high-risk industries may be useful and allow reallocation of sensitized individuals to low-exposure environments, thus lessening the risk of developing clinical diseases [179, 180].

Once OA has been diagnosed, the worker should be removed permanently from further exposure to the offending agent in order to prevent further deterioration and improve the prognosis [179]. Although OR and/or conjunctivitis may precede OA [30], there is little information on the level of risk to develop OA in workers with OR, with only one study having looked at the outcome of workers who have developed OR. Indeed, Karjalainen et al. have shown that these workers have a risk ratio of developing OA between 3.7 and 5.4, depending on the level of certitude of the diagnosis of OR [181]. Therefore, in subjects with OR, removal of exposure will improve the symptoms but simple treatment with H1-antagonists or inhaled corticosteroids may be enough to control the symptoms and allow the worker to continue his job preferably in a much lower exposure environment. Any new case of OA should be considered to represent a sentinel event in the workplace so that proper investigation of other workers is undertaken to detect other cases of OA [150].

As with OA, workers with HP should be removed from the offending agent. Furthermore, it is important to investigate nonaffected workers as well, since they may eventually develop symptoms or disease. For example, when HP caused by inhalation of mollusk shell dust was discovered among employees in a factory, evaluation of the health status of the other factory employees was undertaken. This revealed functional decline in the subjects originally unaffected, despite attempts at improving the occupational environment [182].

In more severe cases of HP, systemic corticosteroids may be needed. When this approach is used, it should be with careful monitoring of X-rays, PFTs, and clinical symptoms. The subject should have slow tapering of the steroids after clinical improvement, as rapid tapering may cause relapse. Although steroids will improve the acute symptoms, there is concern that steroid-treated patients may potentially be at higher risk of disease relapse [183].

As with respiratory disease, drug treatment of occupational dermatoses produce only temporary benefit unless the individual receives no further exposure. Specifically, workers with less than 10% skin involvement are treated with topical steroids and those with more extensive involvement may be treated with oral steroids. The steroids should be tapered and not stopped abruptly, as prematurely stopping steroids can cause a flare of skin symptoms. Protective measures that reduce skin contact, such as appropriate clothing and gloves, may be used if avoidance is impossible. It should not be automatically assumed that such devices are impervious to all materials. Workers have had better outcomes of their OD when they have received hands-on instructions on the measures needed to improve the dermatitis. However, if these measures do not improve or resolve the dermatitis, the worker should be withdrawn from exposure.

Conclusions

Exposure to a wide variety of food-derived and food-associated materials encountered in the workplace is associated with development of OA, HP, rhinitis/conjunctivitis, and dermatitis in sensitized individuals. The number of causative agents will undoubtedly continue to rise as new agents are introduced into the workplace and as physician awareness of these conditions continues to grow. Relatively little is known about the prevalence and incidence, importance of host factors, treatment, or prognosis of the occupational diseases resulting from exposure to these antigens in the food industry.

The examples described in this chapter are but a few of the wide array of food-associated occupational hypersensitivity reactions. New agents causing occupational hypersensitivities are being reported. With globalization of world markets and a continuing increase of individuals employed in the food industry, it is essential for the clinician to keep abreast of any new reactions when diagnosing a new or unusual occupational reaction. For example, a particular interest is the development of genetically modified (GM) crops that may contain novel proteins to which no prior human exposure has occurred. Although most efforts at food safety analysis are directed at ingestion of foods by consumers, particularly those developed through biotechnology, it is possible that such novel proteins could also cause occupationally related allergic reactions in food workers. Although this is unlikely to occur due to the low expression levels of such foods containing novel proteins, such a possibility should be considered whenever occupational reactions occur in industries growing/processing foods developed by biotechnology or using ingredients that have been similarly altered [184].

References

1. US Bureau of Labor Statistics. Available at www.bls.gov (Last accessed June 9, 2013).
2. Tarlo SM, Balmes J, Balkissoon R, et al. Diagnosis and management of work-related asthma: American College of Chest Physicians Consensus Statement. *Chest* 2008; 134(3 Suppl.):1S–41S.
3. Brooks SM, Weiss MA, Bernstein IL. Reactive airways dysfunction syndrome (RADS). Persistent asthma syndrome after high level irritant exposures. *Chest* 1985; 88(3):376–384
4. Tarlo SM, Broder I. Irritant-induced occupational asthma. *Chest* 1989; 96(2):297–300.
5. Moscato G, Vandenplas O, Van Wijk RG, et al. EAACI position paper on occupational rhinitis. *Respir Res* 2009; 10:16.
6. Pepys J. Hypersensitivity diseases of the lungs due to fungi and organic dusts. *Monogr Allergy* 1969; 4:1–147.
7. Patel AM, Ryu JH, Reed CE. Hypersensitivity pneumonitis: current concepts and future questions. *J Allergy Clin Immunol* 2001; 108(5):661–670.
8. Nicholson PJ, Llewellyn D, English JS. Evidence-based guidelines for the prevention, identification and management of occupational contact dermatitis and urticaria. *Contact Dermat* 2010; 63(4):177–186.
9. Seaton A. Surveillance of work related and occupational respiratory disease: SWORD. *Thorax* 1991; 46:548.
10. Gannon PF, Burge PS. The SHIELD scheme in the West Midlands Region, United Kingdom. Midland Thoracic Society Research Group. *Br J Ind Med* 1993; 50(9):791–796.
11. Provencher S, Labreche FP, De Guire L. Physician based surveillance system for occupational respiratory diseases: the experience of PROPULSE, Quebec, Canada. *Occup Environ Med* 1997; 54(4):272–276.
12. Matte TD, Hoffman RE, Rosenman KD, Stanbury M. Surveillance of occupational asthma under the SENSOR model. *Chest* 1990; 98:173S-178S.
13. Global initiative for asthma. *Global strategy of asthma management and prevention.* Updated 2011. Available at www.ginasthma.org (Last accessed December 31, 2011).
14. Schiller JS, Lucas JW, Ward BW, Peregoy JA. Summary Health Statistics for U.S. Adults: National Health Interview Survey, 2010. National Center for Health Statistics. *Vital Health Stat 10* 2012; (252):1–207.
15. Balmes J, Becklake M, Blanc P, et al. American Thoracic Society statement: occupational contribution to the burden of airway disease. *Am J Respir Crit Care Med* 2003; 167(5):787–797.
16. Blanc PD, Toren K. How much adult asthma can be attributed to occupational factors? *Am J Med* 1999; 107(6):580–507.
17. Bakerly ND, Moore VC, Vellore AD, Jaakkola MS, Robertson AS, Burge PS. Fifteen-year trends in occupational asthma: data from the Shield surveillance scheme. *Occup Med (Lond)* 2008; 58(3):169–174.
18. Folletti I, Forcina A, Marabini A, Bussetti A, Siracusa A. Have the prevalence and incidence of occupational asthma and rhinitis because of laboratory animals declined in the last 25 years? *Allergy* 2008; 63(7):834–841.
19. Vandenplas O, Lantin AC, D'Alpaos V, et al. Time trends in occupational asthma in Belgium. *Respir Med* 2011; 105(9):1364–1372.
20. Paris C, Ngatchou-Wandji J, Luc A, et al. Work-related asthma in France: recent trends for the period 2001–2009. *Occup Environ Med* 2012; 69(6):391–397.
21. Jones RN, Hughes JM, Lehrer SB, et al. Lung function consequences of exposure and hypersensitivity in workers

who process green coffee beans. *Am Rev Respir Dis* 1982; 125(2):199–202.

22. Kaye M, Freedman SO. Allergy to raw coffee—an occupational disease. *Can Med Assoc J* 1961; 84:199–202.
23. Gautrin D, Cartier A, Howse D, et al. Occupational asthma & allergy in snow crab processing in Newfoundland and Labrador. *Occup Environ Med* 2010; 67(1):17–23.
24. Herxheimer H. The skin sensitivity to flour of baker's apprentices. A final report of a long term investigation. *Acta Allergol* 1973; 28(1):42–49.
25. Musk AW, Venables KM, Crook B, et al. Respiratory symptoms, lung function, and sensitisation to flour in a British bakery. *Br J Indust Med* 1989; 46:636–642.
26. Smith TA, Lumley KP. Work-related asthma in a population exposed to grain, flour and other ingredient dusts. *Occup Med* 1996; 46(1):37–40.
27. Talini D, Benvenuti A, Carrara M, Vaghetti E, Martin LB, Paggiaro PL. Diagnosis of flour-induced occupational asthma in a cross-sectional study. *Respir Med* 2002; 96(4):236–243.
28. Slavin RG. Update on occupational rhinitis and asthma. *Allergy Asthma Proc* 2010; 31(6):437–443.
29. Cartier A, Malo JL, Forest F, et al. Occupational asthma in snow crab-processing workers. *J Allergy Clin Immunol* 1984; 74(3 Pt. 1):261–269.
30. Malo JL, Lemière C, Desjardins A, Cartier A. Prevalence and intensity of rhinoconjunctivitis in subjects with occupational asthma. *Eur Respir J* 1997; 10(7):1513–1515.
31. Vandenplas O, Delwiche JP, Evrard G, et al. Prevalence of occupational asthma due to latex among hospital personnel. *Am J Respir Crit Care Med* 1995; 151(1):54–60.
32. Saary MJ, Kanani A, Alghadeer H, Holness DL, Tarlo SM. Changes in rates of natural rubber latex sensitivity among dental school students and staff members after changes in latex gloves. *J Allergy Clin Immunol* 2002; 109(1):131–135.
33. Liebers V, Hoernstein M, Baur X. Humoral immune response to the insect allergen Chi t I in aquarists and fish-food factory workers. *Allergy* 1993; 48:236–239.
34. Gross N. Allergy to laboratory animals: epidemiologic, clinical, and physiologic aspects, and a trial of cromolyn in its management. *J Allergy Clin Immunol* 1980; 66:158–165.
35. Grant IW, Blyth W, Wardrop VE, Gordon RM, Pearson JC, Mair A. Prevalence of farmer's lung in Scotland: a pilot survey. *Br Med J* 1972; 1(799):530–534.
36. Tao BG, Shen YE, Chen GX, et al. An epidemiological study on farmer's lung among hay grinders in Dafeng County. *Biomed Environ Sci* 1988; 1(1):13–18.
37. Marx JJ, Guernsey J, Emanuel DA, Merchant JA, Morgan DP, Kryda M. Cohort studies of immunologic lung disease among Wisconsin dairy farmers. *Am J Ind Med* 1990; 18(3):263–268.
38. Fenclova Z, Pelclova D, Urban P, Navratil T, Klusackova P, Lebedova J. Occupational hypersensitivity pneumonitis reported to the Czech National Registry of Occupational Diseases in the period 1992–2005. *Ind Health* 2009; 47(4):443–448.
39. Peltonen L, Wickstrom G, Vaahtoranta M. Occupational dermatoses in the food industry. *Derm Beruf Umwelt* 1985; 33(5):166–169.
40. Veien NK, Hattel T, Justesen O, Norholm A. Causes of eczema in the food industry. *Derm Beruf Umwelt* 1983; 31(3):84–86.
41. Dickel H, Kuss O, Schmidt A, Kretz J, Diepgen TL. Importance of irritant contact dermatitis in occupational skin disease. *Am J Clin Dermatol* 2002; 3(4):283–289.
42. Hjorth N, Roed-Petersen J. Occupational protein contact dermatitis in food handlers. *Contact Dermat* 1976; 2(1):28–42.
43. Cronin E. Dermatitis of the hands in caterers. *Contact Dermat* 1987; 17(5):265–269.
44. Smith TA. Occupational skin conditions in the food industry. *Occup Med (Lond)* 2000; 50(8):597–598.
45. Cherry N, Meyer JD, Adisesh A, et al. Surveillance of occupational skin disease: EPIDERM and OPRA. *Br J Dermatol* 2000; 142(6):1128–1134.
46. Williams JD, Lee AY, Matheson MC, Frowen KE, Noonan AM, Nixon RL. Occupational contact urticaria: Australian data. *Br J Dermatol* 2008; 159(1):125–131.
47. McDonald JC, Beck MH, Chen Y, Cherry NM. Incidence by occupation and industry of work-related skin diseases in the United Kingdom, 1996–2001. *Occup Med (Lond)* 2006; 56(6):398–405.
48. Cullinan P, Lowson D, Nieuwenhuijsen MJ, et al. Work related symptoms, sensitisation, and estimated exposure in workers not previously exposed to flour. *Occup Environ Med* 1994; 51(9):579–583.
49. Baur X, Chen Z, Liebers V. Exposure–response relationships of occupational inhalative allergens. *Clin Exp Allergy* 1998; 28(5):537–544.
50. Houba R, Heederik D, Doekes G. Wheat sensitization and work-related symptoms in the baking industry are preventable. An epidemiologic study. *Am J Respir Crit Care Med* 1998; 158(5 Pt. 1):1499–1503.
51. Nicholson PJ, Cullinan P, Taylor AJ, Burge PS, Boyle C. Evidence based guidelines for the prevention, identification, and management of occupational asthma. *Occup Environ Med* 2005; 62(5):290–299.
52. Douglas JDM, McSharry C, Blaikie L, Morrow T, Miles S, Franklin D. Occupational asthma caused by automated salmon processing. *Lancet* 1995; 346(8977):737–740.
53. Bauer A, Bartsch R, Hersmann C, et al. Occupational hand dermatitis in food industry apprentices: results of a 3-year follow-up cohort study. *Int Arch Occup Environ Health* 2001; 74(6):437–442.
54. Bernstein DI. Genetics of occupational asthma. *Curr Opin Allergy Clin Immunol* 2011; 11(2):86–89.
55. Camarena A, Juarez A, Mejia M, et al. Major histocompatibility complex and tumor necrosis factor-alpha polymorphisms in pigeon breeder's disease. *Am J Respir Crit Care Med* 2001; 163(7):1528–1533.
56. Holst R, Moller H. One hundred twin pairs patch tested with primary irritants. *Br J Dermatol* 1975; 93(2):145–149.
57. Hulbert WC, Walker DC, Jackson A, Hogg JC. Airway permeability to horseradish peroxidase in guinea pigs: the repair phase after injury by cigarette smoke. *Am Rev Respir Dis* 1981; 123(3):320–326.

58. Adisesh A, Gruszka L, Robinson E, Evans G. Smoking status and immunoglobulin E seropositivity to workplace allergens. *Occup Med (Lond)* 2011; 61(1):62–64.

59. McSharry C, Anderson K, McKay IC, et al. The IgE and IgG antibody responses to aerosols of Nephrops norvegicus (prawn) antigens: the association with clinical hypersensitivity and with cigarette smoking. *Clin Exp Immunol* 1994; 97(3):499–504.

60. Jeebhay MF, Robins TG, Miller ME, et al. Occupational allergy and asthma among salt water fish processing workers. *Am J Ind Med* 2008; 51(12):899–910.

61. Zetterström O, Osterman K, Machado L, Johansson S. Another smoking hazard: raised serum IgE concentration and increased risk of occupational allergy. *BMJ* 1981; 283:1215–1217.

62. Holt P. Immune and inflammatory function in cigarette smokers. *Thorax* 1987; 42:241–249.

63. Murin S, Bilello KS, Matthay R. Other smoking-affected pulmonary diseases. *Clin Chest Med* 2000; 21(1):121–137.

64. Hagiwara E, Takahashi KI, Okubo T, et al. Cigarette smoking depletes cells spontaneously secreting Th(1) cytokines in the human airway. *Cytokine* 2001; 14(2):121–126.

65. Dangman KH, Storey E, Schenck P, Hodgson MJ. Effects of cigarette smoking on diagnostic tests for work-related hypersensitivity pneumonitis: data from an outbreak of lung disease in metalworkers. *Am J Ind Med* 2004; 45(5):455–467.

66. Arima K, Ando M, Ito K, et al. Effect of cigarette smoking on prevalence of summer-type hypersensitivity pneumonitis caused by Trichosporon cutaneum. *Arch Environ Health* 1992; 47(4):274–278.

67. Renstrom A, Malmberg P, Larsson K, Larsson PH, Sundblad BM. Allergic sensitization is associated with increased bronchial responsiveness: a prospective study of allergy to laboratory animals. *Eur Respir J* 1995; 8(9):1514–1519.

68. Chan-Yeung M, Lam S. Occupational asthma. *Am Rev Respir Dis* 1986; 133:686–703.

69. O'Neil CE, Salvaggio JE. The pathogenesis of occupational asthma. In: Kay AB (ed.), *The Allergic Basis of Asthma. Balliere's Clinical Immunology and Allergy*. Philadelphia, PA: W.B. Saunders Co, 1988; pp. 143–175.

70. Cartier A. The role of inhalant food allergens in occupational asthma. *Curr Allergy Asthma Rep* 2010; 10(5):349–356.

71. Guarneri F, Barbuzza O, Vaccaro M, Galtieri G. Allergic contact dermatitis and asthma caused by limonene in a labourer handling citrus fruits. *Contact Dermat* 2008; 58(5):315–316.

72. Quirce S, Bernstein DI, Malo JL. High-molecular-weight protein agents. In: Bernstein IL, Chan-Yeung M, Malo JL, Bernstein DI (eds), *Asthma in the Workplace and Related Conditions*. New York: Taylor & Francis Group, 2006; pp. 463–479.

73. Tonini S, Perfetti L, Pignatti P, Pala G, Moscato G. Occupational asthma induced by exposure to lima bean (*Phaseolus lunatus*). *Ann Allergy Asthma Immunol* 2012; 108(1):66–67.

74. Malo JL, L'Archeveque J. Asthma in reaction to two occupational agents in the same workplace. *Thorax* 2011; 66(11):1008.

75. Cartier A, Lemière C, Malo JL. Occupational asthma (OA) to lactoserum in a baker. *J Allergy Clin Immunol* 2005; 115:s29.

76. Jensen A, Dahl S, Sherson D, Sommer B. Respiratory complaints and high sensitization rate at a rennet-producing plant. *Am J Ind Med* 2006; 49(10):858–861.

77. Sikora M, Cartier A, Aresery M, Wild L, Lehrer SB. Occupational reactions to food allergens. In: Metcalfe DD, Sampson HA, Simon RA (eds). *Food Allergy. Adverse Reactions to Foods and Food Additives*, 4th edn. Malden, MA: Blackwell Publishing, 2008; pp. 223–250.

78. van Kampen V, Merget R, Baur X. Occupational airway sensitizers: an overview on the respective literature. *Am J Ind Med* 2000; 38(2):164–218.

79. Malo JL, Chan-Yeung M. Appendix. In: Bernstein IL, Chan-Yeung M, Malo JL, Bernstein DI (eds), *Asthma in the Workplace and Related Conditions*. New York: Taylor & Francis Group, 2006; pp. 825–866.

80. Siracusa A, Desrosiers M, Marabini A. Epidemiology of occupational rhinitis: prevalence, aetiology and determinants. *Clin Exp Allergy* 2000; 30(11):1519–1534.

81. van den Bosch JM, van Toorn DW, Wagenaar SS. Coffee worker's lung: reconsideration of a case report. *Thorax* 1983; 38(9):720.

82. Minamoto K, Harada K, Wei QJ, Wei CN, Omori S, Ueda A. Occupational allergic contact dermatitis from mioga (Zingiber mioga rosc.) in greenhouse cultivators. *Int J Immunopathol Pharmacol* 2007; 20(2 Suppl. 2) :31–34.

83. Williams JD, Moyle M, Nixon RL. Occupational contact urticaria from Parmesan cheese. *Contact Dermat* 2007; 56(2):113–114.

84. Williams J, Roberts H, Tate B. Contact urticaria to olives. *Contact Dermat* 2007; 56(1):52–53.

85. Yanagi T, Shimizu H, Shimizu T. Occupational contact dermatitis caused by asparagus. *Contact Dermat* 2010; 63(1):54.

86. Ackermann L, Aalto-Korte K, Jolanki R, Alanko K. Occupational allergic contact dermatitis from cinnamon including one case from airborne exposure. *Contact Dermat* 2009; 60(2):96–69.

87. Guarneri F. Occupational allergy to cinnamal in a baker. *Contact Dermat* 2010; 63(5):294.

88. Kiec-Swierczynska M, Krecisz B, Chomiczewska D, Swierczynska-Machura D, Palczynski C. Occupational allergic contact dermatitis caused by basil (*Ocimum basilicum*). *Contact Dermat* 2010; 63(6):365–367.

89. Wantke F, Simon-Nobbe B, Poll V, Gotz M, Jarisch R, Hemmer W. Contact dermatitis caused by salami skin. *Contact Dermat* 2011; 64(2):111–114.

90. FAO Fisheries and Aquaculture Department. *The State of World Fisheries and Aquaculture*. Rome: Food and Agriculture Organization of the United Nations, 2010.

91. Lehrer SB. Seafood allergy. Introduction. *Clin Rev Allergy* 1993; 11(2):155–157.

92. De Besche A. On asthma bronchiale in man provoked by cat, dog and different other animals. *Acta Med Scand* 1937; 92(1–3):237–255.

93. Malo JL, Cartier A. Occupational reactions in the seafood industry. *Clin Rev Allergy* 1993; 11(2):223–240.

94. Jeebhay MF, Cartier A. Seafood workers and respiratory disease: an update. *Curr Opin Allergy Clin Immunol* 2010; 10(2):104–113.

95. Jeebhay MF, Robins TG, Lehrer SB, Lopata AL. Occupational seafood allergy: a review. *Occup Environ Med* 2001; 58(9):553–562.
96. Macan J, Kanceljak-Macan B, Mustac M, Milkovic-Kraus S. Analysis of dust samples from urban and rural occupational environments in Croatia. *Arh Hig Rada Toksikol* 2005; 56(4):327–332.
97. Centers for Disease Control [CDC]. Asthma-like illness among crab-processing workers-Alaska. *MMWR Morb Mortal Wkly Rep* 1982; 31(8):95–96.
98. Bang B, Aasmoe L, Aamodt BH, et al. Exposure and airway effects of seafood industry workers in northern Norway. *J Occup Environ Med* 2005; 47(5):482–492.
99. Walusiak J, Hanke W, Gorski P, Palczynski C. Respiratory allergy in apprentice bakers: do occupational allergies follow the allergic march? *Allergy* 2004; 59(4):442–450.
100. U.S. Department of Agriculture (2011) *Mushroom Industry Report (94003)*.Available at http://usda.mannlib.cornell.edu/MannUsda/viewDocumentInfo.do?documentID=1395 (Last accessed June 9, 2013).
101. Bringhurst LS, Byrne RN, Gershon-Cohen J. Respiratory disease of mushroom workers; farmer's lung. *J Am Med Assoc* 1959; 171:15–18.
102. Sakula A. Mushroom-worker's lung. *Br Med J* 1967; 3(5567):708–710.
103. Sanderson W, Kullman G, Sastre J, et al. Outbreak of hypersensitivity pneumonitis among mushroom farm workers. *Am J Ind Med* 1992; 22(6):859–872.
104. Tanaka H, Saikai T, Sugawara H, et al. Workplace-related chronic cough on a mushroom farm. *Chest* 2002; 122(3):1080–1085.
105. Lacey J. Allergy in mushroom workers. *Lancet* 1974; 1(7853):366.
106. Lee MW. Hypersensitivity pneumonitis induced by oyster mushroom spores. *J Asthma Allergy Clin Immunol* 1998; 18(1):84–89.
107. Ampere A, Delhaes L, Soots J, Bart F, Wallaert B. Hypersensitivity pneumonitis induced by Shiitake mushroom spores. *Med Mycol* 2012; 50(6):654–657.
108. Michils A, De Vuyst P, Nolard N, Servais G, Duchateau J, Yernault JC. Occupational asthma to spores of Pleurotus cornucopiae. *Eur Respir J* 1991; 4:1143–1147.
109. Tarvainen K, Salonen JP, Kanerva L, Estlander T, Keskinen H, Rantanen T. Allergy and toxicodermia from shiitake mushrooms. *J Am Acad Dermatol* 1991; 24(1):64–66.
110. Tacke J, Schmidt A, Fartasch M, Diepgen TL. Occupational contact dermatitis in bakers, confectioners and cooks. A population-based study. *Contact Dermat* 1995; 33(2):112–117.
111. Lybarger JA, Gallagher JS, Pulver DW, Litwin A, Brooks S, Bernstein IL. Occupational asthma induced by inhalation and ingestion of garlic. *J Allergy Clin Immunol* 1982; 69(5):448–454.
112. Nakamura S, Yamaguchi M, Oishi M, Hayama T. Studies on the buckwheat allergose report 1: on the cases with the buckwheat allergose. *Allerg Immunol (Leipz)* 1974; 20–21(4):449–456.
113. Baur X, Fruhmann G. Allergic reactions, including asthma, to the pineapple protease bromelain following occupational exposure. *Clin Allergy* 1979; 9:443–450.
114. Bousquet J, Campos J, Michel FB. Food intolerance to honey. *Allergy* 1984; 39(1):73–75.
115. Bousquet J, Dhivert H, Clauzel AM, Hewitt B, Michel FB. Occupational allergy to sunflower pollen. *J Allergy Clin Immunol* 1985; 75(1 Pt. 1):70–74.
116. Hoffman DR, Guenther DM. Occupational allergy to avian proteins presenting as allergy to ingestion of egg yolk. *J Allergy Clin Immunol* 1988; 81:484–488.
117. Butcher BT, O'Neil CE, Reed MA, Salvaggio JE, Weill H. Development and loss of toluene diisocyanate reactivity: immunologic, pharmacologic, and provocative challenge studies. *J Allergy Clin Immunol* 1982; 70:231–235.
118. Malo JL, Ghezzo H, D'Aquino C, L'Archeveque J, Cartier A, Chan-Yeung M. Natural history of occupational asthma: relevance of type of agent and other factors in the rate of development of symptoms in affected subjects. *J Allergy Clin Immunol* 1992; 90:937–944.
119. Vandenplas O, Ghezzo H, Munoz X, et al. What are the questionnaire items most useful in identifying subjects with occupational asthma? *Eur Respir J* 2005; 26(6):1056–1063.
120. Malo JL, Ghezzo H, L'Archeveque J, Lagier F, Perrin B, Cartier A. Is the clinical history a satisfactory means of diagnosing occupational asthma? *Am Rev Respir Dis* 1991; 143(3):528–532.
121. Emmett EA. Occupational skin disease. *J Allergy Clin Immunol* 1983; 72(6):649–656.
122. Ramsdale EH, Morris MM, Roberts RS, Hargreave FE. Bronchial responsiveness to methacholine in chronic bronchitis: relationship to airflow obstruction and cold air responsiveness. *Thorax* 1984; 39:912–918.
123. Vandenplas O, Delwiche JP, Jamart J, Vandeweyer R. Increase in non-specific bronchial hyperresponsiveness as an early marker of bronchial response to occupational agents during specific inhalation challenges. *Thorax* 1996; 51(5):472–478.
124. Baur X, Huber H, Degens PO, Allmers H, Ammon J. Relation between occupational asthma case history, bronchial methacholine challenge, and specific challenge test in patients with suspected occupational asthma. *Am J Ind Med* 1998; 33(2):114–122.
125. Gailhofer G, Wilders-Truschnig M, Smolle J, Ludvan M. Asthma caused by bromelain: an occupational allergy. *Clin Allergy* 1988; 18(5):445–450.
126. Cartier A, Malo JL, Ghezzo H, McCants M, Lehrer SB. IgE sensitization in snow crab-processing workers. *J Allergy Clin Immunol* 1986; 78:344–348.
127. Bardy JD, Malo JL, Séguin P, et al. Occupational asthma and IgE sensitization in a pharmaceutical company processing psyllium. *Am Rev Respir Dis* 1987; 135:1033–1038.
128. Lemière C. The use of sputum eosinophils in the evaluation of occupational asthma. *Curr Opin Allergy Clin Immunol* 2004; 4(2):81–85.
129. Di Franco A, Vagaggini B, Bacci E, et al. Leukocyte counts in hypertonic saline-induced sputum in subjects with occupational asthma. *Respir Med* 1998; 92(3):550–557.

130. Chmelik F, doPico G, Reed CE, Dickie H. Farmer's lung. *J Allergy Clin Immunol* 1974; 54(3):180–188.
131. Akira M. High-resolution CT in the evaluation of occupational and environmental disease. *Radiol Clin North Am* 2002; 40(1):43–59.
132. Selman M. Hypersensitivity pneumonitis: a multifaceted deceiving disorder. *Clin Chest Med* 2004; 25(3):531–547, vi.
133. Yoshizawa Y, Ohtani Y, Hayakawa H, Sato A, Suga M, Ando M. Chronic hypersensitivity pneumonitis in Japan: a nationwide epidemiologic survey. *J Allergy Clin Immunol* 1999; 103(2 Pt. 1):315–320.
134. Grubek-Jaworska H, Hoser G, Droszcz P, Chazan R. CD4/CD8 lymphocytes in BALF during the efferent phase of lung delayed-type hypersensitivity reaction induced by single antigen inhalation. *Med Sci Monit* 2001; 7(5):878–883.
135. Popper HH. Which biopsies in diffuse infiltrative lung diseases and when are these necessary? *Monaldi Arch Chest Dis* 2001; 56(5):446–452.
136. Gawkrodger DJ. Patch testing in occupational dermatology. *Occup Environ Med* 2001; 58(12):823–828.
137. Adams RM. *Occupational Skin Disease*, 3rd edn. Philadelphia, PA: W.B. Saunders Co, 1999.
138. Rietschel RL, Fowler JF Jr. *Fisher's Contact Dermatitis*, 5th edn. Lippincott, Williams & Wilkins, 2000.
139. Marks JG Jr, DeLeo VA. Occupational skin disease. In: Marks JG Jr, Elsner P, DeLeo VA (eds), *Contact and Occupational Dermatology*, 3rd edn. St. Louis, MO: Mosby-Year Book, 2002; pp. 239–303.
140. Beltrani VS, Bernstein IL, Cohen DE, Fonacier L. Contact dermatitis: a practice parameter. *Ann Allergy Asthma Immunol* 2006; 97:S1–S38.
141. Burge PS, O'Brien I, Harries M. Peak flow rate records in the diagnosis of occupational asthma due to isocyanates. *Thorax* 1979; 34(3):317–323.
142. Côté J, Kennedy S, Chan-Yeung M. Sensitivity and specificity of PC20 and peak expiratory flow rate in cedar asthma. *J Allergy Clin Immunol* 1990; 85(3):592–598.
143. Perrin B, Lagier F, L'Archeveque J, et al. Occupational asthma: validity of monitoring of peak expiratory flow rates and non-allergic bronchial responsiveness as compared to specific inhalation challenge. *Eur Respir J* 1992; 5(1):40–48.
144. Malo JL, Trudeau C, Ghezzo H, L'Archeveque J, Cartier A. Do subjects investigated for occupational asthma through serial peak expiratory flow measurements falsify their results. *J Allergy Clin Immunol* 1995; 96(5 Pt. 1):601–607.
145. Quirce S, Contreras G, Dybuncio A, Chan-Yeung M. Peak expiratory flow monitoring is not a reliable method for establishing the diagnosis of occupational asthma. *Am J Respir Crit Care Med* 1995; 152(3):1100–1102.
146. Leroyer C, Perfetti L, Trudeau C, L'Archeveque J, Chan-Yeung M, Malo JL. Comparison of serial monitoring of peak expiratory flow and FEV1 in the diagnosis of occupational asthma. *Am J Respir Crit Care Med* 1998; 158(3):827–832.
147. Moscato G, Godnic-Cvar J, Maestrelli P. Statement on self-monitoring of peak expiratory flows in the investigation of occupational asthma. Subcommittee on Occupational Allergy of European Academy of Allergy and Clinical Immunology. *J Allergy Clin Immunol* 1995; 96(3):295–301.
148. Anees W. Use of pulmonary function tests in the diagnosis of occupational asthma. *Ann Allergy Asthma Immunol* 2003; 90(5 Suppl. 2):47–51.
149. Burge PS, Moscato G, Johnson A, Chan-Yeung M. Physiological assessment: serial measurements of lung function and bronchial responsiveness. In: Bernstein IL, Chan-Yeung M, Malo JL, Bernstein DI (eds), *Asthma in the Workplace and Related Conditions*. New York: Taylor & Francis Group, 2006; pp. 199–226.
150. Tarlo SM, Boulet LP, Cartier A, et al. Canadian Thoracic Society. Guidelines for occupational asthma. *Can Respir J* 1998; 5(4):289–300.
151. Cartier A, Bernstein IL, Burge PS, et al. Guidelines for bronchoprovocation on the investigation of occupational asthma. Report of the Subcommittee on Bronchoprovocation for Occupational Asthma. *J Allergy Clin Immunol* 1989; 84(5 Pt. 2):823–829.
152. Bérubé D, Cartier A, L'Archeveque J, Ghezzo H, Malo JL. Comparison of peak expiratory flow rate and FEV1 in assessing bronchomotor tone after challenges with occupational sensitizers. *Chest* 1991; 99:831–836.
153. Weytjens K, Malo JL, Cartier A, Ghezzo H, Delwiche JP, Vandenplas O. Comparison of peak expiratory flows and FEV1 in assessing immediate asthmatic reactions due to occupational agents. *Allergy* 1999; 54(6):621–625.
154. Perrin B, Cartier A, Ghezzo H, et al. Reassessment of the temporal patterns of bronchial obstruction after exposure to occupational sensitizing agents. *J Allergy Clin Immunol* 1991; 87:630–639.
155. Davies R, Green M, Schoefield N. Recurrent nocturnal asthma after exposure to grain dust. *Am Rev Respir Dis* 1976; 114:1011–1019.
156. Cockcroft DW, Hoeppner VH, Werner GD. Recurrent nocturnal asthma after bronchoprovocation with Western Red Cedar sawdust: association with acute increase in non-allergic bronchial responsiveness. *Clin Allergy* 1984; 14:61–68.
157. Hytonen ML, Sala EL, Malmberg HO, Nordman H. Acoustic rhinometry in the diagnosis of occupational rhinitis. *Am J Rhinol* 1996; 10:393–397.
158. Uzzaman A, Metcalfe DD, Komarow HD. Acoustic rhinometry in the practice of allergy. *Ann Allergy Asthma Immunol* 2006; 97(6):745–751.
159. Bourke SJ, Dalphin JC, Boyd G, McSharry C, Baldwin CI, Calvert JE. Hypersensitivity pneumonitis: current concepts. *Eur Respir J Suppl* 2001; 32:81s–92s.
160. Ameille J, Descatha A. Outcome of occupational asthma. *Curr Opin Allergy Clin Immunol* 2005; 5(2):125–128.
161. Becklake MR, Malo JL, Chan-Yeung M. Epidemiological approaches in occupational asthma. In: Bernstein IL, Chan-Yeung M, Malo JL, Bernstein DI (eds), *Asthma in the Workplace and Related Conditions*. New York: Taylor & Francis Group, 2006; pp. 37–86.
162. Hudson P, Cartier A, Pineau L, et al. Follow-up of occupational asthma caused by crab and various agents. *J Allergy Clin Immunol* 1985; 76:682–688.
163. Malo JL, Cartier A, Ghezzo H, Lafrance M, McCants M, Lehrer SB. Patterns of improvement in spirometry, bronchial

hyperresponsiveness, and specific IgE antibody levels after cessation of exposure in occupational asthma caused by snow-crab processing. *Am Rev Respir Dis* 1988; 138(4):807–812.

164. Côté J, Kennedy S, Chan-Yeung M. Outcome of patients with cedar asthma with continuous exposure. *Am Rev Respir Dis* 1990; 141:373–376.
165. Lemière C, Cartier A, Malo JL, Lehrer SB. Persistent specific bronchial reactivity to occupational agents in workers with normal nonspecific bronchial reactivity. *Am J Respir Crit Care Med* 2000; 162(3):976–980.
166. Dewitte JD, Chan-Yeung M, Malo JL. Medicolegal and compensation aspects of occupational asthma. *Eur Respir J* 1994; 7(5):969–980.
167. Gassert TH, Hu H, Kelsey KT, Christiani DC. Long-term health and employment outcomes of occupational asthma and their determinants. *J Occup Environ Med* 1998; 40(5):481–491.
168. Piirila PL, Keskinen HM, Luukkonen R, Salo SP, Tuppurainen M, Nordman H. Work, unemployment and life satisfaction among patients with diisocyanate induced asthma—a prospective study. *J Occup Health* 2005; 47(2):112–118.
169. Malo JL, Boulet LP, Dewitte JD, et al. Quality of life of subjects with occupational asthma. *J Allergy Clin Immunol* 1993; 91:1121–1127.
170. Miedinger D, Lavoie KL, L'Archeveque J, Ghezzo H, Zunzunuegui MV, Malo JL. Quality-of-life, psychological, and cost outcomes 2 years after diagnosis of occupational asthma. *J Occup Environ Med* 2011; 53(3):231–238.
171. Leigh JP, Romano PS, Schenker MB, Kreiss K. Costs of occupational COPD and asthma. *Chest* 2002; 121(1):264–272.
172. Moscato G, Dellabianca A, Perfetti L, et al. Occupational asthma: a longitudinal study on the clinical and socioeconomic outcome after diagnosis. *Chest* 1999; 115(1):249–256.
173. Groenewoud GC, de GH, Van Wijk RG. Impact of occupational and inhalant allergy on rhinitis-specific quality of life in employees of bell pepper greenhouses in the Netherlands. *Ann Allergy Asthma Immunol* 2006; 96(1):92–97.
174. Braun SR, doPico GA, Tsiatis A, Horvath E, Dickie HA, Rankin J. Farmer's lung disease: long-term clinical and physiologic outcome. *Am Rev Respir Dis* 1979; 119(2):185–191.
175. Zacharisen MC, Schlueter DP, Kurup VP, Fink JN. The long-term outcome in acute, subacute, and chronic forms of pigeon breeder's disease hypersensitivity pneumonitis. *Ann Allergy Asthma Immunol* 2002; 88(2):175–182.
176. Tarlo SM, Liss GM. Prevention of occupational asthma—practical implications for occupational physicians. *Occup Med (Lond)* 2005; 55(8):588–594.
177. Baur X. Are we closer to developing threshold limit values for allergens in the workplace? *Ann Allergy Asthma Immunol* 2003; 90(5 Suppl. 2):11–18.
178. Hendrick DJ. Management of occupational asthma. *Eur Respir J* 1994; 7(5):961–968.
179. Nicholson PJ, Newman Taylor AJ, Oliver P, Cathcart M. Current best practice for the health surveillance of enzyme workers in the soap and detergent industry. *Occup Med (Lond)* 2001; 51(2):81–92.
180. Sarlo K. Control of occupational asthma and allergy in the detergent industry. *Ann Allergy Asthma Immunol* 2003; 90(5 Suppl. 2):32–34.
181. Karjalainen A, Martikainen R, Klaukka T, Saarinen K, Uitti J. Risk of asthma among Finnish patients with occupational rhinitis. *Chest* 2003; 123(1):283–288.
182. Orriols R, Aliaga JL, Anto JM, et al. High prevalence of mollusc shell hypersensitivity pneumonitis in nacre factory workers. *Eur Respir J* 1997; 10(4):780–786.
183. Kokkarinen JI, Tukiainen HO, Terho EO. Effect of corticosteroid treatment on the recovery of pulmonary function in farmer's lung. *Am Rev Respir Dis* 1992; 145(1):3–5.
184. Bernstein JA, Bernstein IL, Bucchini L, et al. Clinical and laboratory investigation of allergy to genetically modified foods. *Environ Health Perspect* 2003; 111(8):1114–1121.

3 Adverse Reactions to Foods: Diagnosis

20 IgE Tests: *In Vitro* Diagnosis

Kirsten Beyer
Charité Universitätsmedizin Berlin, Klinik für Pädiatrie m.S. Pneumologie und Immunologie, Berlin, Germany

Key Concepts

- The presence of food allergen-specific IgE determines the sensitization to a specific food. Sensitization can, but may not result in clinical reactions.
- The level of food allergen-specific IgE correlates with the likelihood of clinical reactivity for several foods, such as peanut, cow's milk, hen's egg, and fish. Therefore, quantitative measurement of food allergen-specific IgE can be used to obtain diagnostic decision points that help to reduce the requirement of an oral food challenge test. However, these diagnostic decision points are population, age, and disease specific.
- For some food allergens, such as peanut and wheat, measurement of specific IgE to individual food allergens (components) and not crude allergen extracts appears to be superior. Cross-reactivity between different food allergens needs to be taken into account.
- Food allergy is a dynamic process with the majority of children becoming tolerant over time; monitoring food allergen-specific IgE seems helpful in predicting the likelihood of oral tolerance development.
- Measurement of specific IgE antibodies to allergenic peptides seems to enable the prediction of the natural course of the disease.

Introduction

The majority of food-allergic reactions are IgE mediated [1]. Therefore, in addition to patient history, the diagnostic workup of suspected food allergy should include the detection of IgE antibody responses *in vivo* and/or *in vitro* [2]. However, the presence of food allergen-specific IgE does not always correlate with clinical reactivity. Generally, *in vitro* methods have the advantage of being safe, and drug interference (e.g., antihistamines) does not play a role. In the past several years, technological advances have provided new laboratory tools for the quantitation of allergen-specific IgE antibodies in serum [3]. Today, automated and quantitative allergen-specific IgE assays are available and open to improved diagnostic methods. In addition to the measurement of IgE antibodies to crude food allergen extracts, detailed analyses of sensitization profiles to individual allergens and allergenic peptides are possible. This concept has been defined as "component-resolved diagnostics" [4]. Moreover, microarray techniques have been adapted in which purified native and recombinant allergens, as well as allergenic peptides, are spotted onto surface-modified glass slides to permit extensive panels of specific IgE measurements to be performed on small quantities of patient serum. Although the double-blind, placebo-controlled food challenge (DBPCFC) still remains the gold standard in food allergy diagnosis, the procedure is time consuming, costly, and places a great deal of stress on the patient. Therefore, *in vitro* tests for prediction of the outcome of oral food challenge tests and the persistence of the food-allergic disorders are under development. The latter is especially important to children who would benefit from specific immunotherapy for food allergy when it is available in the future.

Common diagnostic test methods for the quantitative measurement of food allergen-specific IgE

Common concepts

Over the past decades, the methods of IgE detection have improved drastically. From the first-generation IgE antibody assays that were only semiquantitative and labor

Food Allergy: Adverse Reactions to Foods and Food Additives, Fifth Edition. Edited by Dean D Metcalfe, Hugh A Sampson, Ronald A Simon and Gideon Lack.

intensive to today's quantitative and automated allergen-specific IgE assays, there are several assay methods on the market for the detection of food allergen-specific IgE [3]. Generally, these assays use a liquid or solid phase to capture the allergenic component. Commonly, these allergenic components are allergen extracts of a complex nature and contain allergenic and nonallergenic molecules. Three of the most commonly used systems are the Phadia ImmunoCAP System (Thermo Fisher Scientific, Uppsala, Sweden), HYCOR Ultra-Sensitive EIA (Agilent Technologies) and the Immulite System (Siemens Healthcare Diagnostics). A recent evaluation of these three methods showed that all three allergen-specific IgE assays displayed excellent analytic sensitivity, precision, reproducibility, and linearity [5]. However, the different systems offer different units that are not comparable with one another, thus making direct comparison of results for the physician difficult [6].

Interpretation of food allergen-specific IgE

Food allergen-specific IgE concentrations in the serum have been correlated with patient histories and the outcome of oral food challenge tests to generate probability curves that depict the likelihood of patients with a particular food allergen-specific IgE level reacting to the food. In the same way, several groups have described diagnostic decision points for food allergen-specific serum IgE concentration for several foods (Table 20.1) such as, peanut, hen's egg, cow's milk, and fish [7–10, 12–16]. These diagnostic decision points are meant to reduce the requirement for oral food challenge tests. In most of these publications about diagnostic decision points for food allergy, the Phadia CAP System was used. Recently, an extension of food allergen-specific IgE ranges from the ImmunoCAP to the IMMULITE systems has been published [17]. The results are showing that IgE antibody levels to hen's egg, cow's milk, and peanut from both assays for each of the three food specificities were highly correlated [17]. For milk and peanut, the IgE antibody levels for individuals who either passed or failed a food challenge were not significantly different between the assay methods; however, the numbers of patients studied were small. Because the small sample size of egg white-challenged patients was even too small, no statistical analysis was performed [17]. However, an earlier study failed to show a similar high correlation between the various systems [6].

Moreover, it has been observed that the diagnostic decision points varied among the different study populations [18]. Moreover, they appear to be age dependent [8] and might be different in regard to the presence of atopic dermatitis. Importantly, patients with food allergen-specific IgE levels in the undefined area need to undergo an oral food challenge test. Owing to the lack of strong correlation between the food allergen-specific IgE levels and the clinical reactivity of the patients, diagnostic decision points for some foods, such as wheat and soy, could not be established. It appears that the crude allergen extracts used in the tests are not optimal.

Hen's egg

Sampson et al. determined the potential utility of the CAP System fluorescent-enzyme immunoassay (FEIA) in the diagnosis of IgE-mediated food hypersensitivity. In this retrospective analysis of 196 children and adolescents with atopic dermatitis and food allergy, food-specific IgE concentrations were established that could predict clinical reactivity to various food allergens with 95% certainty [19]. One hundred and twenty-three of these children suffered from hen's egg allergy. For hen's egg, a diagnostic level of IgE, which could predict clinical reactivity in this population with 95% certainty, was identified as 6 kU_A/L. The 90% specificity value was 7 kU_A/L.

To determine the utility of these 95% predictive decision points in the evaluation of food allergy, a study was carried out 4 years later [7]. Sera from 100 children and adolescents referred for evaluation of food allergy were analyzed

Table 20.1 Proposed diagnostic decision points for various foods and age groups.

Allergen	Age group	Population	Food-specific IgE	PPV	Reference
Hen's egg	Children and adolescence	USA	7 kU_A/L	98	[7]
	Children and adolescence	German	13 kU_A/L	95	[8]
	<2 years	Spain	0.35 kU_A/L	94	[9]
	<1 year	German	11 kU_A/L	95	[8]
Cow's milk	Children and adolescence	USA	15 kU_A/L	95	[7]
	Children and adolescence	German	–	95	[8]
	<1 year	Spain	5 kU_A/L	95	[10]
Peanut	Children and adolescence	US	14 kU_A/L	100	[7]
	Children and adolescence	UK	15 kU_A/L	92	[11]
	Children and adolescence	France	57 kU_A/L	100	[9]

PPV, positive predictive value.

for food-specific IgE antibodies by using the Phadia CAP System FEIA. Of these children, 75 had hen's egg allergy, one-third of them were diagnosed through DBPCFC, and two-thirds by patient's history. Hen's egg-specific IgE values were compared with history and food challenges to determine the efficacy of previously established decision points in identifying patients with increased probability of clinical reactivity. On the basis of the previously established 95% predictive decision points and the 90% specificity value for hen's egg, 95% of food allergies diagnosed in this prospective study were correctly identified by quantifying serum hen's egg-specific IgE concentrations.

Using the same IgE detection method, a similar study was carried out later among a German population. In this study, 227 children underwent an oral food challenge test with hen's egg. The 95% decision point among this German population with 13.0 kU_A/L was similar to the one in the United States, thus confirming the results in a large number of children [8]. In addition, age differences have been observed with lower diagnostic decision points in children younger than 1 year of 11.0 kU_A/L. Another study by the same group showed that the proposed cutoff level of 12 kU_A/L IgE would identify children above this level correctly as hen's egg allergic [20]. Moreover, it was shown that the level of hen's egg-specific IgG or IgG4 did not add any additional information in the diagnostic procedure of hen's egg allergy [20]. Similarly, Boyano et al. performed a prospective study among 81 children younger than 2 years with suspected egg allergy. Specific IgE antibodies were quantified using the Phadia CAP System. The group found that a level of >0.35 kU_A/L for specific IgE antibodies to egg white predicted the existence of reaction in 94% of the cases [13], giving a much lower level of specific antibodies than reported in other studies.

Cow's milk

Diagnostic decision points for cow's milk have been described by several authors. In most of these publications, the Phadia CAP System was used. In parallel with their studies on hen's egg allergy, Sampson et al. retrospectively studied 106 children and adolescents with atopic dermatitis and cow's milk allergy [19]. For cow's milk, a diagnostic level of IgE, which could predict clinical reactivity in this population with .95% certainty, was identified as 32 kU_A/L. The 90% specificity value was 15 kU_A/L. Four years later in their study, to determine the utility of this 95% predictive decision points in a prospective evaluation of food allergy [5], sera from 62 children and adolescents with cow's milk allergy were investigated. One-third of the patients with cow's milk allergy were diagnosed through DBPCFC and two-thirds by patient's history. On the basis of the previously established 95% predictive decision points and the 90% specificity value for cow's milk, 95% of food allergies diagnosed in this prospective study were correctly identified by quantifying serum cow's milk-specific IgE concentrations.

Similar to hen's egg, age-specific difference appears to occur. In a prospective study carried out in Spain on 170 patients younger than 1 year, different cutoff points of the specific IgE for cow's milk were analyzed [10]. The group concluded that 2.5 and 5 kU_A/L had a positive predictive value (PPV) of 90% and 95%, respectively. Later, another study was carried out among a German population using the Phadia CAP System. In this study, 398 children underwent the oral food challenge test with cow's milk [8]. A correlation between the challenge outcome and the cow's milk-specific IgE levels has been observed; however, in contrast to the populations of Spain and the United States, a 95% diagnostic decision could not be established. The 90% predicted probability gave a much higher value of 89 kU_A/L than observed in other studies. However, age differences have also been observed with lower diagnostic decision points of 26 kU_A/L in children younger than 1 year.

A study from Spain compared the clinical performance of the Immulite 2000 in the diagnosis of cow's milk allergy with that of UniCAP [21]. The authors concluded that both methods were similarly effective in diagnosing cow's milk allergy; however, cutoff levels chosen for the Immulite had to be higher than that for the UniCAP. Similar results were observed in another recent study from the United States [17]. The usage of the cow's milk-specific IgE in the diagnosis of cow's milk allergy depends also on the clinical setting that is available [22].

Peanut

For peanut allergy, diagnostic levels of IgE, which could predict clinical reactivity in a US population with 95% certainty, were identified as 15 kU_A/L [7, 19]. These data were confirmed a little later in a UK study that observed 136 children undergoing peanut challenges. The authors found that a peanut-specific IgE >15 kU_A/L had a predictive value of 92% for a positive challenge [11]. Rance studied 363 children in France. According to DBPCFC results, 177 children were allergic to peanut and 186 were not. The authors found that the specific IgE concentrations of 57 kU_A/L or greater were associated with a PPV of 100% [9]. A publication from Australia showed recently that by using the previously published 95% PPV of 15 kU_A/L for peanut-specific IgE, a corresponding specificity of 98% was found in their study cohort of 200 randomly selected infants [23].

Tree nuts

To date, not many studies have focused on the determination of diagnostic decision points for tree nut allergy. In one study, the 95% predicted probability for walnut-specific IgE was found to be 18.5 kU_A/L. The usage of this decision point gave a specificity of 98% but a sensitivity of only 17%. The positive and negative predictive values (NPV) were 99% and 56%, respectively [24]. Similarly, Ridout et al. studied 56 patients with the focus on Brazil nut allergy. Of these patients, 43% were diagnosed based on their history, whereas the remaining patients were challenged. The authors concluded from their data that a serum-specific IgE to Brazil nut of 3.5 kU_A/L may require an oral challenge to determine the risk of a Brazil nut-allergic reaction [25]. Most recently, a study on the diagnostic value of hazelnut allergy tests were performed to analyze data of 151 children who underwent DBPCFC for hazelnut [26]. One of the methods used was the ImmunCAP (Thermo Fisher Diagnostics). Some years ago this commercial hazelnut CAP with the crude allergen extracts had been supplemented with Cor a 1. The authors stated that in general the specific IgE of $\geq$0.35 kU_A/L for hazelnut was a moderate predictor for hazelnut allergy. The supplementation of Cor a 1 decreased the PPV from 41% to 38% and increased the NPV from 91% to 100% for sIgE of $\geq$0.35 kU_A/L. The maximum reached PPV was 73% for sIgE cutoff of 26 kU_A/L [26].

Wheat

The performance characteristics of the CAP System FEIA for wheat appears to be poor [7, 16, 19]. No correlation between the outcome of oral food challenges and the level of wheat-specific serum IgE has been observed [8]. A diagnostic decision point could not be established. This suggests that the allergen extracts used in the tests are not optimal for diagnosis of wheat allergy. Not only IgE to the water-/salt-soluble fraction of wheat, but also IgE antibodies to the water-insoluble fractions appear to play a role in wheat allergy [27]. The common measurements, however, are using the water-/salt-soluble fractions.

Soy

Similar to wheat allergy, the performance characteristics of the CAP System FEIA for soy were poor [7, 16, 19]. Diagnostic decision points could not be established [8].

Fish

For fish allergy, a diagnostic level of IgE that can predict clinical reactivity in a U S population with 95% certainty was identified as 20 kU_A/L [7,19]. The major allergens are parvalbumins [28]. However, the problem of serological and clinical cross-reactivity between different fish species has not yet been solved.

Measurement of food-specific IgE over time

There are still conflicting views on whether the initial level of serum food-specific IgE and the changes over time predict the development of clinical tolerance [18, 29, 30–32]. Niggemann et al. concluded from their study of 74 children with atopic dermatitis and various food allergies that specific IgE in serum, although very helpful at the time of first diagnosis, cannot predict whether a child becomes tolerant after a period of avoidance [32]. In contrast, Vanto et al. prospectively studied 95 infants with immediate reactions and 67 with delayed reactions (up to the age of 4 years) to cow's milk [31]. Cow's milk allergy was assessed annually by cow's milk challenges. They were able to show that milk-specific IgE in the serum in children with persistent food allergies appears to have higher levels of milk-specific IgE antibodies initially and are useful prognostic indicators of the development of tolerance to cow's milk in infants with cow's milk allergy. Moreover, recent data showed a relationship between the decrease in food allergen-specific IgE levels, over a specific time period between two challenges, and the development of tolerance [29]. A greater decrease in specific IgE levels over a shorter period of time indicated a greater likelihood of tolerance development. Use of these likelihood estimates could aid clinicians in the prognosis of food allergy and in timing of subsequent food challenges, thereby decreasing the number of premature and unnecessary food challenges.

Total IgE

Considering that food allergy is often the beginning of an "allergic march" and is associated with other atopic diseases in many cases, one must take the total IgE into account and should interpret specific IgE levels differently in patients with high total IgE levels compared to those with low levels [33]. This may be especially true for children with atopic dermatitis, who frequently show very high total IgE levels and sensitivity to numerous allergens, often without clinical relevance. However, it was recently shown that the additional determination of total IgE in food allergy is of no advantage. Mehl et al. analyzed 992 controlled oral food challenges performed among 501 children and evaluated the utility of the ratio of specific IgE/total IgE compared with specific IgE alone in diagnosing symptomatic food allergy. There was no benefit for the additional determination of total IgE compared with specific IgE alone for cow's milk, hen's egg, wheat, or soy [33].

Component-resolved diagnosis with individual food allergens and allergenic peptides

Common concepts

Currently, most diagnostic tests for measurement of food allergen-specific IgE are based on allergen extracts containing a mixture of allergenic and nonallergenic molecules.

Through recent advances in proteomics, identification of new allergens for several foods can be performed. Allergen panels from various sources are now available, and detailed analyses of sensitization profiles in individual patients are possible. This concept has been defined as "component-resolved diagnostics" [4]. The various allergenic components such as the individual allergens from peanut (e.g., Ara h 1, Ara h 2, Ara h 3, and Ara h 8) can be measured in a similar way as the crude allergen extracts using quantitative platforms (e.g., Phadia ImmunoCAP). Simultaneous measurement of hundreds of allergens is possible using microarray-based systems (e.g., Phadia ImmunoCAP ISAC) (see section Protein microarray). However, up to now, these systems provide only semiquantitative results. Observations indicate that molecular analysis of allergen sensitization patterns may serve to enhance the prognostic power of IgE antibody-based allergy diagnostics. Some of the most important findings in regard to peanut, tree nut, cow's milk, hens' egg, and wheat allergy are described below.

Protein microarray

The latest technology trend is toward microarrays, where crude or purified native and recombinant allergens can be spotted in microdot arrays on silica chips or surface-modified glass slides to permit extensive panels of specific IgE measurements to be performed with small quantities of serum [3]. A rapid development in the area of protein microarray technology has occurred [34]. In one of the first studies, Hiller et al. printed 94 purified or recombinant aero- and food-allergens on surface-modified glass slides and reacted them with individual sera from 20 patients. The performance of the allergen microarray was assessed in regard to reproducibility and correlation with skin prick testing or recognition of allergens spotted onto nitrocellulose under conditions of allergen excess. The authors concluded from their study that the allergen microarray allows the determination and monitoring of allergic patients' IgE reactivity profiles to large numbers of disease-causing allergens by using single measurements and minute amounts of serum. This method may change the established practice in allergy diagnosis, prevention, and therapy [35].

Similarly, Kim et al. evaluated the usage of protein microarray [36]. House dust mite, egg white, milk, soybean, and wheat were used as allergens, and human serum albumin as negative control. Sensitivity and clinical efficacy of the protein chip were evaluated. Comparisons between microarray-based immunoassays and the Phadia CAP System showed a good correlation for food- and aero-allergens [36].

Microarray assays have several advantages when compared with the currently used *in vitro* determination of IgE. The test can screen hundreds of allergens in parallel with the requirement of only minute amounts of serum. Therefore, the test is attractive especially among pediatric patients. Moreover, microarray assays require much less allergen than currently used in *in vitro* tests. This is important for the use of individual purified or recombinant allergens that are usually more expensive and difficult to obtain. Although these technologies hold promise, their diagnostic performance requires further assessment once their technical details have been optimized. Potential abuses of this newer IgE antibody technology include the use of allergosorbent specificities that lack validation [3].

Measurement of peptide-specific IgE

IgE-binding epitopes have been identified for numerous food allergens including allergens in peanut [37–39], cow's milk [40–43], hen's egg [44–47], wheat [48, 49], soy [50], tree nuts [51], fish [52], and shellfish [53, 54]. However, their importance in the clinical course of allergic diseases or their roles in cross-reactivity are still not well understood. Generally, *in vitro* cross-reactivity in IgE-binding assays does not correlate well with clinical significance, and currently there is no tool on hand to predict whether a Brazil nut-allergic patient would also react to cashew nut.

In cow's milk allergy, differences in the epitope recognition patterns have been observed between younger children, who are likely to outgrow their allergy, and older patients with persistent cow's milk allergy, which suggested that epitope specificity of IgE antibody responses might predict the clinical outcome of cow's milk allergy [42]. Using SPOTs-membrane technology and sera from 10 patients with persistent and 10 patients with transient cow's milk allergy, "informative" IgE-binding epitopes have been identified that were not recognized by any of the patients with transient cow's milk allergy, but showed binding by most of the patients with persistent allergy [55]. Recently, a larger study of 74 patients with challenge-proven cow's milk allergy confirmed that the presence of IgE antibodies to distinct allergenic epitopes of cow's milk proteins can be used as a marker of persistent cow's milk allergy [56]. Importantly, the peptides used were linked to the matrix of a commercial system for IgE measurement. Similar to cow's milk allergy, measurement of peptide-specific IgE seems to be a valuable parameter in predicting the clinical reactivity in peanut allergy [57]. Until recently, epitope analysis was carried out with protein digests or SPOTs membrane-based immunoassays. These methods are time consuming and require large quantities of patient sera. Therefore, similar to protein microarrays, peptide microarrays have been developed recently for the analysis of IgE-binding epitopes [58, 59]. Using this newly developed method, Shreffler et al. showed that qualitative difference in epitope diversity might provide prognostic information about food-allergic patient [59].

Interpretation of specific IgE to individual components and allergenic peptides

Egg

A recent review showed that molecular diagnosis of hen's egg allergy is promising as measurement of specific IgE antibodies to individual egg white components seems to predict different clinical patterns of egg allergy [60]. Specific IgE to ovomucoid has been identified as a risk factor for persistent allergy and could indicate reactivity to extensively heated (baked) egg. Ovomucoid- and ovalbumin-IgE-binding epitope profiling could also help distinguish different clinical phenotypes of egg allergy. Particularly, egg-allergic patients with IgE antibodies reacting against sequential epitopes tend to have more persistent allergy. However, despite the fact that molecular-based technologies are showing promising results, none of these tests is ready to be used in clinical practice and oral food challenge remains the standard for the diagnosis of egg allergy [60].

Milk

In contrast to hen's egg allergy, a recent review on molecular diagnosis of cow's milk allergy concluded that molecular methods of diagnosis do not afford greater precision than specific IgE determinations performed so far [61]. The problem is that component recognition pattern heterogeneity is observed in different areas. Therefore, further clinical studies seem to be essential to correlate useful molecular diagnostics and biological markers with disease and patient profiles. The authors concluded that oral food challenge remains the reference standard for the diagnosis of cow's milk allergy until such markers are found and validated in different age groups [61].

Peanut and tree nuts

Component-resolved diagnostics seem very promising in the diagnosis of peanut allergy. In a recent study by Nicoplaou et al., marked differences in the pattern of component recognition between children with peanut allergy and peanut-tolerant children were detected using component-resolved diagnostics [62]. The peanut component Ara h 2 which is a 2S albumin belonging to the seed storage protein family was the most important predictor of clinical allergy. Similar results were observed by Codreanu et al. comparing 166 patients with peanut allergy and 61 pollen-sensitized subjects without peanut allergy [63]. In another study from Australia by Dang et al., these results have been confirmed recently in 200 infants [23]. These studies from the United Kingdom, France, and Australia suggest that detection of Ara h 2-specific IgE may accurately discriminate peanut-allergic patients from tolerant individuals. However, as recently highlighted in a review, the pattern of allergenic component recognition in peanut-sensitized patients from different populations or geographical areas varies, reflecting different pollen and dietary exposures [64]. In the United States, peanut-allergic patients are commonly sensitized to Ara h 1–3, in Spain to Ara h 9, and in Sweden to Ara h 8 [64, 65]. Similar results, as those seen with peanut allergy, were found in Brazil nut allergy, where sensitization to Ber e 1, which is a 2S albumin belonging to the seed storage protein family, was seen to correlate with the clinical expression of the allergy [66].

Similar to the measurement of specific IgE to individual peanut allergens, measurement of peptide-specific IgE seems to be a valuable parameter in predicting the clinical reactivity in peanut allergy [67]. A most recent study developed a novel diagnostic approach that could predict peanut allergy with high accuracy by combining the results of a peptide-microarray immunoassay and bioinformatic methods [68]. In this study, it has been shown that individuals with peanut allergy had significantly greater IgE binding and broader epitope diversity than did peanut-tolerant individuals. By using machine learning methods, four peptide biomarkers were identified and prediction models were developed that can predict the outcome of DBPCFC with high accuracy by using a combination of the biomarkers.

Wheat

For wheat allergy, measurement of specific IgE to individual wheat allergens appears to be diagnostically superior to measuring whole wheat extract [69–71]. The fact that wheat allergen w-5 gliadin correlates well with oral challenge results, as shown recently [69], also points in this direction.

Food allergen-specific IgE and the atopic march

Food allergy is one of the first manifestations of the "atopic march," as many of these children will develop asthma and allergic rhinitis later in life. It has been shown that early sensitization to hen's egg is a valuable marker for subsequent allergic sensitization to allergens that cause asthma and allergic rhinitis later in life [72].

References

1. Niggemann B, Reibel S, Roehr CC, et al. Predictors of positive food challenge outcome in non-IgE-mediated reactions to food in children with atopic dermatitis. *J Allergy Clin Immunol* 2001; 108:1053–1058.

2. Eigenmann PA, Oh JW, Beyer K. Diagnostic testing in the evaluation of food allergy. *Pediatr Clin North Am* 2011; 58(2):351–362, ix.
3. Hamilton RG, Adkinson NF. In vitro assays for the diagnosis of IgE-mediated disorders. *J Allergy Clin Immunol* 2004; 114:213–225.
4. Lidholm J, Ballmer-Weber B, Mari A, Vieths S. Component-resolved diagnostics in food allergy. *Curr Opin Allergy Clin Immunol* 2006; 6:234–240.
5. Hamilton RG. Proficiency survey-based evaluation of clinical total and allergen-specific IgE assay performance. *Arch Pathol Lab Med* 2010; 134(7):975–982.
6. Wang J, Godbold JH, Sampson HA. Correlation of serum allergy (IgE) tests performed by different assay systems. *J Allergy Clin Immunol* 2008; 121:1219–1224.
7. Sampson HA. Utility of food-specific IgE concentrations in predicting symptomatic food allergy. *J Allergy Clin Immunol* 2001; 107:891–896.
8. Celik-Bilgili S, Mehl A, Verstege A, et al. The predictive value of specific immunoglobulin E levels in serum for the outcome of oral food challenges. *Clin Exp Allergy* 2005; 35:268–273.
9. Rance F, Abbal M, Lauwers-Cances V. Improved screening for peanut allergy by the combined use of skin prick tests and specific IgE assays. *J Allergy Clin Immunol* 2002; 109:1027–1033.
10. Garcia-Ara C, Boyano-Martinez T, Diaz-Pena JM, et al. Specific IgE levels in the diagnosis of immediate hypersensitivity to cows' milk protein in the infant. *J Allergy Clin Immunol* 2001; 107:185–190.
11. Roberts G, Lack G. Diagnosing peanut allergy with skin prick and specific IgE testing. *J Allergy Clin Immunol* 2005; 115:1291–1296.
12. Sporik R, Hill DJ, Hosking CS. Specificity of allergen skin testing in predicting positive open food challenges to milk, egg and peanut in children. *Clin Exp Allergy* 2000; 30:1540–1546.
13. Boyano MT, Garcia-Ara C, Diaz-Pena JM, et al. Validity of specific IgE antibodies in children with egg allergy. *Clin Exp Allergy* 2001; 31:1464–1469.
14. Hill DJ, Hosking CS, Reyes-Benito LV. Reducing the need for food allergen challenges in young children: a comparison of in vitro with in vivo tests. *Clin Exp Allergy* 2001; 31:1031–1035.
15. Sampson HA. Improving in-vitro tests for the diagnosis of food hypersensitivity. *Curr Opin Allergy Clin Immunol* 2002; 2:257–261.
16. Perry TT, Matsui EC, Conover-Walker MK, Wood RA. The relationship of allergen-specific IgE levels and oral food challenge outcome. *J Allergy Clin Immunol* 2004; 114:144–149.
17. Hamilton RG, Mudd K, White MA, Wood RA. Extension of food allergen specific IgE ranges from the ImmunoCAP to the IMMULITE systems. *Ann Allergy Asthma Immunol* 2011; 107(2):139–144.
18. Niggemann B, Rolinck-Werninghaus C, Mehl A, et al. Controlled oral food challenges in children—when indicated, when superfluous? *Allergy* 2005; 60:865–870.
19. Sampson HA, Ho DG. Relationship between food-specific IgE concentrations and the risk of positive food challenges in children and adolescents. *J Allergy Clin Immunol* 1997; 100:444–451.
20. Ahrens B, Lopes de Oliveira LC, Schulz G, et al. The role of hen's egg-specific IgE, IgG and IgG4 in the diagnostic procedure of hen's egg allergy. *Allergy* 2010; 65(12):1554–1557.
21. Prates S, Morais-Almeida M, Matos V, et al. In vitro methods for specific IgE detection in cow's milk allergy. *Allergol Immuno-pathol (Madr)* 2006; 34:27–31.
22. Fiocchi A, Schunemann HJ, Brozek J, et al. Diagnosis and Rationale for Action against Cow's Milk Allergy (DRACMA): a summary report. *J Allergy Clin Immunol* 2010; 126(6):1119–1128.
23. Dang TD, Tang M, Choo S, et al. Increasing the accuracy of peanut allergy diagnosis by using Ara h 2. *J Allergy Clin Immunol* 2012; 129(4):1056–1063.
24. Maloney JM, Rudengren M, Ahlstedt S, Bock SA, Sampson HA. The use of serum-specific IgE measurements for the diagnosis of peanut, tree nut, and seed allergy. *J Allergy Clin Immunol* 2008; 122(1):145–151.
25. Ridout S, Matthews S, Gant C, et al. The diagnosis of Brazil nut allergy using history, skin prick tests, serum-specific immunoglobulin E and food challenges. *Clin Exp Allergy* 2006; 36:226–232.
26. Masthoff LJ, Pasmans SG, van Hoffen E, et al. Diagnostic value of hazelnut allergy tests including rCor a 1 spiking in double-blind challenged children. *Allergy* 2012; 67(4):521–527.
27. Battais F, Richard C, Szustakowski G, et al. Wheat flour allergy: an entire diagnostic tool for complex allergy. *Allergy Immunol (Paris)* 2006; 38:59–61.
28. Wild LG, Lehrer SB. Fish and shellfish allergy. *Curr Allergy Asthma Rep* 2005; 5:74–79.
29. Shek LP, Beyer K, Jones M, Sampson HA. Determination of food-specific IgE levels over time can be used to predict the development of tolerance in cow's milk and hen's egg allergy. *J Allergy Clin Immunol* 2004; 114(2):387–391.
30. Boyano-Martinez T, Garcia-Ara C, Diaz-Pena JM, Martin-Esteban M. Prediction of tolerance on the basis of quantification of egg white-specific IgE antibodies in children with egg allergy. *J Allergy Clin Immunol* 2002; 110:304–309.
31. Vanto T, Helppila S, Juntunen-Backman K, et al. Prediction of the development of tolerance to milk in children with cow's milk hypersensitivity. *J Pediatr* 2004; 144:218–222.
32. Niggemann B, Celik-Bilgili S, Ziegert M, et al. Specific IgE levels do not indicate persistence or transience of food allergy in children with atopic dermatitis. *J Investig Allergol Clin Immunol* 2004; 14:98–103.
33. Mehl A, Verstege A, Staden U, et al. Utility of the ratio of food-specific IgE/total IgE in predicting symptomatic food allergy in children. *Allergy* 2005; 60:1034–1039.
34. Schweitzer B, Kingsmore SF. Measuring proteins on microarrays. *Curr Opin Biotechnol* 2002; 13:14–19.
35. Hiller R, Laffer S, Harwanegg C, et al. Microarrayed allergen molecules: diagnostic gatekeepers for allergy treatment. *FASEB J* 2002; 16:414–416.
36. Kim TE, Park SW, Cho NY, et al. Quantitative measurement of serum allergen-specific IgE on protein chip. *Exp Mol Med* 2002; 34:152–158.

37. Rabjohn P, Helm EM, Stanley JS, et al. Molecular cloning and epitope analysis of the peanut allergen Ara h 3. *J Clin Invest* 1999; 103:535–542.
38. Stanley JS, King N, Burks AW, et al. Identification and mutational analysis of the immunodominant IgE binding epitopes of the major peanut allergen Ara h 2. *Arch Biochem Biophys* 1997; 342:244–253.
39. Burks AW, Shin D, Cockrell G, et al. Mapping and mutational analysis of the IgE-binding epitopes on Ara h 1, a legume vicilin protein and a major allergen in peanut hypersensitivity. *Eur J Biochem* 1997; 245:334–339.
40. Busse PJ, Jarvinen KM, Vila L, et al. Identification of sequential IgE-binding epitopes on bovine alpha(s2)-casein in cow's milk allergic patients. *Int Arch Allergy Immunol* 2002; 129:93–96.
41. Jarvinen KM, Chatchatee P, Bardina L, et al. IgE and IgG binding epitopes on alpha-lactalbumin and beta-lactoglobulin in cow's milk allergy. *Int Arch Allergy Immunol* 2001; 126:111–118.
42. Chatchatee P, Jarvinen KM, Bardina L, et al. Identification of IgE and IgG binding epitopes on beta- and kappa-casein in cow's milk allergic patients. *Clin Exp Allergy* 2001; 31:1256–1262.
43. Chatchatee P, Jarvinen KM, Bardina L, et al. Identification of IgE- and IgG-binding epitopes on alpha(s1)-casein: differences in patients with persistent and transient cow's milk allergy. *J Allergy Clin Immunol* 2001; 107:379–383.
44. Mine Y, Rupa P. Fine mapping and structural analysis of immunodominant IgE allergenic epitopes in chicken egg ovalbumin. *Protein Eng* 2003; 16:747–752.
45. Mine Y, Wei ZJ. Identification and fine mapping of IgG and IgE epitopes in ovomucoid. *Biochem Biophys Res Commun* 2002; 292(4):1070–1074.
46. Zhang JW, Mine Y. Characterization of IgE and IgG epitopes on ovomucoid using egg-white-allergic patients' sera. *Biochem Biophys Res Commun* 1998; 253:124–127.
47. Honma K, Kohno Y, Saito K, et al. Allergenic epitopes of ovalbumin (OVA) in patients with hen's egg allergy: inhibition of basophil histamine release by haptenic ovalbumin peptide. *Clin Exp Immunol* 1996; 103:446–453.
48. Battais F, Mothes T, Moneret-Vautrin DA, et al. Identification of IgE-binding epitopes on gliadins for patients with food allergy to wheat. *Allergy* 2005; 60:815–821.
49. Matsuo H, Kohno K, Morita E. Molecular cloning, recombinant expression and IgE-binding epitope of omega-5 gliadin, a major allergen in wheat-dependent exercise-induced anaphylaxis. *FEBS J* 2005; 272:4431–4438.
50. Helm RM, Cockrell G, Connaughton C, et al. A soybean G2 glycinin allergen 2. Epitope mapping and three-dimensional modeling. *Int Arch Allergy Immunol* 2000; 123:213–219.
51. Robotham JM, Teuber SS, Sathe SK, Roux KH. Linear IgE epitope mapping of the English walnut (*Juglans regia*) major food allergen, Jug r 1. *J Allergy Clin Immunol* 2002; 109:143–149.
52. Untersmayr E, Szalai K, Riemer AB, et al. Mimotopes identify conformational epitopes on parvalbumin, the major fish allergen. *Mol Immunol* 2006; 43:1454–1461.
53. Ayuso R, Lehrer SB, Reese G. Identification of continuous, allergenic regions of the major shrimp allergen Pen a 1 (tropomyosin). *Int Arch Allergy Immunol* 2002; 127:27–37.
54. Reese G, Ayuso R, Carle T, Lehrer SB. IgE-binding epitopes of shrimp tropomyosin, the major allergen Pen a 1. *Int Arch Allergy Immunol* 1999; 118:300–301.
55. Jarvinen KM, Beyer K, Vila L, et al. B-cell epitopes as a screening instrument for persistent cow's milk allergy. *J Allergy Clin Immunol* 2002; 110:293–297.
56. Beyer K, Jarvinen KM, Bardina L, et al. IgE-binding peptides coupled to a commercial matrix as a diagnostic instrument for persistent cow's milk allergy. *J Allergy Clin Immunol* 2005; 116:704–705.
57. Beyer K. Characterization of allergenic food proteins for improved diagnostic methods. *Curr Opin Allergy Clin Immunol* 2003; 3:189–197.
58. Shreffler WG, Beyer K, Chu TH, et al. Microarray immunoassay: association of clinical history, in vitro IgE function, and heterogeneity of allergenic peanut epitopes. *J Allergy Clin Immunol* 2004; 113:776–782.
59. Shreffler WG, Lencer DA, Bardina L, Sampson HA. IgE and IgG4 epitope mapping by microarray immunoassay reveals the diversity of immune response to the peanut allergen, Ara h 2. *J Allergy Clin Immunol* 2005; 116:893–899.
60. Caubet JC, Kondo Y, Urisu A, Nowak-Wegrzyn A. Molecular diagnosis of egg allergy. *Curr Opin Allergy Clin Immunol* 2011; 11(3):210–215.
61. Fiocchi A, Bouygue GR, Albarini M, Restani P. Molecular diagnosis of cow's milk allergy. *Curr Opin Allergy Clin Immunol* 2011; 11(3):216–221.
62. Nicolaou N, Poorafshar M, Murray C, et al. Allergy or tolerance in children sensitized to peanut: prevalence and differentiation using component-resolved diagnostics. *J Allergy Clin Immunol* 2010; 125(1):191–197.
63. Codreanu F, Collignon O, Roitel O, et al. A novel immunoassay using recombinant allergens simplifies peanut allergy diagnosis. *Int Arch Allergy Immunol* 2011; 154(3):216–226.
64. Nicolaou N, Custovic A. Molecular diagnosis of peanut and legume allergy. *Curr Opin Allergy Clin Immunol* 2011; 11(3):222–228.
65. Vereda A, van Hage M, Ahlstedt S, et al. Peanut allergy: clinical and immunologic differences among patients from 3 different geographic regions. *J Allergy Clin Immunol* 2011; 127(3):603–607.
66. Pastorello EA, Farioli L, Pravettoni V, et al. Sensitization to the major allergen of Brazil nut is correlated with the clinical expression of allergy. *J Allergy Clin Immunol* 1998; 102:1021–1027.
67. Beyer K, Ellman-Grunther L, Jarvinen KM, et al. Measurement of peptide-specific IgE as an additional tool in identifying patients with clinical reactivity to peanuts. *J Allergy Clin Immunol* 2003; 112:202–207.
68. Lin J, Bruni FM, Fu Z, et al. A bioinformatics approach to identify patients with symptomatic peanut allergy using peptide microarray immunoassay. *J Allergy Clin Immunol* 2012; 129(5):1321–1328.

69. Palosuo K, Varjonen E, Kekki OM, et al. Wheat omega-5 gliadin is a major allergen in children with immediate allergy to ingested wheat. *J Allergy Clin Immunol* 2001; 108:634–638.
70. Palosuo K. Update on wheat hypersensitivity. *Curr Opin Allergy Clin Immunol* 2003; 3:205–209.
71. Mittag D, Niggemann B, Sander I, et al. Immunoglobulin E-reactivity of wheat-allergic subjects (baker's asthma, food allergy, wheat-dependent, exercise-induced anaphylaxis) to wheat protein fractions with different solubility and digestibility. *Mol Nutr Food Res* 2004; 48:380–389.
72. Nickel R, Kulig M, Forster J, et al. Sensitization to hen's egg at the age of twelve months is predictive for allergic sensitization to common indoor and outdoor allergens at the age of three years. *J Allergy Clin Immunol* 1997; 99:613–617.

21 *In Vivo* Diagnosis: Skin Testing and Challenge Procedures

Scott H. Sicherer

Division of Allergy and Immunology, Department of Pediatrics, Icahn School of Medicine at Mount Sinai, New York, NY, USA

Key Concepts

- The medical history is the cornerstone for establishing an accurate diagnosis of food allergy.
- Skin prick tests determine sensitization (presence of food-specific IgE) and provide significant diagnostic value when considered in the context of the medical history.
- Increasingly larger skin test wheals are associated with increasing risks for clinical reactions.
- Skin prick tests may offer specific advantages over *in vitro* methods that detect food-specific IgE.
- Response to elimination diets may provide presumptive evidence of food-related disease.
- The oral food challenge, in particular when double-blind and placebo-controlled, is the most definitive modality available to diagnose a food-related illness.

Introduction

An accurate food allergy diagnosis relies upon obtaining an informative medical history, performing appropriate supporting diagnostic tests and interpreting them in the context of the medical history, and decision making in regard to undertaking physician-supervised oral food challenges (OFCs) [1]. This chapter focuses upon skin prick tests (SPTs) and OFCs, *in vivo* modalities that provide immediate diagnostic information that is crucial in the evaluation of an individual with suspected food allergy, as well as the medical history and results of trial elimination diets. The OFC is the primary diagnostic procedure that can most definitively diagnose an adverse reaction to food. The results of an OFC do not depend upon the immunopathology of an adverse reaction to a food, whether the problem is due to intolerance, a pharmacologic response, or an allergic (immunologic) reaction mediated by IgE antibodies or cellular reactions. While potentially definitive, OFCs carry risks because severe reactions may be induced. The clinician, therefore, must also rely upon patient histories and a number of additional tests to help determine the likelihood of a true allergy or adverse reaction to food, and, therefore, whether an OFC is warranted. These additional tests include the medical history, results of elimination diets and, when appropriate, tests for food-specific IgE antibodies. For allergic reactions that are mediated by IgE antibody, the tests most familiar to the allergist are the SPTs, a focus of this chapter, and the determination of serum food-specific IgE antibodies (Chapters 8 and 20), and possibly patch tests (Chapter 22). Numerous additional tests may be needed in various clinical scenarios (e.g., stool culture, endoscopy with biopsy, pH probe, breath hydrogen) and general approaches are reviewed in Chapter 24. In addition, refinements on currently available tests, clinical evaluations of proposed tests (e.g., patch tests with food), and additional novel tests are under investigation to improve and expand the diagnostic armamentarium. Despite the potential for inaccurate histories and various limitations of *in vitro* and *in vivo* tests, the OFC can provide a final diagnostic answer, with the double-blind, placebo-controlled OFC (DBPCFC) being the "gold standard" for the diagnosis of food hypersensitivity.

Skin prick tests

Tests to detect food-specific IgE antibody are central to identify or exclude foods responsible for immediate-type, and some chronic disease-inducing food allergic reactions (e.g., atopic dermatitis and eosinophilic gastroenteropathies) [1–3]. The most familiar, convenient,

Food Allergy: Adverse Reactions to Foods and Food Additives, Fifth Edition. Edited by Dean D Metcalfe, Hugh A Sampson, Ronald A Simon and Gideon Lack.

and commonly used method is prick-puncture skin testing. The intradermal form of allergen skin testing was introduced by Blackley [4] over 100 years ago, and the prick test was described by Lewis and Grant in 1924 [5]. The SPT technique is simple, but specific variations exist [3, 6]. While the patient is off antihistamines for an appropriate length of time, a device such as a needle, bifurcated needle, probe, or lancet is used to puncture the epidermis through an extract of a food. Appropriate positive (histamine) and negative (saline-glycerine) controls are also placed. The test site is examined 10–20 minutes later. A local wheal and flare response indicates the presence of food-specific IgE antibody. A mean wheal diameter 3 mm or greater compared to a saline control is generally considered positive [7, 8], but interpretation will be discussed in more detail below. The test would be expected to be negative for food reactions that are not mediated by IgE antibodies, such as several of the infantile gastrointestinal disorders including food protein-induced enterocolitis syndrome and proctocolitis. Clearly, the SPT is an invaluable screening tool for the allergist. However, the clinician using SPTs for the diagnosis of food hypersensitivity must be aware of the utility and limitations of the test in order to use it to the best advantage for clinical and research purposes.

Technical considerations

Skin test results are influenced by variables such as test reagents, type of skin test device, location of test placement, patient factors, and methods of measuring results [3, 6]. The selection of skin test reagent is of primary importance. Unfortunately, standardized food extracts are not currently available despite a clear, long-standing recognition for the need [7, 8]. Commercial extracts are usually prepared as glycerinated extracts of 1:10 or 1:20 dilution. With the lack of standardized extracts, it is well-recognized that variations exist in allergen distribution and concentration between lots and manufacturers [9, 10]. The problem of protein stability must also be considered. An example demonstrating the lability of certain food extracts is the evaluation of food allergy in pollen-food syndrome (oral allergy syndrome to fresh fruits and vegetables). Patients may react to the uncooked, but not the cooked form of the food and this may similarly be reflected in skin test results as commercial extracts may lack the ability to display the labile proteins involved [11]. For the evaluation of allergy to fresh fruits and vegetables, and possibly other foods, many authorities have suggested the use of fresh foods (e.g., fresh milk, egg white, fruits, and vegetables) [12]. The SPT can be performed using liquid foods, by creating an in-house extract, or using a prick–prick technique (pricking the fruit and then the patient, thereby transferring the juice) [13]. Since it is not convenient to have in hand a variety of fresh fruits for testing, freezing can be undertaken with little impact on results [14]. Presumably, such in-house reagents are more concentrated and this may increase sensitivity, a possible deficit in some circumstances, and may increase the risk for side effects from the test itself. The impact of allergen concentration on wheal size is somewhat tempered by the fact that wheal size increases by a factor of approximately 1.5 for each logarithmic increase in concentration [15]. Another concern is the potential irritant effect of foods such as pineapple, berries, spices, kiwi, mustard, and tomato [3]. Histamine content of foods such as eggplant may also result in false-positive responses [16]. Interestingly, it may be possible to determine scromboid fish poisoning by testing with the actual fish meat that caused a reaction, if it is still available after the meal [17].

The device used for pricking the skin, and the technique used with any given device, may also influence the results [6]. A variety of devices are on the market for introducing the allergen into the epidermis. The more the penetration, the more likely there will be a response and so the area and depth to which the allergen is introduced is pertinent. Therefore, the configuration of the device, the pressure applied by the operator, and the time over which pressure is applied must be considered [18]. Test results also vary according to the location on the body on which they are placed. For example, the back is ~20% more reactive than the arm [19]. Studies that evaluate histamine reactivity indicate that wheals become detectable in early infancy and increase in size with age until adulthood [20, 21]. These physical and patient variables become relevant when comparing study results, and for clinical decision making. In practice, consistency of materials and procedures and review of precision (coefficient of variation should be <20% for wheal diameter) should be undertaken by comparing repeated tests by personnel administering them. Various single and multi-headed devices are available, with significant differences in all areas of device performance among all devices examined. In one study, multi-headed devices were judged more painful than single devices and had larger reactions on the back, whereas single devices had larger reactions on the arms [22]. Topical anesthetics used to reduce pain are not typically needed because the procedure is only mildly uncomfortable; if they were used, they would reduce the axon reflex responsible for the flare response but not affect the wheal [23].

The results of SPTs can be affected by variations, such as the timing at which they are read and the manner in which they are measured and reported. The histamine test peaks at 10 minutes while allergen wheal size generally peaks at 15–20 minutes [6]. One suggested method of measurement is to determine the greatest wheal (or flare) diameter, its perpendicular maximum diameter, and to determine the mean of these two measurements [6]. However, many researchers report the longest diameter, which is less time consuming to measure but presents, on average, a higher

Table 21.1 Aspects that impact sensitivity of skin prick tests (SPTs).

Feature	Correlation with sensitivity
Extract concentration	Direct
Device used	Variable
Pressure applied during application	Direct
Location	Back > volar aspect arm
Reporting progressively larger reaction sizes (e.g., wheal 4 mm instead of 3 mm) as categorically positive	Inverse

value than the mean diameter. Presenting the result in millimeters is preferred, with additional presentation of the size of the histamine and saline controls for comparison; reporting the test as a grade (i.e., 1+, 2+) is not recommended [6]. The measurement of the saline control is typically subtracted from the allergen and histamine results to account for dermographism. Thus, a positive test, reflecting specific IgE, is generally regarded as one with a mean wheal diameter at least 3 mm greater than the saline control. When comparing studies that report skin test results, care is needed because a variety of methods employed may not be directly comparable. Despite the numerous potential confounding variables involved in the SPT procedure, the clinical utility is excellent. Technical issues that can impact SPT sensitivity are summarized in Table 21.1.

Diagnostic value

The ability of a test to indicate the presence or absence of disease depends upon intrinsic characteristics of the test itself and also features of the population on which it is being applied. The SPT is excellent for detecting food-specific IgE antibody and when it is negative, it is highly likely that there is none and that no IgE-antibody-mediated allergic reaction would occur to the tested food (excellent negative predictive accuracy, NPA). However, this conclusion, when considering the individual patient, depends strongly upon the prior probability of true allergy, a concept discussed further below. A negative result does not exclude the possibility of cell-mediated allergic reactions or intolerance. It is important to appreciate that the presence of IgE to a food indicates sensitization, but does not equate with clinical reactions. There is often (~50%) clinically inconsequential sensitization, which is why the medical history is key in selecting and properly interpreting test responses. For example, skin testing to peanut in the general population (no selection for allergy) performed in the United States showed that 8% had a positive SPT [24], yet population-based studies of reported allergy to peanut show that at approximately 0.8% are allergic [25]. Therefore, in unselected patients, one could conclude that approximately 90% of positive tests are "false positive."

The sensitivity and specificity of a test provide information about its ability to identify a known condition. Sensitivity refers to the proportion of patients with an illness who test positive, and for IgE-mediated food allergy, the sensitivity of the SPT is usually high (>80%). Specificity refers to the proportion of individuals without the disorder who test negative, and for IgE-antibody-mediated food allergy, specificity of the SPT is usually lower than the sensitivity but usually better than 50% [12, 26, 27]. Sensitivity and specificity are impacted by intrinsic properties of the test, but the clinical question of import to the physician concerns the probability that a patient has food allergy if the test is positive (positive predictive accuracy, PPA) or does not have food allergy if the test is negative (NPA). The predictive accuracy is impacted by the prevalence of the disorder in the population being tested (or as applied to the individual, the prior probability that the person being tested has the disorder). In studies using referred patients with an increased probability of disease, and a definition of positive SPT as one with a mean wheal diameter of 3 mm or greater, SPTs have an excellent NPA (~90%) but the PPA is on the order of only 50% [12, 26, 27].

The definition used to indicate a positive test (or degree of positive) will additionally impact the PPA and NPA. For example, increasing skin test size correlates directly with increasing IgE antibody and the risk of clinical reactions. Therefore, if one were to analyze skin test sizes (rather than just labeling them categorically as positive or negative at a mean wheal size of 3 mm), there would be variation in sensitivity and specificity with each incremental change in size. In general, as the definition of a positive test requires a larger wheal, specificity increases and sensitivity decreases. Receiver operator curves are used to display the association of test size defined as positive with sensitivity and specificity that must be determined experimentally (Figure 21.1). The uppermost left quadrant on the curve would be the point where combined maximum sensitivity and specificity could be achieved. Similarly, as "cutoff" for positive increases, so does PPA while the NPA simultaneously decreases. Since these indices of predictive value are population dependant, the predictive value drops (illness is overestimated) when results obtained in a referral center (high prevalence) are applied to unselected individuals. Using test reagents of varying concentrations and determining an end point titration may add predictive value, but is more labor intensive and requires more study [28].

An additional way of considering the meaning of a test is to consider the chance that a person with food allergy would have a positive test compared to the chance that one without food allergy would have a negative test. This ratio is termed a likelihood ratio. This ratio is independent of population prevalence, but in order to use it for predicting food allergy, one must have a sense for pretest probability in the individual tested (i.e., the impact is similar to population prevalence of disease on PPA and NPA). If one knows the likelihood ratio of a skin test and the

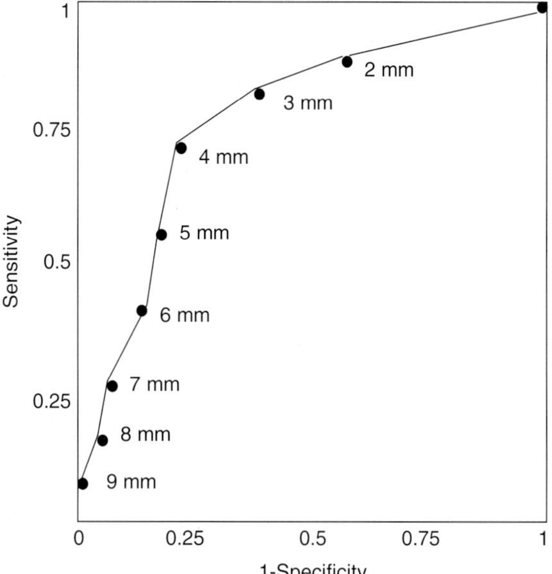

Figure 21.1 A receiver operator curve showing a hypothetical experiment in which SPT sensitivity and specificity were determined for various wheal sizes. When different skin test sizes are considered as a positive "cutoff", there is a trade-off between sensitivity and specificity. The single point at which sensitivity and specificity is maximized is the one closest to the upper left corner (4 mm in this example). When the skin test size meets and exceeds 9 mm in this example, there is 100% specificity and all patients would be expected to react to this food.

pretest probability of food allergy, it is possible to calculate a posttest probability by multiplying the likelihood ratio by the pretest probability [29]. While specific data are not worked out for most foods, the concept is clinically vital to appreciate and underscores the importance of a careful history. Consider, for example, three individuals: one had three severe allergic reactions to egg requiring epinephrine, another has atopic dermatitis and no history of a reaction to egg, and a third sometimes has headaches when he eats egg. Each patient is tested by SPT to egg white and has a 4 mm wheal. The meaning of a 4 mm wheal to egg when there has been recurrent anaphylaxis to egg is that it confirms reactivity because the pretest probability is high. In a chronic condition like atopic dermatitis, a modest size skin test may reflect clinical reactivity in only about half of patients (depending also upon age) and may be a relevant positive in this scenario needing confirmation by other means. The test result in the situation of isolated headaches is most likely of no clinical concern as the pretest probability is essentially zero. Considering again the patient with multiple episodes of egg-related anaphylaxis, if there were no wheal to egg the clinician would not be likely to trust the result because the pretest probability is so high and the correct course of action would be to repeat the test and consider a supervised OFC if the test were negative. These features underscore the importance of considering the medical history when evaluating test results. Likelihood ratios can be calculated for increasing skin test wheal sizes which in turn can assist in broadening the ability to predict reactions in various clinical scenarios, but more studies are needed to provide reliable data for a large number of foods [30]. Such data would be particularly helpful for the interpretation of skin tests performed to foods with homologous proteins (see Chapters 4 and 25) in persons who have a bona fide allergy to one of a group of related foods.

It has been observed by some investigators that particularly large SPTs may have 100% positive predictive value. This concept was demonstrated in a study [30] showing that for young infants, reactions to egg, milk, and peanut were certain to occur if the skin test wheal was ≥8 mm for cow milk and peanut and ≥7 mm for egg. The scenario reflects increasing likelihood ratio with increasing sizes of skin tests (likelihood ratios over 12.5 for all three allergens with wheals 6 mm or greater in the referral population). This result requires replication in further studies. These investigators [31] also evaluated children 4 months to 19 years of age referred for suspected nut allergy with a single lancet technique and commercial extracts (except whole food for sesame and pistachio) and compared skin test sizes to food challenge outcomes. Positive challenges were associated (>95% accuracy) with wheal sizes ≥8 mm for cashew, hazel, walnut, and sesame. Correlation was poor for almond, pistachio, pecan, and Brazil nut though fewer subjects were tested.

When considering the clinical use of such study results, it is also important to consider the variables mentioned previously concerning method of interpretation, skin test device, reagents, study population, and so on. Table 21.2 summarizes predictive values from skin tests from representative international studies [30, 32–37]. As indicated in Table 21.2, the populations differed, but included various groups with an elevated prior probability of allergy. It is important to recognize that skin test sizes reflecting "100% specificity," or diagnostic value, varied by the study. The clinical utility of SPTs is maximized when two decision point wheal sizes are considered in the interpretation: one with high NPA and another with high PPA. When considered together, this may reduce the need for further evaluations (e.g., OFC).

Risks of SPTs

SPTs are typically considered of low risk because allergen exposure is minute and a generalized systemic allergic reaction is rare [6]. In a review of a database of 34 905 skin tests to foods in 1138 patients, the systemic reaction rate was 0.008% and there were no severe reactions [38]. Devenney et al., [39] identified six infants with generalized reactions representing a rate of 521 per 100 000 tested children or 6522 per 100 000 tested infants. All of the

Table 21.2 Predictive value of skin tests from various studies.

Allergen	Age	Skin test wheal (mm)	Probability of reaction/reaction rates (%)	Comments	Reference
Milk	Median 3 years	8	~100	Australia, referred for suspected allergy, lancet technique, commercial extracts, wheal diameter open OFC	30
	<Age 2 years	6	~100	Same as above	
	Median 3 years	0	~15	Same as above	
	Median 22 months	12.5	95	Germany, all OFC, suspected allergy, 87% AD, fresh foods, mean wheal diameter, lancet technique	32
Egg	Mean 5 years	0	20	United States, children without recent egg reaction and serum IgE typically below 2.5 kIU/l, bifurcated needle, commercial extract, mean wheal diameter	33
		3	50	As above	
		9	90	As above	
	Median 3 years	7	~100	Australia, referred for suspected allergy, lancet technique, commercial extracts, wheal diameter open OFC	30
	<Age 2 years	5	~100	Same as above	
	Median 22 months	13	95	Germany, all OFC, suspected allergy, fresh foods, mean wheal diameter, lancet technique	32
	Under age 16 years	9	95	Spain, prior diagnosis of egg allergy, extract, lancet, mean diameter	34
Peanut	Median 3 years	8	~100	Australia, referred for suspected allergy, lancet technique, commercial extracts, wheal diameter open OFC	30
	<Age 2 years	4	~100	Same as above	
	Mean 7 years	8	~95	United Kingdom, mixed suspected allergy, ages 1–16 years, lancet technique, extract, longest diameter	35
		3	~50	As above	
		0	~13	As above	
	Median 40 months	3	~15	Australia, sensitized but no ingestion, extract, lancet, mean diameter	36
		7	~50		
		13	~95		

OFC, oral food challenge; AD, atopic dermatitis.

reactions identified were in infants under 6 months of age and they were tested with fresh foods rather than extracts. Indeed, prick testing with fresh extracts appears to carry more risks [40]. There is one fatality associated with skin prick testing; an adult with food allergy and asthma with a recent exacerbation was tested to 90 foods at one time and experienced a fatal respiratory arrest [41]. In general, these studies support the notion that SPTs are low risk but caution is needed for infants, use of undiluted extracts, and to avoid excessive numbers of tests. The physician performing allergy tests should appreciate the low but possible risk of anaphylaxis and be prepared to identify and treat reactions. Intradermal allergy skin tests with food extracts give an unacceptably high false-positive rate, have been associated with systemic reactions including fatal anaphylactic reactions, and should not be used [1, 42].

Advantages and pitfalls of skin tests and future diagnostic possibilities

A recent literature review evaluating SPT and serum food-specific IgE test results against OFC outcomes concluded that the two manners of testing gave similar diagnostic utility [43]. However, it is clear that there are situations where one test is positive and another is negative [44]. There are several possible reasons for this outcome including procedure error and having different allergens represented in different test formats. As has been indicated for venom testing [45], it may be prudent to perform both serum IgE and SPT to a food to improve sensitivity when suspicion of reactions are high based upon history. In addition, it has been suggested, when suspicion of allergy is high and before proceeding to OFC, to follow a negative SPT performed with a commercial extract with a fresh extract of the same food. Presumably this procedure is more sensitive because labile proteins are displayed, compared to commercial extracts, and proteins that may not have been represented during aqueous extraction in creating a commercial extract may be presented as well [46]. For example, Hauswirth and Burks [47] described a patient with systemic anaphylaxis to banana whose commercial, but not fresh extract, skin testing was positive. Another example is that oil-based allergens in sesame may not be represented well in water-based extracts. Recently, a contact test with sesame oil was shown to overcome this limitation in some cases [48]. Allergy to mammalian meats caused by reactivity to galactose-alpha-1,3 galactose may require testing with fresh meats, serum tests to the alpha-gal moiety, or skin tests to cetuximab, which has the same sugar moiety [49, 50].

The *in vitro* tests for detection of serum food-specific IgE antibodies are also very sensitive and specific, but may not display the very same allergen profile as the skin tests. The tests can therefore be used in a complementary fashion when needed. For example, Knight et al. [33] challenged children to egg when their serum AGE concentrations to egg white was favorable, approximately 50%, to pass an OFC, for example, around 2 kIU/l. The size of the wheal to a commercial egg extract SPT correlated with the outcome of the food challenges: 20% of those with a negative skin test reacted to OFC while 90% with a wheal size of 9 mm reacted.

Improvement in the diagnostic accuracy of SPTs for the future will require additional studies to better characterize the test utility over a broad spectrum of disease, patient age, and types of foods. Standardization of commercial extracts is needed, but development of extracts using bioengineered or extracted components may also prove beneficial. Test results currently do not correlate well with severity of a reaction or level of patient sensitivity, but diagnosis using specific proteins to which IgE binding is associated with severe reactions may allow future diagnosis that is more sensitive and specific with additional predictive value in regard to severity [51–54].

Additional diagnostic steps prior to OFCs

An OFC can determine whether a specific food triggers disease, but it is time consuming and carries risk. Therefore, additional diagnostic steps are taken to determine if an OFC would be of utility and, if so, additional consideration about risks/benefits are considered prior to proceeding. To determine a diagnosis and to determine whether an OFC is needed for a diagnosis requires consideration of patient history, test results, the immunopathology of the disorder under consideration, the physical examination, and the results of elimination diets [55]. These diagnostic steps are considered in more detail in Chapter 24. Specific information about diagnostic tests such as determination and interpretation of serum IgE (Chapters 8 and 20), and the atopy patch test (Chapter 22) are described elsewhere. Here, the specific components of the history and physical examination that are of import for diagnosing food allergy will be described. The value and limitations of diet diaries and elimination diets will be explained. Lastly, decisions about undertaking an OFC and the type of OFC will be reviewed. Specific details about undertaking an elimination diet and performing an OFC will be described in Chapter 23.

The history and physical examination

The history and physical examination are undertaken prior to the selection of any diagnostic tests. The clinician must consider from the history whether the complaints are likely to be associated with food allergy, intolerance, or toxic effects, or not related to foods whatsoever. Furthermore, the physician is interested in constructing *a priori* assessments of the chance that foods are playing a role, which foods may be involved, and whether the pathophysiology, if it is related to a hypersensitivity reaction, is IgE-antibody-mediated, cell mediated, or a combination. The physical examination may confirm atopic dermatitis, growth problems, urticaria, and other symptoms of atopic disease, or may exclude them. A careful history should focus upon the following: the symptoms attributed to food ingestion (type, acute vs. chronic), the food(s) involved, consistency of reactions, the quantity of food required to elicit symptoms, the timing between ingestion and onset of symptoms, the most recent reaction/patterns of reactivity, the manner in which the food was prepared (raw, cooked), potential contamination with known allergens, and any ancillary associated activity that may play a role (i.e., exercise, alcohol ingestion). The importance of these queries, many of which are self-evident, derive from various observations about food allergic reactions. For example, consistent reactions raise prior probability that a suspect food is causal. If a food is an infrequent part of the diet, it is more likely a culprit than a food eaten often. Proteins may be altered through cooking resulting in variations in reaction. Sometimes a rather large amount of a food needs to be ingested for a reaction to occur or ancillary activities such as exercise or ingestion of medications is required [1, 6, 55, 56]. A person with a prior known allergy may have reacted to contamination of their food with a known allergen rather than have developed a new allergy, so careful discussion is required. Details about the meal may disclose nuances of note. Consider, for example, an allergic reaction to ingestion of fish in a person where fish allergic reactions have not been consistent. Canned tuna and salmon are typically tolerated by those who react to fish that is not canned, though allergy to canned tuna is also described [57]. Various fish preparation methods (e.g., canning vs. frying vs. eating raw) may have different outcomes on protein allergenicity for different types of fish [58]. Use of antacids (concomitant medications) may reduce digestion and may result in reactions despite prior tolerance [59]. The part of the fish ingested can have different levels of the major allergen, such that dark or red muscle may lack the allergen compared to white muscle [60, 61]. Lastly, allergy to parasites in fish, specifically to anisakis simplex, represents another potential confounding diagnostic issue [62–65]. A thorough history is needed to appropriately address these possibilities.

It is convenient, and possibly quite illuminating, to have patients keep a symptom diary and chart the foods they consume with and without symptoms and also to collect ingredient labels from the foods they eat. For example, they may chart 3–7 days of meals and snacks, showing the time of ingestions, the amount eaten, brands, preparation methods, and any symptoms. The accuracy and diagnostic utility of such records has not been evaluated [1]. To improve the quality of the information, patients/families should be reminded to record all foods and medications ingested, as they may be prone to neglect beverages, snacks, medications, and condiments. The information gathered from the general history, physical examination, and diet records are used to determine the best mode of diagnosis or may lead to dismissal of the problem from the history alone.

In the case of acute reactions following the isolated ingestion of a particular food with classical food allergic symptoms, such as acute urticaria or anaphylaxis, the history may clearly implicate a particular food and a positive test for specific IgE antibody would be confirmatory and exclude the need for OFC. In the context of an acute reaction to a food to which IgE has been detected, elimination is not considered diagnostic, but rather for purposes of treatment. If the ingestion was of mixed foods and the causal food was uncertain (i.e., a meal with five ingredients), the history may help to eliminate some of the foods. For example, foods frequently ingested without symptoms are generally excluded as potential triggers when evaluating symptoms associated with acute reactions. Tests for food-specific IgE antibodies may help to further narrow the possibilities.

Diagnostic elimination diets

In chronic disorders such as atopic dermatitis, eosinophilic gastroenteropathies, or asthma, it is more difficult to pinpoint causal food(s) [2, 66]. The history is helpful, but since these disorders have a waxing and waning course, and considering limitations in diagnostic laboratory tests, false associations to food ingestions are common. The evaluation of these disorders may require a period of dietary elimination to observe for symptom resolution. This period of trial diet requires selection of foods to be eliminated (based usually on history, test results, epidemiology of the disorder, etc.). The diet trial could be confounded if additional therapies are simultaneously undertaken (e.g., steroids for eosinophilic gastrointestinal disorders, an improved skin care regiment for atopic dermatitis). Therefore, it is usually prudent to alter one variable at a time. Chronic symptoms should resolve during a period of elimination and if they do, OFCs may be needed to determine which food(s) were causing the chronic symptoms. If symptoms do not resolve, then the eliminated foods are not causal. Elimination of foods to which IgE antibodies are demonstrable, but to which acute reactions are not observed, may carry a risk of loss of a desensitized state, where reintroduction later can trigger more evident acute reactions (e.g., urticaria, anaphylaxis) [67, 68]. The frequency of this occurrence is unknown and the length of time for elimination to warrant this concern is currently unclear, but the risk should be considered in decisions to begin dietary trials. Additional details about elimination diets are provided in Chapter 23.

Oral food challenges

OFCs are typically undertaken to identify a causal food when allergy is otherwise unclear (e.g., tests are equivocal or irrelevant), to monitor for resolution of an allergy, or for research purposes. OFC is usually the only means to evaluate disorders or complaints where ancillary tests are irrelevant. For example, the evaluation of reactions to food dyes and preservatives usually requires OFCs. Similarly, patients may attribute a host of medical complaints to food ingestion in disorders that are not proven to be pathophysiologically linked to food allergy (e.g., arthritis, fatigue, behavioral problems). In all of the circumstances where chronic complaints are involved, the OFC is capable of revealing or excluding relationships to foods. Such determinations are crucial because patients may undertake unnecessary dietary alterations that can have nutritional and social consequences [69, 70]. Overall, the approach to diagnosis in chronic disorders, where most readily available diagnostic tests are of limited value, requires elimination diets and OFCs to confirm suspected associations.

In regard to undertaking an OFC when there is supporting evidence of allergy, the decision requires consideration of risk, nutritional need, social need, and other factors. When performed under proper conditions, the procedure is generally safe [71]. The issues to consider when deciding whether to undertake an oral challenge, and what challenge setting (e.g., open, single, or double-masked) are summarized in Table 21.3. Diagnostic tests considered in this chapter and elsewhere, results of elimination diets, and historical points are central to decision making. There are settings in which oral challenges may be optional or contraindicated. Severe anaphylaxis to an isolated ingestion, with a positive test for specific IgE antibody to the causal food is one example of a relative contraindication for oral challenge. On the other hand, in some circumstances, even a patient with this

Table 21.3 Issues to consider for undertaking an OFC.

Category	Variables	Factors
Indication to challenge	Probability to pass (risks)	History, physical examination, test results, nature of allergen, natural history of disease
	Needs (benefits)	Social Nutritional
Challenge type	Open	Numerous foods to screen, disorder with objective symptoms, allowance for bias
	Single-blind	Less prone to bias than open
	DBPCFC	Least prone to bias, most definitive approach for subjective symptoms
Challenge location	Home	Adding foods in chronic or behavioral disorders with no risk of acute/severe reactions
	Office	Challenges at low risk for severe reaction
	Hospital/ICU	Challenges that are more likely to elicit reactions requiring medical intervention

DBPCFC, double-blind, placebo-controlled oral food challenge.

convincing history may require a challenge; for example, if enough time has passed and laboratory indices are favorable for the possibility that tolerance has developed. If the food being eliminated is not nutritionally or socially important (e.g., star fruit), then challenge may be unwarranted. These same may apply if several members of a food family are being eliminated, but the food family is not a major part of the diet (e.g., elimination of all tree nuts when an allergy to one is certain). An evaluation of the history and test results may allow an assessment of a probability a challenge would be tolerated. Depending upon patient preferences and physician judgment, the decision to proceed may vary. For example, an estimation of an 80% risk of a reaction to peanut for a 2 year old is not as likely to result in a decision to challenge as it might be for a 16 year old. Overall, a variety of safety and social issues should be considered.

There are three general modalities to perform OFC and their selection depends upon various considerations [72–75]. Challenges can be done "openly" with the patient ingesting the food in its natural form, "single-blind" with the food masked and the patient unaware if the test substance contains the target food or, DBPCFC where neither patient nor physician knows which challenges contain the food being tested [55]. In the latter two formats, the food must be hidden in some way, such as in another food or opaque capsules. When challenges are undertaken for research purposes, the DBPCFC is the preferred format because there is the least chance for bias from either the patient or physician who must monitor for symptoms. The false-positive and false-negative rate for the DBPCFC, based primarily on studies in children with atopic dermatitis, is 0.7% and 3.2%, respectively [76, 77]. Because the food is masked, it is sometimes difficult to provide meal sized portions in a foods' natural state. To help exclude false negatives, it has long been suggested to include an open feeding under supervision of a meal size portion of the tested food prepared in its usual manner as a follow-up to any negative DBPCFC [77]. Increasing the number of challenges (additional placebo and true foods) helps to diminish the possibility of a random association, but this can be a very labor-intensive approach [78, 79].

There are several factors that weigh in deciding which type of challenge to use, and DBPCFC, a labor-intensive format, may not be the initial choice. Although the open challenge is most prone to bias, it is easy to perform since no special preparation is needed to mask the food. Indeed, if the patient tolerates the ingestion of the food, there is little concern about bias. It is only when symptoms, especially subjective ones, arise that the issue of bias come into play. Therefore, open challenges are a good option for screening when several foods are under consideration and if a food is tolerated, nothing further is needed. If there is a reaction to an open challenge used in the clinical setting, and there is concern that the reaction may not have been physiological, the format could be altered to include blinding and controls. Single-blind challenges help to alleviate patient bias and may be an option to increase efficiency (since a second placebo arm is not always needed). Additional information about undertaking OFC is presented in Chapter 23.

Summary

In vivo tests are primary tools among the armamentarium available to the clinician for the diagnosis of adverse reactions to foods. The medical history, perhaps supplemented with diet records, is the cornerstone of diagnosis. Skin testing is safe, cost-effective, and when properly performed and interpreted, highly informative for the diagnosis of IgE-antibody-mediated disorders. Elimination diets may provide presumptive evidence of a food-responsive disease. OFCs are the most definitive test available for the final confirmation of these disorders. While oral challenges are time consuming and may elicit severe reactions, they can be safely and efficiently performed with the proper preparation and remain the mainstay of diagnosis for clinical and research settings.

References

1. Boyce JA, Assa'ad A, Burks AW, et al. Guidelines for the diagnosis and management of food allergy in the United States: report of the NIAID-sponsored expert panel. *J Allergy Clin Immunol* 2010; 126(6 Suppl.):S1–S58.

2. Liacouras CA, Furuta GT, Hirano I, et al. Eosinophilic esophagitis: updated consensus recommendations for children and adults. *J Allergy Clin Immunol* 2011; 128(1):3–20.
3. Henzgen M, Ballmer-Weber BK, Erdmann S, et al. Skin testing with food allergens. Guideline of the German Society of Allergology and Clinical Immunology (DGAKI), the Physicians' Association of German Allergologists (ADA) and the Society of Pediatric Allergology (GPA) together with the Swiss Society of Allergology. *J Dtsch Dermatol Ges* 2008; 6(11):983–988.
4. Blackley C. *Hay Fever: Its Causes, Treatment and Effective Prevention, Experimental Researches*, 2nd edn. Balliere; London, 1880.
5. Lewis T, Grant R. Vascular reactions of the skin to injury. *Heart* 1924; 11:209–265.
6. Bernstein IL, Li JT, Bernstein DI, et al. Allergy diagnostic testing: an updated practice parameter. *Ann Allergy Asthma Immunol* 2008; 100(3 Suppl. 3):S1–S148.
7. American Academy of Allergy, Asthma and Immunology (AAAAI). The use of standardized allergen extracts. *J Allergy Clin Immunol* 1997; 99(5):583–586.
8. The European Academy of Allergology and Clinical Immunology. Position paper: allergen standardization and skin tests. *Allergy* 1993; 48(14 Suppl.):48–82.
9. Hefle SL, Helm RM, Burks AW, Bush RK. Comparison of commercial peanut skin test extracts. *J Allergy Clin Immunol* 1995; 95(4):837–842.
10. Herian AM, Bush RK, Taylor SL. Protein and allergen content of commercial skin test extracts for soybeans. *Clin Exp Allergy* 1992; 22:461–468.
11. Asero R. Detection and clinical characterization of patients with oral allergy syndrome caused by stable allergens in Rosaceae and nuts. *Ann Allergy Asthma Immunol* 1999; 83(5):377–383.
12. Ortolani C, Ispano M, Pastorello EA, Ansaloni R, Magri GC. Comparison of results of skin prick tests (with fresh foods and commercial food extracts) and RAST in 100 patients with oral allergy syndrome. *J Allergy Clin Immunol* 1989; 83:683–90.
13. Dreborg S. Skin tests in the diagnosis of food allergy. *Pediatr Allergy Immunol* 1995; 6(Suppl. 8):38–43.
14. Begin P, Des RA, Nguyen M, Masse MS, Paradis J, Paradis L. Freezing does not alter antigenic properties of fresh fruits for skin testing in patients with birch tree pollen-induced oral allergy syndrome. *J Allergy Clin Immunol* 2011; 127(6):1624–1626.
15. Dreborg S. Diagnosis of food allergy: tests in vivo and in vitro. *Pediatr Allergy Immunol* 2001; 12(Suppl. 14):24–30.
16. Kumar MN, Babu BN, Venkatesh YP. Higher histamine sensitivity in non-atopic subjects by skin prick test may result in misdiagnosis of eggplant allergy. *Immunol Invest* 2009; 38(1):93–103.
17. Kelso JM, Lin FL. Skin testing for scombroid poisoning. *Ann Allergy Asthma Immunol* 2009; 103(5):447.
18. Nelson HS, Rosloniec DM, McCall LI, Ikle D. Comparative performance of five commercial prick skin test devices. *J Allergy Clin Immunol* 1993; 92(5):750–756.
19. Nelson HS, Knoetzer J, Bucher B. Effect of distance between sites and region of the body on results of skin prick tests. *J Allergy Clin Immunol* 1996; 97(2):596–601.
20. Menardo JL, Bousquet J, Rodiere M, Astruc J, Michel FB. Skin test reactivity in infancy. *J Allergy Clin Immunol* 1985; 75(6):646–651.
21. Skassa-Brociek W, Manderscheid JC, Michel FB, Bousquet J. Skin test reactivity to histamine from infancy to old age. *J Allergy Clin Immunol* 1987; 80(5):711–716.
22. Carr WW, Martin B, Howard RS, Cox L, Borish L. Comparison of test devices for skin prick testing. *J Allergy Clin Immunol* 2005; 116(2):341–346.
23. Sicherer SH, Eggleston PA. EMLA cream for pain reduction in diagnostic allergy skin testing: effects on wheal and flare responses. *Ann Allergy Asthma Immunol* 1997; 78(1):64–68.
24. Arbes SJ Jr, Gergen PJ, Elliott L, Zeldin DC. Prevalences of positive skin test responses to 10 common allergens in the US population: results from the third National Health and Nutrition Examination Survey. *J Allergy Clin Immunol* 2005; 116(2):377–383.
25. Sicherer SH, Muñoz-Furlong A, Godbold JH, Sampson HA. US prevalence of self-reported peanut, tree nut, and sesame allergy: 11-year follow-up. *J Allergy Clin Immunol* 2010; 125(6):1322–1326.
26. Eigenmann PA, Sampson HA. Interpreting skin prick tests in the evaluation of food allergy in children. *Pediatr Allergy Immunol* 1998; 9(4):186–191.
27. Majamaa H, Moisio P, Holm K, Kautiainen H, Turjanmaa K. Cow's milk allergy: diagnostic accuracy of skin prick and patch tests and specific IgE. *Allergy* 1999; 54(4):346–351.
28. Tripodi S, Businco AD, Alessandri C, Panetta V, Restani P, Matricardi PM. Predicting the outcome of oral food challenges with hen's egg through skin test end-point titration. *Clin Exp Allergy* 2009; 39(8):1225–1233.
29. Fagan TJ. Letter: nomogram for Bayes theorem. *N Engl J Med* 1975; 293(5):257.
30. Sporik R, Hill DJ, Hosking CS. Specificity of allergen skin testing in predicting positive open food challenges to milk, egg and peanut in children. *Clin Exp Allergy* 2000; 30(11):1541–1546.
31. Ho MH, Heine RG, Wong W, Hill DJ. Diagnostic accuracy of skin prick testing in children with tree nut allergy. *J Allergy Clin Immunol* 2006; 117(6):1506–1508.
32. Verstege A, Mehl A, Rolinck-Werninghaus C, et al. The predictive value of the skin prick test weal size for the outcome of oral food challenges. *Clin Exp Allergy* 2005; 35(9):1220–1226.
33. Knight AK, Shreffler WG, Sampson HA, et al. Skin prick test to egg white provides additional diagnostic utility to serum egg white-specific IgE antibody concentration in children. *J Allergy Clin Immunol* 2006; 117(4):842–847.
34. Dieguez MC, Cerecedo I, Muriel A, et al. Utility of diagnostic tests in the follow-up of egg-allergic children. *Clin Exp Allergy* 2009; 39(10):1575–1584.
35. Roberts G, Lack G. Diagnosing peanut allergy with skin prick and specific IgE testing. *J Allergy Clin Immunol* 2005; 115(6):1291–1296.
36. Johannsen H, Nolan R, Pascoe EM, et al. Skin prick testing and peanut-specific IgE can predict peanut challenge outcomes in preschool children with peanut sensitization. *Clin Exp Allergy* 2011; 41(7):994–1000.

37. Wainstein BK, Studdert J, Ziegler M, Ziegler JB. Prediction of anaphylaxis during peanut food challenge: usefulness of the peanut skin prick test (SPT) and specific IgE level. *Pediatr Allergy Immunol* 2010; 21(4 Pt. 1):603–611.
38. Codreanu F, Moneret-Vautrin DA, Morisset M, et al. The risk of systemic reactions to skin prick-tests using food allergens: CICBAA data and literature review. *Eur Ann Allergy Clin Immunol* 2006; 38(2):52–54.
39. Devenney I, Falth-Magnusson K. Skin prick tests may give generalized allergic reactions in infants. *Ann Allergy Asthma Immunol* 2000; 85(6 Pt. 1):457–460.
40. Pitsios C, Dimitriou A, Kontou-Fili K. Allergic reactions during allergy skin testing with food allergens. *Eur Ann Allergy Clin Immunol* 2009; 41(4):126–128.
41. Bernstein DI, Wanner M, Borish L, Liss GM. Twelve-year survey of fatal reactions to allergen injections and skin testing: 1990–2001. *J Allergy Clin Immunol* 2004; 113(6):1129–1136.
42. Sampson HA, Rosen JP, Selcow JE, et al. Intradermal skin tests in the diagnostic evaluation of food allergy. *J Allergy Clin Immunol* 1996; 98(3):714–715.
43. Chafen JJ, Newberry SJ, Riedl MA, et al. Diagnosing and managing common food allergies: a systematic review. *J Am Med Assoc* 2010; 303(18):1848–1856.
44. Sicherer SH, Wood RA, Stablein D, et al. Immunologic features of infants with milk or egg allergy enrolled in an observational study (Consortium of Food Allergy Research) of food allergy. *J Allergy Clin Immunol* 2010; 125(5):1077–1083.
45. Moffitt JE, Golden DB, Reisman RE, et al. Stinging insect hypersensitivity: a practice parameter update. *J Allergy Clin Immunol* 2004; 114(4):869–886.
46. Leduc V, Moneret-Vautrin DA, Tzen JT, Morisset M, Guerin L, Kanny G. Identification of oleosins as major allergens in sesame seed allergic patients. *Allergy* 2006; 61(3):349–356.
47. Hauswirth DW, Burks AW. Banana anaphylaxis with a negative commercial skin test. *J Allergy Clin Immunol* 2005; 115(3):632–633.
48. Alonzi C, Campi P, Gaeta F, Pineda F, Romano A. Diagnosing IgE-mediated hypersensitivity to sesame by an immediate-reading "contact test" with sesame oil. *J Allergy Clin Immunol* 2011; 127(6):1627–1629.
49. Commins SP, James HR, Kelly LA, et al. The relevance of tick bites to the production of IgE antibodies to the mammalian oligosaccharide galactose-alpha-1,3-galactose. *J Allergy Clin Immunol* 2011; 127(5):1286–1293.
50. Jacquenet S, Moneret-Vautrin DA, Bihain BE. Mammalian meat-induced anaphylaxis: clinical relevance of anti-galactose-alpha-1,3-galactose IgE confirmed by means of skin tests to cetuximab. *J Allergy Clin Immunol* 2009; 124(3):603–605.
51. Shreffler WG, Beyer K, Chu TH, Burks AW, Sampson HA. Microarray immunoassay: association of clinical history, in vitro IgE function, and heterogeneity of allergenic peanut epitopes. *J Allergy Clin Immunol* 2004; 113(4):776–782.
52. Astier C, Morisset M, Roitel O, et al. Predictive value of skin prick tests using recombinant allergens for diagnosis of peanut allergy. *J Allergy Clin Immunol* 2006; 118(1):250–256.
53. Schocker F, Luttkopf D, Scheurer S, et al. Recombinant lipid transfer protein Cor a 8 from hazelnut: a new tool for in vitro diagnosis of potentially severe hazelnut allergy. *J Allergy Clin Immunol* 2004; 113(1):141–147.
54. Asero R, Jimeno L, Barber D. Component-resolved diagnosis of plant food allergy by SPT. *Eur Ann Allergy Clin Immunol* 2008; 40(4):115–121.
55. Nowak-Wegrzyn A, Assa'ad AH, Bahna SL, Bock SA, Sicherer SH, Teuber SS. Work Group report: oral food challenge testing. *J Allergy Clin Immunol* 2009; 123(6 Suppl.):S365–S383.
56. American College of Allergy, Asthma, & Immunology. Food allergy: a practice parameter. *Ann Allergy Asthma Immunol* 2006; 96(3 Suppl. 2):S1–S68.
57. Kelso JM, Bardina L, Beyer K. Allergy to canned tuna. *J Allergy Clin Immunol* 2003; 111(4):901.
58. Chatterjee U, Mondal G, Chakraborti P, Patra HK, Chatterjee BP. Changes in the allergenicity during different preparations of Pomfret, Hilsa, Bhetki and mackerel fish as illustrated by enzyme-linked immunosorbent assay and immunoblotting. *Int Arch Allergy Immunol* 2006; 141(1):1–10.
59. Untersmayr E, Poulsen LK, Platzer MH, et al. The effects of gastric digestion on codfish allergenicity. *J Allergy Clin Immunol* 2005; 115(2):377–382.
60. Lim DL, Neo KH, Goh DL, Shek LP, Lee BW. Missing parvalbumin: implications in diagnostic testing for tuna allergy. *J Allergy Clin Immunol* 2005; 115(4):874–875.
61. Kobayashi A, Tanaka H, Hamada Y, Ishizaki S, Nagashima Y, Shiomi K. Comparison of allergenicity and allergens between fish white and dark muscles. *Allergy* 2006; 61(3):357–363.
62. Asturias JA, Eraso E, Moneo I, Martinez A. Is tropomyosin an allergen in Anisakis? *Allergy* 2000; 55(9):898–899.
63. Sastre J, Lluch-Bernal M, Quirce S, et al. A double-blind, placebo-controlled oral challenge study with lyophilized larvae and antigen of the fish parasite, Anisakis simplex. *Allergy* 2000; 55(6):560–564.
64. Baeza ML, Rodriguez A, Matheu V, et al. Characterization of allergens secreted by Anisakis simplex parasite: clinical relevance in comparison with somatic allergens. *Clin Exp Allergy* 2004; 34(2):296–302.
65. Daschner A, Pascual CY. Anisakis simplex: sensitization and clinical allergy. *Curr Opin Allergy Clin Immunol* 2005; 5(3):281–285.
66. Sicherer SH, Sampson HA. Food hypersensitivity and atopic dermatitis: pathophysiology, epidemiology, diagnosis, and management. *J Allergy Clin Immunol* 1999; 104(3 Pt. 2):S114–S122.
67. Flinterman AE, Knulst AC, Meijer Y, Bruijnzeel-Koomen CA, Pasmans SG. Acute allergic reactions in children with AEDS after prolonged cow's milk elimination diets. *Allergy* 2006; 61(3):370–374.
68. David TJ. Anaphylactic shock during elimination diets for severe atopic dermatitis. *Arch Dis Child* 1984; 59:983–986.
69. Roesler TA, Barry PC, Bock SA. Factitious food allergy and failure to thrive. *Arch Pediatr Adolesc Med* 1994; 148(11):1150–1155.
70. Sicherer SH, Noone SA, Muñoz-Furlong A. The impact of childhood food allergy on quality of life. *Ann Allergy Asthma Immunol* 2001; 87(6):461–464.

71. Mankad VS, Williams LW, Lee LA, LaBelle GS, Anstrom KJ, Burks AW. Safety of open food challenges in the office setting. *Ann Allergy Asthma Immunol* 2008; 100(5):469–474.
72. Sicherer SH. Food allergy: when and how to perform oral food challenges. *Pediatr Allergy Immunol* 1999; 10(4):226–234.
73. Bock SA, Sampson HA, Atkins FM, et al. Double-blind, placebo-controlled food challenge (DBPCFC) as an office procedure: a manual. *J Allergy Clin Immunol* 1988; 82:986–997.
74. Niggemann B, Rolinck-Werninghaus C, Mehl A, Binder C, Ziegert M, Beyer K. Controlled oral food challenges in children—when indicated, when superfluous? *Allergy* 2005; 60(7):865–870.
75. Bindslev-Jensen C. Standardization of double-blind, placebo-controlled food challenges. *Allergy* 2001; 56(Suppl. 67):75–77.
76. Caffarelli C, Petroccione T. False-negative food challenges in children with suspected food allergy. *Lancet* 2001; 358(9296):1871–1872.
77. Sampson HA. Use of food-challenge tests in children. *Lancet* 2001; 358(9296):1832–1833.
78. Briggs D, Aspinall L, Dickens A, Bindslev-Jensen C. Statistical model for assessing the proportion of subjects with subjective sensitisations in adverse reactions to foods. *Allergy* 2001; 56(Suppl. 67):83–85.
79. Chinchilli VM, Fisher L, Craig TJ. Statistical issues in clinical trials that involve the double-blind, placebo-controlled food challenge. *J Allergy Clin Immunol* 2005; 115(3):592–597.

22 Atopy Patch Testing for Food Allergies

Von Ta & Kari Nadeau
Division of Immunology and Allergy, Stanford Medical School, Stanford, CA, USA

Key Concepts

- In addition to specific serum IgE and skin prick test (SPT), atopy patch testing (APT) may be helpful in unclear and discrepant diagnostic situations.
- APT represents a possible manner of diagnosing delayed type allergic reactions.
- Clinical relevance of a positive APT is still to be proven by standardized outcome definitions.
- APT has been applied to both IgE associated (atopic dermatitis and allergic eosinophilic esophagitis) and non-IgE associated conditions (food protein-induced enterocolitis syndrome (FPIES)).
- The diagnostic gold standard for suspected food allergy is still a double-blinded placebo-controlled oral food challenge (DBPCFC).

Introduction

Atopy patch testing (APT) for food is another type of skin testing that involves the topical application of a food-containing solution to the skin for 48 and 72 hours, and aims to elicit cutaneous cell-mediated immune responses after prolonged skin contact with the allergens. APT with food allergens may be useful in cases of moderate or severe persistent atopic eczema with unknown trigger factors. APT may identify patients with food sensitivities despite negative specific IgE; however, clinical history and symptoms should be used in conjunction with any APT test result before a change in management occurs for the patient. There are currently no standardized reagents, application methods, or guidelines for interpretation. In the diagnosis of non-IgE mediated food allergy, further trials are needed to determine the role of APT.

History

The first experimental study on patch testing was published in 1937 by Rostenberg and Sulzberger, and in 1982, Mitchell et al. demonstrated that skin reactions occurred in patients with atopic dermatitis after applying aeroallergens or food allergens [1]. A Finnish group later reported a possible role for APT in food allergy [2]. The authors proposed that skin prick test (SPT) and specific IgE might reflect early clinical reactions to the offending food (clinical symptoms within 2 hours), while APT might have a predictive capacity for late-phase clinical reactions during a double-blinded placebo-controlled oral food challenge (DBPCFC) [2–5].

A general problem is that prior studies on APT with food have mostly been studied in infants and children since food allergy plays a larger role in this age group. There is no age limit for carrying out APT and many studies have been undertaken on infants from the age of 3 months [6], but the value of APT seems to be highest in children less than 2 years old [7].

History: atopic dermatitis

When standard treatment with topical steroid and emollients become ineffective in treating atopic dermatitis, food allergy needs to be ruled out as a possible potentiating cause. Eczema can be worsened by ingestion of certain foods, and identification of the offending allergen is important since unnecessary elimination of certain foods can be harmful to a child's health [8]. APT may prevent these unnecessary restricted diets among children with atopic dermatitis [9].

Food Allergy: Adverse Reactions to Foods and Food Additives, Fifth Edition. Edited by Dean D Metcalfe, Hugh A Sampson, Ronald A Simon and Gideon Lack.

APT has been described as a method of high sensitivity and specificity in diagnosing delayed onset reactions such as atopic dermatitis unlike SPT, which diagnoses immediate food hypersensitivity. There is clear correlation between a positive APT and delayed type, and between a positive SPT and immediate type of reactions to food. This is evident in a study where 11% of the subjects with atopic dermatitis had an isolated immediate reaction to food, while 49% had a delayed type reaction [10]. In another study, APT results were positive in 89% of children with delayed-onset reactions, despite frequently negative SPT responses [2].

Specific IgE, SPT, and APT do not have power alone, but the combination enables better understanding of atopic dermatitis. One of the early studies by Niggemann et al. examined the utility of APT in children with atopic dermatitis by comparing specific IgE, SPT, and APT diagnostic methods to DBPCFC. The APT was positive in 55% of patients with a positive DBPCFC, whereas specific IgE was positive in 85%. However, in 21 patients who experienced delayed symptoms, APT was superior to specific IgE and SPT [9]. Another study found that combining these diagnostic tests reduced the need for oral food challenges in children with atopic dermatitis [11]. Specifically, combining the APT with specific IgE test gave values of 100% for cow milk and 94% for hen egg [11]. Another study showed that sensitivity of late-phase clinical reactions was 76% and specificity was 95% for the APT, corresponding values for the SPT were 58% and 70%, and for the specific IgE were 71% and 29%, respectively [9]. Other studies investigating the APT with cow milk [12,13], wheat [14], and peanut [15] reported similar findings.

APT is found to be a more sensitive method than SPT in diagnosing cow milk allergy in children under 2 years of age with atopic dermatitis, with 60% sensitivity and 97% specificity for the APT versus 41% and 99% for the SPT, thus confirming the role of the APT in increasing the chances of early detection of food allergy in infants [12, 16]. With regard to peanut allergy, SPT reactivity proved to be higher in patients older than 12 years old whereas APT reactivity for peanut allergy was more frequent and sensitive in children younger than 6 years old [15]. Thus, APT for peanuts represents a useful integration of standard testing modality for the diagnosis of peanut allergy in atopic dermatitis patients. Another study also found APT specificity to be higher than that for specific IgE or SPT for all four allergens evaluated: hen egg, cow milk, wheat, and soy [17]. The study included 437 children of whom 90% had atopic dermatitis. SPT, specific IgE, and APT reactions were evaluated, and the authors also noted that SPT was not only unpleasant for younger children, but eczematous involvement of the test area also made SPT testing challenging in children with atopic dermatitis. Even though the benefits of SPT include instant results and low cost, the specificity of APT was higher [17]. Similarly, a study by Stromberg et al. found APT to be a more statically significant sensitive test than SPT in diagnosing wheat and rye [7].

Not all studies concur with the findings above. Studies such as that by Vanto, concluded that APT added only a small predictive value to the standard SPT and specific IgE in diagnosing suspected food-related symptoms [17]. A prospective clinical study that evaluated the value of APT in 135 children less than 3 years old with atopic dermatitis also could not find enough support for the current addition of APT to the standardized allergy workup for this age group [18]. Despite the discordance, a majority of the studies support the use of APT to significantly increase the chances of early detection of food allergy in infants [12,13, 19]. Thus, APT can significantly enhance accuracy in diagnosing food allergy in young children with atopic dermatitis and is of help in identifying elimination diets.

APT is time consuming and demands a highly experienced evaluator. For daily clinical practice, APT does not seem to add enough information to justify its routine inclusion in the diagnostic workup of suspected food-related symptoms [17]. The role of APT in clinical practice also remains controversial because it is not standardized. While APT has a higher sensitivity and specificity for indentifying foods that cause delayed reactions, it is not proposed as a single screening test in patients with atopic dermatitis and should be used in addition to SPT and specific IgE—these results should be confirmed with a DBPCFC. In patients with atopic eczema, they often will have a negative SPT and specific IgE, but will have a positive APT [12]; further research studies are needed to determine the usefulness of SPT in atopic dermatitis.

History: eosinophilic esophagitis

Eosinophilic esophagitis is increasing in incidence in the United States and Australia [20–24]. APT has been increasingly recognized as a diagnostic method for children with eosinophilic esophagitis. Current data on APT indicate 79% sensitivity and 91% specificity in subjects with gastrointestinal symptoms without skin involvement. APT has a higher sensitivity than SPT, which is consistent with the predominant delayed type of allergy [25].

One study compared the utility of SPT and APT. With the use of current positive predictive values and sensitivity for all the foods, combining SPT and APT correctly identified the correct diet in 70% of the population with resolution of symptoms and biopsy specimens [20]. Other studies also validated the use of APT, particularly in combination with SPT; it correctly identifies diets for subjects and results in the resolution of symptoms and normalization on esophageal biopsies in more than 95% of the patients [22–24].

The sensitivity of APT for diagnosing eosinophilic esophagitis increased significantly when fresh foods were used for testing rather than commercial food extracts [21]. The specificity of APT was high regardless of the preparation used for testing. The results of APT with fresh food versus commercial food extract for cow milk, and hen egg were 64% versus 6%, and 84% versus 5% respectively.

In one study, 26 children with biopsy-proven eosinophilic esophagitis were investigated by SPT and APT and a 6-week elimination diet was initiated on the basis of these results. Out of the 26 children, 8 showed full resolution of symptoms and 6 showed partial resolution [20]. The authors concluded that the combination of SPT and APT could identify potential causative foods that might contribute to the pathogenesis of eosinophilic esophagitis [20]. The same group reported in a follow-up study in 146 patients with biopsy proven eosinophilic esophagitis that symptoms improved after elimination diets directed by APT and SPT with cow milk, hen egg, and soy [26]. Some studies showed differing results. One study found that combining SPT and APT resulted in a high success rate for food elimination in eosinophilic esophagitis with the exception of milk [27]. The APT negative predictive value was 55%, unacceptably low, suggesting that a negative test to milk on APT did not rule out milk triggering eosinophilic esophagitis [27]. The study showed that up to 20% of the foods involved for each episode would not have been identified if APT was not used [28]. APT in eosinophilic esophagitis seems to be, not only a low cost method, but also very reliable to examine food allergies in adult eosinophilic esophagitis patients.

History: food protein-induced enterocolitis syndrome

Food protein-induced enterocolitis syndrome (FPIES) is thought to be due to a non-IgE mediated food allergy syndrome where traditional allergy testing is not useful because tests for specific IgE and SPT are routinely negative. The only method to confirm the diagnosis of FPIES is an oral challenge, which is not without risks. In a study by Fogg, they evaluated whether APT accurately predicted the results of the oral challenge. Twenty-eight children suspected of food allergy related gastrointestinal symptoms underwent diagnostic SPT, serum IgE, APT, and oral food challenge [29]. The children were divided into two groups: children with cow milk allergy and children without cow milk allergy. The study showed that APT was accurate in diagnosing delayed type reactions in children with gastrointestinal symptoms [30]. A positive APT was demonstrated in 70% of children with cow milk allergy in comparison with 9.1% of children with negative results of oral food challenge. Of the 16 cases of FPIES, the APT was positive to the suspected food; however, the APT was positive in five instances where the oral food challenge was negative. Importantly, there were no patients with a negative APT that had FPIES.

However, there are several limitations to this study; one of which has been referred to multiple times is that food allergens APT is not currently a standardized test. This makes performance and interpretation of the test user dependent. Another critique of this study is that the oral food challenges were not blinded. While DBPCFC is ideal, it was thought that oral challenges were sufficient to diagnose FPIES as these symptoms are not subjective [31]. Based on the results of this study, APT is recommended in patients who have a clinical history suggestive of FPIES, and if APT is negative, an oral food challenge is to be completed.

Pathogenic mechanisms

APT has received interest in recent years as a possible model for studying the pathogenic mechanism of atopic dermatitis. The pathogenic mechanism involved in the APT has not yet been studied in detail. The close macroscopic and microscopic similarities between the specimens from APT sites and lesioned skin of patients with atopic dermatitis indicate that APT may be a valid model to study allergic inflammation in atopic dermatitis [16]. In particular, in food-sensitive atopic dermatitis, T-cells play an important role as reported in recent studies [32, 33]. In line with the previous findings, earlier clinical investigations indicate that positive APTs (with T-cell infiltration of the skin) correlate with clinical late-phase responses [9]. Published data indicate that patients with atopic eczema and late-phase reaction have elevated levels of interleukin, tumor necrosis factor-alpha, interferon gamma.

Another study showed that APT reactions are associated with T-lymphocyte-mediated allergen-specific immune responses [34]. A recent investigation demonstrated that the chemokine pattern (CXCR3 activating chemokines) in skin biopsies can be used to distinguish between allergic and irritant patch test reactions [6].

Performance method

The APT is performed epicutaneously, but instead of using typical type IV allergens (such as metals or perfumes), typical immediate type I allergens (aeroallergens or foods) are used. Over the years, several technical procedures aimed to increase the permeability of the tested skin have also been explored. These procedures include sodium lauryl sulfate application, stripping and abrasion, but these procedures were abandoned as they proved unnecessary and difficult to standardize [35]. Today, APT is performed on non-lesioned, untreated skin, usually the back [9].

The European Task Force on Atopic Dermatitis (ETFAD) developed a standardized APT technique. APT is carried out in a similar manner to conventional patch tests. Twelve millimeter aluminum cups are used to cover filter paper on which one drop (50 mL) of the foodstuff preparation has been applied [36]. Even though the ETFAD and Niggemann et al. advise the use of a large cup, 12 mm for APT with food even in infants and small children [37], some investigators find good correlation between APT results using 8 mm cups. The lack of standardization limits the usefulness of APT, and DBPCFC remains the gold standard for diagnosing food allergy [38].

Several commercial preparations are available but less so for food allergens [39]. In a study by Niggemann et al., the food allergens tested were diluted at 1/10, in order to eliminate false positives induced by irritation. The authors found as many positive reactions with the APT diluted at 10% as for the nondiluted APT, but with stronger reactions for the latter. The raw food items were placed on undiluted blotting paper because native fresh foods are preferred over food extracts. For aeroallergens, commercially available extracts may be used; in most studies petrolatum is used as a vehicle. While the use of a negative control, for example saline, is recommended, a positive control would be helpful to use in a standard method.

More recently, an atopy patch test for cow's milk has been developed in a ready-to-use form and is available in pharmacies (Diallertest). One study compared the ready-to-use APT, the Diallertest, with the Finn Chamber. The study compared the ready-to-use form and involved 49 children who underwent APT testing followed by a milk elimination diet for 4–6 weeks and open cow's milk challenge. The basis of the test relies on the ability to provide to the skin intact protein molecules to be solubilized through the sole sweat secretion. This technique exhibits several advantages compared with the Finn Chamber APT, both in terms of practical ease and standardization. The amount of milk deposited on the patch is constant and easily measurable. When applied, the device delivers to the skin the total amount of milk deposited on the patch, whereas in any other kind of testing, the exact amount of food delivered to the skin is difficult to assess. For example, when present in the form of pureed food, only a part of the food comes in close contact with the skin, and when the food is deposited on a blotting paper, a large amount remains inside the paper. It is likely that standardization of APTs requires not only standardizing the amount of antigen deposited in the device but also the amount of antigen able to reach the reactive cells. A positive result was seen in 22 (44.8%) versus 13 (26.5%) patients with the ready-to-use and the comparator APTs, respectively. The ready-to-use APT exhibited a good sensitivity and specificity, with no side effects [5] but its sensitivity seemed to be higher [5]. Diallertest exhibited a significantly higher sensitivity (76% versus 44%) and test accuracy (82% versus 63%) than the Finn Chamber. Several studies confirm the high sensitivity and specificity for APT, 79% and 91%, respectively [5, 25, 30].

Table 22.1 Assessment of the APT.

Allergic	Irritative
Jagged margin	Sharp margin
Marked erythema	No or mild erythema
Papules, infiltration	Bulla, necrosis
Crescendo phenomenon	Decrescendo phenomenon
Persistent reaction	Short duration

Interpretation of APT

The interpretation of an APT on food allergens is still subjective and not standardized. The cups are removed at the end of the 48-hour occlusion period, and 24 hours later reactions are classified as positive or negative (Table 22.1). Unfortunately, the reading of the APT is highly dependent on the experience of the evaluator.

The application sites should be checked after 15 minutes for immediate local reactions. Especially with egg, contact urticaria may occur and uncomfortable pruritus may make it necessary to stop the APT. Apart from local urticaria (Table 22.1), side effects are rare; systemic side effects have not been reported.

One study proposed a standardized interpretation of the APT after having investigated the sensitivity, specificity, and predictive values for each skin sign in relation to the oral food challenge outcome [40]. The authors classify the APT reaction as positive if there is erythema plus clear infiltration/papules [40]. A further important criterion is the so-called "crescendo" or "decrescendo" reaction: while an allergic site shows a "crescendo" of erythema and infiltration, that is increasing erythema and infiltration at the test site, a skin irritation response characteristically tends to clear between 48 and 72 hours.

The reading of the APT should result in a clear yes or no answer. A grading system does not seem to be helpful in daily decisions. Table 22.2 shows the grading system as defined by the ETFAD. Likewise, Heine et al. also published

Table 22.2 European Task Force on Atopic Dermatitis (ETFAD) grading for atopy patchy test reading.

–	Negative
?	Only erythema, questionable
+	Erythema, infiltration
++	Erythema, few papules (up to 3)
+++	Erythema, papules from 4 to < many
++++	Erythema, many or spreading papules
+++++	Erythema, vesicles

Source: From Reference 41.

Table 22.3 Conditions necessary before carrying out APT.

No current outbreak of the disease, no pregnancy
No application of corticosteroids on the APT site for the previous 7 days
No phototherapy treatment on the APT site for the previous 4 weeks
No oral corticosteroids
No cyclosporine or oral tacrolimus
No antihistamine

Source: From References 4 and 36.

that the number of papule formation and skin duration were positive predictors for food allergy. In fact, they found that seven or more papules with skin duration were 100% specific and predictive for predicting the outcome of DBPCFC [40]. Only reactions which are palpable and infiltrated are classed as positive, according to the international criteria for reading patch tests, amended by the ETFAD (Table 22.2) [42]. Reactions in babies and children are generally more severe than those of adults because their thinner skin increases the penetration of allergens.

The occurrence of secondary effects during APT is infrequent (7.9% of cases) [20]. The reactions observed are moderate and most often localized to the site of application of the APT. One study aimed to examine the reproducibility of APT results. The low reproducibility rate of APT results and the poor intertest agreement using allergens from different suppliers show that much work remains to make the APT a reliable tool. The reproducibility rate was 56.3% [43].

Avoidance prior to APT

A few studies have investigated the possible modulation of the APT by an anti-inflammatory skin treatment: both glucocorticosteroids and tar reduce the macroscopic outcome of the APT reaction and the influx of inflammatory cells [44]. The practical consequence is that the APT should be performed on skin with no previous local treatment. No information is available concerning the implications of treatment with oral antihistamines, although no influence would be expected on the basis of the pathogenic mechanisms of the T-cell-mediated late-phase reaction of the APT, but erythema may be decreased. Therefore, antihistamines should be withdrawn at least 72 hours prior to the APT (Table 22.3).

The prior precautions concerning concomitant treatments are summarized in Table 22.3 [4]. The influence of antihistamines on APT results has not been clearly determined, but stopping their use at least 72 hours before carrying out the tests is recommended [36].

Unanswered questions

Despite some advances in the efforts to standardize the APT [19], there are still several unanswered questions [36]. While it could be shown that 12-mm cups are superior to 6-mm cups [45], that the occlusion time of 48 hours is preferable to 24 hours [46], and that age (within childhood) does seem to play an important role [47], it is not clear whether the APT works only in children with atopic dermatitis or also in other clinical conditions. Unpublished data point to a considerably higher sensitivity in children with atopic dermatitis compared with those without. Furthermore, it is not known whether APT is able to predict the development of tolerance after a period of elimination of the corresponding food. In regards to FPIES, an important question for future studies is whether APT reverts to negative when a patient outgrows FPIES. Finally, it is unclear whether the APT itself can lead to sensitization of children who would not otherwise be sensitized.

Conclusion

A positive SPT seems to reflect early reactions to food challenges [11], whereas the APT has a possible diagnostic efficacy for late-phase clinical reactions [11]. To date, APT with foods is not well standardized and various methods in preparing the test materials are likely to cause conflicting results. Until validation data are available, APT testing should be used with other clinical diagnostic tests. Further research is needed to determine the exact role of APT in diagnosing food allergic disorders.

References

1. Mitchell E, Chapman M, Pope F, et al. Basophils in allergen-induced patch test sites in atopic dermatitis. *Lancet* 1982; 1:127–130.
2. Isolauri E, Turjanmaa K. Combined skin prick and patch testing enhances identification of food allergy in infants with atopic dermatitis. *J Allergy Clin Immunol* 1996; 97:9–15.
3. Kekki OM, Turjanmaa K, Isolauri E. Differences in skin-prick and patch-test reactivity are related to the heterogeneity of atopic eczema in infants. *Allergy* 1997; 52:755–759.
4. Breuer K, Heratizadeh A, Wulf A, et al. Late eczematous reactions to food in children with atopic dermatitis. *Clin Exp Allergy* 2004; 34:817–824.
5. Kalach N, Soulaines P, de Boissieu D, et al. A pilot study of the usefulness and safety of a ready to use atopy patch test versus a comparator during cow's milk allergy in children. *J Allergy Clin Immunol* 2005; 116:1321–1326.
6. Flier J, Boorsma DM, Bruynzeel DP, et al. The CXCR3 activating chemokines IP-10, Mig, and IP-9 are expressed in allergic but not in irritant patch test reactions. *J Invest Dermatol* 1999; 113:574–578.
7. Stromberg L. Diagnostic accuracy of the atopy patch test and skin-prick test for the diagnosis of food allergy in young children with atopic eczema/dermatitis syndrome. *Acta Paediatr* 2002; 91:1044.

8. Jesenak M, Banovcin P. Atopy patch test in diagnosis of food allergy in children with atopic dermatitis. *Acta Medica* 2006; 49:199–201.
9. Niggemann B, Reibel S, Wahn U. The atopy patch test (APT)—a useful tool for the diagnosis of food allergy in children with atopic dermatitis. *Allergy* 2000; 55:281–285.
10. Rokaite R, Labanauskas L, Vaideliene L. Role of the skin patch test in diagnosing food allergy in children with atópica dermatitis. *Medicina* 2004; 40:1081–1087.
11. Roehr C, Reibel S, Ziegert M, et al. Atopy patch test together with level of specific IgE reduces the need for oral food challenges in children with atopic dermatitis. *J Allergy Clin Immunol* 2001; 107:548–553.
12. Majamaa H, Moisio P, Holm K, et al. Cow's milk allergy: diagnostic accuracy of skin prick and patch tests and specific IgE. *Allergy* 1999; 54:346–351.
13. Vanto T, Juntunen-Backman K, Kalimo K, et al. The patch test, skin prick test, and serum milk-specific IgE as diagnostic tools in cow's milk allergy in infants. *Allergy* 1999; 54:837–842.
14. Majamaa H, Moisio P, Holm K, Turjanmaa K. Wheat allergy: diagnostic accuracy of skin and patch test and specific IgE. *Allergy* 1999; 54:851–856.
15. Seidenari S, Giusti F, Bertoni L, Mantovani L. Combined skin prick and patch testing enhances identification of peanut-allergic patients with atopic dermatitis. *Allergy* 2003; 58:495–499.
16. Langeveld-Wildschut EG, Thepen T, Bihari IC, et al. Evaluation of the atopy patch test and the cutaneous late-phase reaction as relevant models for the study of allergic inflammation in patients with atopic eczema. *J Allergy Clin Immunol* 1996; 98:1019–1027.
17. Mehl A, Rolinck-Werninghaus C, Staden U, et al. The atopy patch test in the diagnostic work-up of suspected food related symptoms in children. *J Allergy Clin Immunol* 2006; 118:923–929.
18. Devillers A, de Waard-van der Spek F, Mulder P, et al. Delayed and immediate type reaction in the atopy patch test with food allergens in young children with atopic dermatitis. *Pediatr Allergy Immunol* 2009; 20:53–58.
19. Turjanmaa K, Darsow U, Niggemann B, et al. Present status of the atopy patch test. *Allergy* 2006; 61:1377–1384.
20. Spergel JM, Brown-Whitehorn T, Beausoleil JL, et al. The use of skin prick tests and patch tests to identify causative foods in eosinophil esophagitis. *J Allergy Clin Immunol* 2007; 119:509–511.
21. Canani RB, Ruotolo S, Auricchio L, et al. Diagnostic accuracy of the atopy patch test in children with food allergy-related gastrointestinal symptoms. *Allergy* 2007; 62:738–743.
22. Liacouras C, Spergel J, Ruchelli E et al. Eosinophilic esophagitis: a 10 year experience in 381 children. *Clin Gastroenterol Hepatol* 2005; 3:1198–1206.
23. Gupte A, Draganov P. Eosinophilic esophagitis. *World J Gastroenterol* 2009; 15:17–24.
24. Asaa'd A. Eosinophilic gastrointestinal disorders. *Allergy Asthma Proc* 2009; 30:17–22.
25. De Boissieu D, Waguet JC, Dupont C. The atopy patch test for detection of cow's milk allergy with digestive symptoms. *J Pediatr* 2003; 142:203–205.
26. Spergel JM, Andrews T, Brown-Whitehorn TF, et al. Treatment of eosinophilic esophagitis with specific food elimination diet directed by a combination of skin prick and patch tests. *Ann Allergy Asthma Immunol* 2005; 95:336–343.
27. Spergel J, Brown-Whitehorn T, Beausoleil J, et al. Predictive values for skin prick test and atopy patch test for eosinophilic esophagitis. *J Allergy Clin Immunol* 2007; 119:509–511.
28. Tobledo M, Castellano A, Cimbollek S, et al. Defining the role of food allergy in a population of adult patients with eosinophilic esophagitis. *Inflamm and Allergy* 2010; 9:257–262.
29. Fogg MI, Brown-Whitehorn TA, Pawlowski NA, Spergel JM. Atopy patch test for the diagnosis of food protein-induced enterocolitis syndrome. *Pediatr Allergy Immunol* 2006; 17:351–355.
30. Cudowska B, Kaczmarski M. Atopy patch test in the diagnosis of food allergy in children with gastrointestinal symptoms. *Advances in Medical Sciences* 2010; 55:153–160.
31. Niggemann B, Rolinck-Werninghaus C, Mehl A, et al. Controlled oral food challenges in children-when indicated, when superfluous? *Allergy* 2005; 60:865–870.
32. Beyer K, Niggemann B, Nasert S, et al. Severe allergic reactions to foods are predicted by increases of CD41CD451RO1 T cells and loss of L-selectin expression. *J Allergy Clin Immunol* 1997; 99:522–529.
33. Beyer K, Renz H, Wahn U, Niggemann B. Changes in blood leucocyte distribution during double-blind, placebo-controlled food challenges in children with atopic dermatitis and suspected food allergy. *Int Arch Allergy Immunol* 1998; 116:110–115.
34. Wistokat-Wülfing A, Schmidt P, Darsow U, et al. Atopy patch test reactions are associated with T lymphocyte-mediated allergen-specific immune responses in atopic dermatitis. *Clin Exp Allergy* 1999; 29:513–521.
35. Heinemann C, Schliemann-Willers S, Kelterer D, et al. The atopy patch test-reproducibility and comparison of different evaluation methods. *Allergy* 2002; 57:641–645.
36. Niggemann B. Evolving role of the atopy patch test in the diagnosis of food allergy. *Curr Opin Allergy Clin Immunol* 2002; 2:253–256.
37. Niggemann B. The role of the atopy patch test (APT) in diagnosis of food allergy in infants and children with atopic dermatitis. *Pediatr Allergy Immunol* 2001; 12 Suppl. 14:37–40.
38. Bindslev-Jensen C, Ballmer-Weber BK, Bengtsson U, et al.; European Academy of Allergology and Clinical Immunology. Standardization of food challenges in patients with immediate reactions to foods—position paper from the European Academy of Allergology and Clinical Immunology. *Allergy* 2004; 59(7):690–697.
39. Nosbaum A, Hennino A, Berard F, et al. Patch testing in atopic dermatitis patients. *Eur J Dermatol* 2010; 20:563–566.
40. Heine R, Verstege A, Mehl A, et al. Proposal for a standardized interpretation of the atopy patch test in children with atopic dermatitis and suspected food allergy. *Pediatr Allergy Immunol* 2006; 17:213–217.
41. Darsow U, Laifaoui J, Kerschenlohr K, et al. The prevalence of positive reactions in the atopy patch test with aeroallergens and food allergens in subjects with atopic eczema: a European multicenter study. *Allergy* 2004; 59:1318–1325.

42. Keskin O, Tuncer A, Adaliogly G, et al. Evaluation of the utility of atopy patch testing, skin prick testing, and total and specific IgE assays in the diagnosis of cow's milk allergy. *Ann Allergy Asthma Immunol* 2005; 94:553–560.
43. Turjanmaa K, Darsow U, Niggemann B, Rancé F, Vanto T, Werfel T. EAACI/GA2LEN position paper: present status of the atopy patch test. *Allergy* 2006; 61:1377–1384.
44. Langeveld-Wildschut EG, Riedl H, Thepen T, et al. Modulation of the atopy patch test reaction by topical corticosteroids and tar. *J Allergy Clin Immunol* 2000; 106:737–743.
45. Niggemann B, Ziegert M, Reibel S. Importance of chamber size for the outcome of atopy patch testing in children with atopic dermatitis and food allergy. *J Allergy Clin Immunol* 2002; 110:515–516.
46. Rancé F. What is the optimal occlusion time for the atopy patch test in the diagnosis of food allergies in children with atopic dermatitis? *Pediatr Allergy Immunol* 2004; 15:93–96.
47. Perackis K, Celik-Bilgili S, Staden U, et al. Influence of age on the outcome of the atopy patch test with food in children with atopic dermatitis. *J Allergy Clin Immunol* 2003; 112:625–627.

23 Elimination Diets and Oral Food Challenges

Scott H. Sicherer

Division of Allergy and Immunology, Department of Pediatrics, Icahn School of Medicine at Mount Sinai, New York, USA

Key Concepts

- Diagnostic elimination diets are undertaken to provide presumptive evidence that disorders or symptoms are food-responsive.
- Prolonged diagnostic elimination diets may carry risks of nutritional deficiencies or loss of a state of desensitization.
- The oral food challenge, in particular when double-blind and placebo-controlled, is the most definitive modality available to diagnose a food-related illness.
- An oral food challenge may induce anaphylaxis.
- Decisions about when and how to undertake an oral food challenge requires consideration of benefits (nutritional, social) and risks.
- Performance of an oral food challenge requires preparation and consideration concerning dosing, when to stop a challenge and treat a reaction, and how to instruct patients about introducing or avoiding a food following a challenge.

Introduction

The oral food challenge (OFC) is a definitive diagnostic test used to determine if a food is tolerated. The double-blind, placebo-controlled OFC (DBPCFC) is considered the "gold standard" of diagnosis [1–3]. The OFC can be performed to evaluate any type of an adverse reaction, and so it is valid for determination of food allergy, intolerance, and for pharmacologic reactions to foods. Steps taken to determine the need for an OFC are explained in Chapters 21 and 24. Special considerations regarding food challenges for food protein-induced enterocolitis syndrome (FPIES) are described in Chapter 18 and for adverse reactions to food additives in Chapter 28. Here, the technique of performing an OFC will be described, including a review of risks and benefits, selection of challenge location, challenge procedures, challenge preparation, dosing, monitoring, and aftercare. OFCs typically follow a period of dietary elimination undertaken either as treatment of a known or likely allergy, or as a diagnostic trial to determine if a condition is food-responsive. Procedural issues in undertaking a diagnostic elimination diets will be described here as well.

Historical background

The typical diet includes several meals and snacks distributed throughout the day. Since the frequency of food intake is high, any sudden adverse physiological event or chronic illness could incorrectly be ascribed to food. Once a patient makes an erroneous association between a food and a symptom, it may be difficult to dissuade the patient from their notion of cause and effect. In a paper published in 1950, Graham and colleagues [4] performed experiments that would be difficult to undertake today for ethical reasons. Subjects with strong beliefs regarding their reactions to foods were given water by nasogastric tube, told they were receiving the test food, were given the test food, and advised that the water was being instilled. Reactions to the tests correlated with suggestion. To address subject bias, masked ingestions were introduced by Loveless in several studies in the 1950s [5, 6]. In an accompanying editorial, Lowell [7] emphasized the need for blinded challenges to demonstrate cause–effect relationships in the evaluation of adverse reactions to foods. Charles May is credited with bringing DBPCFCs into routine clinical practice and research use [8]. Today,

Food Allergy: Adverse Reactions to Foods and Food Additives, Fifth Edition. Edited by Dean D Metcalfe, Hugh A Sampson, Ronald A Simon and Gideon Lack.

DBPCFCs are a fundamental tool for research and clinical care. However, for most routine clinical purposes, OFCs can be performed without masking/placebos [1].

Food elimination diets

When food hypersensitivity is under consideration as a cause for a chronic disease such as atopic dermatitis or eosinophilic gastroenteropathy, a diagnostic elimination diet is often required before undertaking OFCs [9, 10]. Another reason for dietary elimination prior to a food challenge may be to avoid a suspected or known trigger of reactions. Conceptually, there are three types of elimination diets (Table 23.1), and the type selected for a particular patient will depend upon the clinical scenario being evaluated. The first type involves the elimination of one or several foods from the diet. This may be the obvious course of action when an isolated ingestion of a food (i.e., peanut) causes a sudden acute reaction and there is a positive test for IgE to the food. However, eliminating one or a few suspected foods from the diet when the diagnosis is not so clear (asthma, atopic dermatitis, chronic urticaria) can be a crucial step in determining if food is causal in the disease process. If symptoms persist, the eliminated food(s) is (are) excluded as a cause of symptoms. The length of trial depends upon the type of symptoms, but 1–6 weeks is usually the time interval required. A brief dietary trial should suffice for disorders with frequent acute reactions, while longer trials may be required to allow chronic inflammation to subside.

Table 23.1 Types of elimination diets used to evaluate the role of adverse food reactions in chronic disease.

Diet	Description/target	Example
Specific food(s)	**1.** Targeted diet to one or several suspected foods **2.** May be therapeutically necessary as final treatment	Elimination of egg in toddler with atopic dermatitis Elimination of food dyes and preservatives in child with chronic urticaria
Oligoantigenic/ selected foods	Palatable, balanced diet devised according to patient preferences, but eliminating a large group of common or suspected allergens (e.g., egg, milk, peanut, seafood, etc.)	Allow chicken, broccoli, squash, sweet potato, rice, corn, beets, cooked apple and pear, sugar, salt, and vegetable oil for 6 weeks in patient with reflux and atopic dermatitis
Elemental	Amino acid based formula (or, less ideally, an extensive hydrolysate) as sole nutrition	An 8-week trial to evaluate resolution of eosinophilic gastroenteropathy in a child who failed an elimination diet of 12 foods

Table 23.2 Example elimination diet.

Pick one meat	Chicken or lamb
Pick one grain substitute[a]	Corn or rice
Pick three vegetables (cooked)	Broccoli, sweet potato[a], carrot, squash, string bean
Pick three fruits	Apple, pear, peach, plum, banana
Consider supplement	"Complete" hypoallergenic formula

[a]Allows for variety of textures (breads, pastas, sweet potato chips/mashed, pancakes)

The second type of diet consists of eliminating a larger number of foods suspected as causing a chronic problem (usually including those that are common epidemiologically as causes of food-allergic reactions as described above) and possibly providing the patient with a list of "allowed foods." This "oligoantigenic" diet is useful for evaluation of chronic disorders when a larger number of foods are suspected [9]. This approach is relevant for atopic dermatitis or eosinophilic gastroenteropathies. An example of such a diet is given in Table 23.2, but individualization is almost always needed. The advantage of this diet is that a nutritionally balanced, palatable diet is maintained while most possible causal foods are removed. The primary disadvantage is that, if symptoms persist, the cause could still be attributed to foods left in the diet. For finicky eaters, it may be helpful to assess exactly what foods are favorites, and try to allow foods of low risk that are enjoyed by the patient and can be used for meals and snacks.

The most limited type of diet is an elemental diet, in which calories are obtained from an amino acid based formula. A variation is to include a few foods likely to be tolerated (however, this adds the possibility that persistent symptoms are caused by these foods). Unfortunately, except for the most severe disorders that warrant its use [11], this is a severe diet to impose and is extremely difficult to maintain in patients beyond infancy. In extreme cases, nasogastric feeding of the amino acid based formula can be achieved, although most patients can tolerate the taste of these formulas with gradual introduction or the use of flavoring agents provided by the manufacturers. This diet may be required when the diets mentioned above fail to resolve symptoms, but suspicion for food-related illness remains high.

Information concerning strict adherence to the diet must be carefully reviewed. Errors are common [12]. Patients and families must be educated about label reading, cross-contamination, and the fact that the food protein, as opposed to sugar or fat, is the ingredient being eliminated (for example, lactose-free milk contains cow's milk protein) [13]. If there is no improvement with elimination, then the foods eliminated are not likely to be a cause of the complaints. However, it is crucial to ensure that the diet was followed as prescribed before concluding that the result was negative. If resolution of symptoms is achieved, OFCs may be warranted as a next step in identifying which foods from among those eliminated are or are not tolerated.

There are potential risks when undertaking elimination diets. Elimination diets are usually required for just a few weeks and so nutritional deficiencies are not likely but must be considered if elimination is prolonged [14]. If multiple foods were eliminated and symptoms resolved, a patient or family may wish to maintain the prescribed diet. In this case, the nutritional adequacy of the diet, now being followed long term for treatment rather than diagnosis, should be assessed (see Chapter 39). An additional risk is that elimination of foods to which IgE antibodies were identified and which were associated with chronic inflammatory disease, may result in loss of a desensitized state, leading to an acute reaction such as anaphylaxis or urticaria upon reintroduction [15, 16]. The frequency of this occurrence and the length of time of elimination associated with loss of desensitization are unknown. However, the risk should be considered when undertaking prolonged elimination trials. Finally, food avoidance diets carry burdens on social activities, affecting quality of life [17]. Therefore, nutritional, social, and immunologic risks warrant evaluations, including OFCs, to ensure the diet being followed is the least restrictive.

Table 23.3 Examples of considerations in the pre-, intra- and postchallenge periods.

Decision/step	Examples of considerations
Decision to perform OFC	• Risk assessment (history, tests) • Importance of food (social, nutritional, age)
Decision to perform open or masked procedure	• Potential for bias • Past symptom pattern • Past ambiguous result to open challenge
Challenge location (e.g., office, hospital)	• Severity of past reactions • Risk of a positive challenge • Comorbid conditions
Patient preparation	• Informed consent • Motivation and emotional considerations • Comfort with procedure • Healthy for procedure • Stable baseline/quiescent atopic disease • Off interfering medications
Dosing	• Starting dose • Dose progression • Preparation for dosing adjustments during test
Challenge preparation	• Manner of preparation (heating, food matrix) • Preparation of masked challenge, as indicated
Stopping	• Objective symptoms • Persistent subjective symptoms
Postchallenge care	• Positive: Review of avoidance/treatment • Negative: Review of reintroduction

Oral food challenges

OFCs are performed to determine allergy or tolerance to a food for clinical purposes or to monitor response to treatment in research studies. A number of considerations are needed during the pre-, intra- and postchallenge periods (Table 23.3). Chapter 21 defines the parameters under which an OFC is typically undertaken, and the factors that may be considered in deciding upon open, single-, or double-blind and placebo-controlled challenges. Briefly, this process requires consideration of the likelihood that a food will be tolerated, which typically derives from the past history and test results.[3] Additional consideration includes assessment of nutritional, social, and emotional factors that may indicate the need for, or deferral of an oral challenge. The DBPCFC is considered the "gold standard" for diagnosing food allergy, and is often mandatory for research studies [18, 19]. Any test, however, can have limitations. The false-positive and false-negative rates for the DBPCFC, based primarily on studies in children with atopic dermatitis, are 0.7% and 3.2%, respectively [20, 21]. To help exclude false negatives, it has long been suggested to include an open feeding under supervision of a meal-sized portion of the tested food prepared in its usual manner as a follow-up to any negative DBPCFC [8, 22, 23]. When one is evaluating subjective symptoms, there is a greater likelihood that false-positive or false-negative determinations would occur. Increasing the number of challenges (additional placebo and true foods) helps to diminish the possibility of a random association, but this can be a very labor-intensive approach [24, 25]. While the DBPCFC can elucidate the relationship of symptoms to foods, it is not specific for food hypersensitivity. Any adverse reaction to food (intolerance, pharmacologic effect) can potentially be evaluated, so demonstration of an immunological explanation is still needed to label a reaction as a food allergy [2]. Oral challenges are almost the only methodology to adequately evaluate reactions to food additives (coloring and flavoring agents and preservatives) [26, 27]. The same can be said for symptoms not likely to be associated with food allergy (behavior, etc.). The key role of the OFC in management was demonstrated by Fleischer et al. [28], who evaluated 125 children avoiding foods for various reasons. Following OFCs, they were able to return over 85% of the avoided foods to the diet. Unfortunately, it appears that many opportunities to perform OFCs are missed due to aspects of the procedure (time, lack of staff, space), reimbursement, or concerns about safety [29]. Many of these concerns can and should be overcome to address the need for improving patient care through using this procedure [3].

This chapter focuses upon factors pertinent to undertaking the OFC, including presenting the concept to a patient/family and considering risks/benefits, making a risk assessment for choosing an appropriate location for a challenge and selecting a dosing schedule, preparing challenge materials, preparing to treat a reaction, how to monitor for symptoms and to decide when to discontinue a challenge and treat symptoms, and how to instruct families following the procedure.

Discussing the procedure with a patient

The challenge procedure, its risks and benefits must be discussed with the family/patient. As described in Chapter 21, numerous factors are considered including the assessment of the odds for tolerating (a negative test) or reacting to the food (a positive test), the nutritional/social need for the food, and the ability of the patient to cooperate with the challenge. Patients should understand that the test is being done to determine if the food is safe for them to ingest, but also that should they tolerate the food, it should be added to the diet following a successful challenge. Persons who tolerated a food challenge to peanut, for example, but did not incorporate the food into the diet, appear to be at risk to redevelop reactions [30, 31]. Although an OFC may be used to determine threshold of reactivity, it is not routinely performed for clinical purposes in persons expected to react, simply to define a safe threshold (although this may be a research goal or a conclusion based upon the results of a specific OFC). In addition, since challenges are stopped when symptoms develop, they do not reflect severity of reactions from exposures due to accidental ingestion. Risks include anaphylaxis, though no deaths have been reported from physician supervised OFCs. Risks and benefits also include emotional ones. Following review of risks and benefits, informed consent should be documented.

Deciding upon a challenge location

If a challenge is undertaken, a risk assessment is needed to determine a safe location/setting in which to undertake the challenge. In rare circumstances, the food may be administered without physician supervision at home. For example, if vague complaints or ones not usually associated with food allergy (headache, behavioral issues) are being evaluated and there is no risk of an acute anaphylactic reaction, and especially when symptom onset is perceived to be delayed, foods (even in a DBPCFC structure) could be added at home. Similarly, if many foods were eliminated for a chronic, non-IgE-mediated disease and acute reactions are not a concern, adding the previously tolerated food back to the diet at home for observation of recurrence of chronic symptoms is reasonable, because doing so would not likely cause a severe reaction. On the other hand, whenever there is an even remote potential for an acute and/or severe reaction, physician supervision is mandatory.

Except in the uncommon circumstances described previously, OFCs are undertaken under direct medical supervision. A physician or trained health-care worker evaluates symptoms during a challenge. The decision to undertake a supervised challenge includes, but is not limited to, the evaluation of disorders that include a potential for severe reactions. The next issue at hand is whether the challenge is considered of "low risk" and can be done in an office setting, or should be conducted in a location with heightened capabilities for the management of severe anaphylaxis (e.g., hospital, intensive care unit). Whether intravenous access should be established before commencing the challenge must also be considered. The decisions about challenge location and whether to secure intravenous access before commencing a challenge are based upon the same types of data evaluated for the consideration of food allergy in the early diagnostic process: the history (severity of prior reactions, history of reactions to the test food, etc.), prick skin test results, and serum food-specific IgE tests [3]. The higher the probability of a reaction, the more likely a physician may wish to undertake the procedure in a more highly monitored (e.g., hospital) setting. Additional consideration is given to the potential severity of a reaction, should one occur. For consideration in this regard are comorbid conditions (such as asthma), the type of food (e.g., risk of causing a severe reaction), severity of prior reactions, a history of reacting to small doses, etc. In any setting, it must be appreciated that oral challenges can elicit severe, anaphylactic reactions, so the physician must be comfortable with this potential and be prepared with emergency medications and equipment to promptly treat such a reaction no matter where the test is undertaken. In the office setting, such preparations are similar to those recommended in the context of offices that administer allergens by injection for immunotherapy [3, 18].

If the challenge is considered "high risk" (e.g., positive test for IgE, previous severe reaction, asthmatic patient), then it is best to perform it in a very controlled setting (e.g., hospital). In high-risk challenges, it may also be prudent to have intravenous access before commencing challenges. One research group reviewed their record with 349 food challenges in children with atopic dermatitis and recommended intravenous access for challenges when the history indicated a prior need for medical intervention or when particular tests for IgE antibody indicated a fairly high risk for reactions [32]. A study by Perry et al. [33] reviewed risks of OFCs in children typically assessed to have a 50% risk or less of a reaction prior to challenge. Of the 584 challenges completed, 253 (43%) were positive to: milk (90), egg (56), peanut (71), soy (21), and wheat (15). Of patients who failed, there were 197 (78%)

cutaneous, 108 (43%) gastrointestinal, 66 (26%) oral, 67 (26%) lower respiratory, and 62 (25%) upper respiratory reactions. Despite presumptions about certain foods causing more severe (e.g., peanut) reactions than others (e.g., egg, milk) there was no difference between foods in the severity of failed challenges or the type of treatment required to reverse symptoms. In a report of 701 OFCs performed in 521 patients in an outpatient setting, among children with a median age of 5.7 years, 18.8% were positive [34]. Patients were generally selected for OFC based upon having an estimated 50% or better chance of having a negative test. Most (57%) reactions were cutaneous and 88% were treated with antihistamines alone. Twelve of 132 reactions were treated with epinephrine, with one patient receiving two doses. In another review of OFCs performed primarily in an inpatient research unit [35], 436 of 1273 (34%) were positive and epinephrine was administered for 11% of the positive challenges (3.9% of challenges in total). There was only one biphasic reaction. There were no life-threatening respiratory or cardiovascular symptoms. These observations underscore the need for preparation to treat severe reactions whenever undertaking an OFC, but also suggest that the procedure is safe when performed with appropriate caution and preparation.

FPIES can result in hypotension and should be performed with caution, possibly with intravenous access in a hospital setting [3, 36]. This cell-mediated disorder results in a symptom complex of poor growth and profuse vomiting and diarrhea with or without microscopic blood in the stool while the causal food(s) are part of the diet [36]. When severe, reactions may include lethargy, dehydration, and hypotension, and may be complicated by acidosis and methemoglobinemia.

Preparing the patient for the challenge and baseline assessments

Patients must be given specific preparatory instruction before undertaking the challenge. Patients avoid the suspected food(s) for at least 2 weeks, antihistamines are discontinued according to their elimination half-life, and chronic asthma medications are reduced as much as possible before undertaking the challenge. Beta-agonists are eliminated for a relevant time period before challenges are undertaken. Medications, such as beta-blockers that may interfere with treatment, should be substituted as possible. The patient should be examined carefully prior to challenge to confirm that they are not already having chronic symptoms, and to determine their "baseline." It would not be prudent to undertake a challenge in an individual with, for example, mild wheezing for both the ability to judge a reaction and for safety concerns. Patients should be queried about any symptoms they have been experiencing that could confuse the interpretation of a food challenge, such as urticaria or rhinitis. It is prudent to avoid performing challenges if a patient recently had an exacerbation of asthma, particularly one requiring oral steroids. For some diseases (i.e., severe atopic dermatitis) hospitalization may be necessary to treat acute disease and establish a stable baseline prior to challenges. The patient should avoid food or drink for about 4 hours prior to challenge, though for young children or infants, clear fluids may be allowed. Patients with cardiac or respiratory disorders that may compromise them during anaphylaxis or treatment of anaphylaxis may need additional clearance or precautions (medication adjustment, slower dosing, deferral of OFC, etc.).

Decisions on dosing

Despite attempts and discussions to make a uniform international protocol for performing OFCs, no consensus has been reached and many published studies use variations on a general theme [18, 23, 37–39]. In all challenges, the food is given in gradually increasing amounts. This is for safety reasons. For most IgE-mediated reactions, the author and colleagues [40] give a total of 8–10 g of the dry food or 100 ml of wet food (double amount for meat/fish) in gradually increasing doses at 10–15 minute intervals over about 90 minutes, followed by a larger, meal-sized portion of food a few hours later. The doses may be distributed, for example, in portions such as (0.1%, 0.5%), 1%, 4%, 10%, 20%, 20%, 20%, 25%. However, researchers and clinicians have used a variety of other challenge regimens (lower starting doses, variations in the degree of dosing increases, different time intervals, etc.) with good success [37–39, 41–43]. The dosing interval may be increased or doses repeated either because the observer is unsure of the symptoms, or to more closely mimic the history of reactions. In the latter situation, doses may be administered over days if the history indicates that several days of ingestion were required to trigger symptoms.

The starting dose to select varies among studies, but clinical correlation may be helpful. To put this in perspective, it is reported that highly sensitive cow's-milk-allergic patients may react to trace milk contamination (e.g., 8.8–14 ppm) in commercial products, but these are generally not patients with a profile conducive to oral challenges [44,45]. In a study of adult peanut-allergic patients undergoing DBPCFCs, 50 mg of peanut was generally the lowest dose that elicited objective reactions (one patient experienced subjective symptoms at only 100 μg of peanut) [46]. We reviewed challenge data for 513 positive challenges to six common allergenic foods in children with atopic dermatitis [40]. Starting doses were usually 500 mg, but at the physician's discretion, starting doses were sometimes 100 mg or 250 mg. The percentage of children reacting at the first dose (500 mg or less) was as follows: egg (49%), milk (55%), soy (28%), wheat (25%), peanut (26%), and fish

(17%). Twenty-six milk challenges and 22 egg challenges were positive at a first dose of 250 mg; three milk challenges and seven egg challenges were positive at a first dose of 100 mg. Eleven percent of the reactions that occurred on first dose were severe. The dose to elicit a reaction was not predictable with PST size or IgE antibody concentration, as was also observed in the study by Perry [33]. Based upon these results, starting doses of 100 mg or less were recommended. To be particularly cautious, one could argue for starting doses that begin under the thresholds reported to induce reactions. Unfortunately, the published thresholds vary by logarithmic differences among studies and data are not available for most foods. To avoid first-dose reactions, based upon suggestions for challenges to determine thresholds of reactivity, an OFC would begin with doses of 3–10 μg [47, 42], although such dosing is not typically easily determined in routine clinical settings. Some workers begin challenges by placing the food extract on the lower lip for 2 minutes (labial food challenge), and observing for local or systemic reactions in the ensuing 30 minutes [41]. The development of a contiguous rash of the cheek and chin, edema of the lip with conjunctivitis or rhinitis, or a systemic reaction is considered a positive test. Negative labial challenges are generally followed by an OFC. However, the validity of labial challenges has not been thoroughly investigated.

Dosing regimens for FPIES are slightly different [36, 48]. Food challenges for this non-IgE-mediated syndrome are typically performed with 0.15–0.6 g/kg of the causal protein (usually cow's milk or soy), and reactions of profuse vomiting typically begins 2–4 hours after the ingestion and are accompanied by a rise in the absolute neutrophil count of over 3500 cells/mm^3. Additionally there may be diarrhea and thrombocytosis [49].

Making and administering the challenge food

The successful administration of OFCs to young children requires a great deal of preparation, ingenuity, and patience. Young children may become stubborn and refuse to ingest the challenge food. Prior planning with the family to select palatable or familiar forms of challenge foods or vehicles to hide foods in if the challenge is masked can be helpful in improving the experience. For example, milk protein may be mixed and hidden in soy frozen dessert products. Having additional challenge vehicles, for example liquid and solid forms of the challenge substance, readily at hand may prevent delays. Allowing the use of well-cleansed utensils and dinnerware that are familiar to the child (e.g., a favorite cup or plate) makes the challenge more natural appearing. Diversions such as toys, games, or videotapes are helpful. Since splattered or drooled food can elicit a local skin reaction from direct skin contact (but not necessarily from ingestion), it is helpful to have wet napkins on hand and straws for liquid challenges.

Table 23.4 Equipment and common foods to stock for use in creating masked food challenges.

Equipment	Common allergens	Useful carrier agents
Paper plates, cups utensils	Peanut flour, peanut butter	Proprietary formulas (hydrolyzed casein, amino acid)
Mixing bowls	Powdered egg white	
Scale	Powdered/fresh milk	Baby foods (squash, carrot, potato)
Mortar/pestle	Soy milk, soy flour	
Blender	Wheat breads, flour	Apple sauce
Microwave	Nuts	Juices

Similarly, when performing OFCs with children, it is better to feed them rather than to let them feed themselves and risk splattering.

The set up for a DBPCOFC is more complicated than what is needed for open or single-blind challenges. Although the procedure is more labor intensive, it can be carried out in an office setting if the challenge is not high risk [12]. The procedure still introduces graded doses, but in this case either a challenge food or a "placebo" food is administered. The aid of a "third party" is needed to prepare the challenges so that the observer and patient are kept unaware whether a true or placebo challenge is being undertaken. A "coin flip" can be used by the third party to randomize the order of administration. The food is hidden either in another food or in opaque capsules. Suggestions for materials to have on hand for creating masked challenges are shown in Table 23.4. It is beneficial to stretch the imagination in trying to best mask foods, especially foods with strong odors. Creating meals that definitively mask taste is often difficult and to do it well requires studies of successful test foods, by tasting panels [50–52]. Several tested recipes have been published [53]. This procedure of validating masking of challenges may be warranted for challenges performed for research purposes. To prevent false associations, it has been calculated that multiple challenges may be needed, with several feedings of both the placebo and the allergen being tested, but this procedure has practical limitations [25].

For masking taste, it is easiest to use opaque capsules, but oral symptoms are then bypassed and some patients are unable to ingest enough capsules. Bypassing oral symptoms by using capsules could theoretically result in stronger reactions, should multiple capsules begin to discharge their contents more closely in time than expected [54] and this approach is falling into disfavor. It is often easier to mask liquid into liquid and to use powder or dehydrated forms of foods that can be folded into solid vehicles. Certain flavoring agents such as mint can also help to mask odors. It is important to select vehicles that are clearly tolerated by the patient. If a gritty food is being hidden in a vehicle, then a similarly gritty food should be added as placebo to the carrier vehicle. For example, oat as an allergen mixed in apple sauce may be matched to corn meal in apple sauce. It is also important to appreciate that certain preparation methods (canning, dehydration) may alter the allergens. Examples include canning of fish [55] or using apple sauce compared to raw apple. Baked products with egg or milk (or even cheese) may be tolerated by persons who react to the less heated forms (e.g., French toast, yogurt) because the extensive heating alters the proteins [56, 57]. Depending upon the exact circumstances, an open challenge with a meal-sized portion of the food prepared in its natural state for consumption following a negative DBPCFC is essential to confirm that the food that the individual will be consuming will be tolerated. It is preferable not to use fatty foods as vehicles during OFCs since they can delay gastric absorption [58, 59].

Depending upon the particular food hypersensitivity disorder under consideration, timing of dose administration can be adjusted. For example, when evaluating potentially IgE-antibody-mediated reactions, two challenges may be performed on a single day with 2–4 hours between challenges (one is placebo, one is active—so one food is tested each day). The practice of interspersing placebo and active food proteins during a single challenge (i.e., random ordering of sequential doses that may or may not contain the causal protein) should be discouraged, since it can be difficult to determine if a reaction shortly after a particular dose, possibly a placebo dose, was actually a delayed response from an active dose administered previously.

Open or single-blind food challenges are typically used clinically instead of DBPCFC to screen for reactions, unless bias is suspected, subjective symptoms are the expected outcome, or delayed reactions are being evaluated. These open challenges are less labor- and time-intensive than DBPCFC and objective reactions are usually reliable, although there remains a greater likelihood to obtain a false-positive open OFC compared to DBPCFC [60]. Ambiguous results of open or single-blind challenges can be confirmed using a DBPCFC. A negative DBPCFC is followed, usually a few hours later, with a meal-sized portion of the food prepared in its natural form to ensure it is tolerated.

Monitoring and stopping a challenge/treatment

Challenges should be performed with appropriate monitoring equipment and emergency treatment medications, equipment, and oxygen immediately available. [3] Medication doses (e.g., epinephrine, steroids, antihistamines, H_2 blockers, glucagon, vasopressors, etc.) should be precalculated by patient weight. The physician or health-care worker records the dose given, the time of administration, and any symptoms that arise during the challenge [18]. Forms for recording vital signs, skin, respiratory, gastrointestinal, and cardiovascular examinations have been published [3, 18, 19]. Frequent assessments are made for symptoms affecting the skin, gastrointestinal tract, and/or respiratory tract, for example prior to each dose. With children, early indications of a reaction can include subtle signs such as moving the tongue in the mouth to rub an itchy palate, or ear pulling due to referred pruritus. While some families believe increased physical activities (hyperactivity) are a sign of food allergy, a common early response for children as they begin to experience a reaction is that they become suddenly quiet or assume a fetal position as a prodrome to more objective symptoms. Children with atopic dermatitis may develop a maculopapular rash in predilection areas of eczema. Objective monitoring can be done with peak flow or spirometry. Internationally accepted rules for stopping an OFC are lacking. One large study in infants used predetermined objective stopping criteria of a reaction within 2 hours that included three or more persistent (5 minutes) noncontact urticarial lesions or facial edema, or vomiting or respiratory/cardiovascular symptoms; less than 2% with a negative day 1 OFC had reactions on subsequent days, and the procedure was generally safe [61]. In general, challenges are terminated when a reaction becomes apparent and medications are given as needed. Judgment is required to decide upon discontinuing a challenge, continuing, or modifying the dose or timing for subjective symptoms. Generally, antihistamines are given at the earliest sign of a reaction with epinephrine and other treatments given if there is progression of symptoms or any potentially life-threatening symptoms, but this is open to the judgment of the supervising staff, who must take the patient's history into consideration. In some cases, families or individuals may question whether it is necessary to treat the symptoms at all, or may even ask to proceed with more doses to see "how bad" the reaction could be. This is not advisable for obvious safety reasons and also because the reactions are not likely to reflect what a subsequent exposure may cause in an uncontrolled setting.

Patients may be observed for 1–2 hours or longer as clinically indicated after a negative OFC. Though most reactions occur promptly, it is possible to have late-onset symptoms. Observation may be longer if the history indicates prior delayed reactions or if prior reactions were severe. If a reaction was treated, the patient should be observed 2–4 hours or longer past resolution of symptoms depending upon the features/severity of the symptoms. During that period, repeated assessments are made and additional therapies used as indicated.

Postchallenge care

There are several issues that need to be addressed when an OFC results in a reaction. The disappointment engendered should be openly discussed. Sometimes patients or families can be partly consoled to know that their hard work at avoidance was necessary and successful. Patients often wish to know if future reactions could be severe, a question whose answer may not be related to the result of the challenge because dosing is gradual rather than sudden and possibly high during accidental exposures. In some cases, it may be apparent that patients were not symptomatic with small exposures during the challenge and may have a margin for error in terms of potential accidental exposures. Patients and families may also inquire as to the possibility that the challenge could "boost" or prime their allergy. While there are no published data to clearly support or refute this concern, the OFC is ultimately the only way to know whether the food is tolerated, and is performed clinically when risk assessments are favorable for passing, thus making this concern essentially moot. A plan for reevaluation with laboratory tests and OFCs should be discussed depending upon the usual natural course for the food in question and patient-specific determinants such as age and other food allergies. Review of food avoidance measures is also helpful, and a reevaluation of any nutritional impact that avoidance may have engendered should be undertaken. An opportunity can be taken to review emergency management.

Patients with a negative challenge often need additional counseling about how to introduce or reintroduce the food. In some cases, a remaining fear could result in continued avoidance. In a study of 71 children, 25% reported not reintroducing the food for reasons including fears about persisting allergies, and observing skin rashes [62]. There may also be concerns about redeveloping the food allergy, a situation that is quite rare. However, the patient should be counseled about the small risk of a reaction despite a negative test, as described above. Patients with remaining food allergies must be cautioned specifically about any increased risk of exposure to an allergen that is commonly associated with the food that they are now able to ingest. For example, a patient with milk and egg allergy who passes an OFC to wheat must be warned to carefully check wheat products, now new to the patient that may often also contain milk and egg. When there are no remaining food allergies, patients may be loathe to discontinue carrying epinephrine, and this should be discussed as well with consideration for a period of continued availability to reduce stress, or ensure the allergy is entirely resolved.

Summary

Elimination diets are used as treatment of a known food allergy or for diagnosis to provide presumptive evidence of causality. OFCs provide a definitive means to determine whether a food is causal of symptoms. The safety of the procedure is ensured by careful gradual dosing, close monitoring, promptly discontinuing administration, and providing treatment in the event of symptoms, and providing continued monitoring and therapy as indicated until symptoms resolve. The DBPCFC is considered the "gold standard" for diagnosing a food allergy.

References

1. Boyce JA, Assa'ad A, Burks AW, et al. Guidelines for the diagnosis and management of food allergy in the United States: report of the NIAID-sponsored expert panel. *J Allergy Clin Immunol* 2010; 126(6 Suppl):S1–S58.
2. Sicherer SH, Teuber S. Current approach to the diagnosis and management of adverse reactions to foods. *J Allergy Clin Immunol* 2004; 114(5):1146–50.
3. Nowak-Wegrzyn A, Assa'ad AH, Bahna SL, et al. Work Group report: oral food challenge testing. *J Allergy Clin Immunol* 2009; 123(6 Suppl):S365–S383.
4. Graham DT, Wolf S, Wolff HG. Changes in tissue sensitivity associated with varying life situations and emotions; their relevance to allergy. *J Allergy* 1950; 21:478–86.
5. Loveless MH. Milk allergy: a survey of its incidence; experiments with a masked ingestion test. *J Allergy* 1950; 21:489–499.
6. Loveless MH. Allergy for corn and its derivatives: experiments with a masked ingestion test for its diagnosis. *J Allergy* 1950; 21:500–509.
7. Ingelfinger FJ, Lowell FC, Franklin W. Gastrointestinal allergy. *N Engl J Med* 1949; 241:303.
8. May CD. Objective clinical and laboratory studies of immediate hypersensitivity reactions to food in asthmatic children. *J Allergy Clin Immunol* 1976; 58(4):500–515.
9. Liacouras CA, Furuta GT, Hirano I, et al. Eosinophilic esophagitis: updated consensus recommendations for children and adults. *J Allergy Clin Immunol* 2011; 128(1):3–20.
10. Sicherer SH. Food allergy: when and how to perform oral food challenges. *Pediatr Allergy Immunol* 1999; 10(4):226–234.
11. Liacouras CA, Spergel JM, Ruchelli E, et al. Eosinophilic esophagitis: a 10-year experience in 381 children. *Clin Gastroenterol Hepatol* 2005; 3(12):1198–1206.
12. Joshi P, Mofidi S, Sicherer SH. Interpretation of commercial food ingredient labels by parents of food- allergic children. *J Allergy Clin Immunol* 2002; 109(6):1019–1021.
13. Sicherer SH, Vargas PA, Groetch ME, et al. Development and validation of educational materials for food allergy. *J Pediatr* 2012; 160(4):651–656.
14. Isolauri E, Sutas Y, Salo MK, et al. Elimination diet in cow's milk allergy: risk for impaired growth in young children. *J Pediatr* 1998; 132(6):1004–1009.
15. David TJ. Anaphylactic shock during elimination diets for severe atopic dermatitis. *Arch Dis Child* 1984; 59:983–986.
16. Flinterman AE, Knulst AC, Meijer Y, et al. Acute allergic reactions in children with AEDS after prolonged cow's milk elimination diets. *Allergy* 2006; 61(3):370–374.
17. Lieberman JA, Sicherer SH. Quality of life in food allergy. *Curr Opin Allergy Clin Immunol* 2011; 11(3):236–242.
18. Bock SA, Sampson HA, Atkins FM, et al. Double-blind, placebo-controlled food challenge (DBPCFC) as an office

procedure: a manual. *J Allergy Clin Immunol* 1988; 82:986–997.
19. American College of Allergy, Asthma, & Immunology. Food allergy: a practice parameter. *Ann Allergy Asthma Immunol* 2006; 96(3 Suppl 2):S1–68.
20. Sampson HA. Food allergy: diagnosis and management. *J Allergy Clin Immunol* 1999; 103(6):981–989.
21. Caffarelli C, Petroccione T. False-negative food challenges in children with suspected food allergy. *Lancet* 2001; 358(9296):1871–1872.
22. Metcalfe D, Sampson H. Workshop on experimental methodology for clinical studies of adverse reactions to foods and food additives. *J Allergy Clin Immunol* 1990; 86:421–442.
23. Niggemann B, Wahn U, Sampson HA. Proposals for standardization of oral food challenge tests in infants and children. *Pediatr Allergy Immunol* 1994; 5(1):11–13.
24. Briggs D, Aspinall L, Dickens A, et al. Statistical model for assessing the proportion of subjects with subjective sensitisations in adverse reactions to foods. *Allergy* 2001; 56 (Suppl 67):83–85.
25. Chinchilli VM, Fisher L, Craig TJ. Statistical issues in clinical trials that involve the double-blind, placebo-controlled food challenge. *J Allergy Clin Immunol* 2005; 115(3):592–597.
26. Wilson BG, Bahna SL. Adverse reactions to food additives. *Ann Allergy Asthma Immunol* 2005; 95(6):499–507.
27. Simon RA. Adverse reactions to food additives. *Curr Allergy Asthma Rep* 2003; 3(1):62–66.
28. Fleischer DM, Bock SA, Spears GC, et al. Oral food challenges in children with a diagnosis of food allergy. *J Pediatr* 2011; 158(4):578–583.
29. Pongracic JA, Bock SA, Sicherer SH. Oral food challenge practices among allergists in the United States. *J Allergy Clin Immunol* 2012; 129(2):564–566.
30. Busse PJ, Nowak-Wegrzyn AH, Noone SA, et al. Recurrent peanut allergy. *N Engl J Med* 2002; 347(19):1535–1536.
31. Fleischer DM, Conover-Walker MK, Christie L, et al. Peanut allergy: recurrence and its management. *J Allergy Clin Immunol* 2004; 114(5):1195–1201.
32. Reibel S, Rohr C, Ziegert M, et al. What safety measures need to be taken in oral food challenges in children? *Allergy* 2000; 55(10):940–944.
33. Perry TT, Matsui EC, Conover-Walker MK, et al. Risk of oral food challenges. *J Allergy Clin Immunol* 2004; 114(5):1164–1168.
34. Lieberman JA, Cox AL, Vitale M, et al. Outcomes of office-based, open food challenges in the management of food allergy. *J Allergy Clin Immunol* 2011; 128(5):1120–1122.
35. Jarvinen KM, Amalanayagam S, Shreffler WG, et al. Epinephrine treatment is infrequent and biphasic reactions are rare in food-induced reactions during oral food challenges in children. *J Allergy Clin Immunol* 2009; 124(6):1267–1272.
36. Sicherer SH. Food protein-induced enterocolitis syndrome: case presentations and management lessons. *J Allergy Clin Immunol* 2005; 115(1):149–156.
37. Bindslev-Jensen C. Standardization of double-blind, placebo-controlled food challenges. *Allergy* 2001; 56(Suppl 67):75–77.
38. Rance F, Deschildre A, Villard-Truc F, et al. Oral food challenge in children: an expert review. *Eur Ann Allergy Clin Immunol* 2009; 41(2):35–49.
39. Keil T, McBride D, Grimshaw K, et al. The multinational birth cohort of EuroPrevall: background, aims and methods. *Allergy* 2010; 65(4):482–490.
40. Sicherer SH, Morrow EH, Sampson HA. Dose-response in double-blind, placebo-controlled oral food challenges in children with atopic dermatitis. *J Allergy Clin Immunol* 2000; 105(3):582–586.
41. Rance F, Dutau G. Labial food challenge in children with food allergy [see comments]. *Pediatr Allergy Immunol* 1997; 8(1):41–44.
42. Taylor SL, Hefle SL, Bindslev-Jensen C, et al. A consensus protocol for the determination of the threshold doses for allergenic foods: how much is too much? *Clin Exp Allergy* 2004; 34(5):689–695.
43. Skamstrup HK, Vestergaard H, Stahl SP, et al. Double-blind, placebo-controlled food challenge with apple. *Allergy* 2001; 56(2):109–117.
44. Gern J, Yang E, Evrard H, Sampson H. Allergic reactions to milk-contaminated "non-dairy" products. *N Engl J Med* 1991; 324:976–979.
45. Laoprasert N, Wallen ND, Jones RT, et al. Anaphylaxis in a milk-allergic child following ingestion of lemon sorbet containing trace quantities of milk. *J Food Prot* 1998; 61(11):1522–1524.
46. Hourihane JB, Kilburn SA, Nordlee JA, et al. An evaluation of the sensitivity of subjects with peanut allergy to very low doses of peanut protein: a randomized, double-blind, placebo-controlled food challenge study. *J Allergy Clin Immunol* 1997; 100(5):596–600.
47. Crevel RW, Ballmer-Weber BK, Holzhauser T, et al. Thresholds for food allergens and their value to different stakeholders. *Allergy* 2008; 63(5):597–609.
48. Powell G. Food protein-induced enterocolitis of infancy: differential diagnosis and management. *Compr Ther* 1986; 12(2):28–37.
49. Mehr S, Kakakios A, Frith K, et al. Food protein-induced enterocolitis syndrome: 16-year experience. *Pediatrics* 2009; 123(3):e459–e464.
50. Huijbers GB, Colen AA, Jansen JJ, et al. Masking foods for food challenge: practical aspects of masking foods for a double-blind, placebo-controlled food challenge. *J Am Diet Assoc* 1994; 94(6):645–649.
51. Vlieg-Boerstra BJ, Bijleveld CM, Van Der HS, et al. Development and validation of challenge materials for double-blind, placebo-controlled food challenges in children. *J Allergy Clin Immunol* 2004; 113(2):341–346.
52. Vassilopoulou E, Douladiris N, Sakellariou A, et al. Evaluation and standardisation of different matrices used for double-blind placebo-controlled food challenges to fish. *J Hum Nutr Diet* 2010; 23(5):544–549.
53. Vlieg-Boerstra BJ, Herpertz I, Pasker L, et al. Validation of novel recipes for double-blind, placebo-controlled food challenges in children and adults. *Allergy* 2011; 66(7):948–954.
54. Sampson HA, Leung DY, Burks AW, et al. A phase II, randomized, double-blind, parallel-group, placebo-controlled

oral food challenge trial of Xolair (omalizumab) in peanut allergy. *J Allergy Clin Immunol* 2011; 127(5):1309–1310.

55. Bernhisel-Broadbent J, Strause D, Sampson HA. Fish hypersensitivity. II: Clinical relevance of altered fish allergenicity caused by various preparation methods. *J Allergy Clin Immunol* 1992; 90:622–629.
56. Kim JS, Nowak-Wegrzyn A, Sicherer SH, et al. Dietary baked milk accelerates the resolution of cow's milk allergy in children. *J Allergy Clin Immunol* 2011; 128(1):125–131.
57. Lemon-Mule H, Sampson HA, Sicherer SH, et al. Immunologic changes in children with egg allergy ingesting extensively heated egg. *J Allergy Clin Immunol* 2008; 122(5):977–983.
58. Grimshaw KE, King RM, Nordlee JA, et al. Presentation of allergen in different food preparations affects the nature of the allergic reaction—a case series. *Clin Exp Allergy* 2003; 33(11):1581–1585.
59. Teuber SS. Hypothesis: the protein body effect and other aspects of food matrix effects. *Ann NY Acad Sci* 2002;964:111–116.
60. Venter C, Pereira B, Voigt K, et al. Comparison of open and double-blind placebo-controlled food challenges in diagnosis of food hypersensitivity amongst children. *J Hum Nutr Diet* 2007; 20(6):565–579.
61. Koplin JJ, Tang ML, Martin PE, et al. Predetermined challenge eligibility and cessation criteria for oral food challenges in the HealthNuts population-based study of infants. *J Allergy Clin Immunol* 2012; 129(4):1145–1147.
62. Eigenmann PA, Caubet JC, Zamora SA. Continuing food-avoidance diets after negative food challenges. *Pediatr Allergy Immunol* 2006; 17(8):601–605.

24 General Approach to Diagnosing Food Allergy and the Food Allergy Guidelines

Jonathan O'B. Hourihane[1] & Hugh A. Sampson[2]

[1]Department of Paediatrics and Child Health, University College of Cork, Ireland
[2]Translational Biomedical Sciences, Jaffe Food Allergy Institute Department of Pediatrics, Icahn School of Medicine at Mount Sinai New York, NY, USA

Key Concepts

- A careful, detailed clinical history is the cornerstone for the evaluation and diagnosis of food allergy.
- Both focused *in vivo* (skin prick tests) and *in vitro* tests (quantitative allergen-specific IgE levels) provide strong supplemental information for the diagnosis of food allergy, but alone are not diagnostic.
- The blinded oral food challenge remains the "gold standard" for the diagnosis of food allergy.
- Novel *in silico* approaches, that is, algorithms incorporating clinical and laboratory data, appear to improve the clinicians ability to predict the outcome or oral food challenges.

The recently published NIAID-sponsored Guidelines on the diagnosis and management of food allergy are a major step forward in the systematic management of these common and complicated conditions, which cause symptoms that vary from minor urticaria to fatal anaphylaxis. The evidence on which many clinical practices are based has been evaluated and graded. The guidelines give support for specialists and generalists in managing conditions that can cause physical, social, and psychological deficits to affected individuals and their families, and have also identified other areas in which clinicians and academics must work to improve the evidence base of their specialty [1].

Why is it important to systematically diagnose food allergy?

Food is the major external (nongenetic) determinant of long-term health in the developed world. Population-based surveys suggest a 10-fold overestimation of those who suspect they have a food allergy compared to those in whom food allergy can be formally confirmed by OFC. This confirmation based on studies with relatively small number of people who completed the food challenge protocols has, however, been confirmed in meta-analyses [2].

Many generally well adults suffer transient or low-grade symptoms that may not be specific (e.g., headache, abdominal bloating, or cramps). In the absence of an adequate alternative explanation, they may seek an external and therefore excludable/avoidable cause for their symptoms. Food is an obvious place to start. For adults this may be a minor lifestyle modification that does not result in substantial nutritional consequences. However, infants and young children, who must have optimal nutrition to grow properly, may not adequately achieve growth milestones if their diet is restricted because calorie, nutrient, and micronutrient sources are not adequately substituted [3]. It is a basic tenet of food allergy care that food elimination diets should only be undertaken under the supervision of experienced professional physicians and dieticians/nutritionists and the use of diagnostic elimination diets (see Chapter 39) must be short term in duration and not indefinite.

NIAID has defined food allergy as an immune-mediated adverse reaction to foods, in contrast to food intolerances, where an immune mechanism cannot be demonstrated (see Figure 24.1). Knowledge of this scheme allows clinicians to focus on relevant parts of an allergy-focused clinical history and to reassure families about dietary concerns and worries that they may have, but which may not be justified.

In conjunction with the NIAID-sponsored guidelines, the Royal College of Paediatrics and Child Health in the United Kingdom has produced Allergy Care Pathways [4]

Food Allergy: Adverse Reactions to Foods and Food Additives, Fifth Edition. Edited by Dean D Metcalfe, Hugh A Sampson, Ronald A Simon and Gideon Lack.

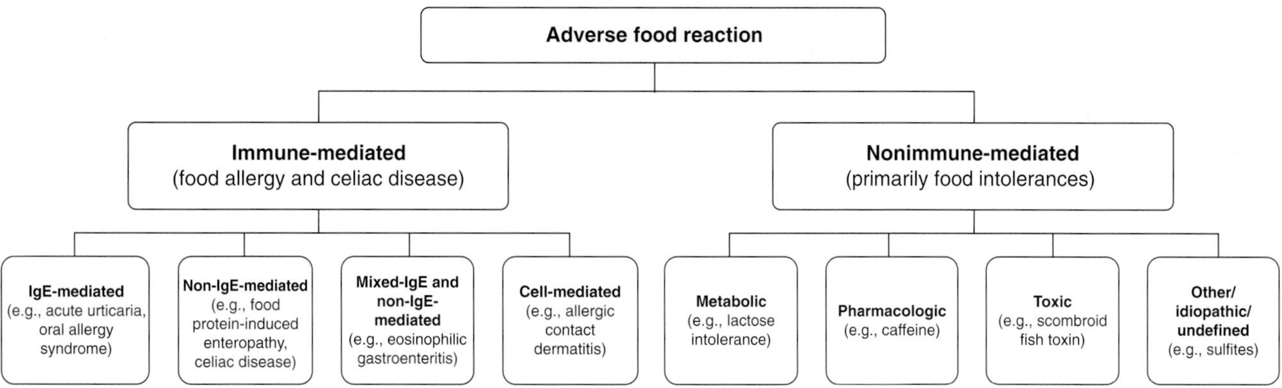

Figure 24.1 NIAID nomenclature of adverse food reactions. From Reference 1.

and the United Kingdom's National Institute of Clinical Excellence (NICE) has produced food allergy guidelines [5], which further facilitate systematic diagnosis in support of these families. Both sets of documents emphasize the primary role of the carefully taken medical history and physical examination as the basis for a proper diagnosis of food allergy. Both documents also make emphatic recommendations about the undesirability of indiscriminate use of screening tests.

A carefully taken clinical medical history will establish whether a food is likely to be responsible for the symptoms described, if the underlying mechanisms are kept in mind (see Table 24.1).

Food allergic reactions can be IgE-mediated or non-IgE-mediated. It is common to find both mechanisms at play in one person after a single exposure to a known allergen. For example, cow's milk causing both immediate urticaria and delayed exacerbation of atopic dermatitis; or for a single person to have IgE-mediated reactions to one food, for example, cow's milk, causing anaphylaxis, but non-IgE-mediated reactions to another food, for example, wheat, causing atopic dermatitis and diarrhea.

Most physicians would recognize that facial urticaria within 5 minutes of eating a known food allergen such as scrambled eggs or peanut butter is likely to be due to that food being allergenic for that person. Most physicians will also recognize that headache or flushing after consumption of alcohol is a direct, predictable, and common pharmacological effect of alcohol rather than an unusual allergy to alcohol. Consumption of not-perfectly fresh scombroid fish (e.g., dark meat tuna, albacore, mackerel) may represent an ingestion of a toxic amount of exogenous histamine, causing an allergy-like response.

Food allergy-focused clinical history-taking can help the clinician to decide what the appropriate tests to perform are and what the next steps to take are. Three key questions can deliver a lot of useful information, based on the mechanisms and symptom clusters associated with them (see Table 24.2):

1. What happened?
2. What food?
3. How much food?

What happened?

It is usually not difficult to distinguish between the two allergy-related mechanisms when an allergy-focused clinical history is taken carefully.

IgE-mediated reactions are usually very stereotyped in the symptoms elicited and usually start nearly immediately, with most individuals or their caretakers reporting an onset within 5–10 minutes of consumption. NIAID's definition of anaphylaxis allows for inclusion of symptoms that start within 2 hours after allergen exposure. Our clinical experience is that most IgE-mediated food-allergic reactions during challenge, or during reliably reported reactions in the field, start much closer to the known food allergen consumption, within minutes. However, this 2-hour "outer limit" allows a broad, inclusive definition of anaphylaxis and is useful in a clinical setting, especially when food is the major noniatrogenic trigger in community-based episodes of anaphylaxis [7]. Most IgE-mediated reactions peak within an hour but biphasic reactions are well described and are an unusual but "not-to-be-missed" significant feature of anaphylactic reactions [8]. Urticaria that is ongoing over a 5-day period suggests that food allergy is not the cause, unless continued food allergen ingestion can be identified over the time period of concern.

The requirement for intercellular signaling and cellular recruitment means non-IgE-mediated symptoms start more slowly. Non-IgE-mediated symptoms such as atopic dermatitis, rectal bleeding from colitis, and so on may take 24 hours or more to manifest with a gradual, evolving onset and may take several days to resolve. In contrast, other enteropathic reactions such as the food protein-induced enterocolitis syndromes also have delayed onset, but they then can manifest very suddenly, 2–3 hours after food protein consumption, with dramatic loss of

Table 24.1 Mechanisms of food allergic reactions.

Pathology	Disorder	Key features	Most common causal foods
IgE-mediated (acute onset)	Acute urticaria/angioedema	Food commonly causes acute (20%) but rarely chronic urticaria.	Primarily "major allergens" (see text)
	Contact urticaria	Direct skin contact results in lesions. Rarely this is due to direct histamine release (nonimmunologic).	Multiple
	Anaphylaxis	Rapidly progressive, multiple organ system reaction can include cardiovascular collapse.	Any but more commonly peanut, tree nuts, shellfish, fish, milk, and egg
	Food-associated, exercise-induced anaphylaxis	Food triggers anaphylaxis only if ingestion is followed temporally by exercise.	Wheat, shellfish, and celery most often described
	Oral allergy syndrome (pollen-associated food allergy syndrome)	Pruritus and mild edema are confined to oral cavity and uncommonly progress beyond the mouth (~7%) and rarely to anaphylaxis (1–2%). Might increase after pollen season.	Raw fruit/vegetables; cooked forms tolerated; examples of relationships: birch (apple, peach, pear, carrot), ragweed (melons)
	Immediate gastrointestinal hypersensitivity	Immediate vomiting, pain	Major allergens
Combined IgE- and cell-mediated (delayed onset/chronic)	Atopic dermatitis	Associated with food allergy in ~35% of children with moderate-to-severe eczema	Major allergens, particularly egg, milk
	Eosinophilic esophagitis	Symptoms might include feeding disorders, reflux symptoms, vomiting, dysphagia, and food impaction.	Multiple
	Eosinophilic gastroenteritis	Vary on site(s)/degree of eosinophilic inflammation; might include ascites, weight loss, edema, obstruction	Multiple
Cell-mediated (delayed onset/chronic)	Food protein–induced enterocolitis syndrome	Primarily affects infants; chronic exposure: emesis, diarrhea, poor growth, lethargy; reexposure after restriction: emesis, diarrhea, hypotension (15%) 2 hours after ingestion	Cow's milk, soy, rice, oat, meat
	Food protein–induced allergic proctocolitis	Mucus-laden, bloody stools in infants	Milk (through breast-feeding)
	Allergic contact dermatitis	Often occupational because of chemical moieties, oleoresins. Systemic contact dermatitis is a rare variant because of ingestion	Spices, fruits, vegetables
	Heiner syndrome	Pulmonary infiltrates, failure to thrive, iron deficiency anemia	Cow's milk

Source: Reproduced from Reference 6.

peripheral circulation and hypotension, responding better to resuscitation with fluids than to epinephrine.

What food is suspected?

While the literature shows nearly 200 individual foods have been implicated in food allergic reactions, it has been known for more than two decades that the repertoire of foods that cause IgE-mediated reactions is much narrower than was originally suspected. Ninety-five percent of children with IgE-mediated reactions react to one of the major food allergens, even if the index reaction was to another food. This list of foods, which had originally been informally designated the "big eight," has been extended, and in Europe and Australia there are regulatory requirements for such foods to be labeled when they form part of the ingredient chain [9].

Some foods are associated more strongly with one mechanism than another. Cow's milk and hen's egg commonly cause both urticaria/angioedema (IgE-mediated) and more delayed exacerbations of eczema (non-IgE-mediated). In contrast, peanut almost exclusively causes IgE-mediated symptoms and can rarely be confidently implicated in isolated non-IgE-mediated reactions. Focusing the clinical history taking on the symptoms elicited is more useful than focusing on the food, however, because typical IgE-mediated responses to foods can happen to any food.

Table 24.2 Three key questions in a food allergy focused clinical history.

	IgE-mediated reactions	Cell-mediated/ non-IgE-mediated reactions	Mixed immunological mechanisms	Intolerance reactions
What happened?	Sudden onset, every time eaten Urticaria Angioedema Vomiting Bronchospasm Severe abdominal pain/diarrhea Anaphylaxis	Delayed or gradual onset, 1–24 h, every time eaten Atopic dermatitis Diarrhea	Mixture, every time eaten	Delayed, may not always occur each time eaten Possibly several days of consumption implicated Abdominal cramps, bloating Diarrhea Mood change in young children
What food?[a]	Milk, egg, peanut, tree nuts, fish shellfish, kiwi, (wheat and soya much less commonly)	Milk, egg, wheat, soya	Common allergens as shown and also fruits and cereals in eosinophilic esophagitis Rice, wheat, soya in enterocolitis syndromes	Wheat (must exclude celiac disease) Milk Fruit
How much food?	Small amounts, eaten infrequently or never knowingly eaten	Occasionally small amounts tolerated		Larger amounts often needed to elicit symptoms

[a]Individual foods' allergenicity can vary with cooking method; for example, baked-egg is much less allergenic than less-cooked egg, milk is similar, peanut is more allergenic when dry-roasted.

How much food?

The immunological mechanisms involved in IgE-mediated reactions determine that very small amounts of food can cause reactions and that a reaction will happen every time this food is eaten, if the threshold dose of the allergen is exceeded (see Oral food challenges; Chapter 23). Due to the small amounts of food required to elicit IgE-mediated reactions, it is uncommon for children or adults to be able to eat more than minimum amounts without reactions. However, it is possible in non-IgE-mediated reactions to tolerate small amounts of allergen without developing symptoms. A history of safe consumption of a food on multiple occasions in average daily portions makes a diagnosis of allergy to that food very unlikely [6]. This would lead a discerning clinician to suspect either food intolerance or a separate non-immune-mediated diagnosis (see Figure 24.1). Quantities of food consumed in accidental reactions can be hard to judge unless the portion size can be accurately assessed. A bite can be big or small, depending on the age and appetite of the consumer (see Figure 24.2)

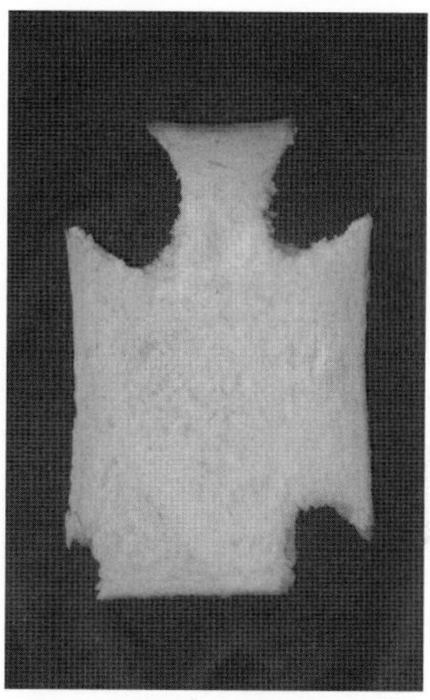

Figure 24.2 Different aged children have different sized bites, which may affect the dose of food allergen consumed. This slice of bread was bitten by four children ranging in age from 9 years (top left) through 7 years (top right) and 3 years (bottom right) down to 23 months (bottom left).

Moving from focused history-taking to focused *in vivo* and *in vitro* testing

No individual symptom or clinically observable sign is pathogenically unique to food allergy and every symptom and sign could be explained on its own, in isolation, by another mechanism. For example, urticaria could be due to contact with stinging nettles or to a bee sting. Angioedema could be due to a viral illness or medications. Hypotension could be due to a syncopal episode. However, the cluster of these exemplar clinical signs in the setting of a routine episode of family life where food is being consumed makes it easier to identify. Nowadays, asking families to use their cell phone or digital cameras to document reactions between office visits has become a mainstay of allergy practice. When a child or adult is newly referred, an experienced clinician can start to drill down into the clinical history to determine what further tests are required.

Most allergists and many nonspecialist clinicians may have access to skin prick tests (SPTs) or to serum food-specific IgE measurements. The limitations and indications for using these are discussed elsewhere (see Chapter 21), but it must be emphasized repeatedly that these tests individually and together have excellent negative predictive values with lower positive predictive values. The interpretation of their positive and negative outcomes is affected by the pretest likelihood of the condition being present in the population tested [10]. In a setting where the prevalence of the condition of interest—in this case food allergy—is low, that is, in a community-based survey where the likely prevalence is known to be less than 10%, even in infants, IgE-focused screening using skin prick testing may only have a positive predictive value of 50% [11, 12]. In contrast, when testing children and adults referred to an allergy clinic (where the likely pretest prevalence is higher), the positive predictive value may reach much higher values such as 80–90% [13](and authors' observations). Using the absolute values of wheals elicited in skin testing have shown that higher readings, for example, 8 mm for peanut are associated with a higher likelihood of confirming the diagnosis on formal challenge and importantly with likely persistence rather than resolution [14].

Skin prick testing is easily performed and with adequate training, is highly reproducible when a single operator performs tests regularly. It is no longer accepted practice to merely report the relative size of the allergen-specific wheal compared to the size of the histamine control (such as "grass 2+", "egg 4+," etc.). Nonetheless, a positive control of 3 mm is the minimum needed to confirm the neurovascular loop in the skin is "active" or intact and is not suppressed by medications, such as long-acting antihistamines. This is to ensure that any negative SPT is a true negative rather than a false negative. Likewise, a negative control must always be used to ensure the absence of dermatographism, which could lead to overinterpretation of SPTs, leading to false-positive test results.

Commercial preparations of the most common food allergens are widely available, and in most cases, results are comparable between different centers that are using the same solutions, despite the recognized limitation that no international standards exist for standardizing reagents for skin prick testing. Methods of measurement and exact techniques can vary, but in general, skin tests are read 15–20 minutes after the initial test is performed. The elicited wheal and flare response usually recedes over a similar time period. More esoteric foods, such as pineapple, sweet corn, and fresh foods, can be used in "prick-to-prick" testing, where the lancet is inserted into the test food before being used for skin testing. The dose introduced in this technique is less predictable than when using commercially prepared solutions, and it is occasionally the case that more significant reactions to skin testing occur with prick-to-prick testing than with skin testing using commercially prepared solutions. The other major indication for prick-to-prick testing is when investigating foods that are known to contain labile/unstable allergens such as fruits (apples, cherries, kiwi; see Chapter 12) for which commercial solutions may not be reliable. The NIAID guidelines explicitly do not recommend the use of intradermal testing due to the absence of standardization and the perceived increased risk of systemic reactions [1].

A major advantage of skin testing over laboratory-based diagnostic tests is the immediacy of the availability of the result and the ability to repeat the test immediately if there are uncertainties about test results at any particular clinic visit (see Table 24.3). While young children may

Table 24.3 Comparison of relative strengths and weaknesses of skin prick testing and *in vitro* allergen-specific IgE testing.

	Skin test	***In vitro* test**
Operator skill	++ Bedside/ office, clinical skills important	++ Lab worker, mostly automated
Cost, per allergen tested	Low	High
Speed of test/speed of result	+/++++	+/–
Standardization of substrate	+	++
Range of substrates	+++++	+ market led
Acceptability to patient		
Child	++ age-related	+/– age-related
Adult	++	+
Inter-test comparison (using same system and technique)	+	+++
Patient/parent recall of test result	+++	+
Storage/retrievability of result	Paper record may be misfiled/lost	Computer record/ standardized lab procedures

become distressed, most children can be tested provided their atopic dermatitis is not extensive. Parents appear to recall SPT results better than the results of blood tests.

The use of *in vitro* allergen-specific IgE testing using serum-based assays has become highly standardized over the last 20 years. Different corporations have developed different technologies and intertest comparisons show sufficient similarities to say they may be broadly similar and sufficient differences to recommend end users (usually clinicians) should familiarize themselves with local test systems and their specific reference ranges for the tests in the laboratory systems they are using [15, 16]; see Chapter 20.

In a situation similar to that relating to skin prick testing, the characteristics of the population being tested affect the interpretation of the tests. Age and atopic dermatitis status are known to influence serum IgE levels significantly. It is often the case, seen in every allergy clinic around the world, that in individuals with atopic dermatitis, allergen-specific IgE levels for commonly allergenic foods can be very elevated, despite either known safe consumption or an absence of supportive clinical history of adverse outcome following exposure to that food. Children and infants with atopic dermatitis may have unnecessarily restricted diets on the basis of such indiscriminate testing and it is strongly discouraged [17]. The allergen-specific IgE levels elicited in this way may even exceed the positive predictive values generated in other tested groups. It is a common scenario for individuals to be referred to allergists with an unconfirmed diagnosis of food allergy based on such indiscriminate testing, performed without sufficient knowledge of the pathogenesis of food allergy, particularly in subjects with atopic dermatitis.

Nonetheless, serum-based allergen-specific IgE testing is a cornerstone of allergy diagnostics in food allergy. Extensive studies in several international centers have shown that allergen-specific serum IgE levels can be used both to positively predict outcomes of formal food challenges and also to more confidently negatively predict the outcome; that is, to correctly identify those who have had negative challenges [13]. More recently, several studies have shown that quantification of food component protein levels may be more predictive of allergic reactivity than the use of the complex food proteins; for example, Ara h 2 for peanut allergy [18–20], Gly m 5 for soybean [21], Cor a 1 in hazelnut allergy [22], and so on.

The earlier studies were from highly referred populations seen in national and supranational referral centers, but these findings have been largely confirmed in other studies. There remains the issue of local, intercenter, and international variation of populations and referral practices, which again leads national and international organizations to encourage allergists to generate their own local data for use when advising individuals about allergen avoidance and when selecting individuals for formal food challenges. However, the "gold standard" diagnostic test is an OFC (see Chapter 23) and many allergists in community practice or in nonspecialist centers do not routinely perform these time-consuming tests and continue to rely on their carefully taken clinical allergy-focused histories and the *in vivo* and *in vitro* test results to make professional, clinical judgments for their patients.

OFCs are now widely standardized and more centers are developing the skill set needed to perform them safely, but it is always necessary to discuss with families that food challenges, even in an expert center, are not risk-free [8, 23]. However, recent studies have shown that a definitive diagnosis of food allergy using OFC has nearly as much positive impact on food allergy-related quality of life when the challenge is "failed," that is, the patient reacts to the food, as when it is "passed," that is, when the food is tolerated, because a major element of parental and child anxiety relating to food allergy is due to the uncertainty about what might happen the next time [24]; see Chapter 44. While long-term studies do show some, but not all, subjects progress from a mild to a more severe manifestation of disease [25–27], it has not proved possible to confidently delineate the factors that could be used early in the allergic march to identify these subjects (who will or may worsen progressively) more accurately.

Using skin and blood tests to follow patients over time

Several leading centers have demonstrated that sequential SPTs and blood tests can be used over time to allow clinicians to better guide families through continuing avoidance diets, if symptoms are not showing improvement, or to point out where a food can be reintroduced. Survival curves can be used to follow patients through childhood and have shown that early and peak values of allergen-specific IgE can be used to prognosticate about resolution or persistence. The Baltimore group have published such data for both egg and milk [28, 29] but again referral bias and patient selection criteria for definitive challenge may be clinic-specific [8, 30]. Combinations of SPTs and specific IgE levels can also be used [31] and the effect of age-related differences in results' predictive values must be considered [32].

Test results may fall from above positive predictive values into the indeterminate/gray zone or they may become completely negative. In this unusual scenario, it might be acceptable for a food to be introduced at home as the risk of a reaction is very low (<5%). It is more often the case that indeterminate/"gray-zone" values (below the 95% positive predictive level but not completely negative) remain low or fall, but do not become negative. In these cases, the clinician must consider the original presentation. Was

	Home challenge	Hospital challenge
High-risk food, possibly persisting	No	Yes
Low-risk food, likely to resolve	Yes	If necessary
Anaphylaxis documented	No	Yes
Biphasic reaction	No	Yes, prolonged observation needed
Asthma status		
Stable	Possibly	Yes
Not stable	No	No
Family attitude to challenge	Competent and confident	Worried

Table 24.4 Considerations in decision to advise challenge of avoided food at home or in hospital.

it genuine anaphylaxis or actually a mild cutaneous reaction? What is the asthma status (unstable asthma should cause OFC to be deferred irrespective of home or hospital location)? What are the family's preferences/worries about doing this? Some families whom clinic staff feel could be supported to introduce the food at home just cannot conceive of doing it and a hospital challenge should be offered. Other more apparently competent families may need a full explanation of the risks involved so that it is not done casually. Other families will never agree to home or hospital challenge, but this is unusual when a productive relationship/dialogue is started with the child and parents early in the child's life (Table 24.4).

Biphasic food allergic reactions are well described but are unusual [8] and special consideration needs to be given to such cases, with a hospital challenge preferable in most such cases, due to the prolonged length of post-challenge supervision/observation needed.

Many factors are involved in determining the outcome of an exposure to a food allergen. These can vary from

Table 24.5 Comparison of three differing approaches to quantification of risk of positive challenge outcome, using clinical and test data available prior to challenge.

	Dunngalvin (2011) [34]	Cianferoni (2012) [35]	Zomer-Kooijker (2012) [36]
Design	1. Retrospective phase, two-center 2. Prospective development phase, single-center 3. Validation phase, single-center	Retrospective, single-center	Prospective single-center
Subjects	Phase 1: 429 Phase 2: 289 Phase 3: 70	983	129
% of challenges positive	Phase 1: 40% Phase 2: 53–58% Phase 3: 50–57%	47%	42%
Foods	Milk, egg, peanut	Milk, egg, peanut	Milk, egg, peanut
Sex	66% male	68% male	63% male
Mean age	7 years	5 years	4.9 years
Clinical factors associated with positive challenge outcome			
Age at challenge	Yes	Yes	No
Index food	Yes	No	Yes
Severity of prior reaction	Yes	Yes, especially non-skin reactions	No
Time to onset of reaction	Not reported	Not reported	Yes
SPT wheal size	Yes	Yes	No
Sp-IgE level	Yes	Yes	Yes
Total IgE	Yes, as Total IgE – specific IgE	Not reported	Not reported
Outcome	Probability score 0–1	Food Challenge Score 0–4	Score 0–10
Area under curve (AUC)/accuracy	AUC 94–97% 97% positive 94% negative	0–1 score >90%accurate for negative challenge 3–4 score 62–92% accurate for anaphylaxis	≤3 unlikely to have positive OFC, ≥9 very likely to have a positive OFC AUC 0.9 97% accuracy overall
Tool developed	Desktop/phone app in development	Simple scoring system	Not reported

SPT, skin prick tests.

one reaction to the next (see Figures 24.3a–24.3c) and this variability may largely account for the inter-reaction variability in severity and outcome that is so unnerving for families and their clinicians. An OFC is designed and intended to minimize the impact of most controllable variables, which is not possible in a community setting.

Skin prick testing and specific IgE testing have been used for many years now to try to predict who will and who will not react in an OFC. However, on their own or even in a simple combination, these two prime pieces of an allergist's diagnostic workup do not suffice, for the reasons outlined above. In addition, not all allergy services routinely perform OFCs as they are time consuming and labor intensive. A history of anaphylaxis is often cited as a reason not to perform a food challenge, despite the known occurrence of resolution in subjects who have been documented to have experienced anaphylactic reactions previously. Our groups and others have explored how patient-based variables and variables relating to the nature of the allergen interact to determine the outcome of an OFC. Bioinformatic approaches involving microarray analysis of diversity of peanut allergy epitope recognition can distinguish peanut allergic and peanut tolerant subjects [33]. Other methods of varying complexity using more widely available or accessible data have been reported (see Table 24.5).

Cianferoni et al. [35] retrospectively reviewed nearly 1000 food challenges in a single unit between 2004 and 2010 and found that four simple factors were associated with a positive/failed OFC: positive-specific IgE, wheal size on SPT, any prior symptoms, and a prior noncutaneous reaction. A simple scoring system showed varying abilities to predict OFC failure for each of the three foods tested. Zomer-Kooijker et al. in Utrecht, the Netherlands, have shown similar data relating to a single year's challenges in a single center [36]. Our group has explored nearly 800 challenges performed utilizing identical protocols in two centers and has prospectively validated the retrospective findings in a separate prospective validation cohort; see Figure 24.4 [34].

Further recent work shows that such analyses can work satisfactorily with incomplete data, and with challenges performed using types of a single food with known differing allergenicity, that is, using boiled, lightly or well cooked egg [37].

While such *in silico* approaches have great promise for all allergists, the need for sound clinical judgment in how and when to perform food challenges will remain and the capacity to perform, supervise, and interpret simple tests, such as SPT and specific IgE and emerging chip-based systems and complex dynamic tests such as OFC will mean clinical allergy remains an area of great academic interest for the foreseeable future.

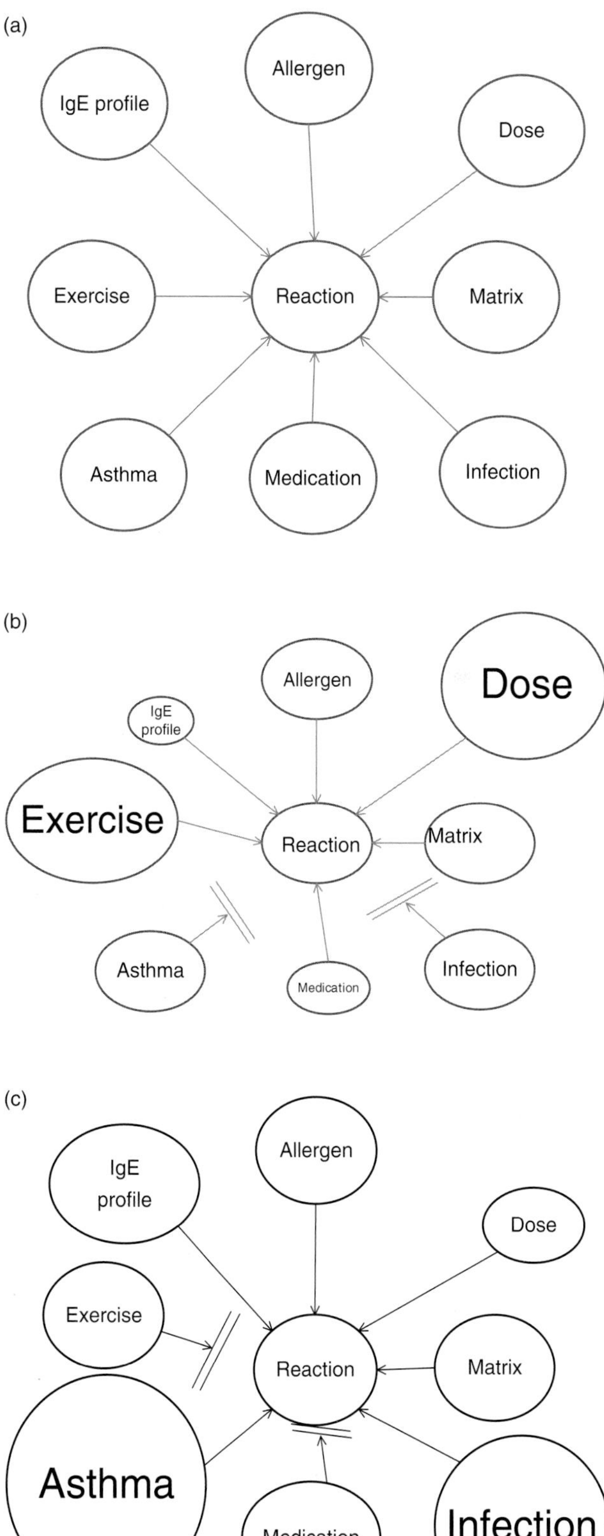

Figure 24.3 (a) All contributing risk factors for reaction severity are equally weighted. (b) Variable weighting of some active and some inactive factors in a food allergic reaction. (c) Factor weighting may change between reactions.

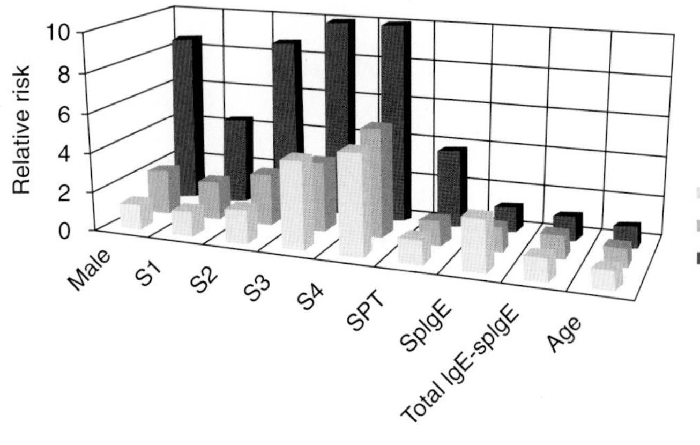

Figure 24.4 Different clinical features contribute differently to the overall relative risk of a positive OFC. S1, single-system symptoms only (skin, oral, or gastrointestinal); S2, upper respiratory and gastrointestinal symptoms or two systems; S3, lower respiratory symptoms or three systems; S4 cardiovascular symptoms or four systems. From data in Reference 34.

References

1. Boyce JA, Assa'ad A, Burks AW, et al. Guidelines for the Diagnosis and Management of Food Allergy in the United States: Report of the NIAID-Sponsored Expert Panel. *J Allergy Clin Immunol* 2010; 126(6):S1–S58.
2. Rona RJ, Keil T, Summers C, et al. The prevalence of food allergy: a meta-analysis. *J Allergy Clin Immunol* 2007; 120(3):638–646.
3. Fox AT, Du Toit G, Lang A, Lack G. Food allergy as a risk factor for nutritional rickets. *Pediatr Allergy Immunol* 2004; 15(6):566–569.
4. Royal College of Paediatrics and Child Health. *Allergy Care Pathways for Children Food Allergy*. London: RCPCH, 2011. Available at www.rcpch ac.uk/allergy/foodallergy
5. Centre for Clinical Practice at NICE (UK). *Food Allergy in Children and Young People: Diagnosis and Assessment of Food Allergy in Children and Young People in Primary Care and Community Settings*. London: National Institute for Health and Clinical Excellence, 2011.
6. Burks AW, Tang M, Sicherer S, et al. ICON: Food allergy. *J Allergy Clin Immunol*. 2012;129(4):906–920.
7. Sampson HA, Muñoz-Furlong A, Campbell RL, et al. Second symposium on the definition and management of anaphylaxis: summary report—Second National Institute of Allergy and Infectious Disease/Food Allergy and Anaphylaxis Network symposium. *J Allergy Clin Immunol* 2006; 117(2):391–397.
8. Jarvinen KM, Amalanayagam S, Shreffler WG, et al. Epinephrine treatment is infrequent and biphasic reactions are rare in food-induced reactions during oral food challenges in children. *J Allergy Clin Immunol* 2009; 124:1267–1272.
9. Directive 2003/89/EC of the European Parliament and the Council of 10 November 2003 amending Directive 2000/13/EC as regards indication of the ingredients present in foodstuffs. *Offic J Eur Union* L 308/15, November 25, 2003.
10. Roberts G, Lack G. Food allergy—getting more out of your skin prick tests. *Clin Exp Allergy* 2000; 30(11):1495–1498.
11. Kagan RS, Joseph L, Dufresne C, et al. Prevalence of peanut allergy in primary-school children in Montreal, Canada. *J Allergy Clin Immunol* 2003; 112(6):1223–1228.
12. Osborne NJ, Koplin JJ, Martin PE, et al. Prevalence of challenge-proven IgE-mediated food allergy using population-based sampling and predetermined challenge criteria in infants. *J Allergy Clin Immunol* 2011; 127(3):668–676. e1–2.
13. Sampson HA. Utility of food-specific IgE concentrations in predicting symptomatic food allergy. *J Allergy Clin Immunol* 2001; 107(5):891–896.
14. Ho MH, Wong WH, Heine RG, Hosking CS, Hill DJ, Allen KJ. Early clinical predictors of remission of peanut allergy in children. *J Allergy Clin Immunol* 2008; 121:731–6.
15. Wang J, Godbold JH, Sampson HA. Correlation of serum allergy (IgE) tests performed by different assay systems. *J Allergy Clin Immunol* 2008; 121(5):1219–1224.
16. Hamilton RG, Mudd K, White MA, Wood RA. Extension of food allergen specific IgE ranges from the ImmunoCAP to the IMMULITE systems. *Ann Allergy Asthma Immunol* 2011; 107(2):139–144.
17. Werfel T, Ballmer-Weber B, Eigenmann PA, et al. Eczematous reactions to food in atopic eczema: position paper of the EAACI and GA^{2}LEN. *Allergy* 2007; 62(7):723–728.
18. Codreanu F, Collignon O, Roitel O, et al. A novel immunoassay using recombinant allergens simplifies peanut allergy diagnosis. *Int Arch Allergy Immunol* 2011; 154(3):216–226.
19. Nicolaou N, Poorafshar M, Murray C, et al. Allergy or tolerance in children sensitized to peanut: prevalence and differentiation using component-resolved diagnostics. *J Allergy Clin Immunol* 2010; 125(1):191–197.
20. Asarnoj A, Movérare R, Östblom E, et al. IgE to peanut allergen components: relation to peanut symptoms and pollen sensitization in 8-year-olds. *Allergy* 2010; 65(9):1189–1195.
21. Holzhauser T, Wackermann O, Ballmer-Weber BK, et al. Soybean (Glycine max) allergy in Europe: Gly m 5 (beta-conglycinin) and Gly m 6 (glycinin) are potential diagnostic markers for severe allergic reactions to soy. *J Allergy Clin Immunol* 2009; 123(2):452–458.
22. Flinterman AE, Akkerdaas JH, Knulst AC, van Ree R, Pasmans SG. Hazelnut allergy: from pollen-associated mild allergy to severe anaphylactic reactions. *Curr Opin Allergy Clin Immunol* 2008; 8(3):261–265.
23. Perry TT, Matsui EC, Conover-Walker MK, Wood RA. Risk of oral food challenges. *J Allergy Clin Immunol* 2004; 114(5):1164–1168.

24. DunnGalvin A, Cullinane C, Daly DA, Flokstra-de Blok BM, Dubois AE, Hourihane JO. Longitudinal validity and responsiveness of the Food Allergy Quality of Life Questionnaire—Parent Form in children 0–12 years following positive and negative food challenges. *Clin Exp Allergy* 2010; 40(3):476–485.
25. Hourihane JO, Kilburn SA, Dean TP, Warner JO. Clinical characteristics of peanut allergy. *Clin Exp Allergy* 1997; 27:634–639.
26. Van der Leek TK, Liu AH, Stefanski K, Blacker B, Bock SA. The natural history of peanut allergy in young children and its association with serum peanut-specific IgE. *J Pediatr* 2000; 137:749–755.
27. Ewan PW, Clark AT. Efficacy of a management plan based on severity assessment in longitudinal and case-controlled studies of 747 children with nut allergy: proposal for good practice. *Clin Exp Allergy* 2005; 35:751–756.
28. Skripak JM, Matsui EC, Mudd K, Wood RA. The natural history of IgE-mediated cow's milk allergy. *J Allergy Clin Immunol* 2007; 120(5):1172–1177.
29. Savage JH, Matsui EC, Skripak JM, Wood RA. The natural history of egg allergy. *J Allergy Clin Immunol* 2007; 120(6):1413–1417.
30. Yanishevsky Y, Daly D, Cullinane C, Hourihane JO'B. Differences in treatment of food challenge-induced reactions reflect physicians' protocols more than reaction severity. *J Allergy Clin Immunol* 2010; 126:182.
31. Shek LP, Soderstrom L, Ahlstedt S, Beyer K, Sampson HA. Determination of food specific IgE levels over time can predict the development of tolerance in cow's milk and hen's egg allergy. *J Allergy Clin Immunol* 2004; 114(2):387–391.
32. Boyano-Martínez T, García-Ara C, Díaz-Pena JM, Martín-Esteban M. Prediction of tolerance on the basis of quantification of egg white-specific IgE antibodies in children with egg allergy. *J Allergy Clin Immunol* 2002; 110(2):304–309.
33. Lin J, Bruni FM, Fu Z, et al. A bioinformatics approach to identify patients with symptomatic peanut allergy using peptide microarray immunoassay. *J Allergy Clin Immunol* 2012; 129(5):1321–1328. e5.
34. DunnGalvin A, Daly D, Cullinane C, et al. Highly accurate prediction of food challenge outcome using routinely available clinical data. *J Allergy Clin Immunol* 2011; 127(3):553–840.
35. Cianferoni A, Garrett JP, Naimi DR, Khullar K, Spergel JM. Predictive values for food challenge-induced severe reactions: development of a simple food challenge score. *Isr Med Assoc J* 2012; 14:24–28.
36. Zomer-Kooijker K, Slieker MG, Kentie PA, van der Ent CK, Meijer Y. A prediction rule for food challenge outcome in children. *Pediatr Allergy Immunol* 2012; 23(4):353–359.
37. DunnGalvin A, Segal LM, Clarke A, Alizadehfar R, Hourihane JOB. Validation of the Cork-Southampton Food Challenge Outcome Calculator in a Canadian sample. *J Allergy Clin Immunol* 2013; 131(1):230–232.

Conflict of interest: Jonathan O'B Hourihane jointly holds, with a colleague and University College, Cork, Ireland, a not-for-profit patent for the computerized calculator discussed in the manuscript.

25 Hidden and Cross-Reacting Food Allergens

Scott H. Sicherer

Division of Allergy and Immunology, Department of Pediatrics, Icahn School of Medicine at Mount Sinai, New York, NY, USA

Key Concepts

- False assumptions of multiple food allergy, or misdiagnoses, may derive from reactions to hidden ingredients, or from positive allergy tests to cross-reactive foods.
- Hidden or unexpected exposure to food allergens may occur from undeclared ingredients, cross-contact with an allergen, or from exposures not expected to carry food proteins, such as kissing, from airborne proteins, or in medications and cosmetics.
- Among related foods, cross-sensitization (positive tests) is more common than clinical cross-reactivity.
- Clinical cross-reactivity is more common (>35%) among tree nuts, fish, shellfish, certain mammalian milks, and certain fruits, than among grains and legumes (<20%).
- Individualization by testing and oral food challenge may be needed to confirm tolerance of potentially cross-reactive foods.

Introduction

The two topics discussed in this chapter, allergic reactions to hidden and cross-reacting food allergens, are ones that may lead to a mistaken conclusion of multiple food allergies. Table 25.1 lists several of the considerations for evaluating possible allergies to multiple foods. Reactions to hidden food allergens that are erroneously attributed to a known ingredient in a culprit food may lead to the false assumption of multiple food allergies or a misdiagnosis. Cross-reactivity may account for reactions to a variety of related foods of plant or animal origin based upon immune reactions toward homologous proteins shared among them. However, immune responses, reflected by positive specific IgE tests to related foods, do not necessarily indicate clinical allergy; therefore, multiple food allergies may erroneously be assumed unless additional testing is undertaken to prove tolerance of related foods that were not already ingested without symptoms. Topics concerning the specific food proteins that frequently account for cross-reactions, oral allergy syndrome (pollen–food cross-reactivity), diagnostic methods, and management of food allergy will not be emphasized here. Rather, this chapter will introduce concepts and provide information to enhance the evaluation of patients with possible multiple food allergy, in regard to hidden and cross-reacting food allergens.

Hidden food allergens

For the purpose of this chapter, the term "hidden food allergens" will refer to a variety of unexpected ways in which an individual may be exposed to food allergens [1]. A "hidden" food allergen may only be unknown to the consumer, not necessarily to a manufacturer or chef who provided the food. The use of peanut flour to thicken tomato sauce or chili is one such example that underscores the importance of maintaining a clear line of communication when an allergic individual is depending upon food provided from a restaurant or other commercial source without ingredient labels. Food proteins can also turn up in many unexpected ways. For example, a teacher may use egg white to make finger paints smoother, or wheat may be an ingredient in modeling clay. Table 25.2 lists the ways in which exposure may occur within the context of hidden food allergens.

Food Allergy: Adverse Reactions to Foods and Food Additives, Fifth Edition. Edited by Dean D Metcalfe, Hugh A Sampson, Ronald A Simon and Gideon Lack.

Table 25.1 Considerations when evaluating patients with apparent multiple food allergies.

Type	Cause	Example
True reactions to multiple food types		
True allergies	True allergic reactions to multiple, diverse food allergens. Usually in highly atopic patients	Reactions to egg, milk, wheat, and soy in one child
Intolerance	Nonimmune-mediated conditions causing adverse reactions when various foods are ingested	Intolerance of fat resulting in gastrointestinal upset to fatty meats; lactase deficiency resulting in symptoms from milk; fructose/sorbitol intolerance resulting in "acidic" diarrhea from multiple fruits
Cross-reactivity	Homologous proteins among foods and between foods and environmental allergens	Pollen allergy syndrome, latex fruit syndrome, pan-allergens in related foods
False assumption of multiple food allergy		
Multiple positive SPTs/RAST	Multiple tests for IgE antibody are positive and reactions are assumed to be related without further evaluation (history, oral challenge)	Atopic individual inappropriately tested to a wide battery of allergens has numerous positive tests and told to avoid all of the foods
Hidden ingredients	Reactions to apparently diverse products because of exposure to a hidden/unexpected source of one or a few previously identified allergens	Milk-allergic child reacts to soy desserts and canned tuna because they contain casein
Unproven tests	Use of unproven/experimental tests that identify multiple problematic foods for potentially vague symptoms	IgG antibody tests identify 43 foods purported to cause weakness in an elderly patient
Psychological	Previous food-allergy-related traumatic event generalizes to increasing numbers of reactions that are based upon psychological triggers	A severely peanut-allergic patient develops paleness and syncope when exposed to a product that she thought contained peanut, but did not
Misperception	Chronic complaints attributed to adverse reactions to a variety of foods without a pathophysiological explanation	Patient with perception that his headaches are triggered by orange foods (carrot, sweet potato, squash, orange soda)

Commercial food products: manufacturing and labeling issues

Consumers with a known food allergy depend upon accurate food label ingredient lists to determine the safety of their food. Sometimes mistakes are apparent from simple misunderstandings: egg substitutes may catch the eye of an egg-allergic consumer who may assume the product is egg free and not realize that egg is clearly labeled as an ingredient. In other cases, there could be labeling errors or mistakes that introduce unintended allergens [2]. The medical literature contains reports of clinical reactions to foods with allergen contamination not declared on the ingredient label for several allergens including egg, milk, and peanut [3–7] and minor ingredients may cause severe reactions [8, 9]. Egg, milk, or fish may be used as processing aids in wines, but allergic reactions appear uncommon [10].

Governmental oversight of manufactured products varies worldwide [11–14]. Labeling laws changed in the United States as the Food Allergen Labeling and Consumer Protection Act (FALCPA) of 2004 came into effect in January 2006. The law requires that the eight major allergens or allergenic food groups—milk, egg, fish, shellfish, tree nuts, wheat, peanut, and soy—be declared on ingredient labels using plain English words. The law requires that the specific type of allergen, in regard to grouped allergens such as nuts, fish, or shellfish, be named. The law still allows terms such as "natural flavor" or "whey" on labels, but plain English must additionally disclose a major allergen. While the law includes the listed eight major allergens/allergenic food groups, additional allergens, for example, garlic, sesame, poppy, and so on, may not be disclosed clearly. For example, the word "spice" may be used for these allergens. Processing aids such as

Table 25.2 Modes of exposure to hidden/unexpected food allergens.

Mode of exposure	Examples
Hidden ingredient in manufactured product	Undeclared ingredient, contaminant, ambiguous label, nonstandard terminology
Nonfood item	Pet food, shampoo, ointment
Medications	Egg, soy, and milk (often in clinically irrelevant concentrations) in a variety of medications (carriers)
Cross-contact	Shared equipment in restaurant/bakery causes contamination
Nonfood allergen found in food	Dust mite contamination of grains
Unexpected exposure route	Skin contact from residual food on table/chair, inhalation of fumes during cooking, exchange of saliva (kissing, shared straws, etc.)

soy lecithin, a fatty derivative of soy which contains a very small amount of soy protein, may now be disclosed. The law acknowledges that certain forms of highly processed oils may not contain any appreciable protein, for example, soy oil. The law is likely to be revised by petition and updates are available from the Center for Food Safety and Applied Nutrition, a branch of the Food and Drug Administration (www.cfsan.fda.gov). The Federal Register (74 FR208) issued a rule that as of January 2011 carmine dye/cochineal extract must be disclosed on ingredient labels; this protein color derived from a dried insect has rarely elicited allergic reactions and anaphylaxis [15]. The US law applies to all types of packaged foods except for meat, egg, and poultry products, and raw agricultural foods such as fruits and vegetables in their natural state. The plain English words used to identify the foods may be placed within the ingredient list or as a separate statement "contains." In regard to soy, terms such as soybean, soy, and soya are considered interchangeable. Labeling laws vary among countries and some have none. Many countries have laws that include more than just the "major" eight food/food groups currently covered by the US laws. For example, the European Union enacted legislation in 2005 requiring that the following allergens not covered in US laws must be listed: rye, barley, oats, celery, mustard, and sesame seeds. Canada requires labeling that is similar to the United States but adds sesame and mustard.

Precautionary or advisory labeling, such as "may contain," are not regulated by the FALCPA legislation. These statements have been used by companies when a particular allergen is not an ingredient of the food, but that allergen may contact or become a part of the food despite good manufacturing processes. Labeling for the possibility of allergen contact is voluntary, and various terms are used at the discretion of the manufacturer such as "processed on shared equipment with..." or "manufactured in a facility that processes...," and many others. Several studies have elucidated the scope of the problem. Unfortunately, advisory labeling is widespread; one study found that 17% of 20 241 US supermarket products had such labeling [16]. Consumers are apt to ignore such labeling: in a study of 174 adolescents, 42% were willing to eat foods labeled "may contain" an allergen [17]. A survey of over 600 parents of food-allergic children revealed a greater comfort level in using products labeled "made in a facility that processes peanut" compared to the term "may contain peanut" [18]. However, in that same study when samples of 179 products with advisory labeling for peanut were assayed, 7% of the products were found to have detectable peanut protein without a relationship to the label terms. Thus, consumers should be educated that risk cannot be stratified according to wording used. Some products may be riskier than others. Milk was detected in 14 of 18 chocolate candies with milk advisory labels [19]. Another study [20] examined products with advisory labeling for milk, egg, or peanut as well as similar products without any advisory declaration. Allergens were detected in 5.3% of products with advisory labeling and 1.9% of products without advisory statements. A higher percentage of foods from small companies were contaminated compared with those from large companies (5.1% vs. 0.75%). Importantly, peanut was not detected in any of the 120 products tested without advisory labels. Most of the time that allergens were detected, the amount was low, possibly below thresholds of reactivity for most patients. However, more studies are needed to define risks and apply those results to labeling regulations regarding the use of advisory statements [21].

Cross-contact

Cross-contact (cross-contamination) refers to having an unintended allergen carried over from an "unsafe" food to one that is purportedly free of the allergen. For example, in the home, a knife used to spread peanut butter could next contact and contaminate jelly. In restaurants, shared grills, pans, food processors, and other equipment used without thorough cleaning between preparations may be a source of cross-contact. Bakeries pose similar problems as shared bowls, mixing equipment, and pans may allow for cross-contact. In ice cream shops, dipping scoops from one flavor to the next can cross-contaminate otherwise safe flavors. In the school setting, cross-contact has been identified as a possible source of inadvertent exposures to peanut and tree nut through shared utensils and cross-contact of foods [22]. A problematic issue of cross-contact, combined with false assumptions by consumers, is demonstrated by "pareve"-labeled products [3]. Pareve is a religious term meaning nondairy and does not ensure absence of milk proteins. These products are often sought out by unknowing milk-allergic consumers and consequently reactions are described to products with this label due to cross-contamination by cow's milk.

Restaurant meals also pose challenges for those with food allergies. The author and colleagues evaluated allergic reactions in peanut- and tree nut-allergic subjects that were associated with restaurants and food from establishments such as bakeries and ice cream shops [23]. Of 5149 voluntary registrants in the US National Peanut and Tree Nut Allergy Registry, 13.7% indicated that they had experienced a reaction in these types of establishments. A review of 156 episodes among 129 randomly selected registrants revealed that 39% of reactions were due to peanut or tree nut hidden in the food and not overtly identifiable to the patron (e.g., in sauces, dressing, egg rolls). In 22% of cases, cross-contact was involved primarily due to the use of shared cooking/serving supplies. There were particular problems regarding cross-contact in desserts, Asian cooking, and buffets. Restaurant personnel may not appreciate risks or understand how to avoid them. A study of 100 restaurant employees in the New York City area showed that only 22% provided correct responses to five questions about food allergy [24]. Misconceptions included believing fryer heat would destroy allergens, that it was safe to consume allergens in small amounts, and that removal of allergen from a finished dish (e.g., picking off nuts) was safe. However, restaurant personnel may indicate comfort with providing a safe meal [24,25]. The lessons learned from the study of reactions in restaurants and food establishments, and concerning reactions from cross-contact and labeling, underscore the need for education of allergic consumers and food providers about these topics [26]. Approaches to management of avoidance are detailed in Chapter 39.

Unexpected sources of food proteins in nonfood items and in medications

Allergenic food proteins may be components of a variety of items not meant for ingestion by humans. For example, pet foods, cosmetics, hair care products, and topical skin care products could contain food proteins (e.g., almond, soy). Reactions to these products applied topically are usually not severe, and some may not have significant protein [27].

Patients with food allergies and their physicians must always consider that a drug (or vaccine) reaction may be induced by a food ingredient in the drug. For example, reaction to carmine dye used in an azithromycin has been described [28]. Additionally, egg protein may be found in influenza and yellow fever vaccines [29, 30], milk protein in the diphtheria, tetanus, and pertussis vaccine [31], and gelatin [32] in a variety of other vaccines. Vaccines that may include gelatin include some of the diphtheria, tetanus, and pertussis vaccines; influenza vaccine; Japanese encephalitis; mumps; measles, mumps, and rubella (MMR); typhoid; varicella; and yellow fever vaccines. Graded dosing might be considered for the yellow fever vaccine or if gelatin-free vaccines are not available. The MMR vaccine is no longer considered to contain appreciable egg protein [33]. The trace amount of egg protein in the inactivated influenza vaccine appears to present little risk and approaches to vaccination have become more liberal with suggestions to vaccinate egg-allergic patients without skin testing to the vaccine and with general anaphylaxis precautions in persons with a possible severe egg allergy [33].

Many other food-related ingredients used in medications have not been well studied in terms of their allergic potential. Pharmaceutical grade lactose is used in many medications and the clinical relevance of possible residual milk protein has not been well established. One report identified milk protein in the lactose used in several dry powdered inhalers used for asthma [34]. Egg or soy lecithin and soy oil are found in a variety of medications; the clinical relevance to most individuals with these allergies remains unexplored, but risk appears very low. [35]

Nonfood allergens in foods

There are case reports of nonfood allergen contamination of foods resulting in allergic reactions. For example, dust mites may contaminate flour mixtures and cause severe reactions when ingested by dust-mite-allergic patients [36, 37]. The use of latex gloves by food handlers has resulted in unexpected reactions when these foods are ingested by latex-allergic individuals [38–40]. Insofar as parasites are not intentionally consumed, it is worthwhile to note that the nematode *Anisakis simplex* that infests fish can induce allergic reactions. This appears to be a problem particularly in Spain and other countries with a high fish consumption and is associated with undercooking [41].

Nonstandard exposure routes to food allergens

There appear to be exceptional cases where topical exposure to foods results in systemic reactions [42]. More commonly, however, topical exposure leads primarily to isolated, local skin reactions [43]. In such cases, residual food proteins on tables and chairs may induce rashes. Although not truly hidden or unexpected, school craft projects using peanut butter (peanut butter-covered pine cone birdfeeders) are commonly responsible for reactions despite school consciousness about avoiding peanut as an ingestant [22]. However, peanut butter appears unlikely to cause serious reactions from air exposure or limited skin contact [44].

Airborne exposure to food allergens is not unexpected in a variety of industrial food-processing settings (e.g., baker's asthma) but is a potential hidden source outside of these settings. There are several published case reports of acute allergic reactions to airborne food particles such as string bean [27], lentil [45], meats [46], and seafood [47] usually during cooking (rapidly boiling milk, frying eggs, steaming soups, sizzling fried seafood, etc.). Reactions have been verified in challenge settings [48]. There are also a few reports concerning peanut reactions to inhalation of peanut dust during commercial airline flights [49, 50]. These reactions are generally isolated to the upper and sometimes lower respiratory tract.

Another source of unintended and unexpected oral exposure is through saliva from an individual who ingested an allergen, for example, through contact during kissing or sharing cups, straws, or utensils. Kissing, in particular passionate kissing, is a common route of exposure. Of 379 allergy patients in the United States with peanut/tree nut/legume or seed allergy, 5.3% reported reactions from kissing [51]. Of 839 food allergy patients in Denmark (self-reported) who recalled possible kissing, 16% reported a reaction [52]. These two reports also support the notion that the food was usually, but not always, recently ingested and that brushing teeth may not be sufficient for removing the allergen. A study was undertaken to determine the time course of peanut protein (a marker protein Ara h 1) in saliva after a meal of peanut butter and possible methods for cleaning [53]. Most (87%) subjects with detectable peanut after a meal had undetectable levels by 1 hour with no interventions. None had detectable levels several hours later following a peanut-free lunch. This result indicates (95% confidence) that 90% would have undetectable Ara h 1 in saliva under these circumstances. There is one case report [54] of a mild reaction to peanut despite a 2-hour wait, brushing teeth, and chewing gum. Food-allergic reactions from blood transfusions carrying food proteins are theoretically possible but not commonly observed, probably because plasma fractions are reduced in packed cell transfusions (which may not be the case for other blood products such as platelets) [55].

Cross-reacting food allergens

When an allergic response is established toward a particular protein, presentation of a homologous form of that protein in another substance may also trigger an allergic response (cross-reaction). Therefore, allergic reactions to multiple foods may follow initial sensitization caused by one food or nonfood allergen such as pollen. The initial sensitization may occur by the oral, cutaneous, or inhaled route. In some cases, distantly related foods or environmental allergens contain common (conserved) homologous (pan-) allergens. To complicate matters further, however, there may be homologous, allergenically important sequences (epitopes) shared even among more distantly related foods that may trigger reactions in some individuals (e.g., seed storage proteins in peanut, sesame, and tree nuts) [56, 57].

Plant-derived proteins responsible for allergy include various families of pathogenesis-related proteins, protease and alpha-amylase inhibitors, peroxidases, profilins, seed storage proteins, thiol proteases, and lectins [58, 59] while homologous animal proteins include muscle proteins, enzymes, and various serum proteins. Remarkably, typical food allergens derive from just these few, out of thousands, of protein families. Over 70% identity in primary sequence is generally needed for cross-reactivity [60]. The biochemical attributes of these proteins will not be discussed here, but the focus will rather be on the clinical relevance of potential cross-reactivity.

IgE binding to a potentially cross-reactive food protein (sensitization demonstrated by skin prick test (SPT) or serum IgE) is not an evidence of clinically relevant allergy to the food. In fact, it is quite common to find food-specific IgE antibody by SPTs or serum tests to foods related to the one causing the index reaction. Bernhisel-Broadbent and colleagues [61] studied 62 children with allergy to at least one legume and found that 79% had serologic evidence of IgE binding to more than one, and 37% bound all six legumes. The scenario is similar for tree nuts [62–64]. In our studies of tree nut-allergic children [62], 92% of 111 patients with peanut and/or tree nut allergy had IgE antibody to more than one tree nut. In all of these cases, however, it is much more common to find that the food to which there is cross-sensitization is actually tolerated when ingested [65]. Factors that determine the clinical appearance of allergy in the face of sensitization are complex and relate to the host (immune response, target organ hyperreactivity) and the allergen (lability, digestibility) [66]. Presumably, these factors also bear upon the clinical relevance of potentially cross-reactive foods. The two main clinical approaches for an individual with an allergy to a particular food within a family of related foods are to avoid the entire family and to confirm tolerance to specific members of that family of foods, allowing consumption of safe food(s). The information to follow may be of particular value in deciding upon the best approach to diagnose potential allergy to cross-reactive foods (the utility of *in vivo* and *in vitro* tests). Unfortunately, comprehensive studies where a patient who is allergic to one member of a food family is challenged to all others are lacking. This is especially true of foods such as tree nuts and seafood that elicit severe reactions. However, decisions to avoid some of these foods as a group may also be based upon concerns about cross-contact or misidentification of the allergens. These are decisions that can be individualized based upon clinical judgment, patient preference, nutritional considerations, and availability of safe foods.

Cross-reactions among specific foods/food families

Legumes

Despite the high rate of cross-sensitization to legumes (beans), clinical cross-reactions are uncommon. Peanut and soy represent two of the most highly allergenic legumes that are dietary staples in North America, and yet the rate of clinical cross-reactivity is low. Bock and Atkins [67] studied 32 children with peanut allergy confirmed by double-blind, placebo-controlled oral food challenges (DBPCFCs) and found that 10 (31%) had a positive skin test to soy, but only 1 (3% of those with peanut allergy) had a clinical reaction to soy. In considering a wider variety of legumes, only 3 (1.8%) of 165 children with atopic dermatitis evaluated with DBPCFCs reacted to more than one legume, despite 19% reacting to at least one [68]. Bernhisel-Broadbent and Sampson [61] specifically addressed the issue of legume cross-reactivity by performing open or DBPCFCs in 69 highly atopic children with at least one positive skin test to a legume. Oral challenges to the five legumes (peanut, soybean, pea, lima bean, and green bean) resulted in 43 reactions in 41 patients (59%). Only 2 of 41 with any one positive challenge reacted to more than one legume (5%).

There are limited data to suggest that particular legumes are more likely than others to trigger reactions and also that the types of beans consumed in various cultures (e.g., lupine used whole or as flour in breads) also impact the rate of cross-reactions. For example, 11 of 24 (44%) French children with peanut allergy [69] had positive skin tests to lupine, and of 8 subjects who underwent DBPCFCs (6 children) or labial challenges (2 children) to lupine, 7 reacted. An elevated risk of co-allergy to peanut and lupine has been noted by other investigators as well [70–72]. As a probable reflection of cultural and geographical influences on the diet, allergy to lentil is more common than to peanut in Spain [73]. Furthermore, of 22 Spanish children with lentil allergy evaluated for reactions to other legumes [74], 6 had a history of reacting to chick pea, 2 to pea, and 1 to green bean. These findings raise suspicion for multiple legume allergies in those reacting to pea, lentil, lupine, or chick pea, but studies in a variety of geographic settings are needed to quantify the risks. While a patient allergic to peanut may have a small chance of other legume allergies, if they react for example to pea, it appears that additional legumes could present a greater risk (chick pea, lentil). The rate of sensitization to multiple legumes is high but as emphasized in Chapters 8, 20, and 21, there is no need to remove a tolerated food from the diet should sensitization be observed.

Tree nuts

Clinical reactions to tree nuts can be severe [75], potentially fatal, and occur from a first apparent exposure to a nut in patients allergic to other nuts [76]. Bock and Atkins [67] performed challenges to one or more nuts in 14 children and at least 2 reacted to multiple nuts (as many as five types). Ewan [75] reported allergy to multiple tree nuts in over a third of 34 patients evaluated for tree nut allergy. Similarly, our group noted that in 54 children with a tree nut allergy, reactions to more than one nut occurred in 37% [62]. Some nut allergens may be homologous and cause reactions (e.g., in pistachio/cashew [77]) while others may be homologous but rarely elicit clinical cross-reactivity (e.g., proteins in coconut and walnut [78]).

Legume/tree nuts/seeds

Co-sensitization to allergenic foods such as peanut, tree nuts, and seeds (sesame, poppy, mustard) is common. In a study of 731 subjects in the United Kingdom, 59% sensitized to peanut were also sensitized to hazelnut and/or Brazil nut [63]. Although clinically significant cross-reacting proteins have not yet been described, it is known that some amino acid sequences (epitopes) are highly homologous among some of the seed storage proteins that constitute the major allergens in these foods [57]. This observation begs the question: is this high rate of concomitant reactivity due to cross-reactivity of IgE antibodies directed against homologous proteins or to co-sensitization to intrinsically allergenic foods among highly atopic patients? Until more data are available, the clinician must consider the age of the patient, history, and sensitization in considering categorical elimination of these allergenic foods. Reactions to seeds such as sesame, mustard, and poppy are being increasingly reported [64, 79–81], and cross-reactivity with foods (hazel, kiwi, other seeds) and pollens is potentially important.

Fish

In a prevalence study in the United States [82], reaction to multiple fish among those with any fish allergy was 67%. Among those with fish allergy ($n = 58$), 19 reported a reaction to only one type, 5 to two types, 13 to three to nine types, and the remainder were uncertain. In serological studies of 10 subjects with codfish allergy, sensitization to salmon was strong while sensitization to halibut, flounder, tuna, and mackerel was lower [83]. To best evaluate clinical cross-reactivity, it would be necessary to perform oral food challenges to multiple types of fish, shellfish, or mollusks in persons allergic to at least one type. The clinical studies concerning fish allergy mirror those of tree nut allergy in that clinical reactions to multiple fish is a common phenomenon, high cross-sensitization rates are even more common, and the allergic reactions tend to be severe [84–86]. The results of several clinical studies are shown in Table 25.3 [84–88]. Regional exposure patterns are relevant. Pascual and colleagues [89] from Spain evaluated the relevance of cross-reactivity among six regionally important species in 79 children with fish allergy where codfish is not a common food. While all subjects had positive skin tests to multiple species, only 31 of 79 (39%) had clinical reactions; hake and whiff had the highest and albacore the lowest reaction rate. Formal studies of fish hypersensitivity have also indicated that fish proteins may be denatured when heated (canned) or lyophilized, and this must be appreciated when considering a history of specific fish that appear to be tolerated in some forms, for example, reactive to salmon but not reactive to canned salmon [90]. Allergy to fish egg is distinct from allergy to fish meat [91].

In summary, a fish-allergic patient is at high risk for reactions to other fish, but may tolerate some fish species, and may therefore deserve further evaluation with supervised oral challenges if desirous of ingesting other fish. The fact that fish allergy can be severe and that cooking/canning and other processing can alter allergenicity must be considered during these evaluations [90].

Table 25.3 Studies of cross-reactivity among fish.

Study population	Design	Results	Reference
Children, US ($n = 10$)	DBPCFC to 4–6 species	3/10 reacted to more than one type	84
Adults, Denmark ($n = 8$)	Proven codfish allergy (DBPCFC) with medical history to other fish	All exposed to plaice (6), herring (5), and mackerel (6) reacted	87
Adults, Denmark ($n = 6$)	Positive DBPCFC to at least one: catfish, cod, snapper and challenged to at least 2.	4/6 reacted to more than one species	85
Children, Norway ($n = 61$)	No formal challenge, exposure 2–8 species	34/61(56%) reacted to all and 27/61 (44%) tolerated some	86
Children, Italy ($n = 20$)	Codfish allergy with natural exposure to other fish	Reaction rates 25–100% (eel, bass, sole, tuna > salmon, sardine, dogfish)	88

Shellfish

The clinical impression is that reactions to multiple Crustaceans are fairly common, but there are few clinical studies addressing this issue. In a prevalence study in the United States [82], reactions to multiple Crustaceans for those with allergy to any was 38%, and for mollusks 49%; only 14% with Crustacean allergy reported a mollusk allergy. In that study, estimation of the rate of allergies to multiple types of seafood was complicated by the fact that not all participants were exposed to all types of seafood and, after a reaction, avoidance of multiple types of seafood was often undertaken. Among those with allergy to shrimp, lobster, and/or crab who indicated specific knowledge of an allergy among these ($n = 232$), 62% indicated allergy to one, 20% to two and 18% to all three types. Among scallops, clams, oysters, and mussels ($n = 67$), 51% reacted to one, 19% to two, 8% to three, and 22% to all four types. Forty-one persons with shellfish allergy (14%) reported an allergy to both one or more Crustaceans and one or more mollusks/bivalves.

The major shared allergenic protein is invertebrate tropomyosin found in Crustaceans (shrimp, crab, lobster) [92–94] and mollusks (oyster, scallop, and squid) [95]. Not surprisingly, the rate of cross-sensitization is high. In 16 atopic, shrimp-allergic patients, >80% had positive SPTs to crab, crayfish, and lobster [96]. Unfortunately, formal clinical studies to determine the rate of clinical reactivity are lacking. In a study of 11 patients with immediate reactions to shrimp ingestion, the reaction rate to lobster, crab, and crayfish was 50–100% per species [97]. On the other hand, there are individuals who react not only to shrimp alone, but are reactive to specific species of shrimp [98].

Also poorly defined is the risk of mollusk allergy for Crustacean- or mollusk-allergic individuals. Lehrer and McCants [99] reported a study of 6 oyster-sensitive, 7 oyster- and Crustacean-sensitive, and 12 Crustacean-sensitive patients in whom serologies were evaluated. Most of the reactions to oyster were isolated to the gastrointestinal tract and not associated with oyster-specific IgE antibody. However, among 19 patients with sensitivity to Crustaceans, 47% had positive IgE tests to oyster, indicating potential cross-reactivity. In another study evaluating nine patients with shrimp anaphylaxis, binding to tropomyosin of 13 Crustaceans and mollusks was universal [95]. These studies only evaluated serologies so the rate of clinical reactivity is unclear, but apparently not high.

Invertebrate tropomyosin is also found in airborne insect allergens found in cockroach and dust mite [100], which raises the possibility of sensitization by the respiratory route. In a report of wheezing induced by snail consumption in 28 patients, inhibition studies indicated that house dust mite sensitization was the likely initial sensitizing event [101].

Overall, Crustacean species represent an increased risk of cross-reactivity with a potential for severe reactions and a potentially high rate of clinical symptoms. However, there are individuals who tolerate most types, so individualization, done cautiously, may be warranted. Allergy to mollusks is less well established and appears less common.

Cereal grains

Wheat, rye, barley, and oat share homologous proteins with grass pollens and with each other [102, 103] and this may account for the high rate of co-sensitization among these foods [102]. Among children with at least one grain allergy undergoing DBPCFCs to multiple grains, 80% were tolerant of all other grains. Caution is warranted, but clinical reactivity to multiple grains appears uncommon and individualization warranted for these common foods.

Avian and mammalian food products

For avian foods such as chicken, sensitization has been described to alpha-livetin found in feathers, egg, and meat [104]. Reactions to chicken meat are often based upon reactivity to this protein (22–32%) [105, 106]. Chicken meat allergy is uncommon [107], but when it occurs in the absence of egg allergy, the risk of reaction to multiple species of avian meats (turkey, pheasant, quail) may be increased. This observation is probably because a meat-specific protein, rather than within-species meat-egg-specific protein, is causally related to reactions [108, 109]. Cross-reactive proteins among various avian eggs are also common [110], but the clinical implications have not been systematically studied. Conversely, allergy to one egg type may not guarantee reactions to others; reactions to duck and goose egg, in the absence of hen's egg allergy, has been described [111].

Some patients with allergy to mammalian milks also react to mammalian meats [112]. This observation may be due to homologous proteins or, more likely, proteins that are identical and are actually residual ones in meat and milk from the same animal. A study employing oral challenges showed that 9.7% of 62 cow's milk-allergic (CMA) children reacted to beef [113]. Heating and other cooking processes can reduce the allergenicity of beef [114], so well-cooked beef is less likely to cause a problem for those with CMA. Reactions to multiple mammalian milks are common among sheep, cow, ewe, buffalo, and goat milks (>90%), but not to donkey, mare, or camel's milk (<~5%) [115]. Cross-sensitization is more common within than between avian and mammalian meats, but clinical correlation with sensitization is generally under 50%, so individualization is also usually warranted [116]. Reactions to multiple mammalian meats may occur due to allergic reactivity to galactose-alpha-1,3-galactose, resulting in delayed anaphylaxis [117].

Fruit

Oral allergy syndrome (pollen–food allergy syndrome) is described elsewhere (Chapter 12) and the focus here will be upon cross-reactions within families of fruits. Several studies have selected patients based upon particular fruit allergies, rather than pollen allergies, and evaluated for reactions to related fruits. Rodriguez and colleagues [118] evaluated 34 adults in Madrid with reported allergy to Rosaceae foods (peach, apple, apricot, almond, plum, pear, and strawberry). Eighty-two percent had positive SPTs and/or food-specific serum IgE to at least one of the foods with a median of five positive foods per patient. Clinical reactivity determined by DBPCFCs was less than 10% for those positive to pear and up to 90% for peach (overall, 35% with a positive skin test reacted to a given food). Multiple fruit allergy was common in the 22 who reacted to at least one fruit (46%). Peach was the dominant allergenic fruit; 46% reactive to peach reacted to another Rosaceae fruit. Pastorello and colleagues [119] studied patients selected for a history of reactions to peach confirmed through open oral food challenges; among 19 evaluated, 63% reacted to at least one other fruit among cherry, apricot, and plum. Of 19 patients with melon allergy confirmed by DBPCFC (of 54 patients suspected), 94% reacted to at least one of the following related fruits: watermelon, avocado, kiwi, chestnut, banana, or peach [120].

Severity of reactions to these foods is an important issue. Pollen-related fruit allergy is usually mild (oral allergy syndrome) and yet in one study 8.7% experienced associated systemic symptoms outside of the gastrointestinal tract [121], 3% at some time experience systemic symptoms without oral symptoms, and 1.7% experienced anaphylactic shock. It is becoming clear why some patients are more likely to experience severe reactions. There is evidence that when fruit allergy develops in the absence of pollen allergy, reactions are directed not only to Bet v 1 or profilins, but also to lipid transfer proteins (LTP) or other components that may indicate a more severe reaction

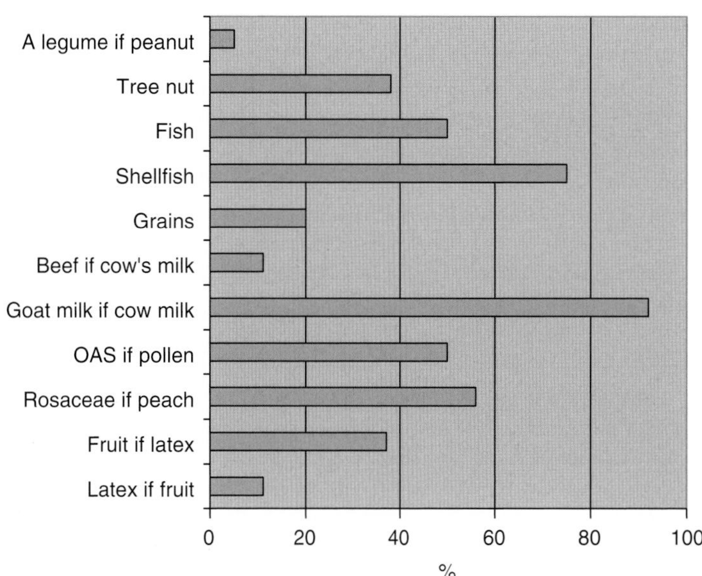

Figure 25.1 The approximate rate of clinical reactivity to at least one other related food. The probability of reacting to related foods varies, depending upon numerous factors (data reviewed in Reference 65). OAS, oral allergy syndrome/pollen–food syndrome.

[122]. Fernández-Rivas and colleagues [123] compared patients with Rosaceae fruit allergy with and without pollenosis and found that systemic reactions occurred in 82% without compared to 45% with pollenosis. Anaphylactic shock was also more common in the former (36% vs. 9%, respectively). Crespo et al. [124] evaluated 65 adults diagnosed with clinical allergy to one or more fruits for allergy to other related foods. Thirty-four of those tested (52%) were found to be clinically allergic to more than one fruit. Food challenges with potential cross-reactive foods uncovered 18 further reactions in 14 (22%) out of 65. Only 8% (18/223) of positive results for allergy tests to potential cross-reactive foods investigated were clinically relevant. Therefore, elimination of related fruits without testing or based on test results could have resulted in unnecessary restriction of 205 foods in the 65 people studied. However, it was worrisome that 18 food reactions in one-fifth (14/65) of patients could have been missed if oral challenges/evaluations were not pursued. The interrelationships of allergy to proteins that are homologous among plant foods, pollens, and even latex [65, 125] represent a diverse risk profile. The clinical lesson is that once a patient experiences more than oral symptoms to a fruit, a careful search by history and/or challenge may be warranted to prove the safety of related fruits. Component testing may add additional insights.

Summary and management

As outlined in each preceding section, there is a high likelihood of sensitization to foods that bear homologous allergens, but clinical reactivity correlates poorly. It is therefore necessary to consider a variety of issues when evaluating a patient for the possibility of multiple food hypersensitivities on the basis of possible cross-reactions. Among these are *a priori* reasoning about likelihood of reactions (Figure 25.1), severity of reactions, social and nutritional importance of the food, and the (poor) predictive value of tests for IgE antibody in this setting. However, for most patients, more foods are being avoided than necessary and the extra effort to prove which foods are or are not tolerated is worthwhile.

References

1. Boyce JA, Assa'ad A, Burks AW, et al. Guidelines for the diagnosis and management of food allergy in the United States: report of the NIAID-sponsored expert panel. *J Allergy Clin Immunol* 2010; 126(6 Suppl.):S1–S58.
2. Vierk K, Falci K, Wolyniak C, Klontz KC. Recalls of foods containing undeclared allergens reported to the US Food and Drug Administration, fiscal year 1999. *J Allergy Clin Immunol* 2002; 109(6):1022–1026.
3. Gern J, Yang E, Evrard H, Sampson H. Allergic reactions to milk-contaminated "non-dairy" products. *N Engl J Med* 1991; 324:976–979.
4. Jones RT, Squillace DL, Yunginger JW. Anaphylaxis in a milk-allergic child after ingestion of milk-contaminated kosher-pareve-labeled "dairy-free" dessert [See comments]. *Ann Allergy* 1992; 68(3):223–227.
5. Enrique E, Cistero-Bahima A, Alonso R, San Miguel MM. Egg protein: a hidden allergen in candies. *Ann Allergy Asthma Immunol* 2000; 84(6):636.
6. Cantani A. Hidden presence of cow's milk proteins in foods. *J Investig Allergol Clin Immunol* 1999; 9:141–145.
7. McKenna C, Klontz KC. Systemic allergic reaction following ingestion of undeclared peanut flour in a peanut-sensitive woman. *Ann Allergy Asthma Immunol* 1997; 79(3):234–236.
8. Cowen DE. Hidden allergens—vehicles and excipients. *Ann Allergy* 1967; 25(3):161–164.
9. Lockey Sr SD. Reactions to hidden agents in foods, beverages and drugs. *Ann Allergy* 1971; 29(9):461–466.
10. Kirschner S, Belloni B, Kugler C, Ring J, Brockow K. Allergenicity of wine containing processing aids: a double-blind, placebo-controlled food challenge. *J Investig Allergol Clin Immunol* 2009; 19(3):210–217.
11. Leitch I, Blair IS, McDowell DA. The role of environmental health officers in the protection of allergic consumers. *Int J Environ Health Res* 2001; 11(1):51–61.
12. Hogendijk S, Eigenmann PA, Hauser C. The problem of hidden food allergens: two cases of anaphylaxis to peanut proteins concealed in a pizza sauce. *Schweiz Med Wochenschr* 1998; 128(29–30):1134–1137.
13. Taylor SL, Hefle SL. Food allergen labeling in the USA and Europe. *Curr Opin Allergy Clin Immunol* 2006; 6(3):186–190.
14. Madsen CB, Hattersley S, Allen KJ, et al. Can we define a tolerable level of risk in food allergy? Report from a EuroPrevall/UK Food Standards Agency workshop. *Clin Exp Allergy* 2012; 42(1):30–37.
15. Greenhawt MJ, Baldwin JL. Carmine dye and cochineal extract: hidden allergens no more. *Ann Allergy Asthma Immunol* 2009; 103(1):73–75.
16. Pieretti MM, Chung D, Pacenza R, Slotkin T, Sicherer SH. Audit of manufactured products: use of allergen advisory labels and identification of labeling ambiguities. *J Allergy Clin Immunol* 2009; 124(2):337–341.
17. Sampson MA, Munoz-Furlong A, Sicherer SH. Risk-taking and coping strategies of adolescents and young adults with food allergy. *J Allergy Clin Immunol* 2006; 117(6):1440–1445.
18. Hefle SL, Furlong TJ, Niemann L, Lemon-Mule H, Sicherer S, Taylor SL. Consumer attitudes and risks associated with packaged foods having advisory labeling regarding the presence of peanuts. *J Allergy Clin Immunol* 2007; 120(1):171–176.
19. Crotty MP, Taylor SL. Risks associated with foods having advisory milk labeling. *J Allergy Clin Immunol* 2010; 125(4):935–937.
20. Ford LS, Taylor SL, Pacenza R, Niemann LM, Lambrecht DM, Sicherer SH. Food allergen advisory labeling and product contamination with egg, milk, and peanut. *J Allergy Clin Immunol* 2010; 126(2):384–385.

21. Ong PY. Are allergy advisory statements helpful to patients with food allergy? *J Allergy Clin Immunol* 2008; 121(2):536–537.
22. Sicherer SH, Furlong TJ, DeSimone J, Sampson HA. The US Peanut and Tree Nut Allergy Registry: characteristics of reactions in schools and day care. *J Pediatr* 2001; 138(4):560–565.
23. Furlong TJ, DeSimone J, Sicherer SH. Peanut and tree nut allergic reactions in restaurants and other food establishments. *J Allergy Clin Immunol* 2001; 108(5 Pt. 1):867–870.
24. Ahuja R, Sicherer SH. Food-allergy management from the perspective of restaurant and food establishment personnel. *Ann Allergy Asthma Immunol* 2007; 98(4):344–348.
25. Bailey S, Albardiaz R, Frew AJ, Smith H. Restaurant staff's knowledge of anaphylaxis and dietary care of people with allergies. *Clin Exp Allergy* 2011; 41(5):713–717.
26. Sicherer SH, Vargas PA, Groetch ME, et al. Development and validation of educational materials for food allergy. *J Pediatr* 2012; 160(4):651–656.
27. Chawla KK, Bencharitiwong R, Ayuso R, Grishina G, Nowak-Wegrzyn A. Shea butter contains no IgE-binding soluble proteins. *J Allergy Clin Immunol* 2011; 127(3):680–682.
28. Greenhawt M, McMorris M, Baldwin J. Carmine hypersensitivity masquerading as azithromycin hypersensitivity. *Allergy Asthma Proc* 2009; 30(1):95–101.
29. Kelso JM. Raw egg allergy—a potential issue in vaccine allergy. *J Allergy Clin Immunol* 2000; 106(5):990.
30. James JM, Zeiger RS, Lester MR, et al. Safe administration of influenza vaccine to patients with egg allergy. *J Pediatr* 1998; 133(5):624–628.
31. Kattan JD, Konstantinou GN, Cox AL, et al. Anaphylaxis to diphtheria, tetanus, and pertussis vaccines among children with cow's milk allergy. *J Allergy Clin Immunol* 2011; 128(1):215–218.
32. Sakaguchi M, Miyazawa H, Inouye S. Specific IgE and IgG to gelatin in children with systemic cutaneous reactions to Japanese encephalitis vaccines. *Allergy* 2001; 56(6):536–539.
33. Greenhawt MJ, Li JT, Bernstein DI, et al. Administering influenza vaccine to egg allergic recipients: a focused practice parameter update. *Ann Allergy Asthma Immunol* 2011; 106(1):11–16.
34. Nowak-Wegrzyn A, Shapiro GG, Beyer K, Bardina L, Sampson HA. Contamination of dry powder inhalers for asthma with milk proteins containing lactose. *J Allergy Clin Immunol* 2004; 113(3):558–560.
35. Murphy A, Campbell DE, Baines D, Mehr S. Allergic reactions to propofol in egg-allergic children. *Anesth Analg* 2011; 113(1):140–144.
36. Erben AM, Rodriguez JL, McCullough J, Ownby DR. Anaphylaxis after ingestion of beignets contaminated with Dermatophagoides farinae. *J Allergy Clin Immunol* 1993; 92(6):846–849.
37. Sanchez-Borges M, Capriles-Hulett A, Fernandez-Caldas E, et al. Mite-contaminated foods as a cause of anaphylaxis. *J Allergy Clin Immunol* 1997; 99(6 Pt. 1):738–743.
38. Franklin W, Pandolfo J. Latex as a food allergen. *N Engl J Med* 1999; 341(24):1858.
39. Schwartz HJ. Latex: a potential hidden "food" allergen in fast food restaurants. *J Allergy Clin Immunol* 1995; 95(1 Pt. 1):139–140.
40. Beezhold DH, Reschke JE, Allen JH, Kostyal DA, Sussman GL. Latex protein: a hidden "food" allergen? *Allergy Asthma Proc* 2000; 21(5):301–306.
41. Daschner A, Pascual CY. Anisakis simplex: sensitization and clinical allergy. *Curr Opin Allergy Clin Immunol* 2005; 5(3):281–285.
42. Tan BM, Sher MR, Good RA, Bahna SL. Severe food allergies by skin contact. *Ann Allergy Asthma Immunol* 2001; 86(5):583–586.
43. Wainstein BK, Kashef S, Ziegler M, Jelley D, Ziegler JB. Frequency and significance of immediate contact reactions to peanut in peanut-sensitive children. *Clin Exp Allergy* 2007; 37(6):839–845.
44. Simonte SJ, Ma S, Mofidi S, Sicherer SH. Relevance of casual contact with peanut butter in children with peanut allergy. *J Allergy Clin Immunol* 2003; 112(1):180–182.
45. Kalogeromitros D, Armenaka M, Galatas I, Capellou O, Katsarou A. Anaphylaxis induced by lentils. *Ann Allergy Asthma Immunol* 1996; 77(6):480–482.
46. Polasani R, Melgar L, Reisman R, Ballow M. Hot dog vapor-induced status asthmaticus. *Ann Allergy Asthma Immunol* 1997; 78:35–36.
47. Taylor AV, Swanson MC, Jones RT, et al. Detection and quantitation of raw fish aeroallergens from an open-air fish market. *J Allergy Clin Immunol* 2000; 105(1 Pt. 1):166–169.
48. Roberts G, Golder N, Lack G. Bronchial challenges with aerosolized food in asthmatic, food-allergic children. *Allergy* 2002; 57(8):713–717.
49. Sicherer SH, Furlong TJ, DeSimone J, Sampson HA. Self-reported allergic reactions to peanut on commercial airliners. *J Allergy Clin Immunol* 1999; 104(1):186–189.
50. Greenhawt MJ, McMorris MS, Furlong TJ. Self-reported allergic reactions to peanut and tree nuts occurring on commercial airlines. *J Allergy Clin Immunol* 2009; 124(3):598–599.
51. Hallett R, Haapanen LA, Teuber SS. Food allergies and kissing. *N Engl J Med* 2002; 346(23):1833–1834.
52. Eriksson NE, Moller C, Werner S, Magnusson J, Bengtsson U. The hazards of kissing when you are food allergic. A survey on the occurrence of kiss-induced allergic reactions among 1139 patients with self-reported food hypersensitivity. *J Investig Allergol Clin Immunol* 2003; 13(3):149–154.
53. Maloney JM, Chapman MD, Sicherer SH. Peanut allergen exposure through saliva: assessment and interventions to reduce exposure. *J Allergy Clin Immunol* 2006; 118(3):719–724.
54. Wuthrich B, Dascher M, Borelli S. Kiss-induced allergy to peanut. *Allergy* 2001; 56(9):913.
55. Jacobs JF, Baumert JL, Brons PP, Joosten I, Koppelman SJ, van Pampus EC. Anaphylaxis from passive transfer of peanut allergen in a blood product. *N Engl J Med* 2011; 364(20):1981–1982.
56. Maloney JM, Rudengren M, Ahlstedt S, Bock SA, Sampson HA. The use of serum-specific IgE measurements for the diagnosis of peanut, tree nut, and seed allergy. *J Allergy Clin Immunol* 2008; 122(1):145–151.

57. Beyer K, Bardina L, Grishina G, Sampson HA. Identification of sesame seed allergens by 2-dimensional proteomics and Edman sequencing: seed storage proteins as common food allergens. *J Allergy Clin Immunol* 2002; 110(1):154–159.
58. Breiteneder H, Ebner C. Molecular and biochemical classification of plant-derived food allergens. *J Allergy Clin Immunol* 2000; 106(1 Pt. 1):27–36.
59. Breiteneder H, Radauer C. A classification of plant food allergens. *J Allergy Clin Immunol* 2004; 113(5):821–830.
60. Aalberse RC. Structural biology of allergens. *J Allergy Clin Immunol* 2000; 106(2):228–238.
61. Bernhisel-Broadbent J, Sampson HA. Cross-allergenicity in the legume botanical family in children with food hypersensitivity. *J Allergy Clin Immunol* 1989; 83:435–440.
62. Sicherer SH, Burks AW, Sampson HA. Clinical features of acute allergic reactions to peanut and tree nuts in children. *Pediatrics* 1998; 102(1):e6.
63. Pumphrey RS, Wilson PB, Faragher EB, Edwards SR. Specific immunoglobulin E to peanut, hazelnut and Brazil nut in 731 patients: similar patterns found at all ages. *Clin Exp Allergy* 1999; 29(9):1256–1259.
64. Vocks E, Borga A, Szliska C, Seifert HU, Burow G, Borelli S. Common allergenic structures in hazelnut, rye grain, sesame seeds, kiwi, and poppy seeds. *Allergy* 1993; 48:168–172.
65. Sicherer SH. Clinical implications of cross-reactive food allergens. *J Allergy Clin Immunol* 2001; 108(6):881–890.
66. Sicherer SH. Determinants of systemic manifestations of food allergy. *J Allergy Clin Immunol* 2000; 106(5 Suppl.):S251–S257.
67. Bock SA, Atkins FM. The natural history of peanut allergy. *J Allergy Clin Immunol* 1989; 83:900–904.
68. Burks AW, James JM, Hiegel A, et al. Atopic dermatitis and food hypersensitivity reactions. *J Pediatr* 1998; 132(1):132–136.
69. Moneret-Vautrin DA, Guerin L, Kanny G, Flabbee J, Fremont S, Morisset M. Cross-allergenicity of peanut and lupine: the risk of lupine allergy in patients allergic to peanuts. *J Allergy Clin Immunol* 1999; 104(4 Pt. 1):883–888.
70. Shaw J, Roberts G, Grimshaw K, White S, Hourihane J. Lupin allergy in peanut-allergic children and teenagers. *Allergy* 2008; 63(3):370–373.
71. Fiocchi A, Sarratud P, Terracciano L, et al. Assessment of the tolerance to lupine-enriched pasta in peanut-allergic children. *Clin Exp Allergy* 2009; 39(7):1045–1051.
72. Peeters KA, Koppelman SJ, Penninks AH, et al. Clinical relevance of sensitization to lupine in peanut-sensitized adults. *Allergy* 2009; 64(4):549–555.
73. Crespo JF, Pascual C, Burks AW, Helm RM, Esteban MM. Frequency of food allergy in a pediatric population from Spain. *Pediatr Allergy Immunol* 1995; 6(1):39–43.
74. Pascual CY, Fernandez-Crespo J, Sanchez-Pastor S, et al. Allergy to lentils in Mediterranean pediatric patients. *J Allergy Clin Immunol* 1999; 103(1 Pt. 1):154–158.
75. Ewan PW. Clinical study of peanut and nut allergy in 62 consecutive patients: new features and associations [see comments]. *BMJ* 1996; 312(7038):1074–1078.
76. Bock SA, Munoz-Furlong A, Sampson HA. Fatalities due to anaphylactic reactions to foods. *J Allergy Clin Immunol* 2001; 107(1):191–193.
77. Willison LN, Tawde P, Robotham JM, et al. Pistachio vicilin, Pis v 3, is immunoglobulin E-reactive and cross-reacts with the homologous cashew allergen, Ana o 1. *Clin Exp Allergy* 2008; 38(7):1229–1238.
78. Teuber SS, Peterson WR. Systemic allergic reaction to coconut (*Cocos nucifera*) in 2 subjects with hypersensitivity to tree nut and demonstration of cross-reactivity to legumin-like seed storage proteins: new coconut and walnut food allergens. *J Allergy Clin Immunol* 1999; 103(6):1180–1185.
79. Asero R, Mistrello G, Roncarolo D, Antoniotti PL, Falagiani P. A case of sesame seed-induced anaphylaxis. *Allergy* 1999; 54(5):526–527.
80. Rance F, Dutau G, Abbal M. Mustard allergy in children. *Allergy* 2000; 55(5):496–500.
81. Derby CJ, Gowland MH, Hourihane JO. Sesame allergy in Britain: a questionnaire survey of members of the Anaphylaxis Campaign. *Pediatr Allergy Immunol* 2005; 16(2):171–175.
82. Sicherer SH, Munoz-Furlong A, Sampson HA. Prevalence of seafood allergy in the United States determined by a random telephone survey. *J Allergy Clin Immunol* 2004; 114(1):159–165.
83. Van Do T, Elsayed S, Florvaag E, Hordvik I, Endresen C. Allergy to fish parvalbumins: studies on the cross-reactivity of allergens from 9 commonly consumed fish. *J Allergy Clin Immunol* 2005; 116(6):1314–1320.
84. Bernhisel-Broadbent J, Scanlon SM, Sampson HA. Fish hypersensitivity. I. In vitro and oral challenge results in fish-allergic patients. *J Allergy Clin Immunol* 1992; 89:730–737.
85. Helbling A, Haydel R, McCants ML, Musmand JJ, El Dahr J, Lehrer SB. Fish allergy: is cross-reactivity among fish species relevant? Double-blind placebo-controlled food challenge studies of fish allergic adults. *Ann Allergy Asthma Immunol* 1999; 83(6 Pt. 1):517–523.
86. Aas K. Studies of hypersensitivity to fish. A clinical study. *Int Arch Allergy Clin Immun* 1966; 29:346–363.
87. Hansen TK, Bindslev JC, Skov PS, Poulsen LK. Codfish allergy in adults: IgE cross-reactivity among fish species. *Ann Allergy Asthma Immunol* 1997; 78(2):187–194.
88. de Martino M, Novembre E, Galli L, et al. Allergy to different fish species in cod-allergic children: in vivo and in vitro studies. *J Allergy Clin Immunol* 1990; 86(6 Pt. 1):909–914.
89. Pascual C, Martin EM, Crespo JF. Fish allergy: evaluation of the importance of cross-reactivity. *J Pediatr* 1992; 121(5 Pt. 2):S29–S34.
90. Bernhisel-Broadbent J, Strause D, Sampson HA. Fish hypersensitivity. II: clinical relevance of altered fish allergenicity caused by various preparation methods. *J Allergy Clin Immunol* 1992; 90:622–629.
91. Gonzalez-De-Olano D, Rodriguez-Marco A, Gonzalez-Mancebo E, Gandolfo-Cano M, Melendez-Baltanas A, Bartolome B. Allergy to red caviar. *J Investig Allergol Clin Immunol* 2011; 21(6):493–494.
92. Daul CB, Slattery M, Reese G, Lehrer SB. Identification of the major brown shrimp (*Penaeus aztecus*) allergen as the muscle protein tropomyosin. *Int Arch Allergy Immunol* 1994; 105:49–55.
93. Leung PS, Chen YC, Gershwin ME, Wong SH, Kwan HS, Chu KH. Identification and molecular characterization of

Charybdis feriatus tropomyosin, the major crab allergen. *J Allergy Clin Immunol* 1998; 102(5):847–852.

94. Leung PS, Chen YC, Mykles DL, Chow WK, Li CP, Chu KH. Molecular identification of the lobster muscle protein tropomyosin as a seafood allergen. *Mol Mar Biol Biotechnol* 1998; 7(1):12–20.
95. Leung PS, Chow WK, Duffey S, Kwan HS, Gershwin ME, Chu KH. IgE reactivity against a cross-reactive allergen in crustacea and mollusca: evidence for tropomyosin as the common allergen. *J Allergy Clin Immunol* 1996; 98(5 Pt. 1):954–961.
96. Daul CB, Morgan JE, Waring NP, McCants ML, Hughes J, Lehrer SB. Immunologic evaluation of shrimp-allergic individuals. *J Allergy Clin Immunol* 1987; 80(5):716–722.
97. Waring NP, Daul CB, deShazo RD, McCants ML, Lehrer SB. Hypersensitivity reactions to ingested crustacea: clinical evaluation and diagnostic studies in shrimp-sensitive individuals. *J Allergy Clin Immunol* 1985; 76:440–445.
98. Morgan JE, O'Neil CE, Daul CB, Lehrer SB. Species-specific shrimp allergens: RAST and RAST-inhibition studies. *J Allergy Clin Immunol* 1989; 83(6):1112–1117.
99. Lehrer SB, McCants ML. Reactivity of IgE antibodies with crustacea and oyster allergens: evidence for common antigenic structures. *J Allergy Clin Immunol* 1987; 80(2):133–139.
100. Wang J, Calatroni A, Visness CM, Sampson HA. Correlation of specific IgE to shrimp with cockroach and dust mite exposure and sensitization in an inner-city population. *J Allergy Clin Immunol* 2011; 128(4):834–837.
101. van Ree R, Antonicelli L, Akkerdaas JH, et al. Asthma after consumption of snails in house-dust-mite-allergic patients: a case of IgE cross-reactivity. *Allergy* 1996; 51:387–393.
102. Jones SM, Magnolfi CF, Cooke SK, Sampson HA. Immunologic cross-reactivity among cereal grains and grasses in children with food hypersensitivity. *J Allergy Clin Immunol* 1995; 96(3):341–351.
103. Donovan GR, Baldo BA. Crossreactivity of IgE antibodies from sera of subjects allergic to both ryegrass pollen and wheat endosperm proteins: evidence for common allergenic determinants. *Clin Exp Allergy* 1990; 20:501–509.
104. Bausela BA, Garcia AM, Martin EM, Boyano MT, Diaz PJ, Ojeda CJ. Peculiarities of egg allergy in children with bird protein sensitization. *Ann Allergy Asthma Immunol* 1997; 78(2):213–216.
105. Bausela BA, Garcia AM, Martin EM, Boyano MT, Diaz PJ, Ojeda CJ. Peculiarities of egg allergy in children with bird protein sensitization. *Ann Allergy Asthma Immunol* 1997; 78(2):213–216.
106. Szepfalusi Z, Ebner C, Pandjaitan R, et al. Egg yolk a-livetin (chicken serum albumin) is a cross-reactive allergen in the bird-egg syndrome. *J Allergy Clin Immunol* 1994; 93:932–942.
107. Bock SA, Sampson HA, Atkins FM, et al. Double-blind, placebo-controlled food challenge (DBPCFC) as an office procedure: a manual. *J Allergy Clin Immunol* 1988; 82:986–997.
108. Kelso JM, Cockrell GE, Helm RM, Burks AW. Common allergens in avian meats. *J Allergy Clin Immunol* 1999; 104(1):202–204.
109. Cahen YD, Fritsch R, Wuthrich B. Food allergy with monovalent sensitivity to poultry meat. *Clin Exp Allergy* 1998; 28(8):1026–1030.
110. Langland T. A clinical and immunological study of allergy to hen's egg white. VI. Occurrence of proteins cross-reacting with allergens in hen's egg white as studied in egg white from turkey, duck, goose, seagull, and in hen egg yolk, and hen and chicken sera and flesh. *Allergy* 1983; 38:399–412.
111. Anibarro B, Seoane FJ, Vila C, Lombardero M. Allergy to eggs from duck and goose without sensitization to hen egg proteins. *J Allergy Clin Immunol* 2000; 105(4):834–836.
112. Martelli A, De Chiara A, Corvo M, Restani P, Fiocchi A. Beef allergy in children with cow's milk allergy; cow's milk allergy in children with beef allergy. *Ann Allergy Asthma Immunol* 2002; 89(6 Suppl. 1):38–43.
113. Werfel SJ, Cooke SK, Sampson HA. Clinical reactivity to beef in children allergic to cow's milk. *J Allergy Clin Immunol* 1997; 99(3):293–300.
114. Fiocchi A, Restani P, Riva E, et al. Heat treatment modifies the allergenicity of beef and bovine serum albumin. *Allergy* 1998; 53(8):798–802.
115. Jarvinen KM, Chatchatee P. Mammalian milk allergy: clinical suspicion, cross-reactivities and diagnosis. *Curr Opin Allergy Clin Immunol* 2009; 9(3):251–258.
116. Ayuso R, Lehrer SB, Tanaka L, et al. IgE antibody response to vertebrate meat proteins including tropomyosin. *Ann Allergy Asthma Immunol* 1999; 83(5):399–405.
117. Commins SP, James HR, Kelly LA, et al. The relevance of tick bites to the production of IgE antibodies to the mammalian oligosaccharide galactose-alpha-1,3-galactose. *J Allergy Clin Immunol* 2011; 127(5):1286–1293.
118. Rodriguez J, Crespo JF, Lopez-Rubio A, et al. Clinical cross-reactivity among foods of the Rosaceae family. *J Allergy Clin Immunol* 2000; 106(1 Pt. 1):183–189.
119. Pastorello E, Ortolani C, Farioli L, et al. Allergenic cross-reactivity among peach, apricot, plum, and cherry in patients with oral allergy syndrome: an in vivo and in vitro study. *J Allergy Clin Immunol* 1994; 94(4):699–707.
120. Rodriguez J, Crespo JF, Burks W, et al. Randomized, double-blind, crossover challenge study in 53 subjects reporting adverse reactions to melon (*Cucumis melo*). *J Allergy Clin Immunol* 2000; 106(5):968–972.
121. Ortolani C, Pastorello EA, Farioli L, et al. IgE-mediated allergy from vegetable allergens. *Ann Allergy* 1993; 71(5):470–476.
122. Ballmer-Weber BK, Hoffmann-Sommergruber K. Molecular diagnosis of fruit and vegetable allergy. *Curr Opin Allergy Clin Immunol* 2011; 11(3):229–235.
123. Fernandez-Rivas M, van Ree R, Cuevas M. Allergy to Rosaceae fruits without related pollinosis. *J Allergy Clin Immunol* 1997; 100(6 Pt. 1):728–733.
124. Crespo JF, Rodriguez J, James JM, Daroca P, Reano M, Vives R. Reactivity to potential cross-reactive foods in fruit-allergic patients: implications for prescribing food avoidance. *Allergy* 2002; 57(10):946–949.
125. Nowak-Wegrzyn A, Sicherer SH. Immunotherapy for food and latex allergy. *Clin Allergy Immunol* 2008; 21:429–446.

26 Controversial Practices and Unproven Methods in Allergy

David R. Scott[1], Jennifer A. Namazy[1], & Ronald A. Simon[1,2]

[1]Division of Allergy, Asthma, and Immunology, Scripps Clinic, San Diego, CA, USA

[2]Department of Molecular and Experimental Medicine, Scripps Research Institute, La Jolla, CA, USA

Key Concepts

- There have been an increasing number of patients who are using complementary therapies for chronic conditions.
- Unproven methods are increasingly being used for the diagnosis and treatment of allergic diseases.
- Unproven methods are procedures or therapies that are not supported by scientific evidence and have no basis in the pathophysiology of allergic disease.
- Inappropriate methods are procedures and therapies that are legitimate but are used inappropriately.
- It is important for the practicing allergist to become familiar with both accepted and unproven practices.

Introduction

The process of diagnosing and treating allergic disease is complex and at times elusive. It requires a thorough history and physical examination and, in certain situations, complementary laboratory tests. Most of the tests which are performed today have undergone rigorous scientific evaluation for proof of effectiveness and safety. They must also have established physiologic significance when used to diagnose a particular disease. Nevertheless, there are a growing number of unconventional, unproven, and inappropriate procedures used by some in order to diagnose allergic disease. Some of these "tests" are legitimate but are misused in their application to the diagnosis of allergy. Other "tests" have no basis in the pathophysiology of allergic disease. It is important for those practicing allergy and immunology to become familiar with all diagnostic procedures. Some may be unsuitable for allergy diagnosis for several reasons. For example, a procedure may be based on an unproven theory. Others are legitimate tests used inappropriately. Some procedures do not have the ability to diagnose any disease. It thus becomes apparent that standardization and controlled evaluation of procedures before their use is imperative for proper patient care. The following information should be useful because there have been an increasing number of patients who are using complementary therapies for chronic conditions. One study found that complementary therapies were usually used alongside conventional treatment [1]. Patients felt empowered to take control over their condition rather than feel dependent on medication [1]. Chiropractors, homeopaths, and acupuncturists are the most commonly seen providers by patients searching for alternative treatments [2]. A survey of food-allergic patients and family members revealed 22% of respondents to have utilized unproven or disproven diagnostic tests (Table 26.1) [3]. These patients may present at the beginning of their search with a multitude of questions regarding a proposed specific diagnostic procedure or they may present having been involved in a questionable, perhaps expensive procedure, resulting in a questionable diagnosis. Each of the primary international allergy specialty societies, including the American Academy of Allergy Asthma and Immunology (AAAAI) [4], European Academy of Allergy and Clinical Immunology (EAACI) [5], Allergy Society of South America (ALLSA) [6], and the Australasian Society of Clinical Immunology and Allergy (ASCIA) [7], has issued position statements regarding several of the diagnostic and therapeutic modalities discussed in this chapter.

Food Allergy: Adverse Reactions to Foods and Food Additives, Fifth Edition. Edited by Dean D Metcalfe, Hugh A Sampson, Ronald A Simon and Gideon Lack.

Table 26.1 Diagnostic tests used by survey participants for food allergy.

Diagnostic modality	Respondents, no. (%) (*N* = 380)
Skin prick test	302 (79.5)
RAST (serum IgE)	292 (76.8)
IgG4	53 (13.9)
Kinesiology	25 (6.6)
Electrodermal	17 (4.5)
Provocation	15 (3.9)
Pulse test	7 (1.8)
Neutralization	3 (0.8)
Sublingual testing	2 (0.5)
Lymphocyte response assay	5 (1.3)
Other[a]	5 (1.3)
Cytotoxic testing	0
Any non-skin prick test/RAST	82 (21.6)

Source: Reprinted from Reference 3 with permission from Elsevier.
RAST, radioallergosorbent testing.
[a]Includes patch testing and unspecified techniques performed by a chiropractor, naturopath, or homeopath.

Definitions

Standard practice is that which is performed by the majority of physicians in the community. It encompasses those procedures and treatments which have been scientifically proven to be effective and safe. Before describing and critiquing the following procedures and therapies, it is important to first attempt to categorize each one. Thus first certain approaches can be considered to be "unproven" and are also at times referred to as "complementary" or "alternative." These types of tests or treatments are those that are not based on any clear rationale based on acceptable allergy pathophysiology, and their effectiveness is not supported by scientific evidence. Although they may appear well constructed they do not seem capable of either diagnosing or treating an allergic disease. Some of these procedures have been loosely adapted from proven methods that are currently available for the diagnosis and treatment of allergic disease. Often one of the reasons why these tests have not been examined scientifically is that their methodology is vague and is often difficult to reproduce. Other procedures are categorized as being "inappropriate." This means that the test itself is a validated test used to diagnose certain conditions; however, in these cases the procedure is being inappropriately applied.

"Controversial" tests

Skin endpoint titration

During the 1940s, Rinkel developed the method of endpoint skin testing [8]. He found that this method was a useful guide in determining a patient's sensitivity and the information found could be used in determining a safe and effective dose for immunotherapy. Variations of this method have been used for both the diagnosis and treatment of inhalant and food allergies.

Method

The procedure involves intradermal testing with 5-fold serial dilutions of extract. A 7-mm whealing response is considered reactive. The endpoint is defined as the weakest dilution that produces a positive skin reaction and initiates a progressive increase in the diameter of the wheals with each stronger dilution tested [9]. The optimal starting dose is usually 0.01–0.02 mL of extract. The optimal therapeutic dose, defined as a dose at which symptoms are controlled on immunotherapy, is reached after the endpoint dilution is given weekly in increasing increments. Rinkel anticipated a relief of patient symptoms at a dose of 0.5 mL of the endpoint dilution.

Conclusion

There have been several trials over the years that have looked at the efficacy of the Rinkel method. Van Metre et al. published several studies which supported the Rinkel method as valid in quantifying skin sensitivity to ragweed pollen and found the method comparable with *in vitro* leukocyte histamine release and radioallergosorbent assay testing (RAST) [10]. While variations of this method of skin testing are being practiced today without any risks, using the results to determine optimal dosing of immunotherapy is questionable. In the opinion of many, most of the time this "dose" is an underestimation resulting in ineffective treatment.

Unproven tests

Applied kinesiology

Kinesiology refers to the science of motion techniques. It is a belief by some that certain diseases, including allergic reactions, may cause a weakening of skeletal musculature. Some believe that by using applied kinesiology one may diagnose allergic disease. This is commonly applied to the diagnosis of food allergy.

Method

Allergens to be tested are placed in stoppered glass bottles. In some cases a glass vial containing a specific allergen is placed on or near the body of the patient, or in other cases, the patient is asked to hold the vial. During allergen "exposure," muscle strength is tested. A positive test is said to be indicated by observed weakening in muscle strength. There are variations to the standard test which include "surrogate" testing in which a relative of the patient undergoes testing for the patient.

Conclusion

In 1988, Garrow [11] published a study of blinded and open challenges of allergen using applied kinesiology and looking at the reproducibility and efficacy of the test. The study reported no significant difference between frequencies of positive reactions to placebo versus allergen. Therefore, at this time, there appears to be no proof of the efficacy or reproducibility of the method of kinesiology in diagnosing food allergy. AAAAI, along with several other internationally recognized allergy societies, has issued expert panel position statements recommending against the use of this technique in diagnosing food allergy [4–7].

Provocative testing and neutralization

Elicitation of a limited reaction by delivering allergen via the transdermal, subcutaneous, intradermal, or bronchial route is a part of an allergy practice. These procedures provide a wealth of information in the diagnosis of several allergic diseases. Such tests include prick and intradermal skin test, intranasal, subconjunctival, oral tests, and methacholine challenge. These approaches differ from provocative testing and neutralization in that standardized preparations and established threshold doses are defined and have undergone repeated scientific validation in studies with both patients and normal controls [12].

The provocation–neutralization method was introduced by Lee in 1961 for the diagnosis of food allergy [13]. Provocation is performed by intradermal, subcutaneous, or sublingual routes. It is currently used to diagnose and treat allergic disease and sensitivities to a wide variety of substances. The items tested are not necessarily those suspected by the history. They can include such chemicals as formaldehyde, phenol, ethanol, and hormones such as progesterone [14].

Method

The patient is given an intradermal/subcutaneous dose of allergen extract using 5-fold serial dilutions (Rinkel method). The patient is observed for 10 minutes and any symptoms are recorded. If the patient remains symptom free then increasing doses of extract are given until symptoms do occur. Once these symptoms occur, the patient is immediately given injections of weaker dilutions of the same extract until symptoms are resolved. This amount of extract is considered the "neutralizing dose" and is then used for future treatment [15].

The technique appears vague and imprecise. There is no generally established validated protocol for performing the provocative testing and neutralization. In addition, there is no consensus on establishing what a positive test is. Symptoms may be quite extensive and nonspecific and may include headache, nasal symptoms, chest symptoms, ear reactions, gastrointestinal reactions, skin eruptions or itching, or general reactions such as fatigue, chills, muscle pain, or drowsiness [16]. There has been no general agreement on the role of wheal diameter in reporting a positive test. Some interpret an increase in wheal size as a further indication of a positive test.

Sublingual provocation testing and neutralization has been advocated by some in the diagnosis and treatment of food allergy. It was first described by Hansel in 1953 [17] as a diagnostic and therapeutic technique. The method consists of placing allergenic extract underneath the tongue and waiting 10 minutes for the appearance of symptoms. If symptoms occur then the patient is given a more dilute solution of the same extract. The neutralizing dose is used as treatment prior to or after eating meals containing the offending food if the food cannot be avoided.

Given the fact that a single item needs to be tested one at a time and requires waiting 10 minutes between each dilution, it comes as no surprise that a single complete provocation–neutralization might take an entire day. Testing multiple items may take many days. Therefore, this test is time consuming and can be costly.

Conclusion

There have been several studies published looking primarily at the efficacy of provocative testing and neutralization. Eight of these studies were double-blinded. Only one study contained a control group. The majority of the studies were not able to demonstrate any benefit from neutralizing solution compared with placebo. Crawford et al. [18] performed a double-blinded study in 61 subjects with a history of reactions to five common foods. The authors were unable to demonstrate reproducibility of results from sublingual food testing. Kailin and Collier [19] in a double-blind study compared neutralizing effects of sublingual or subcutaneous food extracts versus saline placebo. The authors found that in 70% of patients, treatment with saline placebo was "relieving." Draper [20] in a study of 121 patients with inhalant allergy found that only 38% of positive provocation tests correlated with a positive food challenge test. One of the most well-structured double-blind studies was that by Jewett and Greenberg [21]. In this study 18 patients with symptoms previously provoked by intracutaneous testing were tested with food extracts or placebo. The rate of positive responses was similar between placebo and food extracts. This form of testing has also raised concerns regarding patient safety [22, 23]. Teuber reported a case in which anaphylaxis was induced by "neutralizing" injections of milk and wheat in a patient with systemic mastocytosis [23]. In conclusion, overall, these studies fail to confirm the efficacy of provocative testing and neutralization in the diagnosis and treatment of allergic disease.

Neutralization therapy

Neutralization of allergic symptoms is an extension of provocation–neutralization testing described earlier. This type of treatment, also called "relieving therapy," consists of self-administered doses of allergen extract at a concentration that "neutralizes" symptoms provoked during the prior provocation testing [14]. This treatment may be used by some to relieve present symptoms and to prevent anticipated symptoms and for continuous maintenance doses twice weekly. These doses can be given either by injection or sublingually. The patient can change and discontinue or restart treatment as they deem necessary.

Theory

A number of theories have been brought forth to try and explain neutralization of symptoms. A common belief among some practitioners is that this type of therapy induces immunological tolerance. Controlled, double-blind, multicenter studies have reported that sublingual, provocative food testing did not discriminate between placebo controls and food extracts used in neutralization therapy [16]. In addition, there appear to be no long- or short-term studies looking at the efficacy of this therapy.

Conclusion

As a result, since there is no known mechanism for neutralization of symptoms and no clear scientific evidence demonstrating its effectiveness, this form of therapy is not generally recommended in the treatment of allergic conditions such as food allergy.

Cytotoxic leukocyte testing

Also known as "Bryan's" test, this form of allergy testing was adapted by Bryan in the 1960s. Initially designed to help aid physicians in diagnosing allergy, the theory behind the test is that the addition of specific allergen *in vitro* to whole blood or to serum leukocyte suspension will reduce the white blood cell count or result in the death of leukocytes. It has been claimed by some to be useful for the diagnosis of both food and inhalant allergy [24]. The newer ALCAT test currently available functions in a similar way in that it measures volumetric shifts in white blood cells upon incubation with antigens. The blood cells are passed after an incubation period through a narrow channel and are measured by an electronic instrument. The sizes are displayed as either cell diameters or cell volumes. The company claims that their test will identify exactly which foods or chemicals are responsible for triggering a variety of symptoms including joint pain, headaches, asthma, obesity, ADD/hyperreactivity, chronic fatigue among others.

Method

The technique involves collecting the buffy coat from a drop of patient's blood and placing it on a microscope slide coated with dried extract of food or other allergen/substance and then observing microscopically for alteration in the appearance of white blood cells [25]. Once a fair number of white cells have been located, they are rated for degree of destruction. A single sample of blood can be tested to a panel of foods and other substances.

Conclusion

There is no theoretical basis for the cytotoxic test, since there is no evidence for a general cytotoxic mechanism in allergic disease. The test itself is not standardized and has never been shown in controlled trials to be effective in the diagnosis of food or inhalant allergy. Franklin and Lowell [26] reported that there was no significant difference in white blood cell counts in blood exposed to ragweed extract versus saline in ragweed-sensitive individuals. Lieberman et al. [27] could not demonstrate clinical correlation with test results in study patients and found inconsistent results when patients were tested more than once. Benson and Arkins [28] found the test was associated with a high degree of false positives. In regard to ALCAT, one abstract, from the company homepage, assessed the degree of correlation between ALCAT, and the results of oral double-blinded food challenges found an almost 84% correlation between the two tests. However, this small study had some significant limitations and no recent larger studies are available [29].

Electrodiagnosis (Vega testing)

Electrodiagnosis is also known as electroacupuncture according to Voll (EAV), electrodermal screening (EDS), bioelectric functions diagnosis (BFD), or bioenergy regulatory technique (BER) [30]. Some practitioners believe that the presence of specific allergy can lead to a change in the electrical resistance of the skin. These changes are then said to be detectable by Vega machines or bioresonance devices.

Method

In this procedure a sample of food extract is placed in a container in contact with an aluminum plate. This is then placed between the skin of the patient and a galvanometer. Electrical activity of the skin is measured at certain "allergy points." For example, there are certain points on the lower extremities which are said to correspond to food allergy and points on the upper extremities which are said to correspond to inhalant allergies [24]. Children are commonly evaluated by holding the hand of a parent while the parent is tested [7]. These results are entered into a computer which prints a list of allergies for the patient. Children are assessed by testing the parent first, and repeating the test with the parent holding the child's hand.

Conclusion

This type of procedure appeals to those patients who are reluctant to undergo any involved and potentially uncomfortable diagnostic procedures such as skin testing. Also, the use of computers, galvanometers, and "print outs" appears "state of the art" to some patients. Semizzi et al. [31] assessed the accuracy of electrodermal testing in 72 allergic patients compared with healthy controls. They found no significant difference in skin electrical response between the two groups.

Radionics

Method

Radionics is based on the concept that all life forms are submerged in the electromagnetic energy field of the earth. And that a disease will be reflected by changes or "imbalances" in an individual's electromagnetic field said to lie outside the normal electromagnetic spectrum. Practitioners claim to treat disease by restoring normal energy balance. Sometimes the operator is with the patient, and sometimes the operator "connects" with the patient at a distance using an object such as a lock of hair, blood sample, or photograph.

Conclusion

This technique has not been subject to formal study, and there is no published evidence that it is effective for the assessment or treatment of any disorder [7].

Iridology

Method

This is based on the concept that each part of the body is represented by a corresponding part of the iris. A person's state of health is determined by the color, texture, and location of pigment flecks in the eye. Imbalances are treated with dietary supplements or herbal medicines.

Conclusion

Studies have shown that iridologists are unable to distinguish patients with disease from those who are healthy [7, 32].

Body chemical analysis

Some practitioners claim that detection of any amount of inorganic or organic chemical in body fluid may indicate a toxic exposure and may explain the presence of disease. They postulate that certain substances may be toxic to the immune system leading to a state of sensitivity to the environment [8]. Some of these substances include vitamins, drugs, chlorinated hydrocarbons, volatile organic chemicals, pesticides, and metals.

Method

Specific tests include gas chromatographic mass spectrophotometry analysis of body fluids and tissue, quantitation of chemicals in serum and other body fluids, and breath analysis [9].

Conclusion

These procedures are highly sensitive and are able to identify chemicals in virtually every individual, even those who do not report symptoms. This is why a strong clinical correlation is important in conjunction with this type of testing. In certain situations and in certain individuals, it may be appropriate to evaluate for chemical poisoning in order to properly diagnose a disorder. It is important to note that many of the laboratories performing these tests are deficient with respect to quality assurance so, for example, contamination of samples remains a major source of error [9].

Hair Analysis

Method

Hair analysis entails investigating molecular and "energy" patterns of a patient's hair, which supporters claim to be predictive of food sensitivities. A patient typically cuts two to three hairs close to the root and submits samples, which are then analyzed for trace levels of toxins or nutritional imbalances by one of several possible techniques.

Conclusion

There are no published trials evaluating this technique and it lacks a physiologic basis. The AAAAI [4], ASCIA [7], and ALLSA [6] have issued position statements recommending against its use.

Inappropriate tests

IgG antibodies

Immunoglobulin E (IgE) antibody in response to allergens causes the release of mast cell mediators which are important in the immediate-type symptoms of anaphylaxis or atopic disease. Sensitivities to certain allergens can be diagnosed by detecting IgE in the serum by RAST. Many laboratories can test in a similar fashion for the presence of immunoglobulin G (IgG) or, more specifically, IgG4 to certain foods. There are those practitioners who measure circulating IgG antibody reactive with food antigens in diagnosing food allergy. The patient then may receive therapy in the form of elimination and rotation diets. The construct is that while IgG may not be important in the immediate-type reactions to certain foods, it may be important in delayed-type reactions such as depression, apathy, fatigue, myalgias, and gastrointestinal complaints [33]. Diagnosis of delayed-type reactions is challenging and while conventional IgE RAST alone cannot diagnose these types of reactions there are no published double-blind, placebo-controlled studies that demonstrate that such symptoms are related to particular foods as identified using such tests.

IgG antibodies are not known to have a role in the pathogenesis of atopic disease and food allergy. Certain levels of IgG to food antigens as well as other environmental antigens may be found normally and their presence, as of yet, has not been shown to be associated with atopic disease. Therefore, measurement of antigen-specific IgG has not been recommended as a form of diagnosing food allergy in the clinical setting. Manufacturers of IgG testing have been forced to withdraw claims regarding its efficacy [34]. Each of the primary international allergy specialty societies, including the EAACI [5], AAAAI [4], ALLSA [6], and ASCIA [7], has issued position statements recommending against the use of specific IgG antibodies in diagnosing food allergy.

Lymphocyte subset counts

Quantitative counting of leukocytes bearing one or more surface markers known as cluster of differentiation (CD) markers is helpful in the diagnosis of some forms of lymphocyte cellular immunodeficiencies. For example, measuring CD4 lymphocytes is part of the standard procedure for diagnosis and management in human immunodeficiency virus [8]. Lymphocyte subset counts may be labile and nonspecific. Levels may not be elevated in traditional allergic diseases but may be elevated in those with viral illnesses, for example. Use of these tests to diagnose forms of allergy or other presumed immunological disorders is generally considered inappropriate and can lead to inappropriate treatment of a patient.

Pulse test

The pulse test is based on a belief that allergic reactions have an immediate and measurable effect on the sympathetic nervous system. Coca in 1953 reported that tachycardia occurring 5–90 minutes after exposure to a food or inhaled material is a reliable indicator of food allergy [35].

Method

The test dose can be given by any route including injection. A change of 10 bpm is thought to be diagnostic by some, but the procedure has never been standardized. This test has no relationship to the diagnosis of allergic disease.

Unproven therapy

Neutralization therapy

This topic is discussed earlier in the section "Provocation–Neutralization."

Rotation diets

Theory

This particular type of diet recommends that a certain food not be eaten more than once every 4–5 days [9]. Part of the rationale is that if the patient is allergic to most or all foods, by eating them frequently, he or she runs the risk of becoming increasingly sensitized to that food and possibly other foods.

Conclusion

If a patient does have clinical sensitivity to a particular food, then he or she will develop symptoms after contact with that food irrespective of rotation schedule. However, if a patient demonstrates "subclinical sensitivity" to a certain food, that is, no symptoms but evidence of specific IgE by testing, then each exposure to that food will increase sensitivity and likelihood of a future reaction. There are thus no scientific data supporting the efficacy of this type of diet.

Advanced allergy elimination

Theory

This treatment is based on the concept that "allergen" is perceived by the brain as a threat to the body's well-being. Exposure to allergen disrupts the flow of nervous energies from the brain to the body via "meridians," resulting in symptoms [7]. Acupressure is applied to both sides of the spinal column while the patient is in direct contact with the purported allergen.

Conclusion

This approach lacks scientific rationale or published evidence of efficacy.

Orthomolecular therapy

Theory

This refers to the use of supplements and/or vitamins administered in large quantities either parenterally or orally to treat numerous medical and psychiatric conditions [9]. Practitioners of this therapy will commonly measure levels of vitamins in the serum or urine to determine the amount needed for correction. This type of therapy has been used in a wide variety of diseases. For example, antioxidant supplements such as vitamins E and C and glutathione have been used to treat allergic disease based on the theory that allergic inflammation generates free radicals that can cause oxidative damage to tissues [36].

Conclusion

There have been no controlled studies looking at this type of therapy and it is not a recommended treatment of any disease at this time. Large doses of certain vitamins can accumulate in the body and lead to toxic and potentially carcinogenic effects [37].

Reflexology

Theory

Reflexology is based on the belief that various regions of the hands, feet, and ears correspond to specific organs or physiologic systems within the body. Practitioners assert that disease can be diagnosed through palpation of these zones and treatment delivered through strategic application of pressure.

Conclusion

Reflexology lacks reasonable scientific rationale and has no physiologic basis. A recent review of 18 randomized controlled trials of reflexology concluded that there is no quality evidence to support reflexology as a treatment for any medical condition [38].

Mercury amalgam removal

Theory

Silver–mercury amalgam has been used in dental fillings for over 100 years. There have been many claims from physicians and dentists that certain patients may develop sensitivity to this material. Subsequently, it has been blamed for the development of a wide array of symptoms [9]. These claims have led to the removal of these types of fillings.

Conclusion

Sjursen et al. [39] recently reported a prospective randomized study showing improvement in intraoral and general health symptoms 3 years following removal of all amalgam fillings. However, failure to blind the treatment group and the lack of a true control group make the study's validity questionable, especially in the setting of a significant anticipated placebo effect. There remains no sound clinical evidence for the claims that mercury amalgam is responsible for the development of a multiplicity of somatic complaints.

Urine autoinjections

In 1930, Oriel and Barber reportedly found protein-like substances ("proteose") in the urine of allergic individuals during acute exacerbations of allergic disease [40]. Urine obtained from sensitive individuals applied intradermally to those individuals with the same sensitivities resulted in a positive skin test. This was not the case for the same urine applied intradermally in a non-atopic individual [33]. These practitioners felt that these "urine proteins" can be isolated by chemical extraction and given to the patient as a form of therapy in a series of intradermal/subcutaneous injections.

In 1947, the procedure was reintroduced by Plesch [41]. He describes a system of collecting fresh urine from a patient and after sterilization, injecting set amounts intramuscularly. Various reactions would occur within hours of injection and include fever, diarrhea, hypotension, shortness of breath, and vomiting. He found that by performing these injections in patients with various syndromes such as jaundice, allergic disease, gastrointestinal symptoms, and dermatological symptoms there was a decrease in symptoms. There are, however, no controlled studies to support either the efficacy or the safety of the procedure. In fact, in rabbits, urine autoinjection may lead to the formation of autoantibodies to glomerular basement membrane (GBM) and result in nephritis. Although this has not been demonstrated directly in humans, it is possible that receiving these urine autoinjections could induce immune complex disease. It has been established that in humans, anti-GBM antibodies can lead to the development of Goodpasture syndrome. Therefore, at this time, the American Academy of Allergy and Immunology has taken the position that this procedure is unproven, without scientific basis, and potentially dangerous [24].

Inappropriate therapy

Clinical ecology

Clinical ecology is based generally on two concepts. One is that a large number of chemicals and foods can be responsible for illness in the absence of abnormal laboratory tests and physical findings; and the other is that the immune system is functionally depressed as a result of exposure to certain chemicals in the environment [42]. This is not to be confused with toxic illnesses which produce a number of symptoms and abnormal laboratory tests in response to a particular toxin. Those who practice clinical ecology believe that patients with chemical hypersensitivity syndrome, also known as environmental hypersensitivity disorder, or twentieth-century disease, or induced immune dysregulation syndrome, have symptoms which are a result of low-level, long-term exposure to environmental chemicals. The doses which cause these syndromes are far below those established in the general population to cause harmful effects [43]. The agents are sometimes referred to as "incitants" or "offenders," and they include foods, food additives, and synthetic and natural chemicals such as pesticides, detergents, perfumes, vehicle exhaust, and natural gas. Symptoms are often generalized, frequently affecting more than one organ system including the cardiac, gastrointestinal, respiratory, genitourinary, and neurological systems.

Theory
Clinical ecologists [44] have theorized that environmental illness is a result of the development of sensitivity to novel synthetic chemicals. Others believe that these chemicals act as haptens inducing IgG formation and immune complex formation [45]. Environmental illness has also been thought to be the result of a nonspecific autoimmune process. What still needs to be established is a possible mechanism for this disease process; however, there are several concepts that clinical ecologists use to account for patient symptoms. "Total body load" and "chemical overload" draw an analogy between the immune system and a container. The immune system is said to have a limited capacity for handling antigens. Once a patient develops symptoms in response to an environmental antigen this then indicates that the immune system capacity has been exceeded. "Masking" is a concept in which a patient, who is sensitive to a certain food, may eliminate symptoms by eating the food on a regular basis. "Spreading phenomenon" refers to sensitivity to one antigen leading to the development of sensitivity to multiple other antigens [9].

Diagnosis
A detailed history within provocation–neutralization testing remains the mainstay of diagnosing environmental illness by clinical ecologists. Occasionally blood tests looking at immunoglobulin, complement, or specific chemical levels are used to aid in diagnosis.

Treatment
It consists mainly of avoidance measures, elimination diets, neutralization therapy, and, in some cases, as in *Candida* hypersensitivity syndrome, drug therapy.

Anti-*Candida* drugs for *Candida* hypersensitivity syndrome

Theory
Candida albicans is yeast which maintains a role as part of the body's normal flora. There are those who believe that it is this particular organism that is the cause of a condition termed "yeast hypersensitivity syndrome" or "*Candida* hypersensitivity syndrome." Proponents of this hypothesis believe that the syndrome is caused by an overgrowth of *Candida albicans* in the gastrointestinal tract leading to local inflammation as well as a more generalized toxic response. This response is thought to be secondary to a hypersensitivity reaction to a toxin which the organism secretes. As a result, symptoms range from recurrent or persistent candidal infections to chronic gastrointestinal symptoms such as bloating, diarrhea, constipation, and heartburn. Central nervous system symptoms have also been reported including depression, chronic fatigue, and memory problem [9].

Methods
There is no established method of diagnosing this syndrome. Diagnosis is most commonly made by history alone and not with specific laboratory measures. There have been reports of practitioners performing allergy testing in order to document sensitivity to *Candida*.

Treatment
Patients are first warned to avoid broad-spectrum antibiotics and systemic steroids since these medications may potentiate *Candida*. They are given minute doses of oral nystatin until symptoms have resolved. If symptoms persist, treatment can be changed to another anti-candidal drug such as ketoconazole or amphotericin B. In addition to anti-candidal drugs, patients are also started on yeast-free, sugar-free diets. It is thought by some that by eating simple sugars there is an increase in growth of *Candida* in the gut [46]. *Candida* allergy shots are also included in the treatment regimen of some patients.

Conclusion
Books and lay press articles have been published and support groups have been formed, all in the hopes of establishing a connection between yeast and disease. However, a scientific basis for this syndrome has never been established. The reports that do circulate are largely anecdotal. In 1990, Dismukes et al. [47] published the first randomized, double-blind, crossover study looking specifically at the effect of treatment with oral and vaginal nystatin compared with placebo in 42 premenopausal women presumed to have *Candida* hypersensitivity syndrome. Results from their work showed that while nystatin therapy did reduce vaginal symptoms, the efficacy of treatment for systemic symptoms including depression and chronic fatigue was not established. There was no significant reduction in systemic symptoms compared with placebo. Therefore, the study could not establish a therapeutic benefit of nystatin therapy in a patient with *Candida* hypersensitivity syndrome.

Elimination diets

Theory
The elimination of multiple foods has been recommended by some practitioners when multiple food allergies have been discovered on skin testing. This type of diet is also recommended by others who believe that through elimination diets one may "boost" the immune system [9].

Methods
Once the patient is diagnosed with sensitivity to multiple foods, either by unconventional testing or perhaps history,

they are placed on highly restrictive diets in order to prevent further symptoms. Most of the time patients are given supplements of vitamin, minerals, or amino acids [30].

Conclusion

There is no evidence that by eliminating multiple foods one may improve the functioning of the immune system.

In fact, placing patients on such restrictive diets may lead to harmful effects of malnutrition.

Multiple chemical sensitivity syndrome

Theory

Multiple chemical sensitivity (MCS) syndrome or idiopathic environmental intolerances (IEI), as suggested by the WHO/IPCS workshop in 1996, has been used to describe a constellation of symptoms which overlap with those of environmental illness but overall remains a distinct entity. This disorder is characterized by a wide variety of symptoms including somatic, cognitive, and affective symptoms, caused by low-level exposure to environmental chemicals [48]. Symptoms commonly involve almost every major organ system and are thought to result from sensitivity to certain chemicals. Chronic fatigue, depression, headache, and dizziness are commonly reported symptoms. Little is known about the pathophysiology of this condition, but its proponents claim that through certain mechanisms such as disruption of immunological/allergy processes, alterations in nervous system function, changes in biochemical pathways, or changes in neurobehavioral function chemicals cause tissue damage [49]. This may be accomplished through processes such as free radical generation, immune complex formation, or hapten formation.

Methods

Patients with this condition often manifest certain psychological features such as anxiety, depression, somatization, conversion, and phobia [9]. This makes it especially challenging in establishing a diagnosis of MCS. The diagnosis of MCS is, however, made if symptoms cannot be explained by abnormal tests but are associated with a documented environmental exposure. The lack of objective findings of disease such as physical exam and laboratory tests casts doubt on the validity of MCS as a clinical disease.

Critique

The concept of MCSs in the absence of any objective data remains its advocates' greatest challenge. At present, there is no scientific evidence that MCS should be regarded as a true clinical entity, but rather it appears to be based on an association of a wide range of symptoms to a particular or varied number of environmental chemicals.

Clinical ecology is inadequately supported in the literature. Both diagnostics and treatments have not been proven to be of any consistent efficacy or benefit. Das-Munshi et al. [50] performed a systematic review of the literature and found that subjects putatively suffering from MCS were unable to differentiate chemical exposure from control conditions when exposed in a blinded fashion. An additional difficulty in evaluating clinical ecology and environmental disorders is that it is virtually impossible to establish a cause and effect relationship since there is such a varied number of possible "triggers" of symptoms.

Conclusion

Many of the subspecialty groups including the AAAAI and the American College of Physicians have issued position papers looking at several of the above-mentioned procedures and therapies. It was the goal of this chapter to provide definitions of controversial, unproven, and inappropriate procedures and treatments and examples of each so that it might provide insight into remote practices of allergy. By examining each theory and method, we can become more aware of the importance of scientific evidence and standardization of procedures in our daily practice. The history, physical exam, selective skin tests, and appropriate laboratory tests remain the standard of care in first evaluating the allergy patient. However, as we have seen, this may not always be the case. Patients may be asked to undergo rigorous, expensive, invalidated, and even painful testing. They may be given diagnoses and treatments, which may lead to both physical and mental deterioration. We have also seen that many "validated" tests can be misused to diagnose allergic disease. Many supporters of these procedures have misinformed the public by implying that they have been clinically proven. Therefore, it becomes the responsibility of physicians to educate patients regarding such practices of allergy. It also becomes our responsibility to design proper clinical trials to definitively establish the merit or failure of these tests.

References

1. Shaw A, Thompson EA, Sharp D. Complementary therapy used by patients and parents of children with asthma and the implications for NHS care: a qualitative study. *BMC Health Serv Res* 2006; 6:76.
2. Wisniewski JA, Li XM. Alternative and complementary treatment for food allergy. *Immunol Allergy Clin North Am* 2012; 32(1):135–150.
3. Ko J, Lee JI, Muñoz-Furlong A, et al. Use of complementary and alternative medicine by food-allergic patients. *Ann Allergy Asthma Immunol* 2006; 97(3):365–369.
4. Boyce JA, Assa'ad A, Burks AW, et al. Guidelines for the diagnosis and management of food allergy in the United

States: summary of the NIAID-sponsored Expert Panel report. *J Allergy Clin Immunol* 2010; 126(6):1105–1118.
5. Stapel SO, Asero R, Ballmer-Weber BK, et al. Testing for IgG4 against foods is not recommended as a diagnostic tool: EAACI Task Force report. *Allergy* 2008; 63(7):793–796.
6. Motala C, Hawarden D, on behalf of the Allergy Society of South Africa. Diagnostic testing in allergy. *S Afr Med J* 2009; 99(7):531–535.
7. Mullins RJ. *ASCIA Position Statement: Unorthodox Techniques for the Diagnosis and Treatment of Allergy, Asthma, and Immune Disorders*. ASCIA, 2007.
8. Barton M, Oleske J, LaBraico J. Controversial techniques in allergy treatment. *J Natl Med Assoc* 1983; 75:831–834.
9. Van Metre TE Jr. Critique of controversial and unproven procedures for diagnosis and therapy of allergic disorders. *Pediatr Clin North Am* 1983; 30:807–817.
10. Van Metre TE Jr, Adkinson NF Jr, Lichtenstein LM, et al. A controlled study of the effectiveness of the Rinkel method of immunotherapy for ragweed pollen hay fever. *J Allergy Clin Immunol* 1980; 65:288–297.
11. Garrow JS. Kinesiology and food allergy. *BMJ* 1988; 296:1573.
12. Senna G, Passalacqua G, Lombardi C, et al. Position paper: controversial and unproven diagnostic procedures for food allergy. *Eur Ann Allergy Clin Immunol* 2004; 36(4):139–145.
13. Lee CH. A new test for diagnosis and treatment of food allergens. *Buchanan Co Med Bull* 1961; 25:9–12.
14. AAAAI Training Program Directors' Committee. A training program directors' committee report: topics related to controversial practices that should be taught in allergy and immunology training program. *J Allergy Clin Immunol* 1994; 93:955–966.
15. Middleton E Jr, Ellis EF, Yunginer JW, et al. (eds), *Allergy Principles and Practice*, 5th edn. St. Louis, MO: Mosby, 1998.
16. Spector SL. Controversial and unproven techniques. Position statement from the ACCP section on allergy and clinical immunology. *Chest* 1984; 86:132–133.
17. Hansel FK. *Allergy and Immunology in Otolaryngology*. Rochester, MN: American Academy of Ophthalmology and Otolaryngology, 1968.
18. Crawford LV, Lieberman P, Harfi HA, et al. A double-blind study of subcutaneous food testing sponsored by the Food Committee of the American Academy of Allergy. *J Allergy Clin Immunol* 1976; 57:236.
19. Kailin EW, Collier R. "Relieving" therapy for antigen exposure. *J Am Med Assoc* 1971; 217:78–82.
20. Draper LW. Food testing in allergy: intradermal, provocative, or deliberate feeding. *Arch Otolaryngol* 1972; 95:169–174.
21. Jewett DL, Greenberg MR. Placebo responses in intradermal provocation testing with food extracts (abstract). *J Allergy Clin Immunol* 1985; 75:205.
22. Gerez IF, Shek LP, Chng HH, et al. Diagnostic tests for food allergy. *Singapore Med J* 2010; 51(1):4–9.
23. Teuber SS, Vogt PJ. An unproven technique with potentially fatal outcome: provocation/neutralization in a patient with systemic mastocytosis. *Ann Allergy Asthma Immunol* 1999; 82(1):61–65.
24. American Academy of Allergy. Position statements—controversial techniques. *J Allergy Clin Immunol* 1981; 67:333–338.
25. Terr AI. Controversial and unproven diagnostic tests for allergic and immunologic diseases. *Clin Allergy Immunol* 2000; 15:307–320.
26. Franklin W, Lowell FC. Failure of ragweed pollen extract to destroy white cells from ragweed-sensitive patients. *J Allergy* 1949; 20:375.
27. Lieberman P, Crawford L, Bjelland J, et al. Controlled study of the cytotoxic food test. *J Am Med Assoc* 1974; 231:728.
28. Benson TE, Arkins JA. Cytotoxic testing for food allergy: evaluations of reproducibility in correlation. *J Allergy Clin Immunol* 1976; 58:471–476.
29. Fell PJ, Brostoff J, Pasula MJ. *High Correlation of the ALCAT Test Results with Double Blind Challenge in Food Sensitivity* (abstract). Presented at the 45th Annual Congress of the American College of Allergy and Immunology, Los Angeles, CA, 1988.
30. Wuthrich B. Unproven techniques in allergy diagnosis. *J Invest Allergol Clin Immunol* 2005; 15(2):86–90.
31. Semizzi M, Senna G, Crivellaro M, et al. A double-blind, placebo-controlled study on the diagnostic accuracy of an electrodermal test in allergic subjects. *Clin Exp Allergy* 2002; 32(6):928–932.
32. Niggemann B, Gruber C. Unproven diagnostic procedures in IgE-mediated allergic diseases. *Allergy* 2004; 59:806–808.
33. Goldberg BJ, Kaplan MS. Controversial concepts and techniques in the diagnosis and management of food allergies. *Immunol Allergy Clin North Am* 1991; 11:863–884.
34. Advertising Standards Authority (ASA). Available at http://www.asasa.org.za/ResultDetail.aspx?Ruling=4907 (Last accessed June 17, 2013).
35. Coca AF. *Familial Nonreaginic Food Allergy*, 3rd edn. Springfield, IL: Charles C. Thomas, 1953.
36. Levine SA, Reinhardt JH. Biochemical-pathology initiated by free radicals, oxidant chemicals, and therapeutic drugs in the etiology of chemical hypersensitivity disease. *Orthomol Psychiatry* 1983; 12:166.
37. Klein EA, Thompson IM Jr, Tangen CM, et al. Vitamin E and the risk of prostate cancer: the Selenium and Vitamin E Cancer Prevention Trial (SELECT). *J Am Med Assoc* 2011; 306(14):1549–1556.
38. Ernst E. Is reflexology an effective intervention? A systematic review of randomised controlled trials. *Med J Aust* 2009;191(5):263–266.
39. Sjursen TT, Lygre GB, Dalen K, et al. Changes in health complaints after removal of amalgam fillings. *J Oral Rehabil* 2011; 38(11):835–848. doi: 10.1111/j.1365-2842.2011.02223.x
40. Oriel GH, Barber HW. Proteases in urine, excreted in anaphylactic and allergic conditions. *Lancet* 1930; 2:1304.
41. Plesch J. Urine therapy. *Med Press* 1947; 218:128.
42. Terr AI. Clinical ecology. *Ann Intern Med* 1989; 111:168–177.
43. Sparks PJ, Daniell W, Black DW, et al. Multiple chemical sensitivity syndrome: a clinical perspective. I. Case definition, theories of pathogenesis, and research needs. *J Occup Med* 1994; 36:718.
44. Randolph TG. The specific adaptation syndrome. *J Lab Clin Invest* 1956; 48:934.

45. Rea WJ, Bell IR, Suits CW, et al. Food and chemical susceptibility after environmental chemical overexposure: case histories. *Ann Allergy* 1978; 41:101–109.
46. Bennett JE. Searching for the yeast connection. *N Engl J Med* 2002; 323:1766–1767.
47. Dismukes WE, Wade JS, Lee JY, et al. A randomized, double-blind trial of nystatin therapy for the candidiasis hypersensitivity syndrome. *N Engl J Med* 1990; 323:1717–1722.
48. Labarge XS, McCaffrey RJ. Multiple chemical sensitivity: a review of the theoretical and research literature. *Neuropsychol Rev* 2000; 10:183–211.
49. Winder C. Mechanisms of multiple chemical sensitivity. *Toxicol Lett* 2002; 128:85–97.
50. Das-Munshi J, Rubin GJ, Wessely S. Multiple chemical sensitivities: a systematic review of provocation studies. *J Allergy Clin Immunol* 2006; 118(6):1257–1264.

4 Adverse Reactions to Food Additives

27 Asthma and Food Additives

Robert K. Bush[1] & Michelle Montalbano[2]

[1]Division of Allergy, Immunology, Pulmonary, Critical Care, and Sleep Medicine, Department of Medicine, University of Wisconsin School of Medicine and Public Health, Madison, WI, USA
[2]Advanced Allergy and Asthma, PLLC, Silverdale, WA, USA

Key Concepts

- Food additives are an uncommon cause of asthma exacerbations.
- Sulfiting agents can provoke acute and occasionally severe episodes of bronchoconstriction.
- Monosodium glutamate is unlikely to provoke bronchoconstriction.
- Tartrazine has not been definitely shown to cause airflow obstruction.
- A definite diagnosis of food-additive-induced asthma requires properly performed challenges.

Introduction

Food additives are substances added to food products for a wide variety of functions, including coloring, flavoring, nutrient, and antimicrobial purposes. Because additives are typically minor ingredients in food, the intake of additives is usually small. An estimated 23–67% of asthmatics perceive that food additives exacerbate their asthma. However, the prevalence rate of food-additive-induced asthma exacerbations obtained by double-blind, placebo-controlled trials is less than 5%. Because the current therapy for food-additive-induced asthma is avoidance or elimination of inciting agents, a correct diagnosis is imperative to avoid unnecessary dietary restriction. Sulfites, monosodium glutamate (MSG), and tartrazine will be discussed in detail in this chapter.

Evaluating asthma studies

A variety of data are available implicating sulfites, MSG, and tartrazine in asthma exacerbations, but many of the studies are of poor design. Well-designed studies in asthmatic subjects require stable lung function at baseline. When the subjects have wide variability in peak expiratory flow rate (PEFR) or forced expiratory volume in 1 second (FEV1) at baseline, variability seen during the challenge may be related to the substance or a reflection of poor asthma control. If asthma medications are discontinued, the timing in relation to the challenge must be carefully evaluated. For example, antiasthmatic and antiallergic medications that can inhibit a response must be withheld before a challenge. β_2-Agonists are typically withheld the day of the challenge, and cromolyn sodium or antihistamines are withheld for 24 hours or longer prior to the challenge. Asthma controller medications such as theophylline and inhaled or oral corticosteroids may be continued, since they do not interfere with the response.

If rescue medications are given within 3 hours of a challenge, lunch function declines 6 hours after challenge, the decline is more likely due to a waning of medication effect rather than bronchoconstriction from the challenge substance. Consistent timing of challenges is important to exclude confounding due to the physiologic diurnal variability in PEFR. To eliminate observer bias, challenges should be double blinded and placebo controlled.

The method of administration of challenge substance may influence results. For example, some asthmatics

Food Allergy: Adverse Reactions to Foods and Food Additives, Fifth Edition. Edited by Dean D Metcalfe, Hugh A Sampson, Ronald A Simon and Gideon Lack.

respond to oral capsule challenges, while others respond only to challenge with solutions (e.g., sulfites). The route of administration chosen in diagnostic challenges should be tailored to the patient's history.

The reliability of the pulmonary function measure used is another key aspect. The flow-volume loop obtained with spirometry is precise and reproducible, while PEFR is more variable. Criteria used to define positive challenges should be considered.

Duration of subject evaluation following a challenge is also important. For MSG, subjects are evaluated for as few as 2 or as many as 14 hours following challenge. Determining when reactions are most likely to occur and still be linked to the challenge substance will help determine the length of time subjects should be observed.

For sulfites, MSG, and tartrazine, various data are presented and evaluated using the criteria outlined above.

Sulfites

Sulfiting agents have been used in foods for many years. Although sulfites are often added to foods, they occur naturally in certain foods such as mushrooms and Parmesan cheese.

Adding sulfites to foods serves many purposes, for example, inhibition of enzymatic and nonenzymatic browning, antimicrobial actions, and bleaching and as a dough conditioner. Sulfites are also used in pharmaceutical agents, including medications for the treatment of allergic diseases and asthma.

Common forms of sulfites used as food or drug additives include sulfur dioxide (SO_2), inorganic sulfite salts, sodium or potassium metabisulfite ($Na_2S_2O_5$ or $K_2S_2O_5$), sodium or potassium bisulfite ($NaHSO_3$ or $KHSO_3$), and sodium or potassium sulfite ($Na_2S_2O_3$ or $K_2S_2O_3$). Sulfites can react with a variety of food constituents. Dissociable forms of sulfite can serve as reservoirs of "free" sulfites. Irreversibly bound sulfites are removed permanently from the pool of sulfites that may exist in foods.

The form of sulfite present in foods is affected by pH. For example, a low pH favors H_2SO_3, intermediate pH favors HSO_3, and high pH favors SO_3. In solution, especially at an acid pH (saliva, gastric juice) and in the presence of heat (stomach), sulfites are readily transformed into bisulfite and sulfurous acid. These substances may then be volatilized to SO_2, which has been implicated in causing bronchoconstriction.

The estimated prevalence of sulfite sensitivity in adult asthmatics is 3–10% [1], with a higher prevalence in moderate-to-severe persistent asthmatics. Two hundred and three patients initially underwent a single-blind challenge with sulfite-containing capsules [2]. If the single-blind challenges were positive (20% or greater decrease in FEV1 from baseline), a double-blind challenge followed. In the single-blind challenge, 16 of 83 moderate-to-severe persistent asthmatics had a positive response, while only 5 of 120 less severe asthmatics had a positive response. When these results were confirmed with double-blind challenges, three of seven more severe asthmatics and one of five less severe asthmatics had a positive response. The estimated prevalence of sulfite sensitivity in nonsteroid-dependent asthmatics based on the double-blind challenge results was 0.8%. In the more severe asthmatics, the prevalence was higher (8.4%). The estimated prevalence of sulfite sensitivity in the asthmatic population as a whole is less than 3.9% and those with moderate-to-severe persistent asthma are at most risk [2].

The largest group of sulfite-sensitive asthmatics is individuals who respond to ingestion of acidic sulfite solutions. Among these patients, some react to acidic sulfite solution challenge and others do not, a phenomenon perhaps explained by variable inhalation of SO_2. Inhaling as little as 1 ppm SO_2 has been demonstrated to cause bronchoconstriction in asthmatics. In doses of 1–50 ppm, 99% of inhaled SO_2 is absorbed by the upper airway. The resulting bronchospasm may be initiated by stimulation of superficial afferent nerve endings in the larynx or tracheobronchial tree and then mediated by parasympathetic pathways in the bronchi. The mechanism by which sulfites induce asthma symptoms has not yet been fully elucidated [1]. Various hypotheses have been proposed to explain the bronchoconstriction by SO_2: a cholinergic reflex mechanism, an IgE-mediated mechanism, or deficiency of sulfite oxidase. The cholinergic reflex mechanism suggests that inhaled SO_2, such as might occur when swallowing an acidic sulfited beverage, acts on irritant receptors in the lung. This hypothesis is supported by the fact that the response in sulfite-sensitive individuals can be blocked by the administration of anticholinergic drugs, such as inhaled atropine or doxepin, an antihistamine with anticholinergic properties.

Another proposed mechanism is an IgE-mediated mechanism. This mechanism has not yet been proven, but is supported by the presence of positive skin prick tests to sulfites and by anaphylaxis in certain individuals. Sulfite oxidase deficiency has also been proposed as an explanation [1]. Sulfite oxidase metabolizes sulfite (SO_3) to inactive sulfate (SO_4), and a decrease in sulfite oxidase activity has been seen in skin fibroblasts of sulfite-sensitive asthmatics compared with controls, but congenital sulfite oxidase is not associated with asthma.

Although sulfite-induced asthma is typically triggered by the ingestion of a sulfited food, beverage, or drug, inhalation of SO_2 can also be a trigger. Several factors determine the likelihood of an adverse reaction: the nature of the food, the level and form of residual sulfite in the food, and the sensitivity of the patient. Sulfite-sensitive asthmatics are most likely to respond to "free" sulfites. However, the degree of sensitivity these patients have to the various forms of sulfites in foods has yet to be elucidated.

The levels of sulfiting agents in foods are usually expressed as SO_2 equivalents in parts per million (ppm). One part per million equals one microgram per gram. Sulfite salts can release SO_2 under some assay conditions. In the United States, total daily *per capita* intake of sulfites in foods is approximately 6 mg SO_2. The threshold response to challenges with sulfites in sensitive asthmatics is typically between 12 and 30 mg SO_2 equivalents (20 to 50 mg potassium metabisulfite). The levels of sulfites in foods vary (see Chapter 29). The highest levels (up to 1000 ppm) in foods are contained in dried fruits and lemon, lime, grape, and sauerkraut juices. Food processing and preparation may decrease sulfite levels. Therefore, the amounts of sulfite used initially to treat foods will not necessarily reflect residue levels after processing, storage, and preparation. Food processing also differs in various countries, so caution must be used in interpreting reports from other countries that implicate sulfites in eliciting asthma symptoms.

Although the precise mechanism has yet to be elucidated, the bronchoconstriction caused by exposure to sulfites in sensitive asthmatics can be severe and potentially life threatening. Therefore, accurate diagnosis is imperative. But because history does not always correlate with a positive challenge, history alone is insufficient for the diagnosis of sulfite-induced asthma. Skin prick tests and serologic tests are also not reliable in the diagnosis of sulfite-induced asthma. The diagnostic tool with the highest degree of accuracy is a double-blind, placebo-controlled challenge. However, there is no standardized procedure for challenging with sulfiting agents (please see Tables 29.1 and 29.2 for suggested protocols for sulfite challenges). Patients may be challenged with capsules, neutral solutions, or acidic solutions of metabisulfite. A capsule challenge may be preferred, as most exposures are to sulfites in bound form in foods rather than to sulfites in free form, such as in lettuce. Variable thresholds for bronchospastic responses have been seen, from 5 to 200 mg of encapsulated metabisulfite. A challenge with sulfites in solution is optimal for patients who have reacted to beverages such as sulfited wines. In patients with a history of response to particular foods, food challenges are used diagnostically. Challenges, therefore, can be tailored to a patient's history of reaction.

Challenges should be conducted very carefully, with availability of equipment necessary to treat severe bronchospastic or anaphylactic reactions. Because certain drugs can inhibit the response to sulfites, antiasthmatic, and antiallergic medications, such as β_2-agonists, cromolyn, and antihistamines, should be withheld before challenges. β_2-Agonists are typically withheld the day of the challenge, while cromolyn and antihistamines are withheld at least 24 hours prior to the challenge. Theophylline and corticosteroids (inhaled and oral) can be continued, for these drugs do not interfere with sulfite-induced reactions.

Typically, if a single-blind challenge is positive, the results should be confirmed with a double-blind challenge. Randomization of administration of active and placebo challenges should be done, possibly with a third challenge day, to avoid an order effect of challenge. An order effect of challenge has been seen in patients who receive placebo on the first day and do not react, but do react on subsequent challenge days regardless of whether they receive placebo or active challenge.

Given the diagnosis of sulfite-induced asthma with an appropriately performed challenge study and the establishment of a threshold dose of sulfite that provokes asthma, treatment is strict avoidance of sulfite-treated foods and drugs, especially those containing greater than 100 ppm SO_2 equivalents. In the United States, federal regulations require foods and alcoholic beverages containing greater than 10 ppm total SO_2 be labeled. Unlabeled sulfited foods still exist in restaurants, although the use of sulfites in fresh foods such as fruits and vegetables in salad bars has been banned. Residue levels of sulfites in shrimp, which are used to prevent enzymatic browning (black spot formation), are still permitted. Imported table grapes are treated with sulfites to inhibit mold growth, but they must be detained at their port of entry until sulfite residues are no longer detected. Potatoes can be sulfited, so patients with sulfite-sensitive asthma should avoid all potatoes in restaurants, except those baked with intact skins. Sulfite-sensitive asthmatics should avoid sulfite-containing pharmaceutical agents such as certain bronchodilator solutions, subcutaneous lidocaine, and intravenous corticosteroids. Pharmaceutical corporations have eliminated the use of sulfites in many products used for the treatment of asthmatics, although epinephrine contains sulfites as antioxidants because there is no alternative agent. The positive effects of epinephrine overwhelmingly negate any negative effects of sulfites. Epinephrine therefore should *never* be withheld from sulfite-sensitive asthmatics when indicated.

Complete avoidance of sulfites is difficult, and reactions can be severe. Management of reactions includes administration of β_2-agonist medications or nebulized atropine and self-administered epinephrine for severe episodes of sulfite-induced asthma.

Monosodium glutamate

Just as sulfites have been linked to asthma exacerbations in some asthmatics, MSG has also been implicated. Unlike sulfites, however, there is little data to confirm that MSG causes bronchospasm [3].

MSG is a sodium salt of the nonessential amino acid, L-glutamic acid. MSG occurs naturally in a wide variety of foods. MSG exists in free form and bound to proteins and is used as a flavor enhancer in processed foods. In the United States, the average daily intake of MSG is 0.2–0.5 g. As much as 4–6 g might be ingested in a highly seasoned restaurant meal.

Because MSG is perceived as a food chemical likely to cause bronchoconstriction, it is a frequently avoided food item. However, the role of MSG in exacerbating asthma has not been firmly established. Levels of MSG precipitating adverse events are much higher than the usual dietary exposure (2.5–3 g versus 0.2–0.5 daily exposure) and occur in the absence of food.

Thirty-two asthmatic patients with a history of MSG-induced asthmatic reactions were evaluated via single-blind, placebo-controlled oral challenge with MSG. PEFR was followed hourly for 14 hours after oral challenge. Thirteen exhibited significant declines in PEFR. Patients were given placebo on day 1 of the study and then challenged with MSG on days 2 and 3, augmenting the lack of daily controller medications, which were stopped just prior to commencement of the study. Some patients were allowed to have rescue medication within 3 hours of initial challenge, therefore declines in PEFR 6 hours or more after challenge were most likely due to waning effects of β_2-agonist rather than to bronchoconstrictive effects of MSG. The results of this study were not reproduced; a non-blinded challenge was repeated in only one patient [4].

Oral challenges with 1.5 g of MSG in 12 asthmatic patients found no changes in FEV1 that was statistically different from placebo. The number of patients evaluated was small, and subjects were only evaluated for 4 hours after challenge, rather than 12 hours or more as in other studies. This study does suggest that in the usual quantities found in food, MSG is unlikely to induce bronchoconstriction [5].

Another study evaluated 12 asthmatics, all of whom had a history of asthma exacerbation with MSG ingestion. This was a double-blind, placebo-controlled study to evaluate for MSG-induced bronchial hyperresponsiveness. Methacholine challenge was performed before and after oral challenge with MSG. The results of this study were completely negative. This study involved a small number of subjects, and patients were directly monitored for only 4 hours after challenge. Nevertheless, MSG-induced asthma was not demonstrated in this group of adult asthmatics with prior history of asthma symptoms precipitated by MSG [6].

A single-blind, placebo-controlled study evaluated 100 asthmatic patients, 30 of whom reported prior asthma exacerbations with MSG exposure. Subjects were given 2.5 g of MSG, and FEV1 was measured at hourly intervals for 12 hours. No significant drop in FEV1 occurred, and no patients developed asthma symptoms [7].

Table 27.1 Protocol for MSG oral challenge.

Single-blind challenge
Continue maintenance asthma medications
Perform on initial single-blind placebo challenge
- Administer five placebo capsules of 500 mg sucrose each
- Monitor FEV1 hourly
- Failure of placebo challenge is a change in FEV1 by 10%
- If FEV1 remains stable, perform a second placebo challenge, monitoring FEV1 hourly
- Total duration of placebo day: 12 hours

If patients pass the placebo challenge day, perform single-blind challenge with MSG
- Give five capsules MSG totaling 2.5 g
- Monitor FEV1 hourly for total of 12 hours
- Six hours after MSG administered, administer five placebo capsules to maintain a sequence similar to the placebo challenge day
- Positive response is FEV1 drop by 20% (perform double-blind challenge to confirm)

Double-blind challenge
- Continue maintenance asthma medications
- Repeat 12-hour placebo challenge on 1 day
- Request repeat MSG challenge as shown above on another day
- Challenge day (placebo or active) should be in random order

In contrast to the general perception that MSG-induced asthma exists, well-designed studies with oral challenges of MSG clearly have not demonstrated changes in FEV1 or symptoms of asthma. Currently, there is limited evidence that patients with asthma are more at risk for adverse effects from MSG than the general population. Further, avoidance of MSG in patients with chronic asthma may not be beneficial, but additional studies are needed, especially in children [8].

When patients are concerned that a reaction may be occurring to MSG, an oral challenge can be performed (Table 27.1). Maintenance asthma medications should be continued. An initial single-blind, placebo-controlled challenge should be done. FEV1 should be monitored hourly after each five doses of placebo. If the FEV1 changes by more than 10%, the patient has failed the placebo challenge. If the FEV1 is stable (change of less than 10%), a second placebo challenge should be performed and FEV1 monitored hourly for up to 12 hours.

If patients "pass" the placebo challenge day with less than 10% variability in FEV1, a single-blind challenge with MSG should be performed. MSG is given in five 500 mg capsules, totaling 2.5 g. FEV1 is monitored hourly for a total of 12 hours. Five placebo capsules should be given at the 6-hour point to maintain a sequence similar to the placebo challenge day. A positive response is defined as a drop in FEV1 of greater than 20%. If patients have a positive response to a single-blind challenge, a double-blind challenge should be performed.

Tartrazine

Synthetic colorants are often added to foods. One such example is the azo dye tartrazine, also known as FD&C Yellow No. 5. As with MSG, many of the reported studies have design flaws. No well-designed study has corroborated claims that tartrazine provokes asthma exacerbations, for example, lack of baseline asthma stability, withholding of asthma medications, or proper controls [9]. Routine avoidance of tartrazine by asthma patients is usually not necessary [10].

In 194 aspirin-sensitive patients evaluated for tartrazine sensitivity by oral challenge, no cross-sensitivity between aspirin and tartrazine was demonstrated. The authors conclude that reports of tartrazine-induced bronchospasm represent spontaneous asthma coincidentally associated with ingestion of tartrazine, rather than bronchospasm caused by tartrazine. None of the subjects had positive reactions when double-blind, placebo-controlled challenges were performed [11].

While limited in scope, a recent study of 26 atopic adults (including several patients with asthma) who underwent double-blind, placebo-controlled challenges, none reacted to 35 mg of tartrazine [12].

If a patient is concerned about reactions to tartrazine, an oral challenge can be performed (Table 27.2). An initial challenge should involve hourly FEV1 monitoring throughout the challenge. Placebo should be administered first. If FEV1 remains stable after 3 hours, 25 mg tartrazine can be given. If after another 3 hours, FEV1 is still stable, 50 mg tartrazine can be administered. A "conditionally positive" test consists of an FEV1 drop of 25% or more after the 25 or 50 mg dose of tartrazine.

When the initial challenge is positive, a double-blind challenge should be done, using the suspected provoking dose of tartrazine and two placebos. This double-blind challenge should be preceded by a full day of challenge using three doses of placebo administered 3 hours apart. FEV1 should be monitored hourly throughout the placebo challenge and active challenge.

Table 27.2 Protocol for tartrazine oral challenge.

Initial challenge
- Administer placebo first
- Monitor FEV1 hourly
- If FEV1 stable after 3 hours, administer 25 mg tartrazine
- If FEV1 stable after 3 hours, administer 50 mg tartrazine
- A "conditionally positive" test consists of FEV1 drop of 25% or more after the 25 or 50 mg dose tartrazine

Double-blind challenge
- Begin with a full day of placebo challenge using three doses of placebo administered 3 hours apart
- Monitor FEV1 hourly
- On the following day, follow protocol for initial challenge using suspected provoking dose of tartrazine and two placebos

Conclusions

Despite the fact that a multitude of food additives exist, only a few are commonly implicated in asthma: sulfites, MSG, and tartrazine. Of these three, only sulfites have been found to incite bronchoconstriction in some asthmatics, who should avoid sulfite exposure. In contrast, due to the lack of evidence in well-designed studies linking MSG and tartrazine to asthma exacerbation, asthmatic patients need not avoid exposure to MSG or tartrazine if a double-blind, placebo-controlled challenge is negative.

References

1. Vally H, Misso NL, Mad V. Clinical effects of sulphite additives. *Clin Exp Allergy* 2009; 39:1643–1651.
2. Bush RK, Taylor SL, Holden K, et al. Prevalence of sensitivity to sulfiting agents in asthmatic patients. *Am J Med* 1986;. 81:816–820.
3. Williams AN, Woessner KM. Monosodium glutamate "allergy": menace or myth? *Clin Exp Allergy* 2009; 39:640–646.
4. Allen DH, Delohery J, Baker G. Monosodium L-glutamate-induced asthma. *J Allergy Clin Immunol* 1987; 80:530–537.
5. Schwartzstein RM, Kelleher M, Weinberger SE, et al. Airway effects of monosodium glutamate in subjects with chronic stable asthma. *J Asthma* 1987; 24:167–172.
6. Woods RK, Weiner JM, Thein F, et al. The effects of monosodium glutamate in adults with asthma who perceive themselves to be monosodium glutamate-intolerant. *J Allergy Clin Immunol* 1998; 101:762–771.
7. Woessner KM, Simor RA, Stevenson DD. Monosodium glutamate sensitivity in asthma. *J Allergy Clin Immunol* 1999; 104:305–310.
8. Zhou Y, Yang M, Dong BR. Monosodium glutamate avoidance for chronic asthma. *Cochrane Database Syst Rev* 2012; (6):CD004357. doi:10.1002/14651858.CD004357.pub4
9. Gillman A, Douglass JA. What do asthmatics have to fear from food and additive allergy? *Clin Exp Allergy* 2010; 40:1295–1302.
10. Ardern KD, Ram FS. Tartrazine exclusion for allergic asthma. *Cochrane Database Syst Rev* 2001(4):CD000460. doi:10.1002/14651858.CD000460
11. Stevenson DD, Simon RA, Lumry WR, Mathison DA. Adverse reactions to tartrazine. *J Allergy Clin Immunol* 1986; 78:182–191.
12. Pestana S, Moreira M, Olej B. Safety of ingestion of yellow tartrazine by double-blind, placebo-controlled challenge in 26 atopic adults. *Allergol Immunopathol (Madr)* 2010; 38:142–146.

28 Urticaria, Angioedema, and Anaphylaxis Provoked by Food Additives

John V. Bosso[1,2] & David M. Robertson[3,4]

[1]Columbia University College of Physicians and Surgeons, New York, NY, USA
[2]Allergy and Immunology, Nyack Hospital, Nyack, NY, USA
[3]Hampden County Physician Associates, Springfield, MA, USA
[4]Tufts University School of Medicine, Boston, MA, USA

Key Concepts

- Only a small fraction of the thousands of agents added to our foods have been associated with cutaneous and/or anaphylactic hypersensitivity responses.
- Early (pre-1990) literature overestimated the prevalence of such reactions due to dated experimental design.
- Additive-induced urticaria, angioedema, and anaphylaxis are relatively rare.
- Hypersensitivity responses to "natural" additives appear to be primarily IgE mediated, while the mechanism of most reactions to synthetic additives is unclear.
- Chronic idiopathic urticaria/angioedema is rarely associated with food additive hypersensitivity.
- Recommendations for food additive challenge protocols for patients with urticaria, angioedema, and/or anaphylaxis are reviewed in the text.

Between 2000 and 20 000 agents are added to the foods that we consume [1]. These substances include preservatives, stabilizers, conditioners, thickeners, colorings, flavorings, sweeteners, and antioxidants [2]. Despite the multitude of additives known, only a small number have been associated with hypersensitivity reactions. Urticaria, angioedema, and anaphylaxis from food additives should be suspected when adverse reactions after food or beverage consumption occur intermittently, suggesting that the reaction occurs only when an additive is present.

A number of investigators have suggested that urticaria, angioedema, and anaphylaxis related to the ingestion of food additives are relatively common. This apparent misconception is based on several poorly controlled studies, mostly reported before 1990. More recent evidence contradicts this notion, suggesting that the incidence of such reactions is relatively low.

Table 28.1 lists the food and drug additives that have been associated with adverse reactions, the suspected mechanism of reaction, and whether testing for sensitivity has been described. In this chapter, these additives are discussed in detail as they relate to acute and chronic urticaria and angioedema, as well as to anaphylaxis or anaphylactoid reactions. Study design, challenge protocols, and the evidence for elimination diets are also reviewed. Associations between food additives and asthma are discussed in a separate chapter.

Mechanisms of additive-induced urticaria, angioedema, and anaphylaxis

The mechanisms underlying most additive-induced urticaria, angioedema, and anaphylaxis remain unclear. It is likely that multiple mechanisms are responsible for these adverse reactions, given the heterogeneity of chemical structures found among these additives (Fig. 28.1), as well as the variable time course of reported reactions. Possible mechanisms include classic IgE-mediated (type I) hypersensitivity, delayed cell-mediated hypersensitivity, cyclooxygenase (COX) inhibition, direct neural stimulation, and blockade of coagulation pathways.

Immediate (IgE-mediated) hypersensitivity

Naturally derived food colorings, such as annatto and carmine, contain proteins in the 10–100 kDa range, suggesting these colorants can potentially elicit IgE-mediated responses in some atopic individuals. Researchers have demonstrated positive skin prick tests (SPTs), Prausnitz–Küstner test (PK), basophil histamine release assay, IgE radioallergosorbent test (RAST), and immunoblot to carmine [3]. This is likely due to retained insect-derived

Food Allergy: Adverse Reactions to Foods and Food Additives, Fifth Edition. Edited by Dean D Metcalfe, Hugh A Sampson, Ronald A Simon and Gideon Lack.

Table 28.1 Additives associated with adverse reactions, the reported reaction types, and whether skin testing has been described.

	Acute urticaria	Chronic urticaria	Anaphylaxis	Skin testing
Synthetic additives				
FD&C dyes	√	√		√
Azo dyes				
Tartrazine (FD&C Yellow No. 5)	√	√		√
Sunset yellow (FD&C Yellow No. 6)				
Ponceau (FD&C Red No. 4)				
Amaranth (FD&C Red No. 2)				
Non-azo dyes				
Brilliant blue (FD&C Blue No. 1)				
Erythrosine (FD&C Red No. 3)				
Indigotine (FD&C Blue No. 2)				
Sulfites	√		√	√
Sulfur dioxide				
Sodium sulfite				
Sodium/potassium bisulfite	√			√
Sodium/potassium metabisulfite	√		√	√
Parabens	√	Possible		√
p-Hydroxybenzoic acid				
Methyl-, ethyl-, butyl-, and propyl-paraben	√			√
Sodium benzoate	√	Possible		√
Monosodium glutamate (MSG)	√			
Aspartame	√			
Butylated hydroxyanisole (BHA)		√		
Butylated hydroxytoluene (BHT)		√		
Nitrates/nitrites	√	√		
Natural additives (plant/animal sources)				
Annatto	√		√	√
Carmine	√		√	√
Saffron	√		√	√
Mannitol	√		√	√

proteins. Positive SPTs to annatto have also been described [4]. These studies are discussed in more detail below in the section on individual additives.

Only a few reports have suggested IgE-mediated reactions to synthetic additives, notably to sulfites [5, 6] and parabens [7–9]. Due to their small molecular size, most synthetic additives would need to act as haptens to create a response mediated by IgE. Most cases of additive-provoked urticaria are not immediate, with many occurring as late as 24 hours after challenge, suggesting a non-IgE-mediated mechanism.

Delayed (type IV) hypersensitivity

Another suggested mechanism focuses on delayed hypersensitivity. Studies in this area have been few in number and often of dated design. Warrington et al. [10] measured the release of a T-lymphocyte-derived leukocyte-migration inhibition factor (LIF) in response to incubation with tartrazine, sodium benzoate, and aspirin (acetylsalicylic acid) *in vitro* using peripheral blood mononuclear cells from patients with chronic urticaria, with or without associated additive or aspirin sensitivity. Significant production of LIF occurred in response to tartrazine and sodium benzoate in individuals with chronic additive-induced urticaria. Sensitivity to tartrazine, sodium benzoate, and aspirin was determined either by response to elimination diet alone or by challenge-proved sensitivity. In this study, the potential for false-positive reactions on the basis of response to diet alone presented a problem. Essentially no details of the challenge procedures were given.

Valverde et al. [11] studied *in vitro* lymphocyte stimulation in 258 patients with chronic urticaria, angioedema, or both, using a series of food extracts and additives that included tartrazine, benzoic acid, and aspirin. They found positive stimulation (using the lymphocyte transformation test) to additives in 18% of subjects. After the patients were placed on a diet that excluded the offending additives, 62% had total remission of symptoms and 22% had partial remission. The investigators concluded that this response to diet lent credence to the lymphocyte transformation test as an *in vitro* diagnostic test for chronic urticaria and angioedema related to food additives.

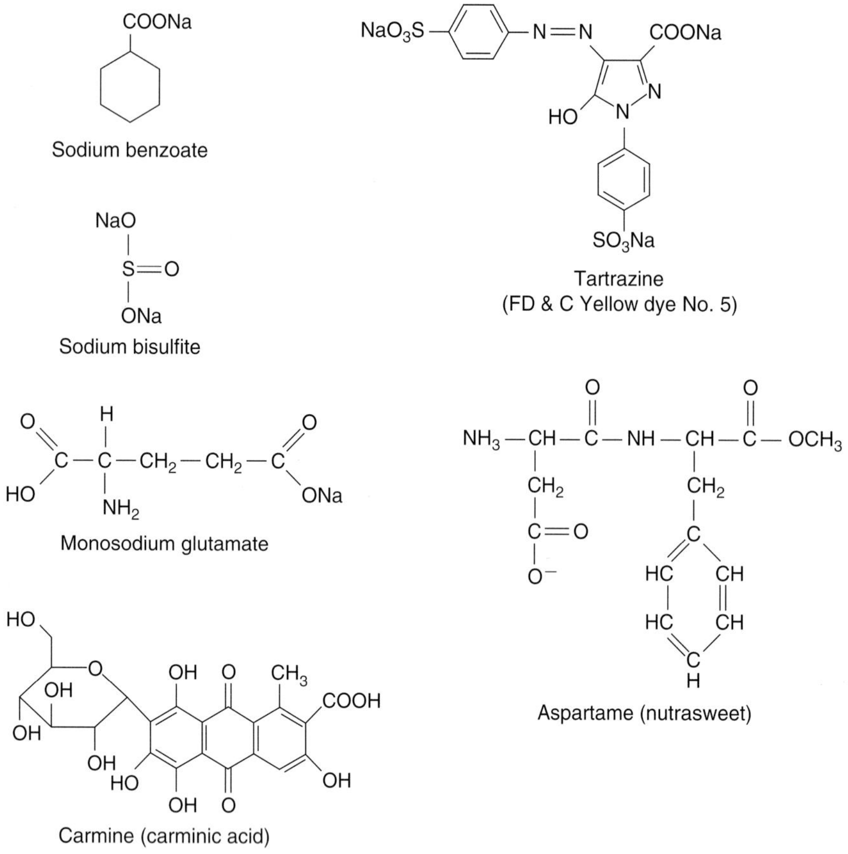

Figure 28.1 Chemical structure of common food additives.

However, no provocation challenges were performed in this study. No definitive conclusions regarding the presence or absence of a delayed-type hypersensitivity mechanism in additive-provoked urticaria appear possible from the studies described above. It seems reasonable to conclude that a reaction with an onset between 30 minutes and 6 hours after exposure to the material in question (most reactions began within the first 6 hours) is not typical of a type IV mechanism.

Cyclooxygenase, aspirin, and tartrazine

Inhibition of COX and the arachidonic acid pathway is suggested as the mechanism of most aspirin sensitivity. Many claims of cross-reactivity between aspirin and tartrazine have been made, with estimates of its incidence in earlier studies ranging from 21% to 100% [12–16]. In a double-blind, placebo-controlled (DBPC) study, with objective reaction criteria and withholding antihistamines for 72 hours prior to challenge, only 1 (4.2%) of 24 patients experienced urticaria after challenge with 50 mg of tartrazine [17]. However, this patient did not react when challenged with 975 mg of aspirin, lending no support to the concept of cross-reactivity. An earlier DBPC crossover challenge with 0.22 μg of tartrazine found sensitivity in 3 (8%) of 38 patients with chronic urticaria and 2 (20%) of 10 patients with aspirin intolerance [15]. This dose of tartrazine is similar to that used to color medication tablets, but remains far less than that typically encountered in the diet. The report did not mention, however, whether antihistamines were withheld during the challenges. No convincing evidence has been found to prove that tartrazine inhibits the enzyme COX in the arachidonic acid cascade.

Neurologically mediated hypersensitivity

Considerable evidence suggests that monosodium glutamate (MSG) has both neuroexcitatory and neurotoxic effects in animals [18] and humans [19], and neurologically mediated urticaria has been described [20]. Several factors, including heat, exercise, and stress, may also induce cholinergic urticaria. This mechanism represents only a theoretical basis for MSG-induced urticaria, possibly via release of cutaneous neuropeptides, and has not been established in controlled studies.

Anticoagulation

In 1986, Zimmerman and Czarnetzki [21] sought to disprove claims by earlier investigators that changes in bleeding time play an important role in diagnosing anaphylactoid reactions to aspirin, other nonsteroidal anti-inflammatory drugs (NSAIDs), and food additives. They measured bleeding time, prothrombin time, and partial thromboplastin times in 10 patients with histories of anaphylactoid reactions to these drugs and various food additives. Challenges were not placebo-controlled, nor were they blinded. Nevertheless, the investigators found no correlation between patients' reactions and the aforementioned coagulation parameters.

Study design for food additive challenges in patients with urticaria/angioedema

It is worth noting that in much of the existing literature examining the role of food additives in urticaria, angioedema, and anaphylaxis, there is broad variability in study design, often making interpretation and comparison between studies difficult. Factors leading to this variability include patient selection, activity of urticaria at the time of enrolment, concomitant medication use (especially antihistamines), reaction criteria, the use of placebo controls, and blinding.

Patient selection

Studies evaluating food additives contributing to urticaria/angioedema have included three types of subjects: (1) all available patients with chronic urticaria, (2) patients with histories suggestive of food additive-provoked urticaria, or (3) patients who have responded to a diet free of commonly implicated additives. The percentage of positive reactors varies depending on the group studied. This variability confounds comparison of results from differing studies.

Activity of urticaria at the time of study

The relative degree of activity or inactivity of urticaria or angioedema at the time of challenge appears to affect the ability to obtain cutaneous responses to food additives. Challenges performed on patients with active urticaria are more likely to yield false-positive results. Challenges performed on patients whose urticaria is in remission, on the other hand, are more likely to yield false-negative results. In a study by Mathison et al., only 1 of 15 patients whose urticaria was in remission experienced a reaction to aspirin, whereas 7 of 10 patients with active urticaria reacted to aspirin [22]. These challenges were performed using objective reaction criteria, and the reactions observed were then compared with baseline observations.

Medications

Several studies make no reference to whether medications—particularly antihistamines—were continued or withheld during a challenge. The following caveats must be considered when interpreting such challenge studies: (1) discontinuation of antihistamines immediately before or within 24 hours of challenge often facilitates more false-positive results. (2) Continuation of antihistamines during challenges may block milder, additive-induced cutaneous responses and, therefore, give more false-negative results. (3) Subjects become increasingly likely to experience breakthrough urticaria as the interval from the last antihistamine dose to the "positive challenge" increases. Such results would be even more confusing if placebo-controlled challenges preceded additive challenges.

Reaction criteria

Often, the experimental design did not incorporate a clear period of baseline observation for later comparison with reaction data. Most challenge studies performed have employed a loosely defined and rather subjective means to define urticarial responses. The reaction criteria might simply consist of "clear signs of urticaria developing within 24 hours." As noted above, the studies by Stevenson et al. [17] and Mathison et al. [22], in contrast, utilized an objective system of scoring urticarial responses.

Placebo controls

Without placebo controls, it is difficult to interpret a positive urticarial challenge response. Nevertheless, a number of reported additive challenge studies do not employ placebo controls. Even in many placebo-controlled studies, the placebo is always the first challenge, followed by aspirin, and finally by an additive. Thus, a spontaneous flare of urticaria would be least likely to coincide with the first placebo challenge. We also question the approach of having only a single placebo in challenge studies that test large numbers of additives. We are of the opinion that a need exists for multiple placebos and randomization of placebo usage in the order of challenges.

Blinding

Among the most important features of any protocol for food additive challenge is a double-blind challenge, because urticaria may be exacerbated by emotional stress [23, 24]. In addition, it is necessary to eliminate observer bias given the subjective nature of positive responses. Open challenges are useful tools for ruling out additive-associated reactions. Positive challenge responses, in contrast, need double-blinded confirmation before they can be accepted as "true positives."

Individual additives in acute urticaria: description, challenges, and testing

An overview of selected additives follows, as well as a brief overview of the challenge and testing literature for each additive or family of additives. The majority of this literature examines acute reactions. Studies examining the role of additives in chronic urticaria frequently address multiple additives simultaneously and are included in a separate section below. For additional information on individual additives, the reader is referred elsewhere in this book.

Tartrazine and food dyes

Dyes approved under the Food, Drug and Cosmetic (FD&C) Act are known as "coal tar" dyes due to their original derivation, though most are now manufactured synthetically. Only a handful of dyes have been clearly associated with clinical reactions, the best known of which is the azo dye tartrazine (FD&C Yellow No. 5). Other clinically significant azo dyes include ponceau (FD&C Red No. 4) and sunset yellow (FD&C Yellow No. 6). Amaranth (FD&C Red No. 2) was banned from use in the United States in 1975 because of claims related to carcinogenicity. Non-azo dyes include brilliant blue (FD&C Blue No. 1), erythrosine (FD&C Red No. 3), and indigotine (FD&C Blue No. 2). A full list of approved dyes is maintained by the US Food and Drug Administration (FDA) [25].

Challenge studies

Murdoch et al. [26] found that at least 2 (8.3%) of 24 patients developed hives after ingesting a panel of four azo dyes, including tartrazine. As previously discussed, Stevenson et al. [17] found that only 1 (4.2%) of 24 aspirin-sensitive subjects undergoing double-blind challenge with 50 mg tartrazine developed urticaria. The tartrazine-sensitive individual identified in Stevenson's study did not react to a blinded challenge with doses of aspirin of as much as 975 mg, suggesting a lack of cross-reactivity between tartrazine and aspirin. In a small (n = 26), DBPC crossover study, Pestana et al. examined the general safety of tartrazine in atopic patients and found no clinical reactions to 35 mg of ingested tartrazine in participants [27]. It appears that tartrazine and other azo dyes rarely induce acute urticaria. The few studies that suggest tartrazine may play a role in chronic urticaria are discussed in the section on chronic urticaria.

Sulfites

Sulfites have been used for centuries to preserve food. In addition, sulfiting agents (including sulfur dioxide and sodium or potassium sulfite, bisulfite, and metabisulfite) are used in the fermentation industry to sanitize containers and to inhibit the growth of undesirable microorganisms. Sulfites act as potent antioxidants and are frequently used to prevent discoloration (browning) and as fresheners.

Many packaged foods, including cellophane-wrapped fruits and vegetables, processed grain foods (crackers and cookies), and citrus-flavored beverages, may contain sulfites. The highest levels occur in foods prone to browning or oxidation: peeled potatoes, dried fruits (apricots and white raisins), shrimp, and other seafoods. Sulfites must be listed as ingredients in prepared and packaged foods or drinks that contain at least 10 ppm SO_2 equivalents. In 1986, the US FDA banned the uses of sulfites on foods marketed as "fresh."

Challenge studies

Reports by Prenner and Stevens [5] and Yang et al. [6] presented single cases of sulfite-provoked anaphylaxis with positive testing (discussed below under "testing"), suggesting an IgE-mediated mechanism in these reactions. Yang et al. performed a single-blind oral challenge on their patient, who responded positively to a 5 mg dose of potassium metabisulfite. No double-blind challenge was performed.

In 1980, Clayton and Busse [28] described a non-atopic female who developed generalized urticaria that progressed to life-threatening anaphylaxis within 15 minutes of drinking wine. Her symptoms were not reproduced by ingestion of other alcoholic beverages or foods. This case may have involved sulfite-provoked urticaria and anaphylaxis.

Habenicht et al. [29] described two patients who experienced several episodes of urticaria and angioedema after consuming restaurant meals. Only one of these individuals underwent a single-blind oral challenge with potassium metabisulfite. Generalized urticaria developed within 15 minutes of the patient receiving a 25 mg challenge dose. No placebo challenge was performed. Avoidance of potential sulfite sources apparently resolved this patient's recurrent symptoms. Similarly, Belchi-Hernandez et al. reported a DBPC challenge that reproduced urticaria after challenge with 25 mg potassium metabisulfite [30]. Skin tests were negative in this subject.

Schwartz reported two patients with symptoms related to ingestion of restaurant salads, who underwent oral challenges with metabisulfite [31]. Symptoms in both patients included weakness, dissociation from the body, dizziness, borderline hypotension, and bradycardia, which are more consistent with vasovagal reactions than with anaphylaxis. Another report described a patient who received less than 2 mL of subcutaneous procaine (Novocaine) with epinephrine administered by her dentist [32]. Within several minutes, she developed flushing, a sense of warmth, and pruritus, followed by scattered urticaria, dyspnea, and anxiety. Skin tests to local anesthetics and sulfite proved negative. Thirty minutes after receiving a single-blind, oral dose of 10 mg of sodium bisulfite, she developed "a sense of fullness in her head, nasal congestion, and a pruritic erythematous blotchy eruption." No respiratory symptoms developed and the investigators did not observe any pulmonary function test abnormalities. This patient was able to tolerate local anesthetics without epinephrine. Importantly, this patient did not describe a history of food-related symptoms. Furthermore, the usual dose of aqueous epinephrine (adrenalin) contains only 0.3 mg of sulfite and local anesthetics contain only as much as 2 mg/mL sulfite. Thus, at usual doses, even in the most sensitive persons, exposure in this form seems unlikely to provoke reactions. The mechanism of this patient's reaction cannot be definitively linked to sulfite and was likely a vasomotor response to epinephrine.

Acute urticaria associated with leukocytoclastic vasculitis and eosinophilia was induced by a single placebo-controlled challenge with 50 mg sodium bisulfite in a subject suffering from recurrent urticaria and angioedema of unclear etiology. Blinded challenges were performed during a symptom-free period, followed by biopsy confirmation of the leukocytoclasis. Conscious avoidance of sulfites reduced the frequency of subsequent reactions dramatically [33].

Two reports have demonstrated the inability to provoke reactions to sulfites in patients with idiopathic anaphylaxis, some of whom had histories of restaurant-associated symptoms [34, 35]. In a study describing food-related skin testing in 102 patients with idiopathic anaphylaxis, only one patient was found to have metabisulfite sensitivity [36]. In addition, Simon et al. performed sulfite-ingestion challenges in 25 patients with chronic idiopathic urticaria/angioedema (CIUA) without a reaction [37]. At present, sulfite-induced urticaria, angioedema, or anaphylaxis appears to be a rare phenomenon.

Skin and serum testing

As mentioned above, Prenner and Stevens reported an anaphylactic reaction in a 50-year-old man minutes after eating a restaurant lunch containing food sprayed with sodium bisulfite [5]. Symptoms included generalized urticaria, pruritus, swelling of the tongue, difficulty swallowing, and tightness in the chest. He responded promptly to treatment with subcutaneous epinephrine. Subsequently, the patient's SPT and an intradermal test gave positive results (with negative controls). The authors were able to demonstrate PK transfer to a non-atopic subject. The patient reported by Yang et al. [6], discussed earlier, had a borderline intradermal skin test, followed by a positive single-blind oral challenge with 5 mg potassium metabisulfite. This patient's cutaneous reactivity was also passively transferred via the PK reaction. However, sulfite challenges in nine other patients with histories of hives related to eating restaurant food were negative. In addition, Sokol and Hydick [38] reported a case of sulfite-induced anaphylaxis that provides evidence for a specific IgE-mediated mechanism. Despite these isolated reports, IgE-mediated immediate hypersensitivity reactions to sulfites (possibly via a hapten mechanism) appear to occur only rarely.

There is limited evidence to suggest a role for basophil activation in sulfite-sensitive urticaria. García-Ortega et al. reported a 56-year-old man with urticaria and facial angioedema following local wine consumption. Skin prick testing with an extended panel of foods, latex, and sodium metabisulfite was negative, but symptoms were reproduced in a DBPC challenge with sodium metabisulfite. Basophil activation tests with 5.21 and 20.8 μg/mL of sodium metabisulfite were positive [39].

Studies measuring serum levels of neutrophil chemotactic factor of anaphylaxis (NCF-A) did not find an increase in this mast cell (MC) mediator post-challenge in subjects with negative metabisulfite skin tests, suggesting that MC degranulation is not associated with non-IgE-mediated sulfite reactions [40]. Cromolyn pretreatment also did not ablate an urticarial reaction in an individual sensitive to potassium metabisulfite [30]. In the overwhelming majority of cases, the mechanisms behind sulfite-provoked urticaria, angioedema, and anaphylaxis (or anaphylactoid reactions) remain unknown.

Parabens and sodium benzoate

Parabens are aliphatic esters of *p*-hydroxybenzoic acid and include methyl-, ethyl-, propyl-, and butyl-parabens. Sodium benzoate is a closely related substance, usually reported to cross-react with these compounds. Parabens are widely used as preservatives in both foods and drugs and are well recognized as causes of severe contact dermatitis. At least three cases of apparent IgE-mediated, paraben-induced urticaria and angioedema have been reported, all with benzoates used as pharmaceutical preservatives [7]. The evaluation of these patients is discussed below under "Skin testing." Michils has also reported one isolated case report of sodium benzoate-induced anaphylaxis [9].

Challenge Studies

Nettis et al. [41] performed DBPC challenges on 47 patients with suspected acute urticaria/angioedema induced by sodium benzoate-containing foods. Only one subject (2%) had a reaction after the ingestion of 75 mg of sodium benzoate without an adverse reaction to placebo, suggesting that even when confronted with suspected historical data on potential reactions to sodium benzoate, true sensitivity rates are quite low.

Skin testing

The three patients mentioned earlier with paraben-induced urticaria and angioedema [7, 8] had positive skin test responses to parabens, but negative results when exposed to the associated drugs minus the paraben preservatives. Interestingly, these subjects could tolerate oral benzoates in their diets without reactions.

Macy et al. [42] reported a series of 287 patients who underwent immediate hypersensitivity skin tests to methylparaben-preserved local anesthetics. Only three patients had positive skin tests. These three individuals underwent skin testing as well as provocative dose testing to 0.1% methylparaben, in addition to local anesthetic without preservative. All three reacted to methylparaben, suggesting this agent as potential cause for local immediate hypersensitivity reactions previously attributed to the local anesthetics themselves.

Monosodium glutamate

Glutamates are salts and anions of the excitatory nonessential amino acid glutamic acid [43]. Glutamate occurs naturally in some foods in significant amounts: 100 g Camembert cheese, for example, contains as much as 1 g MSG. The greatest exposure to MSG in foods, however, occurs through its role as a flavor enhancer. Manufacturers and restaurateurs add MSG to a wide variety of foods and for many years its use has been prevalent in various forms of Asian cooking. As much as 6 g MSG may be ingested in a highly seasoned meal, and a single bowl of wonton soup may contain 2.5 g MSG. MSG may also be found in manufactured meat and chicken products.

MSG has been reported to provoke, within minutes to hours of eating, a syndrome characterized by headache, a burning sensation along the back of the neck, chest tightness, nausea, and sweating. Recently, a trend toward reducing MSG use has emerged, likely in response to consumer dissatisfaction related to this effect.

Challenge studies

Squire described a 50-year-old man with recurrent angioedema of the face and extremities related to ingestion of soup containing MSG [21, 44]. A single-blind, placebo-controlled challenge with the soup base resulted in "a sensation of imminent swelling" within a few hours, with visible angioedema emerging 24 hours after the challenge. In a graded challenge with only MSG, angioedema occurred 16 hours after the challenge with a dose of 250 mg. Avoidance of MSG led to an extended remission. Details of the challenge were not reported, nor was it stated whether medications were withheld during challenges.

Geha et al. [45] challenged 130 patients with self-reported MSG sensitivity in a double-blind, multicenter, placebo-controlled trial, using a fairly large 5 g dose, both with and without accompanying food. It should be noted that the inclusion criteria included many systemic symptoms (e.g., flushing, weakness, headache), but none of the subjects had reported symptoms of urticaria or angioedema. More subjects seemed to react to MSG consumed without food than with food, but the reactions of individual subject were not reproducible on repeat testing in the study, making an underlying immune mechanism unlikely.

Aspartame and other sweeteners

Aspartame is a dipeptide composed of aspartic acid and the methyl ester of phenylalanine. This popular low-calorie artificial sweetener was approved for use in carbonated beverages in 1983 and is 180 times sweeter than sucrose. In addition, it has been implicated in several cases of urticaria and angioedema. As of publication, there have not been similar reports for other natural or artificial sweeteners, including acesulfame potassium (Ace-K), xylitol, sucralose, or extracts of *Stevia rebaudiana*. There is a single case report of saccharine-induced urticaria from 1955 [46], but the lack of additional reports in the intervening 60 years suggests that this is not a common effect.

Challenge studies

Two cases of aspartame-provoked urticaria and angioedema have been reported. Both patients reported the onset of urticaria within 1 hour of ingesting aspartame-sweetened soft drinks. DBPC challenges induced urticaria with doses of aspartame (25–75 mg) that fell below the amount contained in typical 12 oz cans (100–150 mg) [47].

In a multicenter, randomized, placebo-controlled crossover study, Geha et al. [48] challenged 21 subjects with histories of a temporal (minutes to hours) association between aspartame ingestion and urticaria/angioedema. These subjects were identified after an extensive recruiting process spanning 4 years. Only four urticarial reactions were observed: two following aspartame consumption and two following placebo ingestion. Doses ranged as high as 600 mg of aspartame.

Butylated hydroxyanisole and butylated hydroxytoluene

Butylated hydroxyanisole (BHA) and butylated hydroxytoluene (BHT) are antioxidants used in cereals and other grain products. These agents have primarily been implicated in chronic urticaria and are discussed in the section "Food additive sensitivity in chronic idiopathic urticaria/angioedema."

Nitrates/nitrites

Nitrates and nitrites are widely used preservatives. Their popularity stems from both their flavoring and coloring attributes. These agents are found mostly in processed meats such as frankfurters and salami [49].

Challenge studies

Hawkins and Katelaris [50] reported a single case of recurrent anaphylaxis occurring after eating take-out food. DBPC capsule challenge with 25 mg each of sodium nitrate and sodium nitrite resulted in an acute anaphylactic reaction, with hypotension within 15 minutes of the active challenge.

Annatto

Annatto dye is an orange-yellow food coloring extracted from the seeds of the tree *Bixa orellana*, a large fast-growing shrub cultivated in the tropics. It is frequently used in cereals, beverages, cheese, and snack foods. Several case reports of anaphylactic reactions to annatto dye have been documented [4, 51].

Skin testing

Nish et al. [51] reported a case of annatto dye-induced anaphylaxis. SPTs to annatto were strongly positive with negative control results. SDS-PAGE demonstrated two bands in the range of 50 kDa. Immunoblotting showed patient IgE specific for one of these bands while controls showed no binding. Residual or contaminating seed protein was the likely responsible antigen in this rare case.

Revan et al. found 9 (12%) of 77 atopic patients were SPT positive to liquid undiluted annatto [4]. However, only two of these nine subjects had symptomatic annatto allergy: 1 patient with a 4+ SPT had a history of annatto-induced anaphylaxis, and another with a 3+ SPT had angioedema. Only one SPT-positive reactor was challenged and was negative. The negative predictive value (NPV) of SPT in this cohort was 100%; however, the positive predictive value (PPV) was low (22%). Perhaps the undiluted extract was too potent to differentiate between true reactors and an irritant response. Neither patient was challenged, and DBPC challenges are needed to confirm these results.

Carmine

Carmine (or cochineal extract), designated E120 in Europe, is a red colorant derived from the dried bodies of female cochineal insects (*Dactylopius coccus costa*). It is commonly used in cosmetics, textiles, and foods and is responsible for giving the liqueur Campari its characteristic color. As of January 5, 2011, the FDA requires labeling of foods and cosmetics containing carmine [52, 53].

Carmine-induced anaphylaxis was first described in the mid-1990s. Since then, urticaria/angioedema associated with a number of food products containing carmine has also been reported, including Campari-orange liqueur®, Yoplait brand custard style strawberry–banana yogurt, imitation crab meat, Good Humor SnoFruit Popsicles®, and ruby red grapefruit juice [3, 54–56]. In 2009, Greenhawt et al. reported a patient with carmine sensitivity characterized by pruritus and swelling after ingesting generic azithromycin, in which carmine was used to color the tablet [57].

Commercial carmine appears to retain proteinaceous material from the source insects which, when complexed with carminic acid, is likely responsible for IgE-mediated carmine allergy. Liippo and Lammintausta have suggested that sensitization to dust mites and shrimp is common in carmine-sensitive patients, possibly due to similarity in arthropod proteins. Interpretation of this study is limited by a high false-positive rate on carmine skin testing (at least 61%) and need for objective evidence to establish allergy versus sensitization [58].

Skin testing

Evidence for an IgE-mediated mechanism driving anaphylactic episodes associated with carmine-colored foods includes positive SPTs, a positive PK test, a positive basophil histamine release assay, positive IgE RAST studies, and positive SDS-PAGE with IgE immunoblot [3, 54–56]. Using minced cochineal insect extracts, Chung et al. [3] identified several protein SDS-PAGE bands of 23–88 kDa that could induce an IgE-mediated response. The sera from three patients with episodic urticaria/angioedema/anaphylaxis occurring 3–5 hours after ingestion of foods containing carmine recognized these bands on immunoblot, though patient reactivity to specific bands varied. This reactivity was inhibited by carmine.

Specific challenges have not been performed with carmine in any of the above reports, with the exception of Baldwin et al. [55], whose patient showed negative oral challenges to each of the other components of the Good Humor SnoFruit Popsicle, supporting a carmine-induced IgE-mediated reaction.

Saffron

Both saffron spice and saffron color are derived from the dried stigmas and style of the crocus bulb. Saffron color is dark yellow-orange and is used to color soups, bouillabaisse, sauces, rice dishes (paella, "risotto Milanese"), cakes, cheese, and liqueurs [59].

Near-fatal saffron-induced anaphylaxis was reported by Wüthrich [59]. The subject, a 21-year-old atopic farmer, developed violent abdominal cramps, laryngeal edema, and generalized urticaria a few minutes after a meal of saffron rice and mushrooms. This progressed to pulse-less collapse that responded to advanced cardiac life support.

Skin testing

In the earlier patient [59], SPTs to ingredients of the meal were negative except for a strong reaction to saffron. RAST testing to two saffron preparations was positive. SDS-PAGE and immunoblotting showed five IgE-binding bands with molecular weights between 40 and 90 kDa.

Mannitol

Mannitol is a sugar alcohol widely distributed in plants. It is a white, crystalline substance added to processed foods as a thickener, stabilizer, and sweetener. It is also widely used as a drug excipient. In addition, it is widely used as a therapeutic agent for glaucoma, increased intracranial pressure, drug intoxication, and oliguric renal failure [60]. One report of mannitol-induced anaphylaxis has been well described by Hegde and Venkatesh [60]. An individual who demonstrated anaphylactic reactions to mannitol found in pomegranate and cultivated mushroom also experienced severe allergic reactions to mannitol as an excipient in the chewable pharmaceutical cisapride.

Skin testing

In the case above [60], the authors utilized SPTs, serum mannitol-specific IgE by enzyme-linked immunosorbent assay (ELISA), and multiple chemical purification techniques for mannitol separation to demonstrate an immediate hypersensitivity mechanism to mannitol.

Food additive sensitivity in chronic idiopathic urticaria/angioedema

The best available evidence suggests that food additive-associated chronic urticaria/angioedema is rare, though it does occur. Early studies may have overestimated the significance of additives in CIUA due to issues with study design, including a lack of placebo challenges, double-blind challenges, antihistamine use, and lack of standardized scoring. More recent and rigorously designed studies suggest an incidence of 1–3% or less. Additives that have been implicated in CIUA include tartrazine, BHA/BHT, nitrates/nitrites, and possibly parabens/benzoate. We first review studies with multiple additive challenges and then those in which specific additives were examined.

Examples of challenge studies with less stringent design criteria

In one of the earliest additive challenge studies in patients with chronic urticaria, 7 (30.4%) subjects reacted to tartrazine and "4 or 5" (17.4% or 22.7%) reacted to sodium benzoate [61]. Thune and Granholt [62] reported that 20 (21%) of 96 patients reacted to tartrazine, 13 (15%) of 86 reacted to sunset yellow, 5 (71%) of 7 reacted to parabens, and 6 (13%) of 47 reacted to BHA and BHT. Furthermore, in the group of patients with chronic idiopathic urticaria, 62 (62%) of the 100 patients challenged reacted to at least 1 of the 22 different agents used. Neither study was placebo-controlled. Conclusions about the incidence of reactions to a particular agent derived from this study are thus difficult to make.

In a study of 330 patients with recurrent urticaria, Juhlin [63] performed single-blind challenges using multiple additives and a single placebo, which always preceded the additive challenge. He found that one or more positive reactions occurred in 102 (31%) patients tested. Reaction criteria were relatively subjective in this study. In fact, 109 (33%) patients had reactions judged to be "uncertain." Furthermore, if patients reacted to the lactose placebo, retesting involved a wheat starch placebo. Questionable reactors were retested. If the repeat test gave a positive result, the first test was assumed to be positive as well; the same logic applied for negative retesting.

Supramaniam and Warner [64] described 24 of 43 children as reacting to one or more additives used in their double-blind challenge study. No baseline observation period was established. Only one placebo was interspersed among the nine additives used for challenge. There was no mention about whether antihistamines were withheld prior to or during challenges.

In 1985, Genton et al. [65] performed single-blind additive challenges on 17 patients with chronic urticaria or angioedema. The patients were placed on a 14-day elimination diet (free of food additives) before challenge and medications were discontinued at the beginning of the diet. Of the 17 patients in the study, 15 reacted to at least one of the six additives used for the challenge. DBPC challenges were not performed to confirm these results.

Malanin and Kalimo [66] performed prick and scratch skin tests on 91 individuals with CIUA, utilizing a panel of 18 food additives and preservatives. A positive response was defined as a wheal greater than or equal to the size of the histamine control. Sixty-four (26%) subjects had at least one positive skin test as compared with 25 (10%) of 247 non-urticaria control subjects. Ten of the 64 (15.6%) CIUA patients with positive skin tests underwent oral provocation with the additives that were positive on skin test. Only one patient reacted, experiencing an urticarial reaction to benzoic acid. Details of the challenge procedure were not provided and the activity of the patient's urticaria prior to the challenge was not noted.

Examples of challenge studies with more stringent design criteria

At Scripps Clinic and Research Foundation, patients with CIUA underwent single-blinded challenges with a panel of additives (Table 28.2). Positive reactors were confirmed with DBPC challenges. No true positive reactors were identified among more than 100 patients [37]. From these data,

Table 28.2 Suggested maximum doses for additives used in challenge protocols.

Yellow dyes No. 5 and No. 6: 50 mg
Sulfites: 100 mg
MSG: 2.5 g
Aspartame: 150 mg
Parabens/benzoates: 100 mg
BHA/BHT: 250 mg
Nitrates/nitrites: 50 mg

we can conclude with a 95% confidence limit that sensitivity to any of the 11 food and drug additives in patients with CIUA is less than 1%.

Di Lorenzo et al. [67] studied a large series of 838 patients with recurrent chronic idiopathic urticaria for sensitivity to a panel of common food additives. After undergoing historical screenings, all patients had negative food allergen SPTs. After a 4-week food additive-free diet (FAFD), patients were screened with a DBPC mixed additive challenge, consisting of tartrazine, erythrosin, sodium benzoate, *p*-hydroxybenzoate, sodium metabisulfite, and MSG. Positive reactors underwent DBPC single challenges with individual additives with 1-week intervals between challenges. Patients with negative DBPC mixed challenges were used as an additional control group. The incidence of patients with positive histories, clinical response to FAFD, positive DBPC mixed, and DBPC single challenges was only 16 of 838 patients studied (1.9%; 95% CI 1–3%). Twenty-four total reactions occurred in these 16 patients, due to some individuals reacting to multiple agents.

In 1988, Ortolani et al. [68] reported 396 patients with recurrent chronic urticaria and angioedema in follow-up to a study performed in 1984 [69]. DBPC oral food provocations were performed on patients that had experienced significant remissions while following an elimination diet. The diet was maintained, but medications were discontinued during challenges. The report did not describe the timing of discontinuation of medications. On the basis of history alone, 179 patients were considered for an elimination diet for suspected food or food additive intolerance; only 135 patients ultimately participated in the study. Eight (9.2%) of 87 patients with significant improvement on the diet after 2 weeks had positive responses to food challenges. Of the 79 patients with negative responses to food challenges, 72 underwent DBPC oral food additive provocations. Twelve (17%) of these patients experienced positive responses to challenges with one or more additives. Many of these patients reacted to two or three additives. Five (31%) of the 16 patients with positive responses to aspirin challenges gave positive responses to additive challenges; four of these subjects tested positive to sodium salicylate.

The similarity in chemical structure observed between aspirin and sodium salicylate supports the possibility of cross-reactivity between these agents. They differ in that sodium salicylate is a "non-acetylated" salicylate. The doses used (0.4 mg) in the sodium salicylate challenge, however, far exceed the levels encountered in most conventional diets. Furthermore, although it is important in assessing food sensitivity, a patient's history is usually a poor indicator of a possible additive hypersensitivity, because patients are usually unaware of all additives that they consume daily.

Hannuksela and Lahti [70] challenged 44 chronic urticaria patients with several food additives, including sodium metabisulfite, BHA or BHT, β-carotene, and benzoic acid in a prospective, DBPC study. Only 1 (2.2%) of the 44 patients had a positive response to the challenge, reacting positively to benzoic acid. Another patient also reacted to the placebo challenge. All medications were discontinued 72 hours before the first challenge and during the study. Patients were not placed on an additive-free diet prior to the challenge. The challenge dose of metabisulfite was low (9 mg). Similarly, Kellett et al. noted that approximately 10% of 44 chronic idiopathic urticaria patients reacted to benzoates, tartrazine, or both, but 10% of the subjects reacted to placebo challenges [71].

Individual additives implicated in CIUA

Tartrazine

Volonakis et al. [72] performed an extensive analysis of etiologic factors in 226 children with chronic urticaria. Elimination of food additives and DBPC challenges were performed with a panel of four additives (tartrazine, sodium benzoate, nitrates, and sorbic acid) plus aspirin. Three subjects (1.3%) reacted to tartrazine, while there were no reactions to benzoate, nitrate, or sorbic acid.

BHA/BHT

In a DBPC study, Goodman et al. [73] challenged two patients with chronic idiopathic urticaria who experienced remissions following dye- and preservative-elimination diets. Both patients noted significant exacerbations of their urticaria after challenge with BHA and BHT. Subsequent avoidance of foods containing these antioxidants resulted in marked abatement of the frequency, severity, and duration of urticaria episodes. Long-term follow-up revealed urticarial flares after dietary indiscretion, but an otherwise quiescent disease. Yamaki et al. demonstrated that BHT enhances MC degranulation in a mouse model, by increasing the intracellular Ca^+ concentration and PIK3 activity, suggesting a possible mechanism for its role in chronic urticaria [74].

Nitrates/nitrites

Asero [75] reported a case of chronic generalized pruritus without skin eruption that disappeared on an additive-free diet. DBPC challenge with multiple additives resulted in symptom reproducibility within 60 minutes of the 10 mg sodium nitrate challenge. The patient did not react to seven other additives and multiple placebos.

Elimination diets in CIUA

An alternative strategy for investigating additive-induced urticaria involves the elimination of all additives from the diet and the observation of its effects on hives. Unfortunately, there are no reported blinded or placebo-controlled studies of this nature. As noted in a study above, Ortolani [68] found that 87 of 135 participants (64.4%) improved on an additive-free elimination diet.

In uncontrolled studies, Ros et al. [14] reported an additive-free diet to be "completely helpful" in 24% of patients with chronic urticaria; 57% of patients were deemed "much improved," and 19% were "slightly better" or experienced no change in their urticaria. Rudzki et al. [76] reported that 50 (32%) of 158 patients responded to a diet that eliminated salicylates, benzoates, and azo dyes. In a larger study of 140 patients, Magerl et al. found that only 28% of chronic urticaria patients responded to an elimination diet as measured by changes in the urticaria activity score (UAS) and Dermatology Quality of Life Instrument (DQLI), though they used a more restricted diet that eliminated not only food additives but also foods rich in other "pseudoallergens" such as tomatoes, peas, and spinach [77]. These studies did not address the question of which, if any, additives constituted the cause of the problem.

Gibson and Clancy [78] found that 54 (71%) of 76 patients who underwent a 2-week, additive-free diet "responded." They then challenged the responders with individual additives. Although the challenges were controlled, the patients always received the placebo first. No mention was made of whether the challenges were blinded. A diet that eliminated the offending additive was then continued for 6–18 months, followed by repeat challenge. All three patients who initially responded to tartrazine challenge had negative results upon rechallenge, as did one of the four patients with initial responses to benzoate challenges. Thus, despite this approach, the incidence of additive sensitivity in urticaria remains unknown. For providers interested in using an elimination diet for their patients, Di Lorenzo et al. [67] provide an overview of the FAFD used in their study, which is primarily focused on avoiding specific food additives. Magerl et al. provide a more restrictive diet that also excludes specific foods due to possible inherent "pseudoallergens" [77].

Recommendations for food additive challenge protocols in patients with urticaria, angioedema, and/or anaphylaxis

A review of the literature on food and drug additive challenges in patients with urticaria suggests that more rigorously conducted studies are needed. With the use of more objective criteria and stringent design, more meaningful conclusions may be drawn regarding the true incidence of food additive-induced urticaria, angioedema, and anaphylaxis. Our recommendations for future additive challenge protocols in patients with chronic or acute urticaria/angioedema are presented in the following sections.

Patient selection

In view of the ubiquitous and frequent dietary exposure to food and drug additives, the study population should be selected from patients with chronic "idiopathic" urticaria or angioedema, unless the study is intended to examine another defined subgroup of patients with acute or intermittent urticaria, angioedema, and/or anaphylaxis (e.g., patients with a convincingly positive acute history or patients responsive to an elimination diet). The diagnosis of chronic idiopathic urticaria or angioedema should be made in subjects with recurrent urticaria of at least 6 weeks duration without identifiable cause. In addition, appropriate challenges should be conducted to ascertain any physical urticarias. After a negative workup, a patient's urticaria may then be considered idiopathic [79]. It would also seem reasonable to exclude patients with a known antibody against the FcεRI receptor, thyroid peroxidase, or thyroglobulin (chronic autoimmune urticaria).

Activity of urticaria

Chronic urticaria should preferably be in an active phase (e.g., some lesions should have appeared within 1 month prior to challenge), as additives may not only provoke urticaria *de novo*, but also exacerbate ongoing urticaria, as is true with aspirin [22]. The UAS is a widely used scoring tool that can be used to quantify the chronic urticaria activity, using the number of hives and intensity of pruritus [80], yielding a score of 0–6. This instrument is used to generate scores for a single encounter or over a period of time (e.g., the UAS7 is the sum of the UAS over a 7-day period). For patients with an intermittent and/or acute anaphylactic history associated with an additive, challenges should not be conducted for at least 2 weeks time after the acute reaction.

Medications

Antihistamines should be withheld for 3–5 days prior to the challenges, if possible. For patients with intractable chronic symptoms, antihistamines should be tapered to the minimal effective dose. Although corticosteroids are not first-line treatment for chronic urticaria/angioedema, when necessary their use should also be tapered to the minimal effective dose, preferably less than or equal to 10 mg daily.

Food additive-free diet

Patients should be placed on a diet free of all additives included in the challenge protocol at least 1 week prior to the challenge. The FAFD employed by Di Lorenzo et al. is a reasonable guide that can be modified based on specific patient needs [67].

Reaction criteria

Reaction criteria should be as objective as possible. We suggest the "rule of nines," used for assessing thermal burns, as providing a useful method for estimating skin surface area. On each of the 11 divided areas of the body, the investigator assigns a score of 0–4, then derives a total score (0–44 points). A positive urticarial response may be defined as either an absolute increase in the total score of 9 points or an increase of more than 300% from the baseline score determined immediately before challenge. Alternately, for patients with chronic urticaria, Mathias et al. have recently suggested that a change of 9.5–10.5 in the UAS7 (UAS over 7 days) is clinically significant [81]. A positive angioedema response may be defined as a relative increase in size of more than 50% in the body part affected.

Baseline observation

Prior to challenge, baseline skin scores should be recorded at intervals during a period of observation corresponding to the same intervals that will be used during the challenge. The appropriate length of the baseline observation period depends on factors such as the activity of the patient's urticaria, the interval of time between discontinuation of antihistamines and the challenge, and the length of the challenge protocol.

In general, 1 day of pure observation with skin scoring should be followed by 1 day of single-blind placebo challenge with skin scoring, except perhaps in patients who are completely free of hives at challenge. In this instance, 1 day of placebo challenge should be sufficient. Skin scores on those 2 days should not vary by more than 3 points or 30% (whichever is greater) before proceeding to additive and further placebo challenges.

Blinding and placebo controls

Depending on the provider's index of suspicion, screening open challenges may be performed without placebo, as a negative result does not require further confirmation and possible causative agents can be more rapidly excluded in this fashion. However, positive reactors should undergo a subsequent placebo-controlled, preferably double-blinded, protocol.

Placebo-controlled challenges should be conducted in a randomized fashion with, ideally, at least an equal number of placebo and active challenges undertaken. Coded opaque capsules can be used to establish a double-blind protocol, with the code remaining unbroken until the completion of all challenges.

Additive doses

The additive doses used in challenge protocols should reflect natural exposure to each agent. Suggested limits for some common additives are listed in Table 28.2. Starting doses should be individualized on the basis of the patient's history, but usually consist of 1/100 of the maximum dose. Challenges must be performed with informed consent and in a setting where severe reactions may be appropriately treated.

Conclusion

Only a small number of well-designed clinical studies have been conducted in the area of additive-provoked urticaria, angioedema, and anaphylaxis. The true incidence of such reactions remains unknown, although it appears to be relatively rare, despite claims in earlier (pre-1990) additive literature. Most natural additives (carmine, annatto, and saffron) contain source proteins capable of inducing direct IgE-mediated immediate hypersensitivity reactions. In the case of carmine, sensitization may occur through application of carmine-containing cosmetics, as contact urticaria to this natural additive has been described. In the United States, all foods that contain carmine must now be labeled as such.

The case for similar immediate hypersensitivity mechanisms to the synthetic additive group is less compelling. A relatively small number of case reports describing IgE-mediated reactions to sulfites and parabens exist, compared with the overall number of positive challenges reported. Although rare, IgE-mediated paraben reactions can confound the diagnostic evaluation of local anesthetic allergy, given the use of this preservative in multidose vials of these medications.

In terms of chronic urticaria, it is now well accepted that many cases of CIUA have an autoimmune basis, as demonstrated by the presence of autoantibodies directed against the IgE receptor and/or IgE itself or in association with other autoimmune syndromes, most notably thyroid autoimmunity [79]. Most studies attempting to link causation and/or exacerbation of this condition by food or drug additives have been poorly designed. Emerging evidence appears to refute the earlier notion that these additives are frequently associated with chronic urticaria. Guidelines for conducting additive challenges in CIUA, as well as in episodic urticaria/angioedema patients, are reviewed in the text. Further well-designed trials addressing additive-provoked urticaria, angioedema, and anaphylaxis are needed before more complete practice parameters can evolve.

References

1. Collins-Williams C. Intolerance to additives. *Ann Allergy* 1983; 51(2 Pt. 2):315–316.
2. Marmion DM. *Handbook of U.S. Colorants*. Wiley-Interscience, 1991; p. 573.
3. Chung K, Baker JR, Baldwin JL, Chou A. Identification of carmine allergens among three carmine allergy patients. *Allergy* 2001; 56(1):73–77.
4. Revan VB, Gold B, Baldwin JL. Annatto experience with skin testing at a university allergy clinic. Presented at American College Allergy, Asthma, and Immunology Annual Meeting, Abstract P-70, November 2001.
5. Prenner BM, Stevens JJ. Anaphylaxis after ingestion of sodium bisulfite. *Ann Allergy* 1976; 37(3):180–182.
6. Yang WH, Purchase EC, Rivington RN. Positive skin tests and Prausnitz–Küstner reactions in metabisulfite-sensitive subjects. *J Allergy Clin Immunol* 1986; 78(3 Pt. 1):443–449.
7. Nagel JE, Fuscaldo JT, Fireman P. Paraben allergy. *J Am Med Assoc* 1977; 237(15):1594–1595.
8. Aldrete JA. Allergy to local anesthetics. *J Am Med Assoc* 1969; 209(1):113.
9. Michils A, Vandermoten G, Duchateau J, Yernault JC. Anaphylaxis with sodium benzoate. *Lancet* 1991; 337(8754): 1424–1425.
10. Warrington RJ, Sauder PJ, McPhillips S. Cell-mediated immune responses to artificial food additives in chronic urticaria. *Clin Allergy* 1986; 16(6):527–533.
11. Valverde E, Vich JM, García-Calderón JV, García-Calderón PA. In vitro stimulation of lymphocytes in patients with chronic urticaria induced by additives and food. *Clin Allergy* 1980; 10(6):691–698.
12. Juhlin L, Michaëlsson G, Zetterström O. Urticaria and asthma induced by food-and-drug additives in patients with aspirin hypersensitivity. *J Allergy Clin Immunol* 1972; 50(2):92–98.
13. Michaëlsson G, Juhlin L. Urticaria induced by preservatives and dye additives in food and drugs. *Br J Dermatol* 1973; 88(6):525–532.
14. Ros AM, Juhlin L, Michaëlsson G. A follow-up study of patients with recurrent urticaria and hypersensitivity to aspirin, benzoates and azo dyes. *Br J Dermatol* 1976; 95(1):19–24.
15. Settipane GA, Pudupakkam RK. Aspirin intolerance. III. Subtypes, familial occurrence, and cross-reactivity with tartrazine. *J Allergy Clin Immunol* 1975; 56(3):215–221.
16. Settipane GA, Chafee FH, Postman IM, et al. Significance of tartrazine sensitivity in chronic urticaria of unknown etiology. *J Allergy Clin Immunol* 1976; 57(6):541–546.
17. Stevenson DD, Simon RA, Lumry WR, Mathison DA. Adverse reactions to tartrazine. *J Allergy Clin Immunol* 1986; 78(1 Pt. 2):182–191.
18. Bakke JL, Lawrence N, Bennett J, Robinson S, Bowers CY. Late endocrine effects of administering monosodium glutamate to neonatal rats. *Neuroendocrinology* 1978; 26(4):220–228.
19. Allen DH, Van Nunen S, Loblay R, Clarke L, Swain A. Adverse reactions to foods. *Med J Aust* 1984; 141(5 Suppl.):S37–S42.
20. Casale TB, Sampson HA, Hanifin J, et al. Guide to physical urticarias. *J Allergy Clin Immunol* 1988; 82(5 Pt. 1):758–763.
21. Zimmermann RE, Czarnetzki BM. Changes in the coagulation system during pseudoallergic anaphylactoid reactions to drugs and food additives. *Int Arch Allergy Appl Immunol* 1986; 81(4):375–377.
22. Mathison D, Lumry W, Stevenson D, Curd J. Aspirin in chronic urticaria and/or angioedema. Studies of sensitivity and desensitization. *J Allergy Clin Immunol* 1982; 69:135.
23. Kumagai M, Nagano M, Suzuki H, Kawana S. Effects of stress memory by fear conditioning on nerve-mast cell circuit in skin. *J Dermatol* 2011; 38(6):553–561.
24. Malhotra SK, Mehta V. Role of stressful life events in induction or exacerbation of psoriasis and chronic urticaria. *Indian J Dermatol Venereol Leprol* 2008; 74(6):594–599.
25. FDA. (2011) *Color Additives*. US Food and Drug Administration, Center for Food Safety and Applied Nutrition. http://www.fda.gov/ForIndustry/ColorAdditives/; last accessed August 2013.
26. Murdoch RD, Pollock I, Young E, Lessof MH. Food additive-induced urticaria: studies of mediator release during provocation tests. *J R Coll Physicians Lond* 1987; 21(4):262–266.
27. Pestana S, Moreira M, Olej B. Safety of ingestion of yellow tartrazine by double-blind placebo controlled challenge in 26 atopic adults. *Allergol Immunopathol (Madr)* 2010; 38(3):142–146.
28. Clayton DE, Busse W. Anaphylaxis to wine. *Clin Allergy* 1980; 10(3):341–343.
29. Habenicht H, Preuss L, Lovell RG. Sensitivity to ingested metabisulfites: cause of bronchospasm and urticaria. *Immunol Allergy Pract* 1983; 5:243–245.
30. Belchi-Hernandez J, Florido-Lopez JF, Estrada-Rodriguez JL, Martinez-Alzamora F, Lopez-Serrano C, Ojeda-Casas JA. Sulfite-induced urticaria. *Ann Allergy* 1993; 71(3):230–232.
31. Schwartz HJ. Sensitivity to ingested metabisulfite: variations in clinical presentation. *J Allergy Clin Immunol* 1983; 71(5):487–489.
32. Schwartz HJ, Sher TH. Bisulfite sensitivity manifesting as allergy to local dental anesthesia. *J Allergy Clin Immunol* 1985; 75(4):525–527.
33. Wüthrich B, Kägi MK, Hafner J. Disulfite-induced acute intermittent urticaria with vasculitis. *Dermatology (Basel)* 1993; 187(4):290–292.
34. Sonin L, Patterson R. Metabisulfite challenge in patients with idiopathic anaphylaxis. *J Allergy Clin Immunol* 1985; 75(1 Pt. 1):67–69.
35. Meggs W, Atkins F, Wright I. Sulfite challenges in patients with systematic mastocytosis or unexplained anaphylaxis. *J Allergy Clin Immunol* 1985; 75:144.
36. Stricker WE, Anorve-Lopez E, Reed CE. Food skin testing in patients with idiopathic anaphylaxis. *J Allergy Clin Immunol* 1986; 77(3):516–519.
37. Simon R, Bosso J, Daffern R, Ward B. Prevalence of sensitivity to food/drug additives in patients with chronic idiopathic urticaria/angioedema (CIUA). *J Allergy Clin Immunol* 1998; 101:S154–S155.
38. Sokol WN, Hydick IB. Nasal congestion, urticaria, and angioedema caused by an IgE-mediated reaction to sodium metabisulfite. *Ann Allergy* 1990; 65(3):233–238.

39. García-Ortega P, Scorza E, Teniente A. Basophil activation test in the diagnosis of sulphite-induced immediate urticaria. *Clin Exp Allergy* 2010; 40(4):688; author reply 689–690.
40. Sprenger JD, Altman LC, Marshall SG, Pierson WE, Koenig JQ. Studies of neutrophil chemotactic factor of anaphylaxis in metabisulfite sensitivity. *Ann Allergy* 1989; 62(2):117–121.
41. Nettis E, Colanardi MC, Ferrannini A, Tursi A. Sodium benzoate-induced repeated episodes of acute urticaria/angio-oedema: randomized controlled trial. *Br J Dermatol* 2004; 151(4):898–902.
42. Macy E, Schatz M, Zeiger R. Methylparaben immediate hypersensitivity is a rare cause of false positive local anesthetic provocative dose testing. *J Allergy Clin Immunol* 2002; 109:S149.
43. Baad-Hansen L, Cairns B, Ernberg M, Svensson P. Effect of systemic monosodium glutamate (MSG) on headache and pericranial muscle sensitivity. *Cephalalgia* 2010; 30(1): 68–76.
44. Squire EN. Angio-oedema and monosodium glutamate. *Lancet* 1987; 1(8539):988.
45. Geha RS, Beiser A, Ren C, et al. Multicenter, double-blind, placebo-controlled, multiple-challenge evaluation of reported reactions to monosodium glutamate. *J Allergy Clin Immunol* 2000; 106(5):973–980.
46. Stritzler C, Oddo DC. Acute urticaria caused by sensitivity to saccharine. *NY State J Med* 1955; 55(23):3479.
47. Kulczycki A. Aspartame-induced urticaria. *Ann Intern Med* 1986; 104(2):207–208.
48. Geha R, Buckley CE, Greenberger P, et al. Aspartame is no more likely than placebo to cause urticaria/angioedema: results of a multicenter, randomized, double-blind, placebo-controlled, crossover study. *J Allergy Clin Immunol* 1993; 92(4):513–520.
49. Simon RA. Adverse reactions to food additives. *N Engl Reg Allergy Proc* 1986; 7(6):533–542.
50. Hawkins CA, Katelaris CH. Nitrate anaphylaxis. *Ann Allergy Asthma Immunol* 2000; 85(1):74–76.
51. Nish WA, Whisman BA, Goetz DW, Ramirez DA. Anaphylaxis to annatto dye: a case report. *Ann Allergy* 1991; 66(2):129–131.
52. 21 CFR 73.100 (d)(2).
53. 21 CFR 101.22(k)(2).
54. Acero S, Taber AI, Alvarez MJ, Garcia BE, Olaguibel JM, Moneo I. Occupational asthma and food allergy due to carmine. *Allergy* 1998; 53(9):897–901.
55. Baldwin JL, Chou AH, Solomon WR. Popsicle-induced anaphylaxis due to carmine dye allergy. *Ann Allergy Asthma Immunol* 1997; 79(5):415–419.
56. Wüthrich B, Kägi MK, Stücker W. Anaphylactic reactions to ingested carmine (E120). *Allergy* 1997; 52(11):1133–1137.
57. Greenhawt M, McMorris M, Baldwin J. Carmine hypersensitivity masquerading as azithromycin hypersensitivity. *Allergy Asthma Proc* 2009; 30(1):95–101.
58. Liippo J, Lammintausta K. Allergy to carmine red (E120) is not dependent on concurrent mite allergy. *Int Arch Allergy Immunol* 2009; 150(2):179–183.
59. Wüthrich B, Schmid-Grendelmeyer P, Lundberg M. Anaphylaxis to saffron. *Allergy* 1997; 52(4):476–477.
60. Hegde VL, Venkatesh YP. Anaphylaxis to excipient mannitol: evidence for an immunoglobulin E-mediated mechanism. *Clin Exp Allergy* 2004; 34(10):1602–1609.
61. Doeglas HM. Reactions to aspirin and food additives in patients with chronic urticaria, including the physical urticarias. *Br J Dermatol* 1975; 93(2):135–144.
62. Thune P, Granholt A. Provocation tests with antiphlogistica and food additives in recurrent urticaria. *Dermatologica* 1975; 151(6):360–367.
63. Juhlin L. Recurrent urticaria: clinical investigation of 330 patients. *Br J Dermatol* 1981; 104(4):369–381.
64. Supramaniam G, Warner JO. Artificial food additive intolerance in patients with angio-oedema and urticaria. *Lancet* 1986; 2(8512):907–909.
65. Genton C, Frei PC, Pécoud A. Value of oral provocation tests to aspirin and food additives in the routine investigation of asthma and chronic urticaria. *J Allergy Clin Immunol* 1985; 76(1):40–45.
66. Malanin G, Kalimo K. The results of skin testing with food additives and the effect of an elimination diet in chronic and recurrent urticaria and recurrent angioedema. *Clin Exp Allergy* 1989; 19(5):539–543.
67. Di Lorenzo G, Pacor ML, Mansueto P, et al. Food-additive-induced urticaria: a survey of 838 patients with recurrent chronic idiopathic urticaria. *Int Arch Allergy Immunol* 2005; 138(3):235–242.
68. Ortolani C, Pastorello E, Fontana A, et al. Chemicals and drugs as triggers of food-associated disorder. *Ann Allergy* 1988; 60(4):358–366.
69. Ortolani C, Pastorello E, Luraghi MT, Torre Della F, Bellani M, Zanussi C. Diagnosis of intolerance to food additives. *Ann Allergy* 1984; 53(6 Pt. 2):587–591.
70. Hannuksela M, Lahti A. Peroral challenge tests with food additives in urticaria and atopic dermatitis. *Int J Dermatol* 1986; 25(3):178–180.
71. Kellett J, August P, Beck MH. Double-blind challenge tests with food additives in chronic urticaria. *Br J Dermatol* 1984; 111(s26):32.
72. Volonakis M, Katsarou-Katsari A, Stratigos J. Etiologic factors in childhood chronic urticaria. *Ann Allergy* 1992; 69(1): 61–65.
73. Goodman DL, McDonnell JT, Nelson HS, Vaughan TR, Weber RW. Chronic urticaria exacerbated by the antioxidant food preservatives, butylated hydroxyanisole (BHA) and butylated hydroxytoluene (BHT). *J Allergy Clin Immunol* 1990; 86(4 Pt. 1):570–575.
74. Yamaki K, Taneda S, Yanagisawa R, Inoue K-I, Takano H, Yoshino S. Enhancement of allergic responses in vivo and in vitro by butylated hydroxytoluene. *Toxicol Appl Pharmacol* 2007; 223(2):164–172.
75. Asero R. Chronic generalized pruritus caused by nitrate intolerance. *J Allergy Clin Immunol* 1999; 104(5):1110–1111.
76. Rudzki E, Czubalski K, Grzywa Z. Detection of urticaria with food additives intolerance by means of diet. *Dermatologica* 1980; 161(1):57–62.

77. Magerl M, Pisarevskaja D, Scheufele R, Zuberbier T, Maurer M. Effects of a pseudoallergen-free diet on chronic spontaneous urticaria: a prospective trial. *Allergy* 2010; 65(1):78–83.
78. Gibson A, Clancy R. Management of chronic idiopathic urticaria by the identification and exclusion of dietary factors. *Clin Allergy* 1980; 10(6):699–704.
79. Kaplan AP. Clinical practice. Chronic urticaria and angioedema. *N Engl J Med* 2002; 346(3):175–179.
80. Zuberbier T, Bindslev-Jensen C, Canonica W, et al. EAACI/GA2LEN/EDF guideline: definition, classification and diagnosis of urticaria. *Allergy* 2006; 61(3):316–320.
81. Mathias SD, Crosby RD, Zazzali JL, Maurer M, Saini SS. Evaluating the minimally important difference of the urticaria activity score and other measures of disease activity in patients with chronic idiopathic urticaria. *Ann Allergy Asthma Immunol* 2012; 108(1):20–24.

29 Sulfites

Steve L. Taylor[1], Robert K. Bush[2], & Julie A. Nordlee[1]

[1]Food Allergy Research and Resource Program, Department of Food Science and Technology, University of Nebraska, Lincoln, NE, USA

[2]Division of Allergy, Immunology, Pulmonary, Critical Care, and Sleep Medicine, Department of Medicine, University of Wisconsin School of Medicine and Public Health, Madison, WI, USA

Key Concepts

- Sulfites are frequently used food and drug additives.
- Ingestion of sulfite residues has been documented to trigger asthmatic reactions in sensitive individuals.
- Sulfite-induced asthma occurs in less than 5% of asthmatic individuals and those with severe, persistent asthma are at greatest risk.
- The diagnosis of sulfite-induced asthma is best made by blinded oral challenge with assessment of lung function.
- Labeling regulations in the United States alert sulfite-sensitive individuals to the presence of sulfites in foods which must then be avoided.

Introduction

Sulfites or sulfiting agents include sulfur dioxide (SO_2), sulfurous acid (H_2SO_3), and any of several inorganic sulfite salts that may liberate SO_2 under their conditions of use. The inorganic sulfite salts include sodium and potassium metabisulfite ($Na_2S_2O_5$, $K_2S_2O_5$), sodium and potassium bisulfite ($NaHSO_3$, $KHSO_3$), and sodium and potassium sulfite (Na_2SO_3, K_2SO_3). Sulfites have a long history of use as food ingredients, although potassium sulfite and sulfurous acid are not permitted for use in foods in the United States [1]. Sulfites occur naturally in many foods, especially fermented foods such as wines [1]. In addition, sulfites have long been used as ingredients in pharmaceuticals [2, 3].

Over the past 30 years, questions have arisen about the safety of the continued use of sulfites in foods and drugs. These concerns were first voiced following the independent observations in 1981 by David Allen in Australia and Donald Stevenson and Ronald Simon in the United States of the role of sulfites in triggering asthmatic reactions in some sensitive individuals [4–6]. It is now apparent that sulfite sensitivity affects only a small subgroup of the asthmatic population [6–8]. But, concerns remain because sulfite-induced asthma can be severe—even life-threatening—in some sensitive individuals. Accordingly, the use of sulfites in foods and drugs has changed considerably over the years. Sulfites have been replaced in some products, levels have been reduced in others, and the search for effective alternatives continues. Federal regulations have restricted the use of sulfites in certain food products in the United States.

Clinical manifestations of sulfite sensitivity

A host of adverse reactions have been attributed to sulfiting agents, including asthma, anaphylaxis, urticaria, diarrhea, abdominal pain and cramping, nausea and vomiting, pruritis, localized angioedema, difficulty in swallowing, faintness, headache, chest pain, loss of consciousness, "change in body temperature," "change in heart rate," and nonspecific rashes. With the notable exception of the role of sulfites in asthma, the causative role for sulfites in these conditions has not been fully confirmed. For normal individuals, exposure to sulfiting agents appears to pose little risk. Toxicity studies in normal volunteers showed that ingestion of 400 mg of sulfite daily for 25 days had no adverse effect [9].

Nonasthmatic responses on oral exposure to sulfites

Various authors have suggested adverse reactions involving several organ systems following oral exposure to

Food Allergy: Adverse Reactions to Foods and Food Additives, Fifth Edition. Edited by Dean D Metcalfe, Hugh A Sampson, Ronald A Simon and Gideon Lack.

sulfites, but for the most part these effects have not been substantiated by double-blind, placebo-controlled (DBPC) provocation studies. In a preliminary report, Flaherty et al. [10] presented a patient who appeared to have hepatotoxicity as manifested by changes in liver function tests following challenge with potassium metabisulfite. Meggs et al. [11] failed to demonstrate any role for sulfites among eight individuals with systemic mastocytosis. Schwartz [12] described two nonasthmatic subjects who developed abdominal distress and hypotension associated with oral challenge with potassium metabisulfite. Placebo-controlled challenges proved negative, however.

Sulfites have also been implicated as possible causative factors in persistent rhinitis [13]. The role of sulfites was evaluated in a group of 226 patients with persistent rhinitis using DBPC challenges after 1 month on an additive-free diet. Challenges with up to 20 mg of sodium metabisulfite elicited both objective (sneezing, rhinorrhea) and subject (nasal blockage and itching) symptoms in six of 20 individuals who reported improvement in rhinitis on the additive-free diet [13]. A reduction of ≥20% in nasal peak inspiratory flow rate was also observed in these six subjects [13].

Cutaneous adverse reactions suggestive of hypersensitivity responses have been observed but confirmed by challenge in only a few isolated individual cases. Epstein [14] described a patient who developed contact sensitivity, as confirmed by appropriate patch testing, through exposure to sulfiting agents used in a restaurant. Subsequently, several other cases of occupational contact sensitivity of sulfites have been described [15, 16]. The ingestion of sulfites has been reported to elicit urticaria in a very few cases as confirmed by DBPC challenges [17], single-blind challenges [18, 19], or open challenges [20]; in other cases, urticarial responses were not confirmed by oral challenge [21]. Angioedema attributable to the ingestion of sulfiting agents was reported in two of these patients but only urticaria was confirmed by open challenge with potassium metabisulfite [20]. Wuthrich [18] conducted single-blind, placebo-controlled challenges with sodium bisulfite in 245 patients with suspected sulfite sensitivity. Fifty-seven (15%) of the challenges were positive, including 17 patients with urticaria/angioedema, seven patients with rhinitis, and five patients with local anesthetic reactions. Wuthrich et al. [19] reported a case of acute intermittent urticaria with an associated vasculitis due to sulfites based on a placebo-controlled, single-blind challenge. Huang and Fraser [22] presented an individual who developed palmar and plantar pruritis, generalized urticaria, laryngeal edema, and severe abdominal pain with fulminant diarrhea after ingesting sulfiting agents. In a controlled challenge with a local anesthetic containing 0.9 μg of sodium metabisulfite, the patient experienced palmar pruritis but no generalized urticaria. Yao and Bloomberg [23] identified a single patient with urticaria occurring a few hours after oral challenge with a cumulative dose of 390 mg of sodium metabisulfite. Sulfites have also been occasionally implicated in exacerbation of chronic urticaria with the largest trial involving 36 subjects [24]. However, studies of chronic urticaria are often complicated by the underlying condition and breakthrough urticaria occurring if medications are withheld during challenges. The toxicological mechanism involved in these cutaneous reactions has not been elucidated.

Anaphylaxis-like events have been described in several individuals, although appropriate confirmatory testing was only performed in some instances. Prenner and Stevens [25] described a nonasthmatic individual who developed urticaria, pruritis, and angioedema after eating sulfited foods in a restaurant. A single-blind challenge with no placebo controls was conducted with sodium metabisulfite. Some of the symptoms (nausea, coughing, erythema of the patient's skin) were reproduced by this challenge. Clayton and Busse [26] reported a patient who developed anaphylaxis after ingesting wine. An open challenge with wine reproduced the patient's symptoms of urticaria, angioedema, and hypotension. While this patient represents a possible case of sulfite sensitivity, specific testing with sulfites was not conducted, nor was any association with sulfiting agents in wine recognized at that time.

Sokol and Hydick [27] identified a single case of sulfite-induced anaphylaxis presenting with urticaria, angioedema, nasal congestion, and nasal polyp swelling that was later confirmed by multiple, single-blind, placebo-controlled oral challenge trials. The patient, who had a history of similar food-related reactions, also produced a positive skin test to sulfite, and histamine could be released from her basophils following incubation with sulfites. Yang et al. [28] described three patients with systemic anaphylactic symptoms (rhinorrhea with asthma in one, urticaria with asthma in the second, asthma only in the third) confirmed by sulfite challenge. These three patients had positive skin tests to sulfites, and two of the three had positive Prausnitz-Küstner (PK) tests. One individual subsequently died, allegedly after ingestion of sulfited food.

Studies have been undertaken to determine whether sulfiting agent sensitivity frequently causes idiopathic anaphylaxis or chronic idiopathic urticaria [11, 29–31]. Sonin and Patterson [29] conducted sodium metabisulfite challenges on 12 individuals with idiopathic anaphylaxis, nine of whom reported episodes associated with restaurant meals. None of the patients responded to the challenge. One additional patient with CIU and restaurant-associated symptoms was also challenged; this individual also failed to react to the challenge. Meggs et al. [11] studied 25 patients with idiopathic anaphylaxis. Two of the individuals reacted on single-blind challenge; after repeating the sulfite and placebo challenge, one of these patients was subsequently found not to be sulfite sensitive. Another individual appeared to react on repeated challenge and not to placebo. However, institution of a sulfite-free diet had no effect on this patient's subsequent episodes. In a preliminary report on 65 adults with CIU, none reacted to sulfites when appropriately challenged [30]. Using a rigorous blinded, placebo-controlled trial and objective criteria for positive reactions, Simon [31] was unable to demonstrate positive reaction to encapsulated metabisulfite (200 mg maximum dose) in 75 patients with chronic urticaria and/or anaphylaxis with a history suggestive of sulfite sensitivity.

Thus, although many adverse reactions have been ascribed to sulfiting agents, the risk appears to be rather low for the nonasthmatic subject. Properly performed DBPC challenges are necessary to confirm whether sulfite sensitivity was responsible for suspected adverse reactions.

Adverse reactions to sulfites from exposures via other routes

In addition, systemic adverse reactions have been attributed to intravenous, inhalation, and other routes of administration of sulfiting agents contained in pharmaceutical products. While receiving bronchodilator therapy with isoetharine, an asthmatic subject developed acute respiratory failure that required mechanical ventilation [32]. The patient subsequently experienced erythematous flushing with urticaria upon IV administration of metaclopramide that contained a sulfiting agent. In placebo-controlled oral provocation with sodium metabisulfite, this patient developed flushing without urticaria, as well as a significant decrease in pulmonary function. Jamieson et al. [33] performed inhalation challenge in a patient with presumed sulfite sensitivity. This individual experienced intense pruritis, tingling of the mouth, nausea, chest tightness, and a feeling of impending doom. No placebo challenge was undertaken, however. Cutaneous exposure to sulfites can, on rare occasions, apparently elicit contact sensitivity reactions [14–16]. Schmidt et al. [34] posited that sulfiting agents may have caused the appearance of a cardiac arrhythmia in a patient given intravenous dexamethasone. This relationship was never confirmed by appropriate challenge, however. Hallaby and Mattocks [35] attributed central nervous system toxicity to the absorption of sodium bisulfite from peritoneal dialysis solutions. Wang et al. [36] described eight patients who developed chronic neurological defects after receiving an epidural anesthetic agent that contained sodium bisulfite as a preservative. Using an animal model, they demonstrated that the sulfiting agent produced a similar defect. Whether the clinical manifestation in humans was directly attributable to the sodium bisulfite is unknown.

Asthmatic responses on exposure to sulfites through foods and drugs

Although sulfiting agents play a very limited and somewhat controversial role in the causation of nonasthmatic adverse reactions, their role in the causation of bronchospasm and severe asthma is better established. Kochen [37] was among the first to suggest that ingestion of sulfited food can cause bronchospasm. He described a child with mild asthma who repeatedly experienced coughing, shortness of breath, and wheezing when exposed to dehydrated fruits treated with sulfur dioxide that were packaged in hermetically sealed plastic bags. No direct challenge studies were conducted to confirm this observation, however. Single-dose, open challenges without placebo control performed in a group of asthmatics by Freedman [38, 39] suggested that sulfiting agents could trigger asthma. Eight of 14 subjects with a history of wheezing following consumption of sulfited orange drinks were shown to experience changes in pulmonary function upon administration of an acidic solution containing 100 ppm (100 mg/l) of sodium metabisulfite.

The role of sulfite sensitivity in asthma became more widely recognized after reports of Stevenson and Simon [5] and Baker et al. [4]. The initial studies of Stevenson and Simon [5] demonstrated that placebo-controlled oral challenges with potassium metabisulfite could produce significant changes in pulmonary function in certain asthmatics. Their first subjects had severe, persistent asthma. In addition to their asthmatic response, these individuals experienced flushing, tingling, and faintness following sulfite challenges. Baker et al. [4] showed that oral ingestion and intravenous administration of sulfites could cause significant bronchoconstriction to the point of respiratory arrest in two individuals with severe, persistent asthma.

Exposure to sulfiting agents may occur through ingestion and other routes. Sulfur dioxide generated from sulfited foods and drugs may be inhaled. Werth [40] described an asthmatic individual who developed wheezing, flushing, and diaphoresis upon inhaling the vapors released from a bag of dried apricots. The patient did not respond to ingested metabisulfite in capsule form, but reacted to inhalation of nebulized metabisulfite in distilled water. Reports have described several patients who suffered paradoxical responses to the inhalation of bronchodilator solutions. Koepke et al. [41, 42] demonstrated that sodium bisulfite used as a preservative in bronchodilator solutions was capable of producing bronchoconstriction. Other studies from this group [43] confirmed that the concentration of metabisulfite contained in bronchodilator solutions could potentially generate 0.8–1.2 ppm of sulfur dioxide. Four of 10 subjects who tested negative to a capsule challenge with metabisulfite reacted upon inhalation, whereas 10 nonasthmatic controls did not respond.

In addition to sulfiting agents administered intravenously, orally, or via inhalation, patients may respond to the topical application of sulfiting agents. Schwartz and Sher [44] reported an individual who experienced a 25% decrease in FEV_1 after application of one drop of a 0.75 mg/ml potassium metabisulfite solution to the eye. This patient had previously experienced episodes of bronchoconstriction from the use of eye drops containing sulfite preservatives for the treatment of glaucoma.

Asthmatic subjects may develop bronchoconstriction in response to a wide variety of stimuli. Interestingly, a patient has been described [45] who failed to respond to typical triggers of bronchoconstriction, including inhalation of methacholine and cold air hyperventilation, but who nevertheless experienced increased airway resistance and decreased specific airway conductance following oral challenge with potassium metabisulfite. The significance of this response remains unknown, as no changes in other parameters of pulmonary function, including FEV_1, were observed.

The potential for fatal reactions from sulfite exposure has been confirmed [28, 46]. In many instances, individuals who supposedly died from an adverse reactions to sulfite had not undergone appropriate diagnostic challenges. Nonetheless, competent investigators observed that severe bronchoconstriction, hypotension, and loss of consciousness can occur, demonstrating the potential for fatal reactions in some subjects—particularly those with severe, persistent asthma.

Prevalence

Adult populations

The prevalence of adverse reactions to sulfiting agents is not precisely known. Although attempts have been made to establish the prevalence of sulfite sensitivity in asthmatic subjects, the nature of the population studied and use of several different challenge methods in these studies has resulted in some uncertainty regarding the prevalence estimates. Current estimates range from 3% to 10% of asthmatics [7]. Simon et al. [47] examined the prevalence of sensitivity to ingested metabisulfite in a group of 61 adult asthmatics. None indicated a history of sulfite sensitivity. After challenges were conducted with potassium metabisulfite capsules and solutions, a placebo-controlled challenge was used to confirm positive responses. Five of 61 patients (8.2%) experienced a 25% or greater decline in FEV_1 upon challenge.

Koepke and Selner [48] conducted open challenges with sodium metabisulfite in 15 adults with a history of asthma after ingestion of sulfited foods and beverages. One of 15 patients (7%) showed a 28% decline in FEV_1; no confirmatory challenge was conducted. In a larger study by Buckley et al. [49], 134 patients underwent single-blind challenges with potassium metabisulfite capsules. Of these subjects, 4.6% were suspected of having sulfite sensitivity. In these three studies, the population consisted of a large proportion of severe, persistent asthma patients requiring oral steroids for therapy and who were being treated at major referral centers, although sulfite sensitivity was diagnosed in several mild asthmatics as well [6]. Thus, the prevalence estimated from these studies may not be applicable to the asthma population as a whole. Wuthrich [18] challenged 87 suspected, sulfite-sensitive asthmatics (SSAs) with capsules containing sodium bisulfite (5–200 mg doses). Fifteen of 87 asthmatics (17.2%) reacted to these sulfite challenges, but the proportion of patients with severe, persistent asthma in this study population was not determined. Because subjects were selected for suspected sulfite sensitivity, the results of this study cannot be used to assess the prevalence of sulfite sensitivity in the overall population of asthmatics.

In the largest study conducted to date, Bush et al. [7] conducted capsule and neutral solution sulfite challenges in 203 adult asthmatics. None was selected based on a history of sulfite sensitivity. Of these patients, 120 were not receiving oral corticosteroids, while 83 were. Of the patients not receiving oral steroids, only one experienced a 20% or greater decline in FEV_1 after single-blind and confirmatory double-blind challenge. The patients receiving oral steroids had a higher response rate, estimated at approximately 8.4%. The prevalence in the asthmatic population as a whole was less than 3.9%, with patients with severe, persistent asthma appearing to face the greatest risk.

Pediatric population

Limited studies have been conducted in children. Towns and Mellis [50] evaluated 29 children, aged 5.5–14 years, with moderate to severe asthma. Seven subjects had a history suggestive of sulfite sensitivity. Challenges were conducted with placebo on one day and with sequential administration of sodium metabisulfite in capsule and solution form on a second day. Nineteen of 29 subjects showed a decrease in the peak expiratory flow rate varying from 23% to 72%, while peak expiratory flow rates with placebo were either unaffected or dropped 19%. When a 20% decline in peak expiratory flow rate was viewed as a positive response, 66% of these children were considered to be sulfite sensitive. Subsequently, the patients were instructed to avoid sulfited food for 3 months. No overall significant improvement appeared in the patients' asthma as a result of this avoidance diet.

Friedman and Easton [51] studied 51 children, aged 5–17 years. Eighteen of 51 (36%) showed a 20% or greater decrease in FEV_1 when provoked with potassium metabisulfite in an acidic solution, although placebo challenges in these individuals showed only one responder. The severity of asthma was not apparently correlated with the likelihood of a positive sulfite challenge. Steinman et al. [52] evaluated 37 asthmatic children and determined that eight (22%) responded to double-blind challenges of sulfited apple juice with a 20% or greater decline in FEV_1. An additional eight children were considered to experience a reaction to sulfite when the criterion for a positive reaction was changed to a 10% or greater decrease in FEV_1. In contrast, a study by Boner et al. [53] determined that only four of 56 asthmatic children (7%) responded to single-blind challenges with sulfite in capsules and/or solutions. Furthermore, the sulfite-sensitive individuals displayed no additional change in bronchial reactivity as assessed by methacholine challenges conducted after sulfite reactions. In this study, a positive response was defined as a 20% decline in FEV_1.

Whether sulfite sensitivity really occurs more frequently in children has yet to be definitively established. Differences in challenge procedures (capsule vs. acidic beverage solutions) may account for the apparent observation of a higher prevalence in asthmatic children. Nonetheless, the overall prevalence of sulfite sensitivity—particularly in adult asthmatics—is small but significant. Severe, persistent asthmatics, particularly adult asthmatics, appear to be at greatest risk.

Mechanisms

The mechanisms of sulfite sensitivity remain unknown. Depending upon the route of exposure, a number of possible mechanisms have been hypothesized. Asthmatics are known to respond with significant bronchoconstriction upon inhalation of less than 1 ppm of sulfur dioxide [54]. Fine and coworkers [55] demonstrated that bronchoconstriction developed in asthmatics who inhaled sulfur dioxide and bisulfite (HSO_3^-), but not sulfite ($SO_3^=$). Alteration of airway pH itself did not cause bronchoconstriction. Thus, asthmatics may respond differently to various ionic forms of sulfite that are dependent upon pH. Some asthmatics also respond to either oral or inhalation challenge with sulfite, although inhalation appears more apt to produce a bronchoconstrictive response [56]. However, the inhalation of sulfur dioxide or various sulfites may not be the total explanation. Field et al. [57] challenged 15 individuals with increasing concentrations of SO_2 gas or a metabisulfite solution. All 15 subjects reacted to the metabisulfite solution, and 14 of the 15 reacted to inhaled SO_2 with a 20% or greater drop in FEV_1. These investigators concluded that the generation of SO_2 gas cannot fully explain sulfite-induced asthma [57].

Considerable variability has been noted in the response to capsule and acidic beverage challenges with sulfiting agents [58]. When challenged on repeated occasions, the same group of individuals may not consistently experience bronchoconstriction. This variability may provide some clues to understanding of the mechanism of sulfite-induced asthma.

Inhalation during swallowing

In a study of 10 SSA subjects, Delohery et al. [59] demonstrated that all of the subjects reacted to an acidic metabisulfite solution when it was administered as a mouthwash or swallowed. However, none of these subjects reacted when the metabisulfite was instilled through a nasogastric tube. These same individuals did not respond with changes in pulmonary function when they held their breath while swallowing the solution. A control group of 10 non-SSAs showed no response to the mouthwash or swallowing challenge. Delohery et al. [59] hypothesized that some individuals respond to these forms of challenge because they inhale sulfur dioxide during the swallowing process.

Linkage with airway hyperreactivity

Because asthmatics respond to various stimuli (airway irritants) at concentrations lower than normal individuals (i.e., they exhibit airway hyperresponsiveness), attempts have been made to link sulfite sensitivity with airway responsiveness to histamine and methacholine. Such an association has not been established [59, 60]. For example, Australian investigators [57] were unable to demonstrate a relationship between the degree of airway responsiveness to inhaled histamine and the presence of sulfite sensitivity.

In human studies, attempts to block the effect of metabisulfite by agents such as inhaled lysine aspirin, inhaled indomethacin, and inhaled sodium salicylate demonstrated a slight protective effect suggesting a possible role of prostaglandins in the mechanism of sulfite sensitivity [61]. Further, leukotriene receptor antagonists attenuate SO_2-induced bronchoconstriction, implying that leukotriene release may also be involved [62]. Administration of the neutral endopeptidase inhibitor, thiorphan, was shown to enhance the airway response to inhaled sodium metabisulfite challenge in normal individuals [63]. This study suggests that tachykinins may play a role in metabisulfite-induced bronchoconstriction [63]. This mechanism was also supported by observations in guinea pigs that capsaicin-sensitive sensory nerves are involved in sulfite-induced bronchoconstriction [64]. Inhaled magnesium sulfate also has been shown to mildly inhibit inhaled metabisulfite-induced bronchoconstriction, but the mechanism is not known [65].

Refractoriness has been demonstrated to a number of indirect bronchoconstrictor stimuli including metabisulfite. The generation of nitric oxide as a possible explanation for the refractoriness has been investigated in asthmatic subjects undergoing inhaled metabisulfite challenge [66]. Blockage of nitric oxide (NO) had no effect either on the response to metabisulfite per se or the refractory process suggesting that NO is not involved in metabisulfite-induced bronchoconstriction.

Other animal models demonstrated that application of sodium metabisulfite to trachea of anesthetized sheep increased local blood flow and vascular permeability and induced epithelial damage [67]. Sulfite-induced bronchoconstriction in sheep may also involve stimulation of bradykinin B_2 receptors which may subsequently activate cholinergic reflex mechanisms [68].

Our group attempted to induce sulfite sensitivity in a group of 16 asthmatic subjects (unpublished). After the provocative dose of methacholine producing a 20% decrease in FEV_1 was established, a sulfite challenge using an acidic sulfite solution was instigated to identify any sulfite sensitivity. Three of the 16 subjects reacted to the sulfiting agent with a 20% or greater decrease in FEV_1. One week after this challenge, the patients underwent bronchial challenge with an antigen to which they exhibited sensitivity. The following day, the patients returned for a repeat methacholine challenge, followed by a second sulfite challenge 24 hours later. After the antigen challenge, only one additional subject showed a response to sulfiting agent that had not been present before antigen challenge. No significant increase was observed in airway response to methacholine. Thus, this study did not link airway hyperreactivity and sulfite sensitivity. Similar negative results were obtained in a study of asthmatic children [60].

Cholinergic reflux

Because sulfur dioxide may produce bronchoconstriction through cholinergic reflex mechanisms, preliminary studies have examined the effect of atropine and other anticholinergic agents [69]. Inhalation of atropine blocked the airway response to sulfiting agents in three of five subjects and partially inhibited the response in the other two subjects. Doxepin, which possesses both anticholinergic and antihistaminic properties, had protective effects in three of five individuals. In a study on sheep, inhaled metabisulfite induced bronchoconstriction that could be prevented by pretreatment with either ipratropium bromide or nedocromil sodium, but not by chlorpheniramine [68]. Sulfite-induced bronchoconstriction in these sheep was also associated with a ninefold increase in immunoreactive kinins. Consequently, Mansour et al. [68] concluded that sulfite-induced bronchoconstriction in sheep involves stimulation of bradykinin B_2 receptors with subsequent activation of cholinergic mechanisms. Studies in guinea pigs suggest that capsaicin-sensitive sensory nerves may play a role in sulfite-induced bronchoconstriction [64].

Possible IgE-mediated reactions

Adverse reactions to sulfites appear most commonly in atopic individuals, and studies have attempted to identify an immunologic basis for these reactions. Several reports have demonstrated positive skin tests to solutions of sulfiting agents in some sensitive patients. The positive skin tests and other related evidence may point to the existence of an IgE-mediated mechanism in at least some sulfite-sensitive individuals.

Prenner and Stevens [25] observed a positive scratch skin test to an aqueous solution of sodium bisulfite at 10 mg/ml in a patient. This patient also exhibited a dramatic response to intradermal testing at the same concentration. Three nonsensitive control subjects had negative skin tests. The patient of Twarog and Leung [32] also showed a positive intradermal skin test response to an aqueous solution of bisulfite at 0.1 mg/ml whereas controls were negative with concentrations up to 1 mg/ml of the solution. Yang et al. [28] also identified several asthmatic subjects with either positive prick or intradermal skin test to sulfites. Boxer et al. [70] identified two additional cases with positive skin tests who also had positive oral challenges to sulfiting agents. Selner et al. [71] reported positive intradermal and skin prick tests with 0.1 mg/ml and 10 mg/ml potassium metabisulfite solutions, respectively, in an SSA subject. This patient also had a positive intradermal test with a 0.1 mg/ml solution of acetaldehyde hydroxysulfonate, a major bound form of sulfite in wine and other foods [71]. Control subjects had negative skin tests.

Further evidence for an IgE mechanism can be found in positive passive transfer tests (PK transfer). Several investigators have successfully transferred skin test reactivity to nonsensitized subjects with sera from sulfite-sensitive individuals [25, 28, 72]. The effect can be abolished by heating sera to 56°C for 30 minutes [71]. These observations suggest the presence of a serum factor (IgE). However, specific IgE antibodies to sulfiting agents have not been demonstrated [70, 72].

In vitro activation of basophils by metabisulfites has been reported [73]. Sulfiting agents can induce mediator release from human MCs and basophils obtained from some sensitive individuals. Histamine release has been demonstrated in mixed peripheral blood leukocyte studies in sulfite-sensitive individuals [27, 32]. Similarly, Meggs et al. [11] noted a significant rise in plasma histamine levels in two of seven subjects with systemic mastocytosis undergoing a sulfite challenge. No clinical response was observed in these patients, however. In a skin-test-positive individual, sulfite exposure resulted in increased histamine levels in nasal lavage fluid 7.5 minutes after challenge [74]. Similar results were obtained in chronic rhinitis control subjects, although the histamine levels generally fell below those found in patients with sulfite sensitivity [74]. In contrast, other investigators have not been successful or noted inconsistent results in attempting to demonstrate histamine release from the MCs or basophils among sulfite-sensitive individuals [5, 12, 74, 75]. Histamine, per se, may not play a significant role in sulfite-induced airflow obstruction since H_1 receptor antagonists fail to block the response [62].

Indirect evidence for the role of MC mediators in the production of bronchoconstriction due to sulfiting agents has also been found. Freedman [39] mentions that inhaled sodium cromolyn prevented the asthmatic response. In preliminary studies, Simon et al. [69] found that inhaled cromolyn inhibited sulfite-induced asthma in four of six subjects and partially inhibited the response in two other subjects. Schwartz [76] reported that oral cromolyn at a dose of 200 mg blocked an asthmatic response to oral sulfite challenge in a single individual.

Sulfite oxidase deficiency

Simon [75] proposed that a deficiency in sulfite oxidase, an enzyme that metabolizes sulfite to sulfate, may promote sulfite-induced adverse reactions. The skin fibroblasts of six sulfite-sensitive subjects exhibited less sulfite oxidase activity than normal controls. However, the major source of sulfite oxidase activity in humans resides in the liver. In addition, congenital sulfite oxidase deficiency in humans is not associated with asthma [77]. Further investigation will be needed to determine the importance of this suggested mechanism.

Diagnosis

The diagnosis of sulfite sensitivity cannot be established by the patient's history alone. Our group [7] was unable to correlate the presence of a positive sulfite challenge with the patient's history, and vice versa. The diagnosis of sulfite sensitivity should, therefore, be made only in individuals who demonstrate an objective response upon appropriate challenge.

Skin testing—by both prick and scratch methods—has identified some individuals with positive responses [28, 70]. Basophil activation tests may eventually prove useful [73]. In contrast, some individuals who have equally severe bronchospasm or other reactions had negative skin tests.

Diagnostic challenges

Because diagnostic challenges represent the only effective confirmatory technique, and because such challenges may pose significant risk to sensitive subjects, patients must be informed of the risks involved. Physicians instituting such provocation procedures should have available all equipment necessary for the treatment of severe bronchospasm or anaphylaxis, including airway intubation and mechanical ventilation. The end point for objective assessment of reactivity should be ascertained before the challenge begins. Such measures might include changes in airway function in asthmatics or the appearance of urticaria in patients with this type of response. Patients may be challenged with capsules, neutral solutions, or acidic solutions of metabisulfite. Some protocols previously reported in the literature are shown in Tables 29.1 and 29.2 [78].

Table 29.1 Capsule and neutral-solution metabisulfite challenge[a].

Preparing the patient and collecting preliminary data

- Withhold short-acting aerosol sympathomimetics and cromolyn/nedocromil sodium for 8 h and short-acting antihistamines for 24–48 h before pulmonary function testing.
- Measure pulmonary function: forced expiratory volume in 1 s (FEV_1) must be greater than or equal to 70% of predicted normal value and greater than or equal to 1.5 l in adults. (Test contraindicated in patients with an FEV_1 below those levels. Standards for children have not been defined).

Performing the single-blind challenge

- Administer placebo (powdered sucrose) in capsule form. Measure FEV_1.
- Administer capsules containing 1, 5, 25, 50, 100, and 200 mg of potassium metabisulfite at 30-min intervals. Measure FEV_1 30 minutes after administering each dose and if the patient becomes symptomatic.
- If no response, administer 1, 10, and 25 mg of potassium metabisulfite in water–sucrose solution at 30-min intervals. Measure FEV_1 30 min after each dose and if symptoms occur. Positive response is indicated by a decrease in FEV_1 of 20% or more.

Performing the double-blind challenge

- Perform challenge and placebo procedures on separate days, in random order.
- Placebo day: administer only sucrose in capsules and solution. Measure FEV_1 30 min after each dose and if patient becomes symptomatic.
- Challenge day: same protocol as single-blind challenge day.

Source: From Reference 78.
[a]Protocol used in the University of Wisconsin prevalence study [7]. Perform this test only where the capability for managing severe asthmatic reactions exists. Stop challenge sequence after a positive response is obtained.

Table 29.2 Acid-solution metabisulfite challenge[a].

Preparing the patient and collecting preliminary data

- Withhold aerosol sympathomimetics and cromolyn sodium for 8 h and antihistamines for 24–48 h before pulmonary function testing
- Measure pulmonary function: forced expiratory volume in 1 s (FEV_1) must be greater than or equal to 70% of predicted normal value, and greater than or equal to 1.5 l in adults. (Test contraindicated in patients with an FEV_1 below those levels. Standards for children have not been defined).

Performing the bisulfite challenge

- Dissolve 0.1 mg of potassium metabisulfite in 20 ml of a sulfite-free lemonade crystal solution. Have the patient swish the solution around for 10–15 s, then swallow.
- Measure FEV_1 10 minutes after the first dose. Then, administer 0.5, 1, 5, 10, 15, 25, 50, 75, 100, 150[b], and 200[b] mg per 20 ml of the solution at 10-min intervals. Measure FEV_1 10 min after each incremental increase in dose. Positive response is signified by a decrease in FEV_1 of 20% or more.

Source: From Reference 78.

[a]Protocol investigated by the Bronchoprovocation Committee-American Academy of Allergy, Asthma and Immunology. Perform this test only where the capability for managing severe asthmatic reactions exists. Stop challenge sequence after a positive response [78].

[b]Doses in excess of 100 mg are likely to produce nonspecific bronchial reactions in asthmatics due to the high levels of free SO_2 that are generated.

Currently, a capsule challenge is the preferred option as most sulfite exposure is likely to involve bound forms of sulfites in foods rather than solutions.

When conducting challenges in a single-blind fashion, positive results should be confirmed via a double-blind procedure. Moreover, if a placebo day and an active challenge day are conducted on two separate occasions, the possibility of order effects on the results must be considered. For example, if a patient receives placebo on the first day and experiences no response, he or she may experience a reaction on the subsequent challenge day regardless of whether placebo or active challenge with sulfite is administered, because of increased anxiety. To overcome this possibility, the order of administration of active and placebo challenges should be randomized and a third challenge day, either active or placebo, potentially instituted.

Treatment

Avoidance of sulfited foods and drugs

Sulfite-sensitive individuals should avoid sulfite-treated foods [79, 80] and drugs [78, 81] that have been shown to trigger the response. Because individuals may vary in their sensitivity to sulfited foods, it may be necessary to perform challenges with foods containing sulfites to determine which ones the patient can tolerate.

Some bronchodilator solutions, subcutaneous lidocaine, intravenous corticosteroids, and intravenous metaclopramide may pose a risk for sensitive subjects. Many pharmaceutical companies are aware of this possibility, however, and are taking steps to eliminate sulfiting agents from their products. A partial list of sulfited medications appears in Table 29.3. Package inserts for suspect medications should be consulted for the latest information.

Table 29.3 Some antiasthma preparations containing sulfites.

Epinephrine	Adrenalin, Monarch TwinJect™, versus Pharmaceuticals Epi-Pen™, Dey Laboratories Multiple manufacturers
Isoproterenol solutions	Isuprel™, Sanofi-Winthrop Isoproterenol, Elkins-Sinn
Injectable Corticosteroid	Decadron™, Merck Dexamethasone, multiple manufacturers

Use of injectable epinephrine

Although some forms of epinephrine contain sulfite used as a preservative, administration of this drug has not been shown to cause a reaction in sulfite-sensitive individuals. Apparently, epinephrine's action overcomes any adverse effects attributable to the preservative. Thus, patients who are inadvertently exposed to sulfites typically find self-administration of epinephrine useful. Self-injection with an automatic dispenser of epinephrine, delivering 0.3 ml of a 1:1000 solution (0.3 mg) for adults, is available (Epi-Pen, Dey Inc., Napa, CA). A similar device available for children delivers 0.15 ml of a 1:1000 solution of epinephrine.

Use of blocking agents

Limited studies have been conducted with a variety of agents that may block the responses to sulfite, including cromolyn sodium, atropine, doxepin, vitamin B_{12}, inhaled furosemide and leukotriene receptor antagonists [8, 69, 82]. Although these treatments have demonstrated beneficial effects in limited numbers of patients, they remain investigational and cannot be recommended for standard use.

A better understanding of the mechanisms involved in sulfite sensitivity would allow for more specific interventions to treat and perhaps prevent these reactions.

Food and drug uses

Sulfiting agents are added to many different types of foods for several distinct technical purposes (Table 29.4). The key

Table 29.4 Technical attributes of sulfites in foods.

Technical Attribute	Examples of Specific Food Applications
Inhibition of enzymatic browning	Fresh fruits and vegetables[a]
	Salads[a]
	Guacamole[a]
	Shrimp (black spot formation)
	Pre-peeled raw potatoes
Inhibition of nonenzymatic browning	Dehydrated potatoes
	Other dehydrated vegetables
	Dried fruits
Antimicrobial actions	Wines
	Corn wet milling to make cornstarch, corn syrup
Dough conditioning	Frozen pie crust
	Frozen pizza crust
Antioxidant action	No major U.S. applications
Bleaching effect	Maraschino cherries
	Hominy

[a]No longer allowed by the U.S. Food and Drug Administration.

technical attributes of sulfites in foods include the inhibition of enzymatic and nonenzymatic browning, antimicrobial actions, dough-conditioning effects, antioxidant purposes, bleaching applications, and a host of other uses characterized as processing aids [1]. Some uses of sulfites, such as their application to fresh fruits and vegetables (except potatoes) to inhibit enzymatic browning, have now been restricted by Federal regulatory actions in the United States, as will be described later in this chapter. Because of their important technical attributes, sulfites are utilized in an enormous number of specific applications in a wide variety of foods as reviewed elsewhere [1, 83].

Given the wide variety of applications for sulfites in foods, a broad range of use levels and residual sulfite concentrations can be found in foods (Table 29.5). Residual sulfite concentrations in foods can range from undetectable (less than 10 ppm) to more than 2000 ppm (mg SO_2 equivalents per kg of food). Although SSAs vary in their degree of sensitivity to ingested sulfites, all such individuals can tolerate some sulfite. Certainly, the more highly sulfited foods pose the greatest hazard to SSAs.

Sulfites are added to many pharmaceutical products [2, 3]. Table 29.3 contains a list of drugs intended for asthmatics that may contain sulfites. With the increased concern over sulfite-induced asthma, these substances have been removed from some drugs in recent years, especially from drugs intended for asthmatics. Sulfites are used in drugs intended for oral, topical, respiratory, and internal use.

Sulfites have two primary functions as drug ingredients: to prevent the oxidation of active drug ingredients and to prevent nonenzymatic browning, which involves the reactions of reducing sugars with amino acids or amines that

Table 29.5 Estimated total SO_2 level as consumed for some sulfited foods.

>100 ppm	
Dried fruit (excluding dark raisins and prunes)	
Lemon juice (nonfrozen)	
Lime juice (nonfrozen)	
Wine	
Molasses	
Sauerkraut juice	
Grape juice (white, white sparkling, pink sparkling, red sparkling)	
Pickled cocktail onions	
50–99.9 ppm	
Dried potatoes	
Wine vinegar	
Gravies, sauces	
Fruit topping	
Maraschino cherries	
10.1–49.9 ppm	
Pectin	
Shrimp (fresh)	
Corn syrup	
Sauerkraut	
Pickled peppers	
Pickles/relishes	
Corn starch	
Hominy	
Frozen potatoes	
Maple syrup	
Imported jams and jellies	
Fresh mushrooms	
<10 ppm	
Malt vinegar	Sugar (esp. beet sugar)
Dried cod	Gelatin
Canned potatoes	Coconut
Beer	Fresh fruit salad
Dry soup mix	Domestic jams and jellies
Soft drinks	Crackers
Instant tea	Cookies
Pizza dough (frozen)	Grapes
Pie dough	High fructose corn syrup

Source: Adapted from *The Reexamination of the GRAS Status of Sulfiting Agents.* Life Science Research Office, Federation of American Societies for Experimental Biology, January 1985.

can occur in enteral feeding solutions and dextrose solutions. The latter stages of the nonenzymatic browning reaction involve the condensation of quinones. Epinephrine can undergo a similar reaction that diminishes its potency. Consequently, sulfites are routinely added to epinephrine to prevent such condensation reactions.

The usage levels of sulfites in pharmaceutical products vary from 0.1% to 1%, although a few products may contain higher concentrations. Exposure to sulfites via drugs can be high but would be sporadic in most cases. The active ingredients of the drug may, in a few cases, counteract the effects of sulfite in sulfite-sensitive individuals. Until recently, sulfites were common additives in certain bronchodilators but, except in a few rare cases [41], the bronchodilating effect of the active ingredient overwhelms the bronchoconstricting effect of sulfite. As noted earlier, epinephrine easily overwhelms the bronchoconstricting effects of sulfites. Thus, sulfite-containing epinephrine should never be denied to or avoided by an SSA, because it can act as a life-saving antidote [2, 84].

Fate of sulfites in foods

SO_2 and its sulfite salts are extremely reactive in food systems. The wide range of technical attributes of sulfites in foods is a direct result of this reactivity. Thus, these substances often react with a variety of food components. A dynamic equilibrium exists between free sulfites and the many bound forms of sulfite [1]. Thus, the fate of these food additives will vary widely, depending on the nature of each individual food.

SO_2 and the sulfite salts readily dissolve in water and, depending upon the pH of the medium, can exist as sulfurous acid (H_2SO_3), bisulfite ion (HSO_3^-), or sulfite ion ($SO_3^=$) [81]. All of these forms react with a variety of food components with the extent and reversibility of these reactions relating to pH. At acidic pHs (pH of less than 4), SO_2 can be released as a gas from a sulfite-containing food or solution. Thus, sulfites can actually be lost from foods, albeit only under acidic conditions.

Sulfites react readily with food constituents including aldehydes, ketones, reducing sugars, proteins, amino acids, vitamins, nucleic acids, fatty acids, and pigments, to name but a few [1]. The extent of any reaction between sulfite and some food component is dependent on the pH, temperature, sulfite concentration, and reactive components present in the food matrix. An equilibrium always exists between free and bound sulfites, although the reversibility of the reactions varies over a wide range [1, 83]. Some reactions, such as the one between acetaldehyde and sulfite to form acetaldehyde hydroxysulfonate, are virtually irreversible. Other reactions, such as between the anthocyanin pigments of fruits and sulfite, reverse readily. The binding of sulfite by various food constituents diminishes the concentration of free sulfite in the food. While the dissociable, bound forms of sulfite can serve as reservoirs of free sulfite in the food, irreversible reactions tend to remove sulfite permanently from the pool of free sulfite. The desirable actions of sulfites in foods frequently depend on free sulfite, so the concentration of the pool of free sulfite represents a critically important factor in technical effectiveness. Therefore, treatment levels for specific food applications aim to provide an active, residual level of free sulfite throughout the shelf life of the product.

In lettuce, high concentrations of sulfite (500–1000 ppm) were once used to prevent enzymatic browning. Because lettuce consists mostly of cellulose and water, the sulfite had few components with which to react. Consequently, most of the sulfite added to lettuce lingered in the form of free inorganic sulfite [85]. Lettuce is unique in this regard, as most foods contain substances that readily react with sulfites. In most foods, therefore, the bound forms of sulfite would predominate.

A comprehensive discussion of the possible reactions between sulfites and food constituents lies beyond the scope of this chapter. An entire book has been written on the subject of the chemistry of sulfites in foods [83]. Suffice it to say that the fate of sulfites in individual food products is dynamic, extraordinarily complex, and difficult to predict with any degree of precision.

Likelihood of reactions to sulfited foods

Few trials have attempted to evaluate the sensitivity of SSAs to sulfited foods. Based on the suspected mechanisms of sulfite-induced asthma, one might predict that acidic foods and beverages capable of generating SO_2 gas would be more hazardous than other forms of sulfited foods. Clinical challenges with acidic solutions of sulfite in lemon juice or some other vehicle appear to support this conclusion [59, 84]. In all foods, the fate of sulfite may be an important determinant of the degree of hazard faced by the sulfite-sensitive consumer. Little evidence currently exists, however, regarding the hazard levels posed by the various forms of food-borne sulfite. The overall concentration of residual sulfite in the food also represents an important determinant of the likelihood of a reaction.

Clinical challenges have documented several features of sulfite-induced asthma. First, all SSAs exhibit some tolerance for ingested sulfite. The threshold levels vary from one patient to another, ranging from approximately 0.6 mg of SO_2 equivalents (1 mg of $K_2S_2O_5$) to levels greater than 120 mg of SO_2 equivalents (200 mg of $K_2S_2O_5$). Second, clinical challenges have confirmed that free, inorganic sulfite presents a hazard to SSAs. Third, more asthmatics will respond to inhalation of SO_2 or ingestion of acidic sulfite solutions than to ingestion of sulfite in capsules.

From these facts, several predictions can be made about the likelihood of reactions to sulfited foods among SSAs. First, reactions will be more likely and probably more severe to highly sulfited foods such as lettuce, dried fruit, and wines. Certainly, no evidence exists to implicate foods with low levels of residual sulfite (from less than 10 ppm to 50 ppm) in adverse reactions in sensitive individuals [86] [87]. Second, foods containing a higher proportion of free inorganic sulfite may offer greater risks than foods in which the bound forms of sulfite predominate. Sulfited lettuce is certainly the best example of a food with a high proportion of free inorganic sulfite [85]. This prediction assumes, however, that the bound forms of sulfite are less hazardous than free inorganic sulfite—an assumption that has not been clinically established. Finally, one might predict that acidic foods or beverages containing sulfites would pose greater danger than other sulfited foods. Examples of these hazardous foods would include wines, white grape juice, nonfrozen lemon and lime juices, and perhaps lettuce treated with an acidic salad freshener solution. These predictions appear to match the practical experiences of SSAs.

Few experiments have been conducted to test these predictions. Halpern et al. [87] tested 25 nonselected asthmatics with 4 oz of white wine containing 160 mg of SO_2 equivalents per liter. Because patients were not prescreened for sulfite sensitivity, the results of this clinical trial are difficult to evaluate. Only one (4%) of the 25 patients exhibited reproducible symptoms with the wine challenge, however.

Howland and Simon [88] conclusively demonstrated that sulfited lettuce can trigger asthmatic reactions in confirmed SSAs. The five patients in this trial were exposed to 3 oz of lettuce containing 500 ppm of SO_2 equivalents. All of these patients had documented reactions to sulfite ingested in capsule form. Taylor et al. [79] confirmed the reactivity of SSAs to ingestion of sulfited lettuce, including one subject who responded to only acidic solution challenges of sulfite.

In their study, Taylor et al. [79] assessed the sensitivity of eight SSAs to a variety of sulfited foods, including lettuce, shrimp, dried apricots, white grape juice, dehydrated potatoes, and mushrooms. Sulfite sensitivity was confirmed by double-blind, capsule-beverage challenges. Despite the positive double-blind challenges, four of these patients failed to respond to any of the sulfited foods or beverages. The other four patients experienced bronchoconstriction after ingesting sulfited lettuce, although this test was the only positive food challenge for the acidic beverage reactor. Curiously, this patient did not react adversely to a challenge with white grape juice, which is an acidic, sulfited beverage. Two of the remaining three patients also reacted to dried apricots and white grape juice; the third patient did not complete these challenges. Only one of the three patients reacted to challenges with dehydrated potatoes and mushrooms; in the case of dehydrated potatoes, however, her response to multiple double-blind challenges with dehydrated potatoes was not consistent. None of these patients responded to sulfited shrimp.

While these results were somewhat confusing, they illustrated that SSAs will not react equivalently to the ingestion of all sulfited foods. The likelihood of a response could not be predicted on the basis of the dose of residual SO_2 equivalents in the sulfited foods. The nature of the sulfite present in these foods varied widely. In lettuce, the sulfite level is high and free inorganic sulfite predominates [85]. In white grape juice and especially dried apricots, the sulfite level is high, the foods are acidic, and sulfite may be bound to reducing sugars [1, 79]. In dehydrated potatoes, the sulfite level is intermediate, the food is not acidic, and sulfite is typically bound to starch [1, 79]. In mushrooms, the sulfite level is low and variable, but the form of sulfite remains unknown. In shrimp, the sulfite level is intermediate, the food is not acidic, and sulfite is probably bound to protein [1, 79]. The likelihood of a reaction to a sulfited food depends on several factors: the nature of the food, the level of residual sulfite, the sensitivity of the patient, and (perhaps) the form of residual sulfite and the mechanism of sulfite-induced asthma [79].

Avoidance diets

As noted earlier, the most common treatment for individuals with sulfite-induced asthma is the avoidance of sulfite in the diet. Of course, asthmatics with a low threshold for sulfites must take greater care to avoid these substances than individuals with higher thresholds. Certainly, all SSAs should be instructed to avoid the more highly sulfited foods, which are defined as having in excess of 100 ppm of SO_2 equivalents (Table 29.5). Individuals with lower thresholds for sulfite might be advised to remove all sulfited foods from their diets, although adherence to such diets can prove difficult. Packaged foods containing more than 10 ppm residual SO_2 equivalents must declare the presence of sulfites or one of the specific sulfiting agents on their labels. Thus, sulfite-sensitive consumers should be able to avoid significantly sulfited foods by careful perusal of labels. They must also be instructed that the terms sulfur dioxide, sodium or potassium bisulfite, sodium or potassium metabisulfite, and sodium sulfite indicate the presence of sulfites or sulfiting agents. Some sulfite-sensitive individuals may know that they can safely consume certain foods declaring sulfite on the labels because the amount of available sulfite in that particular food falls below their threshold doses. Such patients should be warned that the concentration of residual sulfite in any specific food is variable and that continued consumption might occasionally elicit an adverse reaction. No absolute evidence exists to suggest that sulfite-sensitive individuals need to avoid foods having less than 10 ppm residual SO_2 equivalents.

While the avoidance of sulfited packaged foods is relatively straightforward, restaurant foods pose a more difficult challenge. The FDA has banned sulfite from fresh fruits and vegetables in restaurants, but other sulfited foods in restaurants remain unlabeled. With the banning of sulfites from salad bar items, many of the problems with sulfite-induced asthma in restaurants have disappeared. The major continuing problem is sulfited potatoes. SSAs should be instructed to avoid all potatoes products in restaurants except baked potatoes with the skins intact.

US regulatory agencies have moved to regulate certain uses of sulfites following the discovery of sulfite-sensitive asthma. The FDA initially moved to require the declaration of sulfites on the label of foods when sulfite residues exceeded 10 ppm; similar regulations were enacted with wines. The FDA then banned the use of sulfites from fresh fruits and vegetables other than potatoes. This ban affected lettuce, cut fruits, guacamole, mushrooms, and many other applications, especially the once-common practice of sulfiting fresh fruits and vegetables placed in salad bars. Potatoes remain the sole exception to the ban of sulfite use on fresh fruits and vegetables. Since the FDA has taken these regulatory actions on sulfites, the number of sulfite-induced reactions reported to the FDA has decreased. While, FDA actions have helped to protect sulfite-sensitive individuals from the hazards associated with sulfited foods, FDA has taken no action to limit the use of sulfites in drugs. However, voluntary removal of sulfites from certain drugs has occurred in some instances. Certainly, any regulation is only as effective as its enforcement, so sulfite-sensitive individuals and their physicians should remain alert to avoid inadvertent exposures from both foods and drugs.

Conclusion

Sulfite sensitivity primarily affects a relatively small subgroup of the asthmatic population. The symptoms of sulfite-induced asthma can, on occasion, prove quite severe and even life-threatening. Sulfite sensitivity should ideally be diagnosed with an oral double-blind challenge protocol. Many unknowns remain regarding sulfite-induced asthma, including the mechanism of the illness and the likelihood of reactions to specific sulfited foods. Reactions to sulfited foods certainly derive in part from the concentration of residual sulfite in the food and the degree of sensitivity exhibited by the individual patient. In addition, the form of sulfite in the food and the mechanism of the sulfite-induced reaction may affect the likelihood of a response to a specific sulfited food.

SSAs should be instructed to avoid highly sulfited foods. The FDA and other US Federal regulatory agencies have moved to protect SSAs from unlabeled uses of sulfites in foods. Nevertheless, sulfites continue to be used in many foods and drugs, and sensitive individuals must be cautious to avoid inadvertent exposures.

References

1. Taylor SL, Higley NA, Bush RK. Sulfites in Foods: Uses, Analytical Methods, Residues, Fate, Exposure Assessment, Metabolism, Toxicity, and Hypersensitivity. *Adv Food Res* 1986; 30:1–76.
2. Smolinske SC. Review of parenteral sulfite reactions. *J Toxicol Clin Toxicol* 1992; 30(4):597–606.
3. American Academy of Pediatrics Committee on Drugs. "Inactive" ingredients in pharmaceutical products: update [Subject review]. *Pediatrics* 1997; 99:268–278.
4. Baker GJ, Collett P, Allen DH. Bronchospasm induced by metabisulphite-containing foods and drugs. *Med J Aust* 1981; 2:614–617.
5. Stevenson DD, Simon RA. Sensitivity to ingested metabisulfites in asthmatic subjects. *J Allergy Clin Immunol* 1981; 68(1):26–32.
6. Simon RA. Pulmonary reactions to sulfites in foods. *Pediatr Allergy Immunol* 1992; 3(4):218–221.
7. Bush RK, Taylor SL, Holden K, et al. Prevalence of sensitivity to sulfiting agents in asthmatic patients. *Am J Med* 1986; 81:816–820.
8. Vally H, Misso NL, Madan V. Clinical effects of sulphite additives. *Clin Exp Allergy* 2009; 39:1643–1651.
9. Hotzel D, Muskat E, Bitsch I, et al. Thiamin-mangel und unbedenklichkeit von sulfit fur den menschen. *Int Z Vitaminforsch* 1969; 39:372–383.
10. Flaherty M, Stormont JM, Condemi JJ. Metabisulfite (MBS)-associated hepatotoxicity and protection by cobalbumins (B12). *J Allergy Clin Immunol* 1985; 75:198.
11. Meggs WJ, Atkins FM, Wright R, et al. Failure of sulfites to produce clinical responses in patients with systemic mastocytosis or recurrent anaphylaxis: results of a single-blind study. *J Allergy Clin Immunol* 1985; 76(6):840–846.
12. Schwartz HJ. Sensitivity to ingested metabisulfite: variations in clinical presentation. *J Allergy Clin Immunol* 1983; 71(5):487–489.
13. Pacor ML, Di Lorenzo G, Martinelli N, et al. Monosodium benzoate hypersensitivity in subjects with persistent rhinitis. *Allergy* 2004; 59:192–197.
14. Epstein E. Sodium bisulfite. *Contact Dermatitis* 1970; 7:155.
15. Kaaman AC, Boman A, Wrangsjo K, et al. Contact allergy to sodium metabisulfite: an occupational problem. *Contact Dermatitis* 2010; 63:110–112.
16. Sasseville D, El-Helou T. Occupational allergic contact dermatitis from sodium metabisulfite. *Contact Dermatitis* 2009; 61:244–245.
17. Belchi-Hernandez J, Florido-Lopez F, et al. Sulfite-induced urticaria. *Ann Allergy* 1993; 71:230–232.
18. Wüthrich B (ed.). *Sulfite Additives Causing Allergic or Pseudoallergic Reactions.* Proceedings of the XIVth International Congress of Allergology and Clinical Immunology, October 13–18, 1991, Kyoto. Seattle: Hogrefe & Huber Publishers, 1991.
19. Wüthrich B, Kägi MK, Hafner J. Disulfite-induced acute intermittent urticaria with vasculitis. *Dermatology* 1993; 187:290–292.

20. Habenicht HA, Preuss L, Lovell RG. Sensitivity to ingested metabisulfites: cause of bronchiospasm and urticaria. *Immunol Allergy Pract* 1983; 5:25–27.
21. Riggs BS, Harchelroad FP, Poole C. Allergic reaction to sulfiting agents. *Ann Emerg Med* 1986; 15(1):77–79.
22. Huang AS, Fraser WM. Are sulfite additives really safe? *N Engl J Med* 1984; 311(8):542.
23. Yao L, Bloomberg RJ. Urticaria—a rare presentation of sulfite allergy. *J Allergy Clin Immunol* 2007; 119(Suppl):S206.
24. Jiménez-Aranda GS, Flores-Sandoval G, Gómez-Vera J, et al. Prevalence of chronic urticaria following the ingestion of food additives in a third tier hospital. *Rev Alerg Mex* 1996; 43(6):152–156.
25. Prenner BM, Stevens JJ. Anaphylaxis after ingestion of sodium bisulfite. *Ann Allergy* 1976; 37:180–182.
26. Clayton DE, Busse W. Anaphylaxis to wine. *Clin Allergy* 1980; 10:341–343.
27. Sokol WN, Hydick IB. Nasal congestion, urticaria, and angioedema caused by an IgE-mediated reaction to sodium metabisulfite. *Ann Allergy* 1990; 65:233–237.
28. Yang WH, Purchase ECR, Rivington RN. Positive skin test and Prausnitz-Kuestner reactions in metabisulfite-sensitive subjects. *J Allergy Clin Immunol* 1986; 78(3):443–449.
29. Sonin L, Patterson R. Metabisulfite challenge in patients with idiopathic anaphylaxis. *J Allergy Clin Immunol* 1984; 73(1 Pt 2):136.
30. Simon RA. Additive-induced urticaria: experience with monosodium glutamate (MSG). *J Nutr* 2000; 130:1063S–1066S.
31. Simon RA. Update on sulfite sensitivity. *Allergy* 1998; 53(Suppl 46):78–79.
32. Twarog FJ, Leung DY. Anaphylaxis to a component of isoetharine (sodium bisulfite). *J Am Med Assoc* 1982; 248(16):2030–2031.
33. Jamieson DM, Guill MF, Wray BB, et al. Metabisulfite sensitivity: case report and literature review. *Ann Allergy* 1985; 54:115–121.
34. Schmidt GB, Meier MA, Saldove MS. Sudden appearance of cardiac arrhythmias after dexamethasone. *J Am Med Assoc* 1972; 221:1402–1404.
35. Hallaby SF, Mattocks AM. Absorption of sodium bisulfite from peritoneal dialysis solutions. *J Pharm Sci* 1965; 54:52–55.
36. Wang BC, Hillman DE, Spielholz NI, et al. Chronic neurological deficits and Nescaine-CE—an effect of the anesthetic, 2-chloroprocaine, or the antioxidant, sodium bisulfite? *Anesth Analg* 1984; 63:445–447.
37. Kochen J. Sulfur dioxide, a respiratory tract irritant, even if ingested. *Pediatrics* 1973; 52:145–146.
38. Freedman BJ. Asthma induced by sulphur dioxide, benzoate and tartrazine contained in orange drinks. *Clin Allergy* 1977; 7:407–415.
39. Freedman BJ. Sulphur dioxide in foods and beverages: its use as a preservative and its effect on asthma. *Br J Dis Chest* 1980; 74:128–134.
40. Werth GR. Inhaled metabisulfite sensitivity. *J Allergy Clin Immunol* 1982; 70:143.
41. Koepke JW, Christopher KL, Chai H, et al. Dose-dependent bronchospasm from sulfites in isoetharine. *J Am Med Assoc* 1984; 251(22):2982–2983.
42. Koepke JW, Staudenmayer H, Selner JC. Inhaled metabisulfite sensitivity. *Ann Allergy* 1985; 54(3):213–215.
43. Koepke JW, Selner JC, Dunhill AL. Presence of sulfur dioxide in commonly used broncodilator solutions. *J Allergy Clin Immunol* 1983; 72:504–508.
44. Schwartz H, Sher TH. Bisulfite intolerance manifest as bronchospasm following topical dipirefrin hydrochloride therapy of glaucoma. *Arch Opthamol* 1985; 103:14–15.
45. Schwartz H, Sher TH. Metabisulfite sensitivity in a patient without hyperactive airways disease. *Immunol Allergy Prac.* 1986;8:17–20.
46. Tsevat J, Gross GN, Dowling GP. Fatal asthma after ingestion of sulfite-containing wine. *Ann Intern Med* 1987; 107(2): 263.
47. Simon RA, Green L, Stevenson DD. The incidence of ingested metabisulfite sensitivity in an asthmatic population. *J Allergy Clin Immunol* 1982; 69:118.
48. Koepke JW, Selner JC. Sulfur dioxide sensitivity. *Ann Allergy* 1982; 48:258.
49. Buckley CE III, Saltzman HA, Sieker HO. The prevalence and degree of sensitivity to ingested sulfites. *J Allergy Clin Immunol* 1985;75:144.
50. Towns SJ, Mellis CM. Role of acetyl salicylic acid and sodium metabisulfite in chronic childhood asthma. *Pediatrics* 1984; 73(5):631–637.
51. Friedman ME, Easton JG. Prevalence of positive metabisulfite challenges in children with asthma. *Pediatr Asthma Allergy Immunol* 1987; 1(1):53–59.
52. Steinman HA, Le Roux M, Potter PC. Sulphur dioxide sensitivity in South African asthmatic children. *S Afr Med J* 1993; 83:387–390.
53. Boner AL, Guarise A, Vallone G, et al. Metabisulfite oral challenge: incidence of adverse responses in chronic childhood asthma and its relationship with bronchial hyperreactivity. *J Allergy Clin Immunol* 1990; 85(2):479–483.
54. Boushey HA. Bronchial hyperreactivity to sulfur dioxide: physiologic and political implications. *J Allergy Clin Immunol* 1982; 69(4):335–338.
55. Fine JM, Gordon T, Sheppard D. The roles of pH and ionic species in sulfur dioxide- and sulfite-induced bronchoconstriction. *Am Rev Respir Dis* 1987; 136:1122–1126.
56. Schwartz HJ, Chester EH. Bronchospastic responses to aerosolized metabisulfite in asthmatic subjects: potential mechanisms and clinical implications. *J Allergy Clin Immunol* 1984; 74(4):511–513.
57. Field PI, McClean M, Simmul R, et al. Comparison of sulphur dioxide and metabisulphite airway reactivity in subjects with asthma. *Thorax* 1994; 49:250–256.
58. Lee RJ, Braman SS, Settipane GA. Reproducibility of metabisulfite challenge. *J Allergy Clin Immunol* 1986; 77(1 Pt 2):157.
59. Delohery J, Simmul R, Castle WD, et al. The relationship of inhaled sulfur dioxide reactivity to ingested metabisulfite sensitivity in patients with asthma. *Am Rev Respir Dis* 1984; 130:1027–1032.
60. Boner AL, Benedetti M, Spezia E, et al. Evaluation of the allergenicity of infant formulas in a guinea pig model. *Ann Allergy* 1992; 68:404–406.

61. Wang M, Wisniewski A, Pavord I, et al. Comparison of three inhaled non-steroidal anti-inflammatory drugs on the airway response to sodium metabisulphite and adenosine 5′-monophosphate challenge in asthma. *Thorax* 1996; 51(8):799–804.
62. VanSchoor J, Joos GF, Pauwels RA. Indirect bronchial hyperresponsiveness in asthma: mechanisms, pharmacology, and implications for clinical research. *Eur Respir J* 2000; 16:514–133.
63. Bellofiore S, Caltagirone F, Pennisi A, et al. Neutral endopeptidase inhibitor thiorphan increases airway narrowing to inhaled sodium metabisulfite in normal subjects. *Am J Resp Crit Care Med* 1994; 150:853–856.
64. Bannenberg G, Atzori L, Xue J, et al. Sulfur dioxide and sodium metabisulfite induce bronchoconstriction in the isolated perfused and ventilated guinea pig lung via stimulation of capsaicin-sensitive sensory nerves. *Respiration* 1994; 61(3):130–137.
65. Nannini LJ Jr, Hofer D. Effect of inhaled magnesium sulfate on sodium metabisulfite-induced bronchoconstriction in asthma. *Chest* 1997; 111(4):858–861.
66. Hamad AM, Wisniewski A, Range SP, et al. The effect of nitric oxide synthase inhibitor, L-NMMA, on sodium metabisulfite-induced bronchoconstriction and refractoriness in asthma. *Eur Respir J* 1999; 14:702–705.
67. Wells UM, Hanafi Z, Widdicombe JG. Sodium metabisulphite causes epithelial damage and increases sheep tracheal blood flow and permeability. *Eur Respir J* 1996; 9(5):976–983.
68. Mansour E, Ahmed A, Cortes A, et al. Mechanisms of metabisulfite-induced bronchoconstriction: evidence for bradykinin B2-receptor stimulation. *Journal of Applied Physiology* 1992; 72(5):1831–1837.
69. Simon R, Goldfarb G, Jacobsen D. Blocking studies in sulfite sensitive asthmatics (SSA). *J Allergy Clin Immunol* 1984; 73(1 Pt 2):136.
70. Boxer MG, Bush RK, Harris KE, et al. The laboratory evaluation of IgE antibody to metabisulfites in patients skin test positive to metabisulfites. *J Allergy Clin Immunol* 1988; 82(4):622–626.
71. Selner J, Bush R, Nordlee J, et al. Skin reactivity to sulfite and sensitivity to sulfited foods in a sulfite sensitive asthmatic. *J Allergy Clin Immunol* 1987; 79(1):241.
72. Simon RA, Wasserman SI. IgE mediated sulfite sensitive asthma. *J Allergy Clin Immunol* 1986; 77(1 Pt 2):157.
73. García-Ortega P, Scorza E, Teniente A. Basophil activation test in the diagnosis of sulphite-induced immediate urticaria. *Clin Exp Allergy* 2010; 40:688.
74. Ortolani C, Mirone C, Fontana A, et al. Study of mediators of anaphylaxis in nasal wash fluids after aspirin and sodium metabisulfite nasal provocation in intolerant rhinitis patients. *Ann Allergy* 1987; 59:106–112.
75. Simon RA. Sulfite sensitivity. *Ann Allergy* 1986; 56:281–292.
76. Schwartz HJ. Observations on the use of oral sodium cromoglycate in a sulfite-sensitive asthmatic patient. *Ann Allergy* 1986; 57:36–37.
77. Bindhu PS, Christopher R, Mahadevan A, et al. Clinical and imaging observations in isolated sulfite oxidase deficiency. *J Child Neurol* 2011; 26:1036–1040.
78. Bush RK. Sulfite and aspirin sensitivity: who is most susceptible? *J Respir Dis* 1987; 8:23–32.
79. Taylor SL, Bush RK, Selner JC, et al. Sensitivity to sulfited foods among sulfite-sensitive subjects with asthma. *J Allergy Clin Immunol* 1988; 81(6):1159–1167.
80. Nagy SM, Teuber SS, Loscutoff SM, et al. Clustered outbreak of adverse reactions to a salsa containing high levels of sulfites. *J Food Prot* 1995; 58(1):95–97.
81. Bush RK, Taylor SL, Busse W. A critical evaluation of clinical trials in reactions to sulfites. *J Allergy Clin Immunol* 1986; 78(1):191–202.
82. Añíbarro B, Caballero T, García-Ara MC, et al. Asthma with sulfite intolerance in children: a blocking study with cyanocobalamin. *J Allergy Clin Immunol* 1992; 90(1):103–109.
83. Wedzicha B. *Chemistry of Sulphur Dioxide in Foods*. Barking, UK: Elsevier Applied Science Publishers, 1984.
84. Simon RA. Sulfite sensitivity. *Ann Allergy* 1987; 59:100–105.
85. Martin LB, Nordlee JA, Taylor SL. Sulfite residues in restaurant salads. *J Food Prot* 1986; 49(2):126–129.
86. Taylor SL, Bush RK, Busse WW. The sulfite story. *Assoc Food Drug Off Quart Bull* 1985; 49(4):185–193.
87. Halpern GM, Gershwin ME, Ough C, et al. The effect of white wine upon pulmonary function of asthmatic subjects. *Ann Allergy* 1985; 55:686–690.
88. Howland WC, Simon RA. Restaurant-provoked asthma: sulfite sensitivity? *J Allergy Clin Immunol* 1985; 75(1):145.

30 Monosodium Glutamate

Katharine M. Woessner

Allergy, Asthma and Immunology Training Program, Scripps Clinic Medical Group, San Diego, CA, USA

Key Concepts

- Glutamate is recognized by distinct taste receptors on the tongue as "umami" (savory) along with sweet, sour, salty, and bitter.
- MSG is rapidly and efficiently metabolized by the intestinal mucosa and liver in both adults and infants. Despite high maternal intake of MSG, levels remain low in fetal circulation. Therefore, no limitation for MSG ingestion in pregnant women and infants is recommended.
- MSG has been anecdotally associated with a diverse array of conditions including migraine headache, which have not been validated in carefully controlled challenge studies. Low-MSG diets should not be empirically recommended for migraine sufferers, as there is no science to back up such a recommendation.
- MSG symptom complex (formally the Chinese restaurant syndrome) may occur with high-dose MSG (3 g or more) in the absence of food in some people and is a self-limited condition.
- MSG is generally recognized as safe by the Food and Drug Administration. Numerous studies have failed to show that MSG causes any serious acute or chronic medical problems in the general population.

A 1968 letter to the editors of the *New England Journal of Medicine* by Dr. Robert Kwok describing what he termed the Chinese restaurant syndrome (CRS) with "numbness at the back of the neck ... radiating to both arms and the back, general weakness and palpitation" which he experienced only when dining in Chinese restaurants initiated the public controversy surrounding monosodium glutamate (MSG), which continues to this day [1]. Although Dr. Kwok hypothesized that his symptom complex was due to alcohol in Chinese cooking wine, sodium content, or the flavoring ingredient MSG, attention became focused on MSG. Since the 1960s, the role of MSG has been questioned in not only what has become known as the MSG symptom complex, but also a number of other potential adverse reactions. In addition to the MSG symptom complex, MSG ingestion has been anecdotally associated with asthma, urticaria and angioedema, headache [2], shudder attacks in children, psychiatric disorders, and convulsions. In the four decades since the publication of Dr. Kwok's letter, extensive research has failed to demonstrate a clear and consistent relationship between MSG ingestion and the development of these or any adverse reactions in humans. Despite this, strong suspicion regarding MSG persists in the public arena.

The fifth taste: L-glutamate

Humans can detect four primary tastes: sweet, salty, bitter, and sour. There is also a fifth taste called umami. Umami describes the palatability or deliciousness of a food and has been called a "brothy mouth-watering sensation" [3]. Glutamic acid is a nonessential amino acid that constitutes approximately 20% of dietary proteins. When added to foods in the form of a sodium, potassium, or calcium salt, glutamate enhances the palatability of foods. Ikeda first documented the unique taste- and flavor-enhancing qualities of MSG in 1908 after isolating it from the seaweed *Laminaria japonica*, which has been used for centuries in Japanese cooking as a flavor enhancer [4]. Its characteristic taste, umami, is imparted through its stereochemical structure, monosodium L-glutamate; the D-isomer has no characteristic taste. MSG became widely available in the United States during the 1940s.

MSG is commercially synthesized by taking protein, usually derived from wheat or soy, through an acid wash to

Food Allergy: Adverse Reactions to Foods and Food Additives, Fifth Edition. Edited by Dean D Metcalfe, Hugh A Sampson, Ronald A Simon and Gideon Lack.

Table 30.1 Food labeling of MSG.

Free glutamate	Bound glutamate
MSG	HVP
Monopotassium glutamate	HPP
Glutamic acid	Natural flavorings
Glutamic acid hydrochloride	Flavor(s) or flavoring
Glutamate	Seasoning
	Kombu extract
	Autolyzed yeast extract

isolate amino acids. A neutralizing agent, sodium hydroxide is then added to form the sodium salt of each amino acid. Typically, MSG constitutes 10–30% of the mixture. When other amino acids are present it is referred to as hydrolyzed vegetable protein (HVP). MSG is also produced by fermentation of beetroot pulp or sugarcane. It is then purified to 98% purity. Table 30.1 lists the FDA-approved names of MSG. Since 1986, the FDA has permitted glutamate to be indirectly identified on food labels as HVP, HPP, or HSP [5]. The glutamate salts are used widely in the food manufacturing and restaurant industries and flavor a wide spectrum of foods including crackers, potato chips, canned and dry soups, canned seafood, meats, frozen dinners, salad dressings, and Chinese and other Asian food. When MSG is added to food, the FDA requires "monosodium glutamate" to be listed on the label. Other salts of glutamic acid—such as monopotassium glutamate and monoammonium glutamate—also have to be declared on labels and cannot be lumped together under "spices," "natural flavoring," or other general terms. The salts quickly dissociate in aqueous solution releasing free glutamate.

Normal dietary intake of MSG in the United States is approximately 1 g/day in its free form. An additional 0.55 g/day comes from added MSG. Some foods contain naturally occurring high levels of free glutamate such as tomatoes (0.34% MSG), Parmesan cheese (1.5% MSG), and soy sauce (1.3% MSG) [1, 6]. In the body, the turnover rate for MSG is 5–10 g/h [6]. Glutamate is metabolized in a number of ways, including oxidative deamination, transamination, decarboxylation, and amidation. MSG is readily transaminated to α-ketoglutarate, which is converted to energy by the Krebs cycle [7]. Studies on humans indicate that MSG ingested with meals results in only a very small increase in plasma glutamate concentration when compared with the levels achieved when it is consumed while dissolved in water or consommé [8]. The presence of carbohydrates appears to greatly reduce the levels of free glutamate in plasma after meals, even those containing very high levels of MSG. Even when MSG is administered in large quantities (>30 mg/kg body weight) without food, serum levels are only slightly elevated due to the very efficient metabolism of glutamate in the intestines and liver [6]. Elevated plasma levels due to doses exceeding 5 g of MSG return to basal levels in less than 2 hours [6]. It has been shown that glutamate is the most important oxidative substrate for the intestinal mucosa with glutamate serving as a specific precursor for glutathione serving a protective role for the intestinal mucosa from peroxide damage and from dietary toxins [9–11].

More recent studies have shown a role for L-glutamate in activation of the gut–brain axis and energy homeostasis [12]. Receptors mediating the umami taste, T1Rs and mGluR1, are expressed in the GI mucosa of humans, rats, and mice [13]. Intragastric administration of L-glutamate increases the firing rate of afferent fibers of the vagus nerve in rats and has been shown to increase gastric emptying in humans [14]. Kusano et al. took advantage of these findings and used MSG added to a high-energy protein drink to promote gastric emptying in subjects with functional dyspepsia [15].

Fetal and neonatal exposure to glutamate is likely to be small. Though glutamate can cross the placenta, fetal plasma concentrations do not increase significantly even with maternal ingestion of 100 mg/kg of MSG [16]. Studies by Stegink et al. in pregnant rhesus monkeys showed that it was not until the maternal plasma level of MSG exceeded 2000 μmol/L was there a slight increase in fetal MSG level [17]. These data suggest that transfer of glutamate from the mother to the fetus is unlikely even with very high maternal oral intake. Infants, including premature babies, can metabolize greater than 100 mg of MSG per kilogram body weight administered in infant formulas [18]. Free glutamate is found in breast milk in conjunction with other free amino acids and is among the most prevalent amino acids along with glutamine and taurine [19]. The free glutamate in breast milk is speculated to have a protective role in assuring intestinal growth and supplying functional substrates to the nervous tissue [20].

Monosodium glutamate and neurotoxicity

By the late 1960s, concerns were raised regarding possible neurotoxicity of MSG. Olney reported MSG-induced toxicity in the nervous system of rodents when glutamate was given in large amounts by nondietary routes to neonatal mice [21]. The resulting focal necrosis of the arcuate nucleus of the hypothalamus led to functional alteration of the reproductive capability and body weight regulation in mice. The proposed mechanism for neuronal damage is passage across the blood–brain barrier by glutamate whereby glutamate, as an excitatory transmitter, leads to continuous excitation of the glutaminergic receptors, depleting ATP and leading to cell death. This appears to be a phenomenon to which neonatal mice are particularly susceptible. There have been at least 21 studies looking for effects of MSG-induced neurotoxicity in primates and only two were positive and came from the same laboratory [22, 23]. The threshold blood levels associated with neuronal damage in the mouse are 100–130 μmol/dL in neonates rising to 380 μmol/dL in weanlings and >630 μmol/dL in adult mice [24]. In humans, such levels have not been recorded even after very high bolus doses of MSG. It has been noted by the Joint Food and Agriculture Organization (FAO) of the United Nations and the World Health Organization (WHO) Expert Committee on Food Additives (JECFA) that the oral ED_{50} for production of hypothalamic lesions in the neonatal mouse is ~500 mg MSG/kg body weight by gavage. In humans, the largest palatable dose of MSG is ~60 mg/kg body weight with higher doses causing nausea, making voluntary ingestion of higher doses very unlikely [24].

Neuroendocrine effects of high-dose glutamate administration have been demonstrated in rodents including a reduction in hypothalamic growth hormone releasing hormone (GHRH) release and pituitary growth hormone (GH) secretion as well as an increase in serum leutenizing hormone (LH) levels [6, 23, 25]. Such effects have not been shown in humans and the implications of these findings remain unknown. Acute toxicity of glutamate has been determined with a LD_{50} value of 16–20 g/kg body weight [26]. There is no evidence to date of MSG-associated carcinogenicity or teratogenicity [3, 27–32].

MSG is classified by the FDA as generally recognized as safe (GRAS). The amount of MSG that can be added to foods is limited only by its palatability. JECFA has evaluated MSG and has determined that no numerical limitation is necessary for its use in food [33]. In addition, there was no evidence to support recommendations limiting intake of MSG in pregnant women or infants. However, they did contend that food additives, in general, should not be added to infant foods to be consumed before 12 weeks of age [33]. Around the time of the discovery of MSG-induced neurotoxicity in mice, large amounts of MSG were routinely added to infant formulas in the United States. After these data became available, however, manufacturers of infant formula voluntarily removed MSG from their products.

MSG symptom complex

The controversy surrounding MSG as a food additive first came to light after Dr. Kwok published a letter to the editors in the *New England Journal of Medicine* in 1968 detailing a set of symptoms he experienced when eating at Chinese restaurants [1]. He described the experience of numbness of the back of the neck, general weakness, and palpitations. This set of symptoms became known as CRS. More recently, it has been renamed as the MSG symptom complex. As defined by Settipane, a restaurant syndrome is an adverse reaction to foods occurring within 20 minutes of ingestion, frequently while patients are still dining in restaurants [34]. After Dr. Kwok's letter in 1968, a series of anecdotes implicated MSG as the agent responsible for CRS. In1968, Schaumburg reported on his own experiences, which included tightening of facial muscles, lacrimation, periorbital fasciculations, numbness of the neck and hands, palpitations, and syncope occurring within 20 minutes of eating Chinese food on separate occasions, with symptoms resolving in 45 minutes. He reported having as many as eight experiences per day without sequelae [35]. Over the ensuing 30 years, numerous human challenge studies have been conducted in an attempt to determine the association of MSG with the clinical entity of the MSG symptom complex.

In general, challenge studies with MSG pose great difficulty because of the distinct taste properties of MSG that makes adequate blinding hard to achieve. Interpretation of some reported challenge studies has been hampered by the lack of a food vehicle. As pointed out earlier, the metabolism of MSG is greatly enhanced by the presence of metabolizable carbohydrates, which characterizes most dietary encounters with MSG. Extrapolation of food-free challenges to "in-use" situations may not be valid [36].

In one of the first challenge studies with MSG, Schaumburg et al. found an oral dose–response curve to MSG and concluded that all of the subjects they tested would eventually experience the sensory phenomena if they ingested enough MSG [37]. Double-blind studies by Kenney [38] and Kenney and Tidball [39] identified individuals who experienced symptoms specific to MSG on a relatively regular basis but only when the MSG was given in amounts or concentrations far greater than that normally encountered in a regular diet. Double-blind studies from Italy and the United Kingdom found no difference between the sensation experienced after MSG or placebo [40, 41].

Geha et al. [42, 43] undertook an ambitious multicenter double-blind placebo-controlled (DBPC) challenge study with a crossover design to evaluate reactions allegedly due to MSG in 130 self-identified MSG-sensitive subjects. Their efforts included meeting the criteria set forth by the August 1995 FASEB report on MSG which recommended that in order to confirm the MSG symptom complex, three DBPC challenges that are administered on separate occasions must reproduce the symptoms with ingestion of MSG and produce no response with placebo [44]. In three of their four protocols (A–D), MSG was administered without food. A positive response was defined as the presence of at least 2 of 10 symptoms reported to occur after ingestion of MSG-containing foods. They had 110 subjects who underwent four consecutive 5 g MSG placebo-controlled challenges. Only 2 of the 110 subjects or 1.8% who had previously self-identified themselves to be MSG reactors responded to 5 g of MSG in the four challenges. The data from their study suggest that large doses of MSG given without food may elicit more symptoms than placebo in individuals who believe that they react adversely to MSG. However, neither persistent nor serious effects from MSG ingestion were observed and the frequency of responses was very low [42, 43]. The responses were not observed when MSG was given with food. Their data again confirm the rarity of the MSG symptom complex even among individuals who believe themselves to be MSG sensitive.

Determining the prevalence of MSG sensitivity in the general population has been difficult. Estimating adverse reactions to a particular food ingredient through questionnaires is potentially fraught with subjectivity and bias. This has complicated the estimation of incidence of the MSG symptom complex in the general population. Reif-Lehrer reported that 25% of a population surveyed by questionnaire felt they had experienced MSG-related symptoms [45]. This survey included several leading, closed-ended questions, which likely evoked many false-positive responses. In a 1977 questionnaire survey, Kerr et al. showed that in the Harvard University Medical School community, no one reported experiencing the triad of symptoms in CRS and that 3–7% of subjects could be classified as having experienced "possible Chinese restaurant syndrome" [46]. In a 1979 study, Kerr et al. used a National Consumer Panel to select a representative group to improve the accuracy of extrapolation to the US population at large and found the prevalence of the MSG symptom complex to be 2% [47]. As the clinical studies have shown, the incidence of MSG symptom complex appears to be quite low.

The pathophysiology of the MSG symptom complex remains elusive. It is clearly not the result of an IgE-mediated process. Many theories have been put forth to explain the condition. Ghadimi et al. proposed that the symptoms of the MSG symptom complex are linked to an increase in acetylcholine; this group was able to show an attenuation of symptoms in subjects pretreated with atropine [48]. Gajalakshmi et al. lent further support to this theory when they demonstrated MSG's ability to produce spasmogenic effects on isolated guinea pig ileum; these effects were also blocked by atropine [49]. Glutamic acid is a precursor of acetylcholine, which may account for these findings. Folkers et al. suggested that vitamin B6 deficiency may play a role in the development of the MSG symptom complex [50, 51], while Kenney has suggested that the clinical symptoms result from esophageal dysfunction or reflux esophagitis [39]. More recently, Scher and Scher have proposed that nitric oxide production may be the mediator in the pathogenesis of the MSG symptom complex [52]. Nguyen-Duong in 2001 demonstrated that glutamate-induced vasorelaxation of porcine coronary arteries was potentiated by glycine and proposed that this vasodilatory action might be responsible for the flushing and palpitations associated with the complex [53]. Despite these assorted hypotheses and 30 years of research, the causative mechanism remains unknown.

Asthma

In the early 1980s, several reports suggested that MSG could provoke bronchospasm in asthmatics. In 1981, Allen and Baker reported their experience with two young women who had developed life-threatening asthma after ingesting MSG in meals from Chinese restaurants [54]. The asthma developed 12–14 hours after ingestion of the MSG-containing meals. Allen and Baker performed single-blind oral challenge studies on both patients and found that 2.5 g MSG capsules resulted in asthma 11–12 hours after ingestion. Subsequently in 1987, Allen et al. performed in-hospital, single-blind, placebo-controlled MSG challenges in 32 asthmatic subjects; 14 were suspected MSG reactors by history and 18 were unstable asthmatics with bronchospasm due to aspirin, benzoic acid, tartrazine, or sulfites [55]. As described by Stevenson in 2000, several problems were associated with this study: theophylline was discontinued 1 day prior to placebo challenges, some patients received inhaled bronchodilator therapy within 3 hours prior to their first challenge, bronchospasm was measured by effort-dependent peak expiratory flow rates (PEFR) rather than flow-volume loops, and baseline PEFR exhibited large variations consistent with unstable asthma [56]. Although Allen et al. concluded that 14 patients developed asthma exacerbations 1–12 hours after ingesting MSG, these limiting factors rendered the results difficult to interpret [55]. What was interpreted by the study authors as MSG-provoked asthma may merely have been peak flow variability indicative of underlying active asthma.

Five additional studies attempted to clarify the issue of whether MSG induces bronchospasm in asthmatics using double-blind challenges. Schwartzstein et al. found no exacerbation of asthma from MSG in 12 asthmatics challenged with 25 mg MSG/kg body weight [57]. This study involved mild asthmatics with no history of MSG or Chinese restaurant meal-induced symptoms. In addition, the doses of MSG were lower than those used by Allen and Bakers' 1987 study. In a second study, Moneret-Vautrin published a report of delayed bronchospasm occurring in 2 of 30 asthmatics challenged with MSG [58]. Evidence of bronchoconstriction was defined by a 15% decline in peak flow rate determinations. If the same criteria for bronchospasticity found in the Allen and Baker paper (20% decline from baseline or the "lowest value recorded during placebo single-blind challenge") were applied to Moneret-Vautrin's subjects, the two patients would not fit the definition of a positive response, as the decline was less than 20%.

A third study by Germano et al. reported that 1 of 30 asthmatics during single-blind screening oral challenges with MSG (up to 6 g) experienced a significant reduction in FEV_1 values [59]. However, when the one preliminary reactor was rechallenged with the same dose (6 g MSG), under double-blind, placebo-controlled conditions, the response to MSG challenge was negative. This study was criticized for having only 2 of their 30 asthmatics with a positive history of asthma exacerbations after a Chinese restaurant meal. The report also exists only in abstract form. A 1998 double-blind, placebo-controlled study by Woods et al. [60] challenged 12 asthmatics who reported that MSG caused them to have asthma attacks. They incorporated elaborate controls in their study, including strict dietary avoidance of MSG, home spirometry (PEFR measurements) before and after the challenges, as well as a double-blind, placebo-controlled protocol. The patients were challenged with 1 and 5 g of MSG. The study was completely negative, with none of the subjects reacting at either dose. One minor criticism of this paper is the small number of subjects.

Although it had been previously suggested by Allen et al. that those asthmatics with bronchoconstriction due to food additives or aspirin were more likely to experience MSG-related bronchospasm, a study by Woessner et al. [61] in 1999 demonstrated this not to be the case. In this study, two groups were tested: 30 asthmatics who believed MSG ingestion exacerbated their asthma and 70 subjects with proven aspirin-exacerbated respiratory disease (AERD), a population identified by Allen and Baker as being at high risk for MSG-provoked bronchospasm [55]. Asthma maintenance medications including inhaled and systemic corticosteroids and theophylline were continued, though inhaled β-agonists were not. Patients were enrolled in an in-patient DBPC challenge if their FEV_1 values were at least 70% predicted off on inhaled bronchodilators. The first day consisted of a single-blind placebo day to assess pulmonary baseline. If FEV_1 values varied by 10% or less on placebo day, the patients were challenged with 2.5 g MSG after a low-MSG breakfast. Adverse symptoms and FEV_1 values were recorded during the following 24 hours. Patients whose FEV_1 values decreased by at least 20% next underwent two additional MSG challenges in a blinded, placebo-controlled manner. On initial MSG challenge, only 1 patient of the 30 experienced a decline in FEV_1 of 20% although she remained asymptomatic. She did not have any drop in her FEV_1 on the two subsequent DBPC MSG challenges. None of the 70 AERD patients had a positive MSG challenge.

There does not appear to be any strong evidence that MSG can provoke bronchospasm in asthmatics. Because of the limited number of studies performed to date, further research is needed before any firm claims can be made that MSG provokes bronchospasm.

Urticaria and angioedema

Very few case reports of MSG-induced angioedema or urticaria have appeared in the literature. A report by Squire [62] in *The Lancet* described a 50-year-old man with recurrent angioedema of the face and extremities that was temporally related to the ingestion of a soup mix high in MSG. A single-blind, placebo-controlled challenge with the soup base resulted in angioedema 24 hours after the ingestion. In a graded challenge using only MSG, angioedema was provoked 16 hours after challenge. Avoidance of MSG-containing foods reportedly caused remission of the angioedema episodes.

Though not extensively evaluated, there have been several studies evaluating the role of MSG in urticaria. Genton et al. [63] in 1985 studied 19 subjects with chronic idiopathic urticaria (CIU) for sensitivity to 28 food additives, including MSG. In a single-blind protocol, 4 of the 19 subjects reacted, defined by an increase in urticaria within 18 hours following challenge. In 1986, Supramaniam and Werner [64] evaluated 36 children with asthma or urticaria. There were three reactors in this placebo-controlled study in which one placebo, eight additives, and aspirin were administered at 4-hour increments. Whether the reactions were pulmonary or dermatologic was not specified. A 1998 study in Spain by Botey et al. [65] detailed the workup of five children with angioedema or urticaria who presented for evaluation of possible drug allergy. Particular attention was paid to the dietary history regarding additives including MSG. Following a 2-day diet without known additives, these patients were administered 50 mg MSG orally in a single-blinded fashion: if there was no reaction in 1 hour, an additional 100 mg was given. Three of the five children had recurrence of urticaria at 1, 2, and 12 hours following ingestion; one developed pruritic erythema of the skin at 1 hour; and the fifth developed abdominal pain and diarrhea following ingestion of 50 mg MSG.

Reports in the literature of possible MSG-induced urticaria or angioedema do not clarify whether MSG was the inciting agent. Evaluation of MSG-induced urticaria or angioedema must be approached in a double-blind, placebo-controlled protocol to obtain a clearer picture of the role of MSG in urticaria and angioedema. Simon [66] addressed these concerns in a 2000 report of food additive challenges in 65 patients with chronic urticaria. The subjects initially underwent single-blinded 2.5 g MSG challenges. A baseline urticaria skin score (reminiscent of a burn score) was obtained. This scoring system is based on the "rule of nines" in which the body is divided into areas of 9%. Each of these body areas is then scored on a scale from 0 to 4 (0 = no urticaria; 1 = urticaria involving up to 25% of that surface area; 2 = up to 50% of that area; 3 = urticaria involving up to 75%, and 4 = diffuse urticaria in that area). A score of 9 or a 30% increase in the score from baseline urticaria is considered a positive challenge. Two subjects had positive single-blind challenges. Neither had a positive DBPC MSG challenge. Therefore, as is the case for MSG provoking the MSG symptom complex and bronchospasm, the role in development of urticaria and angioedema is likely to be quite rare.

Headache

Though many people believe they have adverse reactions to foods and food additives, few people have confirmed sensitivity on objective examination. It is not surprising therefore, that MSG has been associated with a myriad of physical and psychiatric complaints. Of all the adverse symptoms thought to be attributable to MSG ingestion, headache was the symptom most often reported to the FDA's Adverse Reaction Monitoring System between 1980 and 1995 [67]. In 1969, Schaumburg et al. [37] performed one of the first formal studies of the symptoms potentially associated with MSG ingestion. Their study suggested that the three main symptoms consisted of a burning sensation, facial pressure or tightness, and chest pain. Headache occurred in a minority of the subjects. Ratner et al. [68] in 1984 described four patients with MSG-related headaches. They were evaluated with double-blind testing consisting of sublingually administered soy sauce with and without 1.5–2 g added MSG. These patients developed recurrent headaches within 15 minutes to 2 hours of sublingual administration of MSG-containing soy sauce but not to "placebo" soy sauce, and reportedly had relief from symptoms with MSG avoidance. No attempt was made to disguise the taste of the two soy sauce formulations. Furthermore, it could be argued that they truly did not have a negative control due to the high glutamate content naturally occurring in soy sauce. Scopp, in 1991, described two chronic headache patients who decreased the frequency of their headaches through MSG avoidance. No objective testing was performed [69]. Yang et al. [70] undertook a placebo-controlled 5 g MSG challenge in self-identified MSG-sensitive subjects. A positive response was two or more index symptoms. The rates of reaction to MSG or placebo were not statistically different in this group of 61 self-identified MSG-sensitive subjects. If the subjects had a positive challenge, they were brought back for blinded placebo-controlled graded MSG challenges. Again, there was a high rate of response to placebo but they did have some patients who developed statistically significant associations of symptoms with MSG such as headache, flushing, muscle tightness, numbness/tingling, and generalized weakness.

Theories regarding the etiology of MSG-induced headache are scarce. Merritt et al. in 1990 found that high concentrations of glutamate caused concentration-dependent contractions of excised rabbit aorta [71]. These authors suggested that a similar vascular response might account for MSG-induced headache. However, there is little data that suggests that MSG can cross the intact blood–brain barrier. More recent work in humans has shown that local injections of high-dose glutamate into the masseter muscle of healthy humans have been found to induce intense but short-lasting pain and increased mechanical sensitivity [72, 73]. Attempts to replicate this with oral administration in healthy male volunteers did not predictably trigger headache or increase pressure pain threshold [74]. Despite a widespread belief that MSG can trigger migraine headaches, there is a striking paucity of literature to support this claim. As a result, low-MSG diets should not be empirically recommended for the chronic headache patient since they are not based in clear scientific fact and are only likely to be an unnecessary burden for these patients.

MSG and the FDA

Because of continuing reports of adverse reactions to MSG, the FDA contracted with FASEB in 1992 to perform a scientific safety review of the effects of glutamates in foods. The FASEB report was submitted in 1995. The MSG symptom complex was defined as an acute, temporary, and self-limiting complex including the following: (1) a burning sensation of the back of neck, forearms, and chest; (2) facial pressure or tightness; (3) chest pain; (4) headache; (5) nausea; (6) upper body tingling and weakness; (7) palpitation; (8) numbness in the back of the neck, arms, and back; (9) bronchospasm (in asthmatics only); and (10) drowsiness. The report concluded that although there was no scientifically verifiable evidence of adverse effects in most individuals exposed to high levels of MSG, there is sufficient documentation to indicate that there is a subgroup of presumably healthy individuals that responds generally within 1 hour of exposure with manifestations of the MSG symptom complex when exposed to an oral dose of MSG of 3 g in the absence of food [75]. This report pointed out that the key data relate to single-dose challenges in capsules or solutions and are limited in their ability to predict adverse reactions resulting from the use of MSG in food. It is well known that carbohydrates greatly modulate the uptake of MSG making extrapolation to real-world experience very difficult. The Hattan memorandum also indicates that the FDA did not consider the evidence regarding the sensitivity of asthmatics to MSG to be compelling and questioned its inclusion in the MSG symptom complex [75].

The FASEB report concludes that there is no evidence to support a role for dietary MSG or other forms of free glutamate in causing or exacerbating serious, long-term medical problems resulting from degenerative nerve cell damage [76]. It was accepted that the neurotoxicologic effects of MSG are limited to animals given very large doses by parenteral, pharmacologic, or other nondietary means.

Conclusion

Overall, the available data on MSG reflect that it is safe for use as a food additive in the population at large. MSG toxicological data have not demonstrated serious nervous system effects in humans. Furthermore, metabolic studies performed in infants and adults have shown ready and rapid utilization of excess glutamate with failure of serum glutamate levels to rise even when very large amounts of MSG were ingested with carbohydrate. The carefully done DBPC studies indicate that MSG ingestion is likely to be without adverse effect even in people suspecting themselves to be MSG reactors [42, 43, 61]. MSG has not been clearly documented to cause bronchospasm, urticaria, angioedema, or migraine headache. It is possible that large doses in excess of 3 g of MSG ingested on an empty stomach and unaccompanied may elicit the MSG symptom complex. This syndrome is likely to be infrequent and transient, resolving without treatment. In conclusion, there is no clear evidence in the current scientific literature documenting MSG as cause of any serious acute or chronic medical problem in the general population.

References

1. Kwok R. Chinese restaurant syndrome. *N Engl J Med* 1968; 278:796.
2. Chinese restaurant syndrome. *Can Med Assoc J* 1968; 99(24):1206–1207.
3. Yamaguchi S. *Fundamental Properties of Umami in Human Taste Sensation*. New York: Marcel Dekker, 1987.
4. Ikeda K. On the taste of the salt of glutamic acid (new seasonings). *J Tokyo Chem Soc* 1909:820–836.
5. Schultz WB. Food labeling; declaration of free glutamate in food. *Fed Regist* 21 CFR Part 101 [Docket No 96N-0244] 1996; 61(178):48102–48110.
6. Filer LJ Jr, Stegink LD. A report of the proceedings of an MSG workshop held August 1991. *Crit Rev Food Sci Nutr* 1994; 34(2):159–174.
7. Meisler A. Biochemistry of glutamate, glutamine and glutathione. In: Filer LJ, Garattini S, Kare MR, Reynolds WA, Wurtman RJ (eds), *Glutamic Acid: Advances in Biochemistry and Physiology*. New York: Raven Press, 1979; pp. 69–84.
8. Stegnik LD, Bell EF, Daabees TT, Anderson DW, Wilbur LZ, Filer LJ. Factors influencing utilization of gylcine, glutamate and aspartate in clinical products. In: Blackburn GL, Grant JP, Young VR (eds), *Amino Acids: Metabolism and Medical Applications*. MA: John Writs, 1983; pp. 123–141.
9. Reeds PJ, Burrin DG, Jahoor F, Wykes L, Henry J, Frazer EM. Enteral glutamate is almost completely metabolized in first pass by the gastrointestinal tract of infant pigs. *Am J Physiol* 1996; 270(3 Pt. 1):E413–E418.
10. Reeds PJ, Burrin DG, Stoll B, Jahoor F. Intestinal glutamate metabolism. *J Nutr* 2000; 130(4S Suppl.):978S–982S.
11. Reeds PJ, Burrin DG, Stoll B, et al. Enteral glutamate is the preferential source for mucosal glutathione synthesis in fed piglets. *Am J Physiol* 1997; 273(2 Pt. 1):E408–E415.
12. Kondoh T, Mallick HN, Torii K. Activation of the gut–brain axis by dietary glutamate and physiologic significance in energy homeostasis. *Am J Clin Nutr* 2009; 90(3):832S–837S.
13. Bezencon C, le Coutre J, Damak S. Taste-signaling proteins are coexpressed in solitary intestinal epithelial cells. *Chem Senses* 2007; 32(1):41–49.
14. Zai H, Kusano M, Hosaka H, et al. Monosodium L-glutamate added to a high-energy, high-protein liquid diet promotes gastric emptying. *Am J Clin Nutr* 2009; 89(1):431–435.
15. Kusano M, Zai H, Hosaka H, et al. New frontiers in gut nutrient sensor research: monosodium L-glutamate added to a high-energy, high-protein liquid diet promotes gastric emptying: a possible therapy for patients with functional dyspepsia. *J Pharmacol Sci* 112(1):33–36.
16. Stegink LD, Filer LJ Jr, Baker GL. Monosodium glutamate: effect of plasma and breast milk amino acid levels in lactating women. *Proc Soc Exp Biol Med* 1972; 140(3):836–841.
17. Stegnik LD, Ptikin RM, Reynolds WA, Filer LJ Jr, Boaz DP, Brummel MC. Placental transfer of glutamate and its metabolites in the primate. *Am J Obstet Gynecol* 1975; 122:70–78.
18. Tung TC, Tung TS. Serum free amino acid levels after oral glutamate intake in infant and adult humans. *Nutr Rep Int* 1980; 22:431–443.
19. Agostoni C, Carratu B, Boniglia C, Riva, E., Sanzini, E. Free amino acid content in standard infant formulas: comparison with human milk. *J Am Coll Nutr* 2000; 19:434–438.
20. Agostoni C, Jochum F, Meinardus P, et al. Total glutamine content in preterm and term human breast milk. *Acta Paediatr* 2006; 95:985–990.
21. Olney JW. Brain lesions, obesity, and other disturbances in mice treated with monosodium glutamate. *Science* 1969; 164(880):719–721.
22. Olney JW, Sharpe LG. Brain lesions in an infant rhesus monkey treated with monosodium glutamate. *Science* 1969; 166:386–388.
23. Olney JW, Sharpe LG, Fergin LD. Glutamate-induced brain damage in infant primates. *J Neuropathol Exp Neurol* 1972; 31:464–488.
24. Walker R, Lupien JR. The safety evaluation of monosodium glutamate. *J Nutr* 2000; 130(4S Suppl.):1049S–1052S.
25. Wakabayashi I, Hatano H, Minami S, et al. Effects of neonatal monosodium glutamate on plasma growth hormone (GH) response to GH-releasing factor in adult male and female rats. *Brain Res* 1986; 372:361–366.
26. Morikyi HIM. Acute toxicity of monosodium L-glutamate in mice and rats. *Pharmacometrics* 1979; 5:433–436.
27. Shibata MA, Tanaka H, Kawabe M, Sano M, Hagiwara A, Shirai T. Lack of carcinogenicity of monosodium L-glutamate in Fischer 344 rats. *Food Chem Toxicol* 1995; 33(5):383–391.
28. Owen G, Cherry CP, Prentice DE, Worden AN. The feeding of diets containing up to 10% MSG to beagle dogs for two years. *Toxicol Lett* 1978; 1:217–219.

29. Ebert AG. Adverse effects of monosodium glutamate. *J Asthma* 1983; 20(2):159–164.
30. Ebert AG. The dietary administration of monosodium glutamate or glutamic acid to c-57 black mice for two years. *Toxicol Lett* 1979; 3:65–70.
31. Ebert AG. The dietary administration of L-monosodium glutamate, DL-monosodium glutamate and L-gluatmic acid to rats. *Toxicol Lett* 1979; 3:71–78.
32. Ishidate M Jr, Sofuni T, Yoshikawa K, et al. Primary mutagenicity screening of food additives currently used in Japan. *Food Chem Toxicol* 1984; 22:623–636.
33. WHO. L-Glutamic acid and its ammonium, calcium, and monosodium and potassium salts. *Toxicological Evaluation of Certain Food Additives. 31st Meeting of the Joint FAO/WHO Expert Committee on Food additives*. New York: Cambridge University Press, 1988; pp. 97–161.
34. Settipane GA. The restaurant syndromes. *N Engl Reg Allergy Proc* 1987; 8(1):39–46.
35. Schaumburg HH, Byck R. Sin cib-syn: accent on glutamate. *N Engl J Med* 1968; 279:105.
36. Tarasoff L, Kelly MF. Monosodium L-glutamate: a double-blind study and review. *Food Chem Toxicol* 1993; 31(12):1019–1035.
37. Schaumburg HH, Byck R, Gerstl R, Mashman JH. Monosodium L-glutamate: its pharmacology and role in the Chinese restaurant syndrome. *Science* 1969; 163(869):826–828.
38. Kenney RA. Placebo controlled studies of human reaction to oral monosodium L-glutamate. In: Filer LJ, Garattini S, Kare MR, Reynolds WA, Wurtman RJ. (eds), *Glutamic Acid: Advances in Biochemistry and Physiology*. New York: Raven Press, 1979; pp. 363–373.
39. Kenney RA, Tidball CS. Human susceptibility to oral monosodium L-glutamate. *Am J Clin Nutr* 1972; 25(2):140–146.
40. Morselli PL, Garattini S. Monosodium glutamate and the Chinese restaurant syndrome. *Science* 1979; 227:611–612.
41. Zanda G, Franciosi P, Tognoni G, et al. A double blind study on the effects of monosodium glutamate in man. *Biomedicine* 1973; 19(5):202–204.
42. Geha RS, Beiser A, Ren C, et al. Multicenter, double-blind, placebo-controlled, multiple-challenge evaluation of reported reactions to monosodium glutamate. *J Allergy Clin Immunol* 2000; 106(5):973–980.
43. Geha RS, Beiser A, Ren C, et al. Review of alleged reaction to monosodium glutamate and outcome of a multicenter double-blind placebo-controlled study. *J Nutr* 2000; 130(4S Suppl.):1058S–1062S.
44. Raiten DJ, Talbot JM, Fisher KD, Raiten DJ, Talbot JM, Fisher KD (eds). *Analysis of Adverse Reactions to Monosodium Glutamate (MSG)*. Bethesda, MD: American Institute of Nutrition, 1995.
45. Reif-Lehrer L. A questionnaire study of the prevalence Chinese restaurant syndrome. *Fed Am Soc Exp Biol* 1977; 36:1617–1623.
46. Kerr GR, Wu-Lee M, El-Lozy M, McGandy R, Stare FJ. Objectivity of food-symptomatology surveys. Questionnaire on the "Chinese restaurant syndrome". *J Am Diet Assoc* 1977; 71(3):263–268.
47. Kerr GR, Wu-Lee M, El-Lozy M, McGandy, R Stare, F. Food symptomatology questionnaires: risks of demand-bias questions and population-based surveys. In: Filer LJ, Garattini S, Kare MR, Reynolds WA, Wurtman RJ (eds), *Glutamic Acid: Advances in Biochemistry and Physiology*. New York: Raven Press 1979; pp. 375–387.
48. Ghadimi H, Kumar S, Abaci F. Studies on monosodium glutamate ingestion. I. Biochemical explanation of the Chinese restaurant syndrome. *Biochem Med* 1971; 5:447–456.
49. Gajalakshmi BS, Thiagarajan C, Yahya GM. Parasympathomimetic effects of monosodium glutamate. *Indian J Physiol Pharmacol* 1977; 21(1):55–58.
50. Folkers K, Shizukuishi S, Willis R, Scudder SL, Takemura K, Longenecker JB. The biochemistry of vitamin B6 is basic to the cause of the Chinese restaurant syndrome. *Hoppe Seylers Z Physiol Chem* 1984; 365(3):405–414.
51. Folkers K, Shizukuishi S, Scudder SL, Willis R, Takemura K, Longenecker JB. Biochemical evidence for a deficiency of vitamin B6 in subjects reacting to monosodium L-glutamate by the Chinese restaurant syndrome. *Biochem Biophys Res Commun* 1981; 100(3):972–977.
52. Scher W, Scher BM. A possible role for nitric oxide in glutamate (MSG)-induced Chinese restaurant syndrome, glutamate-induced asthma, "hot-dog headache", pugilistic Alzheimer's disease and other disorders. *Med Hypotheses* 1992; 38(3):185–188.
53. Nguyen-Duong J. Vasorelaxation induced by L-glutamate in porcine coronary arteries. *J Toxicol Environ Health* 2001; 62:643–653.
54. Allen DH, Baker GJ. Chinese restaurant asthma. *N Engl J Med* 1981; 278:796.
55. Allen DH, Delohery J, Baker G. Monosodium L-glutamate-induced asthma. *J Allergy Clin Immunol* 1987; 80(4):530–537.
56. Stevenson DD. Monosodium glutamate and asthma. *J Nutr* 2000; 130(4S Suppl.):1067S–1073S.
57. Schwartzstein RM, Kelleher M, Weinberger SE, Weiss JW, Drazen JM. Airway effects of monosodium glutamate in subjects with chronic stable asthma. *J Asthma* 1987; 24(3):167–172.
58. Moneret-Vautrin DA. Monosodium glutamate-induced asthma: study of the potential risk of 30 asthmatics and review of the literature. *Allerg Immunol (Paris)* 1987; 19(1):29–35.
59. Germano P, Cohen SG, Hahn B, Metcalfe DD. An evaluation of clinical reactions to monosodium glutamate (MSG) in asthmatics, using a blinded, placebo-controlled challenge. *J Allergy Clin Immunol* 1991; 87:177.
60. Woods RK, Weiner JM, Thien F, Abramson M, Walters EH. The effects of monosodium glutamate in adults with asthma who perceive themselves to be monosodium glutamate-intolerant. *J Allergy Clin Immunol* 1998; 101(6 Pt. 1):762–771.
61. Woessner KM, Simon RA, Stevenson DD. Monosodium glutamate sensitivity in asthma. *J Allergy Clin Immunol* 1999; 104(2 Pt. 1):305–310.
62. Squire EN Jr. Angio-oedema and monosodium glutamate. *Lancet* 1987; 1(8539):988.
63. Genton C, Frei PC, Pecond A. Value of oral provocation tests to aspirin and food additives in the routine investigation of

asthma and chronic urticaria. *J Allergy Clin Immunol* 1985; 76:40–45.
64. Supramaniam G, Werner JO. Artificial food additive intolerance in patients with angio-edema and urticaria. *Lancet* 1986; 2:907–909.
65. Botey J, Cozzo M, Marin A, Eseverri JL. Monosodium glutamate and skin pathology in pediatric allergology. *Allergol Immunopathol (Madr)* 1988; 16(6):425–428.
66. Simon RA. Additive-induced urticaria: experience with monosodium glutamate (MSG). *J Nutr* 2000; 130(4S Suppl.):1063S–1066S.
67. Gray D. Food and Drug Administration Memorandum, glutamate in food. *Fed Regist* 1996; 61(178):48102–48110.
68. Ratner D, Eshel E, Shoshani E. Adverse effects of monosodium glutamate: a diagnostic problem. *Isr J Med Sci* 1984; 20(3):252–253.
69. Scopp AL. MSG and hydrolyzed vegetable protein induced headache: review and case studies. *Headache* 1991; 31(2):107–110.
70. Yang WH, Drouin MA, Herbert M, Mao Y, Karsh J. The monosodium glutamate symptom complex: assessment in a double-blind, placebo-controlled, randomized study. *J Allergy Clin Immunol* 1997; 99(6 Pt. 1):757–762.
71. Merritt JE, Williams PB. Vasospasm contributes to monosodium glutamate-induced headache. *Headache* 1990; 30(9):575–580.
72. Svensson P, Cairns BE, Wang K, et al. Glutamate-evoked pain and mechanical allodynia in the human masseter muscle. *Pain* 2003; 101(3):221–227.
73. Cairns BE, Svensson P, Wang K, et al. Ketamine attenuates glutamate-induced mechanical sensitization of the masseter muscle in human males. *Exp Brain Res* 2006; 169(4):467–472.
74. Baad-Hansen L, Cairns B, Ernberg M, Svensson P. Effect of systemic monosodium glutamate (MSG) on headache and pericranial muscle sensitivity. *Cephalalgia* 2010; 30(1):68–76.
75. Hatten GG. *Evaluation of the Federation of American Societies for Experimental Biology (FASEB) July 1995 Report: Analysis of Adverse Reactions to Monosodium Glutamate (MSG).* Memorandum from the Director of Health Effects Evaluation to Dr Lawrence Lin: HFS-206; 1996.
76. FASEB. *Analysis of Adverse Reactions to Monosodium Glutamate (MSG) Report.* Washington, DC: Life Sciences Research Office, Federation of American Societies for Experimental Biology, 1995.

31 Tartrazine, Azo, and Non-Azo Dyes

Donald D. Stevenson
Division of Allergy, Asthma and Immunology, Scripps Clinic, La Jolla, CA, USA

Key Concepts

- Tartrazine (FD&C Yellow No. 5) is found in many processed foods, drinks, and color-coded pills.
- For the general population tartrazine is safe.
- There are a few patients who developed hives after ingesting tartrazine.
- There are five patients in the world's literature that developed mild asthma after ingesting tartrazine.
- There is no relationship or cross-reactivity between aspirin and tartrazine.
- A few people have contact dermatitis when tartrazine touches their skin.
- Hyperkinesis in children is not caused by tartrazine.

Ten coal tar derivatives are currently accepted under the Food Dye and Cosmetic Act (FD&C) for use as dyes in food, drink, and color coding for capsules and tablets [1]. All of these dyes contain aromatic rings and some contain azo linkages (-N:N-). Azo dyes include tartrazine (FD&C Yellow No. 5) (Fig. 31.1), sunset yellow (FD&C Yellow No. 6), ponceau (FD&C Red No. 4), and carmoisine (FD&C Red No. 2). By contrast the non-azo dyes do not contain the -N:N- linkages. A few examples of non-azo dyes include brilliant blue (FD&C Blue No. 1) (Fig. 31.2), erythrosine (FD&C Red No. 3), and indigotin (FD&C Blue No. 2). Since all of the above dyes are approved for use in humans, they are routinely added to processed food, drinks, and color-coded medications throughout the world. Therefore, the issue is not whether or not we are exposed to these chemicals but rather what harm, if any, do they cause in humans. Some claim that all dyes are harmful and should be banned by regulatory agencies. Others focus on certain subpopulations, as being vulnerable to the adverse effects of dyes. The purpose of this chapter is to review the opinions and relevant data pertaining to this topic. Tartrazine (yellow dye no. 5) may not have any special adverse effects, when compared to the other azo dyes, but it has received the most speculations, theories on adverse effects, and publications. Therefore, a strong emphasis on tartrazine is found in this chapter.

In 1984, Simon reviewed the subject of generalized adverse effects of dietary dyes on the general population and unequivocally took the position that the evidence that azo and non-azo dyes are harmful to humans in general was only speculative [2]. Despite numerous claims that dyes cause disease, reactions, and mental changes, there is no credible evidence to support global claims in the general population. Whether or not there are unusual, perhaps genetically vulnerable, individuals who experience immune or nonimmune reactions to these dyes is a different question which will receive our careful consideration. This chapter is organized into sections dealing with dye-induced urticaria and angioedema reactions, asthma, anaphylaxis, various cutaneous reactions, and hyperkinesis.

Urticaria/angioedema reactions associated with tartrazine and other dyes

In 1959, Lockey described three patients who gave a history of a rash after ingesting yellow color-coded medications [3]. The author conducted unblinded challenges with dilute solutions of tartrazine and concluded that the itching and other subjective complaints, which the patients described over the next few hours, constituted evidence of allergic reactions to tartrazine. In 1972, Juhlin et al. [4] reported a prevalence of tartrazine-associated

Food Allergy: Adverse Reactions to Foods and Food Additives, Fifth Edition. Edited by Dean D Metcalfe, Hugh A Sampson, Ronald A Simon and Gideon Lack.

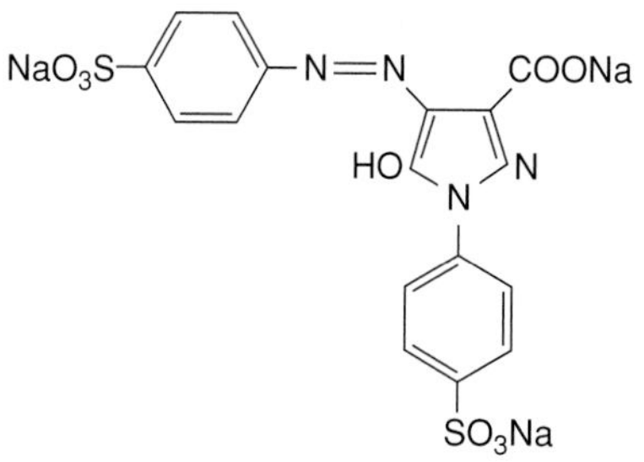

Figure 31.1 An example of an azo dye (tartrazine or FD&C Yellow No. 5). Note azo linkages.

urticaria that ranged between 49% and 100% of subjects who ingested 1–18 mg of tartrazine. During the remainder of the 1970s, other coauthors reported tartrazine-induced urticarial reactions, but the prevalence of reactions was considerably less [5, 6]. A decade after his original reported prevalence of 49% and 100% of tartrazine-induced urticaria, in 1981, Juhlin reported that 18/179 (10%) of patients with chronic urticaria reacted to tartrazine during single-blind challenges [7]. Challenge doses reflected the belief at that time that tiny concentrations of tartrazine (0.1 mg) in color-coded medications were capable of inducing urticarial reactions. During single-blind challenges in patients with chronic urticaria, antihistamines were discontinued before the placebo challenges, which were always conducted first. By challenge day 2 or 3, tartrazine was given when the therapeutic effects of antihistamine would have worn off. The appearance of hives could have been due to timed withdrawal of antihistamine coverage in patients with chronic idiopathic urticaria. It is difficult to understand how the same author could report a prevalence of tartrazine-induced urticaria of 100% in 1972 and, 9 years later in a second population of patients from the same country, report a prevalence of 10%. Even taking into effect the potential, but difficult to carry out, reduction in tartrazine ingestion in the general population, a drop in the reaction rate of 90% seems beyond chance.

Doeglas [8], Thune and Granholt [9], and Gibson and Clancy [10] reported tartrazine-induced urticarial reactions in 21%, 30%, and 34%, respectively, of patient populations with chronic urticaria who underwent single-blind challenges with tartrazine. In the six studies reviewed above, all challenges were single blinded with placebo challenges always given first. Antihistamines were withheld in two studies and no information on the use of or absence of antihistamine treatment was provided for in the other four studies.

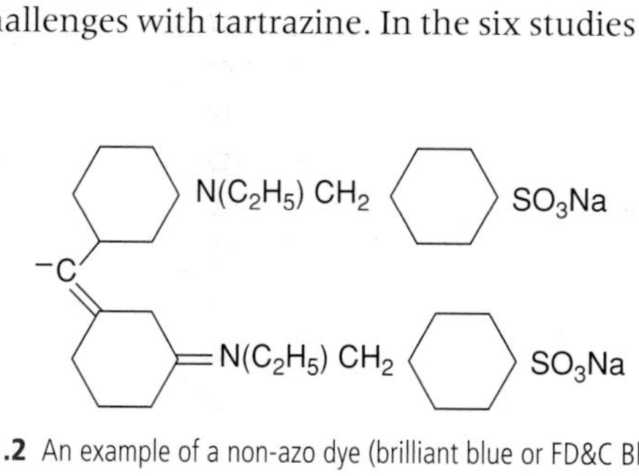

Figure 31.2 An example of a non-azo dye (brilliant blue or FD&C Blue No. 1).

Up through 1976, there were three studies which relied upon double-blind and placebo-controlled oral challenge techniques. In a study by Gibson and Clancy [10], 26/76 (34%) patients with chronic idiopathic urticaria were recorded as having reacted to tartrazine during double-blind placebo-controlled tartrazine challenges. Three of the 26 patients who "reacted" to tartrazine were rechallenged with tartrazine 1 year later and no longer developed hives after ingesting tartrazine. The authors interpreted this change in reactivity to be secondary to the institution of a tartrazine exclusion diet, which the authors and patients believed they were following during the study year. In 1975, Settipane and Pudupakkam [11] conducted double-blind placebo-controlled challenges in 2 patients with chronic urticaria and 18 patients with aspirin-induced urticaria. In one of the two patients with chronic urticaria, ingestion of 0.22 mg of tartrazine correlated with an urticarial flare during a double-blind challenge. In the ASA-induced urticarial patients, 2/18 (11%) experienced a flare of urticaria during double-blind challenges with tartrazine. In a 1976 report, the same authors conducted double-blind tartrazine challenges in 38 patients with chronic urticaria [12]. Of these 38 patients, 10 experienced flares of urticaria after ingesting aspirin. Using tartrazine doses of 0.22 mg during double-blind challenges, reflecting doses in color-coded pills, 3/38 (8%) experienced a flare of urticaria after ingesting these very low doses of tartrazine.

Of the nine studies reviewed, only the last three were double-blind and placebo-controlled. In seven studies, the study population was chronic idiopathic urticaria, including the three double-blinded studies. In the remaining two studies, the study population was never described in enough detail to be known. Antihistamine therapy was withheld in five studies but the timing of withdrawal, relative to the beginning of the challenges, was not stated. The remaining four studies did not provide information about concomitant use of antihistamines during the challenges. The presence or absence of aspirin-induced urticaria in the study populations was not clarified in most studies, with the exception of the studies by Settipane [11, 12]. Nevertheless, in three studies tartrazine-induced urticaria seemed to occur in at least some patients with chronic idiopathic urticaria whose urticaria was not flared by aspirin. Therefore, a linkage between aspirin-induced urticaria and tartrazine-induced urticaria was not established.

In 1986, Stevenson et al. [13] reported the results of tartrazine challenges in 10 patients suspected of having flares of urticaria, which the patients believed were caused by ingestion of tartrazine. None of these patients had chronic idiopathic urticaria and all were classified as having acute intermittent urticaria. Patients had taken antihistamines in the past when urticaria flared. During the challenge study protocol, antihistamines were not ingested by any patients. A screening single-blinded placebo-controlled tartrazine challenge was conducted first, using doses of 25 and 50 mg (approximate dose in tartrazine-colored 8 oz drinks such as Tang and other soft drinks). If this challenge was negative, a double-blind challenge was not conducted. If the screening challenge was associated with a flare of urticaria after ingesting tartrazine doses of either 25 or 50 mg, the protocol called for a confirmatory double-blind challenge. The results of the single-blind challenges were as follows: 1/10 patients broke out in hives 30 minutes after ingesting tartrazine 25 mg. She was rechallenged 5 days later using a double-blind placebo-controlled challenge with 25 mg of tartrazine and two placebos. During this second challenge, her urticaria also flared 30 minutes after ingesting 25 mg of tartrazine. At a later date, she underwent a single-blinded aspirin challenge with doses up to 650 mg and aspirin did not induce urticaria.

In this same study [13], single-blind challenges with tartrazine were conducted in a second group of nine patients with chronic idiopathic urticaria, maintained on daily antihistamines, which were continued during the challenges. After sequential ingestion of tartrazine 25 and 50 mg, hives did not appear in any of the nine patients. Five of these nine patients developed flares of urticaria during challenges with aspirin, despite continuing the same daily antihistamines. Finally, in another group of five aspirin-sensitive urticaria patients, challenges with tartrazine again failed to induce urticarial reactions on the day before ASA challenges induced generalized urticarial reactions. Although the study populations were small, patients were well characterized and, therefore, lent themselves to the following conclusions: it is possible for tartrazine to induce urticarial reactions in occasional patients after ingesting tartrazine. Such urticaria has nothing to do with patients who experience aspirin-induced urticaria. In patients with chronic idiopathic urticaria, aspirin and all NSAIDs that inhibit COX-1 induce urticaria in about a third of this patient population [1]. Evidence that tartrazine causes urticaria in this population of urticaria patients was not apparent in our small study.

In 1998, Simon et al. [14] conducted single-blind oral challenges on 65 patients with chronic idiopathic urticaria who were continuing their antihistamines. A rule of nine burn area was used for scoring any increase in hives during the 4-hour challenge times. None of the patients developed a flare of urticaria after ingesting 50 mg of tartrazine.

Murdoch et al. [15] studied 24 patients who were suspected of having dye-induced urticaria because their urticaria was in remission while consuming a diet free of dyes and additives. During multiple double-blind challenges with a variety of drugs and additives, the following results were recorded. Fifteen of the 24 (63%) did not react to any challenge substance. Four patients experienced urticarial reactions during aspirin challenges, two reacted to sodium benzoate, and three reacted to a panel of azo dyes (tartrazine, sunset yellow, amaranth, and carmoisine). Thus, only 4/24 (17%) reacted to the substances that they were avoiding and to which they believed they were allergic. Furthermore, three of the four subjects were admitted to hospital for more extensive challenge studies. Two of the three experienced urticarial reactions to each of the four dyes on separate days during double-blinded placebo-controlled challenges. The third patient did not react to anything during any of the in-hospital challenges. However, plasma and urine histamine levels were increased during the challenges in all three patients. Simultaneously, prostaglandins were elevated in the urine during all three challenges. It was therefore fascinating to note that even though patient 3 did not have clinical reactions, his plasma and urine histamine rose and elevated prostaglandins were found in the urine only during the active dye exposures. Shock organ responsiveness appeared to be blunted in this patient, even though mediators were formed or released during interactions with the above dyes.

In conclusion, yellow dye no. 5 (tartrazine) and several azo dyes can provoke urticarial reactions in occasional patients who otherwise appear to be normal. Evidence that tartrazine flares hives in patients with chronic idiopathic urticaria has not been forthcoming, and it is inconceivable that tartrazine and other azo dyes are the hidden "cause" of chronic idiopathic urticaria in anyone. Even in the carefully controlled Murdoch study [15], 83% of patients who eliminated dyes and additives in their diet and experienced "improvement" nevertheless did not react to these compounds during double-blind challenges. A theory of cross-reactions between NSAIDs and tartrazine, with respect to the occasional patients with tartrazine-induced urticaria, has not been proven. Therefore, recommendation to discontinue tartrazine in the diet of either chronic idiopathic urticaria or single drug-induced, aspirin-induced urticaria is a waste of the patient's time and not the standard of care.

Asthma associated with tartrazine and other dyes

In 1958, Speer [16] wrote in his book that "agents used in artificial coloring were the cause of asthma in sick children." Data supporting this claim were not presented. In 1967, Chaffee and Settipane [17] discovered a patient who believed that food dyes were worsening her asthma. Using a double-blinded protocol, they introduced a new dye or placebo, each day for 6 days. On the day she ingested tartrazine, coughing occurred. Objective measures of lung function were not obtained and the challenge with tartrazine was not repeated at another time. The possibility of coincidental coughing cannot be excluded in this study.

Samter and Beers attempted to link tartrazine sensitivity to aspirin intolerance [18]. In their first report of 80 asthmatic patients, challenges with unknown doses of tartrazine, using unknown challenge protocols, produced three "reactions" to tartrazine [18]. In their second report, 14/182 (8%) of asthmatic patients were said to have reacted to tartrazine [19]. The report did not indicate how many subjects were aspirin-sensitive, by what criteria this fact was established, and how many of the 14 experienced urticaria or bronchospasm during their tartrazine challenges.

In 1975, Settipane and Pudupakkam conducted double-blind placebo-controlled tartrazine challenges in 20 asthmatic patients [11]. Using small doses of tartrazine (0.44 mg), they reported that 3/20 (15%) experienced a 20% drop in FEV_1 values during challenges with tartrazine. Whether or not asthma medications were withheld during the challenges was not stated.

Stenius and Lemola [20] conducted oral challenge studies using small doses of tartrazine (0.1–10 mg). Following ingestion of tartrazine, 25/114 (22%) unselected asthmatics dropped their peak flow measurements by 20% from baseline values. In the same study, a separate population of 25 aspirin-sensitive asthmatics underwent tartrazine challenges and 12 (50%) reacted with a greater than 20% decline in peak flow values. It is generally agreed that peak flow measurements are less reproducible than timed flow/volume measurements [21, 22]. Most investigators use wedge spirometers and obtain FEV_1 values during repetitive measurements of lung function. This subject was reviewed in detail by Stevenson [23]. During placebo challenges, in patients with hyperirritable airways, FEV_1 values have been documented to decline by as much as 43%. Therefore, it is important to stabilize underlying asthma and demonstrate that the FEV_1 values do not vary by more than 10% during placebo challenges before beginning single- or double-blind challenge studies. Most investigators use a 20% or more decline in FEV_1 as evidence of bronchospasm during challenge studies, assuming that the baseline challenge with placebo was stable. However, in a 1977 report by Freedman [24], a 14% decline in FEV_1 was used as an endpoint and was provided as proof that a tartrazine-induced bronchospastic reactions had occurred.

Spector et al. conducted one of the largest studies investigating the prevalence of tartrazine-induced bronchospasm [25]. In their studies, bronchodilators were withheld for 6–12 hours before beginning double-blind oral challenges with one challenge substance (or placebo) each day during inpatient hospitalizations. A 20% decline in FEV_1 values, when compared to the placebo day, was considered to be evidence of a bronchospastic reaction. Tartrazine challenge doses ranged from 1 to 50 mg. The results of their study are summarized as follows. There were 277 asthmatic patients in their study. All were challenged with aspirin and 44/277 (16%) experienced respiratory reactions and were identified as aspirin-sensitive asthmatics. Of the remaining 233 aspirin-tolerant patients, none experienced a 20% decline on the days they ingested tartrazine. By contrast, when the 44 aspirin-sensitive asthmatics were challenged with tartrazine, 11 (25%) experienced a 20% decline in FEV_1 values. Unfortunately, of the 11 tartrazine reactors, five did not undergo placebo challenges (i.e., did not have a placebo challenge baseline day with proven airway stability before challenges with tartrazine). The authors discontinued controller medications in a group of aspirin-sensitive asthmatics, whose asthma was severe enough to be admitted to National Jewish Hospital and failed to consistently perform baseline placebo challenges. They then noted a 20% decline in FEV_1 values during challenges with tartrazine in 11 patients. Was this change in lung function due to discontinuing anti-asthmatic medications or inherent hyperirritability of the airways or did these patients have tartrazine- and aspirin-induced asthma?

The most revealing study in this area of controversy was performed by Weber et al. [26]. Using standard single-blind oral aspirin challenges, they identified 13 of 44 asthmatic patients as having aspirin-exacerbated respiratory disease (AERD). After challenges with tartrazine, in doses ranging from 2.5 to 25 mg and withholding morning bronchodilators, 7/44 (16%) of the patients experienced a 20% decline in FEV_1 values. Tartrazine challenges were repeated in the same seven patients 1 week later and this time they received their morning bronchodilator medications. During these follow-up challenges, using the same "provoking dose" of tartrazine, FEV_1 values remained steady throughout the testing period. These patients were also challenged with six other azo dyes and did not experience any changes in FEV_1 values. Furthermore, if one took the position that morning bronchodilator treatment prevented the tartrazine reactions, one is faced with the task of explaining why 13/44 (30%) of these patients experienced a 20% or more decline in their FEV_1 values during oral challenges with aspirin while taking the same bronchodilators.

In a study by Vedanthan et al. [27], 49 aspirin-tolerant children and 5 aspirin-sensitive asthmatic children underwent oral challenges with tartrazine. Standard asthma medications, including cromolyn, theophylline, and corticosteroids, were continued during the challenges. None of the subjects reacted to tartrazine. The five aspirin-sensitive asthmatics underwent aspirin challenges and experienced a $>$20% decline in FEV_1 values. Therefore, the endpoint criteria of a 20% or more decline in FEV_1 values, as evidence of induced bronchospasm, was sensitive enough to detect changes in bronchial airways during aspirin challenges. If tartrazine cross-reacted with aspirin, one would have expected this to occur in at least some of the five aspirin-sensitive asthmatic children.

In a study of adult asthmatics by Tarlo and Broder [28], bronchodilators were continued. One of 26 aspirin-tolerant asthmatics experienced a wheezing reaction and a >20% decline in FEV_1 values during a double-blind challenge with tartrazine. The first point of this paper was the disassociation between aspirin sensitivity and tartrazine-induced asthma. Second, the authors stated that elimination of tartrazine from the diet in this one patient did not have any effect on the course of her asthma. This paper is instructive, since the original premise of detecting tartrazine-induced asthma was to then eliminate tartrazine in the diet in order to improve their asthma. Although one patient provides only an anecdotal report, proponents of the theory that "dietary tartrazine causes asthma" and "eliminated tartrazine improves asthma" did not gain support from this patient's clinical course.

In the largest series of aspirin-sensitive asthmatics undergoing tartrazine challenges, Stevenson and his associates were unable to detect tartrazine-induced asthma in any of 150 consecutive patients with proven AERD [13]. The protocol for this study was as follows. All patients were admitted to an inpatient general clinical research center. Regular controller medications were continued. All patients underwent single-blind, placebo-controlled oral challenges with tartrazine 25 and then 50 mg. If the baseline placebo challenge was stable and the FEV_1 values dropped by 20% or more during one of the tartrazine challenges, patients were rescheduled for a repeat double-blind tartrazine challenge at a later date. However, if the single-blind tartrazine challenge was negative, the patient was classified as not having tartrazine-induced asthma. After tartrazine challenges were completed, all 150 patients underwent single-blind oral aspirin challenges on the next day and only those patients with a positive oral aspirin challenge were classified as having AERD and were included in this study. Of the 150 patients, 6 experienced a 20% or more drop in FEV_1 values, compared to placebo challenges, during the single-blind screening challenges with tartrazine. These patients were rechallenged with the same provoking dose of tartrazine in a double-blind placebo-controlled oral challenge protocol at a later date. None of the six reacted to tartrazine during these double-blind challenges. At the time of rechallenge, none of the patients were participating in aspirin desensitization treatment and all were taking the same or less antiasthmatic medications as they were during the first challenge. These studies were extended when another 44 aspirin-sensitive asthmatic patients underwent oral single-blind tartrazine challenges at the same institution [29]. Again, none of the patients reacted to 25 and 50 mg of tartrazine.

A 1986 study from Poland identified tartrazine sensitivity during oral challenges in 16/51 (31%) of aspirin-sensitive asthmatic patients [30]. The authors reported that 5 of the18 aspirin-sensitive asthmatics also experienced reactions (dyspnea) to tartrazine and when these same 5 were desensitized to aspirin they could then take tartrazine without adverse effects. Obviously, there was something radically different about the results of this study and the studies by Stevenson et al. [13, 29.] If the study from Poland was accurate, with a tartrazine cross-challenge rate of 31% [30], Stevenson et al. [13, 29] should have identified 61/194 (31%) tartrazine-sensitive patients in order to equal the percentage identified by this first European study. These two studies are difficult to reconcile even though they were performed in two different populations.

In a large multi-institutional study in Europe, 156 known aspirin-sensitive asthmatic patients underwent screening single-blind oral challenges with tartrazine [31]. Of the 156 participants, 4 (2.6%) reacted to 25 mg of tartrazine with a 25% decline in FEV_1 values during single-blind challenges and were then challenged with the same dose of tartrazine during double-blind challenges. Again, the four patients experienced a 25% decline in FEV_1 values during double-blind tartrazine challenges. A full day of placebo challenges may have been performed for each patient before starting tartrazine single-blind challenges but was not reported in their paper. However, comparative placebo challenges obviously were conducted as part of the double-blind placebo-controlled follow-up challenges. The authors of this study are well-known investigators with extensive experience in conducting oral challenges. The extremely low prevalence of positive single- and double-blind challenge studies with tartrazine (2.6%) in this 1988 European study contrasts sharply with the prevalence in the 1986 study from Poland (31%). Within 2 years, the prevalence of tartrazine sensitivity in Europe dropped by 29%.

What conclusions can be drawn from the literature on this subject? Certainly many of the early studies reporting large numbers of asthmatics with tartrazine-induced reactions were actually measuring spontaneous asthma in patients whose controller medications had been discontinued before the challenges [19]. Most of the high prevalence rates of positive respiratory reactions to tartrazine are simply not credible. Even the very large study by Spector et al. [25] where 11/44 (25%) aspirin-sensitive asthmatics were said to have tartrazine-induced asthma had serious methodological flaws in the performance of the challenges.

Second, there are probably a few patients with reactions to tartrazine, which include urticaria [13] and/or bronchospasm [31]. Whether or not these reactions are IgE mediated is not known but the idea that tartrazine participates in COX-1 inhibiting cross-reactions is impossible because tartrazine does not inhibit cyclooxygenase [32]. Third, the studies with methodological flaws, Samter study in 1968 [19], Spector study in 1979 [25], and the 1986 Polish study [30], provide the bulk of the evidence favoring tartrazine-induced asthma, particularly in the subpopulation of AERD [19]. Since all the NSAIDs that cross-react with aspirin inhibit COX-1 and tartrazine does not inhibit COX-1, there was no reason to suspect cross-reactivity in the first place. Furthermore, the study by Tarlo and Broder [28], where tartrazine induced asthma in an aspirin-tolerant asthmatic, and the two studies by Stevenson and colleagues [13, 29], where tartrazine-induced asthma was not found in 194 consecutive AERD patients, make it impossible to link AERD with the small number of proven tartrazine-induced asthma attacks [31]. In this one well-conducted study, only 4/156 (2.6%) of AERD patients experienced bronchospasm after ingesting tartrazine. Their reported incidence of 2.6% is too low to qualify as a cross-reacting chemical and suggests a different mechanism for tartrazine-induced asthma in an occasional patient with AERD. COX-1-inhibiting NSAIDs cross-react in aspirin-sensitive asthmatics 100% of the time [33] and even the weak inhibitors of COX-1, acetaminophen and salsalate, cross-react 34% and 20%, respectively [34, 35]. There is no other conclusion that makes sense other than that tartrazine-induced IgE-mediated reactions occasionally occur in any asthmatics, even those with AERD. A small chemical, such as tartrazine, requires covalent binding to a carrier protein to become a whole antigen. This makes it difficult to develop tartrazine testing extracts. However, there is a study that almost proves that tartrazine induced a wheal and flare skin test in one patient with anaphylaxis. This case will be described in the next section of this chapter [36].

Finally, with respect to recommendations to patients, it is the standard of care to instruct all aspirin-sensitive asthmatics and chronic urticaria patients to avoid cross-reacting drugs (NSAIDs, acetaminophen, salsalate) [37]. However, to make the same recommendation for tartrazine does not make any sense. Arguably there are only five proven cases of tartrazine-induced asthma in the entire medical literature [28, 31]. Only 4/5 cases were in AERD patients and in an even larger study, where appropriate double-blind and placebo-controlled challenges were conducted, tartrazine-induced bronchospasm did not occur in any of the 194 AERD patients [13, 29]. In an extensive online review of 90 articles on the subject of tartrazine challenges and avoiding tartrazine in the diet of asthmatics, only 18 articles were potentially relevant [38]. None of these articles presented evidence in which either challenge with tartrazine or avoidance of dietary tartrazine altered asthma outcomes in the study subjects. Therefore, my recommendation would be to screen patients on the basis of a tartrazine-associated history and conduct oral challenges with tartrazine in those who gave such a positive history. In those patients who experienced bronchospasm during double-blind placebo-controlled tartrazine challenges, recommending avoidance of tartrazine on a trial basis seems logical. Reporting the results of such a rare occurrence, and potential dietary manipulation, in a letter to the editor would be helpful to the broader allergy community.

Anaphylaxis from ingestion of dyes

There is a case report by Caucino et al. [36] of anaphylaxis after ingesting an estrogen tablet with FD&C Red No. 40 and FD&C Yellow No. 27. A puncture prick test of the skin with a suspension of the ground-up estrogen tablet, including the dyes and other excipients, induced a wheal and flare cutaneous response. Prick test to the estrogen and other excipients was negative. Oral challenges with the two azo dyes were not performed. Another case of anaphylaxis, during a Fleet enema, deduced that the tartrazine in the enema was responsible for the anaphylaxis [39].

Atopic dermatitis and cutaneous reactions to tartrazine

In a small study of 12 children, aged 1–6 years, with atopic dermatitis, multiple double-blinded challenges with tartrazine 50 mg were performed [40]. The 12 children were selected for the study because they had severe and intractable atopic dermatitis and a parental history that tartrazine ingestion caused flares of their dermatitis. In 1/12 children, flares of dermatitis occurred only during the three tartrazine challenges and not when placebos were ingested. Both the symptom scores and the physician observer scores were significantly and consistently increased only after tartrazine challenges. In conclusion, in a sample of 12 patients, with only 1 patient reacting, the chance that three positive challenges with tartrazine and three negative challenges with placebo would occur by chance alone was 0.46. Balanced against the observation that tartrazine sensitivity was probably observed in 1 patient is the fact that for 11/12 atopic children the parents were convinced that tartrazine was a provoking agent when it was not. This is consistent with a desire on the part of parents to fix their child's chronic disease by eliminating something. Since dyes and preservatives are found in many foods, drinks, and color-coded pills, there is a strong chance that a flare of dermatitis will coincidentally occur at the same time as a remembered ingestion of a yellow dye. Advertising this relationship in the lay press further increases the chances that parents will notice yellow dyes as the perceived "cause" of their child's atopic dermatitis. Thus, careful, double challenges with tartrazine and placebos, as in this study, can be useful in steering parents toward a logical dietary elimination. For 11/12 of the parents, attempting to eliminate tartrazine in the diet would have been both difficult and useless.

Contact dermatitis to tartrazine and azo dyes

Azo dyes are skin sanitizers and can induce delayed hypersensitivity reactions of the skin in a small number of patients [41]. Positive patch tests to tartrazine and other azo dyes have been documented in a few patients [42]. Skin contact with azo dyes occurs in workers in the textile industry [43] or in customers who wear clothes that are colored with azo dyes.

Other cutaneous reactions to tartrazine and azo dyes

Reports of purpura after ingestion of tartrazine have been reported [44–46]. In addition, hypersensitivity vasculitis has been documented in patients who were ingesting tartrazine on a regular basis [47]. Discontinuing tartrazine was associated with disappearance of vasculitis in some cases [48].

Hyperkinesis and tartrazine

Hyperkinesis and learning disorders have been attributed to ingestion of tartrazine in children [49, 50]. There is considerable controversy surrounding this subject and some authors do not believe that tartrazine has any effects on either hyperkinesis or learning disorders [51]. In reviewing the literature on this subject the results are inconclusive. This is largely because reports of tartrazine-induced effects on mental function and behavior are plagued by poorly designed studies, imprecise definitions of hyperactivity, and poor reliability of behavioral outcome measures. Furthermore, it has been difficult to define study populations and segregate them from the background noise of a heterogeneous population of children. Placebo effects, as detected by vigilant parents, have consistently reflected parental attitudes and bias in favor of tartrazine as a perceived cause of their child's mental problems. A number of articles, where poorly performed studies of tartrazine and hyperkinesis were reported, were not selected for mention in this review.

Despite this gloomy introduction, there are a few studies that address most of the investigative issues and present a reasonable case in support of occasional children having tartrazine-induced mental effects. Swanson and Kinsbourne [52] conducted oral tartrazine challenges in 40 hyperactive children with up to 150 mg of tartrazine on different days. The performance of the hyperactive children was impaired on the days they received tartrazine but not on the days they received placebos. The control children, without a diagnosis of hyperkinesis, did not experience any differences in behavior on any days, whether ingesting the dye or placebo.

In another study, Rowe examined 220 children referred because of suspected dye-induced behavior problems [53]. After interviewing all 220 children, the author admitted 55 to the study as a core group of suspected tartrazine-induced behavioral disorders. Further screening was then employed by restricting the children's diets to avoid dyes and preservatives over a study period of 6 weeks. At the end of this screening period, 40/55 (73%) of the parents reported improvement in behavior. Of these 40 children, 14 were said to strongly exhibit abnormal behavior, when ingesting foods containing azo coloring. For eight of these highly selected children, the parents agreed to enroll them in a double-blind placebo-controlled crossover challenge study. Each day, the children received placebo, tartrazine, or carmoisine, over a study period of 2 weeks. When the codes were broken, only 2/8 (25%) showed any correlation with ingestion of the dyes and abnormal behavior. The remaining six subjects did experience behavioral changes but such changes occurred on placebo days as well as days when the dyes were given. In summary, of 220 subjects whose parents believed that tartrazine induced behavioral changes, in only 2 subjects did challenges with the dyes correlate with the reported behavioral changes.

The authors extended their studies in a group of 24 patients, selected during challenge studies, from a referral population of 800 children, suspected by their parents of having hyperkinesis secondary to ingestion of tartrazine [54]. A dose–response effect was discovered during double-blind placebo-controlled challenge tests in these 24 study subjects. The minimal dose of tartrazine associated with hyperactivity in affected children was 10 mg per day. However, some children did not become hyperactive until they received larger doses.

The first conclusion was that only a small number of children, suspected of having dye-induced behavioral problems, are actually affected. Second, a dose of at least 10 mg of tartrazine was required before any behavioral changes occurred in the rarely affected children. This makes it impossible to implicate color-coded tablets and capsules where the total dose of dye is <1 mg. Finally, although the evidence is rather persuasive that dye-induced behavioral changes can occur in an occasional child, the claim that most children with behavioral disorders are the victims of dye-induced reactions is not supported by the facts.

Conclusions

Although a few well-designed studies have been conducted, the literature is filled with studies that are not of high quality and yet report dye-induced events, sometimes in large numbers of patients. After sifting through the maze of claims against tartrazine and other azo dyes, the paucity of documented adverse events caused by these dyes is apparent. Except for rare patients who experience mild asthma or urticaria, anaphylaxis, cutaneous vasculitis, and contact dermatitis as a consequence of exposure to dyes, the vast majority of humans tolerate dyes without any problem. In fact the overwhelming majority of claims against dyes are mistaken identity, associations, or misdirected blame.

References

1. Simon RA, Stevenson DD. Adverse reactions to food and drug additives. In: Middleton Jr E, Reed CE, Ellis EF, Adkinson Jr NF, Yunginger JW, Busse WW (eds), *Allergy, Principles and Practice*, vol. 2. St. Louis, MO: Mosby, 1993; pp. 1687–1704.
2. Simon RA. Adverse reactions to drug additives. *J Allergy Clin Immunol* 1984; 74:623–630.
3. Lockey S. Allergic reactions due to FD&C yellow #5 tartrazine, an aniline dye used as a coloring agent in various steroids. *Ann Allergy* 1959; 17:719–725.
4. Juhlin L, Michaelsson G, Zetterstrom O. Urticaria and asthma induced by food and drug additives in patients with aspirin sensitivity. *J Allergy Clin Immunol* 1972; 50:92–102.
5. Michaelsson G, Juhlin L. Urticaria induced by preservatives and dye additives in food and drugs. *Br J Derm* 1973; 88:525–532.
6. Ros A, Juhlin L, Michaelsson G. A follow up study of patients with recurrent urticaria and hypersensitivity to aspirin, benzoates and azo dyes. *Br J Derm* 1976; 95:19–27.
7. Juhlin L. Recurrent urticaria: clinical investigation of 330 patients. *Br J Derm* 1981; 104:369–381.
8. Doeglas H. Reactions to aspirin and food additives in patients with chronic urticaria, including physical urticaria. *Br J Derm* 1975; 93:135–143.
9. Thune P, Granholt A. Provocation tests with antiphlogistica and food additives in recurrent urticaria. *Dermatologica* 1975; 151:360–364.
10. Gibson A, Clancy R. Management of chronic idiopathic urticaria by the identification and exclusion of dietary factors. *Clin Allergy* 1980; 10:699–705.
11. Settipane G, Pudupakkam RK. Aspirin intolerance III: subtypes, familial occurrence and cross-reactivity with tartrazine. *J Allergy Clin Immunol* 1975; 56:215–221.
12. Settipane G, Chafee H, Postman M, Levine MI. Significance of tartrazine sensitivity in chronic urticaria of unknown etiology. *J Allergy Clin Immunol* 1976; 57:541–546.
13. Stevenson DD, Simon RA, Lumry WR, et al. Adverse reactions to tartrazine. *J Allergy Clin Immunol* 1986; 78:182–191.
14. Simon RA, Bosso JV, Daffern PD. Prevalence of sensitivity to food/drug additives in patients with chronic idiopathic urticaria (CIUA). *J Allergy Clin Immunol* 1998; 101:15.
15. Murdoch R, Pollack I, Young E, Lessof MH. Food additive induced urticaria: studies of mediator release during provocation test. *J R Coll Physicians Lond* 1987; 21:262–266.
16. Speer K. The Management of Childhood Asthma. Springfield, IL: Charles C Thomas, 1958; p. 23.
17. Chafee FH, Settipane GA. Asthma caused by FD&C approved dyes. *J Allergy* 1967; 40:65–69.
18. Samter M, Beers RF. Concerning the nature of the intolerance to aspirin. *J Allergy* 1967; 40:281–293.
19. Samter M, Beers RF. Intolerance to aspirin: clinical studies and consideration of its pathogenesis. *Ann Intern Med* 1968; 68:975–983.
20. Stenius BS, Lemola M. Hypersensitivity to acetyl acetic acid (ASA) and tartrazine in patients with asthma. *Clin Allergy* 1976; 6:119–129.
21. Kory R, Hamilton LH. Evaluation of spirometers used in pulmonary function studies. *Am Rev Respir Dis* 1963; 87: 228–236.
22. Fitzgerald M, Smith AA, Gaensler EA. Evaluation of electronic spirometers. *N Engl J Med* 1973; 289:1283–1286.
23. Stevenson DD. Oral challenges to detect aspirin and sulfite sensitivity in asthma. *N Engl Reg Allergy Proc* 1988; 9:135–142.
24. Freedman B. Asthma induced by sulfur dioxide, benzoate and tartrazine contained in orange drinks. *Clin Allergy* 1977; 7:407–411.
25. Spector SL, Wangaard CH, Farr RS. Aspirin and concomitant idiosyncrasies in adult asthmatic patients. *J Allergy Clin Immunol* 1979; 64:500–506.
26. Weber RW, Hoffman M, Raine DA, et al. Incidence of bronchoconstriction due to aspirin, azo dyes, non-azo dyes, and preservatives in a population of perennial asthmatics. *J Allergy Clin Immunol* 1979; 64:32–37.
27. Vedanthan PK, Menon MM, Bell TD, et al. Aspirin and tartrazine oral challenge: incidence of adverse response in chronic childhood asthma. *J Allergy Clin Immunol* 1977; 60:8–13.
28. Tarlo S, Broder I. Tartrazine and benzoate challenge and dietary avoidance in chronic asthma. *Clin Allergy* 1982; 12:303–312.
29. Stevenson DD, Simon RA, Lumry WR, et al. Pulmonary reactions to tartrazine. *Pediatr Allergy Immunol* 1992; 3:222–227.
30. Grzelewska-Rzymowska I, Szmidt M, Kowalski ML, Rozniecki J. Sensitivity and tolerance to tartrazine in aspirin-sensitive asthmatics. *Allergol Immunopathol (Madr)* 1986; 14:31–36.
31. Virchow CH, Szczeklik A, Bianco S. Intolerance to tartrazine in aspirin-induced asthma: results of a multicenter study. *Respiration* 1988; 53:20–23.
32. Gerber JG, Payne NA, Oelz O, et al. Tartrazine and the prostaglandin system. *J Allergy Clin Immunol* 1979; 63:289–294.

33. Stevenson DD, Simon RA. Aspirin sensitivity: respiratory and cutaneous manifestations. In: Middleton E, Reed CE, Ellis EF (eds), *Allergy: Principles and Practice*, vol. 2, 3rd edn. St. Louis, MO: Mosby, 1988; pp. 1537–1554.
34. Settipane RA, Shrank PJ, Simon RA, et al. Prevalence of cross-sensitivity with acetaminophen in aspirin-sensitive asthmatic subjects. *J Allergy Clin Immunol* 1995; 96:480–485.
35. Stevenson DD, Hougham A, Schrank P, et al. Disalcid cross-sensitivity in aspirin sensitive asthmatics. *J Allergy Clin Immunol* 1990; 86:749–758.
36. Caucino J, Armeneka M, Rosensteich DL. Anaphylaxis associated with a change in Premarin dye formulation. *Ann Allergy* 1994; 72:33–35.
37. Stevenson D. Approach to the patient with a history of adverse reactions to aspirin or NSAIDs: diagnosis and treatment. *Allergy Asthma Proc* 2000; 21:25–31.
38. Ardern K, Ram FS. Tartrazine exclusion for allergic asthma. *Cochrane Database Syst Rev* 2001; (4):CD000460. doi:10.1002/14651858.CD000460
39. Trautlein JJ, Mann WJ. Anaphylactic shock caused by yellow dye (FD & C No. 5 and FD & C No. 6) in an enema (case report). *Ann Allergy* 1978; 41:28–29.
40. Devlin J, David TJ. Tartrazine in atopic dermatitis. *Arch Dis Child* 1992; 67:709–711.
41. Theirbach M, Geursen-Reitsma AM, Van Joost T. Sensitization to azo dyes. *Contact Derm* 1992; 27:22–26.
42. Roeleveld C, Van Ketel WG. Positive patch test to the azo dye tartrazine. *Contact Derm* 1976; 2:180–183.
43. Hatch KL, Maibach HI. Textile dye dermatitis. *J Am Acad Dermatol* 1995; 32:631–639.
44. Criep L. Allergic vascular purpura. *J Allergy Clin Immunol* 1971; 48:7–12.
45. Michaelsson G, Pettersson L, Juhlin L. Purpura caused by food and drug additives. *Arch Dermatol* 1974; 109:49–53.
46. Kubba R, Champion RH. Anaphylactoid purpura caused by tartrazine and benzoates. *Br J Dermatol* 1975; 93:61–68.
47. Lowry M, Hudson CF, Callen JP. Leukocytoclastic vasculitis caused by drug additives. *J Am Acad Dermatol* 1994; 30:854–855.
48. Parodi G, Parodi A, Rebora A. Purpuric vasculitis due to tartrazine. *Dermatologica* 1985; 171:62–63.
49. Finegold B. Hyperkinesis and learning disabilities linked to artificial flavors and colors. *Am J Nurs* 1975; 75:797–803.
50. Colins-Williams C. Clinical spectrum of adverse reactions to tartrazine. *J Asthma* 1985; 22:139–143.
51. David T. Reactions to dietary tartrazine. *Arch Dis Child* 1987; 62:119–122.
52. Swanson J, Kinsbourne M. Food dyes affect performance of hyperactive children on a laboratory learning test. *Science* 1980; 207:1485–1491.
53. Rowe K. Synthetic food colourings and hyperactivity: a double blind cross-over study. *Aust Paediatr J* 1988; 24:143–147.
54. Rowe KS, Rowe KJ. Synthetic food coloring and behavior: a dose response effect in a double blind, placebo controlled, repeated measures study. *J Pediatr* 1994; 125:691–698.

32 Adverse Reactions to the Antioxidants Butylated Hydroxyanisole and Butylated Hydroxytoluene

Richard W. Weber
National Jewish Health, University of Colorado Denver School of Medicine, Denver, CO, USA

Key Concepts

- BHA and BHT are phenolic antioxidants commonly added to foods containing fats or oils in regulated concentrations.
- Despite animal toxicology concerns, BHA and BHT have provisional status on the generally recognized as safe (GRAS) list.
- Adverse reactions in humans are best substantiated in the skin.
- Well-documented pulmonary adverse effects have not been reported.
- True reactivity rates are much lower than initially reported due to flawed design in older studies.

Foods containing vegetable or animal fat turn rancid through chemical changes induced by exposure to oxygen, heat, moisture, or the action of enzymes. The rapidity with which rancidity develops depends on the source and storage conditions of the fats or oils. Unsaturated fats have carbon–carbon double bonds in their structure, and these sites are susceptible to the chemical changes causing rancidity. Saturated fats are more resistant. Vegetable oils have more unsaturated fats, but also contain naturally occurring protective antioxidants such as tocopherols. Animal fats are more saturated, but have lower amounts of natural antioxidants, and therefore are at greater risk for spoilage [1, 2]. Similar factors may cause the "browning effect": fruits and vegetables losing their freshness and turning color. Antioxidants block these events and may even restore "freshness" in some cases.

The phenolic antioxidants butylated hydroxyanisole (BHA) and butylated hydroxytoluene (BHT) are used in a large number of foods that contain oil and fat. Other chemicals having antioxidant activity are frequently used in combination with BHA or BHT to enhance their activity: such agents include propyl gallate, citric acid, phosphoric acid, and ascorbic acid. Additionally, there is a group of naturally occurring antioxidant compounds called tocopherols, which have varying amounts of vitamin E action. About eight forms occur naturally in foods such as vegetable oils, cereals, nuts, and leafy vegetables and are used commonly in baked goods, cereals, soups, and milk products.

BHA and BHT are synthetic compounds that did not occur in nature. BHT, also known as 2,6-di-*tert*-butyl-4-methylphenol or 2,6-di-*tert*-butyl-*p*-cresol, is manufactured from *p*-cresol and isobutylene [3]. BHA is a mixture of two isomers, 85% 2-*tert*-butyl-4-methoxyphenol and 15% 3-*tert*-butyl-4-methoxyphenol (see Figure 32.1) [4]. BHT was initially patented in 1947. Originally these substances were developed as antioxidants for petroleum and rubber products, but were discovered to be effective antioxidants for animal fats. Although its use is primarily as an antioxidant, BHA has also been shown to have antimicrobial activity against bacteria including *Pseudomonas aeruginosa, Staphylococcus aureus, Escherichia coli, Salmonella typhimurium*, and several *Bacillus* species, as well as antifungal activity against *Penicillium, Aspergillus*, and *Geotrichum* [5].

In 1949, BHA appeared on the new class IV preservative positive (allowed) list of the Health Protection Branch of Health and Welfare Canada. Usage was restricted to levels under 0.02% [6]. Animal studies from the manufacturers were submitted to the US Food and Drug Administration in 1954 and 1955, and permission for use was granted prior to the 1958 Food Additives Amendment. BHA and BHT were given "generally recognized as safe" (GRAS) status with no further studies required. More recently selected items on the GRAS list have come under scrutiny, and BHA

Food Allergy: Adverse Reactions to Foods and Food Additives, Fifth Edition. Edited by Dean D Metcalfe, Hugh A Sampson, Ronald A Simon and Gideon Lack.

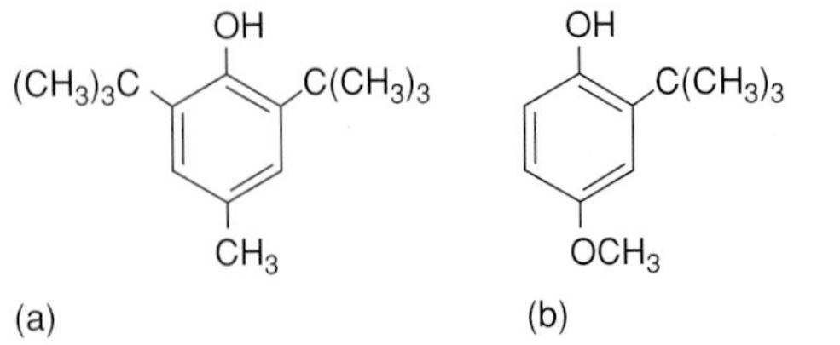

OH $(CH_3)_3C$ $C(CH_3)_3$ CH_3 (a)

OH $C(CH_3)_3$ OCH_3 (b)

Figure 32.1 (a) Butylated hydroxytoluene (BHT, 2,6-di-*tert*-butyl-4-methylphenol). (b) Butylated hydroxyanisole (BHA, 2-*tert*-butyl-4-methoxyphenol). Commercial BHA also contains 15% 3-*tert*-butyl-4-methoxyphenol.

and BHT remain with provisional status. The FDA limits their use in food, either alone or in combination with other antioxidants, to $\leq$0.02% of the total fat and oil content [1].

BHA and BHT are used in breakfast cereals, chewing gum, snack foods, vegetable oils, shortening, potato flakes, granules and chips, enriched rice, and candy to prevent oxidation of unsaturated fatty acids [1]. They are more potent than other antioxidants and have been less expensive than some other agents such as nordihydroguaiaretic acid (NDGA) [6]. BHA is used more than BHT since it is more stable at higher temperatures. BHT may be degraded by visible-light photo-irradiation, especially in the presence of riboflavin (vitamin B_2), where oxygen radicals are generated. BHA is not as negatively affected by the oxygen radicals and maintains its antioxidant activity [7]. Ultra Rice is a type of enriched rice grain, fortified with vitamin A, several B vitamins, iron, and zinc. However, vitamin A in the rice is sensitive to degradation, requiring further research to find suitable antioxidants and stabilizers complying with international food regulations. Best results were found with a combination of BHA and BHT as hydrophobic antioxidants, ascorbic acid as a hydrophilic antioxidant, and citric acid and sodium tripolyphosphate as stabilizers [8].

By 1970, the total amount of BHT used in foods was near 600 000 pounds, twice that used in 1960. By 1976, the total annual production of BHT in the United States was 19.81 million pounds, of which 10.95 million pounds were for nonfood uses and 8.86 million for food use. In addition to human food, BHT is added to animal feeds, such as fish meal in poultry feed [3]. Turkeys are especially susceptible to *Aspergillus* aflatoxin B1, and dietary BHT protects against the deleterious effects of the mycotoxin [9]. Protection is mediated through inhibition of the conversion of aflatoxin B1 to a toxic metabolite [10].

Passive food exposure to these antioxidants also occurs through their use in food-packaging materials like pressure-sensitive adhesives, paper and cardboard, lubricants, and sealing gaskets for food containers [1, 3]. BHA and BHT are also added to various cosmetics and pharmaceuticals. The latter is used in concentrations of 0.0002–0.5%. Skin penetration occurs, but systemic absorption from the skin is considered too low to constitute a risk. The Cosmetics Ingredient Review Expert Panel concluded that BHT is safe as used in cosmetics formulations [11].

The US average daily intake per person of BHT alone was estimated as 2 mg in 1970, while intake in the United Kingdom was estimated at half that rate [3]. With the greater present reliance of the North American diet on processed, packaged foods, more recent daily intakes of BHA and BHT are substantially larger. In 1986, the mean intakes for BHA ranged from 0.13 to 0.39 mg/kg body weight/day. The intake for teenage males was 12.12 mg/person/day, with the average for both sexes of all ages at 7.40 mg/person/day [6]. In 1974, the Joint Food and Agriculture Organization of the United Nation/World Health Organization Expert Committee on Food Additives (JECFA) had recommended 0.5 mg/kg as the acceptable daily intake (ADI) of BHA, BHT, or their sum [4]. A 2000 Netherlands study of older adults reported a mean intake of BHA as 105 μg/day and of BHT as 351 μg/day [12]. Theoretical maximum daily intakes of BHA and BHT in Brazil were estimated using food consumption data and a packaged goods market survey. Estimated BHA consumption ranged from 0.09 to 0.15 mg/kg/day and BHT 0.05 to 0.10 mg/kg/day [13]. Analysis of seven food additives was performed in over 34 000 food samples obtained in Japan by official inspection in 1998 [14]. Assuming a body weight of 50 kg, consumption of BHA and BHT was 0.5% and 0.7% of ADI, respectively. A report from Korea in 2005 used several methods to calculate estimated daily intake of BHA, BHT, and *tert*-butyl hydroquinone (TBHQ). The authors found that average consumption of these three antioxidants ranged from 6 to 14.42% of the ADI established by the JECFA [15]. A study of dietary exposure of children and teenagers in Beirut, Lebanon, utilizing chemical analysis of over 400 foods and beverages with a comparison to food consumption data revealed that the ADI could be exceeded by a fraction of the population, namely children from 9 to 13 years of age [16]. The highest contributors to intake of BHA were bread and biscuits, and BHT was chewing gum. Concentrations of BHA and BHT in fillets of farmed fish obtained from several sources in Norway revealed that consumption of a 300 g fillet of various species would not contribute measurably to the intake of BHA; however, the consumption of a similar fillet of farmed Atlantic salmon would contribute up to 75% of the ADI for BHT [17].

Toxicology

Despite the ease with which these antioxidants passed muster at the FDA, animal toxicology studies have revealed a variety of adverse events. These may well be related to their actions as antioxidants. BHA and BHT act as lipid-soluble chain-breaking agents, delaying lipid peroxidation by scavenging intermediate radicals such as lipid peroxyls [18]. In the process, however, the antioxidant has lost a hydrogen atom, thus becoming a radical. The antioxidant radical is generally less reactive than the peroxyl free radical, but under some circumstances can show pro-oxidant properties, frequently due to interactions with iron ions.

In mice studies, BHA inhibited several microsomal enzymes, but long-term administration also induced specific P450 cytochrome enzymes [19]. In humans, BHA 0.5 mg/kg for 10 days had no appreciable effects on biotransformation capacity [20]. Antipyrine and paracetamol (acetaminophen) metabolism were unaffected. Urinary excretion of BHA metabolites was significantly increased on days 3 and 7 compared to day 1, suggesting either an inhibition of BHA metabolizing enzymes or bioaccumulation of BHA and/or its metabolites in the body.

Single doses of BHT have been shown to induce interstitial pneumonitis and pulmonary fibrosis in mice, while BHA and other antioxidants did not appear to have this action [21]. This BHT effect can be potentiated by oxygen given early but not late [22, 23]. High-dose corticosteroids additionally may significantly worsen lung damage if given early, while late administration may alleviate the injury [24, 25]. Whether the lung injury is mediated through some unique property of BHT, rather than through an antioxidant pathway, is unclear; it does appear that the extent of damage is dependent on several factors interweaving both dose and timing. There are distinct mice strain differences in the chronic response to BHT, part of which may be due to cytochrome P450 conversion of BHT to the more pneumotoxic metabolite *tert*-butyl hydroxylated BHT (BHT-BuOH) [26]. CXBH mice became tolerant to the chronic administration of BHT, while BALB/cBy mice showed a chronic inflammatory process with activated alveolar macrophages and increased lung tumor multiplicity. Acute effects demonstrated two- to fivefold decreases in protein kinase Cα and calpain II (calcium-dependent protease isozyme II).

Impact of dietary antioxidants on cancer prevention has received much scientific and media attention. BHA and BHT have been shown to both protect from and enhance tumor development in different systems. BHT may inhibit tumor induction of carcinogens if given prior, but may promote tumor growth if given after the carcinogen [27]. BHA, BHT, and NDGA have been shown to decrease skin tumor promotion by 12-*O*-tetradecanoylphorbol-13-acetate (TPA), benzoyl peroxide, and ultraviolet light. BHA achieves this result through decreased gene expression of ornithine decarboxylase, an indicator of skin tumor promotion and hyperproliferation [28]. BHT, however, increased the incidence of liver tumors in male C3H mice [29]. The same study showed increased colon cancer in BALB/c mice following one chemical carcinogen, dimethylhydrazine, but not another, methylnitrosourea. BHA, on the other hand, appeared to protect against the acute liver toxicity of a colon-specific carcinogen, methylazoxymethanol acetate [30]. BHA can inhibit growth and induce apoptosis of HeLa cervical cancer cells [31]. This effect was due to caspase activation and glutathione depletion. However, high-dose BHA was shown to produce cancers of the forestomach in rats [6]. Since man does not have a forestomach, and doses used were about 10 000 times higher than likely human consumption, it was felt on review of the data by JECFA that the benefits of BHA outweighed the potential risks [6]. With the usual daily intake of BHA and BHT, the Netherlands Cohort Study found no significant association with stomach cancer risk [12].

In Wistar albino rats, pretreatment with BHT augmented LPS-induced liver toxicity through enhancement of superoxide dismutase activity [32]. The authors commented that while the risk of liver toxicity with the use of BHT alone was low, there could be a higher risk with overconsumption of the additive in endotoxemic settings. BHT may have anti-atherogenic impact. Using a cholesterol-fed rabbit model, Xiu and colleagues showed that BHT prevented decreased blood flow and vessel diameter in the microcirculation [33]. This effect of BHT is mediated through induction of elevated levels of triglycerides [34].

Using human lymphocytes, Klein and Bruser demonstrated BHT cytotoxicity with concentrations >100 μg/mL [35]. At 50 μg/mL, BHT inhibited the mixed lymphocyte reaction, but not PHA stimulation. A synergistic effect of PHA suppression was seen with co-incubation with either cortisol or prednisolone. Using a rat passive cutaneous anaphylaxis (PCA) model, Yamaki and colleagues demonstrated that BHT augmented DNP-specific PCA in a dose-dependent fashion [36]. Additionally, in the presence of BHT, IgE-induced rat RBL2H3 cells released greater amounts of mediators, associated with increased intracellular concentrations of Ca^{2+} and PI3 kinase activation. The authors suggested therefore that BHT could have an impact on allergic diseases.

Asthma/rhinitis

In contrast to the wealth of animal toxicology literature, there are only scattered reports of adverse reactions to BHA and BHT in humans. In 1973, Fisherman and Cohen reported on seven patients with either asthma, vasomotor rhinitis with or without nasal polyps, or the combination, all of whom were suspected of intolerance to BHA and BHT [37]. There were no clinical details given or why BHA and BHT were incriminated. These patients were identified following open challenge with capsule ingestion of 125–250 mg of BHA/BHT and reproduction of symptoms of worsening vasomotor rhinitis, headache, flushing, asthma, conjunctival suffusion, dull retrosternal pain radiating to the back, diaphoresis, or somnolence. No objective measures were noted. BHA/BHT intolerance was additionally documented by a doubling of a Duke earlobe bleeding time (termed by the authors the sequential vascular response) in all cases. No rationale for the effect on the bleeding time was given, other than a supposed similarity to aspirin intolerance. In a follow-up paper the same year dealing with aspirin cross-reactivity, these authors had found 21 patients with intolerance to BHA/BHT via the bleeding time, of whom 17 had clinical symptoms on challenge. No clinical details were given [38].

The following year, in an unsuccessful attempt to duplicate Fisherman and Cohen's initial findings, Cloninger and Novey performed a similar study using oral ingestion of 300–850 mg BHA in five asthmatic and two rhinitic patients [39]. They reported that the baseline earlobe bleeding time was not reproducible in the degree suggested by the previous authors. None of the patients had clinical exacerbations, changes in peak flows, or more than a 50% change in the bleeding times; there was a non-dose-related effect of drowsiness noted in four of the patients. These authors therefore questioned the validity of clinical BHA intolerance as well as the validity and reproducibility of the sequential vascular response. Goodman and colleagues, in a case of well-documented BHA/BHT-induced chronic urticaria (discussed further below), could not demonstrate an effect of either BHA 250 mg or placebo on the earlobe bleeding time in either the patient or two controls [40].

Weber and colleagues found no asthmatic responses (>25% drop in FEV1) in 43 moderately severe perennial asthmatics undergoing single-blind capsule challenges with sequential doses of 125 and 250 mg of BHA and BHT [41]. This was a portion of a larger study where single-blind challenges were validated by subsequent double-blind challenges. Aspirin sensitivity was documented in 44% of the patients and reactivity to *p*-hydroxybenzoic acid, sodium benzoate, and non-azo or azo dyes in 2–5%. The author is aware of two unpublished cases: a drop of pulmonary function following double-blind challenge with BHT 250 mg in a patient with food anaphylaxis and oral allergy syndrome; and cough and drop in PEFR with double-blind BHA challenge in a patient with food allergy. Therefore, at present, there are no published reports of challenges with either BHA or BHT resulting in well-documented, reproducible asthmatic responses.

Urticaria

In 1975, Thune and Granholt reported on 100 patients with recurrent urticaria evaluated with provocative food additive challenges [42]. Sixty-two patients had positive challenges, with two-thirds reacting to multiple substances. Positivity rates for individual dyes, preservatives, or anti-inflammatory drugs ranged from 10% to 30%. Most reactions occurred within 1–2 hours, with a number of them occurring between 12 and 20+ hours. Six of 47 (12.7%) tested to BHA reacted, and 6 of 43 (13.9%) reacted to BHT; it is unclear whether these were the same six patients. Test doses were given in two to three increments, with the total dose of BHA and BHT being 17 mg. The provocative challenges were not blinded, nor did the authors state criteria for a positive challenge.

In 1977, Fisherman and Cohen reported the results of provocative oral or intradermal challenges of a large number of suspected agents on the bleeding time (the "sequential vascular response") in the assessment of 215 patients with chronic urticaria [43]. Medications were withdrawn 12 hours prior to challenge, with the exception of hydroxyzine, which was held for 72 hours. Intolerance was found in 19 patients with challenges of 250–500 mg of BHA and BHT. Slight details of four reactors challenged with 250 mg each of BHA and BHT were included in a table: in addition to doubling of the earlobe bleeding time, two developed nasal congestion, and three had urticaria, although it is not clear whether this was increased over baseline. These authors felt they made a determination of "single or partial etiologies" in 203 of the 215 patients (94.4%), an astounding success rate in a clinical entity known for its resistance to defining a cause. Obviously, the same criticism of the lack of conceivable mechanism and the nonreproducibility of the test in other hands holds for these authors' urticaria evaluations as well as the asthma challenges.

Juhlin mentioned in a review on urticaria in 1977 the results of provocative challenges with a mix of BHA and BHT in 130 urticaria patients [44]. Incremental doses of 1, 10, and 50 mg each of BHA and BHT resulted in nine positive and five probable positive challenges (6.9–10.8%). Details as to the nature of the patients' symptoms, criteria for positive responds, or the blinding of the challenges were not given. Four years later, Juhlin published the results of an evaluation of 330 patients with recurrent urticaria [45]. He used a 15-day single-blind challenge battery of dyes, preservatives, and placebo. Antihistamines were withheld from 4 to 5 days before the commencement of the challenge sequence. Testing was accomplished when patients had "no or slight symptoms." Tests were judged positive if "clear signs of urticaria or angiooedema" occurred within 24 hours. Slightly less than half of the 330 patients (156) received a BHA/BHT challenge with cumulative doses of 1, 10, 50, and 50 mg given (total dose 111 mg). Fifteen percent had positive reactions and 12% had equivocal reactions. Lactose placebo was given in two doses on days 1, 3, 9, and 12, although modifications in the order did occur. Active substances were given in single to six divided doses at hourly intervals. Most patients did not undergo the entire challenge schedule; one-third did not receive a placebo challenge.

Hannuksela and Lahti published their results of an extensive double-blind challenge study in 1986 [46]. They evaluated 44 patients with chronic urticaria of greater than 2 months duration, 91 atopic dermatitis patients, and 123 patients with resolved contact dermatitis. They used wheat starch as their placebo rather than lactose since Juhlin had reported positive responses to lactose placebo. Patients were challenged to sodium metabisulfite 9 mg, benzoic acid 200 mg, BHA and BHA mixture of 50 mg each, and β-carotene and β-apo-carotenal mixture 200 mg each. Positive reactions were repeated 4 days later to validate the response: challenges were rated as positive if the patient responded both times, and as equivocal if the repeat was negative. Of the 44 urticaria patients, none had reproducible positive reactions to BHA/BHT: two responded to the first challenge but not the second 4 days later. The same response occurred with the atopic dermatitis patients: two had equivocal reactions to BHA/BHT. None of the contact dermatitis patients reacted to the antioxidants. One urticaria patient had reproducible responses to the wheat placebo, another to benzoic acid, and one had an equivocal response to metabisulfite. One atopic dermatitis patient had positive reactions to carotenal/carotene, and another had an equivocal reaction to metabisulfite. One contact dermatitis patient had an equivocal reaction to the wheat placebo (second challenge not done). The authors contrasted their results to those of Juhlin and cited challenge differences to explain their lack of responses. They also wondered whether a prolonged refractory period following the initial positive challenges could account for the negative follow-up trials, since they had waited only 4 days. In general, however, the authors felt that ordinary amounts of food additives do not provoke urticaria or influence atopic dermatitis [46].

In 1990, Goodman and colleagues reported the first double-blind placebo-controlled multiple challenge protocol documenting the link of BHA and BHT with chronic urticaria [40]. The demonstration of symptom aggravation did not rest on single challenges: two patients with chronic urticaria and angioedema of 3–4 years duration underwent oral challenges with several agents performed two to three times for verification. The patients had demonstrated improvement on restricted diets, but had lost 20–30 pounds in the process. Both patients were admitted, placed on an elemental diet formula, and observed for 5–7 days to establish an estimate of baseline activity. The patients ranked pruritus severity, and skin lesions were ranked from 0 to 4+ based on the degree of body distribution. Only challenges inducing lesions within 12 hours of ingestion and involving an entire extremity or body area, or generalized, were considered positive. Those occurring within 12–24 hours were considered equivocal. A mixture of 125 mg each of BHA and BHT was given, followed by 250 mg of the mixture, given 2–4 hours later if no major reaction had occurred. One patient was additionally challenged to BHA 250 mg alone. Placebo capsules were either dextrose or lactose. The patients were also challenged to sodium benzoate, *p*-hydroxybenzoic acid, tartrazine, and other azo dyes. Both patients reacted within 1–6 hours to BHA and BHT at all times and did not react to the other additives or placebo on numerous trials. There were no delayed reactions past 6 hours.

Oatmeal that one patient had been routinely ingesting for breakfast contained BHA and BHT. Both patients were placed on diets specifically avoiding BHA and BHT, resulting in sustained diminution of frequency and severity of urticaria. The first patient, at 7 years follow-up, continued to rigidly adhere to his diet and noted exacerbations of his urticaria when unexpected exposures occurred. The other, at 1 year follow-up, also continued to follow his diet, noting only two minor exacerbations, again after ingesting foods containing BHA and BHT. These two episodes lasted under 12 hours and required no medication. Each patient returned to his pre-illness weight and was able to resume his normal occupation.

The first patient assessed had serial plasma determinations throughout the challenge period for CH50, activated C_3 and factor B, and PGE2, PGF2α, and dihydroxyketoPGF2α. Blood was drawn at baseline, and half-hour intervals after the first dose to 2 hours, and hourly intervals until 6 hours after the second dose. After the initial challenges were completed on the first patient, and the code broken, the patient as well as two normal controls underwent an additional double-blind session, using BHA 250 mg and placebo. This was done to evaluate the predictive value of the sequential vascular response test of Fisherman and Cohen. As commented above, this test is an earlobe bleeding time, advanced by those authors as diagnostic in adverse reactions to BHA/BHT, aspirin, and other chemicals. Skin prick tests with serial dilutions of BHA, BHT, sodium salicylate, and OHBA were also performed, which were uniformly negative.

Serial complement and prostaglandin determinations during the challenges were unrewarding. CH50 was seen to decrease 30–35% randomly on both placebo and active compound days. Activated C_3 and factor B were sporadically elevated on four occasions, twice with placebo and once during the pre-challenge baseline period. The prostaglandin levels all decreased as the day progressed, regardless of whether placebo or active compound was given. Therefore, the authors could not demonstrate any changes with positive challenges in the prostaglandins measured. Despite the extensive evaluation, the mechanism of action is uncertain. An immunological process was not supported by the inconsistent changes in complement components, negative immediate skin tests, and lack of vasculitis on biopsy. The strict elimination diets did not totally ablate lesions in either patient. It may be that the antioxidants acted as potentiating agents of an underlying unrelated process, similar to the action of aspirin in chronic urticaria [47]. Serial earlobe bleeding times were all unchanged with both placebo and BHA in the patient and control subjects, despite the patient having a brisk urticarial response to the BHA.

Osmundsen reported a case of contact urticaria due to BHT contained in plastic folders [48]. Contact with the folders on unbroken skin resulted in a strong urticarial reaction within 20 minutes. The patient had positive wheal and flare responses to 1% BHA and BHT in ethanol.

The importance of these antioxidants causing or aggravating chronic urticaria is not clear. The true incidence of urticarial adverse reactions to BHA/BHT is unknown. Identification of provokers in a disease of waxing and waning nature may be difficult. Are reactions truly causally related, or only spontaneous exacerbations of the process? This is especially an issue when a background of urticarial activity persists during challenges. A sharp definition of what constitutes a positive reaction is necessary. Additionally, the observer rating the severity of the reaction must be blinded as well as the subject, since he is also susceptible to expectation bias. The studies of Thune and Granholt [42] and Juhlin fail on both counts [44, 45]. The 13–15% incidence of BHA/BHT reactions reported in these studies is surely an overestimate. Preliminary results of single-blind, placebo-controlled food additive panel challenges at Scripps Clinic have been unrewarding [49]. In evaluating somewhat over 20 chronic urticaria patients, a panel including tartrazine, potassium metabisulfite, monosodium glutamate, aspartame, sodium benzoate, methylparaben, BHA, BHT, and sunset yellow (FD&C Yellow No. 6) has revealed no responders. Additionally, the importance of double-blinding in such studies has been pointed out by Weber and colleagues [41], and reinforced by Stevenson and associates [50]. In the former study, of 15 patients who reacted to dyes or preservatives on open challenge, only three responded under repeat double-blind conditions.

Dermatitis

A variety of non-urticarial skin eruptions have been attributed to food additives. Contact dermatitis may occur to a large number of food additives, especially antioxidants, spices, gums, and waxes. Evidence for such responses can be objectively obtained through patch testing for delayed hypersensitivity.

Tosti and colleagues reported two cases of contact dermatitis due to BHA in topical agents for psoriasis and eczema [51]. Patch testing was positive for BHA but not BHT in both cases. The concentration of BHA in the preparations was 0.1% and 0.2%, respectively. As of their report in 1987, the authors cited 14 cases of BHA contact dermatitis in the literature. Contact sensitivity to latex gloves is an ever increasing problem; one recent report, however, revealed sensitivity not to the usual rubber allergens, but to antioxidants, one being BHA [52]. Acciai and coworkers found one case of contact dermatitis from BHA in a pastry cook during the investigation of 72 caterers with eczema [53]. An evaluation of contact sensitivity in 69 women with pruritus vulvae revealed patch positivity of clinical significance in 40 (58%), one of whom demonstrated sensitivity to BHA (2% in petrolatum) [54]. The importance of these instances of contact sensitivity to food considerations is that in some cases, once the hypersensitivity has been initiated through cutaneous exposure, dermatitis symptoms could be flared by ingestion of the causative agent. Roed-Petersen and Hjorth found four patients with eczematous dermatitis who had positive patch tests to BHA and BHT [55]. Dietary avoidance of the antioxidants resulted in remissions in two of their patients. When challenged with ingestion of 10–40 mg BHA or BHT both patients had exacerbations of the dermatitis.

Cutaneous vasculitis from food additives in chewing gum has been induced by ponceau (FD&C Red No. 4) and also by BHT [56, 57]. The case of acute urticarial vasculitis due to BHT was reported in 1986 by Moneret-Vautrin and associates. Biopsy revealed a heavy perivascular lymphoid infiltrate of the upper dermis, with immunofluorescence revealing IgM, C1q, C_3, C_9, and fibrinogen. Lesions resolved with discontinuation of chewing gum. A series of single-blind challenges showed a reproduction of the lesions with ingestion of BHT and not other ingredients.

Mechanisms

The reports of Roed-Petersen and Hjorth, Osmundsen, and Moneret-Vautrin suggest that certain adverse reactions to BHA and BHT may be mediated through immunological mechanisms in addition to that seen in typical contact-delayed hypersensitivity. Histamine release from leukocytes has been described following ASA, benzoate, BHA/BHT, and azo dyes [58]. The authors studied 12 urticaria patients as well as 18 healthy subjects. BHA and BHT caused histamine release one time each in an urticaria patient, but four healthy subjects reacted to BHT and one to BHA, raising the question of clinical relevance in these *in vitro* tests. These studies suggest that immune effector cells are probably involved in at least some of these adverse effects, and that different mechanisms are operant. The majority of data to date, however, do not support that these are immunologically specific reactions.

Several authors have felt that adverse cutaneous reactions in humans to BHA or BHT were akin to skin lesions induced by aspirin and nonsteroidal anti-inflammatory drugs and represented alterations in the arachidonic acid–prostaglandin cascade. There is no data at present supporting such an action of the phenolic antioxidants. The evaluation of the single patient of Goodman and associates did not reveal obvious perturbations of prostaglandin metabolites despite clinical exacerbation [40]. It appears reasonable that BHA and BHT are acting in these circumstances in a pharmacological manner, but the mode continues to be unclear.

Unsubstantiated effects

In addition to the purported adverse effects of BHA and BHT advanced by Fisherman and Cohen based on the non-reproducible earlobe bleeding time prolongation, these two antioxidants have gained notoriety in the health food lay press in the past as life prolongation agents. Claims for their benefit in increasing life span are apparently based on mice studies performed 25 years ago [3]. Unfortunately, these studies had somewhat contradictory results, and it appears unclear whether the improved life span in the mice could not also be achieved by optimal normal diet. Recommendations have been made for the ingestion of 2 g of BHT daily as a counteragent for disordered nutrition, age-related problems, and genital herpes [4]. As pointed out by Llaurado, however, the dosing recommended by these health food advocates is only an order of magnitude, 10-fold lower, than the lethal concentration noted in certain rat toxicology studies [4]! Obviously, such careless dosing is to be strongly discouraged.

Summary

BHA and BHT are ubiquitous food additives found in a variety of foods, but to a greatest degree in food that contains larger amounts of fats or oils which may become rancid. Additionally, these phenolic antioxidants are also added to plastic or paper products which may come in contact with food items as well as to cosmetics and medicinals which may come in contact with the skin or mucosa. They continue to be widely used despite concerns over animal toxicity studies. Continued provisional status on the GRAS list reflects that the toxicology studies in animals are with greatly larger doses than that utilized in the food industry. Nevertheless, consumption appears to be increasing.

Adverse reactions in humans to date are best substantiated in the skin. Delayed hypersensitivity contact dermatitis through a variety of occupational or medicinal exposures is well documented, but not common. The true incidence of antioxidant sensitivity in chronic urticaria is presently unknown. High reaction rates of adverse reactions to food additives have not been substantiated by carefully done double-blind studies. Despite older European reports suggesting a 1–15% incidence of BHA/BHT intolerance in chronic urticaria patients, this reflects weakness in study design. There appears to be the strong likelihood that a number of positives were due to random fluctuations of disease activity, and not true reactions to the antioxidants or other food additives. To date, there are no convincing published reports of human respiratory adverse responses. Therefore, the true prevalence of adverse reactions to BHA and BHT remains unclear.

Oral challenges, preferably double-blinded, remain the desired approach to verifying suspected adverse reactions to these antioxidants. The recommended schedule used is a truncated incremental challenge. The doses used may be considered high and certainly far exceed an average daily intake. However, such doses are more likely to provide a definitive reaction. Clinical relevance can then be ascertained by elimination of the incriminated agent from the diet. It must be noted that such doses, while appropriate for urticaria evaluations, could be dangerous if one were examining potential asthmatic responses.

Considering the lack of success in identifying causes in chronic urticaria, a search for additive sensitivity is probably warranted, even considering the anticipated low yield. Strict elimination diets or the use of elemental formulas are difficult and poorly tolerated by patients. Open or single-blind challenges could identify possible aggravants, which should then be further authenticated with double-blind testing. The diet restrictions could then be rationally addressed.

References

1. Lecos C. Food preservatives: a fresh report. *FDA Consum* 1984; 4:23–25.
2. Jukes TH. Food additives. *N Engl J Med* 1977; 297:427–430.
3. Babich H. Butylated hydroxytoluene (BHT): a review. *Environ Res* 1982; 29:1–29.
4. Llaurado JG. The saga of BHT and BHA in life extension myths. *J Am Coll Nutr* 1985; 4:481–484.
5. Nanditha B, Prabhasankar P. Antioxidants in bakery products: a review. *Crit Rev Food Sci Nutr* 2009; 49:1–27.
6. Lauer BH, Kirkpatrick DC. Antioxidants: the Canadian perspective. *Toxicol Ind Health* 1993; 9:373–382.
7. Criado S, Allevi C, Ceballos C, García NA. Visible-light promoted degradation of the commercial antioxidants butylated hydroxyanisole (BHA) and butylated hydroxytoluene (BHT): a kinetic study. *Redox Rep* 2007; 12:282–288.
8. Li YO, Lam J, Diosady LL, Jankowski S. Antioxidant system for the preservation of vitamin A in Ultra Rice. *Food Nutr Bull* 2009; 30:82–89.

9. Klein PJ, Van Vleet TR, Hall JO, Coulombe Jr RA. Dietary butylated hydroxytoluene protects against aflatoxicosis in turkeys. *Toxicol Appl Pharmacol* 2002; 182:11–19.
10. Klein PJ, Van Vleet TR, Hall JO, Coulombe Jr RA. Effects of dietary butylated hydroxytoluene on aflatoxin B1-relevant metabolic enzymes in turkeys. *Food Chem Toxicol* 2003; 41:671–678.
11. Lanigan RS, Yamarik TA. Final report on the safety assessment of BHT (1). *Int J Toxicol* 2002; 21:19–94.
12. Botterweck AA, Verhagen H, Goldbohm RA, Kleinjans J, van den Brandt PA. Intake of butylated hydroxyanisole and butylated hydroxytoluene and stomach cancer risk: results from analyses in the Netherlands Cohort Study. *Food Chem Toxicol* 2000; 38:599–605.
13. Maziero GC, Baunwart C, Toledo MC. Estimates of the theoretical maximum daily intake of phenolic antioxidants BHA, BHT, and TBHQ in Brazil. *Food Addit Contam* 2001; 18:365–373.
14. Ishiwata H, Nishijima M, Fukasawa Y. Estimation of inorganic food additive (nitrite, nitrate sulfur dioxide), antioxidant (BHA and BHT), processing agent (propylene glycol) and sweetener (sodium saccharin) concentrations in foods and their daily intake based on official inspection results in Japan in fiscal year 1998. *J Food Hyg Soc Jpn* 2002; 43:49–56.
15. Suh HJ, Chung MS, Cho YH, et al. Estimated daily intakes of butylated hydroxyanisole (BHA), butylated hydroxytoluene (BHT) and tert-butyl hydroquinone (TBHQ) antioxidants in Korea. *Food Addit Contam* 2005; 22:1176–1188.
16. Soubra L, Sarkis D, Hilan C, Verger P. Dietary exposure of children and teenagers to benzoates, sulphites, butylhydroxyanisole (BHA) and butylhydroxytoluene (BHT) in Beirut (Lebanon). *Regul Toxicol Pharmacol* 2007; 47:68–77.
17. Lundebye A-K, Hove H, Måge A, Bohne VJB, Hamre K. Levels of synthetic antioxidants (ethoxyquin, butylated hydroxytoluene and butylated hydroxyanisole) in fish feed and commercially farmed fish. *Food Addit Contam* 2010; 27:1652–1657.
18. Halliwell B, Gutteridge JMC, Cross CE. Free radicals, antioxidants, and human disease: where are we now? *J Lab Clin Med* 1992; 119:598–620.
19. Peng R-X, Lewis KF, Yang CS. Effects of butylated hydroxyanisole on microsomal monooxygenase and drug metabolism. *Acta Pharmacol Sin* 1986; 7:157–161.
20. Verhagen H, Maas LM, Beckers RHG, et al. Effect of subacute oral intake of the food antioxidant butylated hydroxyanisole on clinical parameters and phase-I and phase-II biotransformation capacity in man. *Human Toxicol* 1989; 8: 451–459.
21. Omaye ST, Reddy KA, Cross CE. Effect of butylated hydroxytoluene and other antioxidants on mouse lung metabolism. *J Toxicol Environ Health* 1977; 3:829–836.
22. Williamson D, Esterez P, Witschi H. Studies on the pathogenesis of butylated hydroxytoluene-induced lung damage in mice. *Toxicol Appl Pharmacol* 1978; 43:577–587.
23. Haschek WM, Reiser KM, Klein-Szanto AJP, et al. Potentiation of butylated hydroxytoluene-induced acute lung damage by oxygen: cell kinetics and collagen metabolism. *Am Rev Respir Dis* 1983; 127:28–34.
24. Hakkinen PJ, Schmoyer RL, Witschi HP. Potentiation of butylated-hydroxytoluene-induced acute lung damage by oxygen. Effects of prednisolone and indomethacin. *Am Rev Respir Dis* 1983; 128:648–651.
25. Kehrer JP, Klein-Szanto AJP, Sorensen EMB, Pearlman R, Rosner MH. Enhanced acute lung damage following corticosteroid treatment. *Am Rev Respir Dis* 1984; 130:256–261.
26. Miller ACK, Dwyer LD, Auerbach CE, Miley FB, Dinsdale D, Malkinson AM. Strain-related differences in the pneumotoxic effects of chronically administered butylated hydroxytoluene on protein kinase C and calpain. *Toxicology* 1994; 90: 141–159.
27. Malkinson AM. Review: putative mutagens and carcinogens in foods. III. Butylated hydroxytoluene (BHT). *Environ Mutagen* 1983; 5:353–362.
28. Taniguchi S, Kono T, Mizuno N, et al. Effects of butylated hydroxyanisole on ornithine decarboxylase activity and its gene expression induced by phorbol ester tumor promoter. *J Invest Dermatol* 1991; 96:289–291.
29. Lindenschmidt RC, Tryka AF, Goad ME, Witschi HP. The effects of dietary butylated hydroxytoluene on liver and colon cancer development in mice. *Toxicology* 1986; 38:151–160.
30. Reddy BS, Furuya K, Hanson D, Dibello J, Berke B. Effect of dietary butylated hydroxyanisole on methylazoxymethanol acetate-induced toxicity in mice. *Food Chem Toxicol* 1982; 20:853–859.
31. Moon HJ, Park WH. Butylated hydroxyanisole inhibits the growth of HeLa cervical cancer cells via caspase-dependent apoptosis and GSH depletion. *Mol Cell Biochem* 2011; 349:179–186.
32. Engin AB, Bukan N, Kurukahvecioglu O, Memis L, Engin A. Effect of butylated hydroxytoluene (E321) pretreatment versus L-arginine on liver injury after sub-lethal dose of endotoxin administration. *Environ Toxicol Pharmacol* 2011; 32:457–464.
33. Xiu RJ, Freyschuss A, Ying X, et al. The antioxidant butylated hydroxytoluene prevents early cholesterol-induced microcirculatory changes in rabbits. *J Clin Invest* 1994; 93:2732–2737.
34. Freyschuss A, Al-Schurbaji A, Björkhem I, et al. On the anti-atherogenic effect of the antioxidant BHT in cholesterol-fed rabbits: inverse relation between serum triglycerides and atheromatous lesions. *Biochim Biophys Acta* 2001; 1534:129–138.
35. Klein A, Bruser B. The effect of butylated hydroxytoluene, with and without cortisol, on stimulated lymphocytes. *Life Sci* 1992; 50:883–889.
36. Yamaki K, Taneda S, Yanagisawa R, Inoue K, Takano H, Yoshino S. Enhancement of allergic responses in vivo and in vitro by butylated hydroxytoluene. *Toxicol Appl Pharmacol* 2007; 223:164–172.
37. Fisherman EW, Cohen G. Chemical intolerance to butylated-hydroxyanisole (BHA) and butylated-hydroxytoluene (BHT) and vascular response as an indicator and monitor of drug intolerance. *Ann Allergy* 1973; 31:126–133.
38. Fisherman EW, Cohen GN. Aspirin and other cross-reacting small chemicals in known aspirin intolerant patients. *Ann Allergy* 1973; 31:476–484.

39. Cloninger P, Novey HS. The acute effects of butylated hydroxyanisole ingestion in asthma and rhinitis of unknown etiology. *Ann Allergy* 1974; 32:131–133.
40. Goodman DL, McDonnell JT, Nelson HS, Vaughan TR, Weber RW. Chronic urticaria exacerbated by the antioxidant food preservatives, butylated hydroxyanisole (BHA) and butylated hydroxytoluene (BHT). *J Allergy Clin Immunol* 1990; 86:570–575.
41. Weber RW, Hoffman M, Raine Jr DA, Nelson HS. Incidence of bronchoconstriction due to aspirin, azo dyes, non-azo dyes, and preservatives in a population of perennial asthmatics. *J Allergy Clin Immunol* 1979; 64:32–37.
42. Thune P, Granholt A. Provocation tests with antiphlogistica and food additives in recurrent urticaria. *Dermatologica* 1975; 151:360–367.
43. Fisherman EW, Cohen GN. Chronic and recurrent urticaria: new concepts of drug-group sensitivity. *Ann Allergy* 1977; 39:404–414.
44. Juhlin L. Clinical studies on the diagnosis and treatment of urticaria. *Ann Allergy* 1977; 39:356–361.
45. Juhlin L. Recurrent urticaria: clinical investigation of 330 patients. *Br J Dermatol* 1981; 104:369–381.
46. Hannuksela M, Lahti A. Peroral challenge tests with food additives in urticaria and atopic dermatitis. *Int J Dermatol* 1986; 25:178–180.
47. Moore-Robinson M, Warin RP. Effect of salicylates in urticaria. *Br Med J* 1967; 4:262–264.
48. Osmundsen PE. Contact urticaria from nickel and plastic additives (butylhydroxytoluene, oleylamide). *Contact Dermat* 1980; 6:452–454.
49. Manning ME, Stevenson DD, Mathison DA. Reactions to aspirin and other nonsteroidal anti-inflammatory drugs. *Immunol Allergy Clin N Am* 1992; 12:611–631.
50. Stevenson DD, Simon RA, Lumry WR, Mathison DA. Adverse reactions to tartrazine. *J Allergy Clin Immunol* 1986; 78:182–191.
51. Tosti A, Bardazzi F, Valeri F, Russo R. Contact dermatitis from butylated hydroxyanisole. *Contact Dermat* 1987; 17:257–258.
52. Rich P, Belozer ML, Norris P, Storrs FJ. Allergic contact dermatitis to two antioxidants in latex gloves: 4,4'-thiobis (6-*tert*-butyl-*meta*-cresol) (Lowinox 44S36) and butylhydroxyanisole. Allergen alternatives for glove-allergic patients. *J Am Acad Dermatol* 1991; 24:37–43.
53. Acciai MC, Brusi C, Francalanci S, Giorgini S, Sertoli A. Allergic contact dermatitis in caterers. *Contact Dermat* 1993; 28:48.
54. Lewis FM, Harrington CI, Gawkrodger DJ. Contact sensitivity in pruritus vulvae: a common and manageable problem. *Contact Dermat* 1994; 31:264–265.
55. Roed-Petersen J, Hjorth N. Contact dermatitis from antioxidants: hidden sensitizers in topical medications and foods. *Br J Dermatol* 1976; 94:233–241.
56. Veien NK, Krogdahl A. Cutaneous vasculitis induced by food additives. *Acta Dermatol Venereol* 1991; 71:73–74.
57. Moneret-Vautrin DA, Faure G, Bene MC. Chewing-gum preservative induced toxidermic vasculitis. *Allergy* 1986; 41:546–548.
58. Murdoch RD, Lessof MH, Pollock I, Young E. Effects of food additives on leukocyte histamine release in normal and urticaria subjects. *J Royal Coll Phys Lond* 1987; 21:251–256.

33 Adverse Reactions to Benzoates and Parabens

Raymond M. Pongonis & John M. Fahrenholz
Division of Allergy, Pulmonary, and Critical Care Medicine, Vanderbilt University Medical Center, Nashville, TN, USA

Key Concepts

- Benzoates and parabens are used extensively as chemical preservatives in foods and beverages throughout much of the developed world and have essentially no toxicity at approved concentrations.
- Although investigated frequently in association with chronic urticaria, well-designed studies place the incidence of benzoate- and paraben-induced urticaria/angioedema at 2–3% of all cases.
- Well-designed trials have not provided a conclusive link between persistent asthma and benzoates or parabens.
- Some studies have implicated food additives including benzoates in provoking atopic dermatitis in a minority of patients. A potential mechanism may be via increased production of leukotrienes.
- Anaphylactic-type reactions have been rarely reported with ingested benzoates. Paraben ingestion to our knowledge has not been reported as a potential cause of anaphylaxis.
- A variety of other adverse reactions to benzoates and parabens have been reported ranging from cutaneous vasculitis to rhinitis to hyperactivity in children. Additional studies are needed to confirm these associations.

Benzoic acid and sodium benzoate (benzoates) are widely used as antimycotic agents and antibacterial preservatives in foods and beverages. The methyl, *n*-propyl, *n*-butyl, and *n*-heptyl esters of *para*-hydroxybenzoic acid (collectively referred to as parabens) are utilized as preservatives in a limited number of foods and beverages. Parabens, however, are used extensively as preservatives in pharmaceuticals and cosmetics. Benzoic acid, sodium benzoate, methylparaben, propylparaben, and heptylparaben are approved as direct food additives by the U.S. Food and Drug Administration (FDA) and have generally been recognized as safe (GRAS) status [1].

Benzoates and parabens as food and beverage additives

Benzoates have been used since the early 1900s as preservatives in foods and beverages. Annual consumption worldwide has been estimated at greater than 10 million pounds, making benzoates one of the most commonly used additives. Benzoates have a broad range of antimicrobial activity, exhibit little or no toxicity in the concentrations used for food applications, and are relatively inexpensive to produce.

The chemical structures of benzoic acid and sodium benzoate are shown in Figure 33.1. Benzoic acid is a white crystalline solid with an acidic pH and limited water solubility [2]. Sodium benzoate is a white crystalline powder with alkaline pH that readily dissolves in water [3]. When sodium benzoate is dissolved in acidic solutions, it is partially converted to the free acid. Benzoates appear to be most effective as antimicrobial agents at acidic pH.

Benzoates are widely distributed in nature in the form of the free acid or as simple salts, esters, and amides. They occur naturally in prunes, cinnamon, cloves, tea, anise, and many berries. Raspberries and cranberries contain up to 0.05% by weight [2, 4]. Benzoates as preservatives are found in alcoholic beverages, fruit juices, soft drinks, baked goods, cheeses, gum, condiments, frozen dairy products, relishes, and sugar substitutes to name a few. Orally administered benzoates are rapidly absorbed through the intestine and transported to the liver. Benzoate is converted to a thioester with coenzyme A to form

Food Allergy: Adverse Reactions to Foods and Food Additives, Fifth Edition. Edited by Dean D Metcalfe, Hugh A Sampson, Ronald A Simon and Gideon Lack.

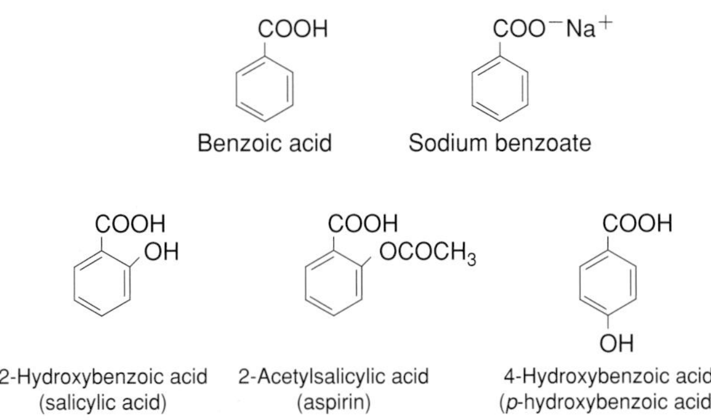

Figure 33.1 Benzoates and closely related conveners.

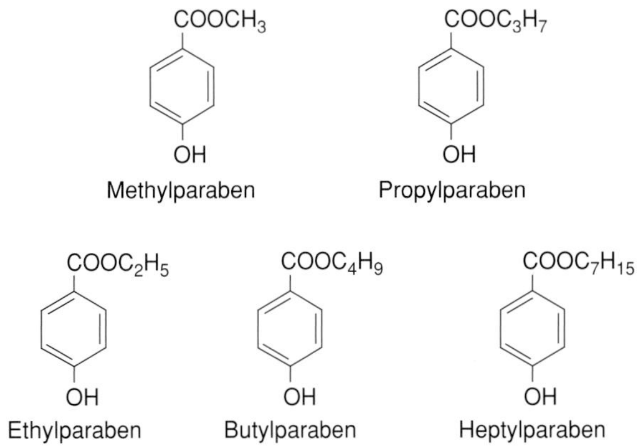

benzoyl-CoA. Benzoyl-CoA then reacts with glycine to form hippuric acid, which is excreted in the urine.

The use of parabens as antimicrobial agents in pharmaceuticals, cosmetics, and food began in Europe in the 1920s and spread to the United States in the 1930s. While primarily used as preservatives in pharmaceuticals and cosmetics, parabens are also approved for use in foods by the FDA, the European Community, the Joint FAO/WHO Expert Committee on Food Additives, and the regulatory agencies of several other countries. Methylparaben and propylparaben are the forms most commonly used as food additives. Parabens are contained in coffee extracts, fruit juices, pickles, sauces, soft drinks, processed vegetables, baked goods, fats and oils, seasonings, sugar substitutes, and frozen dairy products. Concentrations vary between 450 and 2000 ppm. The use limit for parabens as chemical preservatives in foods is 0.1%. Parabens are not described as occurring naturally in nature. Oral administration normally results in rapid absorption and subsequent hydrolyzation to *p*-hydroxybenzoic acid. Glycine, glucuronic acid, and sulfuric acid conjugates are then formed and all are eliminated in the urine [5]. Toxicity studies have demonstrated little or no adverse effects either acutely or chronically at doses far exceeding the current acceptable daily intake of 55 mg/kg/day [6].

The chemical structures of the parabens are shown in Figure 33.2. They are white crystalline or powder solids that have essentially no odor or taste. Bactericidal activity is present over a wide pH range in contrast to the benzoates [7]. Methylparaben has antimicrobial properties against cold-tolerant bacteria and has been used frequently as a preservative in prepared chilled foods [8].

Benzoates, parabens, and associations with chronic urticaria–angioedema

The prevalence of reactions to food additives in the setting of chronic urticaria has been studied frequently. Unfortunately, due to design issues with oral challenge studies in

Figure 33.2 The paraben family of food additives.

this patient population, variable study design, and the lack of adequate controls in many studies, the prevalence of such reactions has not been definitively elucidated. Design considerations in food additive challenge studies are of critical importance. Selection of patients may include, for example, all patients with a history of chronic idiopathic urticaria, only those with histories suggestive of food additive reactions, or only those patients who appeared to improve on an additive-free diet. Depending on the selection criteria, different percentages of positive reactors have been reported. These variables have not been explicitly stated in many reports and add confusion to the already difficult task of comparing studies.

The relative activity or inactivity of the urticaria at the time of challenge appears to be a key factor. In a study by Lumry et al. [9], only 1 of 15 patients whose urticaria was in remission experienced a reaction to aspirin (ASA). However, 7 of 10 patients whose urticaria was active at the time of challenge reacted to ASA. These challenges were performed using semi-quantitative reaction criteria. Reactions were judged in comparison to a baseline observation period in each individual patient.

In most reported studies, a period of baseline observation for comparison with reaction data was never made. Further, most challenge studies report loosely defined criteria for identifying urticarial responses. Other potential confounding factors include discontinuation of medications (particularly antihistamines), timing, and the number of placebo challenges and additive doses. Finally, the importance of the double-blind challenge cannot be overemphasized. A more detailed description of design considerations for oral challenge protocols in chronic urticaria–angioedema can be found elsewhere in this book.

One of the earliest open additive challenge studies in chronic urticaria patients was reported by Doeglas [10]. He observed that "four or five" of 23 patients reacted to sodium benzoate. Placebo-controlled challenges were not performed. Patients with physical urticarias were included.

Thune and Granholt [11] reported that 2 of 32 patients reacted to parabens while 4 of 41 patients reacted to benzoates after oral challenge. Overall, 62 of 100 patients reacted to at least 1 of 22 different additives used in the challenges. Again, placebo controls were not utilized making any firm conclusions difficult to support.

A study performed by Juhlin [12], involved single-blind challenges using multiple additives. The prevalence of benzoate hypersensitivity was reported to be 11% among 172 participants. Overall, one or more positive reactions were observed in 31% of patients. This study utilized only a single administration of placebo, which was always given first, followed by multiple additive challenges. Reaction criteria were subjective and were determined to be "uncertain" in 33% of patients. Previous studies by the same group reported a prevalence range of 44–60% for benzoate hypersensitivity in chronic urticaria patients [13, 14]. Due to study design limitations, firm conclusions are again difficult to support.

Supramaniam and Warner [15] reported that 4 of 27 children with urticaria reacted to sodium benzoate. Overall, 24 out of 43 children reacted to one or more additives. The study did utilize a double-blind challenge design. However, only one placebo was interspersed with nine different additives, and a baseline observation period to determine the relative activity of the chronic urticaria was not utilized. Whether antihistamines were withheld or continued was not mentioned. Genton et al. [16] also reported a significant reaction rate to benzoates in single-blind additive challenges in 17 patients with chronic urticaria and/or angioedema. Among these patients, 5 of 17 reacted to successive doses of sodium benzoate (10, 50, 250, and 500 mg). Urticaria developed in 15 of the 17 patients after at least one of the six additives used. If urticaria or angioedema were "noticed by a physician during the 18-hour period after the test," the challenge was considered positive. All patients considered for the study were observed to have had "sufficient improvement" in their disease while on a 2-week elimination diet (free of additives). Explicit baseline disease activity was not reported.

Ortolani et al. [17] studied 396 patients with chronic urticaria and angioedema. Based on history, 179 patients were considered for treatment with an elimination diet and 135 elected to proceed. Eighty-seven of the 135 patients had an 80% or greater reduction in urticaria symptom scores during the 2-week elimination diet compared to the 2-week baseline observation period. Only 8 of the 87 patients who had improved on the elimination diet had a positive double-blind challenge to foods. Of the 79 patients who did not react to foods, 72 underwent double-blind placebo-controlled (DBPC) oral food additive challenges. Three of the 72 subjects had urticarial reactions with sodium benzoate (60, 410, and 410 mg). Twelve of the 72 patients reacted to one or more additives including tartrazine and sodium metabisulfite. Parabens were not tested.

Hannuksela and Lahti [18] reported 1 of 44 patients reacted to benzoic acid in a DBPC challenge study. One of the 44 patients also reacted to placebo. Several other food additives were tested in this study but no other reactions were observed. In a study with similar design, Kellett et al. [19] reported that 10% of 44 chronic idiopathic urticaria patients reacted to benzoates and/or tartrazine. Ten percent also reacted to placebo.

Simon [20] studied 65 patients with active chronic idiopathic urticaria who continued antihistamines at the minimum effective dosage. Twenty of the participants reported a history of adverse reactions to additives. A baseline urticaria skin score was obtained in each patient using a semi-quantitative method utilizing the "Rule of Nines." Initially, participants were challenged with capsules containing multiple additives (including benzoates and parabens) or placebo in a single-blind fashion. Two of the participants had positive additive reactions. These two individuals were then rechallenged utilizing a DBPC design at least 2 weeks later. Neither of them had a positive reaction. The author concluded with 95% confidence limits that the prevalence of additive sensitivity in patients with active chronic idiopathic urticaria is somewhere between 0% and 3%. A different study by Nettis et al. [21] also found the prevalence of sodium benzoate-induced urticaria/angioedema to be 2%. The Nettis study included 47 patients who had reported episodes of acute urticaria with or without angioedema after ingesting products containing sodium benzoate. The patients underwent skin prick tests for common inhalant and food allergens in addition to measures of serum-specific IgE to common food allergens. Allergy testing revealed five subjects (11%) with at least one positive reaction to an IgE test for food. The patients then underwent DBPC challenges with sodium benzoate. A placebo was given on day 1 followed by either placebo or sodium benzoate 48 hours later on day 3. A washout day was allowed followed by either placebo or sodium benzoate on day 5. The sodium benzoate was given at increasing dosage from 25 to 50 mg and finally 100 mg with 2 hours of time after each dose. The patients were monitored closely but only the appearance of urticaria and/or angioedema were considered positive responses. Only one subject (2%) had a reaction after ingestion of sodium benzoate. The patient had an atopic history but negative IgE tests for food extracts and did not react to placebo. Her reaction consisted of urticarial lesions 40 minutes after ingestion of 50 mg of sodium benzoate. Based on history of prior reactions, the patient underwent DBPC food challenges with suspected foods and all were negative. The patient then agreed to undergo a second confirmatory DBPC challenge 2 weeks later, and again had a positive response to sodium benzoate with urticaria.

This study evaluated patients with a history of acute, not chronic urticarial reactions to food additives and found the prevalence of urticaria/angioedema reactions to sodium benzoate to be very low at 2%.

Several studies have utilized an elimination diet approach in their evaluation of food additive contributions to chronic urticaria. Unfortunately, no blind or placebo studies of this type have been reported. The Ros study [14] reported an additive-free diet to be "completely helpful" in 24% of patients with chronic urticaria. Another 57% of patients were "much improved," 19% were "slightly better" or had experienced "no change." Rudzki et al. [22] observed clinical response to a diet free of salicylates, benzoates, and azo dyes in 50 of 158 patients. These studies did not investigate which particular additive was potentially inducing or exacerbating the urticaria.

Gibson and Clancy [23] reported the use of an elimination diet in 69 patients with chronic idiopathic urticaria (symptoms present for greater than 3 months; physical urticarias excluded). They found that 54 of the patients experienced complete remission within 2–4 weeks of beginning the diet. Challenge studies using multiple additives revealed that 34% reacted to benzoates. An initial placebo tablet was utilized in the challenges; blinding was not mentioned. Twelve patients agreed to rechallenge after remaining in complete remission for 1 year on the elimination diet. Three of the four in this group who had initially reacted to benzoates remained positive to benzoate challenge at 1 year. None of the three patients who had reacted initially to tartrazine remained positive at 1 year.

Ehlers et al. [24] evaluated the response to an elimination diet in 16 children with chronic urticaria (at least 3 months duration). Nine of the 16 children were free of symptoms within 10 days of beginning the diet. An additional three patients "improved considerably." Six of the patients who responded to the diet were challenged in a DBPC fashion. Details of the challenge protocol and criteria for positive reactions were not discussed. Five of the six patients reacted to at least one of the additives. Four of them reacted to multiples additives (three or more). Parabens elicited reactions in three of the six. Benzoic acid caused a reaction in one of the six. The authors suggested that additives appear to play a significant role in pediatric chronic urticaria, a relatively uncommon condition.

Malanin and Kalimo [25] evaluated the utility of skin testing with additives in chronic urticaria patients. Ninety-one subjects were skin tested with 18 food additives. Twenty-four subjects had at least one histamine equivalent positive food additive skin test. Ten of the 24 participants with a positive skin test underwent oral food additive challenges with the suspected additive(s). Only one had a positive challenge (benzoic acid). Overall, significantly more patients with positive skin tests responded to an elimination diet (16 of 18 with positive skin tests versus 17 of 42 with negative skin tests.) The authors proposed non-IgE-mediated skin hyperreactivity as the mechanism for skin test-positive reactions. The pathogenesis of additive reactions is presently unknown.

In summary, oral challenge studies with food additives in the setting of chronic urticaria–angioedema present many design challenges. Meticulously designed studies which utilize DBPC challenge such as the Ortalani study and the Simon study suggest that benzoates and parabens are uncommon provoking or exacerbating factors. In selected patients, a trial of an additive-free diet may be warranted followed by systematic reintroduction of additive-containing foods if significant clinical improvement was observed. DBPC additive challenges could then be utilized to diagnose the particular additive sensitivity if clinically appropriate.

Benzoates, parabens, and associations with asthma

The prevalence of asthmatic reactions to food additives in the general population or select groups such as atopic asthmatics has not been definitively defined. Nevertheless, several studies suggest that such reactions are unusual. Weber and colleagues evaluated aspirin and additive sensitivity in a group of 43 patients with moderate to severe persistent asthma [26]. In the initial single-blind challenges, two showed a positive response (decrease in FEV_1 of 25% or more from baseline) to benzoates and parabens. Only one (2%) of the patients remained positive during double-blind testing. The prevalence of tartrazine sensitivity in this study was 16% during initial open challenges. This fell to 0% during subsequent double-blind challenges. Of note, bronchodilator medication was not withheld in the majority of patients because a number of apparent false-positive reactions had been obtained earlier in the study when these medications were withheld. This study emphasizes the importance of the double-blind challenge and observing a relatively stable baseline FEV_1 prior to the initiation of challenges in patients with persistent asthma.

Tarlo and Broder found only one patient with sodium benzoate hypersensitivity (FEV_1 fall of more than 20% from baseline) among 28 patients with persistent asthma [27]. The protocol utilized a DBPC design and medications were not withheld. Of note, clinical improvement of this patient's asthma was not observed when benzoates were removed from the diet. Osterhalle et al. performed initial open multiple additive challenges in 46 children with persistent asthma [28]. Eleven of the 46 showed positive reactions (FEV_1 decrease greater than 20% of baseline). Confirmatory DBPC challenges gave only three positive responders.

Genton and associates found 1 of 17 asthmatic patients who reacted to sodium benzoate in a single-blind, randomized placebo-controlled study [16]. García et al. reported no reactions to sodium benzoate among 62 patients with steroid-dependent asthma [29]. Not surprisingly, other less rigorously controlled studies have reported more widely varying rates of asthmatic reactions to food additives [30, 31].

Similar to chronic urticaria, some authors have suggested an additive-free diet is useful in selected persistent asthmatic patients [32]. This approach has not been evaluated in published controlled trials.

Benzoates, parabens, and anaphylaxis

Relatively few reports of possible anaphylactic/anaphylactoid reactions have appeared in the medical literature. Given the widespread consumption of these preservatives, one can conclude that such reactions are exceedingly rare. In 1944, Kinsey and Wright reported an "anaphylactoid-type" reaction in an individual 4 hours after he had received a 6 g oral dose of sodium benzoate to evaluate liver function [33]. The following day, identical symptoms of "shock" developed within 4 hours of another 6 g sodium benzoate dose. Michels et al. reported the case of a young woman who developed "flush, angioedema and severe hypotension (systolic blood pressure under 50 mmHg)" 30 minutes after eating a meal containing sodium benzoate as a food preservative [34]. One week earlier she had experienced "generalized itching" after eating cheese, which also contained benzoates. A placebo-controlled challenge with 20 mg of oral sodium benzoate produced urticaria confined to her arms and generalized pruritus. A second challenge, apparently several days later after treatment of a sinus infection, resulted in only "mild localized itching" after ingestion of 160 mg of sodium benzoate. Neither of the above cases provides conclusive evidence of systemic anaphylaxis related to ingested benzoates.

Orally ingested parabens have not (to our knowledge) been reported to cause systemic anaphylaxis. Nagel et al. did report a case of bronchospasm and generalized pruritus associated with administration of intravenous steroids containing parabens in an asthmatic child [35]. Intravenous steroids without paraben preservatives did not induce any symptoms. Skin testing to individual parabens, as well as passive transfer tests, was positive. Skin testing with the steroid preparations with and without parabens provided further evidence of a hypersensitivity reaction induced by the paraben preservatives. Carr [36] reported two cases of hypotension and diffuse macular rash potentially associated with paraben preservatives contained in a topical lignocaine preparation used for intraurethral anesthesia prior to cystoscopy. One of the patients tolerated a preservative-free topical lignocaine preparation 2 months after his initial reaction. No mention was made concerning whether or not the second patient was able to tolerate a preservative-free preparation.

Benzoates, parabens, and dermatitis

The development of contact dermatitis associated with topical parabens used in cosmetics and other skin care products has been reported extensively in the literature dating back to 1940 [5]. A loosely controlled study by Veien et al. [37] evaluated the possibility of oral paraben ingestion as an exacerbating factor in patients with chronic "dermatitis" and contact paraben sensitivity diagnosed by patch testing. Two of 14 patients reported flares of their "usual dermatitis" within 24 hours of ingesting parabens; placebo challenges were negative. These two patients were subsequently followed on an elimination diet for 1– 2 months. Neither the patients nor the physicians noted any significant improvement. Perioral contact urticaria has been reported in association with sodium benzoate in a toothpaste [38]. Overall, reported contact reactions to benzoates are rare in comparison to the parabens.

The potential role of ingested benzoates or parabens in atopic dermatitis has received limited attention in the medical literature. Van Bever et al. [39] investigated the role of food and food additives in 25 children with severe atopic dermatitis. All of the children were hospitalized and received an elemental diet by nasogastric tube. Topical therapy was continued in the hospital setting. All children were reported to be "almost free of active eczema" after 1–2 weeks of the elemental diet and topical therapy. Selective DBPC food and food additive challenges were performed after 1 week of the observed clinical improvement. Six of the children were challenged with sodium benzoate and three "reacted." The reactions consisted of "pruritus and redness of the skin" which had apparently resolved within the 4-hour period of observation post challenge since no "late reactions" were seen. Exacerbations of underlying atopic dermatitis related to challenges were not reported. Any skin findings lasting more than 4 hours were not observed after any food or food additive challenge. Nevertheless, the authors reported that 24 of the 25 children "reacted" to one or more foods, and all children who were challenged with additives "reacted" to at least one. Clearly, reaction criteria were among the major sources of concern within the study. This study has also been criticized because no placebo reactions occurred after 132 placebo challenges. Hannuksela and Lahti had observed equivalent reaction rates between placebo and active substances in patients with chronic urticaria and atopic dermatitis in an earlier study [18].

Worm et al. have performed two carefully designed studies that provide evidence of a link between food additives and atopic dermatitis. In the initial study [40], 50 patients with atopic dermatitis were monitored while eating their usual diet for 4 weeks. Baseline atopic dermatitis skin status scores were obtained using a variation of the Costa method. In phase 2, 41 of the patients followed an elimination diet for 6 weeks. At the end of the dietary intervention phase, 26 of the 41 patients showed an improvement in their skin status scores of greater than 35%. Open oral provocation tests with an additive-rich diet given over a period of 2 days were performed in 24 of the 26 responders (two refused). The open diet challenge resulted in positive reactions (worsening of the Costa score above 10 points within 48 hours) in 19 of the 24 patients. The authors reported no immediate reactions but rather solely late-phase reactions typically occurring between 24 and 48 hours. Ten patients who had not responded to the dietary intervention also underwent the open challenge as a control group. None of the control patients reacted. In 15 of the 19 patients reacting to the open challenge, DBPC oral food additive challenges were performed. The additives given together in a single capsule included sodium benzoate, *p*-hydroxybenzoate, azo dyes, BHA/BHT, and others. Six of 15 patients reacted to the additive challenge given as a single dose followed by a 48-hour observation period. One patient reacted to placebo. Additives were not tested individually.

In the second study [41], the authors set out to determine food-additive-induced sulfidoleukotriene production by leukocytes isolated from the peripheral blood of the group of patients who had positive DBPC oral food additive challenges and to compare these values with both atopic and nonatopic controls. Cysteinyl leukotrienes are potent inflammatory mediators, and studies have shown biologically active amounts of leukotrienes present in the skin of atopic dermatitis patients [42]. The study evaluated three groups of patients. Group A ($n = 10$) included nonatopic donors whereas groups B and C included patients suffering from atopic dermatitis. Group B patients ($n = 9$) were those who had improved Costa skin scores after following an elimination diet for 6 weeks but who did not show a positive response to DBPC food challenge with food additives. Group C patients ($n = 9$) included patients similar to group B except who did react to DBPC food challenge with food additives. Peripheral leukocytes were obtained from each patient of the three groups and incubated with the food additives (food color mix, tartrazine, nitrite, benzoate, metabisulfite, and salicylate) after priming with IL-3. The authors found that baseline sulfidoleukotriene production in the nonatopic group A was significantly lower than that of the atopic groups B and C. No significant baseline differences were noted between atopic groups in this measure. None of the nonatopic group A controls showed increased sulfidoleukotriene production in the presence of any of the food additives used. However, in atopic dermatitis patients with negative food challenges (group B), a modest induction of sulfidoleukotriene production was determined in one patient using tartrazine and two patients using nitrites. Group C patients (atopic dermatitis with positive food challenge) showed seven of the nine patients with increased sulfidoleukotriene production in the presence of different food additives, the most frequent additives implicated being nitrite (5/9 patients), benzoate (4/9), and tartrazine (3/9).

The more recent study assessing for a causative relationship between food additives and adverse dermatologic reactions such as eczema, urticaria, and angioedema and the utility of diagnostic testing in these circumstances was performed in a Korean study by Park et al. [43]. The researchers recruited 54 people at random with a history of atopic disease to undergo skin prick, patch test, and DBPC food challenge to seven different food additives, including sodium benzoate. Of the 54 patients, 5 were positive on either skin prick or patch testing to one of the seven additives. However, these results were not predictive of positivity to oral challenge with a mixture of the seven additives. Interestingly, there was one patient who was positive on skin prick testing to a nonirritating concentration of sodium benzoate and went on to develop urticaria following blinded ingestion of the seven preservative mixtures that included sodium benzoate and did not react to placebo. This was the only such patient and only such additive out of 54 patients and 7 additives that exhibited this direct correlation. An additional patient was positive on skin prick testing to multiple additives, including benzoate, but reacted to both placebo and the additive mixture. In general, the authors concluded that the mixture of seven common food additives did not cause adverse reactions or aggravate atopic dermatitis symptoms in patients with allergic disease.

Miscellaneous reactions

Isolated case reports appear in the literature suggesting symptoms ranging from depression to rhinitis may be related to benzoate ingestion in certain individuals [44]. A study by Pacor et al. [45] enrolled 226 patients with persistent rhinitis categorized as moderate to severe (symptoms present more than 4 days a week and longer than 4 weeks). Patients with asthma, positive skin prick results, a history of smoking, recent corticosteroid use, and other medical conditions were excluded. Each patient underwent a 30-day additive-free diet and recorded daily rhinitis symptom scores. At the end of the diet, each patient was reintroduced to a food additive-rich diet for 15 days, again with daily recording of rhinitis symptom scores.

Finally, each patient then underwent a DBPC food additive challenge with three different doses of each additive including tartrazine, erythrosine, monosodium benzoate, *p*-hydroxybenzoate, sodium metabisulphite, and MSG. Evaluation of the food additive challenge was performed subjectively by patient report of rhinitis symptoms and objectively by nasal peak inspiratory flow rate, where decline of 20% in the flow rate was considered positive. Twenty patients (8.8%) reported statistically significant improvement in their daily rhinitis symptom scores while on the food additive elimination diet, with 6 of these patients (2.6%) reporting no symptoms at all. These same 20 patients showed a positive DBPC food challenge with monosodium benzoate as evidenced by reduction in nasal peak inspiratory flow rate by at least 20%. In this study, monosodium benzoate was the only food additive tested that was found to result in a positive oral challenge. All 20 subjects documented return of their rhinitis symptoms during the food-additive-rich diet.

Cutaneous vasculitis has been reported occasionally in association with sodium benzoate ingestion [44, 46, 47]. In two of these reports the patients also had microhematuria. Challenge tests were reported to be associated with cutaneous vasculitic lesions and the patients improved with dietary intervention. A study by Lunardi et al. evaluated the effects of an elimination diet in five patients with biopsy-proven leukocytoclastic cutaneous vasculitis [47]. Evidence for an associated autoimmune disorder, infection, or neoplastic disease was not found. All patients improved on the elimination diet; four showed complete resolution of their skin lesions. All patients "reacted" to at least one food or food additive. Patients were asked to record skin scores on a daily diary. One of the patients reacted to benzoates. The authors reported that with elimination of the offending foods and/or food additives, no relapses were seen in 2 years of follow-up.

The Melkersson–Rosenthal syndrome is a rare disorder characterized by recurrent or persistent orofacial edema, which typically involves the lips, variable facial paralysis, and lingua plicata (fissuring of the tongue) [48]. The syndrome's etiology is unknown but is reported to be more common in atopic individuals. A few reports have suggested that food additives, including benzoates, may play a role [48–52]. However, another investigation using DBPC challenges in six patients found no evidence of food or food additive sensitivity [53].

There has been some interest in linking the prevalence of hyperactivity in children to food additive intolerance. The initial reports linked hyperactivity to artificial food flavors and colors [54]. A large study of 3-year-old children from the Isle of Wight, UK, attempted to address the possible link between food additives and hyperactivity in children in a population-based study [55]. The study was designed to test the hypothesis that food additives have a pharmacological effect on behavior that is irrespective of other characteristics of the child, specifically hyperactivity at baseline and atopy. Bateman et al. attempted to enroll all children resident on the Isle of Wight with birth dates in a specified date range who were registered with a general practitioner. Phase 1 of the trial involved screening with a behavioral questionnaire and was followed by skin prick testing for atopy (phase 2). A total of 397 children were selected to enter the challenge stage of the trial, phase 3. Based on results of the behavior questionnaire and skin prick testing, the children were divided into four groups: hyperactive/atopic, not hyperactive/atopic, hyperactive/not atopic, and not hyperactive/not atopic. After assessment, each group was subjected to a diet eliminating artificial colorings and benzoate preservatives for 1 week. In the subsequent 3 weeks, the subjects underwent a double-blind crossover study where they received periods of dietary challenge with a drink containing artificial colorings and sodium benzoate or a placebo mixture. Behavior was then assessed by a tester blind to the subjects' dietary status and by parent's ratings. The study found significant reductions in hyperactive behavior during the additive-free diet phase by parental report. There were also significantly greater increases in hyperactive behavior during the additive versus placebo period based on parental reports. There was no correlation with presence or absence of hyperactivity either at baseline or in the presence of atopy. The authors concluded that there is a general adverse effect of artificial food coloring and benzoate preservatives on the behavior of 3-year-old children. However, there are aspects of the study that make it difficult to interpret. There were a significant number of dietary mistakes reported where children consumed products that contained preservatives and/or artificial colorings. Also, research psychologists using validated tests were unable to associate the subjects' hyperactivity with consumption of the additive drink versus placebo. Further study of the relationship between childhood hyperactivity and food additives needs to be carried out before any firm conclusions can be made.

Summary and conclusions

Benzoates and parabens are used extensively as chemical preservatives in foods and beverages in the United States and throughout much of the developed world. These compounds have essentially no toxicity at approved concentrations and considering their widespread consumption are well tolerated. Benzoates and parabens have been investigated frequently in association with chronic urticaria–angioedema. Many studies with less stringent design criteria have implicated these agents, particularly the benzoates, as relatively frequent exacerbating factors. On the other hand, more rigorously designed protocols suggest that these chemicals are unusual provoking or exacerbating agents among urticaria patients.

Asthmatic reactions have also been reported and investigated in association with food additives including benzoates and parabens. Well-designed trials have not provided a conclusive link between persistent asthma and benzoates or parabens.

The association of atopic dermatitis with food additives has received relatively limited attention in the medical literature. No well-designed study has implicated benzoates or parabens individually as pathogenic factors. Studies by Worm et al. using multiple food additives including benzoates provide evidence that at least some of these substances may be provoking factors in a minority of patients and a potential mechanism may be increased production of leukotrienes.

Rarely, anaphylactic-type reactions have been reported with ingested benzoates but definitive evidence of systemic anaphylaxis is lacking. Oral parabens have not been reported as potential causes of anaphylaxis. However, parabens have been implicated in systemic reactions related to their use in pharmaceutical agents, particularly local anesthetic preparations. Other miscellaneous reports have appeared suggesting benzoates as occasional inciting agents in cutaneous vasculitis.

Reports of hyperactivity in children induced by food additives have been present in the literature for several decades, but further study is needed to confirm this association.

References

1. U.S. Food and Drug Administration [FDA]. *Everything Added to Food in the U.S.* Boca Raton, FL: C.K. Smoley, 1993; p. 149.
2. Williams AE. Benzoic acid. In: *Kirk-Othmer Encyclopedia of Chemical Technology*. 1978, New York: Wiley-Interscience, 1978; pp. 778–792.
3. Lueck E. *Antimicrobial Food Additives*. New York: Springer-Verlag, 1980.
4. Juhlin L. Intolerance to food additives. In: Marzulli FM, Maibach HI (eds), *Advances in Modern Toxicology, Dermatotoxicology and Pharmacology*, vol. 4. New York: John Wiley & Sons Inc., 1977; pp. 455–463.
5. Elder RL. Final report on the safety assessment of methylparaben, ethylparaben, propylparaben and butylparaben. *J Am Coll Toxicol* 1984; 3:147–209.
6. Soni MG, Burdock GA, Taylor SL, Greenberg NA. Safety assessment of propyl paraben: a review of the published literature. *Food Chem Toxicol* 2001; 39:513–532.
7. Aalto TR, Foirman MC, Rigler NE. p-Hydroxybenzoic acid esters as preservatives. I. Uses, antibacterial and antifungal studies, properties and determination. *J Am Pharm Assoc* 1953; 42:449–457.
8. Moir CJ, Eyles MJ. Inhibition, injury, and inactivation of four psychotrophic foodborne bacteria by the preservatives methyl p-hydroxybenzoate and potassium sorbate. *J Food Prot* 1992; 55:360–366.
9. Lumry WR, Mathison DA, Stevenson DD, Curd JC. Aspirin in chronic urticaria and/or angioedema: studies of sensitivity and desensitization. *J Allergy Clin Immunol* 1982; 69(Suppl.):135
10. Doeglas HMG. Reactions to aspirin and food additives in patients with chronic urticaria, including the physical urticarias. *Br J Dermatol* 1975; 93:135–144.
11. Thune P, Granholt A. Provocation tests with antiphlogistic and food additives in recurrent urticaria. *Dermatologica* 1975; 151:360–367.
12. Juhlin L. Recurrent urticaria: clinical investigation of 330 patients. *Br J Dermatol* 1981; 104:369–381.
13. Michaelsson G, Juhlin L. Urticaria induced by preservatives and dye additives in food and drugs. *Br J Dermatol* 1973; 88:525–532.
14. Ros AM, Juhlin L, Michaelsson G. A follow-up study of patients with recurrent urticaria and hypersensitivity to aspirin, benzoates and azo dyes. *Br J Dermatol* 1976; 95:19–24.
15. Supramaniam G, Warner JO. Artificial food additive intolerance in patients with angio-oedema and urticaria. *Lancet* 1986; 2:907–909.
16. Genton C, Frei PC, Pecond A. Value of oral provocation tests to aspirin and food additives in the routine investigation of asthma and chronic urticaria. *J Allergy Clin Immunol* 1985; 76:40–45.
17. Ortolani C, Pastorello E, Luraghi MT, Della-Torre F, Bellani M, Zanussi C. Diagnosis of intolerance to food additives. *Ann Allergy* 1984; 53:587–591.
18. Hannuksela M, Lahti A. Peroral challenge tests with food additives in urticaria and atopic dermatitis. *Int J Dermatol* 1986; 25(3):178–180.
19. Kellett JK, August PJ, Beck MH. Double-blind challenge tests with food additives in chronic urticaria. *Br J Dermatol* 1984; 111(Suppl.):32.
20. Simon RA. Additive-induced urticaria: experience with monosodium glutamate. *J Nutr* 2000; 130:1063S–1066S.
21. Nettis E, Colanardi MC, Ferrannini A, Tursi A. Sodium benzoate-induced repeated episodes of acute urticaria/angio-oedema: randomized controlled trial. *Br J Dermatol* 2004; 151(4):898–902.
22. Rudzki E, Czubalski K, Grzywa Z. Detection of urticaria with food additive intolerance by means of diet. *Dermatologica* 1980; 161:57–62.
23. Gibson A, Clancy R. Management of chronic idiopathic urticaria by the identification and exclusion of dietary factors. *Clin Allergy* 1980; 10:699–704.
24. Ehlers I, Niggemann B, Binder C, Zuberbier T. Role of non-allergic hypersensitivity reactions in children with chronic urticaria. *Allergy* 1998; 53:1074–1077.
25. Malanin G, Kalimo K. The results of skin testing with food additives and the effect of an elimination diet in chronic and recurrent urticaria and recurrent angioedema. *Clin Exp Allergy* 1989; 19:539–543.

26. Weber RW, Hoffman M, Raine DA, Nelson HS. Incidence of bronchoconstriction due to aspirin, azo dyes, non-azo dyes, and preservatives in a population of perennial asthmatics. *J Allergy Clin Immunol* 1979; 64:32–37.
27. Tarlo SM, Broder I. Tartrazine and benzoate challenge and dietary avoidance in chronic asthma. *Clin Allergy* 1982; 12:303–312.
28. Osterhalle O, Taudoroff E, Hashr J. Intolerance to aspirin, food-colouring agents and food preservatives in childhood asthma. *Ogeskr Laeger* 1979; 141:1908–1910.
29. Hernandez García J, Negro Alvarez JM, García Sellés FJ, Pagán Alemán JA. Reacciones adversas a conservatanes alimentarios [Article in Spanish]. *Allergol Immunopathol (Madr)* 1986; 14:55–63.
30. Juhlin L, Michaelsson G, Zetterstrom O. Urticaria and asthma induced by food and drug additives in patients with aspirin sensitivity. *J Allergy Clin Immunol* 1972; 50:92–98.
31. Rosenhall L, Zetterstrom O. Asthma provoked by analgesics, cold colorants and food preservatives. *Lakartidningen* 1973; 70:1417–1419.
32. Hodge L, Yan KY, Loblay RL. Assessment of food chemical intolerance in adult asthmatic subjects. *Thorax* 1996; 51:805–809.
33. Kinsey RE, Wright DO. Reaction following ingestion of sodium benzoate in a patient with severe liver damage. *J Lab Clin Med* 1944; 29:188–196.
34. Michels A, Vandermoten G, Duchateau J, et al. Anaphylaxis with sodium benzoate. *Lancet* 1991; 337:1424–1425.
35. Nagel JE, Fuscaldo JT, Fireman P. Paraben allergy. *J Am Med Assoc* 1977; 237:1594–1595.
36. Carr TW. Severe allergic reaction to an intraurethral lignocaine preparation containing parabens preservatives. *Br J Urol* 1990; 66:98.
37. Veien NK, Hattel T, Laurberg G. Oral challenge with parabens in paraben-sensitive patients. *Contact Dermat* 1996; 34:433.
38. Munoz FJ. Perioral contact urticaria from sodium benzoate in a toothpaste. *Contact Dermat* 1996; 35:51.
39. Van Bever HP, Docx M, Stevens WJ. Food and food additives in severe atopic dermatitis. *Allergy* 1989; 44:588–594.
40. Worm M, Ehlers I, Sterry W, Zuberbier T. Clinical relevance of food additives in adult patients with atopic dermatitis. *Clin Exp Allergy* 2000; 30:407–414.
41. Worm M, Vieth W, Ehlers I, Sterry W, Zuberbier T. Increased leukotriene production by food additives in patients with atopic dermatitis and proven food intolerance. *Clin Exp Allergy* 2001; 31(2):265–273.
42. Fauler J, Neumann CH, Tsikas D, et al. Enhanced synthesis of cysteinyl leukotrienes in atopic dermatitis. *Br J Dermatol* 1993; 128:627–630.
43. Park HW, Park CH, Park SH, et al. Dermatologic adverse reactions to 7 common food additives in patients with allergic diseases: a double-blind, placebo-controlled study. *J Allergy Clin Immunol* 2008; 121(4):1059–1061.
44. Wuthrich B. Adverse reactions to food additives. *Ann Allergy* 1993; 71:379–384.
45. Pacor ML, Di Lorenzo G, Martinelli N, Manseuto P, Rini GB, Corrocher R. Monosodium benzoate hypersensitivity in subjects with persistent rhinitis. *Allergy* 2004; 59(2):192–197.
46. Vogt T. Sodium benzoate-induced acute leukocytoclastic vasculitis with unusual clinical appearance. *Arch Dermatol* 1999; 135:726–727.
47. Lunardi C, Bambara LM, Biasi D, Zagni P, Caramaschi P, Pacor ML. Elimination diet in the treatment of selected patients with hypersensitivity vasculitis. *Clin Exp Rheumatol* 1992; 10:131–135.
48. Lamey PJ, Lewis MA. Oral medicine in practice: orofacial allergic reactions. *Br Dent J* 1990; 168:59–63.
49. Patton DW, Ferguson MM, Forsyth A, James J. Oro-facial granulomatosis: a possible allergic basis. *Br J Oral Maxillofac Surg* 1985; 23:235–242.
50. Sweatman MC, Tasker R, Warner JO, Ferguson MM, Micthcell DN. Oro-facial granulomatosis. Response to elemental diet and provocation by food additives. *Clin Allergy* 1986; 16:331–338.
51. Pachor ML, Ubani G, Cortina P, et al. Is the Melkersson-Rosenthal syndrome related to the exposure to food additives? A case report. *Oral Surg Oral Med Oral Pathol* 1989; 67:393–395.
52. McKenna KE, Walsh MY, Burrows D. The Melkersson–Rosenthal syndrome and food additive hypersensitivity. *Br J Dermatol* 1994; 131:921–922.
53. Morales C, Penarrocha M, Bagan JV, Burches E, Pelaez A. Immunological study of Melkersson–Rosenthal syndrome: lack of response to food additive challenge. *Clin Exp Allergy* 1995; 25:260–264.
54. Feingold BF. Hyperkinesis and learning disabilities linked to artificial food flavors and colors. *Am J Nurs* 1975; 75:797–803.
55. Bateman B, Warner JO, Hutchinson E, et al. The effects of a double blind, placebo controlled, artificial food colourings and benzoate preservative challenge on hyperactivity in a general population sample of preschool children. *Arch Dis Child* 2004; 89(6):506–511.

34 Food Colorings and Flavors

Matthew J. Greenhawt & James L. Baldwin
Division of Allergy and Clinical Immunology, Food Allergy Center, University of Michigan Medical School, Ann Arbor, MI, USA

Key Concepts

- Food flavorings and colorings are often derived from potential allergens.
- The overall prevalence of reactions attributable to food colorings and flavorings is thought to be low.
- Carmine/cochineal extract, annatto, and spices are the most commonly implicated agents in this group.
- Current labeling regulations for these agents make identification of potential allergens a difficult task. However, since 2009, the Food and Drug Administration has required labeling of the presence of carmine/cochineal extract in all foods, cosmetics, and prescription drugs.
- Many spices and food flavorings are plant derived and have homologous epitopes to Bet v 1, seed storage proteins, or lipid transfer proteins. However, the prevalence of IgE-mediated reactions to spices and flavorings is low, though Type IV reactions are reported.
- Spices can sometimes be labeled broadly as "spices" and not their actual individual ingredient, depending on whether their use is as an additive or a primary ingredient.

Food colorings and flavors are essential parts of the experience of eating that have existed for centuries. Though their inclusion is often an afterthought in our consumption, ultimately, the colorings and flavorings are at the core of what we enjoy about eating our favorite foods. In many processed foods, coloring and flavoring are inseparable from the food's identity in the eyes of the consumer and the corporate production of the food itself.

The use of both synthetic and biogenic sources for color and flavor is a common practice. Most of these pose no risk of adverse events. However, there is a growing body of medical literature regarding adverse reactions involving food colorings and flavors derived from both synthetic and nonsynthetic sources.

This chapter will discuss nonsynthetic food colorings and flavorings that have been implicated in adverse food reactions. We will review known mechanisms of reaction, treatment strategy, and legislation involved in changing the way that colors and flavors are used in foods. Synthetic color additives are discussed elsewhere in this book.

Food colorings

Background history

According to the United States Food and Drug Administration (FDA), food colorants are any dye, pigment, or substance that imparts color when applied to food. Both synthetic and biogenic sources are used for this purpose [1]. Coloring not only influences one's acceptance of food, but also aids food manufacturing in several ways. Coloring is essential to correct the loss of a product's true color from exposure to light, air, temperature, moisture, or the elements involved in storage. It can be useful in correcting natural variations in color between products, to make them appear more uniform in quality to the consumer, or to enhance and augment an appearance of a natural occurring color. Coloring is also a useful marketing tactic to give otherwise colorless substances identity or to make them appear more festive. Coloring can also be essential to protect vitamins and flavors that can be damaged from direct sunlight [2–4].

There is a lengthy relationship between food coloring and adverse reactions attributed to such coloring. One of the first recorded case reports was from 1848, involving 21 individuals at a public dinner poisoned by copper arsenite, which was used to color a dessert green [4]. By 1900,

Food Allergy: Adverse Reactions to Foods and Food Additives, Fifth Edition. Edited by Dean D Metcalfe, Hugh A Sampson, Ronald A Simon and Gideon Lack.

it was estimated that there were 80 synthetic color additives available for use in foods, but there were no regulations pertaining to the quality and use for these dyes. The Food and Drug Act of 1906 created the first seven dyes "certified" for the use in foods, and established a voluntary certification program for quality and purity. Initial control of this process was under the United States Department of Agriculture (USDA). However, in 1938, authority and responsibility for this process was transferred to the FDA [1–3, 5]. Three separate categories were additionally created to delineate food manufacturing processes from other use of colors: FD&C (Food, Drug, and Cosmetic), D&C (Drug and Cosmetic), and external D&C (External Drug and Cosmetic) [1–3, 5].

There was a paucity of further legislation until the Food Additive Amendment of 1958, which declared that food additives safely in use before 1958 were exempted from obtaining FDA approval. However, in 1960, the Color Additive Amendments to the FDA Act of 1906 created a "provisional" listing for all known colors in use for foodstuff [1–3, 5, 6]. This act required that all previously certified dyes and colors used in food undergo further testing to establish safety before they were re-certified. Manufacturers were given a provisional time allotment in which they could continue using the particular color on the market, while submitting the required data regarding safety to the FDA. Other types of additives were exempted from this act. This act also set limits to usable amounts of color in products, deemed good manufacturing practices [1–3, 5].

Specifically, one section of the 1960 amendment, known as the Delaney Clause, placed a strict prohibition on the use of any amount of a substance shown to be carcinogenic in humans or laboratory animals [1–3, 5, 6]. This clause was applied to additives as well, though they were exempt from the rest of the amendment. The market effect of the 1960 Color Additive Amendments was the reduction of a list of 200 provisionally approved colors to a final list of 90 that were deemed safe for human consumption, after meeting newly applied regulations [1–3, 5, 6]. Colors that did not meet the new standards were removed from the market. Interestingly, the Delaney Clause had a vague definition of safety beyond establishing lack of carcinogenesis, and established no absolute standard for safety beyond "convincing evidence that establishes with reasonable certainty that no harm will result from the intended use of the color additive" [3, 6].

The amendment also designated two distinct classes of colorants: certified and noncertified [1–3, 5–7]. Colors exempt from certification were given this designation if certification was deemed unnecessary in the interest of public health to examine the color batch physical properties, including purity, moisture, residual salts, unreacted intermediates, color impurities, other specified impurities, and presence of heavy metals [5]. Generally, this exemption was applied to a particular color that was from a biogenic source, with a history of use prior to the Amendment, and without complaints of toxicity or allergic reactions to the FDA or its manufacturer [1–3, 5–7]. Colors exempt from FD&C certification are still subject to the standards of the Delaney Clause of the Color Additive Amendment [6]. In reality, there are virtually no restrictions applied to the use of either certified or noncertified colors in food manufacturing. One notable exception is for colors to be used in meat and poultry, which requires additional authorization from the USDA Food Safety Inspection Service (FSIS) above the FDA approval (Figure 34.1 and Table 34.1) [5].

Color additives in the United States are regulated by the Food and Drug Administration Title 21 of the Code of Federal Regulations (CFR) part 73, subpart A (colors not subject to batch certification) and part 74, subpart A (colors subject to batch certification) [8]. As part of this legislation, all certified colors carry an FD&C or D&C color label and have undergone rigorous testing to establish their safety and batch purity, in contrast to their noncertified counterparts, as explained in the previous section. In 1990, the National Labeling and Education Act (NLEA) required that certified color additives must be declared on package labeling as individual ingredients as of July 1, 1991, regardless of their quantity in the item [9]. Biogenic colors were exempt from this requirement and, therefore, may be referred to on labels as "artificial color," "artificial color added," or "color added" [8]. The use of the term "natural color" is not allowed as it could imply that the coloring might be derived from the food item itself, when in fact it is referring to an additive. As will be discussed in detail in the section on carmine, the unique labeling requirements for noncertified colors has become a controversial issue, as there are increasing numbers of case reports of biogenic color-induced hypersensitivity [10, 11]. Since certified colors (azo and non-azo dyes) are discussed in detail elsewhere in this book, henceforth, we will be referring to colors exempt from certification only.

An important distinction of how colors are used in foods and drugs is between dyes and lakes. A color dye is a water-soluble form of color (liquid, powder, or granule) and a lake is a water-insoluble form. Lakes are more stable than dyes and are better for use with fat or oil. Most pharmaceuticals use lakes in their coatings. A major technical advantage of certified colors is that they often require less chemical to produce an intense color, allow for more uniform distribution of color, and do not influence the flavor [1, 2].

Biogenic colors are believed to contain either low molecular weight nonprotein chemicals, most likely acting as haptens when they elicit reactions. Reactions to this class of colorants can be both immunologic and nonimmunologic. There is growing concern that biologic

Table 34.1 Colors exempt from FDA certification (with both US Congressional Federal Register Section designation and European designation).

Color additives approved for use in human food
Part 73, Subpart A: Color additives exempt from batch certification

21 CFR section	Straight color	EEC#	Year approved	Uses and restrictions
73.30	Annatto extract	E160b	1963	Foods generally
73.40	Dehydrated beets (beet powder)	E162	1967	Foods generally
73.75	Canthaxanthin	E161g	1969	Foods generally, NTE 30 mg/lb of solid or semisolid food or per pint of liquid food; may also be used in broiler chicken feed
73.85	Caramel	E150a–d	1963	Foods generally
73.90	-Apo-8′-carotenal	E160e	1963	Foods generally, NTE 15 mg/lb solid, 15 mg/pt liquid
73.95	Carotene	E160a	1964	Foods generally
73.100	Cochineal extract	E120	1969	Foods generally
	Carmine		1967	
73.140	Toasted partially defatted cooked cottonseed flour	–	1964	Foods generally
73.160	Ferrous gluconate	–	1967	Ripe olives
73.165	Ferrous lactate	–	1996	Ripe olives
73.169	Grape color extract	E163?	1981	Nonbeverage food
73.170	Grape skin extract (enocianina)	E163?	1966	Still and carbonated drinks and -ades; beverage bases; alcoholic beverages (restrict 27 CFR parts 4 & 5).
73.200	Synthetic iron oxide	E172	1994	Sausage casings NTE 0.1% (by wt)
73.250	Fruit juice	–	1966	Foods generally
			1995	Dried color additive
73.260	Vegetable juice	–	1966	Foods generally
			1995	Dried color additive, water infusion
73.300	Carrot oil	–	1967	Foods generally
73.340	Paprika	E160c	1966	Foods generally
73.345	Paprika oleoresin	E160c	1966	Foods generally
73.450	Riboflavin	E101	1967	Foods generally
73.500	Saffron	E164	1966	Foods generally
73.575	Titanium dioxide	E171	1966	Foods generally; NTE 1% (by wt)
73.600	Turmeric	E100	1966	Foods generally
73.615	Turmeric oleoresin	E100	1966	Foods generally

Source: Adapted from http://www.fda.gov/downloads/Food/GuidanceComplianceRegulatoryInformation/GuidanceDocuments/FoodLabelingNutrition/UCM301394.pdf, updated September 2006.
NTE, not to exceed.

source contamination in the colorant is the source of IgE-mediated reactions attributed to them [7, 10]. Annatto and carmine/cochineal extract have both been linked to such reactions in the literature [7]. Because these colors are noncertified, it is difficult to ascertain the purity of a particular lot of these dyes. Thus, there could be varying levels of biogenic protein contamination due to technical discrepancies in different batches. There have been a few reports of SDS-PAGE analysis of carmine and cochineal insect protein fractions to determine their allergenicity, but there has been nothing conclusively nor consistently proven in this analysis [12–18]. Thanks to the lobbying efforts of several consumer groups, the labeling requirements for carmine were changed in 2009 [11, 19]. This will be discussed in detail in the section covering carmine. As of this date, lobbying efforts to have annatto's labeling requirements changed have failed.

Biogenic colorants involved in hypersensitivity reactions

Only a few biogenic substances have been linked to allergic-type reactions. These include carmine (cochineal extract), annatto, turmeric, saffron, β-carotenoid, and grape anthocyanins. However, the majority of the literature pertains to carmine, with a small amount pertaining to annatto.

Carmine

Carmine is a red color derived from the female insect *Coccus cacti or Dactylopius coccus costa* [3, 7, 10, 20–22]. This insect

Name	Hue	Common uses
Annatto	Orange	dairy products, popcorn oil, butter mixes, baked goods, icings, snacks, ice cream, salad dressing, yogurts
β-Carotene	Orange	margarine, non-dairy creamers
Beet powder	Purple	ice cream, cake icings, mixes, yogurt, gelatin desserts, fruit chews, frozen products, chewable tablets
Caramel color		dairy foods, drinks, colas, iced tea, cocoa, beer, coffee, icings, cereals, popcorn, gravies, sauces, candies
Carrot oil	Orange	
Carmine	Wine Red	cake icings, hard candy, bakery products, yogurt, ice cream, gelatin desserts, fruit syrups, pet foods, jams/preserves
Fruit juice		beverages, jellies, candy, gelatin desserts, dry mixes, dark chocolate
Paprika	Red-orange	sausage, cheese sauces, gravies, condiments, salad dressings, baked goods, snacks, icings, cereals
Riboflavin	Yellow-orange	
Saffron	Yellow-orange	
Turmeric	Yellow	baked products, dairy products, ice cream, yogurts, cakes, cookies, popcorn, candy, cake icings, cereals, sauces, gelatins
Vegetable juice		

Figure 34.1 Pictorial of the noncertified color additives. Adapted and modified from www.red40.com

is commonly found in Peru, Central America, and the Canary Islands, where it grows as a parasite on the prickly pear cactus *Nopalea coccinellifera*. Its origin in Europe dates back to the 1500s, when Hernando Cortez discovered its use by the Aztecs and brought the cochineal insects back to Spain [23]. The color is produced from the aqueous alcohol extract of the dried, gravid, female insect, resulting in cochineal extract. Cochineal extract contains ~10% carminic acid, a hydroxyanthraquinone, and the rest is the residual insect body. Cochineal extract is acidic, and the color variation from deep red to orange is dependent on the pH. Carmine is produced from the aluminum or calcium–aluminum lake on an aluminum hydroxide substrate of carminic acid. Since the lake is minimally soluble in water, strong acids or bases can be used to make the color more soluble. Commercial preparations of carmine are estimated to contain approximately 20–50% carminic acid, but it is usually diluted to 2–4% for sale. Commercial cochineal extract contains 1.8% carminic acid. Carmine is relatively expensive to produce. It is estimated that it requires 70 000 dried insects to make 1 lb of dye (Figures 34.2 and 34.3) [3, 7, 21].

Carmine was given approval by the FDA for use in food in 1967 and cochineal extract in 1968 [24, 25]. As part of this approval, it was determined that carmine or cochineal extract had no carcinogenic or teratogenic properties in studies on rats. Carmine, as a biogenic color, is not certified, and therefore is exempt from specific declaration on food labels. It is generally labeled as "color added," "artificial color" or "artificial color added," "colored with carmine," "cochineal extract," or "carmine color." In Europe it is designated as E120 by the European Union and may be labeled as "Natural Red No. 4" or CI 75470 (color index). Carmine is also used in cosmetics, where it had been required to be declared as an ingredient since 1977, but in order of its relative weight per volume of cosmetic [3, 7, 8, 10, 26]. Carmine is distinct from and should not be confused with Indigo Carmine (FD&C Blue #2), Cochineal Red (E124), Food Red 7, or Ponceau 4R (Table 34.2).

Most foods colored with carmine contain very low levels that would limit exposure when consumed [7]. However, there are several case reports of hypersensitivity reactions attributed to carmine ranging from anaphylaxis to occupational asthma (see Table 34.3). Though these reports

Carminic acid (1260-17-9)

Carmine (1390-65-4)

Figure 34.2 Chemical structures of carminic acid and carmine.

are uncommon, the actual incidence of these reactions is unknown and was complicated by former labeling regulations that did not require carmine to be explicitly labeled on packaged goods, which made it difficult to suspect reactivity attributable to a substance not listed by name on a label.

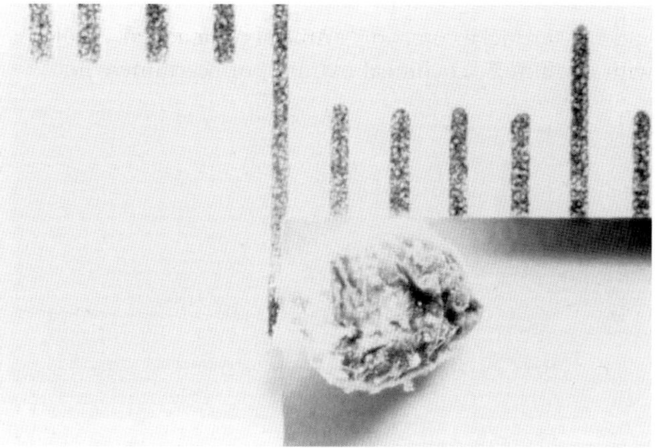

Figure 34.3 The dried *Coccus cacti* insect used to make Carmine (photo of dried cochineal insect).

Table 34.2 Commercial uses of carmine/cochineal extract.

Water-insoluble carmine colors	Water-soluble carmine colors	Water-soluble cochineal
Cosmetics	Yogurt	Beverages
Pharmaceuticals	Ice cream	Yogurt
Dairy products	Fruit-based drinks	Ice cream
Baked goods	Beverages	Fruit fillings
Condiments	Fruit fillings	Puddings
	Puddings	Confections
	Bakery mixes	
	Confections	
	Cosmetics	
	Pharmaceuticals	

Since levels of carmine in food are low, our group (Baldwin et al.) and others have hypothesized another likely route of sensitization (e.g., respiratory or dermatologic). Most of the reported cases involve workers with occupational exposure, or females with a prior history of use of carmine-containing cosmetics [13]. Carmine was approved for use in cosmetics as a noncertified color in 1977 and is the only biogenic color allowed to be used around the eyes [26]. It is plausible that persons using makeup containing carmine can become sensitized through a cutaneous route. Upon reexposure to carmine in food, an IgE-mediated reaction can occur. Similarly, occupational inhalation could cause sensitization in textile or dye workers exposed to high levels of carmine powder in the environment and cause an IgE-mediated reaction upon ingestion of carmine-containing food or beverage. Carminic acid is a low molecular weight molecule and may act as a hapten during sensitization. Protein remnants from the cochineal insects are likely candidate antigens as well. Most authors believe that there is chemical modification of the protein contaminants in the processing of the extracted carminic acid from the insect. Once sensitization occurs, low levels of exposure could result in hypersensitivity. However, no mechanism of sensitization has definitively been proven to date [7, 10, 12, 13, 22].

A current review of published literature revealed 38 reported patient cases of hypersensitivity to carmine. Eleven of these include detailed reports to the FDA under the MedWatch program and the rest reported in the medical literature (Table 34.3). There are no known reports of fatalities related to carmine [10, 12]. The range of symptoms reported includes occupational asthma, extrinsic allergic alveolitis, cheilitis, contact dermatitis, and food allergy manifesting as anaphylaxis, angioedema, bronchospasm, and urticaria. There have been no consistent reports pertaining to time from exposure to symptoms, nor dose required to elicit symptoms [10, 13]. The first case was reported in 1961, involving cheilitis from a lip salve that contained carmine [27]. In 1997, our group successfully

Table 34.3 Known reported cases of carmine hypersensitivity.

Author	Year	Reference	Sex	Atopy	Exposure route	Reaction	Occupation	Prick test	Specific IgE	Immunoblot	Bronchial challenge	Notes
Sarkany et al.	1961	[27]	3 pts	NA	Cutaneous: lip salve	Contact dermatitis		Positive patch test	No	No	No	First known report in medical literature
Burge et al.	1979	[28]	M, M	Both	Inhalation	Bronchospasm	Factory workers	Not performed	Not performed	Not performed	Both positive	
Park et al.	1981	[29]	M	NA	Cutaneous: lip stick	Anaphylaxis	Soldier	Not performed	Not performed	Not performed	Not performed	
Tenabene et al.	1987	[30]	F, M, M	None	Inhalation	Bronchospasm	Spice/food handlers	Female negative, males positive	Not performed	Not performed	All 3 positive	
Quirce et al.	1994	[31]	M, F, M	None	Inhalation	Bronchospasm	Dye factory workers: manufacturer (M), cleaning staff (F), ex-worker (M)	All positive	Manufacturer positive, other 2 negative	Not performed	Positive in manufacturer only	Ex-employee left company because of allergic alveolitis prior to discovery of this problem
Kägi et al.	1994	[32]	F	Yes	Ingestion: Campari-Orange	Anaphylaxis		Positive	Yes–initial RAST negative, class 2 at 1 year later	Not performed	Not performed	First case of reported anaphylaxis due to ingestion
Beaudouin et al.	1995	[33]	F	None	Ingestion: fruit-flavored yogurt	Anaphylaxis		Positive	Not performed	Not performed	Not performed	First positive basophil histamine release test reported
Stücker et al.	1996	[34]	F	None	Inhalation	Bronchospasm	Food factory worker	Positive	Positive	Not performed	Not performed	
Wüthrich et al.	1997	[35]	F, F, F, F, F	3 of 5	Ingestion: alcoholic beverage	Anaphylaxis		All 5 positive	All 5 positive	Not performed	Not performed	
Baldwin et al.	1997	[22]	F	Yes	Ingestion: red popsicle	Anaphylaxis		Positive	Positive (P-K test)	Not performed	Not performed	Only known P-K testing done to carmine. Additionally, this case was reported by patient to FDA MedWatch program
Acero et al.	1998	[14]	M	None	Inhalation and ingestion	Bronchospasm, rhinoconjunctivitis	Spice factory packer, non-manufacturing	Positive	Not performed	Positive (no MW determined)	Positive	
DiCello et al.	1999	[36]	F, F	None	Ingestion: artificial crabmeat, fruit-flavored yogurt	Anaphylaxis		Positive	Not performed	Not performed	Not performed	
Lizaso et al.	2000	[15]	M, F, F	None	Inhalation	Bronchospasm	Dye plant worker, dye plant clerical worker, dye plant chemist	Positive	Not performed	28 and 50 kDa band to pooled serum	All positive	
Chung et al.	2001	[12]	F, F, F	All 3	Ingestion	Anaphylaxis		Positive	Not performed	Pt 1: 28 kDa, 50 kDa; Pt 2: 23 kDa, 50 kDa; Pt 3: 88 kDa	Not performed	No patient sera recognized the same protein bands. Sera also tested to pulverized cochineal insect and had bands recognized, with cochineal insect inhibition of carmine band
Tabar et al.	2003	[37]	F, F	Yes in 1	Inhalation	Bronchospasm	Dye factory clerical worker, dye factory laboratory worker	Positive	Positive	Not performed	Positive	
Anibarro et al.	2003	[16]	M, M	Both yes	Inhalation	Bronchospasm	Both butchers	Positive	Not performed	Both 10 kDa	Positive	
Ferrer et al.	2005	[13]	M	None	Inhalation	Bronchospasm	Spice blender	Positive	Positive	28 kDa	Positive	

Greenhawt et al.	2006	[38]	F	Yes	Ingestion and topical: generic azithromycin, fruit-flavored yogurt, colored pasta, eye makeup	Anaphylaxis, local rash, and angioedema	Office worker	Positive	Not performed	Not performed	Not performed	This is the first case report of exposure from a pharmaceutical source, in a patient with past history of carmine-induced anaphylaxis. She had tolerated the trade named medication before and after the incident, and tested positive to both carmine and the generic tablet coating, which contained a carmine lake
Shaw	2009	[39]	F	NA	Topical	Contact dermatitis	NA	Positive patch test	Not performed	Not performed	Not performed	
Yamakawa et al.	2009	[17]	F, F, F	All 3 yes	Ingestion	Anaphylaxis; angioedema, and pruritus; pruritus and globus sensation	NA	Positive to cochineal but not carmine	Positive to cochineal in patients 1 and 2	Pt 1: 39–45 kDa; pt 2: 40–45 kDa; pt 3: 33–44 kDa	Not performed	Suggestive of difference between cochineal and carmine in protein content
The following 10 case reports were submitted to the FDA under the MedWatch program. All products reported in the table were verified to contain either carmine or cochineal extract												
FDA MedWatch	1997	[10]	F	NA	Ingestion: Tropicana Ruby Red Grapefruit Juice; topical–purple eye shadow	Anaphylaxis; skin rash		Positive				PST positive to the grapefruit juice, Good & Plenty candy, eye shadow also
FDA MedWatch	1997	[10]	F	NA	Ingestion: custard style strawberry banana yogurt	Anaphylaxis		Positive	Serum tryptase of 18			PST positive to yogurt also
FDA MedWatch	1998	[10]	F	NA	Ingestion: SoBe fruit juice	Anaphylaxis		NA				Cochineal extract was declared on the bottle label. Pt was admitted to the hospital for observation
FDA MedWatch	2000	[10]	F	NA	Ingestion: crab soup, yogurt, candy, Ruby Red Grapefruit Juice, pasta salad with artificial crab meat	Anaphylaxis		Positive				
FDA MedWatch	NA	[10]	F	Yes	Ingestion: gelatin-based desert	Eyelid angioedema		Not performed				Pt called case in to the FDA, no workup done
FDA MedWatch	NA	[10]	F	NA	Ingestion: custard style yogurt, multiple cosmetics	Anaphylaxis (to the ingestion)		NA				Pt reports she was treated by an allergist but not specified
FDA MedWatch	NA	[10]	NA	NA	NA	NA		NA				FDA contacted by a law firm to indicate that they were considering implicating carmine in the case of an allergic reaction in a client attributed to carmine
FDA MedWatch	1999	[10]	NA	NA	Ingestion: yoghurt	Anaphylaxis		Positive				
FDA MedWatch	2000	[10]	F	NA	Ingestion, topical: neither specified	NA		NA				Pt informed the FDA that she carries an EpiPen® for treatment when needed
FDA MedWatch	2000	[10]	F	NA	Topical: eyeliner	NA						

showed there was a definitive IgE-mediated reaction in a 27-year-old woman with anaphylaxis to a red-colored ice pop containing carmine by the use of a Prausnitz–Küstner test [22]. Other groups have shown the reactions were IgE mediated through skin prick tests (SPTs), leukocyte histamine release test, RAST or other serum-specific IgE (sIgE) testing, atopy patch testing, and immunoblotting for specific IgE [12–16, 22, 30–39].

Reactions have been reported with two common predominating phenotypes, food hypersensitivity and occupational respiratory disease. In the occupational respiratory disease phenotype, these cases involve predominately males with no atopic background. In the food hypersensitivity phenotype, all case reports have involved females, half of whom were atopic. Two of these females also showed occupational disease features, and some have described prior episodes of itching and burning with application of makeup, suspicious for contact reactions [13]. There have been four distinct reports via the FDA MedWatch program of contact dermatitis, comprising a small third phenotype of reaction [10].

Immunoblot analysis of persons with occupational respiratory disease and food hypersensitivity phenotypes has shown mixed results. Typically, authors have used both carmine and pulverized cochineal insect extract, subjected to SDS-PAGE and column chromatography fractionation to determine protein bands. Subsequent immunoblotting with patient sera has determined IgE-recognized protein bands [10]. However, investigators who have performed these experiments have not found consistent recognition of any particular protein band in either carmine, pulverized cochineal insect, or carminic acid [12–16]. Our group found that commercial carmine could inhibit recognition of pulverized cochineal insect bands, strong evidence that there is insect protein contaminant in the commercial dye [36]. A recent immunoblot study confirmed this finding and inferred that these proteins undergo chemical modification in the commercial processing of carmine [12]. Groups have identified proteins 17, 28, 38, 50, 88, and 40–97 kDa in size. Most recently, a group identified a 335 amino acid cochineal allergen fragment within the 38-kDa band (named CC38K) as the major cochineal allergen [18]. However, there remains no evidence of a universally recognized specific protein band found in carmine or cochineal extract, and there is considerable overlap when examining the reported data [12–18]. Considering that carmine is noncertified and exempt from batch certification, batch-to-batch variability secondary to this regulation might be playing a role in these findings.

Diagnostic investigations to determine IgE-mediated sensitivity to carmine are problematic due to lack of available standardized allergenic extract. Furthermore, the same problem of batch-to-batch variability of the commercially available stock could create reliability problems with development of a standardized SPT carmine extract. For these reasons, in a patient with high suspicion for carmine allergy, we generally recommend a simple SPT using the suspicious foodstuff. If this is positive, then one should attempt to obtain a small aliquot of the dye from that particular food manufacturer for a confirmatory undiluted SPT. If possible, obtaining a small commercial lot of carmine dye would be helpful for future testing, but our experience with this has been difficult, though we were ultimately able to do so. *Most importantly, it has been these authors' experience that the wheal-and-flare reaction to carmine-containing foods and manufacturer-supplied carmine develops slightly later than with other extracts, generally between 20 and 30 minutes* [12, 22, 36, 38]. We do not perform intradermal challenge to carmine, nor do we routinely test pulverized cochineal insect extract. Dried cochineal insects are more readily available than carmine dye, but of course the proteins present in the raw extract lack any of the potential chemical modifications contained in commercially processed carmine. A commercial serum-specific IgE (ImmunoCAP®) test does exist, but its validity has not been determined due to the small frequency of reported events.

Our group published the one study that used passive transfer to prove there was an IgE-mediated reaction, in which we were able to consent a married couple for a Prausnitz–Küstner (P–K) test [22]. This reaction, while exceptionally helpful in determining the presence of an IgE-mediated reaction, is no longer advocated for infection control reasons. Eight authors have described bronchial provocation challenges to carmine, cochineal extract, and carminic acid to measure a 20% decrease in FEV_1 and to determine the dose that caused a 20% drop in FEV_1, or PC_{20} [13–16, 28, 30, 31, 37]. Other diagnostic techniques that have been used in practice include blinded oral challenge [12, 36] and ocular challenge [12, 14, 28, 31].

Persons with hypersensitivity to carmine face two large obstacles. The first is having a provider who can recognize this entity and has the resources to test for it. The second is being able to recognize and avoid products containing carmine. Prior to 2009, the exemption in labeling declaration for noncertified dyes created a potentially dangerous environment for the uninformed consumer [19]. However, since January 5, 2009, in the United States, carmine must be explicitly labeled on packaged foodstuff, and no longer can be referred to as artificial color or color added, and the task of identifying carmine-containing foodstuff within American products has become much easier [11, 40].

Carmine was the focus of a highly successful grass-roots style consumer-driven petition to change the labeling requirements for noncertified dyes [11, 19]. Prior to January 5, 2009, carmine/cochineal extract could be referred to for labeling purposes as "artificial color," "color added," but not "natural color" [24, 25]. This made it exceptionally difficult to identify if carmine was an ingredient and posed danger to the carmine-allergic individual. In 1998, the Center for Science in the Public Interest (CSPI) filed a petition with the FDA to review the labeling policies for carmine and cochineal extract, additionally requesting designation of the insect source for these dyes, formal study to determine the exact antigen in cochineal/carmine to see if it was a key component of the coloring, and to ban the dyes if necessary [10, 19]. This petition was supported by the several known case reports in the medical literature at the time.

In January of 2006, the FDA published a proposed rule to amend the labeling regulations after an in-depth examination of the allergic properties of carmine and cochineal extract [10]. This was prompted after reviewing 11 MedWatch reports of allergic reactions attributed to carmine/cochineal extract and 35 patient case reports in the medical literature, of which most had established the reactions to be IgE mediated (see Table 34.3). The FDA investigation concluded the following [10]:

- Carmine/cochineal extract dye can cause hypersensitivity, but it is a rare event and they were unable to estimate either an incidence or report a conclusive mechanism.
- There is presently no conclusive evidence that there is biologic contamination of the cochineal insect proteins in the dye that cause hypersensitivity, though several groups had discovered distinct protein bands in cochineal extract that were inhibited by carmine. This was based on no conclusive evidence in the medical literature that any one particular protein fraction was recognized universally in affected individuals studied.

The FDA's ultimate recommendation was that although carmine/cochineal extract is a definitive allergen, it posed no harm to the general public and, therefore, did not need to be prohibited from use. Furthermore, they felt there was no need for any further FDA-directed testing to determine if the allergenic fraction is essential to the color. However, they did recognize that requiring specific name declaration of carmine and cochineal extract in products would aid recognition of the allergen in food sources for affected individuals. The FDA ultimately accepted a proposal to amend the Federal Food, Drug, and Cosmetic Act, Title 21, part 73, § 73.100, 73.2087; and part 101, § 101.22 to incorporate the following changes, effective January 5, 2009 [10, 11]:

- Require all foods, including butter, cheese, and ice cream, containing carmine or cochineal extract to label it as such by its "respective or common name," and immediately disallow it to be generically referred to as artificial color or color added.
- Require all cosmetics to declare the presence of carmine.
- Require all prescription drugs to declare the presence of carmine.

Since this legislation officially went into effect, there has been clear labeling of the presence of carmine when used in foods. It is unknown, to date, what the effect has been on deterring inadvertent exposure to carmine in hypersensitive individuals.

This legislation gave carmine/cochineal extract special status not afforded to other similar exempt colorants, in that carmine must be labeled when used for cosmetic purposes, in "professional use" or samples, and in foods such as butter, cheese, and ice cream [41]. Over-the-counter medications had recently been required to declare all inactive ingredients, including any type of color additives, as do non-oral prescription drugs, as part of the Food and Drug Administration Modernization Act [11, 42]. Typically, commercially sold cosmetics for general retail must declare all ingredients in "descending order of predominance," but colors can be declared without respect to predominance [41]. Similarly, foods, prescription drugs, and cosmetics intended for "professional use only" or given as samples/free gifts and not meant for general purchase do not have to specifically declare the presence of any single color additive, by individual name, and instead can use the declaration "artificial color" or "artificial color added" (Professional use cosmetics include salon products, studio products, and camouflaging makeup for disfigurement dispensed by physician.) [24–26]. Foods such as butter, cheese, and ice cream are sometimes exempt from having to declare color additives [41]. Additionally, the labeling for cochineal extract and carmine has been extended to cover alcoholic beverages, and thus is fully comprehensive [43].

Though no study exists to denote the effect of this policy implementation, it is widely believed that this will greatly benefit susceptible patients. Formerly, in the absence of the labeling regulations, very limited knowledge for sensitive individuals about carmine-containing products was available and was limited to a small list of products anecdotally compiled by diagnosing providers, several MedWatch reports to the FDA, and the cases from the medical literature mentioned in this discussion. An example of the difficulty encountered by carmine-allergic patients was encountered by a patient of our center several years ago, who became the index case of carmine hypersensitivity from pharmaceutical exposure in generic azithromycin [38]. Prescription medication is a further source of regulatory frustration with respect to dyes/additives, as it is presently voluntary as to what inactive ingredients are declared on the package insert for prescription drugs [10].

Annatto

Annatto is a natural carotenoid-based color dye made from the seeds of the fruit of *Bixa orellana* tropical bush. The fruit has a pod full of approximately 50 seeds the size of grape seeds, covered in a red-pulp covering that serves as the base material from which the color is made [7, 44]. The major pigment is *cis*-bixin, which gives a red coloration, but upon heating becomes *trans*-bixin, and with further heating breaks down to two compounds. One of these compounds is water soluble for extraction (norbixin) and the other oil soluble (bixin) [7, 44]. In addition to yielding color extracts, it also yields edible vegetable oils and fats. Approximately 10,000 tons are produced each year, mainly in Latin America, Africa, and Asia. Annatto, as the bixin extract, is used as a colorant in fatty dairy products such as butter and margarine, and also leather [7, 44, 45]. As the norbixin extract, it is used as a colorant in cheese. Norbixin is a very strong colorant in small quantities [7,44,45]. Annatto is also used as both a color and flavor in confections, meats, soda, and processed snacks [46]. It has particular use as an additive to butter and cheese flavorings to produce the desired color. It has been used for centuries, dating back to the ancient Aztec and Mayan civilizations, and imported for use later by the Spanish when they conquered Mexico [7, 44, 45].

Annatto is purported to have medicinal properties such as a cure for diabetes (no evidence), as an antimicrobial (partial evidence), and as an antitoxin for snake bites (partial evidence) [45]. As a natural color, it is classified as a noncertified dye under Title 21 CFR § 73.30 [47]. Outside of the United States, it is also labeled as CI Natural Orange No. 4, E160b, bija, rocou, orlean, or achiote.

Annatto has been attributed to allergic reactions, including urticaria, anaphylaxis, angioedema, asthma, and contact dermatitis [48–54]. However, given the long-standing use of this colorant and the paucity of reported reactions, this is likely a rare hypersensitivity [7]. We do not know the actual prevalence of this hypersensitivity. In a 1987 study of the prevalence of food additive intolerances, Young et al. estimated the general population prevalence of hypersensitivity to annatto to be between 0.01 and 0.07 with a 95% confidence interval. This was extrapolated from data on 81 children in a study examining several additives [48].

The first report in the medical literature regarding annatto-provoked hypersensitivity was from a 1978 study in patients with chronic urticaria, in which they were administered a dose of annatto. Though this study was severely flawed because it lacked double-blind placebo controls and took place in patients who had their controlling medications withdrawn, it did suggest that annatto could provoke reactions [49]. A similar study in 1981 in the same population type had identical flaws and similar conclusions [50]. Other attempts at using annatto to provoke symptoms in two open challenges and one double-blind placebo were also either inconclusive or were flawed similarly to the earlier studies [51–53]. However, a 1991 case of a man with anaphylactic shock (urticaria, angioedema, and hypotension) developing within 20 minutes of consuming Fiber One® cereal colored with annatto was the first reported case of anaphylaxis attributed to annatto. The authors were able to demonstrate positive SPTs at 1:1000 dilution and full strength annatto, in the setting of negative SPTs to corn, wheat, and milk. Subsequent SDS-PAGE fractionation of annatto yielded two bands between 50 and 60 kDa, of which the 50 kDa band was recognized by the patient's serum when an immunoblot was performed [54]. There is one report of annatto-induced bronchospasm attributed to a pharmaceutical product containing annatto, but the author did not attempt skin testing or other challenge to prove the suspected association [55]. Specifically *cis*-bixin, but the not norbixin component, has been shown to induce allergic contact dermatitis in mice [56].

There is limited data supporting an IgE mechanism for annatto hypersensitivity. This is based on the fact that there has been only a single case report of positive SPTs and specific protein fractionation and positive immunoblot analysis [54], and that the oral challenge data have not proven conclusive in the multiple trials, as discussed above [49–53]. Much like carmine, the significance of the recognized protein band on immunoblot is suggestive of a protein contamination from the biogenic source as the likely allergenic culprit, and not the actual pigment, but this is based on the interpretation of a single study [45]. Neither carmine nor annatto has been studied further to determine if the pigment fraction is distinct from the protein recognized by IgE of patients with clinical sensitivity. A recent report demonstrated a positive basophil activation test after challenge from annatto-containing Gouda cheese in a patient with suspected IgE-mediated allergy to annatto, and evidence of a positive immunoblot to both Gouda and annatto [57]. In our clinics, we do test annatto with SPTs in patients with a history suspicious for possible annatto-induced hypersensitivity. In such cases, we would recommend a stepwise workup analogous to that described for suspected carmine hypersensitivity. A commercial specific IgE test does exist (Viracor Reference Laboratory, Lenexa, KS; Mayo Medical Laboratories, Rochester, MN) but its validity has not been determined due to the small frequency of reported events.

Other exempt from certification colors causing allergy

Table 34.4 summarizes the major case reports for several other colors to which clinical hypersensitivity reactions have been attributed. However, only a handful of these agents have had any conclusive test results.

Saffron is made from the dried stigmas and styles of the flower of the *Crocus sativus* L. plant [7, 59, 68]. This dark-yellow to dark-orange spice is among the most expensive of all spices. Its color comprises several components, including carthamin, saffron yellow A and B

Table 34.4 Known case reports of hypersensitivity to other noncertified colors besides carmine/cochineal extract.

Coloring	Author	Year	Reference	Reaction	Specific IgE	Study comments
Saffron	Feo et al.	1997	[58]	Bronchospasm, rhinoconjunctivitis	PST, sIgE, bronchial provocation, 15.5 kDa protein band	Case report
	Wuthrich et al.	1997	[59]	Anaphylaxis	PST, sIgE, 40 and 90 kDa protein bands	Case report
	Gomez-Gomez et al.	2010	[60]	Rhinitis	PST; 9.15 and 9.55 kDa protein bands for recombinant allergen	First report of LTP (rCro s 3.01 and 3.02) in spice allergy
Turmeric, curcumin	Vein et al.	1987	[53]	Studied in children with eczema as part of DBPCFC to multiple colorants	Not tested	Study inconclusive as it failed to achieve statistical significance of reactions versus placebo, and results were not reproducible in a second challenge
	Fugelsang et al.	1993, 1994	[51, 52]	Studied as part of open challenge to multiple additives including natural colorants in these two related studies involving children with atopic symptoms	Not tested	Both studies inconclusive. Data in both were confounded as to true cause of observed reactions, as a color mixture was used for testing
Carotenoids	Greenbaum	1979	[61]	Atopic dermatitis, colic, irritability	PST negative, double-blind challenge to vitamin A drops positive	Case report of 9-month-old baby, no causative role of carotenoids confirmed, however
	Juhilin	1981	[50]	Studied in open challenge in patients with chronic angioedema/urticaria	Open study	Poor study design with inconclusive results
	Fugelsang et al.	1993, 1994	[51, 52]	See above		
Anthocyanins (Grape) (*see also References 78–93 for other cases related to grape*)	Pastorello et al.	2003	[62]	Study of 14 patients with history of reaction to grape (11) and wine (3)	Demonstrated that endochitinases 4A and B as the key proteins responsible for allergy to grape but that 4A is responsible for reactions to wine. Also showed the lipid transfer protein had homology to peach lipid transfer protein and 24-kDa protein homologous to the cherry thaumatin-like allergen was a minor allergen	This is one of the first characterizations of grape allergens
No actual reports of grape color extract or grape skin extract causing reactions	Kalogeromitros et al.	2005, 2006	[63, 64]	Case series involving anaphylaxis in 11 patients attributed to grape products including wine, grape leaves, raisins, grape juice, vinegar	PST; sIgE; 9/11 pts HLA-DR11 positive	This is the first study with grape to look at HLA genes to see if there is allergen recognition effect. Additionally, demonstrated that grape and grape product allergy is more prevalent than thought in a Mediterranean population

(*continued*)

Table 34.4 (*Continued*)

Coloring	Author	Year	Reference	Reaction	Specific IgE	Study comments
Paprika (*see also References 86–88 for other cases*)	Jensen-Jarolim et al.	1998	[65]	Study of sera of 11 pts with bell pepper allergy	Showed the expression of Bet v 1 homolog, profilin homolog, and pathogenesis-related protein P23 in many strains of bell peppers. P23 had strong IgE-binding capability	Shows that bell peppers contain Bet v 1 and profilin homologs, and P23. Unlike the Bet v 1 homolog and profilin homolog, the P23-related protein was not destroyed in processing of paprika
No actual cases of allergic reactions attributed to the use of paprika as a color have been reported, but these cases demonstrate that this is theoretically possible	van Toorenenbergen et al.	2000	[66]	Study of sera from three symptomatic greenhouse workers (multiple allergic symptoms) and three food-allergic patients to see if paprika pollen sensitization existed in both groups	sIgE and immunoblot recognized specific IgE to paprika pollen in both patient populations	Recognition of paprika pollen is seen in non-horticultural workers and can be seen in the food-allergic population
	Willerroider et al.	2003	[67]	34 serum-positive patients allergic to bell pepper had serum drawn for cDNA cloning of bell pepper antigen	Used cDNA to clone the profilin protein Cap a 2 in *Capsicum annuum* and showed recognition of patient-specific IgE by immunoblot analysis of a 14 kDa protein	Defines a clinical marker for profilin sensitivity and cross-reactivity in the bell pepper-allergic population

SPT, skin prick test; sIgE, serum-specific IgE (e.g., ImmunoCAP, RAST); kDa, kilo Dalton; LTP, lipid transfer protein; r, recombinant.

(saffron yellow), saffloamine A, ethereal oils (safranal, pinen, cineol), glycosides (picrocrocin), and pectins [68]. It is identified as E164 in Europe, by CI 75100 or as CI Natural Yellow 6. It is most commonly used as both a spice and color in soups, sauces, rice dishes, cakes, cheese, and chartreuse liqueur [7]. An anaphylactic reaction developing 5 minutes after eating a meal with saffron rice and mushroom was reported in a 21-year-old farmer with known OAS, who required emergent resuscitation after developing laryngeal edema, urticaria, oral itching, and gastrointestinal cramping [59]. His SPT was positive to saffron and negative to the other components of the meal; furthermore, an IgE RAST test to both retail saffron and pure saffron revealed specific IgE, and SDS-PAGE fractionation and immunoblotting to this patient's serum produced 40 and 90 kDa bands. However, he also tested positive by skin test and RAST to celery and cooked celeriac, though the reaction was ultimately attributed to saffron [59]. Additionally, another investigator demonstrated occupational disease in 3 saffron workers in a group of 50, 1 with asthma and 2 with rhinoconjunctivitis by history (confirmed with saffron provocation testing), who had positive SPTs and RAST tests to specific saffron pollen [58]. Ten controls from a general allergic population in this area (all were non-saffron workers without history of symptoms attributed to exposure to saffron) also displayed positive prick and RAST tests to saffron pollen. SDS-PAGE immunoblotting to saffron pollen and stamens revealed a 15.5 kDa protein with similarity to profilin in the combined 13 patients that had positive SPTs and RAST scores. In cross-pollen studies, immunoblot inhibition occurred with Lolium, Salsola (Russian thistle), and Olea in 8 of the 13 patients that had a class 3 or greater RAST score. Thus, it was thought that this cross-reactivity could potentate an oral allergy syndrome, though it has not been reported [58]. More recently, lipid transfer proteins (LTP) rCro s 3.01 and rCro s 3.02 were identified as reactive to the serum of six saffron-allergic individuals, which is the first known report of LTP in spice allergy and demonstrates the important emergence of molecular allergy diagnostic testing as a useful tool for testing potential allergy to colorants or spices [60].

Turmeric, an orange-yellow dye made from the ground powder of rhizomes of *Curcuma longa* Linnaeus plant, is a noncertified color additive and spice. Curcumin is responsible for the imparted natural color [7, 69, 70]. It is also labeled as E 100 in Europe, CI #75300, CAS (Chemical Abstract Society) #458-37-7, INS 100(i), and CI Natural

Yellow 3. Turmeric has been used for centuries to enhance taste and has much promise as a potential therapeutic agent for many diseases, mediated through curcuminoid-induced decrease in NF-κB expression [71]. It was studied, along with annatto and several other additives, in the series of oral challenges that were either inconclusive or flawed in their design [51–53]. Thus, no evidence exists that turmeric causes a clinical allergy. However, there have been reports attributing allergic contact dermatitis to turmeric [72]. Evidence has continued to emerge that curcumin is not only immunomodulatory in terms of anti-inflammatory, anti-myeloid, antitumor, and antioxidative properties, but likely protective of the allergic response in animal models [73, 74]. Furthermore, the European Food Safety Authority (EFSA) recently ruled that curcumin is not carcinogenic and that its use at 3 mg/kg of bodyweight per day posed no harmful effects [75].

Carotenoids are another yellow-orange natural color used in butter, cheese, cereal, and other items. It is derived from either biologic or synthetic sources. Carotenoids are vitamin A precursors. The natural coloring is from carotene, but the synthetic version is made from acetone, and is all-*trans* in chemical structure. β-Carotene is an isomer of carotene. A related compound, canthaxanthin, isolated from the edible mushroom *Cantharellus cinnabarinus*, is another carotenoid compound used in food and also available as a synthetic color [7, 68]. Carotenoids are also labeled as CI 40800 and CAS# 514-78-3. These coloring agents have rarely been implicated in causing allergic reactions. Oral challenges to β-carotene were part of the studies discussed in the annatto and turmeric sections that were both flawed in design and inconclusive in determining if any of the additives studied, including carotenoids, caused hypersensitivity [50–52]. However, there is a 1978 case report describing atopic dermatitis, vomiting, colic, and restlessness in an infant being fed a diet with vitamin A drops and foods rich in β-carotene. This author could not prove skin test reactivity to β-carotene, but did show clinical sensitivity to vitamin A drops via a double-blind challenge. Thus, no mechanism for the reactivity of β-carotene was shown in this case [61]. A recent murine study involving B10A mice orally sensitized to ovalbumin found that a diet high in β-carotene was protective of the development of food allergy (both anaphylactic response and IgE development) [76].

Anthocyanins are plant-derived glycosides that, in combination, are responsible for red, blue, or purple color in fruits and vegetables [7, 69]. Anthocyanoids are closely related to flavanols and are produced from the same flavonoid biosynthetic pathway [77]. Grape color extract and grape skin extract are anthocyanin-containing colors that are used as a noncertified color additives, supplied as both an aqueous solution and water-soluble powder [69]. They are also labeled as INS 163 (ii). Grape color extract is made from Concord grapes and is very similar to grape juice, differing, however, in its ratio of anthocyanins, tartrates, malates, sugars, and minerals. The water-soluble color is derived from 3-mono- and 3, 5 di-glucosides of malvidin, delphinidin, cyanidin, and their acylated derivatives. Grape skin extract is made by steeping (aqueous extraction) fresh, de-seeded marc that is residual after pressing grapes into wine or juice. Again, its composition is similar to that of grape juice, but in different proportions [7, 69, 70]. Both grape skin extract and grape color extract are very expensive to produce because the color is found in trace quantities in most flowers, fruits, and vegetables (780–5000 ppm) and is difficult to extract. Anthocyanins are also found in purple corn, black carrot, passion fruit, and other exotic fruits as well. Most of the commercial color comes from either grapes or red cabbage [70]. Internationally, the color is known as E163 (Europe), cyanidin, delphinidin, malvidin, pelargonidin, peonidin, and petunidin.

Grape color extract is used in nonbeverage foods. Grape skin extract is used in carbonated drinks, -ades, beverage bases, and alcohol; additionally, both forms can be found in cherries used in ice cream and yogurt, fruit fillings, and candy/confections [54]. To date, there have been no case reports of allergy to grape skin extract or to grape color extract. Though rare, there are several reported cases and a case series of grape- and grape product (wine)-induced allergic reactions, ranging from anaphylaxis to oral allergy syndrome to exercised-induced anaphylaxis [63, 64, 78–93]. One group found a trend of HLA matching to HLA-DR11 in 9 of 11 patients, and additionally reported extensive cross-reactivity with other fruits (apples, cherries, peaches) [63, 64]. It has been suggested by data in one study that grape products might have a common allergen in endochitinases 4A and B, which are lipid transfer proteins [62]. It is unknown if this protein is present in grape color extract or grape juice extract, but it could be a potential allergen in susceptible individuals if it is found in the extracts [62, 64].

Paprika is a dark red, sweet powder made from dried, ground pods of the bell pepper *Capsicum annuum*. Paprika oleoresin is colored principally from capsanthin and capsorubin, amongst other compounds. They are labeled as CAS # 68917-78-2 and INS 160c. Both paprika and paprika oleoresin are used as a color and a spice in canned goods, vegetable oils, processed meats, salad dressings, snack food coatings, popcorn oil, cheese, and confections [3]. Neither is allowed in cosmetics or drugs [94, 95]. *Capsicum annuum* contains a profilin, Cap a 2, and the pollen of this plant has also been shown to sensitize horticultural workers and provoke IgE-mediated reactions [65–67, 96–98]. Specifically, SDS-PAGE fractionation of paprika and sera immunoblot analysis revealed binding to protein bands at 30 and 60 kDa [66]. There are also certain bell pepper species that express Bet v 1 and profilin homologs and a pathogenesis-related protein P23 that can be key for IgE binding [65, 99]. Despite the presence of profilin and Bet v 1 homologs, and evidence that there is a potential role for *Capsicum annuum* in latex-fruit syndrome, there have been no reported reactions specifically attributed to paprika's use as a color [96]. This is probably because the IgE-binding capacity of the homolog to Bet v 1 and profilin is destroyed in the processing of the color/spice, though P23 has been shown to survive this processing [99]. Its allergenicity as a spice will be discussed later in the chapter.

Beet powder (CAS# 7659-95-2, INS 162, beetroot red, betanine), carrot oil, and toasted partially defatted cooked cottonseed flour have not been implicated in causing clinical allergy when used as a coloring agent. Cottonseed has shown homology to Jug r 1 and Jug r 2 in walnut [71, 100, 101]. Cottonseed has caused anaphylaxis but its derived color has not [102–104]. Beet powder (beet juice base color) is used in fruit preparations, condiments, dairy, sauces, fillings, and candies. Carrot oil has been used in sauces, salad dressings, meat seasoning, pasta, margarine, and other foods. Additionally, titanium dioxide (CAS# 13463-67-7, CI 77891, INS 171, CI Pigment White 6) is also a noncertified dye for use in foods, such as confections, icings, cheese, medications, and cosmetics. It is restricted to 1% total of the product weight. There are no reports of allergy to its use as a colorant [3].

Food flavorings

Food flavorings are a heterogeneous group of supplements added in small quantities to foods to enhance flavor and quality. Flavorings are not primary ingredients because they are present in minute quantity compared to the main ingredients. Flavorings may be synthetic (artificial), natural, or derived from natural sources. The manufacturing process is thought to reduce protein content of naturally derived flavors as protein is separated from the flavorful molecules, and therefore would generally be expected to reduce allergenicity. However, many parent compounds from which these natural flavors are derived may be allergenic [105]. Artificial flavors, products synthesized from aromatic alcohols or terpenes, are used either as solo agents or in combination to mimic natural occurring flavors [106]. The overall incidence of allergy attributed to food flavors is low, and these are rare events, but Type I and IV hypersensitivities have been described [105].

Taste and flavor have a unique biochemistry and neuroproprioception. Flavor perception is a multifactorial sensory input that is integrated into an overall unique experience [107, 108]. It allows us to fully appreciate food while at the same time serving as a warning system against toxins, spoilage, smoke, or other untoward experiences [109]. This sensation has been conserved through our evolution [110]. Taste serves as an upstream trigger for digestive secretions [109]. Taste buds are located in specific areas of the tongue, palate, pharynx, larynx, epiglottis, uvula, and proximal esophagus. These require constant salivary secretions to maintain optimal taste perception [109]. Cranial nerves VII, IX, and X participate in receiving and transmitting signals from taste receptors located within the taste buds when stimulated by a food molecule [109]. This process is transmitted from these receptors through selective ion channels, structure-specific receptors, and G protein-coupled pathways. These signals are ultimately processed in the brainstem nuclei of cranial nerves VII, IX, and X, and the relative rates of signaling along these nerves are interpreted in the brain as a particular flavor [110, 111].

Flavor components are generally considered to be low molecular weight proteins, and thus too small to be considered allergens. Often these are considered volatile components [105]. Many natural flavors we encounter are the end product of chemical reactions that modify the original parent structure to arrive at the molecule that delivers flavor. This may involve heating, fermentation, distillation, concentration, or microencaspulation. The final product becomes a distinct form, such as an essence, powder, crystal, or emulsion. Artificial flavors are often similar in structure but unrelated to the natural component, yet they impart the same taste when we consume these flavors [105]. If a parent compound is allergenic, there is a distinct possibility that the derivative will also be allergenic. Though processing quite often separates the volatile flavoring from the protein, there can still be some contamination of protein allergens. Despite small molecule sizes these particles may become allergenic as haptens. This is typical in Type IV reactions, seen when food has contact with mucosa for a prolonged period of time. It can also be a route of sensitization for Type I reactions as well. Many reactions attributed to flavors are seen in patients with a continual, high concentration occupational exposure [105].

Regulations and definitions

Flavorings are food additives and are regulated by the FDA in the United States, under the Food, Drug, and Cosmetic Act, CFR, Title 21, Part 101, § 101.22 [41]. All ingredients in commercially sold food must be labeled on the package, in descending order of quantity contained in the product. Unlike colors, flavors can be group labeled under the term "artificial and natural flavors" and do not have to be individually declared [41]. This contrast to the regulations for color was initially intended as a protection for corporations in the marketplace to maintain trade secrets (e.g., the formula to Coca-Cola®) [105]. There are several exceptions to this requirement for ingredients widely thought or known to cause reactions, such as sulfites [112]. However, many allergens still are undeclared [105]. This is problematic to the unsuspecting patient.

Flavorings derived from known allergens have produced reactions as "hidden" allergens. "Hidden" allergens are not so much hidden on the label as they are disguised by their true chemical names. One such example is milk, which is often labeled as casein, a milk protein, or when broken down further called hydrolyzed sodium caseinate, a natural flavor derived from milk but conserving its antigenicity [113]. Protein derivatives, prior to 2006, were allowed to be labeled cryptically as their chemical breakdown product, or if they were natural flavors did not have to be specifically labeled at all. The Food Allergen Labeling and Consumer Protection Act of 2004 (FALCPA) now mandates that as of January 1, 2006, all products containing the "common 8" protein allergens (milk, egg, fish, crustacean shellfish, tree nuts, peanuts, wheat, and soy) must explicitly declare these items in the ingredient list in plain English (e.g., contains milk or soy) [114]. This measure is intended to allow patients to clearly identify potential allergens on the labels. These allergens were chosen because they cause approximately 90% of food allergies. However, in cases of factory-level contamination, such as ambient dust or use of the same conveyor belt line for different products, there is no requirement to label products with a "may contain..." statement. Many products do have such a designation, but it is purely voluntary at this point [115]. Recent research has suggested that such advisory labels are often ignored by food-allergic individuals when they do not specifically indicate the definitive presence of a particular ingredient [116–118].

The current definition of a spice, under the United States CFR is "any aromatic substance in the whole, broken, or ground form, except for those substances which have been traditionally regarded as foods... whose significant function in food is seasoning rather than nutritional; that is true to name; and from which no portion of any volatile oil or other flavoring principle has been removed" [41]. Spices are a special category of flavor, as they are derived exclusively from plants. Thus, they potentially harbor antigenicity. They are often used as both ingredients and additives. Spices that are also natural colors can be labeled as "spice and coloring" (e.g., paprika, turmeric, saffron). Spices can otherwise be labeled as spice, or as the actual spice if so desired. "Substances obtained by cutting, grinding, drying, pulping, or similar processing of tissue derived from fruit, vegetable, meat, fish, or poultry... are commonly understood... to be food rather than flavor and should be declared by their common name, meaning garlic powder must be labeled as such" [41].

Of the estimated 2% prevalence of food allergy internationally, spices represent 2% of this total [99]. Spices have been reported to cause anaphylaxis, asthma, and contact dermatitis [72, 99]. Moreover, further confounding prevalence data on spice allergy is the fact that use of certain spices is dictated by cultural and regional dietary preference [99, 119]. Prevalence of allergy to spice might also be influenced by occupational exposure, leading to increased sensitization, as has been noted with saffron and bell pepper workers [58, 120, 121]. As spices are flavors, they are present in minute quantities compared to the other ingredients, but have been known to cause allergy even at the low doses at which they are typically used. There is some question as to whether there is a threshold effect below which allergy cannot occur because the relative concentrations of spices in food are low [99]. However, the European Food Safety Authority (EFSA) issued a statement in 2004 that stated it failed to find sufficient evidence to establish such an intake threshold for spices that are on the food allergen list [122]. Because spices are also used to flavor other commercial products besides edible foods, there have been cases of reactions attributed to spices contained in cosmetics, toothpaste, fragrances, and massage oils [123–133].

Hot spices have some unique properties that make them more susceptible to potentially cause allergy. Piperine, in black pepper, can produce local swelling as a means to inhibit paracellular transport. Capsicum may increase its own paracellular transport across epithelium. Though it has been attributable to inducing occupational rhinitis, capsaicin is presently under investigation as a therapy in nonallergic rhinitis, and in a double-blind, placebo-controlled challenge demonstrated significant 2-week improvement from baseline in total nasal symptom score index, nasal congestion, sinus pressure, sinus pain, and headache versus placebo [134, 135]. Saponin, commonly found in plants, might have a detergent-like effect on gastric epithelium. In general, hotter spices can be sensitizing adjuvants by promoting transport of 70 kDa or smaller molecules, a size previously determined to be relevant for IgE binding and sensitization in spice allergy [99].

Because spices have plant origins, they often contain their parent plant allergens that might survive processing, most commonly the birch pollen allergen Bet v 1 and profilin [136, 137]. In hot spices, the grinding process destroys Bet v 1 (and homologs) and some profilins, but in roasted poppy seed they remain intact [138–141]. Apiaceae and Solanaceae family proteins tend to remain stable through various processing procedures, including roasting, grinding, and even cooking, increasing their allergenic potential in foods that are flavored with these spices [99]. Freezing was shown in certain lyophilized foods to increase the strength of SPTs [55]. Extensive cross-reactivity exists in oral pollen syndrome (oral allergen syndrome), most notoriously as described with celery-mugwort-birch-carrot, the so-called condiment syndrome [99, 136, 137]. The oral

Table 34.5 Reported allergic reactions to spices.

Spice	Family	Allergy	Specific IgE	Bet v 1 homolog	Profilin homolog	Other proteins	Reference
Allspice	*Myrtaceae*	Contact dermatitis	None	None	None		[132, 150]
Anise	*Apiaceae*	Rhinoconjunctivitis, anaphylaxis, angioedema	PST, 12, 12.9–13.7, 15–17.5, 20, 33, 34, 35, 37, 39, 40, 42, 48, 50–70 kDa	Pim a 1	Pim a 2		[139, 149, 151–159]
Basil	*Lamiaceae*	Contact dermatitis	PST, sIgE	None	None		[136, 158, 160–162]
Bay leaf	*Lauraceae*	Contact dermatitis, perioral dermatitis, asthma	PST, sIgE	None	None		[163–166]
Caraway seed	*Apiaceae*	Rhinoconjunctivitis, GI	20, 33, 34, 37, 39, 42, 48 kDa	None	None		[151]
Cardamom	*Zingiberaceae*	Dermatitis	PST	None	None		[167, 168]
Cayenne	*Solanaceae*	Atopic dermatitis, bronchospasm	PST, sIgE	None	None		[145, 146, 166, 169–171]
Celery	*Apiaceae*	Anaphylaxis, OAS, food-dependent exercise-induced anaphylaxis	PST, 30–70 kDa, including 55/58 kDa (Api g 5)	Api g 1	Api g 4		[172–177]
Chervil	*Apiaceae*		None	None	None		None
Chili	*Solanaceae*	Atopic dermatitis, bronchospasm	None	None	See paprika		[145, 146, 166, 169–171]
Chives	*Alliaceae*	Contact dermatitis		None	None		[178]
Cinnamon	*Canellaceae*	Bronchospasm, rhinoconjunctivitis, contact dermatitis, stomatitis, Type IV hypersensitivity	None	None	None		[97, 130, 132, 150, 151, 160, 164, 167–169, 179–196]
Cloves	*Myrtaceae*	Contact dermatitis	None	None	None		[97, 132, 150, 192, 194, 195]
Coriander	*Apiaceae*	Bronchospasm, anaphylaxis, contact dermatitis	PST, sIgE, basophil activation test, 12, 20, 21, 33, 34, 35, 37, 39, 40, 42, 34, 35, 37, 39, 40, 42, 48, ~70 kDa	Cor s 1	Cor s 2		[97, 139, 140, 145, 146, 151, 160, 169, 196–202]
Cumin	*Apiaceae*	Anaphylaxis, contact dermatitis	20, 33, 34, 37, 39, 42, 48, ~70 kDa	Cum c 1	Cum c 2		[139, 151, 152, 196, 203]
Curry	*Umbelliferae* and others	Anaphylaxis, urticaria/pruritus	PST, sIgE, 30 kDa, 90 kDa	NA	NA		[202, 204–206]
Dill	*Apiaceae*	Anaphylaxis, contact urticaria	12, 21, 35, 40 kDa	None	None		[151, 154, 207–210]
Fennel	*Apiaceae*	Rhinoconjunctivitis, bronchospasm, atopic dermatitis	20, 33, 34, 37, 39, 42, 48, 50–70, 65, 75 kDa	Foe v 1	Foe v 2		[139, 151, 153, 171, 196, 211–218]
Fenugreek	*Fabaceae*	Anaphylaxis, urticaria	PST, sIgE, 20–36 kDa, 50–66 kDa, 74 kDa; several minor bands at 14, 43, and 88 kDa	Tri f 4		2S albumin (Tri f 2), 7S vicilin (Tri f 1), 11S legumin (Tri f 3)	[219–222]
Garlic	*Alliaceae*	Contact dermatitis, bronchospasm, rhinitis, anaphylaxis	10, 12, 20, 31–60, 40, 42, 54, 56 kDa (alliin lyase)	None	None		[211, 223–250]
Ginger	*Zingiberaceae*	Contact dermatitis, bronchospasm	14, 23, 34 kDa	None	None		[154, 160, 169, 196, 198, 251]
Jalapeno	*Solanaceae*	Same as chili	None	None	None		[145, 146, 166, 169–171]
Lovage	*Apiaceae*		None	None	None		None
Mace	*Myristicaceae*	Bronchospasm, contact dermatitis	See nutmeg	None	None		[97, 160, 163, 166, 168, 169, 173–175, 251–254]
Marjoram	*Lamiaceae*	Atopic dermatitis, perioral dermatitis	PST, sIgE				[162, 164, 255, 256]
Mustard	*Myrtaceae*	Anaphylaxis, Type IV hypersensitivity, contact urticaria, oral allergy syndrome, asthma	PST, sIgE	None	None	14 kDa (Bra j 1, Sin a 1) seed storage proteins; 20 kDa, 30–40 kDa, 50 kDa Sin a 2 11S globulin in yellow mustard seed	[101, 142, 146, 198, 257–261]

Table 34.5 *(Continued)*

Spice	Family	Allergy	Specific IgE	Bet v 1 homolog	Profilin homolog	Other proteins	Reference
Nutmeg	*Myristicaceae*	Bronchospasm, contact dermatitis	PST, sIgE, histamine release assay	None	None		[97, 160, 163, 166, 168, 169, 173–175, 251–254]
Onion	*Alliaceae*	Anaphylaxis, bronchospasm, contact dermatitis, rhinoconjunctivitis, urticaria	PST, sIgE 12, 15, 43 kDa	None	None	15 kDa lipid transferase	[202, 231, 242, 262–272]
Oregano	*Lamiaceae*	Systemic reactions	PST, sIgE	None	None		[160, 162, 166, 256]
Paprika	*Solanaceae*	Contact urticaria, rhinoconjunctivitis (occupational rhinitis reported to capsaicin)	10, 17, 23 (Cap a 1w = osmotin-like), 24, 28, 29, 30, 32, 36, 40, 46, 69 kDa	None	Cap a 2		[65, 66, 97, 120, 121, 135, 146, 163, 169, 198, 273–283]
Parsley	*Apiaceae*	Angioedema, urticaria	None	Pet c 1	Pet c 2		[212, 242, 284–287]
Pepper	*Piperaceae*	Anaphylaxis, bronchospasm, contact dermatitis	PST, 11.8, 13.6, 14, 25, 28 (GLP), 30, 35, 40, 60 kDa	None	None		[65, 97, 145, 163, 167, 169, 196, 197, 275, 276, 278, 281–283, 288–292]
Pink peppercorns	*Anacardiaceae*	Atopic dermatitis (canine)	None	None	None		[293]
Peppermint	*Lamiaceae*	Contact allergy, anaphylactoid reactions, stomatitis	PST	None	None		[129, 162, 169, 202, 294–299]
Poppy seed	*Papaveraceae*	Anaphylaxis, exercise-induced anaphylaxis	5, 20, 25, 30, 34, 40, 45 kDa	None	None		[138, 141, 300–306]
Rosemary	*Lamiaceae*	Bronchospasm, contact dermatitis	PST, sIgE	None	None		[166, 307, 308]
Saffron	*Iridaceae*	Anaphylaxis, bronchospasm, rhinoconjunctivitis	21 kDa (Cro s 1); rCro s 3.01, rCro s 3.02	None	None	rCro s 3.01 and 3.02 are prolamin family LTPs with homology to Pru p 3	[58–60, 105, 251]
Sage	*Lamiaceae*	Bronchospasm, contact dermatitis	PST	None	None		[160, 162, 309–311]
Savory	*Lamiaceae*	Bronchospasm	PST	None	None		[166]
Sesame seed	*Pedaliaceae*	Anaphylaxis, bronchospasm, rhinitis, urticaria	10, 12, 14, 15–20, 15 (Ses i 5, oleosin), 17 (Ses i 4, oleosin), 25, 29, 32, 34, 45, (Ses i 3, vicilin-type globulin), 45, 52, 30–67, 78 kDa, Ses i 4, Ses i 5	None	None	7 (Ses i 2 2S), 9 kDa (Ses i 1 2S) seed storage proteins	[279, 300, 312–335]
Star anise	*Alliaceae*	Contact dermatitis	None	None	None		[336, 337]
Tarragon	*Asteraceae*	Subglottic edema	28–46, 60 kDa in related mugwort (*Artemisia vulgaris*)	None	None		[334, 338]
Thyme	*Lamiaceae*	Bronchospasm, atopic dermatitis, systemic reactions	PST, sIgE	None	None		[162, 166, 255, 339]
Turmeric	*Zingiberaceae*	Bronchospasm, contact dermatitis	None	None	None		[105, 160, 340–343]
Vanilla	*Orchidaceae*	Atopic dermatitis, contact dermatitis	None	None	None		[128, 131, 193–195, 344, 345]

PST, skin prick test; sIgE, serum-specific IgE (e.g., ImmunoCAP, RAST); kDa, kilo Dalton; LTP, lipid transfer protein; r, recombinant.

allergy syndrome is discussed in full detail elsewhere in this text. Spice allergy in this context would be secondary to a primary pollen allergy sensitization [99]. The cross-reactivity is stronger and more prevalent the more related the spice is to the primary pollen. Molecules such as Bet v 1 (and other PR-10 homologs) and profilins are generally responsible for the cross-reactivity, and therefore it can be inferred that the expression of these proteins in spices is testament to their functional importance in the plant from which the spice is derived. With sesame specifically, there is a seed storage 2S protein, identified in edible seeds and nuts including peanut, that has been identified as binding IgE in both mustard and sesame [99]. Yellow mustard contains an 11S globulin (legumin) with moderate homology to peanut (Ara h 3), hazelnut (Cor a 9), and cashew (Ana o 2) [142]. Other major plant proteins involved in spice allergy include lipid transfer proteins and the cupin 7S globulins (vicilins) [143].

In testing for spice allergy, clinical history is of utmost importance, as spices are minor food ingredients, and thus they might represent a less easy cause of allergic reaction. Based on older data, skin testing, including prick-to-prick method in the absence of commercial extract, has shown more accuracy than RAST testing for specific IgE, though a combination approach is most commonly recommended [144–146]. Naturally, some ingredients in spice, when applied to the skin could be irritants. With both onion and garlic, bronchial provocation tests have been performed in the setting of spice workers [147]. One author described a leukocyte histamine release assay used with several different spices [148]. An exercise challenge was also described for a case of food-dependent exercise-induced anaphylaxis attributable to celery [149]. Also, as was the case with colorants, there is one pharmaceutical-related case, involving anaphylaxis attributable to star anise contained in Oseltamivir (Tamiflu®), in a patient with star anise sensitivity (Table 34.5) [346].

Summary

Food flavorings and colorings are a heterogeneous group of compounds that are often derived from potential allergens. Despite processing, allergenic epitopes or haptens that are recognized by specific IgE or cause Type IV reactions have been reported in the medical literature. Though the overall prevalence of reactions attributable to food colorings and flavorings is unknown it is thought to be low. Although recent legislation has required declaration of carmine/cochineal extract by name on product labels, current labeling regulations continue to make identification of other potential food color and flavor allergens a frustrating process in susceptible individuals.

References

1. Barrows JN, Lipman AL, Bailey CJ. Color additives: FDA's regulatory process and historical perspectives. *Food Saf Mag* 2003; October/November issue. Reprinted on FDA/CSFAN. Available at http://www.fda.gov/downloads/ForConsumers/ConsumerUpdates/ucm048960.pdf (Last accessed July 13, 2013).
2. United States Food and Drug Administration/International Food Information Council Brochure. Food color facts. January 1992 and January 1993. Available at http://www.healthyschools.org/documents/food_dyes-CEH_2-09.pdf (Last accessed July 13, 2013).
3. Hallagan JB, Allen DC, Borzelleca JF. The safety and regulatory status of food, drug and cosmetics colour additives exempt from certification. *Food Chem Toxicol* 1995;33:515–528.
4. Denner WHB. Colorings and preservatives in food. *Hum Nutr Appl Nutr* 1984;38A:435–449.
5. United States Department of Health & Human Services, United States Food & Drug Administration, Center for Food Safety and Applied Nutrition, Food Ingredients and Packing. Summary of color additives listed for use in the United States in foods, drugs, cosmetics, and medical devices, November 2004 (updated 3/10/2006). Available at http://www.fda.gov/forindustry/coloradditives/coloradditiveinventories/ucm115641.htm (Last accessed July 13, 2013).
6. Color Additive Amendments of 1960, Public Law 86-618, 74 Stat. 397.
7. Lucas CD, Hallagan JB, Taylor SL. The role of natural color additives in food allergy. *Adv Food Nutr Res* 2001;43:195–216.
8. 21 CFR parts 73 and 74 (April 1, 2006).
9. 21 CFR § 101.22 (April 1, 2006).
10. 71 FR § 19, 4839–4851 (January 30, 2006).
11. 71 FR 208 (January 5, 2009).
12. Chung K, Baker JR, Baldwin JL, et al. Identification of carmine allergens among three carmine allergy patients. *Allergy* 2001;56:73–77.
13. Ferrer A, Marco FM, Andreu C, et al. Occupational asthma to carmine in a butcher: analysis of the literature on allergy to carmine. *Int Arch Allergy Immunol* 2005;158:243–250.
14. Acero S, Tabar, AI, Alvarez MJ, et al. Occupational asthma and food allergy due to carmine. *Allergy* 1998;53:897–901.
15. Lizaso MT, Moneo I, Garcia BE, et al. Identification of allergens involved in occupational asthma due to carmine dye. *Ann Allergy Asthma Immunol* 2000;84:549–552.
16. Anibarro B, Seoane J, Vila C, et al. Occupational asthma induced by carmine among butchers. *Int Occup Med Environ Health* 2003;16:133–137.
17. Yamakawa Y, Hiroyuki H, Yamakawa T, et al. Cochineal extract-induced immediate allergy. (Letter to the Editor). *J Dermatol* 2009;36:72–74.
18. Ohigaya Y, Arakawa F, Akiyama H, et al. Molecular cloning, expression, and characterization of a major 38-kd cochineal allergen. *J Allergy Clin Immunol* 2009;123:1157–1162.
19. Docket Number 98P-0724. Petition to the United States Food and Drug Administration, Center for Science in the

Public Interest, August 24, 1998. Available at http://www.cspinet.org (Last accessed July 13, 2013).
20. Taylor SL, Dormedy ES. Flavorings and colorings. *Allergy* 1998;53(Suppl 46):80–82.
21. Dweck AC. Natural ingredients for colouring and styling. *Int J Cosmet Sci* 2002;24:1–16.
22. Baldwin J, Chou A, Solomon WR. Popsicle-induced anaphylaxis due to carmine dye allergy. *Ann Allergy Asthma Immunol* 1997;79:415–419.
23. Donkin RA. *Spanish Red: An Ethnogeographical Study of Cochineal and the Opuntia Cactus*, 1977, *American Philosophical Society*. 67, part 5.
24. 21 CFR § 73.111 (April 1, 2006).
25. 21 CFR § 73.2087 (April 1, 2006).
26. 21 CFR § 701.3 (April 1, 2006).
27. Sarkany I, Meara R, Everall J. Cheilitis due to carmine in lip salve. *Trans Ann Rep St John's Hosp Dermatol Soc* 1961;46:39.
28. Burge PS, O'Brien M, Harries MG, et al. Occupational asthma due to inhaled carmine. *Clin Allergy* 1979;9:185–189.
29. Park GR. Anaphylactic shock resulting from casualty simulation. A case report. *J R Army Med Corps* 1981;127:85–86.
30. Tenebene A, Bessot JC, Lenz D, et al. Asthme profesionnel au carmine de cochenille. *Arch Mal Prof* 1987;48:569–571.
31. Quierce S, Cuevas M, Olaguibel JM, et al. Occupational asthma and immunologic responses induced by inhaled carmine among employees at a factory making natural dyes. *J Allergy Clin Immunol* 1994;93:44–52.
32. Kagi MK, Wuthrich B, Johansson SG. Campari-orange anaphylaxis due to carmine allergy. *Lancet* 1994;344:60–61.
33. Beaudouin E, Kanny G, Lambert H, et al. Food anaphylaxis following ingestion of carmine. *Ann Allergy Asthma Immunol* 1995;74:427–430.
34. Stücker W, Roggembuck D, von Kirchbach G. Schweres asthma nach berflicher exposition gegenüber dem lebensmittelfarbstoff kochenille/karmin. *Allegro J* 1996;5:143–146.
35. Wuthrich B, Kagi M, Stucker W. Anaphylaxis reactions to ingested carmine (E120). *Allergy* 1997;52:1133–1137.
36. Dicello MC, Myc A, Baker JR Jr, et al. Anaphylaxis after ingestion of carmine colored foods: two case reports and a review of the literature. *Allergy Asthma Proc* 1999;20(6):377–382.
37. Tabar AI, Alvarez MJ, Acero S, et al. Carmine (E 120) induced occupational asthma revisited. *J Allergy Clin Immunol* 2003;111:415–419.
38. Greenhawt MJ, McMorris MS, Baldwin JL. Carmine dye hypersensitivity masquerading as azithromycin hypersensitivity. *Allergy Asthma Proc* 2009;30:95–101.
39. Shaw DW. Allergic contact dermatitis from carmine. *Dermatitis* 2008;20:292–295.
40. Greenhawt MJ, Baldwin JL. Carmine dye and cochineal extract: hidden allergens no more (perspectives). *Ann Allergy Asthma Immunol* 2009:103:73–75.
41. 21 CFR § 101.22 (April 1, 2006).
42. 21 CFR § 201.1 (April 1, 2006).
43. 77 FR 22485 (April 16, 2011).
44. Galindo-Cuspinera V, Lubran MB, Rankin SA. Comparison of volatile compounds in water- and oil-soluble annatto (*Bixa orellana* L) extracts. *J Agric Food Chem* 2002;50:2010–2015.
45. Giuliano G, Rosati C, Bramley PM. To dye or not to dye: biochemistry of annatto unveiled. *Trends Biochem* 2003;21(12):513–516.
46. 9 CFR § 424.21 (January 1, 2006).
47. 21 CFR § 73.3 (April 1, 2006).
48. Young E, Patel S, Stoneham M, et al. The prevalence of reaction to food additives in a survey population. *J R Coll Physicians Lond* 1987;21:241–247.
49. Mikkelsen H, Larsen JC, Tarding F. Hypersensitivity reactions to food colors with special reference to the natural color annatto extract. *Arch Toxicol Suppl* 1978;(Suppl 1):141–143.
50. Juhlin L. Recurrent urticaria: clinical investigation of 330 patients. *Br J Dermatol* 1981;104:369–381.
51. Fuglsang G, Madsen C, Saval P, et al. Prevalence of intolerance to food additives among Danish school children. *Pediatr Allergy Immunol* 1993;4:123–129.
52. Fuglsang G, Madsen C, Halken S, et al. Adverse reactions to food additives in children with atopic symptoms. *Allergy* 1994;49:31–37.
53. Veien NK, Hattel T, Justesen O, et al. Oral challenge with food additives. *Contact Dermat* 1987;17:100–103.
54. Nish W, Whisman B, Goetz D, et al. Anaphylaxis to annatto dye: a case report. *Ann Allergy* 1991;61:47–52.
55. Van Assendelft AHW. Bronchospasm induced by vanilla and lactose. *Eur J Respir Dis* 1984;65:468–472.
56. Auttachoat W, Germolec DR, Smith MJ, et al. Contact sensitizing potential of annatto extract and its two primary color components, cis-bixin and norbixin, in female BALB/c mice. *Food Chem Toxicol* 2011;49:2638–2644.
57. Ebo DG, Ingelbrecht S, Bridts CH, et al. Allergy for cheese: evidence for an IgE-mediated reaction from the natural dye annatto. *Allergy* 2009;64:1554–1561.
58. Feo F, Martinez J, Martinez A, et al. Occupational allergy in saffron workers. *Allergy* 1997;52(6):633–641.
59. Wuthrich B, Schmid-Grendelmeyer P, Lundberg M. Anaphylaxis to saffron. *Allergy* 1997;52:476–477.
60. Gomez-Gomez L, Feo-Brito F, Rubia-Moraga A, et al. Involvement of lipid transfer proteins in saffron hypersensitivity: molecular cloning of the potential allergens. *J Investig Allergol Clin Immunol* 2010;20:407–412.
61. Greenbaum J. Vitamin A sensitivity. *Ann Allergy* 1979;43:98–99.
62. Pastorello EA, Farioli L, Pravettoni V, et al. Identification of grape and wine allergens as an endochitinase 4, a lipid-transfer protein, and a thaumatin. *J Allergy Clin Immunol* 2003;111(2):350–359.
63. Kalogeromitros DC, Makris MP, Gregoriou SG, et al. Sensitization to other foods in subjects with reported allergy to grapes. *Allergy Asthma Proc* 2006;27:68–71.
64. Kalogeromitros DC, Makris MP, Gregoriou SG, et al. Grape anaphylaxis: a study of 11 adult onset cases. *Allergy Asthma Proc* 2005;26:53–58.
65. Jensen-Jarolim E, Santner B, Leitner A, et al. Bell peppers (*Capsicum annuum*) express allergens (profilin, pathogenesis-related protein P23 and Bet v 1) depending on the

horticultural strain. *Int Arch Allergy Immunol* 1998;116:103–109.

66. van Toorenenbergen AW, Waanders J, Gerth Van Wijk R, et al. Immunoblot analysis of IgE-binding antigens in paprika and tomato pollen. *Int Arch Allergy Immunol* 2000;122:246–250.
67. Willerroider M, Fuchs H, Ballmer-Weber BK, et al. Cloning and molecular and immunological characterisation of two new food allergens, Cap a 2 and Lyc e 1, profilins from bell pepper (*Capsicum annuum*) and tomato (*Lycopersicon esculentum*). *Int Arch Allergy Immunol* 2003;131:245–255.
68. Farrell KT. *Spices, Condiments and Seasoning*, 1985, New York: Van Nostrand Reinhold.
69. Marmion DM. *Handbook of US Colorants: Foods, Drugs, Cosmetics and Medical Devices*, 3rd edn, 1991, New York: John Wiley & Sons, Inc.
70. *Natural Colors* (Brochure), 1999, Warner Jenkinson.
71. Aggarwal BB, Shishodia S. Suppression of the nuclear factor-kappaB activation pathway by spice-derived phytochemicals: reasoning for seasoning. *Ann N Y Acad Sci* 2004;1030:434–441.
72. Brancaccio RR, Alvarez MS. Contact allergy to food. *Dermatol Therapy* 2004;17:302–313.
73. Kurup VP, Barios CS. Immunomodulatory effects of curcumin in allergy. *Mol Nutr Food Res* 2008;52:1031–1039.
74. Srivastava RM, Singh S, Dubey SK et al. Immunomodulatory and therapeutic activity of curcumin. *Int Immunopharmacol* 2011;11:331–341.
75. European Food Safety Authority. Scientific opinion on the re-evaluation of curcumin (E100) as a food additive. *EFSA J* 2010;8:1679.
76. Sato Y, Akiyama H, Matsuoka H, et al. Dietary carotenoids inhibit oral sensitization and the development of food allergy. *J Agric Food Chem* 2010;58:7180–7186.
77. Mattivi F, Guzzon R, Vrhovsek U, et al. Metabolite profiling of grape: flavonols and anthocyanins. *J Agric Food Chem* 2006;54:7692–7702.
78. Eyermann CH. Allergic purpura. *South Med J* 1935;28:341–345.
79. Kahn IS. Fruit sensitivity. *South Med J* 1942;35:858–859.
80. Tuft L, Blumstein G. Studies in food allergy II, sensitization to fresh fruits: clinical and experimental observations. *J Allergy* 1942;13:574–581.
81. Frankland AW, Aalberse RC. Silver birch (Betula) pollen allergy and fresh fruit allergy. *Clin Ecol* 1987;5:55–58.
82. Kivity S, Sneh E, Greif J, et al. The effect of food and exercise on the skin response to compound 40/80 in patients with food-associated exercise-induced urticaria-angioedema. *J Allergy Clin Immunol* 1988;81:1155–1158.
83. Ortolani C, Ispano M, Pastorello E, et al. The oral allergy syndrome. *Ann Allergy* 1988;61:47–52.
84. David TJ. Anaphylactic shock during elimination diets for severe atopic eczema. *Arch Dis Child* 1984;59:983–986.
85. Moyer DB. Utility of food challenges in unexplained anaphylaxis. *J Allergy Clin Immunol* 1990;85:272.
86. Dohi M, Suko M, Sugiyama H, et al. Food-dependent, exercise induced anaphylaxis: a study on 11 Japanese cases. *J Allergy Clin Immunol* 1991;87:34–40.
87. Esteve P, Vega F, Garcia-Quintero MT, et al. IgE-mediated hypersensitivity to white grape. *Allergy* 1993;(Suppl I):14–17, 164.
88. Parker SL, Krondl M, Coleman P. Foods perceived by adults as causing adverse reactions. *J Am Diet Assoc* 1993;93:40–46.
89. Steinman HA, Potter PC. The precipitation of symptoms by common foods in children with atopic dermatitis. *Allergy Proc* 1994;15:203–210.
90. Garcia-Ortiz JC, Cosmes-Martin P, Lopez-Asunsolo A. Melon sensitivity shares allergens with Plantago and grass pollens. *Allergy* 1995;50:269–273.
91. Fernandez-Rivas M, Van Ree R, Cuevas M. Allergy to Rosaceae fruits without related pollinosis. *J Allergy Clin Immunol* 1997;100:728–733.
92. Vaswani SK, Hamilton RG, Carey RN, et al. Anaphylaxis, recurrent urticaria and angioedema from grape hypersensitivity. *J Allergy Clin Immunol* 1998;101:S31.
93. Karakaya G, Kalyanev AF. Allergy to grapes [Letter; Comment]. *Ann Allergy Asthma Immunol* 2000;84(2):265.
94. 21 CFR § 73.340 (April 1, 2006).
95. 21 CFR § 73.345 (April 1, 2006).
96. Wagner S, Radauer C, Hafner C, et al. Characterization of cross-reactive bell pepper allergens involved in the latex-fruit syndrome. *Clin Exp Allergy* 2004;34:1739–1746.
97. van den Akker TW, Roesyanto-Mahadi ID, van Toorenenbergen AW, et al. Contact allergy to spices. *Contact Dermat* 1990;22:267–272.
98. Niinimaki A, Hannuksela M, Makinen-Kiljunen S. Skin prick tests and in vitro immunoassays with native spices and spice extracts. *Ann Allergy Asthma Immunol* 1995;75:280–286.
99. Schöll I, Jensen-Jarolim E. Allergenic potency of spices: hot, medium hot, or very hot. *Int Arch Allergy Immunol* 2004;135:247–261.
100. Teuber SS, Jarvis KC, Dandekar AM, et al. Identification and cloning of a complementary DNA encoding a vicilin-like proprotein, Jug r 2, from English walnut kernel (*Juglans regia*), a major food allergen. *J Allergy Clin Immunol* 1999;104:1311–1320.
101. Teuber SS, Dandekar AM, Peterson WR, et al. Cloning and sequencing of a gene encoding a 2S albumin seed storage protein precursor from English walnut *(Juglans regia)*, a major food allergen. *J Allergy Clin Immunol* 1998;101:807–814.
102. O'Neil, CE, Lehrer SB. Anaphylaxis apparently caused by a cottonseed-containing candy ingested on a commercial airliner [Letter] *J Allergy Clin Immunol* 1989;84(3):407.
103. Malanin G, Kalimo K. Angioedema and urticaria caused by cottonseed protein in whole-grain bread. *J Allergy Clin Immunol* 1988;82(2):261–264.
104. Atkins FM, Wilson M, Bock SA. Cottonseed hypersensitivity: new concerns over an old problem. *J Allergy Clin Immunol* 1988;82(2):242–250.
105. Taylor SL, Dormedy ES. The role of flavoring substances in food allergy and intolerance. *Adv Food Nutr Res* 1998;42:1–44.
106. Kumar A, Rawlings RD, Beaman DC. The mystery ingredients: sweeteners, flavorings, dyes and preservatives in analgesic/antipyretic, antihistamine/decongestants, cough and

cold, antidiarrheal and liquid theophylline preparations. *Pediatrics* 1993;91:927–933.

107. Small DM, Prescott J. Odor/taste integration and the perception of flavor. *Exp Brain Res* 2005;166:345–357.
108. Verhagen JV. The neurocognitive bases of human multimodal food perception: consciousness. *Brain Res Rev* 2006;53:1–16.
109. Bromley SM. Smell and taste disorders: a primary care approach. *Am Fam Physician* 2000;61:427–436, 438.
110. Cullen MM, Leopold DA. Disorders of smell and taste. *Med Clin North Am* 1999;83(1):57–74.
111. Bruch RC, Kalinoski DL, Kare MR. Biochemistry of vertebrate olfaction and taste. *Annu Rev Nutr* 1988;8:21–42.
112. 21 CFR § 101.100 (April 1, 2006).
113. Gern JE, Yank E, Evrard HM, et al. Allergic reactions to milk-contaminated "non-dairy" products. *N Engl J Med* 1991;324:976–979.
114. Food Allergen Labeling and Consumer Protection Act of 2004, Pub. L. No. 108-282, 118 Stat. 905.
115. United States Department of Health and Human Services, Food and Drug Administration, Center for Food Safety and Nutrition. *Guidance for Industry: Questions and Answers Regarding Food Allergens, Including the Food Allergen Labeling and Consumer Protection Act of 2004 (Edition 4)*, October 2006. Available at http://www.cfsan.fda.gov/guidance.html (Last accessed July 13, 2013).
116. Pieretti MM, Chung D, Pacenza R. Audit of manufactured products: use of allergen advisory labels and identification of labeling ambiguities. *J Allergy Clin Immunol* 2009;124:337–341.
117. Barnett J, Muncer K, Leftwich J, et al. Using 'may contain' labeling to inform food choice: a qualitative study of nut allergic consumers. *BMC Public Health* 2011;11:734–742.
118. Sheth SS, Wasserman S, Kagan R, et al. Role of food labels in accidental exposures in food-allergic individuals in Canada. *Ann Allergy Asthma Immunol* 2010:104:60–65.
119. Dalal I, Binson I, Reifen R. Food allergy is a matter of geography after all: sesame as a major cause of severe IgE-mediated food allergic reactions among infants and young children in Israel. *Allergy* 2002;57:362–365.
120. Groenewoud GC, de Jong NW, van Oorschot-van Nes AJ, et al. Prevalence of occupational allergy to bell pepper pollen in greenhouses in the Netherlands. *Clin Exp Allergy* 2002;32:434–440.
121. Vermeulen AM, Groenewoud GC, de Jong NW, et al. Primary sensitization to sweet bell pepper pollen in greenhouse workers with occupational allergy. *Clin Exp Allergy* 2003;33:1439–1442.
122. European Food Safety Authority, Scientific Panel on Dietetic Products, Nutrition, and Allergies. EFSA provides scientific basis for labeling of food allergens: current evidence does not allow determination of intake thresholds (Press Release). March 25, 2004 (updated July 25, 2006).
123. Fisher AA. Dermatitis due to cinnamon and cinnamicaldehyde. *Curr Contact News* 1975;16:383–384.
124. Veien NK, Hattel T, Justesen O, et al. Oral challenge with balsam of Peru in patients with eczema: a preliminary study. *Contact Dermat* 1983;9:75–76.
125. Veien NK, Hattel T, Justesen O, et al. Oral challenge with balsam of Peru. *Contact Dermat* 1985;12:104–107.
126. Veien NK, Hattel T, Justesen O, et al. Reduction of intake of balsams in patients sensitive to balsam of Peru. *Contact Dermat* 1985;3:270–273.
127. Spencer LV, Fowler JF. "Thin Mint" cookie dermatitis. *Contact Dermat* 1988;18(3):185–186.
128. Kanny G, Hatahet R, Moneret-Vautrin DA, et al. Allergy and intolerance to flavouring agents in atopic dermatitis in young children. *Allerg Immunol (Paris)* 1994;26(6):209–210.
129. Sainio EL, Kanerva L. Contact allergens in toothpastes and a review of their hypersensitivity. *Contact Dermat* 1995;33:100–105.
130. Sanchez-Perez J, Garcia-Diez A. Occupational allergic contact dermatitis from eugenol, oil of cinnamon and oil of cloves in a physiotherapist. *Contact Dermat* 1999;41:346–347.
131. Ferguson JE, Beck MH. Contact sensitivity to vanilla in a lip salve. *Contact Dermat* 1995;33:352.
132. Niinimaki A. Delayed-type allergy to spices. *Contact Dermat* 1984;11:34–40.
133. Niinimaki A. Double-blind placebo-controlled peroral challenges in patients with delayed-type allergy to balsam of Peru. *Contact Dermat* 1995;33:78–83.
134. Bernstein JA, Davis BP, Picard JK, et al. A randomized, double-blind, parallel trial comparing capsaicin nasal spray with placebo in subjects with a significant component of nonallergic rhinitis. *Ann Allergy Asthma Immunol* 2011;107:171–178.
135. Nam Y-H, Jin HJ, Hwang E-K, et al. Occupational rhinitis induced by capsaicin. *Allergy Asthma Immunol Res* 2012;4:104–106.
136. Helbling A, Lopez M, Schwartz HJ, et al. Reactivity of carrot-specific IgE antibodies with celery, apiaceous spices, and birch pollen. *Ann Allergy* 1993;70:495–499.
137. Halmepuro L, Lowenstein H. Immunological investigation of possible structural similarities between pollen antigens and antigens in apple, carrot and celery tuber. *Allergy* 1985;40:264–272.
138. Jensen-Jarolim E, Gerstmayer G, Kraft D, et al. Serological characterization of allergens in poppy seeds. *Clin Exp Allergy* 1999;29:1075–1079.
139. Jensen-Jarolim E, Leitner A, Hirschwehr R, et al. Characterization of allergens in Apiaceae spices: anise, fennel, coriander and cumin. *Clin Exp Allergy* 1997;27:1299–1306.
140. Bock SA. Anaphylaxis to coriander: a sleuthing story. *J Allergy Clin Immunol* 1993;91:1232–1233.
141. Gloor M, Kagi M, Wuthrich B. Poppyseed anaphylaxis. *Schweiz Med Wochenschr* 1995;125:1434–1437.
142. Palomares O, Vereda A, Cuesta-Herranz, et al. Cloning, sequencing, and recombinant production of Sin a 2, an allergenic 11S globulin from yellow mustard seeds. *J Allergy Clin Immunol* 2007;119:1189–1196.
143. Breitenender H, Radauer C. A classification of plant food allergens. *J Allergy Clin Immunol* 2004;113:821–831.
144. Muhlemann RJ, Wuthrich B. Food allergies 1983-1987. *Schweiz Med Wochenschr* 1991;121:1696–1700.

145. Niinimaki A, Bjorksten F, Puukka M, et al. Spice allergy: results of skin prick tests and RAST with spice extracts. *Allergy* 1989;44:60–65.
146. Niinimaki A, Hannuksela M. Immediate skin test reactions to spices. *Allergy* 1981;36:487–493.
147. Jimenez-Timon A, Rodriguez Trabado A, Hernandez Arbeiza FJ, et al. Anterior rhinomanometry as a diagnostic test in occupational allergy caused by Liliaceae. *Allergol Immunopathol* 2002;30:295–299.
148. van Toorenenbergen AW, Dieges PH. Demonstration of spice-specific IgE in patients with suspected food allergies. *J Allergy Clin Immunol* 1987;79(1):108–113.
149. Baek C-H, Bae Y-J, Cho S, et al. Food-dependent exercise-induced anaphylaxis in the celery-mugwort-birch-spice syndrome. *Allergy* 2010;65:792–793.
150. Kanerva L, Estlander T, Jolanki R. Occupational allergic contact dermatitis from spices. *Contact Dermat* 1996;35:157–162.
151. Garcia-Gonzalez JJ, Bartolome-Zavala B, Fernandez-Melendez S, et al. Occupational rhinoconjunctivitis and food allergy because of aniseed sensitization. *Ann Allergy Asthma Immunol* 2002;88:518–522.
152. Anliker MD, Borelli S, Wuthrich B. Occupational protein contact dermatitis from spices in a butcher: a new presentation of the mugwort-spice syndrome. *Contact Dermat* 2002;46:72–74.
153. Wüthrich B, Dietschi R. The celery-carrot-mugwort-condiment syndrome: skin test and RAST results. *Schweiz Med Wochenschr* 1985;115:258–264.
154. van Toorenenbergen AW, Huijskes-Heins MI, Leijnse B, et al. Immunoblot analysis of IgE-binding antigens in spices. *Int Arch Allergy Appl Immunol* 1988;86:117–120.
155. Sainte-Laudy J, Vallon C, Guerin JC. Bioclinical interest in the assay of leukotrienes in four cases of sensitization to trophallergens. *Allerg Immunol (Paris)* 1997;29(152):155–156, 159.
156. Eseverri JL, Cozzo M, Castillo M, et al. Round table: immunological urticaria mediated by IgE. *Allergol Immunopathol (Madr)* 1999;27:104–111.
157. Gonzalez-Gutierrez ML, Sanchez-Fernandez C, Esteban-Lopez MI, et al. Allergy to anis. *Allergy* 2000;55:195–196.
158. Romano A, Di Fonso M, Giuffreda F, et al. Diagnostic work-up for food-dependent, exercise-induced anaphylaxis. *Allergy* 1995;50:817–824.
159. Garcia VG, Jane PG, Zavala BB. Aniseed-induced nocturnal tongue angioedema. *J Investig Allergol Clin Immunol* 2007;17:406–408.
160. Futrell JM, Rietschel RL. Spice allergy evaluated by results of patch tests. *Cutis* 1993;52:288–290.
161. Hefle SL, Jeanniton E, Taylor SL. Development of a sandwich enzyme-linked immunosorbent assay for the detection of egg residues in processed foods. *J Food Prot* 2001;64:1812–1816.
162. Benito M, Jorro G, Morales C, et al. Labiatae allergy: systemic reactions due to ingestion of oregano and thyme. *Ann Allergy Asthma Immunol* 1996;76:416–418.
163. Jensen-Jarolim E, Gajdzik L, Haberl I, et al. Hot spices influence permeability of human intestinal epithelial monolayers. *J Nutr* 1998;128:577–581.
164. Farkas J. Perioral dermatitis from marjoram, bay leaf and cinnamon. *Contact Dermat* 1981;7:121.
165. Hausen BM. A 6-year experience with compositae mix. *Am J Contact Derm* 1996;7:94–99.
166. Lemiere C, Cartier A, Lehrer SB, et al. Occupational asthma caused by aromatic herbs. *Allergy* 1996;51:647–649.
167. Meding B. Skin symptoms among workers in a spice factory. *Contact Dermat* 1993;29:202–205.
168. Dooms-Goossens A, Dubelloy R, Degreef H. Contact and systemic contact-type dermatitis to spices. *Dermatol Clin* 1990;8:89–93.
169. Zuskin E, Kanceljak B, Skuric Z, et al. Immunological and respiratory findings in spice-factory workers. *Environ Res* 1988;47:95–108.
170. Settipane GA. Anaphylactic deaths in asthmatic patients. *Allergy Proc* 1989;10:271–274.
171. Rance F, Dutau G. Labial food challenge in children with food allergy. *Pediatr Allergy Immunol* 1997;8:41–44.
172. van der Walt A, Lopata AL, Nieuwenhuizen NE. Work related allergy and asthma in spice mill workers—the impact of processing dried spices on IgE reactivity patterns. *Int Arch Allergy Immunol* 2010;152:271–278.
173. Ebner C, Hirschwehr R, Bauer L, et al. Identification of allergens in fruits and vegetables: IgE cross-reactivities with the important birch pollen allergens Bet v 1 and Bet v 2 (birch profilin). *J Allergy Clin Immunol* 1995;95:962–969.
174. Breiteneder H, Hoffmann-Sommergruber K, O'Riordain G, et al. Molecular characterization of Api g 1, the major allergen of celery *(Apium graveolens)*, and its immunological and structural relationships to a group of 17-kDa tree pollen allergens. *Eur J Biochem* 1995;233:484–489.
175. van Ree R, Voitenko V, van Leeuwen WA, et al. Profilin is a cross-reactive allergen in pollen and vegetable foods. *Int Arch Allergy Immunol* 1992;98:97–104.
176. Vallier P, DeChamp C, Valenta R, et al. Purification and characterization of an allergen from celery immunochemically related to an allergen present in several other plant species: identification as a profilin. *Clin Exp Allergy* 1992;22:774–782.
177. Caballero T, Martin-Esteban M. Association between pollen hypersensitivity and edible vegetable allergy: a review. *J Investig Allergol Clin Immunol* 1998;8:6–16.
178. Roller E, Meller S, Homey B, et al. Contact dermatitis caused by spinach, hedge mustard and chives. *Hautarzt* 2003;54:374–375.
179. Calnan CD. Cinnamon dermatitis from an ointment. *Contact Dermat* 1976;2:167–170.
180. Cohen DM, Bhattacharyya I. Cinnamon-induced oral erythema multiforme-like sensitivity reaction. *J Am Dent Assoc* 2000;131:929–934.
181. De Benito V, Alzaga R. Occupational allergic contact dermatitis from cassia (Chinese cinnamon) as a flavouring agent in coffee. *Contact Dermat* 1999;40:165.
182. Drake TE, Maibach HI. Allergic contact dermatitis and stomatitis caused by a cinnamic aldehyde-flavored toothpaste. *Arch Dermatol* 1976;112:202–203.
183. Goh CL, Ng SK. Bullous contact allergy from cinnamon. *Derm Beruf Umwelt* 1988;36:186–187.

184. Hurlimann AF, Wüthrich B. Eating cinnamon in cinnamaldehyde allergy. *Hautarzt* 1995;46:660–661.
185. Lamey PJ, Lewis MA, Rees TD, et al. Sensitivity reaction to the cinnamonaldehyde component of toothpaste. *Br Dent J* 1990;168:115–118.
186. Ludera-Zimoch G. Case of urticaria with immediate local and generalized reaction to cinnamon oil and benzaldehyde. *Przegl Dermatol* 1981;68:67–70.
187. Magnusson B, Wilkinson DS. Cinnamic aldehyde in toothpaste. 1. Clinical aspects and patch tests. *Contact Dermat* 1975;1:70–76.
188. Miller RL, Gould AR, Bernstein ML. Cinnamon-induced stomatitis venenata. Clinical and characteristic histopathologic features. *Oral Surg Oral Med Oral Pathol* 1992;73:708–716.
189. Nixon R. Cinnamon allergy in a baker. *Australas J Dermatol* 1995;36:41.
190. Speer F. Food allergy: the 10 common offenders. *Am Fam Physician* 1976;13:106–112.
191. Uragoda CG. Asthma and other symptoms in cinnamon workers. *Br J Ind Med* 1984;41:224–227.
192. Warin RP, Smith RJ. Chronic urticaria: investigations with patch and challenge tests. *Contact Dermat* 1982;8:117–121.
193. Salam TN, Fowler JF Jr. Balsam-related systemic contact dermatitis. *J Am Acad Dermatol* 2001;45:377–381.
194. Hjorth N. Eczematous allergy to balsams, perfumes and flavouring agents. *Dan Med Bull* 1961;8:143–144.
195. Hjorth N. Eczematous allergy to balsams, allied perfumes and flavouring agents, with special reference to balsam of Peru. *Acta Derm Venereol Suppl (Stockh)* 1961;41(Suppl 46):1–216.
196. Stager J, Wüthrich B, Johansson SG. Spice allergy in celery-sensitive patients. *Allergy* 1991;46:475–478.
197. van Toorenenbergen AW, Dieges PH. Demonstration of spice-specific IgE in patients with suspected food allergies. *J Allergy Clin Immunol* 1987;79:108–113.
198. van Toorenenbergen AW, Dieges PH. Immunoglobulin E antibodies against coriander and other spices. *J Allergy Clin Immunol* 1985;76:477–481.
199. Suhonen R, Keskinen H, Bjorksten F, et al. Allergy to coriander: a case report. *Allergy* 1979;34:327–330.
200. de Maat-Bleeker F. Etiology of hypersensitivity reactions following Chinese or Indonesian meals. *Ned Tijdschr Geneeskd* 1992;136:229–232.
201. Ebo DG, Bridts Ch, Mertens MH, et al. Coriander anaphylaxis in a spice grinder with undetected occupational allergy. *Acta Clin Belg* 2006;61:152–156.
202. Vermaat H, Smienk F, Rustenmeyer T, et al. Anogenital allergic contact dermatitis, the role of spices and flavor allergy. *Contact Dermat* 2008;59:233–237.
203. Boxer M, Roberts M, Grammer L. Cumin anaphylaxis: a case report. *J Allergy Clin Immunol* 1997;99:722–723.
204. Ohnua N, Yamaguchi Y, Kawakami Y. Anaphylaxis to curry powder. *Allergy* 1998;53:452–454.
205. Bustamante SP, Alvarez-Perea A, DeBarrio M, et al. Allergy to curry: a case report. *Allergol Immunopathol (Madr)* 2011;39:383–385.
206. Yagami A, Nakazawa Y, Suxuki K, et al. Curry spice allergy associated with pollen-food allergy syndrome and latex fruit-syndrome. *J Dermatol* 2009;36:45–49.
207. Chiu AM, Zacharisen MC. Anaphylaxis to dill. *Ann Allergy Asthma Immunol* 2000;84:559–560.
208. Monteseirin J, Perez-Formoso JL, Hernandez M, et al. Contact urticaria from dill. *Contact Dermat* 2003;48:275.
209. Monteseirin J, Perez-Formoso JL, Sanchez-Hernandez MC, et al. Occupational contact dermatitis to dill. *Allergy* 2002;57:866–867.
210. Freeman GL. Allergy to fresh dill. *Allergy* 1999;54:531–532.
211. Schwartz HJ, Jones RT, Rojas AR, et al. Occupational allergic rhinoconjunctivitis and asthma due to fennel seed. *Ann Allergy Asthma Immunol* 1997;78:37–40.
212. Wüthrich B, Hofer T. Food allergy: the celery-mugwort-spice syndrome. Association with mango allergy? *Dtsch Med Wochenschr* 1984;109:981–986.
213. Guin JD, Skidmore G. Compositae dermatitis in childhood. *Arch Dermatol* 1987;123:500–502.
214. Gluck U. Pollinosis and oral allergy syndrome. *HNO* 1990;38:188–190.
215. Gluck U. Neglected allergens. *Ther Umsch* 1992;49:669–673.
216. Gral N, Beani JC, Bonnot D, et al. Plasma levels of psoralens after celery ingestion. *Ann Dermatol Venereol* 1993;120:599–603.
217. Ottolenghi A, De Chiara A, Arrigoni S, et al. Diagnosis of food allergy caused by fruit and vegetables in children with atopic dermatitis. *Pediatr Med Chir* 1995;17:525–530.
218. Asero R. Relevance of pollen-specific IgE levels to the development of Apiaceae hypersensitivity in patients with birch pollen allergy. *Allergy* 1997;52:560–564.
219. Dugue P, Bel J, Figueredo M. Fenugreek causing a new type of occupational asthma. *Presse Med* 1993;22:922.
220. Patil SP, Niphadkar PV, Bapat MM. Allergy to fenugreek (Trigonella foenum graecum). *Ann Allergy Asthma Immunol* 1997;78:297–300.
221. Faeste CK, Namork E, Lindvik H. Allergenicity and antigenicity of fenugreek (Trigonella foenum-graecum) proteins in foods. *J Allergy Clin Immunol* 2009;123:187–194.
222. Faeste CK, Christians U, Egaas E, et al. Characterization of potential allergens in fenugreek (Trigonella foenum-graecum) using patient sera and MS-based proteomic analysis. *J Proteomics* 2010;73:1321–1333.
223. Benes J, Prerovsky K, Rehurek L, et al. Garlic food allergy with symptoms of Ménière's disease. *Cas Lek Cesk* 1966;105:825–827.
224. Mitchell JC. Contact sensitivity to garlic *(Allium). Contact Dermat* 1980;6:356–357.
225. Martinescu E. Contact dermatitis caused by *Allium sativum. Rev Med Chir Soc Med Nat Iasi* 1981;85:541–542.
226. Falleroni AE, Zeiss CR, Levitz D. Occupational asthma secondary to inhalation of garlic dust. *J Allergy Clin Immunol* 1981;68:156–160.
227. Lybarger JA, Gallagher JS, Pulver DW, et al. Occupational asthma induced by inhalation and ingestion of garlic. *J Allergy Clin Immunol* 1982;69:448–454.
228. Couturier P, Bousquet J. Occupational allergy secondary inhalation of garlic dust. *J Allergy Clin Immunol* 1982;70:145.

229. Molina C, Lachaussée R, Jeanneret A, et al. A garlic story. *Presse Méd* 1983;12:1941.
230. Haenen JM. The garlic story. *Presse Méd* 1984;13:745.
231. Lautier R, Wendt V. Contact allergy to Alliaceae. Case report and literature review. *Derm Beruf Umwelt* 1985;33:213–215.
232. Bojs G, Svensson A. Contact allergy to garlic used for wound healing. *Contact Dermat* 1988;18:179–181.
233. Lee TY, Lam TH. Contact dermatitis due to topical treatment with garlic in Hong Kong. *Contact Dermat* 1991;24:193–196.
234. Miyazawa K, Ito M, Ohsaki K. An equine case of urticaria associated with dry garlic feeding. *J Vet Med Sci* 1991;53:747–748.
235. McFadden JP, White IR, Rycroft RJ. Allergic contact dermatitis from garlic. *Contact Dermat* 1992;27:333–334.
236. Burden AD, Wilkinson SM, Beck MH, et al. Garlic-induced systemic contact dermatitis. *Contact Dermat* 1994;30:299–300.
237. Armentia A, Vega JM. Can inhalation of garlic dust cause asthma? *Allergy* 1996;51:137–138.
238. Delaney TA, Donnelly AM. Garlic dermatitis. *Australas J Dermatol* 1996;37:109–110.
239. Anibarro B, Fontela JL, De La Hoz F. Occupational asthma induced by garlic dust. *J Allergy Clin Immunol* 1997;100:734–738.
240. Asero R, Mistrello G, Roncarolo D, et al. A case of garlic allergy. *J Allergy Clin Immunol* 1998;101:427–428.
241. Jappe U, Bonnekoh B, Hausen BM, et al. Garlic-related dermatoses: case report and review of the literature. *Am J Contact Derm* 1999;10:37–39.
242. Perez-Pimiento AJ, Moneo I, Santaolalla M, et al. Anaphylactic reaction to young garlic. *Allergy* 1999;54:626–629.
243. Seuri M, Taivanen A, Ruoppi P, et al. Three cases of occupational asthma and rhinitis caused by garlic. *Clin Exp Allergy* 1993;23:1011–1014.
244. Kyo E, Uda N, Kasuga S, et al. Immunomodulatory effects of aged garlic extract. *J Nutr* 2001;131:1075S–1079S.
245. Pires G, Pargana E, Loureiro V, et al. Allergy to garlic. *Allergy* 2002;57:957–958.
246. Hughes TM, Varma S, Stone NM. Occupational contact dermatitis from a garlic and herb mixture. *Contact Dermat* 2002;47:48.
247. Ghazanfari T, Hassan ZM, Ebrahimi M. Immunomodulatory activity of a protein isolated from garlic extract on delayed type hypersensitivity. *Int Immunopharmacol* 2002;2:1541–1549.
248. Kao SH, Hsu CH, Su SN, et al. Identification and immunologic characterization of an allergen, alliin lyase, from garlic *(Allium sativum). J Allergy Clin Immunol* 2004;113:161–168.
249. Bassioukas K, Orton D, Cerio R. Occupational airborne allergic contact dermatitis from garlic with concurrent type I allergy. *Contact Dermat* 2004;50:39–41.
250. Clement F, Pramod SN, Venkatesh YP. Identity of the immunomodulatory proteins from garlic (Allium sativum) with the major garlic lectins or agglutinins. *Int Immunopharmacol* 2010;10:316–324.
251. Moneret-Vautrin DA, Morisset M, Lemerdy P, et al. Food allergy and IgE sensitization caused by spices: CICBAA data (based on 589 cases of food allergy). *Allerg Immunol (Paris)* 2002; 34:135–140.
252. Sastre J, Olmo M, Novalvos A, et al. Occupational asthma due to different spices. *Allergy* 1996;51:117–120.
253. Allergy to mace. *J Am Med Assoc* 1977;237:1201.
254. Frazier CA. Contact allergy to mace. *J Am Med Assoc* 1976;236:2526.
255. Anderson C, Lis-Balchin M, Kirk-Smith M. Evaluation of massage with essential oils on childhood atopic eczema. *Phytother Res* 2000;14:452–456.
256. Maddocks-Jennings W. Critical incident: idiosyncratic allergic reactions to essential oils. *Complement Ther Nurs Midwifery* 2004;10:58–60.
257. Monreal P, Botey J, Pena M, et al. Mustard allergy. Two anaphylactic reactions to ingestion of mustard sauce. *Ann Allergy* 1992;69:317–320.
258. Jorro G, Morales C, Braso JV, et al. Mustard allergy: three cases of systemic reaction to ingestion of mustard sauce. *J Investig Allergol Clin Immunol* 1995;5:54–56.
259. Gonzalez de la Pena MA, Menendez-Arias L, Monsalve RI, et al. Isolation and characterization of a major allergen from oriental mustard seeds, BrajI. *Int Arch Allergy Appl Immunol* 1991;96:263–270.
260. Menendez-Arias L, Moneo I, Dominguez J, et al. Primary structure of the major allergen of yellow mustard (*Sinapis alba* L.) seed, Sin a I. *Eur J Biochem* 1988;177:159–166.
261. Rance F, Dutau G, Abbal M. Mustard allergy in children. *Allergy* 2000;55:496–500.
262. Van Hecke E. Contact allergy to onion. *Contact Dermat* 1977;3:167–168.
263. Valdivieso R, Subiza J, Varela-Losada S, et al. Bronchial asthma, rhinoconjunctivitis, and contact dermatitis caused by onion. *J Allergy Clin Immunol* 1994;94:928–930.
264. Gastaminza G, Quirce S, Torres M, et al. Pickled onion-induced asthma: a model of sulfite-sensitive asthma? *Clin Exp Allergy* 1995;25:698–703.
265. Kawane H. Bronchial asthma caused by onion. *J Allergy Clin Immunol* 1995;96:568.
266. Singhal V, Reddy BS. Common contact sensitizers in Delhi. *J Dermatol* 2000;27:440–445.
267. Sanchez-Hernandez MC, Hernandez M, Delgado J, et al. Allergenic cross-reactivity in the Liliaceae family. *Allergy* 2000;55:297–299.
268. Arena A, Cislaghi C, Falagiani P. Anaphylactic reaction to the ingestion of raw onion. A case report. *Allergol Immunopathol (Madr)* 2000;28:287–289.
269. Asero R, Mistrello G, Roncarolo D, et al. A case of onion allergy. *J Allergy Clin Immunol* 2001;108:309–310.
270. Perez-Calderon R, Gonzalo-Garijo MA, Fernandez de Soria R. Exercise-induced anaphylaxis to onion. *Allergy* 2002;57:752–753.
271. Hjorth N, Roed-Petersen J. Occupational protein contact dermatitis in food handlers. *Contact Dermat* 1976;2:28–42.
272. Enrique E, Malek T, De Mateo JA, et al. Involvement of lipid transfer protein in onion allergy. *Ann Allergy Asthma Immunol* 2007;98:202.
273. Foti C, Carino M, Cassano N, et al. Occupational contact urticaria from paprika. *Contact Dermat* 1997;37:135.

274. Vega de la Osada F, Esteve Krauel P, Alonso Lebrero E, et al. Sensitization to paprika: anaphylaxis after intake and rhinoconjunctivitis after contact through airways. *Med Clin (Barc)* 1998;111:263–266.
275. Leitner A, Jensen-Jarolim E, Grimm R, et al. Allergens in pepper and paprika. Immunologic investigation of the celery-birch-mugwort-spice syndrome. *Allergy* 1998;53:36–41.
276. Ebner C, Jensen-Jarolim E, Leitner A, et al. Characterization of allergens in plant-derived spices: Apiaceae spices, pepper (Piperaceae), and paprika (bell peppers, Solanaceae). *Allergy* 1998;53:52–54.
277. Willerroider M, Fuchs H, Ballmer-Weber BK, et al. Cloning and molecular and immunological characterisation of two new food allergens, Cap a 2 and Lyc e 1, profilins from bell pepper *(Capsicum annuum)* and tomato *(Lycopersicon esculentum)*. *Int Arch Allergy Immunol* 2003;131:245–255.
278. Gallo R, Cozzani E, Guarrera M. Sensitization to pepper *(Capsicum annuum)* in a latex-allergic patient. *Contact Dermat* 1997;37:36–37.
279. Beyer K, Bardina L, Grishina G, et al. Identification of sesame seed allergens by 2-dimensional proteomics and Edman sequencing: seed storage proteins as common food allergens. *J Allergy Clin Immunol* 2002;110:154–159.
280. Winek CL, Markie DC, Shanor SP. Pepper sauce toxicity. *Drug Chem Toxicol* 1982;5:89–113.
281. Spuzic V, Spuzic I, Djordjevic S, et al. The role of paprika in the appearance of allergic manifestations. *Acta Allergol* 1962;17:516–520.
282. Rogov VD. Toxicoderma caused by sweet red pepper. *Vestn Dermatol Venerol* 1985:53–54.
283. Gallo R, Roncarolo D, Mistrello G. Cross-reactivity between latex and sweet pepper due to prohevein. *Allergy* 1998;53:1007–1008.
284. Hannuksela M, Lahti A. Immediate reactions to fruits and vegetables. *Contact Dermat* 1977;3:79–84.
285. Kauppinen K, Kousa M, Reunala T. Aromatic plants–a cause of severe attacks of angioedema and urticaria. *Contact Dermat* 1980;6:251–254.
286. Dechamp C, Deviller P. Rules concerning allergy to celery (and other Umbellifera). *Allerg Immunol (Paris)* 1987;19:112–114, 116.
287. Vallet G. Allergy to market garden plants: artichoke, celery, parsley. *Concours Med* 1964;86:3603–3606.
288. Arias Irigoyen J, Talavera Fabuel A, Maranon Lizana F. Occupational rhinoconjunctivitis from white pepper. *J Investig Allergol Clin Immunol* 2003;13:213–215.
289. Maillard H, Drouet M, Sabbah A. Allergy associated with pepper and latex: new cross-reaction? *Allerg Immunol (Paris)* 1995;27:292–294.
290. Tucke J, Posch A, Baur X, et al. Latex type I sensitization and allergy in children with atopic dermatitis. Evaluation of cross-reactivity to some foods. *Pediatr Allergy Immunol* 1999;10:160–167.
291. Dikensoy O, Bayram NG, Filiz A. Severe asthma attack in a patient with premenstrual asthma: hot pepper is the possible trigger. *Respiration* 2001;68:227.
292. Gimenex L, Zacharisen M. Severe pepper allergy in a young child. *WMJ* 2011;110:138–139.
293. Mueller RS, Bettenay SV, Tideman L. Aero-allergens in canine atopic dermatitis in southeastern Australia based on 1,000 intradermal skin tests. *Aust Vet J* 2000;78:392–399.
294. Morton CA, Garioch J, Todd P, et al. Contact sensitivity to menthol and peppermint in patients with intra-oral symptoms. *Contact Dermat* 1995;32:281–284.
295. Andersen KE. Contact allergy to toothpaste flavors. *Contact Dermat* 1978;4:195–198.
296. Mooller NE, Skov PS, Norn S. Allergic and pseudo-allergic reactions caused by penicillins, cocoa and peppermint additives in penicillin factory workers examined by basophil histamine release. *Acta Pharmacol Toxicol (Copenh)* 1984;55:139–144.
297. Wilkinson SM, Beck MH. Allergic contact dermatitis from menthol in peppermint. *Contact Dermat* 1994;30:42–43.
298. Rogers SN, Pahor AL. A form of stomatitis induced by excessive peppermint consumption. *Dent Update* 1995;22:36–37.
299. Dooms-Goossens A, Degreef H, Holvoet C, et al. Turpentine-induced hypersensitivity to peppermint oil. *Contact Dermat* 1977;3:304–308.
300. Vocks E, Borga A, Szliska C, et al. Common allergenic structures in hazelnut, rye grain, sesame seeds, kiwi, and poppy seeds. *Allergy* 1993;48:168–172.
301. Richter J, Susicky P. Latex allergy. *Cesk Slov Oftalmol* 2000;56:129–131.
302. Kutting B, Brehler R. Exercise-induced anaphylaxis. *Allergy* 2000;55:585–586.
303. Frantzen B, Brocker EB, Trautmann A. Immediate-type allergy caused by poppy seed. *Allergy* 2000;55:97–98.
304. Kalyoncu AF, Stalenheim G. Allergy to poppy seed. *Allergy* 1993;48:295.
305. Crivellaro M, Bonadonna P, Dama A, et al. Severe systemic reactions caused by poppy seed. *J Investig Allergol Clin Immunol* 1999;9:58–59.
306. Braun W, Kovary PM. Poppy seed allergy. *Z Hautkr* 1988;63:344.
307. Armisen M, Rodriguez V, Vidal C. Photoaggravated allergic contact dermatitis due to Rosmarinus officinalis cross-reactive with Thymus vulgaris. *Contact Dermat* 2003;48:52–53.
308. Fernandez L, Duque S, Sanchez I, et al. Allergic contact dermatitis from rosemary (*Rosmarinus officinalis* L.). *Contact Dermat* 1997;37:248–249.
309. Zuskin E, Kanceljak B, Schacter EN, et al. Respiratory function and immunologic status in workers processing dried fruits and teas. *Ann Allergy Asthma Immunol* 1996;77:417–422.
310. Katial RK, Lin FL, Stafford WW, et al. Mugwort and sage (Artemisia) pollen cross-reactivity: ELISA inhibition and immunoblot evaluation. *Ann Allergy Asthma Immunol* 1997;79:340–346.
311. Golec M, Skorska C, Mackiewicz B, et al. Immunologic reactivity to work-related airborne allergens in people occupationally exposed to dust from herbs. *Ann Agric Environ Med* 2004;11:121–127.

312. Pastorello EA, Pompei C, Pravettoni V, et al. Lipid transfer proteins and 2S albumins as allergens. *Allergy* 2001;56(Suppl 67):45–47.
313. Malish D, Glovsky MM, Hoffman DR, et al. Anaphylaxis after sesame seed ingestion. *J Allergy Clin Immunol* 1981;67:35–38.
314. Kanny G, De Hauteclocque C, Moneret-Vautrin DA. Sesame seed and sesame seed oil contain masked allergens of growing importance. *Allergy* 1996;51:952–957.
315. Wolff N, Cogan U, Admon A, et al. Allergy to sesame in humans is associated primarily with IgE antibody to a 14 kDa 2S albumin precursor. *Food Chem Toxicol* 2003;41:1165–1174.
316. Steurich F. Allergy to sesame seeds. *Pneumologie* 1989;43:710–714.
317. Kagi M, Wüthrich B. Falafel-burger anaphylaxis due to sesame seed allergy. *Lancet* 1991;338:582.
318. Chiu JT, Haydik IB. Sesame seed oil anaphylaxis. *J Allergy Clin Immunol* 1991;88:414–415.
319. Keskinen H, Ostman P, Vaheri E, et al. A case of occupational asthma, rhinitis and urticaria due to sesame seed. *Clin Exp Allergy* 1991;21:623–624.
320. James C, Williams-Akita A, Rao YA, et al. Sesame seed anaphylaxis. *N Y State J Med* 1991;91:457–458.
321. Kagi MK, Wüthrich B. Falafel burger anaphylaxis due to sesame seed allergy. *Ann Allergy* 1993;71:127–129.
322. Eberlein-Konig B, Rueff F, Przybilla B. Generalized urticaria caused by sesame seeds with negative prick test results and without demonstrable specific IgE antibodies. *J Allergy Clin Immunol* 1995;96:560–561.
323. Alday E, Curiel G, Lopez-Gil MJ, et al. Occupational hypersensitivity to sesame seeds. *Allergy* 1996;51:69–70.
324. Perkins MS. Peanut and nut allergy: sesame allergy is also a problem. *Br Med J* 1996;313:300.
325. Sporik R, Hill D. Allergy to peanut, nuts, and sesame seed in Australian children. *Br Med J* 1996;313:1477–1478.
326. Kolopp-Sarda MN, Moneret-Vautrin DA, Gobert B, et al. Specific humoral immune responses in 12 cases of food sensitization to sesame seed. *Clin Exp Allergy* 1997;27:1285–1291.
327. Stern A, Wüthrich B. Non-IgE-mediated anaphylaxis to sesame. *Allergy* 1998;53:325–326.
328. Asero R, Mistrello G, Roncarolo D, et al. A case of sesame seed-induced anaphylaxis. *Allergy* 1999;54:526–527.
329. Pajno GB, Passalacqua G, Magazzu G, et al. Anaphylaxis to sesame. *Allergy* 2000;55:199–201.
330. Senti G, Ballmer-Weber BK, Wüthrich B. Nuts, seeds and grains from an allergist's point of view. *Schweiz Med Wochenschr* 2000;130:1795–1804.
331. Levy Y, Danon YL. Allergy to sesame seed in infants. *Allergy* 2001;56:193–194.
332. Fremont S, Zitouni N, Kanny G, et al. Allergenicity of some isoforms of white sesame proteins. *Clin Exp Allergy* 2002;32:1211–1215.
333. Morisset M, Moneret-Vautrin DA, Kanny G, et al. Thresholds of clinical reactivity to milk, egg, peanut and sesame in immunoglobulin E-dependent allergies: evaluation by double-blind or single-blind placebo-controlled oral challenges. *Clin Exp Allergy* 2003;33:1046–1051.
334. Uvitsky IH. Sensitivity to sesame seed. *J Allergy* 1951;22:377–378.
335. Pastorello EA, Varin E, Farioli L, et al. The major allergen of sesame seeds *(Sesamum indicum)* is a 2S albumin. *J Chromatogr B Biomed Sci Appl* 2001;756:85–93.
336. Rudzki E, Grzywa Z. Sensitizing and irritating properties of star anise oil. *Contact Dermat* 1976;2:305–308.
337. Rudzki E, Grzywa Z, Krajewska D, et al. New contact allergens and allergen sources. *Arch Immunol Ther Exp (Warsz)* 1978;26:735–738.
338. Kurzen M, Bayerl C, Goerdt S. Occupational allergy to mugwort. *J Dtsch Dermatol Ges* 2003;1:285.
339. Mackiewicz B, Skorska C, Dutkiewicz J, et al. Allergic alveolitis due to herb dust exposure. *Ann Agric Environ Med* 1999;6:167–170.
340. Olive-Perez A, Granel Tena C. Asthma caused by culinary spices. *Allergol Immunopathol (Madr)* 1992;20:85–86.
341. Hata M, Sasaki E, Ota M, et al. Allergic contact dermatitis from curcumin (turmeric). *Contact Dermat* 1997;36:107–108.
342. Li C, Li L, Luo J, et al. Effect of turmeric volatile oil on the respiratory tract. *Zhongguo Zhong Yao Za Zhi* 1998;23:624–625, inside back cover.
343. Lamb SR, Wilkinson SM. Contact allergy to tetrahydrocurcumin. *Contact Dermat* 2003;48:227.
344. Reus KE, Houben GF, Stam M, et al. Food additives as a cause of medical symptoms: relationship shown between sulfites and asthma and anaphylaxis; results of a literature review. *Ned Tijdschr Geneeskd* 2000;144:1836–1839.
345. Beyer AV, Gall H, Peter RU. Immediate-type hypersensitivity to vanilla. *Allergologie* 1999;22 433–436.
346. Hirschfeld G, Weber L, Renkl A, et al. Anaphylaxis after Oseltamivir (Tamiflu®) therapy in a patient with sensitization to star anise and celery-carrot-mugwort-spice syndrome. *Allergy* 2008;63:243–244.

5 Contemporary Topics in Adverse Reactions to Foods

35 Pharmacologic Food Reactions

Timothy J. Franxman & James L. Baldwin
Division of Allergy and Clinical Immunology, University of Michigan, Ann Arbor, MI, USA

Key Concepts

- Naturally occurring or added food substances can result in pharmacologic or drug-like activity.
- Pharmacologic food reactions tend to be dose dependent.
- Pharmacologic food reactions can be mistaken for food allergy.
- Concomitant medications may alter the propensity to elicit pharmacologic food reactions.

Introduction

Many foods contain a variety of either naturally occurring or added components that have pharmacologic or drug-like activity [1]. When consumed in moderation, however, only a small number of substances have been identified that account for the majority of clinically apparent adverse pharmacologic reactions to foods. This chapter focuses on the most common substances implicated in pharmacologic reactions to foods and discusses their mechanisms and strategies for prevention and treatment.

Pharmacologic food reactions have been defined as adverse reactions to foods or food additives that result from naturally derived or added chemicals that produce drug-like or pharmacologic effects in the host [2]. Unlike type I-allergic food reactions, which affect only a selected group of atopic patients, pharmacologic food reactions can potentially be elicited in a wider, more diverse group of individuals. The dose or quantity of food necessary to elicit a clinically apparent reaction typically varies among individuals and even in the same individual over time. Pharmacologic food reactions depend on metabolic differences, concurrent medication usage, food freshness, and food preparation.

Vasoactive amines

The vasoactive amines include dopamine, histamine, norepinephrine, phenylethylamine, serotonin, tryptamine, and tyramine. All of these low-molecular-weight molecules are synthesized by decarboxylation of naturally occurring amino acids. The role of biogenic amines as a cause of adverse reactions to foods has recently been called into question [3]. It is true that dietary amines do not appear to elicit clinical symptoms when ingested in moderate quantities. However, when circumstances arise that result in excessive intake of a biogenic amine or inhibition of metabolic processing to inactive products, clinical consequences will be seen.

Histamine

The diamine histamine is perhaps the best-known vasoactive amine. Because of histamine's significant contribution to the pathophysiology of atopic disease, histamine-induced pharmacologic food reactions are frequently confused with food-allergic reactions.

Synthesis

Histamine is synthesized in nature by the decarboxylation of its amino acid precursor histidine. This synthesis is catalyzed by the enzyme histidine decarboxylase and other enzymes that are widely distributed in nature. The most important example of histamine causing pharmacologic effects by ingestion of food is scombroid fish poisoning which will be discussed further [4, 5].

Food Allergy: Adverse Reactions to Foods and Food Additives, Fifth Edition. Edited by Dean D Metcalfe, Hugh A Sampson, Ronald A Simon and Gideon Lack.

Table 35.1 Physiologic responses elicited by histamine.

Responses mediated by H1 receptors
Smooth muscle contraction
Increased vascular permeability
Mucous gland secretion
Responses mediated by H2 receptors
Gastric acid secretion
Inhibition of basophile histamine release
Inhibition of lymphokine release
Responses mediated by H1 and H2 receptors
Vasodilation
Hypotension
Flush
Headache
Tachycardia

Physiologic effects

Histamine mediates its effects on tissues through H1 and H2 receptors. The subsequent tissue responses to histamine, summarized in Table 35.1, can present following any type I hypersensitivity. A clinically similar physiologic response can be noted in non-IgE-dependent pharmacologic food reactions in which histamine is either present in the food ingested or released from tissue stores due to some intrinsic histamine-releasing ability of the food ingested. The IgE- and non-IgE-dependent histamine-mediated events both occur within minutes of ingestion of the culpable food and are clinically indistinguishable. Adverse responses to histamine, including abdominal cramping, flushing, headache, palpitations, and hypotension, appear to be roughly dose dependent. Ingestion of 25–50 mg of histamine may precipitate headache, whereas 100–150 mg may induce flushing [6]. These values are only rough estimates, however, and scombroid toxicity has been described with ingestion of as little as 2.5 mg of histamine [7].

Metabolism

The duration of histamine's effect depends on its metabolism. In normal physiology, conversion of histamine to its major inactive metabolites by either histamine methyltransferase or diamine oxidase (DAO) generally occurs rapidly [8, 9]. Figure 35.1 shows the two routes of histamine metabolism. Prolonged binding of histamine from normal dietary sources to H1 and H2 receptors is uncommon, and symptoms rarely occur with such incidental ingestions. When large ingestions of histamine occur (e.g., scombroid poisoning), however, the metabolic capacity is temporarily exceeded and a multitude of histamine-mediated effects are observed. Experimental administration of large oral quantities of histamine yields similar clinical responses [10].

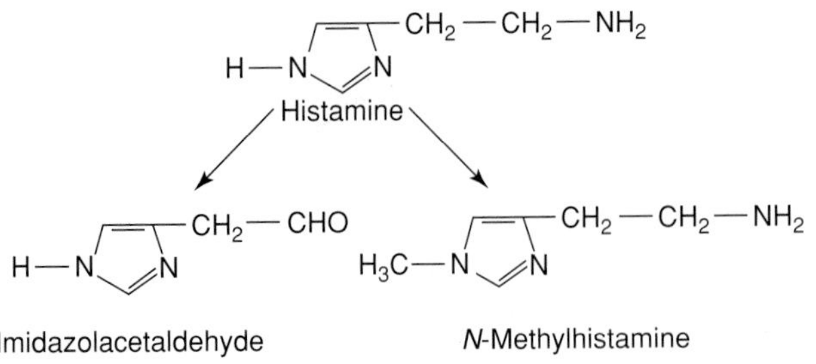

Figure 35.1 Histamine metabolism.

Although methylation appears to be the primary route for metabolism of histamine administered by both the oral and intravenous routes, DAO is important as well. DAO is present in the intestinal mucosa in almost all mammalian species examined [11]. Ingestion of a histamine-containing meal along with ingestion of drugs that inhibit DAO can produce histamine-induced symptoms. Isoniazid is a potent DAO inhibitor and, when combined with a histamine-containing meal, has resulted in severe histamine-induced symptoms [12–14]. *In vitro* experiments have shown a number of drugs (e.g., chloroquine, pentamidine, clavulanic acid, dobutamine, pancuronium, imipenem, and others) to be potent human intestinal mucosal DAO inhibitors. The *in vivo* clinical relevance of these findings remains uncertain [15].

Histamine-containing foods

Certain foods are generally accepted as having higher histamine content than others [16, 17]. Three cheeses (Parmesan, Blue, and Roquefort), two vegetables (spinach and eggplant), two red wines (Chianti and Burgundy), yeast extract, and scombroid fish have histamine content adequate to raise postprandial 24-hour urinary histamine levels [16]. For this reason, dietary histamine restrictions are recommended for patients undergoing 24-hour urinary histamine determinations.

The histamine content in red wines is commonly cited as one of the possible causes of wine intolerance. The symptoms most often reported by susceptible individuals include flushing of the face, headache, nasal congestion, and/or respiratory distress. A French study, however, found no significant difference in the occurrence of adverse reactions in wine-intolerant individuals who underwent two double-blind provocation tests, one with a wine poor in histamine (0.4 mg/L) and one with a wine rich in histamine (13.8 mg/L) [18]. The histamine-rich wine also contained higher levels of other biogenic amines including tyramine, ethylamine, putrescine, and phenylethylamine [18]. This suggests that the histamine content of wine may not be directly linked to adverse reactions to wines. It is also interesting to note that fermented cheeses contain amounts of histamine that are much greater than those found in wines, yet signs typical of intolerance to histamine have rarely been reported after ingestion of cheeses [19].

Several symptoms generally attributed to monosodium glutamate (MSG) resemble those associated with histamine toxicity. Using a radio enzymatic assay technique, the histamine content of several common Asian dishes, condiments, and basic ingredients was measured. Although the amount of histamine in individual food portions was determined to fall below the level generally thought necessary to induce symptoms, consumption of multiple portions could result in ingestion of enough histamine to produce symptoms [19].

Scombroid poisoning

Histamine poisoning from ingestion of foods with high histamine content is well documented. The prototype for this kind of histamine toxicity is scombroid poisoning. Marine bacteria such as *Morganella morganii*, *Klebsiella pneumoniae*, and *Photobacterium phosphoreum* generate histamine from histadine through a chemical reaction involving histadine decarboxylase. This gene was cloned from *P. phosphoreum* and sequenced by Morii et al. in 2006 [20]. Improperly refrigerated scombroid fish (e.g., tuna, mackerel, skipjack, and bonito) and nonscombroid fish (e.g., mahimahi, bluefish, amberjack, herring, sardines, marlin, and anchovies) develop an enriched histamine content through this bacterial action.

Ingestion of such fish causes a clinical picture bearing strong resemblance to anaphylaxis. Symptoms generally begin within an hour of ingestion and include flushing, sweating, nausea, vomiting, abdominal cramps, diarrhea, headache, palpitations, urticaria, dizziness; a metallic, sharp, or peppery taste; and, in severe cases, hypotension and bronchospasm [7, 21]. Diagnosis is made by clinical history. Laboratory confirmation of scombroid is established by sampling the muscle of the suspected meal and finding a histamine level over 50 ppm [22].

A recent report by Ricci et al. suggests serum tryptase levels may help delineate allergic reactions from scombroid poisoning. The article analyzed 10 cases of scombroid poisoning and 50 cases of allergic anaphylaxis and noted that serum tryptase levels were elevated in each of the anaphylaxis cases, while the cases suggestive of scombroid poisoning exhibited normal tryptase levels. This observation is consistent with the belief that anaphylaxis is mediated by histamine from intrinsic mast cell (MC) degranulation (resulting in concomitant tryptase release) while scombroid symptoms are attributed directly to the effects of extrinsic histamine consumption [23]. Treatment of scombroid poisoning is supportive and includes H1 and H2 receptor blockade. Prevention of scombroid poisoning can be achieved by proper handling and refrigeration of fish. Improper warming between the time that the fish is caught and when it is prepared can lead to histamine production sufficient to cause poisoning [4, 24, 25].

The US Food and Drug Administration (FDA) recognizes the issue of scombroid poisoning and has conducted a study to base recommendations regarding fish handling to prevent histamine formation. Mahimahi, skipjack, and yellowfin tuna were tested for the formation of histamine after storage. At 26°C, over 12 hours of incubation was required before a histamine concentration of 50 ppm was reached; however at 35°C, 50 ppm of histamine was formed by 9 hours [24]. In the literature, levels from 2.5 to 250 mg of histamine per 100 g of fish have been reported in most cases of scombroid poisoning. The US FDA has established a hazard concentration for histamine poisoning of greater than 450 mg per 100 g of tuna [21]. Despite more stringent legislation and guidelines put forth by the FDA, outbreaks of scombroid poisoning continue to occur.

Histamine-releasing foods

Some foods without significant histamine content may contain substances capable of triggering degranulation of tissue MCs, with resultant histamine release. Substances thought to be responsible for this histamine-releasing activity include enzymes in foods, such as trypsin, and other agents from both animal and vegetable sources, such as peptone. Foods with this unproven intrinsic histamine-releasing capacity include egg whites, crustaceans, chocolate, strawberries, ethanol, tomatoes, and citrus fruits [26].

Monoamines

Synthesis

Naturally occurring amino acids are converted into vasoactive monoamines by a number of microorganisms that possess amino acid decarboxylases necessary for this conversion. For example, tyrosine is the precursor for both dopamine and tyramine, phenylalanine is the precursor for phenylethylamine, and tryptophan is the precursor for serotonin. Amine production by these microorganisms varies depending on a variety of different conditions, including pH, temperature, and sodium chloride content [26].

Metabolism

The vasoactive monoamines are metabolized by the enzyme monoamine oxidase (MAO), which includes two subtypes: MAO-A and MAO-B. The genes for both MAO-A and MAO-B have been mapped to the short arm of the X chromosome (Xp11.23) [27] and appear to be derived from a duplication of a common ancestral gene [28]. MAO is found in a variety of tissues, where it is localized to the outer membrane of mitochondria. It catalyzes the oxidative deamination of a variety of neurotransmitters as well as the monoamines of dietary significance. Dopamine and tyramine can be metabolized by both MAO-A and MAO-B. The polar amines (serotonin, epinephrine, and norepinephrine) are metabolized primarily by MAO-A, whereas the nonpolar amine phenylethylamine metabolizes primarily by MAO-B [29].

Patients with rare deletions in their MAO-A gene have increased levels of serotonin, epinephrine, and norepinephrine detectable in their urine, whereas MAO-B-deficient subjects have increased urinary phenylethylamine levels [30]. Although no studies have examined pharmacologic food reactions in these individuals, it is interesting to note that the MAO-A-deficient individuals clinically have problems with impaired impulse control, including a propensity toward stress-induced aggression. MAO-B-deficient individuals do not seem to have clinically apparent disturbances in their behavior [30]. Although the reasons for these clinical differences are not known, it may be that raised serotonin levels in MAO-A-deficient individuals have a disruptive effect on the developing brain [30].

Specific monoamines

Tyramine

Many fermented foods contain tyramine derived from the bacterial decarboxylation of tyrosine. Foods with particularly high levels of tyramine include Camembert and Cheddar cheeses, yeast extract, wine (especially Chianti), pickled herring, fermented bean curd, fermented soybean, soy sauces, miso soup, and chicken liver. Smaller but still detectable amounts are present in avocados, bananas, figs, red plums, eggplant, and tomato [31–33].

Although tyramine exerts an indirect sympathomimetic effect by releasing endogenous norepinephrine [34], dietary tyramine usually does not cause detectable clinical effects. However, it is suggested to be responsible for adverse clinical effects involving migraine headache and the hypertensive crisis experienced by patients receiving concurrent treatment with MAO inhibitors. Foods and beverages containing tyramine have been linked to headache in some patients with food-induced migraine. In one study employing double-blind, placebo-controlled (DBPC) challenges in 45 patients with food-induced migraine, 75 (80%) of 94 tyramine (125 mg) challenges evoked a migraine, whereas only 5 (8%) of 60 placebo challenges were followed by migraine [35]. Several other studies, however, have failed to demonstrate a relationship between migraines and tyramine [36, 37]. Two trials have examined the effect of a low-tyramine diet on the frequency of migraine headaches in pediatric and adult populations. Neither study was able to find a difference in headache indices between high-tyramine and regular diets [38]. Although dietary tyramine has not been proven to cause migraines, it is possible that there is a subgroup of migraine patients that are hypersensitive to the effects of dietary tyramine because of a deficiency in MAO and conjugating enzymes [39].

As noted earlier, ingestion of foods and beverages containing large quantities of tyramine can lead to headache and hypertensive crisis in patients being treated with MAO inhibitors [32]. Normally, MAO found in the gastrointestinal (GI) tract and liver readily metabolizes dietary monoamines prior to their release into the systemic circulation. When MAO inhibitors block MAO function, however, exogenous dietary monoamines are absorbed and release endogenous norepinephrine. The resulting pressor effect is linked to palpitations, severe headache, and hypertensive crisis. These episodes can be averted by avoiding foods rich in tyramine and other monoamines. Treatment involves slow intravenous administration of the α-adrenergic antagonist phentolamine, which is given until blood pressure stabilizes.

Dopamine

Dopamine exerts both an indirect sympathomimetic effect, by releasing endogenous norepinephrine, and a direct sympathomimetic effect, by interacting with α- and β_1-adrenergic receptors. Although tyramine in foods and beverages accounts for the majority of MAO inhibitor-associated hypertensive crises, dopamine present in fava beans or broad beans can also precipitate such a crisis. Avoidance of those foods is recommended for patients taking MAO inhibitors [32].

Phenylethylamine

Like the other monoamines, phenylethylamine may be found in several fermented foods and beverages, especially Gouda and Stilton cheeses and red wine. Unlike the other monoamines, however, phenylethylamine is also found in chocolate [31, 40]. Several mechanisms have been implicated in producing phenylethylamine's action [41, 42]. It appears likely that phenylethylamine, like tyramine, exerts primarily an indirect sympathomimetic effect by releasing endogenous norepinephrine. Consequently, phenylethylamine has been implicated in both food-induced migraine and MAO inhibitor-associated hypertensive crisis [43].

Serotonin (5-hydroxytryptamine)

Serotonin is found in highest concentrations (3.0 mg/g) in certain fruits, vegetables, and nuts, including banana, kiwi, pineapple, plantain, plum, tomato, walnuts, and hickory nuts [31, 44]. Serotonin is present in moderate amounts (0.1–3.0 mg/g) in avocados, dates, grapefruit, cantaloupe, honeydew melon, black olives, broccoli, eggplant, figs, spinach, and cauliflower [44]. The only nonplant foods with significant amounts of serotonin are certain mollusks, especially octopus [31].

Serotonin acts on at least two distinct receptors and a variety of cell types. Its actions are complex and exhibit wide species and receptor variability. Two major effects attributed to serotonin are skeletal muscle vasodilation with flushing and both intracranial and extracranial vasoconstriction. Although these effects are often seen with endogenous serotonin production from carcinoid tumors, dietary serotonin does not appear to produce any immediate clinical symptoms, even in patients concurrently taking MAO inhibitors. In fact, oral feeding of serotonin equivalent to as many as 30 bananas failed to elicit clinical symptoms [45]. The urinary excretion of the major metabolite of serotonin, 5-hydroxyindoleacetic acid (5-HIAA), increases following ingestion of large amounts of serotonin. In this circumstance, a false diagnosis of carcinoid tumor may be entertained. Consequently, patients collecting 24-hour urine for 5-HIAA measurement should avoid serotonin-containing foods.

Methylxanthines

The three dietary methylxanthines are caffeine, theophylline, and theobromine. All are methylated derivatives of xanthine, which is a dioxypurine. Theobromine is extremely weak physiologically when compared to beverages and foods that contain caffeine. Theophylline is present in only very small amounts in these foods and beverages, and theobromine is only present in significant amounts in chocolate products. Consequently, caffeine accounts for most of the adverse responses from dietary methylxanthine consumption. This section will, therefore, focus on dietary caffeine and its effects.

Physiologic effects

By far the most common physiologic effect of the methylxanthines involves stimulation of the central nervous system (CNS). The methylxanthines also exert effects on the cardiovascular, respiratory, GI, renal, and musculoskeletal systems [46]. These effects are outlined in Table 35.2.

Table 35.2 Physiologic effects of the methylxanthines.

Central nervous system:
Psychostimulation (anxiety, insomnia)
Cardiovascular:
Increased contractility, blood pressure, pulse
Increased cerebrovascular resistance
Respiratory:
Relaxation of respiratory smooth muscle
Increased diaphragm contractility
Renal:
Diuretic effect
Gastrointestinal:
Decreased lower esophageal sphincter pressure; increased gastric secretion, nausea
Skeletal muscle:
Increased contractility

Mechanism of action

The mechanism of action of the methylxanthines has been studied in various systems [46], and at least three have been suggested. Initial investigations focused on the ability of these agents to inhibit the enzyme phosphodiesterase. In many systems, however, it appears that under physiologic conditions this mechanism plays a minor role at best. In the CNS, the methylxanthines appear to act as adenosine antagonists, producing excitation by blocking adenosine's inhibitory effects. In addition, caffeine has been shown to compete for excitation by blocking adenosine's inhibitory effects. Finally, caffeine has been shown to compete for binding at the benzodiazepine site of central chloride channels, causing excitation by limiting activation of these channels [47].

Absorption, distribution, and metabolism

The three dietary methylxanthines are readily absorbed from the GI tract and distributed throughout body water. They are extensively metabolized in the liver, primarily to uric acid derivatives that are, in turn, excreted in the urine. Females taking oral contraceptives have significantly slower rates of catabolism of caffeine than females not taking oral contraceptives and males [46]. In addition, fluoroquinolones impair caffeine and theophylline metabolism, resulting in increased serum concentrations [48].

Methylxanthine-containing foods

The methylxanthine content of foods and beverages has been widely studied via high-performance liquid chromatography (HPLC) [46, 49]. Rough estimates of the quantities of the methylxanthines are given in Table 35.3. These values may fluctuate widely, depending on the variety of foods and their preparation. For example, Robusta coffee blends yield higher caffeine content in general than Arabica blends [46]. Furthermore, brewing times and methods can alter the caffeine content by 100% in certain teas and coffees [46].

Adverse effects of caffeine

As noted, caffeine exerts pharmacologic effects on a variety of organ systems. Consequently, adverse pharmacologic reactions to caffeine-containing foods and beverages are manifested in many ways. Large quantities of coffee and tea are known to produce clinical symptoms that mimic anxiety and panic disorders [54]. In a blinded, placebo-controlled trial of caffeine consumption in patients diagnosed as having panic disorder or agoraphobia with

Table 35.3 Methylxanthine content of food and beverages.

Beverage	Volume	Caffeine (mg)	Theobromine (mg)
Soft drinks		30–99	0
Coca-cola	12 oz	33.9	0
Diet coke	12 oz	46.3	0
Coke zero	12 oz	35.8	0
Cherry coke	12 oz	34.4	0
Pepsi	12 oz	38.9	0
Diet Pepsi	12 oz	36.7	0
Pepsi one	12 oz	57.1	0
Cherry Pepsi	12 oz	39.7	0
Tab	12 oz	48.1	0
Faygo cola	12 oz	41.7	0
Shasta cola	12 oz	42.9	0
RC cola	12 oz	45.2	0
Diet RC	12 oz	47.3	0
Dr. Pepper	12 oz	42.6	0
Diet Dr. Pepper	12 oz	44.1	0
Vault citrus	12 oz	70.6	0
Mountain Dew	12 oz	54.8	0
Diet Mt. Dew	12 oz	55.2	0
Mt. Dew Code Red	12 oz	54.3	0
Mellow Yellow	12 oz	49.5	0
Sunkist	12 oz	40.6	0
Diet Sunkist	12 oz	41.5	0
Big Red	12 oz	34.0	0
Barq's Root Beer	12 oz	22.4	0
A&W Cream Soda	12 oz	28.6	0
A&W Root Beer	12 oz	0	0
7UP	12 oz	0	0
Sprite	12 oz	0	0
Tea			
Black tea	6 oz	14–61	0–4
Green tea	6 oz	15–41	0
Coffee			
Black coffee	6 oz	30–95	0
Black coffee decaff	6 oz	2	0
Chocolate drinks			
Chocolate milk	8 oz	5–8	181–278
Hot chocolate	6 oz	3–5	92–99
Chocolate milkshake	12 oz	4	128
Energy drinks			
Red bull	16 oz	160	0
Rockstar	16 oz	160	0
Monster	16 oz	Not listed	0
Full Throttle	16 oz	141	0
5-Hour Energy	2 oz	207	0
Sweets			
Milk chocolate chips	1 cup	34	345
Baking chocolate	1 oz	13	453

Sources: USDA [50]; Higgins et al. [51]; Chin et al. [52]; Chou et al. [53]; www.mayoclinic.com

panic attacks and in normal controls, caffeine produced significantly greater increases in subject-related anxiety, nervousness, fear, nausea, palpitations, restlessness, and tremors in patients compared with controls [55]. Furthermore, these effects were correlated with plasma caffeine levels and were reported to resemble those experienced during panic attacks. The only somatic effect that differed significantly from baseline in the normal controls was an increase in tremors [55]. In addition, caffeine abstention has been reported to reduce the frequency of panic attacks in this patient population [56]. A central adenosine receptor dysfunction in patients with panic attacks has been proposed as an explanation for their increased sensitivity to caffeine [57].

Two cases of caffeine-induced urticaria reported in the literature were diagnosed by DBPC [58, 59]. Although the mechanism remains obscure, both cases were inhibited by pretreatment with terfenadine, suggesting mediator release and H1 receptor stimulation in the pathogenesis of the reactions.

Capsaicin

The genus *Capsicum* encompasses many species, including chili peppers, red peppers, paprika, Tabasco pepper, and Louisiana long pepper. Capsicum peppers have been used for centuries by cultures around the world to enhance the flavor of relatively bland foodstuffs, as well as for its medicinal and irritant properties. Although more than 100 volatile compounds are present in capsicum oleoresin, capsaicin is the most important biologically active compound and is used most frequently for its pharmacotherapeutic benefits [60]. About 70% of the irritant effect of these foods that accounts for their "hot" sensation derives from their capsaicin content [61].

Capsaicin's initial irritant action is mediated by release of the neurosecretory compound substance P from nociceptive nerve fibers. Substance P depolarizes neurons to produce vascular dilation, smooth muscle stimulation, and pain. Repeated exposure to capsaicin results in blockage of substance P synthesis, diminishing the neurons' ability to transmit pain. This process is the basis on which capsaicin creams are used for painful conditions such as rheumatoid arthritis, osteoarthritis, diabetic neuropathy, postherpetic neuralgia, postmastectomy pain syndrome, and reflex sympathetic dystrophy [60]. Novel uses for capsaicin continue to be developed. A recent clinical trial demonstrated that intranasal capsaicin, when used continuously over 2 weeks, rapidly and safely improves symptoms in rhinitis subjects with a significant nonallergic rhinitis (NAR) component [62].

The most common adverse effect associated with capsaicin is the "burning" oral sensation associated with its ingestion. In this instance, capsaicin binds strongly through its lipophilic side chain to the lipoproteins of oral mucosal receptors. To hinder this strong interaction and "cool the burn," a lipophilic phosphoprotein such as casein (present in milk, nuts, chocolate, and some beans) is more effective than cold water [63]. A case of plasma cell gingivitis has also been attributed to oral exposure to capsaicin [64].

Adverse pharmacologic effects associated with capsaicin have also been reported in several tissues following exposure by different routes. Gastric installation has been shown to cause significant increases in gastric acid and pepsin secretion, as well as mucosal microbleeding and exfoliation [65]. Nausea vomiting, abdominal pain, and perforated viscus with peritonitis have been reported following ingestion of multiple peppers at a single sitting [66, 67]. Inhalation has been reported to result in cough in occupationally exposed capsicum-processing workers [68] and in laryngospasm [69]. Involvement with the eyes causes pain, tearing, erythema, and blepharospasm; this effect has led to use of "pepper sprays" to ward off would-be attackers. Both acute and chronic dermatologic manifestations can also occur when handling capsicum. Possible acute effects include skin irritation, erythema, and burning pain without vesiculation. In chronic exposures, severe dermatitis with vesiculation can occur [70].

Ethanol

Ethanol, the most widely abused pharmacologic substance in the world, exerts diverse effects on several body systems. The most prominent effects of ethanol consumed in moderate amounts involve the CNS. Ethanol can also act as a peripheral vasodilator and diuretic. It exerts its effects on the brain by dissolving in neuronal plasma membranes, thereby altering the movement of chloride and calcium ions involved in regulation of electrical signals and neurotransmitter release. Ethanol's diuretic effect is thought to relate to its ability to inhibit posterior pituitary secretion of antidiuretic hormone [71]. Both the diuretic and CNS effects of ethanol are well known and not commonly mistaken for allergic reactions. The histamine-releasing ability of ethanol was discussed earlier. Consequently, this section will focus on other responses to ethanol that depend on its peripheral vasodilator properties, sometimes mistaken for ethanol "allergy."

The mechanism of ethanol-induced peripheral vasodilation remains incompletely understood. Both direct effects, possibly mediated through increases in nitric oxide synthase activity [72, 73], and centrally mediated effects [74] have been suggested. Both normal individuals and those with metabolic deficiencies can experience ethanol's vasodilator effects. In normal subjects, nasal congestion with increases in upper airway resistance [75] and mild cutaneous flushing reactions have been noted within minutes of ethanol ingestion. Alcohol sensitivity is a symptom complex that can consist of cutaneous flushing, tachycardia, hypotension, somnolence, nausea, and vomiting. This response is thought to be mediated by increased levels of acetaldehyde resulting from diminished or inhibited aldehyde dehydrogenase (ALDH) enzymatic activity. It can occur following ethanol interaction with disulfiram, metronidazole, griseofulvin, quinacrine, hypoglycemic sulfonylureas, phenothiazines, or phenylbutazone in normal individuals or in individuals deficient in one of the mitochondrial isoenzymes of ALDH, designated ALDH2.

ALDH2 deficiency is common in certain Asian groups (affecting about 50% of Chinese, Japanese, and Koreans) and has been reported to protect against alcoholism [76, 77]. It appears only rarely among non-Asian ethnic groups. The inactive ALDH2 allele is dominant, so that both homozygotes and heterozygotes exhibit ALDH2 deficiency and alcohol sensitivity. Affected individuals experience symptoms to varying degrees within minutes of ingestion, responding with elevations in serum cortisone [78]. Extreme cases of ethanol sensitivity presenting with coma have been reported [79]. Treatment is supportive. A cutaneous ethanol patch test has been suggested as a more reliable indicator of the ALDH2 phenotype than self-reported ethanol-induced flushing [80].

Myristicin

The spice nutmeg is derived from the dried fruit of the nutmeg tree (*Myristica fragrans*). Taken in moderation as a flavoring for foods, nutmeg is innocuous. Consumption of large quantities can precipitate psychosis, however. The active ingredient in nutmeg thought to be responsible for this adverse effect is myristicin. Structurally, myristicin is similar to mescaline (Fig. 35.2) [81]. It has been proposed that myristicin may be metabolized *in vivo* to an amphetamine-like compound with effects similar to those of lysergic acid diethylamide (LSD) [82]. It remains unclear whether myristicin or one or more metabolites accounts for its psychoactive properties, as synthetic myristicin does not always precipitate hallucination [83]. Some investigators questioned nutmeg's psychoactive properties and have reviewed various medicinal uses of this spice [84]. One tablespoon of grated nutmeg (roughly 7 g) contains about 2% myristicin by weight [85]. Symptoms generally appear 3–8 hours after ingesting more than one tablespoon. The most prominent effects involve the CNS and cardiovascular system. Apprehension, fear of impending death, anxiety, and visual hallucinations accompanied by regular tachycardia are common [86, 87]. Patients may also experience palpitations, nausea, vomiting, and chest pressure. Because dry mouth, fever, cutaneous flushing, and blurred vision

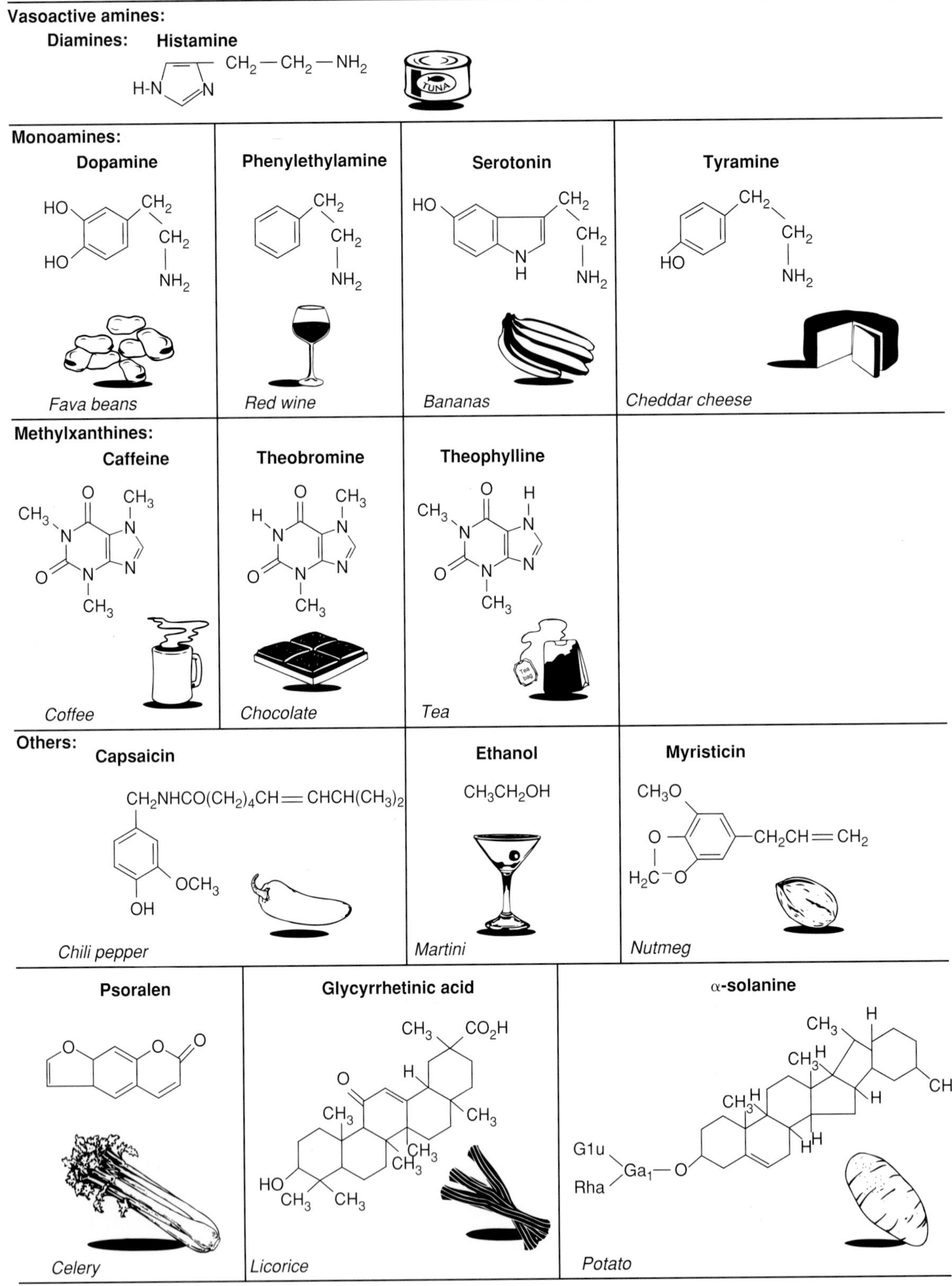

Figure 35.2 Endogenous substances responsible for pharmacologic food reactions (vasoactive amines and others).

can occur, acute nutmeg intoxication is sometimes mistaken for anticholinergic intoxication. One differentiating physical examination feature is that myristicin usually, although not always, causes miosis rather than mydriasis [88, 89].

Treatment for acute nutmeg intoxication is supportive. Emesis induction of an unknown ingestion is controversial. Many patients ingesting a toxic quantity of nutmeg are nauseated and will vomit spontaneously. Activated charcoal with sorbitol may decrease the systemic absorption, thereby mitigating the duration and severity of symptoms. Various psychotropics have also been employed, including diazepam and haloperidol for anxious and hallucinogenic features [34, 88].

Psoralen

Psoralens are naturally occurring compounds belonging to a group of compounds known as furocoumarins. Furocoumarins are tricyclic hydrocarbons consisting of a furan ring condensed on benzopyrone (Fig. 35.2) [90]. Synthetic psoralens are used commonly for the treatment of certain dermatologic diseases, including psoriasis. In PUVA (psoralen 1 ultraviolet A radiation), therapy patients receive psoralen with the addition of UVA light which causes the photoaddition of psoralen to pyrimidine bases of DNA, resulting in a cross-linking between DNA strands [90]. PUVA-induced cross-linking of DNA is thought to mediate the observed antiproliferative effects of psoralen on psoriasis. Sunlight with addition of psoralen also leads to the generation of reactive oxygen species, free radicals that can damage cell membranes, cytoplasmic constituents, and cell nuclei, resulting in a photodermatitis [90]. Naturally occurring psoralens have been found to be present in celery, parsley, limes, lemons, and parsnips. Celery field workers and handlers frequently develop photosensitization problems as a result of celery furanocoumarins [91]. Photocontact dermatitis of the skin has also been demonstrated to occur following external contact with the fig tree (*Ficus carica*) in conjunction with exposure to the sun. Contact with the fig leaf sap and shoot sap is required in fig-induced photodermatitis; the fruit sap does not contain significant amounts of psoralen [92].

Patients exposed to food psoralens typically develop clinical symptoms within 24 hours of skin contact with furocoumarins. The initial presentation usually includes sunburn, linear bullae, and/or blisters, which may persist for up to 1 week. Hyperpigmentation usually follows and may remain for several weeks to months [93]. In children, phytophotodermatitis may be confused with child abuse [93]. Awareness of this condition in pediatric patients may prevent an unpleasant situation when questioning parents or caretakers, as well as unnecessary diagnostic procedures. Most cases of photodermatitis do not require treatment. Marked pain and discomfort may be treated with cool, moistened dressings for several days. Topical corticosteroids may also be used, and in severe cases the use of systemic steroids has been recommended [93]. The use of aspirin and other prostaglandin inhibitors has been proposed but there is no scientific evidence that this therapy is helpful [93]. The prognosis is usually excellent, although severe, life-threatening burns occur rarely.

Solanine and chaconine

α-solanine and α-chaconine are general terms used to describe the glycosidic alkaloids present in the common potato (*Solanum tuberosum*). Structurally, these glycoalkaloids are complex molecules consisting of three sugars attached to a nitrogen-containing steroidal skeleton (Fig. 35.2) [94] [95]. Potato plant synthesis of glycoalkaloids is thought to be a defense mechanism against fungus growth on potatoes; the compound α-solanine has been shown to be fungitoxic and is synthesized at cut (wound) surfaces [95]. The production of α-solanine is also stimulated by mechanical injury, by exposure to light in the field (green potatoes) or in the marketplace, and with aging of the potato [95]. In addition to its fungicidal properties, glycoalkaloids are also moderate inhibitors of specific and nonspecific cholinesterases. The highest total glycoalkaloid levels in the potato plant are present in the foliage, blossoms, and sprouts, followed by the peel, potato sprouts, and the tuber flesh. The US Department of Agriculture (USDA) potato-breeding program has an accepted guideline for glycoalkaloid content in commercial potatoes at below 200 mg/g fresh weight [95]. Unfortunately, the level of glycoalkaloid under certain weather conditions can rise too far above that level. Several outbreaks of illness have been traced to the consumption of potatoes with glycoalkaloid contents ranging from 100 to 400 mg/g [95].

The symptoms of glycoalkaloid poisoning may occur 2–20 hours after a meal. They can include vomiting, diarrhea, and severe abdominal pain, and more severe cases present with neurologic symptoms, including headaches, dizziness, drowsiness, confusion, visual disturbances, dilated pupils, and weakness, sometimes followed by unconsciousness. The vital signs include fever, rapid weak pulse, low blood pressure, and rapid respiration—not unlike the vitals seen in patients experiencing anaphylaxis [96]. Recovery from glycoalkaloid poisoning is usually complete, but coma and death have been reported in cases of severe poisoning. Pharmacokinetic differences in interindividual metabolism have been demonstrated, suggesting that some subjects may be more susceptible than others to the adverse effects of glycoalkaloids [97].

Baking, boiling, or microwaving does not affect the α-solanine content of potatoes. The contents are only slightly reduced by frying. Fried potato peels are a source of large quantities of solanine. In one study, fried potato peels had glycoalkaloid levels that ranged from 1390 to 450 mg/g, which is more than 7 times the upper safety limit [95].

Treatment of glycoalkaloid poisoning is mostly supportive once a history of potato consumption has been obtained. The best way to avoid poisoning is to avoid excessive potato consumption, especially the eating of potato peels. One simple test of glycoalkaloid levels is to chew a small piece of the raw peel. Potato skins with levels of total glycoalkaloid higher than 100 mg/g of tuber cause a slow developing, hot burning, persistent irritation of the sides of the tongue and back of the mouth. Potato skins that contain more than 200 mg/g give an immediate burning sensation [95].

Glycyrrhetinic acid

Glycyrrhetinic acid is the pharmacologically active constituent of licorice that is extracted from the sweet root of the plant *Glycyrrhiza glabra* (Fig. 35.2) [98]. The use of licorice dates back to at least 1000 BC when stores of the root were placed in the tombs of Egyptian pharaohs. Its therapeutic activity for a wide variety of ailments was extolled in the writings of the ancient Greeks, Romans, and Chinese [99]. More recently, licorice has been shown to have the pharmacologic properties of a gastric mucosal protectant and anti-inflammatory agent [99]. The largest consumer of licorice in the United States is the tobacco industry for use as a conditioning and flavoring agent. Licorice cures tobacco and thus has been used for a century in cigars, pipe tobacco, cigarettes, and chewing tobacco [100].

When licorice is ingested habitually or in excess, patients develop symptoms that share most of the clinical and biochemical features of primary hyperaldosteronism. Clinical manifestations include those of sodium retention (pulmonary and peripheral edema, breathlessness, and hypertension) and hypokalemia (cardiac dysrhythmias, polyuria due to nephrogenic diabetes insipidus, proximal myopathy, lethargy, paresthesias, muscle cramps, headaches, and tetany) [98, 101]. Biochemical markers for excessive activation of mineralocorticoid receptors in the distal renal tubules include hypokalemic alkalosis and suppression of plasma renin activity [98]. It is thought that glycyrrhetinic acid acts by inhibiting renal 11-b-hydroxysteroid dehydrogenase activity thereby diminishing the conversion of cortisol to cortisone and resulting in high renal levels of cortisol [102]. Because cortisol binds to mineralocorticoid receptors with the same affinity as aldosterone, there is a resulting hypermineralocorticoid effect of cortisol [102].

Treatment of patients with licorice-induced hypermineralocorticoidism includes the administration of spironolactone, which acts as a competitive inhibitor of mineralocorticoid receptors. Since most sodium is reabsorbed in the proximal renal tubules, concomitant administration of a thiazide diuretic, which blocks reabsorption of sodium proximal to the distal portion of the nephron, is required for maximal diuretic effect. The suppression of 11-b-hydroxysteroid dehydrogenase activity, as well as many of the changes in electrolyte balance, may persist for almost 2 weeks after licorice intake is discontinued. The prolonged suppression of 11-b-hydroxysteroid dehydrogenase activity appears to be due to the continued action of glycyrrhetinic acid, because as urinary glycyrrhetinic acid levels fall, the suppression of 11-b-hydroxysteroid dehydrogenase activity is reversed [98]. Unfortunately it takes 2–4 months following cessation of licorice consumption for the function of the renin–aldosterone system to return completely to normal [102].

Oleocanthal

Extra-virgin olive oil is composed of phenolic compounds of the secoiridoid family [103]. In 2005, Beauchamp et al. discovered that the characteristic pungency of olive oil is attributed to one of its phenolic compounds. The dialdehydic form of deacetoxy-ligstroside aglycone that was identified as the substance responsible for the bitter taste of olive oil was called oleocanthal (oleo- for olive, canth- for sting, and al- for aldehyde) by the authors [104]. Oleocanthal has been shown to mimic the pharmacology of ibuprofen. Although structurally different, both molecules are oropharyngeal irritants and oleocanthal has the ability to inhibit the same cyclooxygenase (COX) enzymes in the inflammatory pathway as ibuprofen. Thus, oleocanthal is a naturally occurring anti-inflammatory that inhibits prostaglandin synthesis [104–106]. Like ibuprofen, both enantiomers of oleocanthal cause a dose-dependent inhibition of COX-1 and COX-2 activities, but it has no effect on lipoxygenase *in vitro* [104].

In addition to their COX activity, both oleocanthal and ibuprofen selectively and robustly activate transient receptor potential channel A1 (TRPA1), an ion channel that plays an important role in signaling and has been implicated in the initiation of the cough response. TRPA1-selective agonists generate action potentials from bronchopulmonary C-fibers, thereby eliciting nocifensor reflex responses [107–109]. Oleocanthal in olive oil gives a pungency and irritation of the throat causing cough and throat clearing in humans via TRPA1 receptors [110]. This oleocanthal-induced cough can be misinterpreted as an allergic rather than a pharmacologic reaction to olive oil.

Oleocanthal represents about 10% of the total phenolic compounds in olive oil, and in "extra-virgin" olive oil the concentration usually ranges between 100 and 300 mg/kg [103]. Beauchamp suggested that a diet consisting of 50 g of olive oil per day would equate to a daily intake of 9 mg of oleocanthal. This corresponds to about 10% of the standard dose of ibuprofen; however, some feel that even this modest intake would be enough to elicit anti-inflammatory effects that may account for the health benefits attributed to the Mediterranean diet [104]. Other sources suggest that daily consumption of olive oil is far less than 50 g per day in these diets. De Lorenzo estimates that many consuming a "Mediterranean diet" consume less than 0.9 mg/day [103, 111].

Oleocanthal has been shown to be heat stable when exposed to temperatures up to 240°C for up to 90 minutes [112]. There is no available data on the absorption or biotransformation of oleocanthal after olive oil ingestion; therefore the bioavailability of oleocanthal *in vivo* is yet to be determined and the anti-inflammatory actions observed *in vitro* have not been substantiated [112].

Because of the pharmacologic similarities between oleocanthal and ibuprofen there is a theoretical risk that olive oil consumption could illicit symptoms consistent with aspirin-exacerbated respiratory disease (AERD). There have been no documented reports of such clinical manifestations. Case reports of allergic reactions attributed to olive oil typically describe symptoms of contact dermatitis. Literature review shows no reports of IgE-mediated food allergy symptoms after olive oil consumption.

References

1. Sapeika N. *Food Pharmacology*. Springfield, IL: Charles C. Thomas, 1969.
2. Metcalfe DD. Food hypersensitivity. *J Allergy Clin Immunol* 1984; 73(6):749–762.
3. Jansen SC, van Dusseldorp M, Bottema KC, et al. Intolerance to dietary biogenic amines: a review. *Ann Allergy Asthma Immunol* 2003; 91(3):233–240.
4. Hughes JM, Merson MH. Current concepts fish and shellfish poisoning. *N Engl J Med* 1976; 295(20):1117–1120.
5. Geiger E. Role of histamine in poisoning with spoiled fish. *Science* 1955; 121(3155):865–866.
6. Motil KJ, Scrimshaw NS. The role of exogenous histamine in scombroid poisoning. *Toxicol Lett.* 1979;3:219–222, 232.
7. Morrow JD, Margolies GR, Rowland J, et al. Evidence that histamine is the causative toxin of scombroid-fish poisoning. *N Engl J Med* 1991; 324(11):716–720.
8. Green JP, Prell GD, Khandelwal JK, et al. Aspects of histamine metabolism. *Agents Actions* 1987; 22(1–2):1–15.
9. Schayer RW. The metabolism of histamine in various species. *Br J Pharmacol Chemother* 1956; 11(4):472–473.
10. Sjaastad O. Fate of histamine and N-acetylhistamine administered into the human gut. *Acta Pharmacol Toxicol* 1966; 24(2):189–202.
11. Kusche J, Schmidt J, Schmidt A, et al. Diamine oxidases in the small intestine of rabbits, dogs and pigs: separation from soluble monoamine oxidases and substrate specificity of the enzymes. *Agents Actions* 1975; 5(5):440–441.
12. Senanayake N, Vyravanathan S. Histamine reactions due to ingestion of tuna fish (*Thunnus argentivittatus*) in patients on anti-tuberculosis therapy. *Toxicon* 1981; 19(1):184–185.
13. Uragoda CG, Kottegoda SR. Adverse reactions to isoniazid on ingestion of fish with a high histamine content. *Tubercle* 1977; 58(2):83–89.
14. Miki M, Ishikawa T, Okayama H. An outbreak of histamine poisoning after ingestion of the ground saury paste in eight patients taking isoniazid in tuberculous ward. *Intern Med* 2005; 44(11):1133–1136.
15. Sattler J, Lorenz W. Intestinal diamine oxidases and enteral-induced histaminosis: studies on three prognostic variables in an epidemiological model. *J Neural Transm Suppl* 1990; 32:291–314.
16. Feldman JM. Histaminuria from histamine-rich foods. *Arch Intern Med* 1983; 143(11):2099–2102.
17. Malone MH, Metcalfe DD. Histamine in foods: its possible role in non-allergic adverse reactions to ingestants. *N Engl Reg Allergy Proc* 1986; 7(3):241–245.
18. Kanny G, Gerbaux V, Olszewski A, et al. No correlation between wine intolerance and histamine content of wine. *J Allergy Clin Immunol* 2001; 107(2):375–378.
19. Chin KW, Garriga MM, Metcalfe DD. The histamine content of oriental foods. *Food Chem Toxicol* 1989; 27(5):283–287.
20. Morii H, Kasama K, Herrera-Espinoza R. Cloning and sequencing of the histidine decarboxylase gene from *Photobacterium phosphoreum* and its functional expression in *Escherichia coli*. *J Food Prot* 2006; 69(8):1768–1776.
21. US FDA. Defect action levels for histamine in tuna: availability of a guide. *Fed Reg* 1982; 47:487.
22. Chegini S, Metcalfe DD. Contemporary issues in food allergy: seafood toxin-induced disease in the differential diagnosis of allergic reactions. *Allergy Asthma Proc* 2005; 26(3):183–190.
23. Ricci G, Zannoni M, Cigolini D, et al. Tryptase serum level as a possible indicator of scombroid syndrome. *Clin Toxicol (Phila)* 2010; 48(3):203–206.
24. Staruszkiewicz WF, Barnett JD, Rogers PL, et al. Effects of on-board and dockside handling on the formation of biogenic amines in mahimahi (*Coryphaena hippurus*), skipjack tuna (*Katsuwonus pelamis*), and yellowfin tuna (*Thunnus albacares*). *J Food Prot* 2004; 67(1):134–141.
25. Gellert GA, Ralls J, Brown C, et al. Scombroid fish poisoning. Underreporting and prevention among noncommercial recreational fishers. *West J Med* 1992; 157(6):645–647.
26. American Academy of Allergy and Immunology Committee on Adverse Reactions to Foods. *Adverse Reactions to Foods.* US Department of Health and Human Services, 1984.
27. Lan NC, Heinzmann C, Gal A, et al. Human monoamine oxidase A and B genes map to Xp. 11.23 and are deleted in a patient with Norrie disease. *Genomics* 1989; 4(4):552–559.

28. Grimsby J, Chen K, Wang LJ, et al. Human monoamine oxidase A and B genes exhibit identical exon-intron organization. *Proc Natl Acad Sci USA* 1991; 88(9):3637–3641.
29. Kanazawa I. Short review on monoamine oxidase and its inhibitors. *Eur Neurol* 1994; 34(Suppl 3):36–39.
30. Lenders JW, Eisenhofer G, Abeling NG, et al. Specific genetic deficiencies of the A and B isoenzymes of monoamine oxidase are characterized by distinct neurochemical and clinical phenotypes. *J Clin Invest* 1996; 97(4):1010–1019.
31. Marley E, Blackwell B. Interactions of monoamine oxidase inhibitors, amines, and foodstuffs. *Adv Pharmacol Chemother* 1970; 8:185–349.
32. Food interacting with MAO inhibitors. *Med Lett Drugs Ther* 1989; 31(785):11–12.
33. Da Prada M, Zurcher G. Tyramine content of preserved and fermented foods or condiments of Far Eastern cuisine. *Psychopharmacology (Berl)* 1992; 106(Suppl):S32-S34.
34. Raiteri M, Levi G. A reinterpretation of tyramine sympathomimetic effect and tachyphylaxis. *J Neurosci Res* 1986; 16(2):439–441.
35. Smith I, Kellow AH, Hanington E. A clinical and biochemical correlation between tyramine and migraine headache. *Headache* 1970; 10(2):43–52.
36. Moffett A, Swash M, Scott DF. Effect of tyramine in migraine: a double-blind study. *J Neurol Neurosurg Psychiatry* 1972; 35(4):496–499.
37. Ziegler DK, Stewart R. Failure of tyramine to induce migraine. *Neurology* 1977; 27(8):725–726.
38. Martin VT, Behbehani MM. Toward a rational understanding of migraine trigger factors. *Med Clin North Am* 2001; 85(4):911–941.
39. Millichap JG, Yee MM. The diet factor in pediatric and adolescent migraine. *Pediatr Neurol* 2003; 28(1):9–15.
40. Chaytor JP, Crathorne B, Saxby MJ. The identification and significance of 2-phenylethylamine in foods. *J Sci Food Agric* 1975; 26(5):593–598.
41. Zeller EA, Mosnaim AD, Borison RL, et al. Phenylethylamine: studies on the mechanism of its physiological action. *Adv Biochem Psychopharmacol* 1976; 15:75–86.
42. Sabelli HC, Borison RL. 2-Phenylethylamine and other adrenergic modulators. *Adv Biochem Psychopharmacol* 1976; 15:69–74.
43. Sandler M, Youdim MB, Hanington E. A phenylethylamine oxidising defect in migraine. *Nature* 1974; 250(464):335–337.
44. Feldman JM, Lee EM. Serotonin content of foods: effect on urinary excretion of 5-hydroxyindoleacetic acid. *Am J Clin Nutr* 1985; 42(4):639–643.
45. Crout JR, Sjoerdsma A. The clinical and laboratory significance of serotonin and catechol amines in bananas. *N Engl J Med* 1959; 261(1):23–26.
46. Spiller GA. Overview of the methylxanthine beverages and foods and their effect on health. *Prog Clin Biol Res* 1984; 158:1–7.
47. Craig CR, Stitzel RE. *Modern Pharmacology*. Boston, MA: Little, Brown & Co, 1997; pp. 383–385.
48. Marchbanks CR. Drug-drug interactions with fluoroquinolones. *Pharmacotherapy* 1993; 13(2 Pt 2):23S–28S.
49. Terada H, Sakabe Y. High-performance liquid chromatographic determination of theobromine, theophylline and caffeine in food products. *J Chromatogr* 1984; 291:453–459.
50. USDA. *USDA Nutrient Database for Standard Reference*, Release 23, 2010.
51. Higgins JP, Tuttle TD, Higgins CL. Energy beverages: content and safety. *Mayo Clin Proc* 2010; 85(11):1033–1041.
52. Chin JM, Merves ML, Goldberger BA, et al. Caffeine content of brewed teas. *J Anal Toxicol* 2008; 32(8):702–704.
53. Chou KH, Bell LN. Caffeine content of prepackaged national-brand and private-label carbonated beverages. *J Food Sci* 2007; 72(6):C337–C342.
54. Greden JF. Anxiety or caffeinism: a diagnostic dilemma. *Am J Psychiatry* 1974; 131(10):1089–1092.
55. Charney DS, Heninger GR, Jatlow PI. Increased anxiogenic effects of caffeine in panic disorders. *Arch Gen Psychiatry* 1985; 42(3):233–243.
56. Bruce MS, Lader M. Caffeine abstention in the management of anxiety disorders. *Psychol Med* 1989; 19(1):211–214.
57. Nutt D, Lawson C. Panic attacks. A neurochemical overview of models and mechanisms. *Br J Psychiatry* 1992; 160:165–178.
58. Pola J, Subiza J, Armentia A, et al. Urticaria caused by caffeine. *Ann Allergy* 1988; 60(3):207–208.
59. Quirce Gancedo S, Freire P, Fernandez Rivas M, et al. Urticaria from caffeine. *J Allergy Clin Immunol* 1991; 88(4):680–681.
60. Cordell GA, Araujo OE. Capsaicin: identification, nomenclature, and pharmacotherapy. *Ann Pharmacother* 1993; 27(3):330–336.
61. Mack RB. Capsicum annum. Another revenge from Montezuma. *N C Med J* 1994; 55(5):198–200.
62. Bernstein JA, Davis BP, Picard JK, et al. A randomized, double-blind, parallel trial comparing capsaicin nasal spray with placebo in subjects with a significant component of nonallergic rhinitis. *Ann Allergy Asthma Immunol* 2011; 107(2):171–178.
63. Henkin R. Cooling the burn from hot peppers. *J Am Med Assoc* 1991; 266(19):2766.
64. Serio FG, Siegel MA, Slade BE. Plasma cell gingivitis of unusual origin. A case report. *J Periodontol* 1991; 62(6):390–393.
65. Myers BM, Smith JL, Graham DY. Effect of red pepper and black pepper on the stomach. *Am J Gastroenterol* 1987; 82(3):211–214.
66. Bartholomew LG, Carlson HC. An unusual cause of acute gastroenteritis. *Mayo Clin Proc* 1994;69(7):675–676.
67. Landau O, Gutman H, Ganor A, et al. Post-pepper pain, perforation, and peritonitis. *J Am Med Assoc* 1992; 268(13):1686.
68. Blanc P, Liu D, Juarez C, et al. Cough in hot pepper workers. *Chest* 1991; 99(1):27–32.
69. Rubin HR, Wu AW, Tunis S. WARNING—inhaling tabasco products can be hazardous to your health. *West J Med* 1991; 155(5):550.
70. Burnett JW. Capsicum pepper dermatitis. *Cutis* 1989; 43(6):534.

71. Craig CR, Stitzel RE. *Modern Pharmacology*. Boston, MA: Little, Brown & Co, 1994; pp. 451–457.
72. Greenberg SS, Xie J, Wang Y, et al. Ethanol relaxes pulmonary artery by release of prostaglandin and nitric oxide. *Alcohol* 1993; 10(1):21–29.
73. Davda RK, Chandler LJ, Crews FT, et al. Ethanol enhances the endothelial nitric oxide synthase response to agonists. *Hypertension* 1993; 21(6 Pt 2):939–943.
74. Malpas SC, Robinson BJ, Maling TJ. Mechanism of ethanol-induced vasodilation. *J Appl Physiol* 1990; 68(2):731–734.
75. Robinson RW, White DP, Zwillich CW. Moderate alcohol ingestion increases upper airway resistance in normal subjects. *Am Rev Respir Dis* 1985; 132(6):1238–1241.
76. Crabb DW, Dipple KM, Thomasson HR. Alcohol sensitivity, alcohol metabolism, risk of alcoholism, and the role of alcohol and aldehyde dehydrogenase genotypes. *J Lab Clin Med* 1993; 122(3):234–240.
77. Yoshida A. Genetic polymorphisms of alcohol metabolizing enzymes related to alcohol sensitivity and alcoholic diseases. *Alcohol Alcohol* 1994; 29(6):693–696.
78. Wall TL, Nemeroff CB, Ritchie JC, et al. Cortisol responses following placebo and alcohol in Asians with different ALDH2 genotypes. *J Stud Alcohol* 1994; 55(2):207–213.
79. Lerman B, Bodony R. Ethanol sensitivity. *Ann Emerg Med* 1991; 20(10):1128–1130.
80. Yu PH, Fang CY, Dyck LE. Cutaneous vasomotor sensitivity to ethanol and acetaldehyde: subtypes of alcohol-flushing response among Chinese. *Alcohol Clin Exp Res* 1990; 14(6):932–936.
81. Sapeika N. Pharmacodynamic action of natural food. *World Rev Nutr Diet* 1978; 29:115–123.
82. Mack RB. Toxic encounters of the dangerous kind. The nutmeg connection. *N C Med J* 1982; 43(6):439.
83. Farnsworth NR. Nutmeg and epena snuff: differing hallucinogens. *Am J Psychiatry* 1979; 136(6):858–859.
84. Van Gils C, Cox PA. Ethnobotany of nutmeg in the Spice Islands. *J Ethnopharmacol* 1994; 42(2):117–124.
85. Archer AW. Determination of safrole and myristicin in nutmeg and mace by high-performance liquid chromatography. *J Chromatogr* 1988; 438(1):117–121.
86. Abernethy MK, Becker LB. Acute nutmeg intoxication. *Am J Emerg Med* 1992; 10(5):429–430.
87. Brenner N, Frank OS, Knight E. Chronic nutmeg psychosis. *J R Soc Med* 1993; 86(3):179–180.
88. Payne RB. Nutmeg intoxication. *N Engl J Med* 1963; 269:36–39.
89. Ahmad A, Thompson HS. Nutmeg mydriasis. *J Am Med Assoc* 1975; 234(3):274.
90. Lauharanta J. Photochemotherapy. *Clin Dermatol* 1997; 15(5):769–780.
91. Beier RC. Natural pesticides and bioactive components in foods. *Rev Environ Contam Toxicol* 1990; 113:47–137.
92. Zaynoun ST, Aftimos BG, Abi Ali, et al. *Ficus carica*; isolation and quantification of the photoactive components. *Contact Derm* 1984; 11(1):21–25.
93. Watemberg N, Urkin Y, Witztum A. Phytophotodermatitis due to figs. *Cutis* 1991; 48(2):151–152.
94. Hopkins J. The glycoalkaloids: naturally of interest (but a hot potato?). *Food Chem Toxicol* 1995; 33(4):323–328.
95. Ware GW. *Reviews of Environmental Contamination and Toxicology*. New York: Springer-Verlag, 1990.
96. Slanina P. Solanine (glycoalkaloids) in potatoes: toxicological evaluation. *Food Chem Toxicol* 1990; 28(11):759–761.
97. Mensinga TT, Sips AJ, Rompelberg CJ, et al. Potato glycoalkaloids and adverse effects in humans: an ascending dose study. *Regul Toxicol Pharmacol* 2005; 41(1):66–72.
98. Walker BR, Edwards CR. Licorice-induced hypertension and syndromes of apparent mineralocorticoid excess. *Endocrinol Metab Clin North Am* 1994; 23(2):359–377.
99. Shibata S. A drug over the millennia: pharmacognosy, chemistry, and pharmacology of licorice. *Yakugaku Zasshi* 2000; 120(10):849–862.
100. Davis EA, Morris DJ. Medicinal uses of licorice through the millennia: the good and plenty of it. *Mol Cell Endocrinol* 1991; 78(1–2):1–6.
101. Robinson HJ, Harrison FS, Nicholson JT. Cardiac abnormalities due to licorice intoxication. *Pa Med* 1971; 74(3):51–54.
102. Farese RV Jr, Biglieri EG, Shackleton CH, et al. Licorice-induced hypermineralocorticoidism. *N Engl J Med* 1991; 325(17):1223–1227.
103. Fogliano V, Sacchi R. Oleocanthal in olive oil: between myth and reality. *Mol Nutr Food Res* 2006; 50(1):5–6.
104. Beauchamp GK, Keast RS, Morel D, et al. Phytochemistry: ibuprofen-like activity in extra-virgin olive oil. *Nature* 2005; 437(7055):45–46.
105. Breslin PA, Gingrich TN, Green BG. Ibuprofen as a chemesthetic stimulus: evidence of a novel mechanism of throat irritation. *Chem Senses* 2001; 26(1):55–65.
106. Cicerale S, Breslin PA, Beauchamp GK, et al. Sensory characterization of the irritant properties of oleocanthal, a natural anti-inflammatory agent in extra virgin olive oils. *Chem Senses* 2009; 34(4):333–339.
107. Geppetti P, Patacchini R, Nassini R, et al. Cough: the emerging role of the TRPA1 channel. *Lung* 2010; 188(Suppl 1):S63-S68.
108. Nassenstein C, Kwong K, Taylor-Clark T, et al. Expression and function of the ion channel TRPA1 in vagal afferent nerves innervating mouse lungs. *J Physiol* 2008; 586(6):1595–1604.
109. Belvisi MG, Dubuis E, Birrell MA. Transient receptor potential A1 channels: insights into cough and airway inflammatory disease. *Chest* 2011; 140(4):1040–1047.
110. Peyrot des Gachons C, Uchida K, Bryant B, et al. Unusual pungency from extra-virgin olive oil is attributable to restricted spatial expression of the receptor of oleocanthal. *J Neurosci* 2011; 31(3):999–1009.
111. De Lorenzo A, Alberti A, Andreoli A, et al. Food habits in a southern Italian town (Nicotera) in 1960 and 1996: still a reference Italian Mediterranean diet? *Diabetes Nutr Metab* 2001; 14(3):121–125.
112. Lucas L, Russell A, Keast R. Molecular mechanisms of inflammation. Anti-inflammatory benefits of virgin olive oil and the phenolic compound oleocanthal. *Curr Pharm Des* 2011; 17(8):754–768.

36 The Management of Food Allergy

Maria Laura Acebal[1], Anne Muñoz-Furlong[2], & Hugh A. Sampson[3]

[1]Food Allergy Research & Education, Washington, DC, USA
[2]The Food Allergy & Anaphylaxis Network, Fairfax, VA, USA
[3]Translational Biomedical Sciences, Jaffe Food Allergy Institute Department of Pediatrics, Icahn School of Medicine at Mount Sinai, New York, NY, USA

Key Concepts

- Complete allergen avoidance is key to managing food allergy and preventing allergic reactions.
- Individuals with food allergies must be vigilant about reading all ingredient labels, every time, to prevent accidental ingestion. Precautionary statements, that is, "may contain," have frustrated food-allergic consumers, who should be instructed to avoid products with these labels.
- Even traces of food allergens can cause severe reactions, therefore the issue of cross-contact in food manufacturing practices, restaurants, and even home cooking presents challenges for families managing food allergies.
- Having a family member with a food allergy has a significant impact on the quality of life of the entire family.
- Patients at high risk for anaphylaxis include teens and young adults, who engage in risk-taking behaviors.
- With roughly two students in every classroom, schools must have written guidelines in place to care for students with food allergies and staff should be trained to recognize and treat anaphylactic emergencies. Epinephrine is the medication of choice for management of anaphylactic reactions.
- Dining with food allergies requires heightened vigilance. Reactions in restaurants are caused by a number of factors.
- Air travel can be daunting for individuals managing food allergies, particularly peanut allergy. Advance planning and coordination with the airline is recommended.

Introduction

Allergic reactions to foods encompass a spectrum of symptoms ranging from mild to life-threatening to fatal anaphylactic reactions. The relationship of a food to a reaction may be very clear, as in an acute IgE-mediated reaction following peanut ingestion. In such cases, elimination of the food should prevent the onset of symptoms. The overall contribution of a food to the production of atopic dermatitis or eosinophilic gastroenteritis may be less understood, however, and elimination of the offending antigen may not necessarily result in complete resolution of the disease.

For patients who have food allergies, avoidance of the offending food is the key to preventing an allergic reaction. Unfortunately, complete avoidance is difficult to achieve, because food allergens can be hidden in other foods. Therefore, all patients need written instructions for emergency management of a reaction. Treatment of food allergy may include attempts to prevent sensitization, medications to prevent or palliate symptoms associated with ingestion of the antigen, and possibly oral immunotherapy, a recent development.

This chapter covers topics on the management of food allergies in the day-to-day life of patients. For patients looking for additional resources on the clinical aspects of food allergy, including diagnosis and treatment, an excellent referral is the lay summary of the "Guidelines for the Diagnosis and Management of Food Allergy in the United States" (December 2011), National Institute of Allergy and Infectious Diseases, NIH. This document was specifically created for the public and highlights the information most important to patients, families, and caregivers, in order for them to work in partnership with their healthcare provider and to empower them to successfully manage food allergies (*Guidelines for the Diagnosis and Management of Food Allergy in the United States: Summary for Patients, Families, and Caregivers. Available at:* http://www.niaid.nih.gov/topics/foodAllergy/clinical/Documents/FaguidelinesPatient.pdf).

Food Allergy: Adverse Reactions to Foods and Food Additives, Fifth Edition. Edited by Dean D Metcalfe, Hugh A Sampson, Ronald A Simon and Gideon Lack.

Allergen avoidance

The best strategic approach to the management of true food hypersensitivity is complete avoidance of the allergen. It is critical to provide patients with adequate information about the allergen, including the types of food in which it may be found and the various terms that are used to identify the allergen on an ingredient statement.

Allergen identification

Close to 200 foods have been reported as causing an allergic reaction [1]. However, the foods most commonly implicated in food-allergic patients in the United States are egg, peanut, milk, soy, wheat, fish, shellfish, tree nuts (pecans, almonds, walnuts, pistachio nuts, cashews, hazelnuts, Brazil nuts, etc.), and sesame seed. Although avoidance of the offending food with careful menu planning and label reading would appear reasonably possible, it is actually quite challenging. The literature is replete with reports of accidental exposures of food-sensitive individuals to the very antigen they are striving to avoid, and a recent prospective study of 512 preschool children reported 1171 reactions over a 3-year period, that is, an annualized reaction rate of 0.81 [2]. Even minute quantities of an allergen may provoke serious reactions in extremely sensitive patients. The following discussion identifies potential problem areas and provides suggestions for educating patients in avoidance strategies.

Label reading

Food-allergic individuals should read the ingredient label on all foods. This step ought to be repeated every time they shop, because ingredients may change without warning. Label reading for some can take as much as 2 hours each time they go to the grocery store. Ingredient statements should also be read for bath products and cosmetics, as some contain extracts from common food allergens such as almonds or milk. Pet food sometimes contains wheat, eggs, milk, or peanuts. Children have had a reaction after being licked by a dog that had ingested food containing a food allergen. Because toddlers may eat things they find on the floor, including pet food, extra care and attention should be given when selecting pet food. Medications, such as dry powder inhalers [3] may contain allergens, further emphasizing the need for ingredient label reading for all products all the time.

To minimize the chance of missing an allergen, families report reading the ingredient label three times: at the store, before they put the groceries away at home, and before they serve the food to the allergic child. Some say they only noticed the allergen during the third reading, thus justifying to themselves the need for this extra-cautious approach. Others read the label backwards, from the last ingredient to the first, to ensure careful scrutiny.

It is also important to understand kosher rules and markings in order to make label reading easier. A "D" indicates that a product contains dairy products, even if its presence is not disclosed in the ingredient statement. Products that list a "D" on the front label but may not list milk in the ingredient statement include some brands of tuna, sliced bread and bread sticks, breakfast cereals, cookies, imitation butter flavor, pancake syrup, pretzels, fruit snacks, cake mixes, and frostings. The designation "D.E." (dairy equipment) on a label signifies that the product was manufactured on equipment also used to produce dairy-containing food. As a result, the product might contain trace amounts of milk protein [4].

"Pareve" or "Parve" on a label indicates that a rabbinical agency has determined that the product does not contain dairy. However, under Jewish law, a food product may contain a small amount of milk and still meet religious specifications for "pareve" [5]. Anaphylaxis has been reported in milk-sensitive children after ingestion of pareve-labeled food [4]. As a result, products labeled "pareve" may not be safe for those with milk allergy.

An important food allergen labeling law that changed the landscape for families in the United States managing food allergies took effect on January 1, 2006. The *Food Allergen Labeling and Consumer Protection Act of 2004* (FALCPA; Pub. L. No. 108-282, Title II, §202(1)(B), 118 Stat. 905 [codified as amended in scattered sections of 21 U.S.C.]) mandates that packaged food items must declare, in plain language, the presence of a major food allergen: (1) in the ingredient list; (2) via a "contains *allergen*" statement; or (3) by use of a parenthetical statement following a scientific ingredient term, for example, "albumin (egg)." In the case of fish, shellfish, and tree nuts, the specific type must be listed, for example, salmon, shrimp, cashew. A "major food allergen" is defined as peanuts, tree nuts, milk, egg, wheat, soy, fish, and crustacean shellfish (FALCPA §§202(2)(A), 203(a)). These eight allergens are commonly referred to as "the top eight" allergens.

The labeling requirements of FALCPA also apply to allergens in colorings, flavorings, and spices. Previously, allergens were simply listed under collective terms such as "Natural Flavors."

Before the implementation of FALCPA, to properly avoid the food to which they were allergic, patients had to learn all the scientific and technical names for foods that may have appeared on food labels. For example, the presence of milk protein may have been indicated as *whey* or *ammonium caseinate* and eggs as *albumin* or *globulin* (Table 36.1). Joshi reported that of 91 sets of parents participating

Table 36.1 Partial list of synonyms for common food allergens.

Milk protein
Ammonium caseinate
Casein
Curds
Whey
Ghee
Non-dairy
Soy protein
Edamame
Shoyu sauce
Wheat protein
Semolina
Cracker meal
Peanuts
Valencias
Monkey nut
Groundnut
Beer nuts

in a label-reading study in an allergy clinic, less than 10% of those avoiding milk were able to spot the "milk words" on a label, only 54% of those avoiding peanuts correctly identified peanuts on a label, and just 22% correctly identified soy [5]. Ninety percent of the parents with near-perfect scores in label reading were members of the Food Allergy & Anaphylaxis Network (FAAN), supporting the need for proper education of label reading for patients and their families. Today, these terms are still relevant for products not covered by FALCPA, but with the potential for the inclusion of a food allergen as an ingredient, namely cosmetics, bath products, lotions, pet foods, and medicines. For the top eight allergens, FALCPA mandates that their "plain English" and not their scientific name be used on a packaged food ingredient label.

FAAN (Fairfax, VA: 800-929-4040, www.foodallergy.org) provides wallet-size laminated cards to make identifying the presence of allergens easier. These "how to read a label" cards contain lists of synonyms and ciphers under which milk, egg, wheat, peanut, soy, shellfish, and tree nuts may masquerade. The cards are updated as new terms are identified.

While FALCPA greatly simplified the task of food label reading for the top eight allergens, the law has certainly not solved all of the issues related to allergen labeling.

Advisory labeling or "may contain" statements, the use of which has proliferated in recent years, are not covered at all by FALCPA. These allergen advisory statements are voluntary; as a result, manufacturers have their own criteria for when and what statement to use on a product. Examples of these statements include "may contain peanuts"; "processed in a facility that also processes nuts"; "manufactured in a plant that also processes milk, eggs, and wheat"; and "manufactured on shared equipment with nuts."

Many patients report frustration at their diminishing food choices as the proliferation of products with these advisory statements appears on the market; others have chosen to ignore these statements completely. This should be discouraged. The food industry indicates that these labeling messages are designed to alert patients that there is a chance the product may contain the allergen listed on the advisory statement. The FDA has notified the industry that these allergen advisory statements are not to be used in place of good manufacturing practices (Shank FR. Notice to manufacturers: *Label Declaration of Allergenic Substances in Foods*. 6 October 1996. US Food and Drug Administration Center for Food Safety and Applied Nutrition). Until there are set guidelines or regulations for the conditions under which these statements may be used, it is best to err on the side of caution and avoid these products. A study by Hefle et al. found that 2 of 51 (4%) products labeled as "may contain," 3 of 57 (5%) products labeled as being produced on "shared equipment," and 7 of 68 (10%) of those labeled as being produced in a "shared facility" in fact contained the food allergen [6]. These investigators also found an increasing disregard for such labels by food-allergic patients.

Another remaining labeling loop hole is the use of the term "non-dairy" in food that contains milk-derived proteins such as casein or caseinates. Examples of foods listed as non-dairy that may contain milk include coffee whiteners, whipped toppings, and imitation cheeses. A number of reactions have occurred to children whose family members believed "non-dairy" to mean "no dairy" and did not read the ingredient statement on the back of the package.

A labeling practice that may pose a threat to patients is the listing of the food allergen as the last ingredient. Patients have reported ingesting products with the allergen as the last ingredient. Having suffered no reaction, the patients determine that the ingredient is not present or that they are no longer allergic. Neither can be assumed. In one case, a young teen consumed a baked good that listed peanut flour as the last ingredient, allegedly telling her friend that she had done this before without having a reaction. Unfortunately, the product did contain peanuts and she died a short time later from the reaction.

Patients are advised to call the food manufacturer if they have difficulty interpreting a food label. To get the information they are looking for, patients must be as specific as possible, for example, ask "Does this product contain soy?" rather than "What does the 'may contain' statement mean?" Most large manufacturers will provide the specific allergen information. Companies who do not or cannot provide this are to be avoided. Imported foods may pose a risk, even though such foods are required to follow US labeling regulations. Labeling standards in other countries are not as strict as those in the United States, and US distributors often do not take responsibility for tracking down

Table 36.2 Unexpected sources of common allergens.

Food	Ingredient
Worcestershire sauce	Anchovies, sardines
Soy sauce	Wheat
Imitation butter flavor	Milk protein
Water-added ham, deli meats, some sausages, and hot dogs	Milk or soy
Sweet and sour sauce	Wheat or soy
Sorbet	Egg
Sweet potato puree	Peanut
Pizza	Egg
Low-fat peanut butter	Soy
Pet food[a]	Eggs, wheat, milk, peanuts, and soy
Cosmetic and bath products	Milk, tree nut, egg, wheat
Imitation crab legs	Wheat, fish, egg
Barbeque flavor potato crisps	milk
Pesto sauce	Peanuts, pistachio, walnut, pine nuts

[a]Toddlers may sample pet food off the floor.

ingredient information from foreign sources. Most of the products that cause reactions to individuals with peanut or tree nut allergy are desserts or bakery products [7, 8]. It is prudent for patients to avoid these types of products unless they are prepared in their home.

Some foods may appear to be so straightforward that the patient may not feel it necessary to scrutinize the ingredient label for allergens. Alternatively, the food product may be considered so unlikely to contain an allergen that the label is never reviewed (Table 36.2). Ingredient labels should be reviewed for all products.

Lists of commercially prepared "safe" foods are a popular request of busy parents looking for shortcuts in label reading. Manufacturers change ingredients without warning, making these lists potentially dangerous. A list of "safe" products can quickly become outdated and the incorrect information on the list can lead to a reaction, particularly since these lists are often copied and shared with caregivers, teachers, and others and old lists may not be retrieved and replaced. In one example, a school and day care center published such a list and included a "peanut and tree nut safe" donut shop. Months later the establishment introduced a nut-containing product made on shared equipment with "plain" donuts. In another case, the parent of a child with milk allergy provided a list of safe products. The mother forgot to update the list when some of the products were reformulated to contain milk. The school staff was uncertain about whether the product or the mother's list was safe.

Occasionally, a manufacturer makes a labeling or packaging error by including an undeclared allergen in a product, putting a product in the wrong packaging, or using an outdated label with incomplete ingredient information. Recalls due to undeclared allergens were the leading cause of food recalls in early 2011, according to FDA enforcement reports. These situations pose a special hazard to those with food allergies. The FDA requires products whose labels are incorrect to be recalled from the market. To quickly get the word out to the allergic community when these situations arise, FAAN has developed a Special Allergy Alert System. Information about the mistake, product name, code, and other criteria are sent via e-mail and placed on FAAN's web site (www.foodallergy.org). All patients who have food allergies should be encouraged to sign up for these free special allergy alert notices.

Cross-contact

Even with careful labeling, concealed allergens may still adulterate a food. Cross-contact can occur during the processing of foods thereby introducing an unintended food allergen into the product. These situations are handled differently by food manufacturers since advisory labeling or "may contain" statements on ingredient labels are purely voluntary and not mandated by FALCPA. Although production lines are cleaned thoroughly between each product run, mistakes are sometimes made. It has been reported that some dark chocolate may be manufactured on the same line as milk-containing products (e.g., milk chocolate), making contact with milk allergens possible.

Granola bars are often produced on the same line as products that contain peanuts or a variety of nuts, which could allow the granola bars to become contaminated with substances not listed on the label. One product can sometimes incorporate a stray ingredient from another product. For example, small pieces of peanuts or nuts can remain in the equipment after thorough cleaning and become dislodged during the next production run.

Various types of nut butter, including peanut butter, are commonly run on the same production line, allowing contamination of subsequent products. Ice cream containing nuts may be sieved to remove the nuts so that the base can be used for another flavor of ice cream. This policy may result in unsuspected contamination with nut allergen. Food industry experts now recommend that companies put "like into like" when reusing materials. Although large manufacturers heed this advice, small companies may not.

In addition to packaged foods, other potential sources of cross-contact may occur in the grocery store. Bulk food bins may be used for a variety of products with little or no cleaning of the bins in between each changeover, and shoppers may inadvertently transfer a scoop from one bin to another. Cheese is often sliced on the same equipment as deli meats, making cross-contact possible. It is common practice to place various types of donuts, croissants, and muffins together in display cases, where they are likely to come into contact with one another or where the same serving tool is used for all.

Avoiding these types of high-risk foods will help minimize the patient's chances of suffering an accidental ingestion of the food to which they are allergic.

Sources of cross-contact

Production/manufacturing lines
Deli slicers
Bulk food bins
Bakery display cases
Serving utensils and ice cream scoops
Buffet-style restaurants

Cooking

Families must learn how to adapt recipes and make appropriate allergy-safe substitutions. Often the entire family elects to follow the restricted diet and avoids bringing the allergen into the home, so that home can be a safe place for the child. This also minimizes the amount of cooking needed and the chances for cross-contact between allergen-containing and allergen-free foods.

Some families choose to bring the allergen into the home and use it as an opportunity to role-play situations that the child may encounter outside of the home. These families often have designated areas of the pantry and refrigerator for the allergen-free foods; some place stickers on all foods: green stickers to indicate "safe" foods and red stickers symbolizing "unsafe" foods. This strategy helps the child and other family members avoid unsafe foods. Other families have used colored dishes, spoons, and glasses for the allergic child, thus keeping food allergy top-of-mind at all times.

If the allergen is present in the home, extra care should be taken during cooking. The allergen-free meal may be prepared first, covered, and removed from the cooking area to be sure it is not accidentally contaminated with the allergen. One mother reported causing a reaction in her milk-allergic son after mistakenly using the same serving spoon for his food after using it to serve cheese-containing food to the rest of the family.

Keeping an extra supply of "safe" foods ready ensures that there is always something available for the allergic child especially on harried days or when a babysitter or other family member takes over the cooking responsibility.

There is no one way to manage food allergies; each family must decide what strategies work best for them. Their decisions will have to be revisited as the child ages and takes more control of his or her food allergy management.

Day-to-day management

All ingredient labels must be read—including foods, medications, bath and beauty products, and pet foods
Patients should avoid eating food with "may contain"-type warnings
Lists of "safe foods" quickly become out of date and should be discouraged
Food allergens can appear in unexpected places; patients should be on alert at all times
Desserts and bakery products cause the majority of peanut and tree nut reactions
Cross-contact between allergens can occur during manufacturing, storing, or cooking

Psychosocial impact

The constant vigilance required to avoid a reaction can be a source of stress to the family. In a study of the impact of food allergy on the quality of life, Sicherer reported that childhood food allergy has a significant impact on general health perception, had an emotional impact on parents, and placed limitations on family activities [9]. Marklund showed similar results in a Swedish study of children aged 8–9 years. Both studies noted that families managing multiple food allergies or food allergy and other atopic diseases such as eczema experienced more stress and worry than families with only one food allergen to avoid. The Swedish study reported that the ability of families to get along is higher in families with food allergy. This may be, in part, because they must work together to keep the allergic family member safe [10]. A study of the daily impact of food allergy on children by Bollinger reported that food allergy causes stress in the family and affects meal preparation. Ten percent of the respondents reported homeschooling their child because of the food allergy [11].

Stress on the family may come from a number of sources. Parents may have to work around family members or friends who do not believe food allergies are dangerous and who attempt to slip some of the restricted food to the child in an attempt to "prove" their theory to the child's parents. Relatives may also express skepticism about the potential for cross-contact to cause a reaction or mistakenly think that "just one taste" of the allergen is harmless.

In the school setting, children with food allergies can be the targets of class bullies. Some have had reactions as a result of this bullying. In one case, a child was sprayed with milk and suffered an allergic reaction. In another, classmates threatened a student who was allergic to peanuts by telling him they were going to shove a peanut down his throat. In their study about bullying, Sicherer and coworkers reported that more than 30% of children with food allergies reported being bullied, teased, or harassed because of their food allergy [12]. Schools have a responsibility to keep all children safe and to hold those who harass or tease others accountable.

Sometimes, a family that has adjusted to living with food allergy may experience a setback when their child has a reaction. If the parent served the food that caused the reaction, the parent may experience guilt or lose confidence in their ability to care for their child. Children who have suffered a severe reaction sometimes develop eating disorders. Some only eat one or two foods for long periods of time after a reaction. Others become withdrawn and extremely fearful, not trusting anyone else to read the ingredient label on their behalf. It is not uncommon for these children to experience panic attacks. Their siblings may also express anxiety, fearing that their brother or sister will die; some become jealous of the attention the parents give to the "at-risk" child.

Mothers of young children who have been diagnosed with food allergies have a unique set of stressors. Frequently they report feeling guilty for causing their child's food allergies, particularly children that have been breastfed. These feelings are more intense in families where the mother reports eating peanuts or tree nuts while pregnant or nursing and the child subsequently develops a peanut or tree nut allergy. Mothers should be reassured and not be made to feel guilty about past diet decisions. Mothers also express remorse for the pain their child may have suffered before a diagnosis was made.

Parents need to know how serious a reaction could be and what they should do if one were to occur. Statements such as "You worry too much" minimize the potential seriousness of food allergy. However, statements such as "This child is so allergic he won't be safe in school and must be homeschooled" or "This is the worst case I've ever seen" create an atmosphere of fear and dread. Some parents become so fearful they cannot function; they homeschool their child and minimize contact with others in an effort to avoid a possible deadly reaction. Parents need to have a healthy balance of education and caution from their physician.

Messages that empower the parents ultimately benefit the child. The family must work to find a balance for their child between safety and social normalcy. Knowing that there are millions of students with food allergies across the country who participate in class activities, team sports, recreational camps, sleepovers, and so on shows parents that food allergies are manageable and they need not restrict their child's social activities. Allowing the child to be part of the decision-making for food allergy management builds confidence in the child and prepares the child to successfully manage his or her food allergies later in life.

It is clear that food allergies affect the entire family. The psychological impact on the family can be intense, will change according to family events, and will differ among the parents, siblings, and the child who is allergic.

A follow-up visit with a physician and a registered dietitian (if recommended) a month or so after diagnosis and after severe allergic reactions may provide families the opportunity to ask questions and get information for handling situations that may have come up since the diagnosis. Parents who find their fears are impeding their day-to-day activities or whose children are showing signs of acute stress should be encouraged to speak with a professional counselor.

The psychosocial impact of food allergies

Food allergy can create stress
Food allergy can help build family unity in some families
Children can be the target of harassment/bullying
After a reaction, children and parents can become withdrawn and fearful
Children can develop eating disorders after a reaction
Parents sometimes feel guilty for creating their child's food allergy
Food allergy can limit family activities
Parents need information that empowers them and educates them
Food allergy impacts the entire family

Teens and young adults: high-risk patients

Studies of fatal food-induced anaphylactic reactions have shown that high-risk patients include adolescents and young adults with food allergy (particularly peanut or tree nut allergy) and asthma. In a study of 32 fatal food allergy reactions, the largest study of its kind, 17 (54%) of the fatalities involved individuals aged 10 to 19 years [7]. This age group poses unique challenges: teens generally spend more time away from home in the company of their friends; often do not carry their prescribed epinephrine (EpiPen®, or Adrenaclick®); try to treat anaphylaxis with asthma inhalers; and tend to go off alone when a reaction occurs.

In a study on risk-taking behaviors of adolescents and young adults affected by food allergy, 54% of the subjects indicated they purposefully ingested a potentially unsafe food; 42% indicated a willingness to eat a food labeled "may contain"; and only 61% reported that they "always" carry their self-injectable epinephrine. However, upon further query, it appears that the rate of carrying medications changes according to the social event or even the type of clothing they are wearing. Many teens reported carrying medication when going to a restaurant (84%), less than half (43%) do so when involved in sports. Wearing tight clothes (53%) or hanging out with friends (57%) were other reasons for not carrying medications [13].

In one tragic fatal anaphylaxis case, a teen went to the restroom alone and was discovered some time later by his friends. He was found clutching his asthma inhaler. There have been several publicized deaths of teens where anaphylaxis was mistaken for an asthma attack and therefore epinephrine was not administered or administered too late. It is important to stress to patients that if there is ever any doubt, the correct course of action is to administer epinephrine [14]. In another case, a teen collapsed in front of her friends, who stood by and watched not knowing how to help.

These tragedies point to some critical lessons. Adolescents and young adults should be given specific information for managing their food allergies in a variety of new situations. They must be reminded that epinephrine is the medication of choice for handling a severe reaction, and that reactions are never planned. Teens want their friends to know about their food allergy, but they prefer to have the school staff educate them [13]. FAAN's *Be a PAL: Protect a Life from Food Allergies* program and the *Friends Helping Friends* video/DVD are designed to simplify this educational task. There are several epinephrine autoinjector holders on the market, which will make it easier for teens, especially boys, to carry their prescribed epinephrine.

FAAN's *Stories from the Heart: A Collection of Essays from Teens with Food Allergies (Volumes I and II)* is a good resource for teaching teens that their concerns are universal and that they can learn from what others have done to balance their food allergies and active social calendar. Available on the FAAN website (www.foodallergy.org) along with many other products for teens and young adults, these resources provide teens and their friends with a tech-savvy outlet to secure information and support they need.

Adolescents and adults are high-risk patients

- Often spend time away from home with friends
- Exhibit risky behavior such as purposefully ingesting an allergen
- May not always carry their prescribed epinephrine
- Often confuse asthma and anaphylaxis symptoms and mistakenly use asthma inhalers to treat anaphylaxis

Management of food allergy at school

Food allergy affects an estimated 6–8% of young children, which equates to about 1 in 13, or roughly 2 students in every classroom [15]. In a school setting, one child's food allergy is likely to impact the child's friends and, in some cases, the entire class. Often, classmates avoid the food to which their friend is allergic so they can all eat together at lunch. In other cases, educators request that parents not send in peanut- or nut-containing products for class celebrations. Some, particularly teachers of young children, designate their classroom to be food free.

In a survey of 400 elementary school nurses, 44% reported an increase in children with food allergies in their schools over the last 5 years; only 2% reported a decrease. More than one-third of the nurses reported having 10 or more students with food allergies [16].

As food allergy continues to increase in the school setting, educators should institute school-wide policies to promote food allergy safety at lunch time, during class celebrations and field trips, and more.

Elementary schools frequently designate a "peanut- or milk-free" table in the cafeteria; others allow the children to eat in the library or another room outside the cafeteria with a few friends. Parents often fear that the smell of peanut butter will cause their child to have a life-threatening or fatal reaction. As a result, many demand that the school issue a peanut ban to keep their child safe. However, in a study by Simonte et al. to determine if casual contact with peanut butter would cause anaphylaxis, none of the patients (some of whom reported having reacted to the smell of peanut butter) experienced anaphylaxis from smelling peanut butter or from skin contact with peanut butter [17]. Some of the patients experienced local erythema, local pruritus, and a single hive following contact with peanut butter; however, they did not require medication.

Educators and parents are often concerned about removing peanut allergens from desks, tables, hands, and other surfaces. Investigators sampled a variety of cleaners' ability to remove peanut residue. Perry et al. tested a number of cleaning products and reported that plain water, Formula 409® cleaner, Lysol sanitizing wipes, and Target brand cleaner with bleach were most effective in removing peanut residue. Dishwashing liquid was ineffective [18].

Hand washing and the use of hand wipes are also a common practice in schools, particularly in elementary grades, to remove peanut residue. Perry's group found the following to be most effective: Tidy Tykes wipes, Wet Ones antibacterial wipes, liquid soap, bar soap. Of note, water and hand sanitizer did not remove peanut from hands [18].

In an effort to control the risks, some schools provide nonfood treats (pencils, stickers, etc.) in lieu of food, while others require that foods sent in for class celebrations must be commercially prepared and contain preprinted ingredient statements or request that the student's parents send in "safe" snacks for their child. Many schools hold yearly "in-service" training sessions, whereby appropriate staff members (teachers, aides, coaches, etc.) are instructed in recognizing an allergic reaction and administering autoinjectable epinephrine.

Nonetheless, food allergy reactions frequently occur in the school setting. In a telephone survey of 80 schools, Nowak-Wegrzyn et al. reported that 39% had at least one reaction to a food in the previous 2 years [19]. Some of the reactions in school are severe or fatal [7, 20, 21]. In spite of this, Nowak-Wegrzyn reported that 30% of 132 students with food allergies did not have physician's instructions or medication at school at the time of their reaction [19].

Reactions in schools are common, in part, because food is everywhere: in the cafeteria, in the classroom, on the playground, on the school bus, and so on. Foods used in school projects or class celebrations [21, 22] have caused reactions, as have treats exchanged with well-meaning friends who believe the food to be safe [23]. In response, some schools have implemented a "no food trading" policy to prevent these types of reactions.

Two studies have shown that 25% of reactions in schools are first-time reactions [21, 22]. Thus, it is critical that school staff learn the symptoms of a reaction and have a plan in place to administer epinephrine and get help quickly. Lack of written emergency action plans and insufficient staff training in the recognition of symptoms have been attributed to a delay in treatment of a reaction in some cases [24]. It is recommended that children with food allergies have a written plan for handling a reaction and for managing their food allergy day to day, on file at the school.

The development of the day-to-day plan should be a collaborative effort, with input from the child's teachers, the school principal, the school nurse, the child's physician, and the child's parents. Often, the written plan takes the form of an Individualized Health Care Plan ("IHP"), recommended by the National Association of School Nurses (NASN). Some parents choose to implement with the school another type of written plan known as a "504 Plan," based on the protections afforded to students with the disabilities under Section 504 of the Rehabilitation Act of 1973 (discussed in more detail later).

Whichever written plan a student uses, at a minimum, it should contain a one-page emergency action plan for use during an anaphylactic emergency. FAAN's *Food Allergy Action Plan* (Fig. 36.1) is a popular tool employed by schools throughout the country. This document (available in English and Spanish for free download at www.foodallergy.org) contains crucial information: the signs and symptoms of a reaction; directions for treatment; emergency contact information; an indication of which school staff members have received food allergy training; and directions for administering autoinjectable epinephrine.

The *School Food Allergy Program* (SFAP), produced by FAAN for school staff, includes a staff education program on a CD-ROM called Safe@School® and a binder filled with practical information and standardized forms. The SFAP, which has been distributed to tens of thousands of schools across the United States, was developed in conjunction with NASN, the National School Boards Association, the National Association of Elementary School Principals, and the National Association of Secondary School Principals. It is supported by the Anaphylaxis Committee of the American Academy of Allergy, Asthma & Immunology and NASN.

Managing food allergies at school:

There is no "one-size-fits-all" approach

A written management plan will help ensure the student's safety at school

School staff should be trained to recognize and treat a reaction and how to reduce the risk of allergen exposure

Lack of a written emergency action plan and quick access to epinephrine are believed to be a factor in fatal food allergy reactions

Schools are taking a number of approaches to managing food allergies, including no food trading, designated cafeteria seating, and food-free celebrations

A school-wide food allergy management plan should consider all places where food is found and develop a plan to minimize risks of a reaction

Figure 36.1 Food allergy action plan.

Another important resource for educators is *How to C.A.R.E™ for Students with Food Allergies: What Educators Should Know*, available at www.allergyready.com. This state-of-the-art online course, developed by FAAN, the Food Allergy Initiative, Anaphylaxis Canada, the Canadian Society of Allergy and Clinical Immunology, and Leap Learning Technologies, provides a comprehensive tutorial on managing anaphylaxis in schools and is available free of charge on the web.

Epinephrine is the medication of choice for managing an anaphylactic reaction. A review of epinephrine use in Massachusetts schools indicated that in one-fifth of the cases, the allergic reaction occurred outside the school building on the playground, traveling to and from school, and on field trips. Clearly, anaphylactic reactions in schools are not uncommon events and are not confined primarily to the cafeteria [22]. To protect students, states throughout the country have changed laws and regulations to allow students, with a physician and parent's permission, to carry their own epinephrine throughout the school day.

It is important to differentiate between a student's right to self-carry medication and a student's ability to self-inject. In the United States, students at any age have the legal right, with a physician and parent's permission, to carry their own epinephrine. Most pediatricians, however, would not expect to transfer the primary responsibility of recognizing an anaphylactic reaction and treating that reaction with epinephrine to their patients until at least the age of 12–14 years, and even recognize that the assessment is dependent on a variety of patient readiness factors [25].

Although it does sometimes happen, no school should turn away a child solely because of the child's food allergies. Children with life-threatening food allergies are considered *disabled* under federal civil rights laws, such as Section 504 (of the Rehabilitation Act of 1973) and the Americans with Disabilities Act (ADA). Under these laws, schools must address the health and safety needs of the child and must provide accommodations to ensure that the child participates fully and equally in all normal facets of the school day. There are many resources, including government agencies such as the Office for Civil Rights within the US Department of Justice, available to assist families, if they encounter discrimination at school because of their child's food allergies.

It is important to note that there is no "one-size-fits-all" approach to managing food allergies in the school setting. There are many different ways to keep children with food allergies safe at school. The important requirement is that schools develop an approach, write it down, educate all stakeholders on this school-wide food allergy management plan, and then enforce its measures consistently.

Eating away from home

When food is consumed that is not personally prepared and served in one's home, the risk of encountering a hidden allergen increases. As an example, a peanut-sensitive teenager made her own jam sandwich while on a camping trip. She was not aware that the knife had been used earlier to spread peanut butter and had been wiped but not washed. She died minutes after eating the sandwich. Another individual suffered a reaction after eating ice cream that should not have contained nuts. It was later discovered that the wait staff mistakenly put the wrong flavor ice cream on the child's ice cream cone.

Food-allergic patients must be on heightened alert when dining away from home. Common ingredients can appear in unexpected places, for example, eggs in meat loaf or peanut butter in meat sauce. Convincing the wait staff that food allergies are real and that it is critical that they give accurate information about ingredients are just some of the obstacles patients must be prepared to address.

From the restaurateur's perspective, high staff turnover and part-time staff make training or standardization of food allergy policies difficult to implement. When dining in a restaurant, patients should address food allergy queries to the restaurant manager. The manager is often more seasoned and less distracted than harried wait staff, increasing the chances that the patient will receive accurate information (FAAN).

Furlong et al. reported that reactions in restaurants were caused by a number of factors: the food-allergic individual not telling the wait staff about the food allergy; cross-contact between foods (primarily from shared ice cream equipment, cooking surfaces, and serving utensils); and establishment error (e.g., switching ingredients and not notifying the wait staff). Half of the reactions were caused by allergens in unexpected places, for example, in sauces, dressings, or egg rolls. Desserts accounted for 43% of the reactions, followed by entrées (35%), appetizers (13%), and other (9%) [21].

There are some simple strategies for avoiding a reaction in a restaurant setting. Individuals who are allergic to peanuts or tree nuts should not eat in Chinese, Thai, Indian, or other Asian-type restaurants. These ingredients are commonly used in many dishes and cross-contact between foods during meal preparation and cooking is likely. Peanut-allergic individuals have reported reactions after eating Mexican food. These restaurants are now using peanut butter in some dishes, an example being enchilada sauce.

Patients who are allergic to fish or shellfish should avoid eating at seafood restaurants. The fryer oil, grill, and other cooking areas are likely to contain small amounts of fish or shellfish protein that could come into contact with the fish-free meal. Some individuals are so sensitive to a food that simply breathing the aerosolized protein in steam can cause a severe or even fatal reaction. A shrimp-sensitive woman is said to have suffered fatal anaphylaxis within minutes after a waiter in a restaurant walked past her carrying a sizzling shrimp dish.

Buffet-style service offers another potentially high risk for cross-contact. The food is often placed in serving dishes that are close to each other and small amounts of one food may fall into another serving dish; diners often dip one spoon into several dishes. Finally, dishes and their ingredients are rarely identified. One woman learned after she had a reaction that the food she ate contained walnuts. Another family tragically lost their 18-year-old son after he ate a dessert containing peanuts at a hotel buffet.

While eating in a quick-serve or fast-food restaurant, it is not prudent to assume that what is safe in one restaurant will necessarily be safe in another. Although food preparation at chain restaurants is usually standardized, regional differences may exist in products served or ingredients used. Franchise owners may not follow corporate policy regarding separation of various foods during cooking and preparation.

When eating in restaurants, individuals with food allergies will minimize the chance for an allergic reaction if they identify themselves to the wait staff and manager, ask questions about ingredients used, cooking methods (i.e., whether the grill is greased with butter), the use of "secret ingredients," and ask for advice on selecting menu items. Patients should order simply prepared foods with as few ingredients as possible, for example, a baked potato without the toppings.

As an example, a peanut-sensitive teenager died after eating an egg roll at an Asian restaurant. He apparently had asked the waiter if any of the food was cooked in peanut oil and was assured that the restaurant did not use any peanut oil. He may not have inquired about the use of peanut butter, which the restaurant used in its egg rolls. It is imperative that food-allergic patients make their food allergy known to the manager and staff of food service establishments. As a rule, if the patient has any doubt about whether his or her questions and concerns are being taken seriously, the individual should eat elsewhere.

To discreetly and consistently convey information to the restaurant staff, some patients prefer to use a "chef card" (Fig. 36.2). These personalized cards usually include the list of synonyms for the allergen, a caution about food preparation, and the symptoms of a reaction (to convey the seriousness of the food allergy, some use a brightly colored laminated card; others have business cards printed with this information).

When it comes to menu selection, avoidance of high-risk foods on a menu, such as sauces and desserts, foods prepared in a pastry covering, combination foods (such as stews), and fried foods, may help patients avoid an allergic reaction.

Surprise use of allergens include

Almonds in dressings for chicken entrees, sauces used on fresh fruit and in baked goods.

Eggs used to create foam for toppings on specialty coffee drinks, as a binder in meatballs or meatloaf, and as a glaze on baked goods.

Peanut butter used to thicken chili, Mexican salsa, spaghetti sauce, hot chocolate, and brown gravy. It has also been used as the "glue" to hold egg rolls and rice krispie treats together, to add crunch and texture to pie crusts and cheesecakes, and to add flavor to brownies.

Nuts and other toppings are often accidentally dropped into containers of ice cream. Furthermore, the scoopers for the various flavors are often placed in a common tub of water, and therefore may contain protein from all of the different flavors.

It is a common industry policy for restaurants to cook several types of foods in the same deep-fat fryer. This can pose a risk to the allergic individual who has no way of knowing what other foods were fried in that cooking oil. In one case, an individual with a fish allergy reacted to French fries that had been cooked in the same oil as the fish.

In spite of their precautions, however, mistakes can occur in the kitchen during meal preparation as well. Several reactions have occurred after the kitchen staff simply removed the allergen rather than making a new dish. To avoid this risk, if a food-allergic individual is served an allergen-containing dish at a restaurant (a cheeseburger instead of a plain burger), the individual should keep the original dish at their table to ensure that a new dish is prepared.

New state legislation that took effect on February 1, 2011, offers important support for food-allergic patients choosing to dine out at restaurants. Several other states are also considering similar legislation. The Massachusetts Food Allergy Awareness in Restaurants Act requires restaurants to post a food allergy awareness poster in the staff area and include a notice on menus and menu boards that reads "Before placing your order, please inform your server if a person in your party has a food allergy."

The new law also includes food allergy training for certified food protection managers via video, along with an accompanying training manual, FAAN's *Welcoming Guests with Food Allergies*, as well as allergen awareness training for required certified food protection managers (The United States *Food Allergy Awareness in Restaurants Act*, 105 CMR 590 et seq.).

Sample chef card
To the chef:
WARNING! I am allergic to peanuts. In order to avoid a life-threatening reaction, I must avoid the following ingredients:
Artificial nuts
Beer nuts
Cold pressed, expelled, or extruded peanut oil
Groundnuts
Mandelonas
Mixed nuts
Monkey nuts
Nut pieces
Peanut
Peanut butter
Peanut flour
Please ensure any utensils and equipment used to prepare my meal, as well as prep surfaces, are thoroughly cleaned prior to use. Thanks for your cooperation.

Figure 36.2 Sample chef card.

Dining away from home

Selection of low-risk restaurants is key for minimizing the chances of an allergic reaction.

Avoiding desserts, sauces, fried foods, and foods in covered pastry will help minimize the chance of an accidental ingestion of an allergen.

Individuals can use a "chef card" to identify themselves to the wait staff in restaurants.

If an order is incorrect, the allergic individual should keep it until a new dish is served.

Buffets offer a tremendous risk for cross-contact with allergens and are best avoided.

Special occasions

Preparation, planning ahead, and minimizing risks are the key ingredients for success during special occasions such as birthday parties, family gatherings, vacations, and air travel.

Before attending a birthday party or visiting a relative's house, the hostess should be alerted of the food allergy. Some families prefer to bring their own "safe" food for their peace of mind. For vacations, many seek lodging with kitchens so they can prepare the child's meals themselves. Those that choose this option often bring food with them or ship staples such as bread and cereals to their vacation destination. For sleepaway camps, the options may include providing the child's food or reviewing the menu to determine what foods the child can eat. Careful attention should be given to ensure that camp staff and counselors are trained to recognize and treat allergic reactions and that any camp activities requiring children to be in remote areas ensure emergency medical services are available if needed.

Regarding air travel, the best policy is to avoid eating any food served by the airline, as ingredient lists are not usually available and the meals are prepared in large warehouses with many opportunities for mistakes or cross-contact to occur. Some families of children with peanut allergy request peanut-free flights. No airline can guarantee a peanut-free flight. There may be peanut ingredients in meals; other passengers may carry peanuts on the plane with them. Some airlines will serve a non-peanut snack upon request, others make no such accommodations. Families would do well to check with the airline when booking their flights, confirm the arrangements before the trip, and keep in mind that airlines may change their policy without warning. As a precaution, all families should keep their child's medications stored in a carry-on bag, and be prepared to treat a reaction should one occur.

According to the Transportation Security Administration (TSA), passengers are permitted to bring self-injectable epinephrine on board, provided that the medication features a professionally printed label identifying the medication or the manufacturer's name. FAAN recommends that patients carry additional documentation such as a doctor's note and the prescription label from the pharmacy. A sample doctor's note is available on the FAAN web site.

When traveling outside the United States, other problems may arise. In some parts of Europe, for example, product labels do not have to list all ingredients and emergency services differ from country to country. FAAN's booklet *Dining Out and Traveling with Food Allergy* includes information and advice for managing meals while traveling (FAAN; Munoz-Furlong, 1994). It is also helpful to translate a chef's card into the language spoken in the country patients are traveling to. Note that many countries that speak the same language may use different words for food allergens. For example, though Spanish is spoken in both countries, in Argentina a peanut is known as "maní," whereas in Mexico it is called "cacahuate."

References

1. Hefle SL, Nordlee JA, Taylor SL. Allergenic foods. *Crit Rev Food Sci Nutr* 1996; 36(Suppl):S69–S89.
2. Fleischer DM, Perry TT, Atkins D, et al. Allergic reactions to foods in preschool-aged children in a prospective observational food allergy study. *Pediatrics* 2012; 130(1):e25–e32.
3. Nowak-Wegrzyn A, Shapiro GG, Beyer K, et al. Contamination of dry powder inhalers for asthma with milk proteins containing lactose. *J Allergy Clin Immunol* 2004; 113(3):558–560.
4. Gern J, Yang E, Evrard H, et al. Allergic reactions to milk-contaminated "non-dairy" products. *N Engl J Med* 1991; 324:976–979.
5. Joshi P, Mofidi S, Sicherer SH. Interpretation of commercial food ingredient labels by parents of food-allergic children. *J Allergy Clin Immunol* 2002; 109(6):1019–1021.
6. Hefle SL, Furlong TJ, Niemann L, et al. Consumer attitudes and risks associated with packaged foods having advisory labeling regarding the presence of peanuts. *J Allergy Clin Immunol* 2007; 120(1):171–176.
7. Bock SA, Munoz-Furlong A, Sampson HA. Fatalities due to anaphylactic reactions to foods. *J Allergy Clin Immunol* 2001; 107(1):191–193.
8. Furlong TJ, DeSimone J, Sicherer SH. Peanut and tree nut allergic reactions in restaurants and other food establishments. *J Allergy Clin Immunol* 2001; 108(5):867–870.
9. Sicherer SH, Noone SA, Munoz-Furlong A. The impact of childhood food allergy on quality of life. *Ann Allergy Asthma Immunol* 2001; 87(6):461–464.
10. Marklund B, Ahlstedt S, Nordstrom G. Health-related quality of life among adolescents with allergy-like conditions - with emphasis on food hypersensitivity. *Health Qual Life Outcomes* 2004; 2:65.
11. Bollinger ME, Dahlquist LM, Mudd K, et al. The impact of food allergy on the daily activities of children and their families. *Ann Allergy Asthma Immunol* 2006; 96(3):415–421.
12. Lieberman JA, Weiss C, Furlong TJ, et al. Bullying among pediatric patients with food allergy. *Ann Allergy Asthma Immunol* 2010; 105(4):282–286.
13. Sampson MA, Munoz-Furlong A, Sicherer SH. Risk-taking and coping strategies of adolescents and young adults with food allergy. *J Allergy Clin Immunol* 2006; 117(6):1440–1445.
14. Sicherer SH, Simons FE. Self-injectable epinephrine for first-aid management of anaphylaxis. *Pediatrics* 2007; 119(3):638–646.
15. Gupta RS, Springston EE, Warrier MR, et al. The prevalence, severity, and distribution of childhood food allergy in the United States. *Pediatrics* 2011; 128(1):e9–e17.

16. Weiss C, Munoz-Furlong A, Furlong TJ, et al. Impact of food allergies on school nursing practice. *J Sch Nurs* 2004; 20(5):268–278.
17. Simonte SJ, Ma S, Mofidi S, et al. Relevance of casual contact with peanut butter in children with peanut allergy. *J Allergy Clin Immunol* 2003; 112(1):180–182.
18. Perry TT, Conover-Walker MK, Pomes A, et al. Distribution of peanut allergen in the environment. *J Allergy Clin Immunol* 2004; 113(5):973–976.
19. Nowak-Wegrzyn A, Conover-Walker MK, Wood RA. Food-allergic reactions in schools and preschools. *Arch Pediatr Adolesc Med* 2001; 155(7):790–795.
20. Sampson HA, Mendelson LM, Rosen JP. Fatal and near-fatal anaphylactic reactions to food in children and adolescents. *N Engl J Med* 1992; 327:380–384.
21. Sicherer SH, Furlong TJ, Desimone J, et al. The US peanut and tree nut allergy registry: characteristics of reactions in schools and day care. *J Pediatr* 2001; 138:560–565.
22. McIntyre CL, Sheetz AH, Carroll CR, et al. Administration of epinephrine for life-threatening allergic reactions in school settings. *Pediatrics* 2005; 116(5):1134–1140.
23. Bock SA, Munoz-Furlong A, Sampson HA. Further fatalities caused by anaphylactic reactions to food, 2001-2006. *J Allergy Clin Immunol* 2007; 119(4):1016–1018.
24. Sampson HA, Munoz-Furlong A, Campbell RL, et al. Second symposium on the definition and management of anaphylaxis: summary report—second National Institute of Allergy and Infectious Disease/Food Allergy and Anaphylaxis Network Symposium. *Ann Emerg Med* 2006; 47(4):373–380.
25. Simons E, Sicherer SH, Simons FE. Timing the transfer of responsibilities for anaphylaxis recognition and use of an epinephrine auto-injector from adults to children and teenagers: pediatric allergists' perspective. *Ann Allergy Asthma Immunol* 2012; 108(5):321–325.

37 The Natural History of Food Allergy

Robert A. Wood

Pediatric Allergy and Immunology, Johns Hopkins University School of Medicine, Baltimore, MD, USA

Key Concepts

- The natural history of food allergy is generally positive.
- Natural history varies widely from one food to another.
- Peanut, tree nuts, fish, and shellfish allergies tend to be most persistent.
- Natural history varies widely for individual foods from one individual to another.
- Regular follow-up is important to monitor food-allergic patients over time.

Introduction

The natural history of food allergy refers to both the acquisition of allergic sensitivities and their natural course over time. Food allergy most often begins in the first 1–2 years of life with the process of sensitization, by which the immune system responds to specific food proteins, most often with the development of allergen-specific immunoglobulin E (IgE). Over time, most food allergy is lost, although allergy to some foods is more often long lived. For example, while most milk and egg allergy is outgrown, most peanut and tree nut allergies are not. This chapter will review the development of food allergy and the natural history of food sensitivities over time.

When considering the natural history of food allergy, it is critical that the criteria used to define food allergy be carefully considered. Some studies report solely on rates of sensitization while others focus on clinical reactivity to specific foods. The definition of clinical reactivity is also not consistent between studies, with some relying solely on parental reports of food reactions, while others utilize food challenges and other more objective evidence of true food allergy. These details are important in that a history of an adverse food reaction, or even evidence of sensitization, does not necessarily mean that a patient will exhibit a clinical reaction upon exposure to that food. The specific criteria used to diagnose food allergy may therefore have a significant impact on the results of these studies, especially those used to measure the prevalence of food allergy.

Studies on the development of food allergy

Most food allergy is acquired in the first 1–2 years of life. The prevalence of food allergy overall, and of allergy to specific foods, is uncertain because studies vary in methodological approaches. Estimates of food allergy prevalence are highest when based upon self-report alone, fall somewhat when sensitization data are added, and are most accurate when detailed evaluations, including oral food challenges, are included in the evaluation. Food allergy has been estimated in various studies to affect as few as 1–2% and as many as 10% of the population in developed countries [1–8], although most agree that the prevalence of food allergy peaks at 5–8% at 1 year of age and then falls progressively until late childhood or adolescence, after which the prevalence remains stable at about 3–4%. In this section studies on the development of food allergy will be reviewed.

Bock prospectively followed 480 children, recruited from a single pediatric practice, for the development of food allergy from birth through the age of 3 years [9]. Foods that were suspected of causing adverse reactions were eliminated from the diet and then reintroduced in either open or blinded challenges at regular intervals. Limited allergy testing was performed, so it was not possible to characterize the proportion of reactions that were IgE mediated. Overall, 28% of the children were reported to

Food Allergy: Adverse Reactions to Foods and Food Additives, Fifth Edition. Edited by Dean D Metcalfe, Hugh A Sampson, Ronald A Simon and Gideon Lack.

have an adverse food reaction and the reactions were confirmed by challenge in 8%. Eighty percent of these reactions occurred in the first year of life and the majority of the foods could be successfully reintroduced into the diet within 1 year of the onset of the allergy.

Another prevalence study was conducted in Finland in a cohort of 866 children who were followed for the occurrence of food allergy at ages 1, 2, 3, and 6 years [10]. The diagnosis of food allergy was based on a history of either rash or vomiting and all suspected reactions were confirmed by elimination and home rechallenge. Allergy testing was not otherwise conducted. Based on these criteria, the prevalence of adverse food reactions was 19% at age 1, 22% at age 2, 27% at age 3, and 8% at age 6 years. In order of prevalence, the foods most commonly implicated at all ages were citrus fruits, tomato, egg, strawberry, and fish.

An even larger cohort study was recently conducted in Norway [11–13]. For the first part of the study, a population-based cohort of 3623 children was followed from birth until the age of 2 years [3], during which parents completed questionnaires regarding adverse food reactions at 6-month intervals. The cumulative incidence of adverse food reactions was 35% by age 2 years, with milk being the single food item most commonly incriminated at 11.6%. The duration of the reactions was overall short, with approximately two-thirds of the reactions resolving within 6 months of their onset.

In the second phase of the study, those children who had persistent complaints of milk or egg allergy underwent a more detailed evaluation at the age of 2–2.5 years [12, 13], including skin testing and open and double-blind oral challenges. The point prevalence of cow's milk and egg allergy or intolerance at the age of 2.5 years were estimated to be 1.1% and 1.6%, respectively. Most milk reactions were not IgE mediated and only 33% of parental reports of adverse milk reactions were confirmed, while most egg reactions were IgE mediated and 56% of parental reports were confirmed.

Host and Halken sought to determine the prevalence of milk allergy by prospectively following 1749 Danish children from birth through age 3 years [14]. The children were carefully evaluated by history, milk elimination, oral challenge, and skin tests or radioallergosorbent tests (RASTs). Milk allergy was suspected in 117 children (6.7%) and confirmed in 39 (2.2%). Of those, 21 had IgE-mediated allergy and the remaining 18 were classified as non-IgE-mediated. All milk allergy developed in the first year of life and most of the allergic children were able to tolerate milk by age 3 years (56% by age 1, 77% by age 2, and 87% by age 3 years). All children with non-IgE-mediated allergy were tolerant by age 3, compared to 75% with IgE-mediated allergy. Also of note, of those with IgE-mediated allergy, 35% had other food allergies by age 3 and 25% had other food allergies by age 10 years [15]. Those children were also more likely to develop inhalant allergies over time.

Tariq and colleagues followed a cohort of children for the development of peanut and tree nut sensitization through the age of 4 years [16]. All children born on the Isle of Wight in a 1-year period were recruited and evaluated at ages 1, 2, and 4 years. Fifteen (1.2%) of the 1218 children were sensitized to peanut or tree nuts. Thirteen were sensitive to peanut and six had had allergic reactions to peanut (0.5% of the population), while one child each had had a reaction to hazelnuts and cashews.

One final study of importance followed the development of sensitization to common food allergens in a large cohort of children, without clinical confirmation of food sensitivity. Two hundred and sixteen children from a birth cohort of 4082 children in the Multicenter Allergy Study conducted in Germany were assessed for food-specific IgE at 1, 2, 3, 5, and 6 years of age [17]. The overall annual incidence rates for food sensitization decreased from a peak of 10% at age 1 to 3% at age 6 years. Sensitization to egg and milk was most common at all ages, followed by wheat and soy. This study also found that there was a high rate of aeroallergen sensitization in children who began with food sensitivities, especially to egg [18, 19]. Remarkably, if a child had both a positive family history of allergy and an egg-specific IgE level above 2 kU_A/L at the age of 12 months, there was a 78% positive predictive value and a 99% specificity for the development of inhalant allergen sensitivity by the age of 3 years [18].

Several points are worth emphasizing from these studies. First, suspected food allergy is extraordinarily common in early childhood, with at least one-fourth of all parents reporting one or more adverse food reactions. Second, adverse food reactions can be confirmed in 5–10% of young children with a peak prevalence at around 1 year of age. Third, most food allergy is lost over time. And finally, children who begin with one food allergy, especially if it is IgE mediated, have a very high chance of developing additional food allergies, as well as inhalant allergies. It is therefore critical that children with food allergy be identified as early as possible, both to initiate an appropriate diet for their existing allergies and to consider preventative measures that may help to reduce their chance of developing additional food allergies, as well as asthma and allergic rhinitis.

Studies on the loss of food allergy

Most food allergy is indeed lost over time. The process of outgrowing food allergies, by which a patient becomes completely tolerant to a food that had previously caused a reaction, varies a great deal for different foods and among individual patients. In the study by Bock described above [9], almost all of the adverse food reactions had been lost by the age of 3 years. Among these, there were 11 children with confirmed milk allergy and 14 children with probable milk allergy, all of whom were able to tolerate milk by the age of 3 years. The median duration of adverse reactions to milk was in fact only 9 months. In a second study by Bock, nine children who had had severe reactions to milk, egg, and/or soy at 2–15 months of age were followed for 3–9 years [20]. Over time, three of the nine children were able to fully tolerate the offending food, four could tolerate small amounts, and two continued to have reactions with small exposures.

Dannaeus and Inganas followed 82 children between the ages of 6 months and 14 years with a variety of food allergies for a period of 2–5 years [21]. Of the 12 children who were allergic to milk, 4 developed complete tolerance, 7 had reduced sensitivity, and only 1 remained unchanged by the completion of their follow-up. Fifty-five children had egg allergy, of whom 20 developed complete tolerance, 24 had reduced sensitivity, and 11 remained unchanged. The results were very different for fish and peanut/tree nut allergy, with only 5 of 32 patients with fish allergy and 0 of 35 patients with peanut or tree nut allergy developing tolerance.

Sampson and Scanlon followed a group of 75 patients between the ages of 3 and 18 years with atopic dermatitis and food allergy that had been diagnosed by skin testing, RASTs, and double-blind, placebo-controlled food challenges (DBPCFCs) [22]. Patients were rechallenged yearly to each of the foods that had previously elicited a positive challenge and after 1 year, 19 of the 75 had lost all food allergies, including 15 of 45 patients allergic to one food and 4 of 21 allergic to two foods. A total of 38 of 121 specific food sensitivities had been lost after 1 year. After 2 years, an additional 4 of 44 patients lost their food allergy, while none of the 20 patients rechallenged after 3 years had a negative challenge. The results for specific foods after 1–2 years of follow-up are represented in Table 37.1,

Table 37.1 The persistence or loss of specific food sensitivities over 1–2 years in children with atopic dermatitis.

		Challenge	
Allergen	Total	Positive (%)	Negative (%)
Egg	59	45 (76)	14 (24)
Milk	21	17 (81)	4 (19)
Soy	10	5 (50)	5 (50)
Wheat	6	4 (67)	2 (33)
Peanut	10	8 (80)	2 (20)
Other	15	5 (33)	10 (66)

Source: Reproduced from Reference 21 with permission from Blackwell Publishing.

showing that egg allergy had been lost in 24%, milk in 19%, soy in 50%, wheat in 33%, and peanut in 20%. In a similar study by Sampson, follow-up data were provided on 40 of 113 patients with food allergy and atopic dermatitis 1–2 years after their original diagnosis [23]. In that study, egg allergy had been outgrown in 14 of 20 patients (30%), compared to 4 of 7 with milk allergy (57%), 1 of 4 with wheat allergy (25%), and 2 of 3 with soy allergy (67%).

Shek et al. monitored food-specific IgE levels in 88 patients with egg allergy and 49 patients with cow's milk allergy (CMA) who also underwent repeated DBPCFCs [24]. Twenty-eight of the 66 egg-allergic and 16 of the 33 milk-allergic patients lost their allergy over time. For egg, the decrease in serum IgE (IgE) levels was significantly related to the probability of developing clinical tolerance, with the duration between challenges having an influence. For milk, there was also a significant relationship between the decrease in IgE levels and the probability of developing tolerance to milk but no significant contribution with regard to time. Stratification into two age groups, those below 4 years of age and those above 4 years of age at the time of first challenge, had an effect, with the younger age group being more likely to develop clinical tolerance in relation to the rate of decrease in IgE. The median food IgE level at diagnosis was significantly less for the group developing tolerance to egg, and a similar trend was seen for milk allergy.

Milk allergy

The natural history of milk allergy has been most extensively studied [25–35]. However, as summarized in Table 37.2, the results of these studies do not provide a completely clear and consistent picture.

Dannaeus and Johansson followed 47 infants with milk allergy for 6 months to 4 years [26]. In children with immediate-type, IgE-mediated reactions, 29% developed complete tolerance to milk over the course of the study, compared to 74% of those with delayed-type, non-IgE-mediated reactions. The trend for non-IgE-mediated milk allergy to be outgrown more quickly than IgE-mediated allergy has been demonstrated in most studies, including the study by Host and Halken [14], in which the vast majority of all children were milk tolerant by age 3.

A series of studies on milk allergy have been published by Hill and colleagues [27–30]. In their first natural history study [27], 47 children from 3 to 66 months of age with challenge-confirmed milk allergy were followed for a median of 16 months (range 6–39 months). Overall, 38% of the children were able to tolerate milk by the

Table 37.2 Studies on the natural history of milk allergy.

Reference	*N*	Age at diagnosis	Duration of follow-up	Percent tolerant at completion of study: IgE-mediated (or immediate-type) reactions	Percent tolerant at completion of study: Non-IgE-mediated (or delayed-type) reactions
Dannaeus and Johansson [26]	47	14 days to 20 months	6 months to 4 years (mean 28 months)	29%	74%
Host and Halken [14]	39	0–12 months	Up to age 3 years	76%	100%
Hill [30]	47	3–66 months	6–39 months (mean 16 months)	40%	38%
Bishop et al. [29]	100	1–98 months (median 16 months)	5 years	67%	86%[a]
Hill et al. [30]	98	4–100 months (median 24 months)	6–73 months (mean 24 months)	22%	59%
James and Sampson [35]	29	3–14 years (median 3 years)	3 years	38%	NA
Saarinen et al. [31]	116	Mean 7 months	Up to 8.6 years	85%	100%
Skripak et al. [33]	807	1–209 months (median 13 months)	4–285 months (median 55 months)	19% at age 4, 42% at age 8, 79% at age 16	NA
Elizur et al. [32]	54	0–12 months	48–60 months	54%	NA

[a]Combines immediate and late reactors.

completion of the study. When the children were divided into groups based on having immediate, intermediate, or late milk reactions, tolerance occurred in 40%, 42%, and 25%, respectively. Milk-specific IgE, IgA, IgM, and IgG levels were measured and no specific immunologic changes were clearly associated with the development of milk tolerance.

In the second study from this group, a cohort of 100 children with challenge-confirmed milk allergy were followed for 5 years [29]. Overall, milk tolerance had occurred in 28% of patients by age 2, 56% by age 4, and 78% by age 6 years. When the children were again divided into groups based on having immediate, intermediate, or late reactions, tolerance had occurred by the completion of the study in 67%, 87%, and 83%, respectively. Adverse reactions to other foods were also common in this cohort, occurring to egg in 58%, soy in 47%, and peanut in 34%. Most children also developed one or more other atopic diseases, such that at the completion of the study 40% had asthma, 43% had allergic rhinitis, and 21% had eczema.

A final study from this group followed 98 children with milk allergy for a median of 2 years (range 6–72 months) [30]. In this study, the children were divided into two groups: 69 had IgE antibodies to milk with immediate-type reactions and 29 had delayed-type reactions. Over the period of follow-up, 15 of 69 (22%) with IgE-mediated disease developed tolerance, compared to 17 of the 29 (59%) with non-IgE-mediated reactions. For those children with IgE-mediated milk sensitivity, the development of tolerance was associated with lower milk-specific IgE levels at the time of diagnosis and at study completion, as well a significant reduction in their milk skin test reactivity. However, it is also important to note that 8 of the 15 who developed tolerance still had strong positive skin tests at that time.

In the largest prospective study to date, Saarinen et al. followed 118 children diagnosed with milk allergy from a birth cohort study of over 6000 children [31]. Eighty-six (73%) had IgE-mediated milk and of those 51% had become tolerant by age 2 years and 85% were tolerant at age 8.6 years. All children with IgE-negative CMA were tolerant by age 5 years. By age 8.6 years, children with IgE-positive CMA more frequently had asthma, rhinoconjunctivitis, atopic eczema, and sensitization to any allergen than control subjects. They concluded that IgE-mediated milk allergy often persists to school age and is a risk factor for other atopy, while non-IgE-mediated milk allergy is a benign infantile condition.

In a prospective cohort study from Israel, 54 infants with IgE-CMA were identified from a population of 13 019 children followed from birth [32]. Diagnosis of IgE-mediated CMA was based on history, skin prick tests, and oral food challenges when indicated. Allergic infants were followed for 48–60 months, with 31 children (57.4%) recovering from their CMA during the study period. Most infants (70.9%) recovered within the first 2 years. Risk factors for persistence included a reaction to <10 mL of milk on food challenge, larger skin test wheal size, and an age of ≤30 days at the time of first reaction.

In the largest overall study to date, our group retrospectively collected data on 807 patients with IgE-mediated milk allergy [33]. Patients were considered to have become tolerant if they passed a challenge, or experienced no reactions in the past 12 months and had a CM- IgE level, 3 kU_A/L. Using that definition, the rates of resolution were 19% at age 4, 42% by age 8, 64% by age 12, and 79% by age 16 years. Patients with persistent allergy had higher CM-IgE levels at all ages up to age 16 years. The highest CM-IgE for each patient, defined as "peak" CM-IgE, was found to be highly predictive of outcome. Of note, some patients developed tolerance during adolescence, indicating that follow-up and reevaluation of CMA patients is an important component of their care.

Several studies have focused specifically on the immunologic changes associated with the development of milk tolerance. From a group of 80 milk-allergic children, James and Sampson reported on a subset of 29 who were followed for a minimum of 3 years [35]. Evaluations included annual DBPCFCs, skin tests, and measurement of casein-specific and b-lactoglobulin-specific IgE, IgG, IgG1, and IgG4 antibody concentrations. All children had specific IgE to milk as well as positive skin tests and 80% had atopic dermatitis. The median age at the time of study entry was 3 years with a range from 1 month to 11 years. Of the 29 children, 11 (38%) developed tolerance at a median age of 7 years. In those who became tolerant to milk-specific IgE and IgE/IgG ratios to both milk proteins were lower initially and decreased significantly over time.

Three additional studies focused on antibody responses to milk proteins and the development of milk tolerance [36–38]. In the first study, IgE- and IgG-binding epitopes on a_{s1}-casein were identified using the sera of 24 milk-allergic children, and the patterns of epitope recognition were analyzed to determine if they might help predict the natural history of milk allergy. When comparing epitope recognition of patients with persistent milk allergy to younger children likely to outgrow their allergy, they found that two IgE-binding regions were recognized by all of the older children with persistent milk allergy but none of the younger children. In the second study, a similar analysis was performed of IgE- and IgG-binding epitopes on b- and k-casein in milk-allergic patients. Three IgE-binding regions on b-casein and six on k-casein were recognized by the majority of patients in the older age group but none of the younger patients. In the third study, the binding of IgE, IgG4, and IgA antibodies to sequential epitopes derived from five major milk proteins was measured with a peptide microarray-based immunoassay. They found that IgE epitope-binding patterns were stable over time in patients with persisting CMA, whereas binding decreased in patients who recovered early. Among patients who recovered early, the signal of IgG4 binding increased and that of IgE decreased over time. IgE and IgG4 binding to a panel of a_{s1}-, a_{s2}-, b-, and k-casein regions predicted outcome with significant accuracy. In addition to a more clear definition of the antibody responses to specific milk proteins/epitopes, these studies suggest that it may eventually be possible to develop clinical tests, in essence of epitope-specific IgE levels, that may help to identify children at risk for more persistent milk allergy.

A summary of studies on the natural history of milk allergy is presented in Table 37.2. As one examines this information, a somewhat confusing picture emerges. For example, in the study by Host and Halken [14], which in many ways is the best study on milk allergy yet performed, 76% of those with IgE-mediated milk allergy and 100% of those with non-IgE-mediated milk allergy were milk tolerant by the age of 3 years. These numbers are far higher than those presented in the other studies. The only numbers that approach those are from the study by Bishop et al. [29], although it took until age 6 for 78% of those children to become milk tolerant. The differences in these studies are almost certainly a result of selection biases. The study by Host and Halken was a population-based study that would therefore include all degrees of milk sensitivity, whereas the other studies included children who were under the care of an allergy specialist, indicating that they may have had a more severe form of milk allergy. For the primary care physician, it is therefore likely that the more optimistic numbers will be correct, while the allergist might expect a slower rate of loss of milk allergy in their patients over time, as well as a higher percentage of patients with persistent milk allergy.

A final issue relevant to the natural history of milk allergy relates to the recent findings that a large number of children with milk allergy can tolerate milk that has been extensively heated, sometimes only in small quantities but in others even in concentrated forms [39], [40]. This is presumed to relate to the fact that children who outgrow their milk allergy have milk-specific IgE antibodies primarily directed against conformational epitopes which are largely destroyed by high temperature. Nowak-Wegrzyn et al. challenged 100 children with milk allergy to baked milk and found that 68 tolerated extensively heated milk only, 23 reacted to heated milk, and 9 tolerated both heated and unheated milk [39]. Heated milk-reactive subjects had significantly larger skin prick test wheals and higher milk-specific and casein-specific IgE levels than other groups. At 3 months, subjects ingesting heated milk products had significantly smaller skin prick test wheals and higher casein-IgG4 compared with baseline. A subsequent study from the same group provided additional information on the immunologic changes associated with baked milk ingestion, as well its effects on natural history

[40]. They found that subjects who incorporated dietary baked milk developed significant increases in milk-specific IgG4 and were far more likely than the comparison group to become unheated milk tolerant.

Egg allergy

With regard to the natural history of egg allergy, Ford and Taylor followed 25 children from 7 months to 9 years of age (median 17 months) with challenge-confirmed egg allergy for 2–2.5 years [41]. Egg allergy resolved in 11 of 25 (44%) and persisted in the other 14. Skin tests were negative or diminished in size in those who lost their egg reactivity compared to those with ongoing reactivity. This is similar to the 36% of children in the Dannaeus study [21] who became egg tolerant, although they also reported that an additional 44% had become less sensitive over time. The largest prospective study of the natural history of egg allergy is from a Spanish cohort of 58 children, in which 50% of egg-allergic children developed tolerance by age 4–4.5 years [42].

In a retrospective review in 52 of 881 patients from a tertiary referral clinic, the rate of egg allergy resolution was slower than in the studies mentioned above [43]. Egg allergy resolution, defined as passing an egg challenge or having an egg IgE level <2 kU_A/L and no symptoms in 12 months, occurred in 11% of patients by age 4, 26% by age 6, 53% by age 10, and 82% by age 16. Risk factors for persistence of egg allergy were a high initial level of egg IgE, the presence of other atopic disease, and the presence of an allergy to another food.

As with milk, several recent studies have focused on differences in reactivity to extensively heated and less heated egg. Clark et al. conducted a longitudinal study assessing the rate of resolution to well-cooked egg, compared with uncooked egg in 95 children whose median age of allergy onset was 12 months [44]. Tolerance was gained twice as rapidly to well-cooked than uncooked egg (median 5.6 vs. 10.3 years), with nearly one-third tolerating well-cooked egg by age 3 and two-thirds by age 6.

Lemon-Mulé et al. reported baked egg challenges in 117 patients with a history of egg allergy and found that 64 tolerated heated egg, 23 tolerated regular egg, and 27 reacted to heated egg [45]. Heated egg-reactive subjects had larger skin test wheals and greater egg white-specific, ovalbumin-specific, and ovomucoid-specific IgE levels compared with heated egg- and egg-tolerant subjects. Continued ingestion of heated egg was associated with decreased skin test wheal diameters and ovalbumin-specific IgE levels and increased ovalbumin-specific and ovomucoid-specific IgG4 levels. A subsequent study from the same group found that egg-specific IgE to IgG4 ratios best predicted those patients who tolerated heated egg [46].

Peanut allergy

Until recently, the dogma had been that peanut allergy is rarely, if ever, outgrown and studies had in fact suggested that that was the case. For example, Bock followed 32 children, 1–14 years of age, with challenge-confirmed peanut allergy over a period of 2–14 years and found that 24 had had accidental peanut exposures/reactions and no patients appeared to outgrow their allergy [47].

Evidence that a subset of children with peanut allergy may indeed lose their sensitivity was first reported by Hourihane et al. [48]. They evaluated 230 children with a diagnosis of peanut allergy and performed oral challenges in 120. A total of 22 children between the ages of 2 and 9 years had a negative challenge, equaling 18% of those challenged or 9.8% of the total group. They found that a negative challenge was associated with a smaller skin test size and fewer allergies to other foods compared to those with persistent peanut allergy.

Spergel et al. retrospectively reviewed 293 patients with a diagnosis of peanut allergy [49]. All families were offered a peanut challenge to confirm their diagnosis and a total of 33 children between the ages of 18 months and 8 years with a convincing history of peanut allergy and a positive skin test were actually challenged. Of those, 14 passed their challenge and were felt to have resolved their peanut allergy. None of the five patients with a history of peanut anaphylaxis developed tolerance, compared to 9 of 17 with a history of urticaria and 4 of 10 with a history of atopic dermatitis. In addition, those developing tolerance had significantly smaller skin test responses than the 19 with a positive challenge.

Skolnick et al. performed a detailed evaluation of 223 children with a diagnosis of peanut allergy [50], including an oral peanut challenge in those who had not had a reaction in the past year and who had a peanut-specific IgE (PN-IgE) of 20 kU_A/L. As shown in Table 37.3, 97 children were not challenged because they were considered to still be peanut allergic based on either a history of a recent reaction or a PN-IgE level of 20 kU_A/L [51], and an additional 41 children were eligible to be challenged but declined. Of the 85 children who were challenged, 48 (21.5% of the total group) passed the challenge and were felt to have outgrown their peanut allergy. The PN-IgE level was the best predictor of a negative challenge, with 61% of those with a PN-IgE level of 5 kU_A/L and 67% with a level of 2 kU_A/L passing their challenge. The presence of other atopic diseases and the severity of initial peanut reactions did not predict the probability of losing peanut allergy, and even one patient who had had severe anaphylaxis with his initial reaction outgrew his allergy.

A study by Vander Leek et al. focused on children with persistent peanut allergy [52]. Eighty-five children with

Table 37.3 Characteristics of patients with persistent and resolved peanut allergy.

	Passed challenge (*N* = 48)	Failed challenge (*N* = 37)	Unable to be challenged (*N* = 97)	Refused challenge (*N* = 41)	Total (*N* = 223)
Age at diagnosis					
Range	8 months to 12 years	6 months to 4 years	2 months to 10 years	8 months to 15 years	2 months to 15 years
Median (years)	1.5	1.5	1.5	2	1.5
Current age (years)					
Range	4–17.5	4–13	4–20	4–16.5	4–20
Median	6	6.5	7	7	6.5
PN-IgE at diagnosis[a]					
Range	0.35–52.9	1.8–24.4	4.5–100	0.64–100	0.35–100
Median	2.2	2.91	100	6.27	19.8
Current PN-IgE[a]					
Range	0.35–20.4	0.35–18.2	16.8–100	0.35–16.9	0.35–100
Median	0.69	2.06	100	4.98	10.7

Source: From Reference 50.

[a]PN-IgE refers to peanut-specific IgE level in kU_A/L. A level of 0.35 is considered negative and any level over 100 is reported as 100.

peanut allergy were studied, including 55 who were followed for at least 5 years. Among those patients, 58% who had been followed for 5 years and 75% who had been followed for at least 10 years had had at least one reaction due to an accidental exposure. In addition, the majority of these reactions were more severe than initial reactions and 52% included potentially life-threatening symptoms. Severe reactions were associated with higher PN-IgE levels compared to those with purely cutaneous reactions. The only positive note from this study was that four children did outgrow their peanut allergy.

One final study by Neuman-Sunshine et al. examined 782 patients with persistent peanut allergy with a median duration of follow-up of 5.3 years [53]. The rate of accidental exposures was just 4.7%/year. Reaction severity did not change with repeated exposures. More severe reactions were associated with higher PN-IgE levels but not with age, sex, or asthma.

Peanut allergy is therefore likely to be lifelong for most but not all patients. Given the fact that a substantial minority of patients do appear to lose their sensitivity over time, it is appropriate to reevaluate children with peanut allergy on a regular basis. Those patients who have not had reactions in the past 1–2 years and who have a low PN-IgE level should be considered for an oral challenge in a supervised setting. Some patients may outgrow their peanut allergy into adulthood [54] but overall patients who are still peanut allergic by adolescence are unlikely to lose their allergy and regular retesting is not likely to be of value.

One additional issue in the natural history of peanut allergy relates to the potential for the recurrence of the allergy in some patients with resolved peanut allergy. Busse et al. first reported such recurrences and estimated a recurrence rate of 14% after 3 of their 21 patients had recurrences [55]. Each of these patients reported consuming peanut intermittently in small amounts after passing a food challenge to peanut, and then reacquired their allergy 1–2 years later. Next, Fleischer et al. surveyed 64 patients who had outgrown their peanut allergy to see whether patients ate peanut products since passing their challenge, what types of peanut containing foods they ate, and how frequently they ate them, and whether there were any allergic reactions to peanuts [56]. They found that although 97% had eaten peanut since passing their challenge, ongoing aversion to peanut is common, with 70% of patients eating peanut infrequently and in small amounts. Two of the 64 patients had suspicious allergic reactions to peanut.

Because of concerns that more patients might have had recurrences and did not know it because of their ongoing peanut avoidance, Fleischer et al. invited all patients from their center who had outgrown peanut allergy to undergo reevaluation, including questionnaires, skin tests, peanut-specific IgE levels, and DBPCFCs [57]. Of 68 patients, 47 continued to tolerate peanut, of which 34 ingested concentrated peanut products at least once per month and 13 ate peanut infrequently or in limited amounts but passed a DBPCFC. The status of 18 patients was indeterminate because they ate peanut infrequently or in limited amounts and declined to have a DBPCFC. The overall recurrence rate was 7.9 (95% CI 1.7–21.4). They concluded that children who outgrow peanut allergy are at risk for recurrence, and this risk is significantly higher for patients who continue to largely avoid peanut after resolution of their allergy. Based on these findings, they recommended that patients eat peanut frequently and carry epinephrine indefinitely until they have demonstrated ongoing peanut tolerance.

Tree nuts allergy

The study by Dannaeus [21] did include 26 patients with tree nut allergy, none of whom lost their sensitivity in a 2–5-year follow-up. Fleischer et al. evaluated 278 patients with tree nut allergy, defined as a history of reaction on ingestion and evidence of tree nut-specific IgE or positive tree nut-specific IgE level but no history of ingestion [58]. If all current tree nut-specific IgE levels were $<10\,kU_A/L$, DBPCFCs were offered. One hundred and one of the 278 (36%) had a history of acute reactions, 12 (12%) of whom had reactions to multiple tree nuts and 73 (63%) of whom had a history of moderate-to-severe reactions. Nine of 20 patients who had previously reacted to tree nuts passed challenges, so that 9 (8.9%; 95% CI 4–16) of 101 patients with a history of prior tree nut reactions outgrew their allergy. Fourteen of 19 who had never ingested tree nuts but had detectable tree nut-specific IgE levels passed challenges. One hundred and sixty-one did not meet the challenge criteria, and 78 met the criteria but declined challenges. Fifty-eight percent with tree nut-specific IgE levels of $5\,kU_A/L$ or less and 63% with tree nut IgE levels of $2\,kU_A/L$ or less passed challenges. They concluded that approximately 9% of patients outgrow tree nut allergy, including some who had prior severe reactions.

Other foods

A retrospective review of 133 patients with soy allergy was reported from tertiary referral clinic [59]. The median age at the initial visit was 1 year and the median duration of follow-up was 5 years. Kaplan–Meier analysis predicted resolution of soy allergy in 25% by age 4, 45% by age 6, and 69% by age 10. By age 6, tolerance to soy developed in 59% of children with a peak soy IgE level of $<5\ kU_A/L$, 53% with a peak soy IgE level of 5–9.9, 45% with a peak soy IgE level of 10–49.9, and18% with a peak soy IgE level of $>50\ kU_A/L$.

A similar retrospective study was also conducted on 103 patients with IgE-mediated wheat allergy which found resolution rates of 29% by age 4, 56% by age 8, and 65% by age 12 [60]. Higher wheat IgE levels were associated with poorer outcomes and the peak wheat IgE level recorded was a useful predictor of persistent allergy, although many children with even the highest levels of wheat IgE outgrew their allergy. The median age of resolution of wheat allergy was approximately 6.5 years in this population but in a significant minority of patients, wheat allergy persisted into adolescence.

As was noted above in a number of studies, adverse reactions to fruits, vegetables, and other cereal grains are typically very short lived [9, 10, 21]. While some children do have severe, IgE-mediated allergies to these foods that may persist over time, for most children they can be successfully reintroduced into the diet within a period of 6–12 months. Many of these may in fact represent intolerances or irritant reactions than true allergy as well.

On the contrary, although actual studies are limited, it has been appreciated that allergies to fish, shellfish, and seeds are usually not outgrown. The study by Dannaeus [21] did include 32 children with fish allergy, of whom 5 became tolerant. One additional study followed 11 patients with shrimp allergy over a 2-year period and found that there were no significant changes in allergen-specific antibody levels over that period of time [61]. The limited data available suggest that sesame allergy, similar to peanut and tree nut allergies, is more likely to persist, with reported rates of resolution ranging from 20% to 30% [62–64].

Food allergy in adults

Most study on the natural course of food allergy has logically involved children. The most common food sensitivities in adults include peanut, tree nuts, fish, and shellfish, all of which are most often lifelong. These allergies are most common in adulthood both because of their persistent nature and because of the fact that most shellfish allergy actually develops in adulthood.

One study focused on the natural history of food allergies in adults [65]. Twenty-three adults with allergies to a variety of foods underwent baseline DBPCFCs, in which clear reactions in 10 patients to a total of 13 foods were identified. They were then placed on strict dietary avoidance of the offending food for 1–2 years and rechallenged. Five (38%) of the 13 previously offending foods were well tolerated, including milk in two patients and wheat, egg, and tomato in one patient each. The two patients with nut allergy continued to react, as did two patients with milk allergy and one patient each with allergies to potato, garlic, and rice.

Another study examined adults with peanut allergy, including patients with an onset of peanut allergy in both early childhood and adulthood [54]. Of the 35 patients studied, 8 passed a DBPCFC to peanut, suggesting that at least select patients with peanut allergy should be monitored into adulthood for the possibility of resolution.

Follow-up of the food-allergic child

It is imperative that food-allergic children undergo regular follow-up. This is necessary to monitor growth and to reassess signs and symptoms of ongoing food allergy, adherence to the recommended avoidance diet, and objective measures of food allergy. Any reactions that have occurred need to be reviewed with particular attention to how the reaction might have been prevented and whether the treatment provided was appropriate.

All children with food allergy should also be reevaluated at regular intervals to determine if the allergy has been outgrown. This typically should be done annually, although for some food allergies a shorter or longer interval might be appropriate. For example, an infant with adverse reactions to fruits or vegetables might deserve reevaluation after 3–6 months whereas an older child who clearly has persistent peanut or tree nut allergy may no longer need repeat testing, although regular follow-up is still important to review avoidance procedures and treatment protocols. In some instances, exposures may have occurred with little or no reaction, suggesting that the allergy may have resolved and that the food might be reintroduced into the diet.

The reevaluation process may include skin testing, measurement of specific IgE levels, and/or oral food challenges, depending on the specific clinical scenario. It is very important to note, however, that a positive skin test or IgE level does not necessarily mean that the food allergy has not been outgrown, since these tests can remain positive even when the patient is no longer clinically sensitive. Quantitative IgE levels have increasingly become the test of choice to monitor food allergies over time and to help guide decisions about the timing of oral food challenges. In the end, a food challenge will usually be necessary to prove that an allergy has been outgrown. These must be performed with caution because severe reactions may at times occur even when the testing suggested that the food allergy had most likely been outgrown.

Until an allergy has been outgrown, it has traditionally been recommended that a strict avoidance diet be maintained. While this is essential to prevent reactions, the previous impression that strict avoidance increases the chance of outgrowing a food allergy, and may even hasten the process, has come under increasing question. In fact, there is very little data to support this notion [35, 60] and it is clear that some children rapidly outgrow their food allergies without strict avoidance, while others fail to lose their allergies even with the most stringent diet. There is now also increasing evidence to suggest that exposure to the food to which one is allergic may actually hasten the resolution of the allergy. This is particularly the case for milk and egg, for which it has been shown that extensive heating renders the allergens less potent—and completely tolerable—for a majority of milk- and egg-allergic individuals [39,40, 45,46, 66]. While comprehensive data are not available, studies to date do suggest that exposure to the baked forms of milk and egg are likely to hasten the resolution of the allergy, even to the uncooked food. Clear recommendations regarding the optimal introduction of baked milk and egg, and the need for strict avoidance of other foods, are not yet available, although many centers do now routinely challenge milk- and egg-allergic patients to baked products. If tolerated, this can vastly improve a patient's quality of life and may even lead to a quicker resolution of the allergy. However, this is not without risk and the entire process needs to be carefully monitored.

Conclusions

An understanding of the natural history and prevention of food hypersensitivity is extremely important to the management of food-allergic patients. Although the various studies on these topics are not completely consistent, there are trends in the data that provide several clear messages. First, food allergy is very common. Second, the vast majority of food allergy has its onset in the first 1–2 years of life. Third, most food allergy is outgrown, although there are notable exceptions to this generally positive outcome. Fourth, food allergy is often the first of the atopic diseases, with most children going on to develop respiratory allergies over time.

It is also important to stress the importance of making early, accurate diagnoses of childhood food allergy. Only this will allow for the initiation of the key elements necessary for the care of the food-allergic patient, including education about avoidance diets and the development of emergency care plans for the treatment of allergic reactions. Avoidance diets are complex and require detailed education, without which the child will be at risk for accidental reactions. In addition, measures that might help to prevent the development of additional food allergies, as well as inhalant allergies, should be initiated at the time of the initial diagnosis.

References

1. Boyce JA, Assa'ad A, Burks AW, et al. Guidelines for the diagnosis and management of food allergy in the United States: report of the NIAID Sponsored Expert Panel. *J Allergy Clin Immunol* 2010; 126:S1–S58.
2. Rona RJ, Keil T, Summers C, et al. The prevalence of food allergy: a meta-analysis. *J Allergy Clin Immunol* 2007; 120:638–646.
3. Zuidmeer L, Goldhahn K, Rona RJ, et al. The prevalence of plant food allergies: a systematic review. *J Allergy Clin Immunol* 2008; 121:1210–1218.e4.
4. Osborne NJ, Koplin JJ, Martin PE, et al. Prevalence of challenge-proven IgE-mediated food allergy using population-based sampling and predetermined challenge criteria in infants. *J Allergy Clin Immunol* 2011; 127:668–676.

5. Liu AH, Jaramillo R, Sicherer SH, et al. National prevalence and risk factors for food allergy and relationship to asthma: results from the National Health and Nutrition Examination Survey 2005–2006. *J Allergy Clin Immunol* 2010; 126:798–806.
6. Branum AM, Lukacs SL. Food allergy among children in the United States. *Pediatrics* 2009; 124:1549–1555.
7. Luccioli S, Ross M, Labiner-Wolfe J, Fein SB. Maternally reported food allergies and other food-related health problems in infants: characteristics and associated factors. *Pediatrics* 2008; 122(Suppl. 2):S105–S112.
8. Chafen JJ, Newberry SJ, Riedl MA, et al. Diagnosing and managing common food allergies: a systematic review. *J Am Med Assoc* 2010; 303:1848–1856.
9. Bock SA. Prospective appraisal of complaints of adverse reactions to foods in children during the first 3 years of life. *Pediatrics* 1987; 79:683–688.
10. Kajosaari M. Food allergy in Finnish children aged 1 to 6 years. *Acta Paediatr Scand* 1982; 71:815–819.
11. Eggesbo M, Halvorsen R, Tambs K, Botten G et al. Prevalence of parentally perceived adverse reactions to food in young children. *Pediatr Allergy Immunol* 1999; 10:122–132.
12. Eggesbo M, Botten G, Halvorsen R, Magnus P. The prevalence of CMA/CMPI in young children: the validity of parentally perceived reactions in a population-based study. *Allergy* 2001; 56:393–402.
13. Eggesbo M, Botten G, Halvorsen R, Magnus P. The prevalence of allergy to egg: a population-based study in young children. *Allergy* 2001; 56:403–411.
14. Host A, Halken S. A prospective study of cow milk allergy in Danish infants during the first 3 years of life. Clinical course in relation to clinical and immunological type of hypersensitivity reaction. *Allergy* 1990; 45:587–596.
15. Host A, Halken S, Jacobsen HP, et al. The natural course of cow's milk protein allergy/intolerance [abstract]. *J Allergy Clin Immunol* 1997; 99:S490.
16. Tariq SM, Stevens M, Matthews S, et al. Cohort study of peanut and tree nut sensitisation by the age of 4 years. *BMJ* 1996; 313:514–517.
17. Kulig M, Bergmann R, Klettke U, et al. Natural course of sensitization to food and inhalant allergens during the first 6 years of life. *J Allergy Clin Immunol* 1999; 103:1173–1179.
18. Nickel R, Kulig M, Forster J, et al. Sensitization to hen's egg at the age of 12 months is predictive for allergic sensitization to common indoor and outdoor allergens at the age of 3 years. *J Allergy Clin Immunol* 1997; 99:613–617.
19. Kulig M, Bergmann R, Niggermann B, et al. Prediction of sensitization to inhalant allergens in childhood: evaluating family history, atopic dermatitis and sensitization to food allergens. *Clin Exp Allergy* 1998; 28:1397–1403.
20. Bock SA. Natural history of severe reactions to foods in young children. *J Pediatr* 1985; 107:676–680.
21. Dannaeus A, Inganas M. A follow-up study of children with food allergy. Clinical course in relation to serum IgE- and IgG- antibody levels to milk, egg, and fish. *Clin Allergy* 1981; 11:533–539.
22. Sampson HA, Scanlon SM. Natural history of food hypersensitivity in children with atopic dermatitis. *J Pediatr* 1989; 115:23–27.
23. Sampson HA, McCaskill CC. Food hypersensitivity and atopic dermatitis: evaluation of 113 patients. *J Pediatr* 1985; 107:669–675.
24. Shek LP, Soderstrom L, Ahlstedt S, et al. Determination of food specific IgE levels over time can predict the development of tolerance in cow's milk and hen's egg allergy. *J Allergy Clin Immunol* 2004; 114:387–391.
25. Businco L, Benincori N, Cantani A, et al. Chronic diarrhea due to cow's milk allergy. A 4- to 10-year follow-up study. *Ann Allergy* 1985; 55:844–847.
26. Dannaeus A, Johansson SGO. A follow-up of infants with adverse reactions to cow's milk. *Acta Paediatr Scand* 1979; 68:377–382.
27. Hill DJ, Firer MA, Ball G, Hosking CS. Recovery from milk allergy in early childhood: antibody studies. *J Pediatr* 1989; 114:761–766.
28. Hill DJ, Firer MA, Shelton MJ, Hosking CS. Manifestations of milk allergy in infancy: clinical and immunologic findings. *J Pediatr* 1986; 109:270–276.
29. Bishop JM, Hill DJ, Hosking CS. Natural history of cow milk allergy: clinical outcome. *J Pediatr* 1990; 116:862–867.
30. Hill DJ, Firer MA, Ball G, Hosking CS. Natural history of cows' milk allergy in children: immunological outcome over 2 years. *Clin Exp Allergy* 1993; 23:124–131.
31. Saarinen KM, Pelkonen AS, Makela MJ, Savilahti E. Clinical course and prognosis of cow's milk allergy are dependent on milk-specific IgE status. *J Allergy Clin Immunol* 2005; 116:869–875.
32. Elizur A, Rajuan N, Goldberg MR, et al. Natural course and risk factors for persistence of IgE-mediated cow's milk allergy. *J Pediatr* 2012; 161:482–487.
33. Skripak J, Matsui EC, Mudd K, Wood RA. The natural history IgE-mediated cow's milk allergy. *J Allergy Clin Immunol* 2007; 120:1172–1177.
34. Host A, Jacobsen HP, Halken S, Holmenlund D. The natural history of cow's milk protein allergy/intolerance. *Eur J Clin Nutr* 1995; 49:S13–S18.
35. James JM, Sampson HA. Immunologic changes associated with the development of tolerance in children with cow milk allergy. *J Pediatr* 1992; 121:371–377.
36. Chatchatee P, Jarvinen K-M, Bardina L, et al. Identification of IgE- and IgG-binding epitopes on a_{s1}-casein: differences in patients with persistent and transient cow's milk allergy. *J Allergy Clin Immunol* 2001; 107:379–383.
37. Chatchatee P, Jarvinen K-M, Bardina L, et al. Identification of IgE-and IgG-binding epitopes on b- and k-casein in cow's milk allergic patients. *Clin Exp Allergy* 2001; 31:1256–1262.
38. Savilahti EM, Rantanen V, Lin JS, et al. Early recovery from cow's milk allergy is associated with decreasing IgE and increasing IgG4 binding to cow's milk epitopes. *J Allergy Clin Immunol* 2010; 125:1315–1321.
39. Nowak-Wegrzyn A, Bloom KA, Sicherer SH, et al. Tolerance to extensively heated milk in children with cow's milk allergy. *J Allergy Clin Immunol* 2008; 122:342–347.
40. Kim JS, Nowak-Węgrzyn A, Sicherer SH, et al. Dietary baked milk accelerates the resolution of cow's milk allergy in children. *J Allergy Clin Immunol* 2011; 128:125–131.

41. Ford RP, Taylor B. Natural history of egg hypersensitivity. *Arch Dis Child* 1982; 57:649–652.
42. Boyano-Martínez T, García-Ara C, Díaz-Pena JM, Martín-Esteban M. Prediction of tolerance on the basis of quantification of egg white-specific IgE antibodies in children with egg allergy. *J Allergy Clin Immunol* 2002; 110:304–309.
43. Savage JH, Matsui EC, Skripak JM, Wood RA. The natural history of egg allergy. *J Allergy Clin Immunol* 2007; 120:1413–1417.
44. Clark A, Islam S, King Y, et al. A longitudinal study of resolution of allergy to well-cooked and uncooked egg. *Clin Exp Allergy* 2011; 41:706–712.
45. Lemon-Mulé H, Sampson HA, Sicherer SH, Shreffler WG, Noone S, Nowak-Wegrzyn A. Immunologic changes in children with egg allergy ingesting extensively heated egg. *J Allergy Clin Immunol* 2008; 122:977–983.
46. Caubet JC, Bencharitiwong R, Moshier E, et al. Significance of ovomucoid- and ovalbumin-specific IgE/IgG(4) ratios in egg allergy. *J Allergy Clin Immunol* 2012; 129:739–747.
47. Bock SA, Atkins FM. The natural history of peanut allergy. *J Allergy Clin Immunol* 1989; 83:900–904.
48. Hourihane JO, Roberts SA, Warner JO. Resolution of peanut allergy: case-control study. *BMJ* 1998; 316:1271–1275.
49. Spergel JM, Beausoleil JL, Pawlowski NA. Resolution of childhood peanut allergy. *Ann Allergy Asthma Immunol* 2000; 85:473–476.
50. Skolnick HS, Conover-Walker MK, Barnes-Koerner C, et al. The natural history of peanut allergy. *J Allergy Clin Immunol* 2001; 107:367–374.
51. Sampson HA, Ho DG. Relationship between food specific IgE concentrations and the risk of positive food challenges in children and adolescent. *J Allergy Clin Immunol* 1997; 100:444–451.
52. Vander Leek TK, Liu AH, Stefanski K, et al. The natural history of peanut allergy in young children and its association with serum peanut-specific IgE. *J Pediatr* 2000; 137:749–755.
53. Neuman-Sunshine DL, Eckman JA, Keet CA, et al. Natural history of persistent peanut allergy. *Ann Allergy Asthma Immunol* 2012; 108:326–331.
54. Savage JH, Limb SL, Brereton NH, Wood RA. The natural history of peanut allergy: extending our knowledge beyond childhood. *J Allergy Clin Immunol* 2007; 120:717–719.
55. Busse PJ, Nowak-Wegrzyn AH, Noone SA, et al. Recurrent peanut allergy. *N Engl J Med* 2002; 347:1535–1536.
56. Fleischer DM, Conover-Walker MK, Christie L, et al. The natural progression of peanut allergy: resolution and the risk of recurrence. *J Allergy Clin Immunol* 2003; 112:183–189.
57. Fleischer DM, Conover-Walker MK, Matsui EC, Wood RA. Peanut allergy: recurrence and its management. *J Allergy Clin Immunol* 2004; 114:1195–1201.
58. Fleischer DM, Conover-Walker MK, Matsui EC, Wood RA. The natural history of tree nut allergy. *J Allergy Clin Immunol* 2005; 116:1087–1093.
59. Savage JH, Kaeding AJ, Matsui EC, Wood RA. The natural history of soy allergy. *J Allergy Clin Immunol* 2010; 125:683–686.
60. Keet CA, Matsui EC, Dhillon G, et al. The natural history of wheat allergy. *Ann Allergy Asthma Immunol* 2009; 102:410–415.
61. Daul CB, Morgan JE, Lehrer SB. The natural history of shrimp-specific immunity. *J Allergy Clin Immunol* 1990; 86:88–93.
62. Cohen A, Goldberg M, Levy B, et al. Sesame food allergy and sensitization in children: the natural history and long-term follow-up. *Pediatr Allergy Immunol* 2007; 18:217–223.
63. Aaronov D, Tasher D, Levine A, et al. Natural history of food allergy in infants and children in Israel. *Ann Allergy Asthma Immunol* 2008; 101:637–640.
64. Agne PS, Bidat E, Agne PS, et al. Sesame seed allergy in children. *Eur Ann Allergy Clin Immunol* 2004; 36:300–305.
65. Pastorello EA, Stocchi L, Pravettoni V, et al. Role of elimination diet in adults with food allergy. *J Allergy Clin Immunol* 1989; 84:475–483.
66. Huang F, Nowak-Węgrzyn A. Extensively heated milk and egg as oral immunotherapy. *Curr Opin Allergy Clin Immunol* 2012; 12:283–292.

38 Prevention of Food Allergy

Gideon Lack & George Du Toit

Department of Paediatric Allergy, King's College London Clinical Lead for Allergy Service Guy's and St Thomas' NHS Foundation Trust St Thomas' Hospital London, UK

Key Concepts

- Despite a trend towards delayed weaning, food allergies have increased in the past decades.
- Exclusive breast-feeding for the first three months of life may have a protective effect on allergy outcomes, but not, specifically food allergies.
- There is no consistent evidence to support exclusive breast-feeding beyond three months of age as a means to prevent food allergy or atopic disease.
- Hydrolyzed formulae in high-risk infants may reduce symptoms of eczema but not food allergy.
- There is a need for randomized controlled studies to test novel prevention strategies such as oral tolerance induction.

Introduction

The prevalence of IgE-mediated food allergy (FA) appears to have increased over the past two decades with approximately 3–6% of children in the developed world being affected [1, 2]. The increase in FA is best described for peanut allergy (PA) [3–5]. For example, in the United Kingdom three sequential studies (cohorts born 1989–2000) demonstrate an increase in the prevalence of PA from 0.6% to 1.8% over the last 10 years [4]. There are similar findings in the United States where Sicherer et al. looked at changes in the prevalence of PA and tree nut allergy. They compared three large telephone surveys enquiring about PA and tree nut allergy in 5300 households. These cross-sectional surveys were conducted in 1997, 2002, and 2008. They showed a significant increase in PA and tree nut allergy, particularly in children less than 18 years of age. The prevalence of PA increased from 0.4% in 1997 to 0.8% in 2002 and 1.4% in 2008 ($p <$ 0.0008). Although these studies rely on self-report rather than objective testing, the same methodology was used for all three surveys. The increase reported is similar to that seen in other studies using objective measures, such as skin testing [5, 6]. It should be noted that knowledge about the epidemiology of FA is limited and inaccurate as most studies documenting the prevalence of peanut, milk, and egg allergies are performed in Western countries; there are no published international surveys defining FA on a broader scale with the consequence that our knowledge of FA in the developing world is limited and based mainly on case series. Nonetheless, FA is now considered a public health concern as the condition is associated with significant morbidity and occasional mortality. Known risk factors for the development of allergy include family history, male sex (at least in childhood), ethnicity, and genetic polymorphisms. While genetic factors are clearly important in the development of FA, the increase in FA has occurred over a short period of time and is therefore unlikely to be due to germ line genetic changes alone. It seems plausible therefore that one or more environmental exposures may, through epigenetic changes, result in the interruption of the "default immunologic state" of tolerance to foods. Strategies are therefore required for the prevention of FA: primary prevention strategies seek to prevent the onset of IgE-sensitization; secondary prevention seeks to interrupt the development of FA in IgE-sensitized children; and tertiary prevention seeks to reduce the expression of "end organ" allergic disease in children with established FA.

This chapter does not seek to replicate the many reviews in this field. Rather it aims to highlight the important conclusions derived from these reviews and focuses on novel strategies that help advance contemporaneous thinking in this field.

Food Allergy: Adverse Reactions to Foods and Food Additives, Fifth Edition. Edited by Dean D Metcalfe, Hugh A Sampson, Ronald A Simon and Gideon Lack.

Methodological challenges

In this section we examine the methodological aspects that complicate the interpretation of the many studies performed in the field of allergy prevention (summarized in Table 38.1).

Numerous studies have assessed different strategies for the prevention of FA. Despite this extensive body of work, findings have generally proved ineffective. The fact that no single intervention or combination of interventions is able to repeatedly demonstrate a strong protective effect against FA reflects either on the interventions themselves or, alternatively, the study methods used to measure them.

A major limitation of many FA prevention studies lies in the study design, with few nutritional studies being randomized due to the necessary ethical restrictions that surround randomization of infants to anything but breast milk.

A second major limitation of studies in this field is the phenotypic description of FA, particularly for young children. Few studies make use of food challenge procedures. While the determination of tolerance is adequately determined by an open food challenge, the gold standard for the determination of FA is the Double-Blind Placebo-Controlled Food Challenge (DBPCFC). Such challenges are laborious and not without risk. In addition, entry-level oral challenges cannot be performed in those children assigned to the avoidance arm of food intervention studies. A certain diagnosis of FA in infants at the time of enrolment or exit from studies is therefore seldom certain. This limitation is particularly problematic for the diagnosis of cow's milk allergy (CMA), which is a common and frequently studied childhood allergy associated with both immediate-onset IgE-mediated and delayed-onset non-IgE-mediated reactions.

The most frequently used surrogate marker for the determination of FA is the outcome of IgE sensitization (determined by skin prick test (SPT) results and/or specific-IgE determination). Although IgE-mediated FA requires the state of "sensitization," the majority of children who are sensitized to foods are not food allergic. Methodological differences in determining sensitization can lead to markedly different study outcomes. For example, in the Australian Health Nuts study [7], 9% of a birth cohort of 2848 1-year-old infants had challenge-proved IgE-mediated egg allergy. However, this high prevalence of egg allergy arises due to the use of raw egg-white extract to perform both SPTs and oral challenges. Unsurprisingly, they then found that only 19.7% of children with raw egg-white allergy reacted during a baked egg challenge. This results in a baked egg prevalence of 2.2%, which is similar to other epidemiologic surveys considering the prevalence of baked egg allergy.

Eczema is also a commonly used surrogate for FA. Whereas eczema has been shown to be a risk factor for the development of FA, not all food allergic children have eczema [8, 9]. Hence, although eczema is strongly associated with FA, the two are not synonymous, as evidenced by studies that demonstrate an improvement in eczema but not FA. In addition, most studies that report an effect on eczema do not assess the severity of the eczema. Mild eczema has been shown to run a transient course when compared with moderate-to-severe eczema [10]. It may therefore be that studies that claim to prevent eczema are actually treating eczema (i.e., tertiary prevention) in children who entered the study with FA. Alternatively, study effects may be limited to the transient disease of mild eczema. Similar limitations apply to the diagnosis of asthma and rhinoconjunctivitis.

Additional limitations of the surrogate markers used for the diagnosis of FA include inconsistencies in nomenclature and difficulties in accurately diagnosing these conditions in infants and young children. For example, different terms are used to describe the "eczematous" condition. This results not only in disease misclassification, but may describe different immunological conditions. Indeed, the role of atopic sensitization in childhood eczema remains obscure as it is neither a prerequisite nor a uniform cause of the disease.

Nutritional studies are prone to selection bias and reverse causality. Such bias may arise when atopic families—if aware of public health recommendations, or if early-onset eczema is noted, are increasingly motivated to alter dietary practices, either in their own diet, or in the diet of their infants. The effects of reverse causality are highlighted in various studies and for different allergic outcomes. For example, in the Avon Longitudinal Study of Parents and Children (ALSPAC), a history of an allergic reaction to peanut was associated with prolonged breast-feeding [8]. However, when adjusted for infantile eczema by regression analysis, there was no effect of breast-feeding on the development of PA.

Childhood FAs are dynamic with the general trend being for resolution of many, but not all, during the first decade of life. This is also true for mild eczema and select asthma phenotypes. Study planning needs to take these natural histories into account prior to assessing for long-term study outcomes.

Observational studies (as most studies in this field are) are vulnerable to bias from both unmeasured and unknown sources. In an ideal world, study hypothesis would therefore only be assessed by RDBPC studies. The inclusion of a placebo in nutritional studies is not always practical or safe. Randomized controlled studies in infants testing the early or delayed introduction of a food or foods, cannot practically incorporate a placebo in the control group. It is also difficult (e.g., shrimp) or

Table 38.1 Methodological issues known to complicate the interpretation of studies aimed at the prevention of food allergy.

Issue	Problem	Recommended approach
Study design	The majority of studies in this field are observational studies.	RCTs represent the gold standard of clinical medicine, especially when findings are replicated and shown to be consistent in further meta-analyses. Positive RCT results are however easier to interpret than negative studies. Given that the pathogenesis of FA is likely to be multifactorial we need to differentiate between necessary and sufficient causality.
Reverse causality	Early signs of suspected allergic disease (such as eczema) will result in altered feeding patterns.	If possible, trials should adopt RDBPC methodologies for food challenging.
Randomization	There are necessary ethical restraints that limit randomization to dietary interventions. This is especially so for studies involving infant milks.	Breast-feeding should always be encouraged. Studies that wish to assess the effect of complementary feeds should randomize within the breast-fed group.
Blinding of dietary interventions	Blinding of specific dietary interventions may not be possible due to safety concerns or practical limitations, for example, breast-feeding.	It may not always be possible to have a placebo arm to infant nutritional studies.
Determination of food allergy	Few studies make use of the oral food challenges (OFC) for the diagnosis of FA. The diagnosis of FA is therefore often inadequate both at study entry and exit. Too many studies rely exclusively on the presence of specific-IgE (as determined by skin prick testing and/or specific-IgE).	Aim to perform oral challenges in all participants. For children who do not undergo OFC's, *a priori* diagnostic algorithms are required that will then reach a diagnosis through the combination of history, examination, skin prick testing, and specific-IgE determination.
Surrogate markers	Eczema, rhinitis, and asthma are often used as surrogate markers of FA.	As above.
Natural history of food allergy	Tolerance is anticipated for many, but not all, childhood food allergies.	Account for natural remission rate of a disease before assessing for a study effect.
Nomenclature	There is insufficient consensus within the allergy community with respect to the terminology of common allergic conditions.	Consensus with respect to the allergy nomenclature of common allergic disorders will greatly facilitate research in this field.
Allergy diagnosis	There is little consensus within the allergy community with respect to the ideal diagnostic criteria to be used for common allergic conditions, particularly, in early childhood. For example, many studies refer to generic terms such as "allergy" or "atopy." Definitions for each of these conditions are open to great variability.	Consensus with respect to the diagnosis of common allergic disorders is desperately required between specialist allergy organizations.
Determination of diet	The determination of food consumption is usually by retrospective Food Frequency Questionnaire (FFQ). FFQs are prone to many forms of bias.	Use should be made of prospective food diaries that have been validated for context, language, and consistency.
Dietary variables and measurement thereof	Few dietary analyses consider all variables; these include age of introduction, quantity ingested (individual and cumulative), frequency of exposure, variability of allergens, allergen processing, and concomitant breast-feeding at time of commencing complementary feeds.	Well-designed validated tools are required in order to accurately record all dietary variables.
Definitions: weaning	Use of the term "weaning" is not consistent and is usually limited to the introduction of solid foods only.	Adopt the term "complementary feeding" which incorporates any nutrient-containing food or liquid other than breast milk given to young children during the period of complementary feeding.
High-risk markers	Many studies are aimed at high-risk atopic populations. However, such populations are difficult to define.	Studies should include entire study populations (i.e., both low- and high-risk). At-risk populations should be defined *a priori*. Better high-risk markers are required.
Separation of specific effects when interventions are combined	Multiple interventions are often studied at different time points. For example, probiotic administration may be to mother (during pregnancy and/or breast-feeding) and/or newborn infant. This makes it difficult to determine the specific effect of each intervention at each time point.	Preliminary proof-of-concept studies need to separate the effects of each intervention.
Introduction of complementary feeds is associated with multiple variables	The early cessation of breast-feeding and introduction of complementary feeds has been associated with cultural, socioeconomic factors as well as specific factors such as maternal age, formula feeding, and maternal smoking.	Regression analysis should control for as many relevant confounders as possible, especially, in observational studies. This highlights the need for randomized controlled trials.
Monitoring adherence	Monitoring of adherence to interventions, particularly dietary interventions, is difficult.	Better tools for monitoring dietary adherence are required.

impossible (e.g., breast-feeding) to blind certain nutritional interventions.

Above all, study interventions should be safe for both mother and child. Safety concerns have nonetheless arisen in select studies. For example, dietary interventions have been noted to compromise fetal and maternal wellbeing [11] and studies using probiotics have shown increased rates of sensitization and allergic outcomes in separate studies [12, 13].

Prevention studies are often aimed at high-risk families. The high-risk population is however difficult to define. For example, ~10% of children without an allergic first-degree relative develop allergic disease, compared with 20–30% with single allergic heredity (parent or sibling) and 40–50% with double allergic heredity [14]. In addition, the definition of the term "atopy" is inconsistent.

Many interventions are introduced to both mother and child. This complicates the understanding of specific study effects as it is unclear whether the immunological effects were achieved pre- or postnatally or whether effects should be attributed to a single or multiple factors.

The determination of dietary intake is usually performed by Food Frequency Questionnaires (FFQs). FFQs are known to be subject to substantial forms of bias. FFQs do not always assess all relevant dietary variables, such as age of introduction, recurrence of exposure, quantity (single and cumulative) of exposure, variability of allergens consumed, and allergen processing. In addition, it is often difficult to disguise those questions which relate to the specific food/s of interest. Prospective food diaries are cumbersome as they demand detailed information and effort by parents.

It is difficult to measure food allergen exposures which occur via routes other than the oral route, for example, through an abraded skin barrier. For example, the nursing mother who ingests peanut butter is also likely to transfer this allergen to the infant through kiss and touch contact [15, 16]. In addition, it is often the nursing mother who determines consumption patterns within the household, which further increases (or decreases) the opportunity for environmental food allergen exposure to foods that the mother likes (or dislikes). A different problem arises if the intervention is one of avoidance as the elimination of one or more foods from the diet is likely to impact the diet. Such changes may be anticipated and therefore measured, or unknown and missed.

Onset of sensitization and food allergy

It remains unclear as to when prevention strategies should be implemented. It is therefore important to determine whether sensitization occurs *in utero*. Prerequisites for the development of FA (particularly in genetically susceptible individuals) are thought to include allergen exposure, uptake, recognition, and processing. The fact that *in utero* sensitization to foods is possible is suggested by the early clinical presentation of IgE-mediated FAs. This is usually apparent within the first year of life. For example, in a large population-based sample of 12-month-old infants in Australia, using predetermined food challenge criteria, to measure outcomes, high rates of sensitization to foods were found; for example, any peanut sensitization, 8.9% (95% CI, 7.9–10.0); raw egg white, 16.5% (95% CI, 15.1–17.9); sesame, 2.5% (95% CI, 2.0–3.1); cow's milk, 5.6% (95% CI, 3.2–8.0); and shellfish, 0.9% (95% CI, 0.6–1.5). The prevalence of challenge-proven PA was 3.0% (95% CI, 2.4–3.8); raw egg allergy, 8.9% (95% CI, 7.8–10.0); and sesame allergy, 0.8% (95% CI, 0.5–1.1) [17]. Likewise, non-IgE-mediated food-induced immunological reactions such as cow's milk protein induced colitis may also present in infancy [18].

There is some data that food and aeroallergens can be transmitted via the placenta [19]. However, two large birth cohort studies were unable to demonstrate measurable food specific-IgE in cord blood, even in those children who subsequently developed FAs or sensitization [8, 20].

Summary. Although possible on theoretical grounds, there is no evidence to support the hypothesis that sensitization and allergy to foods commence *in utero*.

Maternal diet (during pregnancy and/or breast-feeding) and the prevention of food allergy

In this section, we examine the effect of maternal diet during pregnancy and/or lactation on the development of FA.

There are three studies that assess the effects (with respect to allergy prevention) of maternal dietary avoidance of one or more common food allergens during pregnancy [21–23]. In a Cochrane review, Kramer et al. [24], assessed the evidence for allergy prevention through prescribing an antigen avoidance diet during lactation. They included four trials involving 334 women. Their findings suggested a protective effect of maternal antigen avoidance on the incidence of atopic eczema during the child's first 12–18 months of life. There was no effect on asthma or rhinitis. They however also noted the methodological challenges in three of the trials and argued for caution in applying these results. Most importantly, one trial reported that a restricted diet (egg and CMP) during pregnancy was associated with both maternal and fetal nutritional compromise.

In a recent cross-sectional study [25] the relevant route of peanut exposure in the development of allergy was evaluated. Maternal peanut consumption during pregnancy, breast-feeding, and the first year of life was captured by using a questionnaire; additionally, peanut consumption among all household members was quantified. The median weekly household peanut consumption in the patients with PA was significantly increased (18.8 g, n = 5133) compared with that seen in control subjects without allergy (6.9 g, n = 5150) and high-risk control subjects (1.9 g, $n = 5160$, $p < 0.0001$). A dose–response relationship was observed between environmental (non-oral) peanut exposure and the development of PA. Although maternal peanut consumption during pregnancy was increased in the mothers of peanut allergic children, this relationship was no longer significant after adjustment for household exposure. These findings suggest that high levels of environmental exposure to peanut during infancy can promote sensitization, whereas low levels appear protective in atopic children. Early oral exposure to peanut in infants with high environmental peanut exposure might have had a protective effect against the development of PA. This supports the hypothesis that peanut sensitization occurs as a result of environmental exposure. This contrasts with a study by Sicherer et al. [26] based on the National Institutes of Health Consortium Food Allergy Research study that enrolled 503 high-risk atopic infants. In this study, frequent peanut consumption in pregnancy was associated with specific-IgE levels to peanut of greater than 5 kU/L (Odd Ratio (OR), 2.9; 95% CI, 1.7–4.9). Although this study reports that peanut present in the home at the time of assessment did not influence sensitization to peanut, the presence of peanut was recorded as a dichotomous variable, and thus detailed household consumption and environmental exposure were not quantifiable.

Until recently, the American Academy of Pediatrics recommended that infants whose family history placed them at an increased risk of atopy should avoid peanuts during the first three birthdays and common food allergens until the first (milk), second (egg), or third (tree nuts and fish) birthdays [27]. According to these recommendations, mothers should avoid peanuts during pregnancy and breast-feeding, and additional allergens during lactation. In the United Kingdom, similar recommendations were in place with respect to peanut avoidance [28]. However, more recently, these recommendations were withdrawn by the American Academy of Pediatrics [29]. The more recent position is that "current evidence does not support a major role for maternal dietary restrictions during pregnancy or lactation . . . There is also little evidence that delaying timing of the introduction of complementary foods beyond 4–6 months of age prevents the occurrence of atopic disease." Similarly, the UK recommendations on dietary exclusion were rescinded in 2008 [30].

There are no studies that assess effects of modifying maternal diet during lactation only. There are however studies that modify the maternal diet during pregnancy or both pregnancy and lactation; these have not shown a protective role against infant FA through maternal dietary avoidance of cow's milk, egg, and fish during either pregnancy and/or breast-feeding. In addition, the ALSPAC study showed no effect of maternal peanut consumption in pregnancy or lactation on the development of immunologic or clinical reaction to peanuts on follow-up at 4–6 years of age [8].

Breast milk contains low concentrations of dietary proteins, which are present in maternal serum. Indeed, β-lactoglobulin is found in the breast milk of 95% of mothers consuming cow's milk during lactation. Whether at-risk infants are protected by the many beneficial immunological properties of breast milk or put at risk by this low dose allergen exposure is an ongoing debate. There are studies that modify the maternal diet during both pregnancy and lactation. Neither the study by Hattevig et al. [10] nor the study by Herman et al. [31] demonstrates a protective role against infant FA through maternal dietary avoidance of cow's milk, egg, and fish during either pregnancy or both pregnancy and lactation. The study by Herman et al. did however note effects for eczema.

Summary. Manipulation of the maternal diet during pregnancy and/or breast-feeding has not consistently been shown to exert protective effects on the development of allergy; however preventative effects are noted for eczema. Such strategies carry the risk of nutritional compromise for both mother and child.

Complementary infant feeding and the prevention of food allergy

In this section we examine the effect of complementary feeding on the development of FA.

The WHO now recommends that the term "weaning" be replaced by the term "complementary feeding" which incorporates any nutrient-containing food or liquid other than breast milk. Most studies in this field consider weaning to be the introduction of solid foods only. However, the biophysical properties of allergens are complex and there is no reason to believe that the allergenic potential of liquid feeds is different from that of solid or semisolid feeds. For example, both cow's milk and hen's egg allergy are common childhood allergies despite being ingested as liquid and solid, respectively. An infant who is breast-fed while receiving cow's milk formula supplementation is no more or less weaned than a breast-fed infant who is fed rice cereal mixed with expressed breast milk. It is therefore arbitrary to restrict the usage of the term "weaning" to solids and valuable lessons may become apparent when including studies which assess all "complementary foods" irrespective of the food "medium."

Breast milk provides a rich and favorable source of immune-regulating substances and possesses numerous other qualities that have the capability of directly influencing allergic disease expression. For example, breast milk regulates food antigen absorption and processing which may delay or prevent the development of FA. Breast milk has also been shown to decrease lower respiratory tract infections (LRTIs) in the first year of life and LRTIs are known risk factors for the development of asthma. That the rates of breast-feeding, worldwide, is initiated in only 60–80% of newborns and exclusive breast-feeding rates remain below WHO targets.

There are numerous health care specialist allergy organizations that offer advice with respect to infant feeding in at-risk infants [32–37]. While there is consensus that breast milk remains unchallenged as the milk of choice for all infants, advice with respect to the duration of exclusive breast-feeding, and the avoidance of common food allergens differs between organizations.

Studies that support a protective effect of breast-feeding over cow's milk formulae date back to the 1930s when Grulee and Sanford demonstrated a protective effect of breast-feeding on the development of eczema in the first 12–48 months of life in a large ($n \approx 20\,000$) observational study [38]. Not all of the observational studies that followed supported these early findings. In a 2007 review by the Pediatric Section of the European Academy of Allergy and Clinical Immunology, Muraro et al. [39] suggested an overall protective effect (for at-risk children) of exclusive breast-feeding during the first 3 months of life on atopic eczema and asthma, but not childhood allergic rhinitis.

Brew et al. [40] recently combined data from two cohorts, the Childhood Asthma Prevention Study (CAPS) from Australia and the Barn Allergi Miljo Stockholm cohort from Sweden, that had reported different findings on the association between breast-feeding and asthma. For this analysis, the definitions for breast-feeding, asthma, and allergy were harmonized. Subjects were included if they had at least one parent with wheeze or asthma and had a gestational age of more than 36 weeks (combined $n = 882$). Breast-feeding had no effect on the prevalence of sensitization to inhaled allergens in this cohort with a family history of asthma, but was a risk factor for sensitization to cow's milk, peanuts, and eggs in the CAPS cohort at 4 or 5 years and in the combined cohort at 8 years. There was no evidence to support the existence of reverse causality in either cohort.

While exclusive breast-feeding for 3 months may protect against the development of allergy taken in the context of the numerous studies done in this field, the consensus however is that prolonged exclusive breast-feeding beyond 3 months of age has not been shown to consistently protect against the development of FA or atopy. Kramer et al. [41] performed a WHO commissioned systematic review of the available evidence concerning the effects of exclusive breast-feeding for 6 months vs. exclusive breast-feeding for 3–4 months followed by mixed breast-feeding (complementary liquid or solid foods with continued breast-feeding) to 6 months, on eczema, asthma, and other atopic outcomes. This extensive review covers 20 independent, observational studies. They were unable to establish evidence for a significant reduction in the risk of atopic eczema, asthma, or other atopic outcomes amongst those infants who were exclusively breast-fed for 6 months compared with those exclusively breast-fed for 3–4 months followed by mixed feeding.

It is therefore surprising that the WHO recommendations use the justification of reduction in atopy to support exclusive breast-feeding for the first 6 month of the infant's life. While there are other beneficial health effects of prolonged exclusive breast-feeding, prevention of allergy does not provide a justification.

There are only two randomized studies looking at the introduction of CMP formula against exclusive breast-feeding on the development of FA and atopy. Lucas et al. [42] in a large ($n = 777$) randomized interventional study of premature infants, compared the effects of human breast milk, standard preterm formula, and nutrient-enriched preterm formula. Interestingly, at 18 months after term there was no overall difference in the incidence of food-allergic reactions between dietary groups, although a subgroup effect was noted for the group of infants with a family history of atopy. Similarly, in a large ($n = 1693$) randomized intervention study of term infants, De Jong et al. [43] found that early (first 3 days of life) high-dose exposure to CMP (as frequently occurs in nurseries) was not associated with an increase in allergic disease or symptoms. In addition, no increase in sensitization or allergy to CMP was found between the groups up to 5 years of age.

There are indeed some observational studies that demonstrate an increased risk in the development of allergic disorders in breast-fed infants. In a large ($n = 1037$ children) observational study, Sears et al. [44] followed up children until 21 years of age. They found that breast-feeding (for at least 4 weeks) did not protect against childhood atopy and asthma. Indeed, significantly more breast-fed children were atopic to common aeroallergens at the age of 13 than non-breast-fed children. Breast-feeding also increased the likelihood of asthma at the ages of 9 and 21 years. Findings were similar when breast-feeding was considered over longer periods (8–12 weeks). Exclusive breast-feeding did not offer any protection against atopy and there was even a suggestion that the risk of atopy was increased. Likewise, in the large Multicentre Allergy Study (MAS) observational birth cohort ($n = 1314$ infants born in 1990), Bergman et al. [45] found that each month of breast-feeding elevated the risk of developing atopic eczema in the first 7 years by approximately 3%. It was noted however, that breast-feeding persisted for longer if at least one parent had eczema, the mother was older, did not smoke in pregnancy, or the family had a high social status. Reverse causality could not be ruled out in this study.

Interestingly, there has, since 1975, been a significant trend in developed countries towards the later introduction of solid foods. For example, in the United Kingdom, the proportion of infants given solids by 8 weeks of age has decreased, 49% in 1975, 24% in 1980 and 1985, and 19% in 1990 [46]. It is interesting that this decrease to a third of what it was has coincided with a threefold increase in allergy in children [47]. Reasons for differences in weaning are complex and early weaning has been associated with cultural, socioeconomic, as well as specific factors such as maternal age, formula feeding, and maternal smoking. All of these factors need to be controlled for in study analyses.

A review of the evidence for the relationship between the early (defined as less than 4 months of age) introduction of solid foods to infants and the development of allergic disease was performed by Tarini et al. [48]. Thirteen studies met their criteria for review, of which only one was a controlled study. Studies were not limited to at-risk study populations. They concluded that there was insufficient evidence to suggest that, on its own, the early introduction of solids to infants was associated with an increased risk of asthma, FA, or allergic rhinitis. They noted the consistent association between the persistence of eczema and the introduction of solid foods before 4 months of age that is supported by long-term follow-up studies and the dose-dependent nature of the association.

Fergusson et al. [49] is the only study to report an increased risk of persistent eczema with the early introduction of solids. They reported a 2.9 times greater risk of chronic or recurrent eczema amongst children fed four or more solids before 4 months of age compared with those not fed solids before 4 months of age. This difference was still apparent at 10 years of age. When they assessed the effect of exposure to individual foods such as cow's milk, egg, cereals, vegetables, meat products, or fruit they found no increased risk of developing atopic dermatitis (AD). Zutavern et al. [50] conducted a large multicenter study that controlled for the effects of reverse causality while assessing for the effect of early life diet on allergy outcomes. They found no evidence of a protective effect of late introduction of solids on the development of preschool wheezing, transient wheezing, atopy, or eczema. There was no evidence for a protective effect of the delayed introduction of solids beyond 4 months of age on the development of sensitization to foods. On the contrary, there was a statistically significant increased risk of eczema in relation to late introduction of egg and milk. The late introduction of egg was also associated with a non-significant increased risk of preschool wheezing.

Although exclusive breast-feeding does not have proven effects in the prevention of allergy, there have been numerous studies examining the protective effects of different types of formulae especially CMP hydrolysates as a substitute for breast milk where the mother is unable to or chooses not to breast-feed. There are several studies and a meta-analysis of the evidence for the role of infant formula in the prevention of allergic disease in high-risk infants who are unable to be breast-fed. The Cochrane review by Osborn et al. [51] found no evidence to support feeding with a hydrolyzed formula for the prevention of allergy compared with exclusive breast-feeding. For high-risk infants who are unable to be completely breast-fed, they found limited evidence that prolonged feeding with a hydrolyzed formula compared with a cow's milk formula reduced infant and childhood allergy and infant CMA. The general consensus among the reviews is that the use of hydrolyzed milk formula in at-risk infants offers at least some protection against allergic disease, and in particular eczema. These findings are reflected in the recommendations of specialist allergy organizations [32–36, 52].

The German Infant Nutritional Interventional (GINI) study [53, 54], and the Melbourne Allergy Cohort Study [55], are two of the largest studies on this topic. The GINI Study is a large ($n = 2252$) randomized multicenter study in which Von Berg et al. allocate high-risk infants to one of four milks: cow's milk formula (CMF), partially hydrolyzed whey formula (pHW-F), extensively hydrolyzed whey formula (eHW-F), or extensively hydrolyzed casein formula (eHC-F). A significant reduction in the incidence of AD was achieved at 1 and 3 years with the eHC-F and the pHW-F. The greater reduction in eczema at 1 year of age in high-risk children with a pHW-F and eHC-F rather than with an eHW-F is difficult to explain. In this study, hydrolyzed formula did not protect against wheezing. The clinical benefits demonstrated by the GINI study are convincing. However, it remains unclear whether dietary modification has truly prevented allergic disease. The GINI study [53, 54] was not able to clearly define the end point of FA by DBPCFC as many parents declined. The reduction in eczema could therefore either be due to the primary prevention of eczema through dietary modification or alternatively, reflect the beneficial effect of removing CMP from the diet of infants with concomitant eczema and milk allergy. More recently, Lowe et al. [55] report on a single-blind randomized trial on the effects of soy or partially hydrolyzed whey formula (pHWF) compared with CMF on allergy risk in 620 infants with a family history of allergy and found no group difference at the of age 2 years for cumulative incidence of any allergic manifestation (CMF, 48.7%; soy, 54.5%; pHWF, 53.4%), eczema, or FA. They found no evidence to support recommending the use of pHWF at weaning for the prevention of allergic disease in high-risk infants. Both studies failed to demonstrate a beneficial effect of pHWF for allergic manifestations, eczema, asthma, or allergic rhinitis with intention-to-treat analysis. The only area in which the results of these studies diverge is on the per-protocol analysis within the first year of life. Per-protocol analyses are not protected (from bias) by the randomization process. Furthermore, a per-protocol analysis of the Lowe data does not confirm the findings of the GINI analysis. When all studies have their data integrated in a review such as the Cochrane review, these findings will become clearer.

Soy formulae have long been used as CMF alternatives. In a recent Cochrane review, Osborn et al. [56] found three studies which met their inclusion criteria. They concluded that, on current evidence, the use of soy formulae could not be recommended for the prevention of allergy or food intolerance in at-risk infants. No study demonstrated an increase in soy allergy. There is also no evidence to support the use of "other" mammalian milks for the prevention of FA.

Summary. There is some evidence of a protective effect against the development of allergy in high-risk infants when exclusively breast-feeding for the first 3 months of life. There is no convincing effect noted beyond 3 months of life in both high-risk infants and normal infants. Some studies suggest that prolonged exclusive breast-feeding may increase the risk of allergies, although reverse causality may be an explanation. The use of CM-hydrolysates in high-risk infants shows amelioration of eczema—but not FA—at 1 year and 3 years of age (in the GINI study) but not the Melbourne Allergy Cohort Study. There is no evidence that hydrolyzed formulae prevent against the development of other allergies There is no evidence to support the use of Soy formula or "other" mammalian milk formula for the prevention of allergy.

Combined maternal and infant dietary measures and the prevention of food allergy

It seems intuitive that of all dietary interventions aimed at the prevention of FA the combined approach should offer the greatest hope as it covers many routes of allergen exposure at immunologically vulnerable time points.

In a Cochrane review, Kramer et al. [24] assessed the evidence for the prevention of allergic disease through maternal dietary antigen avoidance during pregnancy or lactation, or both. Their analysis found that the prescription of an antigen avoidance diet to a high-risk woman during pregnancy was unlikely to substantially reduce her child's risk of atopic disease.

There were two randomized studies that adopted a multi-intervention approach. Zeiger et al. [57] in a study of 165 mother/infant pairs randomized participants to either a prophylactic group (maternal avoidance of cow's milk, egg, and peanut during the last trimester of pregnancy and lactation; and infants diet free of cow's milk until the age of 1 year and using a hydrolysate formula as supplement; egg until the age of 2 years; and peanut and fish until the age of 3 years) or a control group (following standard feeding practice). Findings demonstrate a significant reduction in cow's milk sensitization and eczema before the age of 2 years but no significant reduction in FA, AD, allergic rhinitis, asthma, any atopic disease, lung function, food or aeroallergen sensitization, or serum-IgE level at 7 years of age. No difference in SPT or specific-IgE testing was shown for the other food allergens tested, including peanut, which was the most common skin test-positive food allergen at 7 years of age. This indicates that the beneficial effect of the dietary interventions was mainly in reducing CMA.

Arshad et al. [58] in a study of 120 infants randomized participants to either a prophylactic group (breast-fed with mother on a low allergen diet or given an extensively hydrolyzed formula and House Dust Mite reduction) or a control group (who followed standard UK Department of Health (DoH) advice). Findings demonstrate a reduction in allergic disease (asthma, atopy, rhinitis, and eczema) at least for the first 8 years of life in the prophylactic group. Repeated measurement analysis, adjusted for all relevant confounding variables, confirmed a preventive effect on asthma, AD, rhinitis, and atopy. The protective effects were primarily observed in the subgroup of children with persistent disease (symptoms at all visits) and in those with evidence of allergic sensitization. Study powering did not allow for the assessment of FA at 8 years of age, but earlier transient effects were noted.

Summary. There are randomized trials that adopt a multi-intervention approach (dietary modification of both maternal diet—during pregnancy and/or lactation—and infant diet) that have demonstrated a reduction in allergic disease. While findings in one study were transient and no longer observed at 7 years of age, in a second study, the effects in allergy reduction were still observed at 8 years of age. The effects with respect to a reduction in FA appear to predominantly apply to CMA. Caution is required prior to the recommendation of such interventions due to the potential for nutritional compromise in both mother and child.

Routes of sensitization, cross sensitization, and oral tolerance induction

Until recently, preventive strategies have focused on oral exposure to foods. However, the oral route of exposure is not the only route, as exposure to food allergens may occur through aerosolized allergen exposure (e.g., fish and milk cooking vapors) or via the skin. The ALSPAC study [8] followed a large cohort of children (n = 13 971) from birth; the results of this study showed a positive association between PA and eczema, and an even greater association with an oozing or crusting skin rash. They also found an increased use of skin preparations using peanut oil in children with PA (this was limited to cutaneous rather than oral exposure). The observations support the occupational health findings in adults that sensitization may occur through contact with the skin, particularly through abraded skin. There is a molecular basis for the increased skin permeability seen in patients with eczema: the loss-of-function or missense mutations in the gene encoding FLG. This protein has been recognized as the strongest genetic contributor to eczema and is important for epidermal differentiation, desquamation, and barrier function [59–62]. FLG deficiency is also associated with increased transepidermal water loss; importantly, this measurable functional impairment of the skin barrier precedes the development of eczema [63]. In the positive studies 14–56% of cases of eczema carry one or more FLG null mutations and the presence of an FLG null allele represents a 1.2- to 13-fold increased risk of AD [64]. Furthermore, TH2 inflammation in the skin of patients with eczema reduces FLG gene expression [65]. It has been suggested that low-dose exposure to environmental food proteins on tabletops, hands, and dust can occur [66]. Such food proteins can penetrate the disrupted skin barrier and are taken up by Langerhans cells leading to TH2 responses and IgE production by B cells [67].

There is a significant body of evidence in animal models that a single oral dose of antigen is sufficient to induce oral tolerance [68–70]. This phenomenon has been demonstrated for different antigens and in different experimental models. The data is consistent, uniformly showing that a single dose of oral protein administration effectively causes immunological tolerance and prevents the expression of related clinical disease.

Poole et al. [71] in a large prospective cohort study in Colorado ($n = 1612$) found an association between age at initial exposure to cereal grains and the development of wheat allergy. Their date suggested that delaying introduction of cereal grains until after 6 months was not protective against development of wheat allergy, but that it may in fact increase the child's risk of wheat allergy. This study excluded children with celiac disease (positive tissue transglutaminase autoantibodies) and controlled for family history of allergy, prior FA, breast-feeding duration, and whether the child was breast-fed when first exposed to cereals.

Koplin et al. [72] assessed the impact of timing of introduction of egg using data from the Health Nuts study. They found that the later introduction of egg into the diet was associated with higher rates of egg allergy, with the adjusted odds ratio for introduction of egg after 12 months being 3.4 (95% CI, 1.8–6.5) compared with introduction at 4–6 months of age. Interestingly, introduction of cooked egg, such as scrambled, baked, or fried, was more protective than introducing egg in baked goods, with the risk of egg allergy in infants who had cooked egg introduced into their diet at 4–6 months being five times lower than those infants who had cooked egg introduced into their diet at the normally recommended time of 10–12 months of age after adjusting for confounding factors. In contrast, there was no protective effect amongst infants who were first introduced baked egg into their diet between 4 and 6 months presumably because a lower dose exposure did not confer a beneficial effect against egg allergy.

Katz et al. [73], in a large-scale, population-based prospective study, sought to determine the prevalence and risk factors for the development of CMA. In a prospective study, the feeding history of 13 019 infants was obtained by means of telephone interview (95.8%) or questionnaire (4.2%). Infants with probable adverse reactions to milk were examined, skin prick tested, and underwent oral challenges. The cumulative incidence for IgE-mediated CMA was 0.5% (66/13 019 patients). The mean age of CMP introduction was significantly different ($p < 0.001$) between the healthy infants (61.6 ± 92.5 days) and those with IgE-mediated CMA (116.1 ± 64.9 days). Only 0.05% of the infants who were started on regular CMP formula within the first 14 days versus 1.75% who were started on formula between the ages of 105 and 194 days had IgE-mediated CMA ($p < 0.001$). The odds ratio was 19.3 (95% CI, 6.0–62.1) for development of IgE-mediated CMA among infants with exposure to CMP at the age of 15 days or more ($p < 0.001$). This raises the question as to whether very early exposure to CMP as a supplement to breast-feeding might promote tolerance.

There are no interventional studies that examine the potential role of oral tolerance induction to foods in childhood. There is one adult human study that showed that feeding keyhole limpet hemocyanin (KLH), resulted in immunological tolerance to KLH antigen [74]. Ecological data suggests that African, Asian, and Middle Eastern countries[75] where peanuts are consumed throughout pregnancy and early childhood enjoy low rates of PA compared with Western, industrialized societies such as the United Kingdom and United States where PA is high despite peanut avoidance during pregnancy and infancy. However, differential predisposition to atopy due to both genetic and environmental factors could explain these differences.

It has been suggested that early introduction of foods, such as peanut, can lead to tolerance and protect against the development of FA. These theories are currently being tested in two RCTs. The Learning Early About Peanut Allergy study [76] involves 640 high-risk children who were enrolled at age 4–10 months. Each child was randomly assigned to one of the two approaches: avoidance or consumption. Children in the avoidance group completely avoid eating peanut-containing foods; in the consumption group parents are asked to feed their child a peanut snack three times per week (equivalent to about 6 g of peanut protein per week). The proportion of each group with PA by 5 years of age will be used to determine which approach, avoidance or consumption, works best for preventing PA. The study will reach completion in 2013.

The Enquiring About Tolerance study [77] is a Randomized Controlled Trial (RCT) investigating the effect of early introduction of complementary foods together with breast-feeding. Infants taking part in the study (n = 11 302) are being recruited from the general population and randomized to one of two groups. One group (n = 5651) introduces six allergenic foods from 3 months of age alongside continued breast-feeding, with screening to check for pre-existing FA (early introduction group). The other group (n = 5651) follows present UK government weaning advice (i.e., aim for exclusive breast-feeding for 6 months (standard weaning group)). The children will be monitored until 3 years of age to determine whether early diet has an effect in reducing the prevalence of FA determined by DBPCFCs. Interventional studies clearly represent an advantage over observational studies in the determination of the role of early food and micronutrient exposure in the development of allergies.

There are observational studies to other foods that lend weight to the hypothesis of tolerance induction through early oral exposure. A large observational cohort of children, by Poole et al.[71] demonstrated that delaying the initial exposure to cereal grains until after 6 months may increase the risk of developing IgE-mediated wheat allergy. In a population-based observational study by Saarinen et al. [78], fish and citrus allergy were determined at 3 years of age by oral food challenge. They then found no difference in the cumulative incidence of fish and citrus allergy at 3 years of age between children with fish introduced early or late (after 1 year old of age).

Summary. Recent observational and animal studies raise the question of whether sensitization to food antigens may occur via the cutaneous route. There is a body of literature in animal models that demonstrates the effect of tolerance induction following early high-dose food allergen consumption. Human trials are awaited.

Unpasteurized milk, probiotics, and prebiotics

In general, allergies are associated with a Western lifestyle. The hygiene hypothesis [79] proposes that the lack of early childhood exposure to infectious agents, gut flora, and parasites increases susceptibility to allergic diseases by modulating immune system development, although limited data for the hygiene hypothesis exist with respect to FA.

Exposure to food proteins in the gastrointestinal tract might require an optimal microenvironment if the necessary conditions for the induction of tolerance are to be met (e.g., immune factors, such as cytokines, antibodies, regulatory T cells (the function of which might depend on vitamin D), and bacterial colonization).

The mode of delivery has been investigated in relation to FA outcomes. A Norwegian birth cohort study found that birth by means of caesarean section was associated with a sevenfold increased risk of parental perceived reactions to eggs, fish, or nuts.[80, 81] A recent meta-analysis found six studies that showed a mild effect of caesarean delivery, increasing the risk of FA or food atopy (OR, 1.32; 95% CI, 1.12–1.55) [82]. However, it should be noted that in a large recent study evaluating 503 infants, the mode of delivery at birth bore no relationship to sensitization or FA, as determined by specific-IgE levels in young infants [26].

Observations from rural environments suggest an inverse association between consumption of farm-produced dairy products and the prevalence of allergic disease. Waser et al. [83] conducted a cross-sectional multicenter study that demonstrated that the consumption of farm milk might offer protection against asthma and allergy. These associations were independent of farm-related co-exposures and other farm-produced products, but were not independently related to any allergy-related health outcome. Similarly, Perkin et al. [74] conducted a two-stage cross-sectional study that demonstrated that unpasteurized milk might be a modifiable influence on allergic sensitization in children. The effect was seen in all children, independent of farming status.

Other strategies have sought to alter the commensal gut flora either directly through the administration of living microorganisms (probiotics), or indirectly through the provision of non-digestible, growth-enhancing substrates (prebiotics). That the gut microbiota play a role in tolerance induction is suggested by studies in germfree mice where oral tolerance cannot be induced [84].

There are many variables between studies performed in this field; these include probiotic strain and viability, dose, and duration. In addition, not all studies treat both mother (during pregnancy and/or breast-feeding) and child. Hence, clinical trial results from one probiotic strain in one population cannot be automatically generalized to other strains or to different populations. There is also great variability with respect to patient groups recruited in trials to date. Boyle et al. [85] published a review in 2005 of the evidence for the use of probiotics in the management of allergic disease. They found evidence for the use of probiotics in the treatment of eczema, but the level of evidence regarding the role of probiotics for the prevention of eczema, was "weak."

More recently, Kukkonene et al. [86] in a large randomized trial (n = 925) assessed the combined role of prebiotics (galacto-oligosaccharides) and probiotics (four bacterial strains) in the prevention of allergic disease in a high-risk population. They randomized pregnant women to probiotic or placebo for 2–4 weeks before delivery; their infants received the same intervention or a placebo for 6 months. Results indicate that the prebiotic–probiotic combination treatment, when compared with placebo, showed no effect on the cumulative incidence of allergic disease at 2 years of age. However, the prebiotic–probiotic combination treatment did reduce eczema and atopic eczema (in both IgE-sensitized and non-IgE-sensitized children). Taylor et al. [13] randomized high-risk newborns ($n = 231$) to either receive *Lactobacillus acidophilus* or placebo daily for the first 6 months of life. They were unable to demonstrate a significant difference in eczema between the groups at 6 and 12 months of age, and found that the proportion of children with positive SPTs and eczema was significantly higher in the probiotic group.

Pelucci et al. [87] recently published their findings of a meta-analysis updated to October 2011 of dietary supplementation with probiotics versus placebo; primary outcomes were incidence of AD and IgE-associated AD. Differences in rates of FA were not assessed. They identified 18 publications based on 14 studies. Their meta-analysis demonstrated that probiotic use decreased the incidence of AD (RR = 0.79 (95% CI = 0.71–0.88)). Studies were fairly homogeneous (I = 24.0%). The corresponding RR of IgE-associated AD was 0.80 (95% CI = 0.66–0.96). This meta-analysis therefore provides evidence in support of a moderate role of probiotics in the prevention of AD and IgE-associated AD in infants. The favorable effect was similar regardless of the time of probiotic use (pregnancy or early life) or the subject(s) receiving probiotics (mother, child, or both).

Whether the probiotic-induced microbiota changes—and associated clinical effects—persist after the administration ceases remains unclear. For example, in a study by Kalliomaki et al. [12, 88] initial findings at 4 years of age suggested a reduction in eczema, rhinitis, and asthma; however at 7 years of age, the overall risk for developing eczema remained lower in the LGG- probiotic group while allergic rhinitis and asthma were more common. Interestingly, both the Kukkonene et al. and Kalliomaki et al. studies find the preventive effect on eczema not to be associated with IgE changes [12, 86].

Boyle et al. [89] recently highlighted the known and theoretical safety concerns of probiotics; these include infection, deleterious metabolic activities, immune deviation, excessive immune stimulation, and microbial resistance.

It has been shown that infant formulae that are fortified with prebiotics can bias the microbiota to more closely resemble that of breast milk (the so called "bifidogenic" effect). The clinical relevance of these prebiotic-induced changes remains unclear.

Summary. Observational studies suggest that the consumption of unpasteurized milk may reduce the prevalence of allergic sensitization and disease. There are safety concerns regarding unpasteurized milk and this cannot therefore be recommended for the prevention of FA. Although some studies do show that the use of probiotics (and in one study a mixture of both pro- and prebiotics) reduces eczema, these effects are not consistent in all studies and are not associated with a reduction in atopy. Currently neither prebiotics nor probiotics can be recommended as a strategy to prevent FAs or other allergic disease, and safety concerns need to be considered.

Nutritional supplements

There are ecological observations that note that the geographical distribution of allergy prevalence is linked with regional dietary practices [90]. In recent years, there has been a focus on the role of vitamins, antioxidants, fruits, and vegetables, as well as fatty acid intake on the prevention or treatment of allergies.

Fatty acids

Dietary lipids, especially n-3 and n-6 long-chain polyunsaturated fatty acids (LCPUFA) regulate immune function, and may modify the adherence of microbes in the mucosa thereby contributing to host–microbe interactions. There are data arguing that reduction in consumption of animal fats and a corresponding increase in the use of margarine and vegetable oils have led to the increase in allergies. Proponents of this hypothesis argue that there has been an increase in the consumption of v-6 polyunsaturated fatty acids, such as linoleic acid, and through reduced consumption of oily fish, there has been a reduction in v-3 polyunsaturated fatty acids, such as eicosapentaenoic acid [91]. v-6 Fatty acids lead to the production of prostaglandin E2 (PGE2), whereas v-3 fatty acids inhibit synthesis of PGE2. PGE2 reduces IFN-g production by T lymphocytes, thus resulting in increased IgE production by B lymphocytes.

There are studies in this field that demonstrate a positive effect with respect to the prevention of allergies; however outcomes are inconsistent. Peat et al. [92] randomized 616 high-risk pregnant mothers (at 36 weeks gestation) to either an intervention group (omega-3-fatty acid supplementation and house dust mite reduction measures) or placebo. They demonstrated a reduction in the outcomes for dust mite sensitization and cough (in atopic children only) for infants in the intervention group. No significant differences in wheeze were found with either intervention. There was however limited perinatal intervention in this study. Kull et al. [93] in a large prospective birth cohort assessed for the effect of fish (a rich source of omega-3 fatty acids) consumption on allergy outcomes in a large prospective birth cohort. After controlling for confounding factors (parental allergy and early onset eczema or wheeze), regular fish consumption during the first year of life was associated with a reduced risk of allergic sensitization to foods by age 4. It is unclear whether such an effect could be explained by oral tolerance induction to food proteins or whether omega-3 fatty acids could have a generic antiallergic effect. Negative study findings include those by Almqvist et al. [94], who conducted a large ($n = 516$) randomized, placebo controlled trial in high-risk children and found that dietary fatty acids (in the first 5 years of life) did not reduce the risk of asthma or allergic disease at 5 years of age.

A systematic review (published 2009) identified 10 reports satisfying the inclusion criteria for a meta-analysis on the influence of v-3 and v-6 oils on allergic sensitization [95]. The study concludes that "supplementation with Omega 3 and Omega 6 oils is unlikely to play an important role in the strategy for the primary prevention of sensitization or allergic disease."

Palmer et al. [96] more recently sought to determine whether dietary n-3 LCPUFA supplementation of pregnant women with a fetus at high risk of allergic disease reduces IgE-associated eczema or FA at 1 year of age. This was a follow-up of infants at high hereditary risk of allergic disease in the Docosahexaenoic Acid to Optimize Mother Infant Outcome (DOMInO) randomized controlled trial. The mothers of 706 infants at high hereditary risk of developing allergic disease were participating in the DOMInO trial. The intervention group ($n = 368$) was randomly allocated to receive fish oil capsules (providing 900 mg of n-3 LCPUFA daily) from 21 weeks' gestation until birth; the control group ($n = 338$) received matched vegetable oil capsules without n-3 LCPUFA. No differences were seen in the overall percentage of infants with IgE-associated allergic disease between the n-3 LCPUFA and control groups, although the percentage of infants diagnosed as having atopic eczema (i.e., eczema with associated sensitization) was lower in the n-3 LCPUFA group (26/368 (7%) vs. 39/338 (12%); unadjusted RR 0.61 (95% CI 0.38–0.98, $p = 0.04$); adjusted RR 0.64 (95% CI 0.40–1.02, $p = 0.06$)). Fewer infants were sensitized to egg in the n-3 LCPUFA group (34/368 (9%) vs 52/338 (15%); unadjusted RR 0.61 (95% CI 0.40–0.91, $p = 0.02$); adjusted RR 0.62 (95% CI 0.41–0.93, $p = 0.02$)), but no difference between groups in IgE-associated FAwas seen. In summary, n-3 LCPUFA supplementation in pregnancy did not reduce the overall incidence of IgE-associated allergies in the first year of life, although atopic eczema and egg sensitization were lower.

Despite these conflicting findings, many infant formulae are supplemented with LCPUFA's such as arachidonic acid and docosahexaenoic acid.

Vitamins

Dietary vitamins have potent immune-modulating effects. There are epidemiologic and immunologic data that suggest that either excessive vitamin D or, conversely, vitamin D deficiency results in increased allergies. It has been possible to study the effect of vitamin supplementation in young children with respect to allergy outcomes, as many countries advocate routine vitamin supplementation during early childhood. Separate studies in Finland [97] and the United States [98], observed an increased association between vitamin D supplementation in infancy and atopic disease. However, study outcomes were restricted to rhinitis in adulthood in the first study, and select subgroups in the second study; asthma in black children and FAs (as defined by a medical professional) in the exclusively formula-fed population. The first observations were derived from farming communities in Germany in which less vitamin D supplementation was used in foods and a lower prevalence of allergies in children were found. Allergies increased, coinciding with vitamin D supplementation intervention programs to prevent rickets in childhood [99]. Likewise, two independent cohort studies by Milner et al. [98] and Hypponen et al. [100] showed that infants who had vitamin D supplementation were at increased risk of FA. Conversely, the vitamin D deficiency hypothesis argues that inadequate vitamin D (predominantly caused by inadequate sunlight associated with more time indoors) is responsible for the increase in asthma and allergies. The study by Camargo et al. [101] found a strong north–south gradient for EpiPen (Dey, Napa, Calif) prescriptions in the United States. Northernmost states were prescribing 8 to 12 EpiPen self-injectors per 1000 population, whereas the southern states were prescribing 3 per 1000 population. This gradient persisted despite a multivariate analysis. There was an inverse association between EpiPen prescription and the incidence of melanoma in the population, suggesting that this north–south effect was due to sunlight exposure. Recent findings by Vassalo et al. [102] show that season of birth is a risk factor for FA and that infants born during the winter had a higher risk of FA. Another study by Nwaru et al. [103] shows that maternal intake of vitamin D during pregnancy was associated with a decreased risk of food sensitization.

Kull et al. [104] in a large ($n = 4089$) prospective birth cohort investigated the association between the supplementation of vitamins A and D (administered in either a water or peanut-oil based vehicle) during the first year of life and the outcome of allergic disease up to 4 years of age. Children supplemented with vitamins A and D in the water-soluble vehicle during the first year of life had an almost twofold increased risk of asthma, food hypersensitivity (determined by parental questionnaire), and sensitization (to common food and airborne allergens) at the age of 4 years, when compared with those receiving vitamins in peanut oil. There are various possible explanations for these findings. Vitamin A and/or D may protect against the risk of developing allergy; the study findings would then hinge on better absorption of vitamin A and D from the oil-based vehicle than from a water-based vehicle. Alternatively, vitamin A and/or D may actually increase the risk of the development of allergic disease; the absorption of vitamin A and/or D would then need to be superior when the vitamins were administered in the water-based vehicle. Systemic uptake was unfortunately not measured in this study. It is not known how the rates of allergy in the two study groups compare with children who had not received vitamin supplementation at all (less than 2% of children in this cohort did not receive vitamin supplementation). It may also be that vitamin A and/or D has no effect on allergy outcomes and the effects observed are due to the use of peanut oil itself. However, the fatty acids in peanut oil are strongly biased towards the pro-inflammatory omega-6 fatty acids in a ratio of omega-6:omega-3 fatty acids of 34:1. Were this effect to be significant, a higher rate of allergy would have been expected in the group of children who received the oil-based supplement. It is therefore difficult to interpret these findings.

Antioxidants and trace elements

Antioxidants are free radical scavengers shown to decrease inflammatory processes. The antioxidant hypothesis suggests that the decrease in consumption of fresh fruit and vegetables (containing antioxidants, such as vitamin C, vitamin E, β-carotene, selenium, and zinc) in some countries, for example, the United Kingdom, might account for an increase in allergies. There are however conflicting dietary trends in these countries; although the intake of some antioxidants has increased, the intake of others has decreased. There is epidemiologic, animal, molecular, and immunologic evidence suggesting associations between antioxidants and asthma and a reduced number of studies on AD and allergic rhinitis [105]. There are no interventional studies that assess the effect of antioxidant supplementation on the prevention of FA; however, ecological observations suggest that the higher intake of fresh fruit and vegetables in certain European countries is associated with a decreased prevalence of FA [90]. In addition, preliminary findings from the ALSPAC cohort suggest that low cord blood selenium and iron may be associated with a higher subsequent risk of persistent wheeze and eczema [106].

Overnutrition

The coinciding trend in increasing atopy with increasing childhood obesity has been well studied, especially in the context of asthma. Obesity induces an inflammatory state associated with an increased risk of atopy and theoretically could lead to an increased risk of FA. A recent study by Visness et al. [107] demonstrated that atopy (as defined by any positive specific-IgE measurement) was increased in obese children compared with normal-weight children. This association was driven primarily by allergic sensitization to foods (OR for food sensitization, 1.59; 95% CI, 1.28–1.98). Increased C-reactive protein levels as a measure of inflammation were associated with total IgE levels, atopy, and food sensitization.

Summary. Randomized controlled studies provide conflicting results with respect to LCPUFA supplementation for the prevention of allergy. Studies that show a positive effect do so for different allergic disease outcomes. Observational studies that examine the effect of vitamins A and D supplementation during the first year of life suggests an increased rate of sensitization and allergy at 4 years of age, but only when administered in a water-soluble vehicle. It remains unclear as to why vitamin A and D supplementation in different vehicles should exert different clinical effects.

Ecological observations, and preliminary studies, suggest that the higher intake of foods rich in antioxidants may confer protection against allergy outcomes. There is data to support an association between obesity and allergic sensitization to foods. Although the role of nutritional supplements for the prevention of allergy is interesting, further randomized interventional studies are required.

Conclusions

The natural history of FA suggests "plasticity" within the developing immune system as many common FAs (such as egg and milk allergy) are outgrown. Indeed, the switch from a state of allergy to tolerance may even occur during the first few years of life. Turcanu et al. [108] demonstrated that the resolution of PA was accompanied by a reversal of the Th2- to Th1-skewed, allergen-specific, immune response. These findings are encouraging as it raises the possibility that immune responses are susceptible to prevention strategies.

The conventional wisdom is that early exposure to allergenic food proteins during pregnancy, lactation, or infancy leads to FAs, and that, prevention strategies should aim to eliminate allergenic food proteins during these periods of "immunologic vulnerability", especially in high-risk subgroups. However the evidence does not support this and there are data suggesting that environmental food allergen exposure may lead to allergic sensitization and that early consumption of food antigens could induce tolerance. There is some evidence to support the use of dietary interventions in high-risk pregnant and/or lactating women, especially for the outcome of atopic eczema. Such interventions may however compromise maternal and fetal nutrition. Exclusive breast-feeding for at least the first 3 months of life offers some protection against allergic disease in high-risk infants. The protective effect of exclusive breast-feeding beyond 4 months of age remains uncertain. For high-risk infants who are not exclusively breast-fed, or where supplementation of breast-feeding is required, the use of hydrolyzed formula may offer some protection against the development of eczema. The findings of dietary interventions such as LCPUFAs, antioxidants, pre- and probiotics and vitamin supplementation, are unconvincing, inconsistent, or not adequately tested. There are safety concerns surrounding some of the interventions trialed to date.

Future studies will need to overcome the methodological challenges detailed in this chapter, many of which are unique to this field of research. Better markers are required to identify high-risk populations, as not all children who develop FA are born to atopic families. With current advances in the field of gene-environment interactions, it may also be that future studies need to focus their interventions at specifically-defined groups of children, whose genotyping identifies them at being at risk of (or protected from) specific environmental exposures.

Finally, in order for the field of FA prevention to significantly advance, strategies will need to be put to the test using rigorous study design methodologies.

References

1. Sicherer SH, Sampson HA. Food allergy. *J Allergy Clin Immunol* 2006; 117:S470–S475.
2. Rona RJ, Keil T, Summers C, et al. The prevalence of food allergy: a meta-analysis. *J Allergy Clin Immunol* 2007; 120:638–646.
3. Grundy J, Matthews S, Bateman B, Dean T, Arshad SH. Rising prevalence of allergy to peanut in children: data from 2 sequential cohorts. *J Allergy Clin Immunol* 2002; 110:784–789.
4. Hourihane JO, Aiken R, Briggs R, et al. The impact of government advice to pregnant mothers regarding peanut avoidance on the prevalence of peanut allergy in United Kingdom children at school entry. *J Allergy Clin Immunol* 2007; 119:1197–1202.
5. Sicherer SH, Munoz-Furlong A, Sampson HA. Prevalence of peanut and tree nut allergy in the United States determined by means of a random digit dial telephone survey: a 5-year follow-up study. *J Allergy Clin Immunol* 2003; 112:1203–1207.
6. Sicherer SH, Munoz-Furlong A, Godbold JH, Sampson HA. US prevalence of self-reported peanut, tree nut, and sesame allergy: 11-year follow-up. *J Allergy Clin Immunol* 2010; 125:1322–1326.
7. Osborne NJ, Koplin JJ, Martin PE, et al. Prevalence of challenge-proven IgE-mediated food allergy using population-based sampling and predetermined challenge criteria in infants. *J Allergy Clin Immunol* 2011; 127:668–676.
8. Lack G, Fox D, Northstone K, Golding J. Factors associated with the development of peanut allergy in childhood. *N Engl J Med* 2003; 348:977–985.
9. Hill DJ, Hosking CS. Food allergy and atopic dermatitis in infancy: an epidemiologic study. *Pediatr Allergy Immunol* 2004; 15:421–427.
10. Hattevig G, Kjellman B, Siqurs N, et al. The effect of maternal avoidance of eggs, cow's milk, and fish during lactation on the development of IgE, IgG, and IgA antibodies in infants. *J Allergy Clin Immunol* 1990; 85:108–115.
11. Zeiger RS. Food allergen avoidance in the prevention of food allergy in infants and children. *Pediatrics* 2003; 111:1662–1671.
12. Kalliomaki M, Salminen S, Poussa T, Isolauri E. Probiotics during the first 7 years of life: a cumulative risk reduction of eczema in a randomized, placebo-controlled trial. *J Allergy Clin Immunol* 2007; 119:1019–1021.
13. Taylor AL, Dunstan JA, Prescott SL. Probiotic supplementation for the first 6 months of life fails to reduce the risk of atopic dermatitis and increases the risk of allergen sensitization in high-risk children: a randomized controlled trial. *J Allergy Clin Immunol* 2007; 119:184–191.
14. Sigurs N, Hattevig G, Kjellman B, et al. Appearance of atopic disease in relation to serum IgE antibodies in children followed up from birth for 4 to 15 years. *J Allergy Clin Immunol* 1994; 94:757–763.
15. Maloney JM, Chapman MD, Sicherer SH. Peanut allergen exposure through saliva: assessment and interventions to reduce exposure. *J Allergy Clin Immunol* 2006; 118:719–724.
16. Nolan RC, de Leon MP, Rolland JM, Loh RK, O'Hehir RE. What's in a kiss: peanut allergen transmission as a sensitizer? *J Allergy Clin Immunol* 2007; 119:755.
17. Osborne NJ, Koplin JJ, Martin PE, et al. Prevalence of challenge-proven IgE-mediated food allergy using population-based sampling and predetermined challenge criteria in infants. *J Allergy Clin Immunol* 2011; 127:668–676.
18. du Toit G, Meyer R, Shah N, et al. Identifying and managing cow's milk protein allergy. *Arch Dis Child Educ Pract Ed* 2010; 95:134–144.
19. Vance GH, Lewis SA, Grimshaw KE, et al. Exposure of the fetus and infant to hens' egg ovalbumin via the placenta and breast milk in relation to maternal intake of dietary egg. *Clin Exp Allergy* 2005; 35:1318–1326.
20. Arshad SH, Kurukulaaratchy RJ, Fenn M, Matthews S. Early life risk factors for current wheeze, asthma, and bronchial hyperresponsiveness at 10 years of age. *Chest* 2005; 127:502–508.
21. Falth-Magnusson K, Kjellman NI. Allergy prevention by maternal elimination diet during late pregnancy—a 5-year follow-up of a randomized study. *J Allergy Clin Immunol* 1992; 89:709–713.
22. Falth-Magnusson K, Kjellman NI. Development of atopic disease in babies whose mothers were receiving exclusion diet during pregnancy—a randomized study. *J Allergy Clin Immunol* 1987; 80:868–875.

23. Lilja G, Dannaeus A, Foucard T, et al. Effects of maternal diet during late pregnancy and lactation on the development of atopic diseases in infants up to 18 months of age—in-vivo results. *Clin Exp Allergy* 1989; 19:473–479.
24. Kramer MS, Kakuma R. Maternal dietary antigen avoidance during pregnancy or lactation, or both, for preventing or treating atopic disease in the child. *Cochrane Database Syst Rev* 2006; (3):CD000133. doi:10.1002/14651858.CD000133.pub2
25. Fox AT, Sasieni P, du Toit G, Syed H, Lack G. Household peanut consumption as a risk factor for the development of peanut allergy. *J Allergy Clin Immunol* 2009; 123:417–423.
26. Sicherer SH, Wood RA, Stablein D, et al. Maternal consumption of peanut during pregnancy is associated with peanut sensitization in atopic infants. *J Allergy Clin Immunol* 2010; 126:1191–1197.
27. American Academy of Pediatrics. Committee on Nutrition. Hypoallergenic infant formulas. *Pediatrics* 2000; 106(2 Pt 1):346–349.
28. Committee on Toxicity of Chemicals in Food, Consumer Products and the Environment [COT]. (2000) *Adverse Reactions to Food and Food Ingredients*, Chapter 11, pp. 91–97. Available at http://cot.food.gov.uk/pdfs/adversereactionstofood.pdf (Last accessed July 11, 2013).
29. Greer FR, Sicherer SH, Burks AW. Effects of early nutritional interventions on the development of atopic disease in infants and children: the role of maternal dietary restriction, breastfeeding, timing of introduction of complementary foods, and hydrolyzed formulas. *Pediatrics* 2008; 121:183–191.
30. Committee on Toxicity of Chemicals in Food, Consumer Products and the Environment [COT]. (2008) *Statement on the Review of the 1998 COT Recommendations on Peanut Avoidance*. Available at http://cot.food.gov.uk/pdfs/cotstatement200807peanut.pdf (Last accessed March 22, 2012).
31. Herrmann ME, Dannemann A, Gruters A, et al. Prospective study of the atopy preventive effect of maternal avoidance of milk and eggs during pregnancy and lactation. *Eur J Pediatr* 1996; 155:770–774.
32. World Health Organization. (2001) *Global strategy for infant and young child feeding: the optimal duration of exclusive breastfeeding*. Fifty-Fourth World Health Assembly. Provisional agenda item 13.1.1, Geneva, Switzerland.
33. Department of Health. Committee on the Toxicity of Chemicals in Food, Consumer products and the Environment [COT], (1998) Peanut Allergy, pp. 35–37.
34. Fiocchi A, Assa'ad A, Bahna S, et al. Food allergy and the introduction of solid foods to infants: a consensus document. Adverse Reactions to Foods Committee, American College of Allergy, Asthma and Immunology. *Ann Allergy Asthma Immunol* 2006; 97:10–20.
35. Gartner LM, Morton J, Lawrence RA, et al. Breastfeeding and the use of human milk. *Pediatrics* 2005; 115:496–506.
36. Prescott SL, Tang ML. The Australasian Society of Clinical Immunology and Allergy position statement: summary of allergy prevention in children. *Med J Aust* 2005; 182:464–467.
37. Host A, Koletzko B, Dreborg S, et al. Dietary products used in infants for treatment and prevention of food allergy. Joint Statement of the European Society for Paediatric Allergology and Clinical Immunology (ESPACI) Committee on Hypoallergenic Formulas and the European Society for Paediatric Gastroenterology, Hepatology and Nutrition (ESPGHAN) Committee on Nutrition. *Arch Dis Child* 1999; 81:80–84.
38. Grulee CG, Sanford HN. The influence of breast and artificial feeding on infantile eczema. *J Pediatr* 1930; 9:223–225.
39. Muraro A, Dreborg S, Halken S, et al. Dietary prevention of allergic diseases in infants and small children. Part III: Critical review of published peer-reviewed observational and interventional studies and final recommendations. *Pediatr Allergy Immunol* 2004; 15:291–307.
40. Brew BK, Kull I, Garden F, et al. Breastfeeding, asthma, and allergy: a tale of two cities. *Pediatr Allergy Immunol* 2012; 23: 75–82.
41. Kramer MS, Kakuma R. The optimal duration of exclusive breastfeeding: a systematic review. *Adv Exp Med Biol* 2004; 554:63–77.
42. Lucas A, Brooke OG, Morley R, Cole TJ, Bamford MF. Early diet of preterm infants and development of allergic or atopic disease: randomised prospective study. *BMJ* 1990; 300:837–840.
43. De Jong MH, Scharp-Van Der Linden VT, Aalberse R, Heymans HS, Brunekreef B. The effect of brief neonatal exposure to cows' milk on atopic symptoms up to age 5. *Arch Dis Child* 2002; 86:365–369.
44. Sears MR, Greene JM, Willan AR, et al. Long-term relation between breastfeeding and development of atopy and asthma in children and young adults: a longitudinal study. *Lancet* 2002; 360:901–907.
45. Bergmann RL, Diepgen TL, Kuss O, et al. Breastfeeding duration is a risk factor for atopic eczema. *Clin Exp Allergy* 2002; 32:205–209.
46. CoMA working group on the weaning diet. Weaning and the weaning diet. Report of the Working Group on the Weaning Diet of the Committee on Medical Aspects of Food Policy. Page 13 of DH Report on Health and Social Subjects 45 Weaning and The Weaning Diet. 1994. London.
47. Asher MI, Montfort S, Bjorksten B, et al. Worldwide time trends in the prevalence of symptoms of asthma, allergic rhinoconjunctivitis, and eczema in childhood: ISAAC Phases One and Three repeat multicountry cross-sectional surveys. *Lancet* 2006; 368:733–743.
48. Tarini BA, Carroll AE, Sox CM, Christakis DA. Systematic review of the relationship between early introduction of solid foods to infants and the development of allergic disease. *Arch Pediatr Adolesc Med* 2006; 160:502–507.
49. Fergusson DM, Horwood LJ, Shannon FT. Early solid feeding and recurrent childhood eczema: a 10-year longitudinal study. *Pediatrics* 1990; 86:541–546.
50. Zutavern A, von Mutius E, Harris J, et al. The introduction of solids in relation to asthma and eczema. *Arch Dis Child* 2004; 89:303–308.
51. Osborn DA, Sinn J. Primary prevention with hydrolysed formula: does it change natural onset of allergic disease? *Clin Exp Allergy* 2010; 40(4):534–535.
52. Host A, Koletzko B, Dreborg S, et al. Dietary products used in infants for treatment and prevention of food allergy. Joint Statement of the European Society for Paediatric Allergology

and Clinical Immunology (ESPACI) Committee on Hypoallergenic Formulas and the European Society for Paediatric Gastroenterology, Hepatology and Nutrition (ESPGHAN) Committee on Nutrition. *Arch Dis Child* 1999; 81:80–84.

53. Von, BA, Koletzko S, Grübl A, et al. The effect of hydrolyzed cow's milk formula for allergy prevention in the first year of life: the German Infant Nutritional Intervention Study, a randomized double-blind trial. *J Allergy Clin Immunol* 2003; 111:533–540.
54. Von BA, Koletzko S, Fillipiak-Pitroff B, et al. Certain hydrolyzed formulas reduce the incidence of atopic dermatitis but not that of asthma: three-year results of the German Infant Nutritional Intervention Study. *J Allergy Clin Immunol* 2007; 119:718–725.
55. Lowe AJ, Hosking CS, Bennett CM, et al. Effect of a partially hydrolyzed whey infant formula at weaning on risk of allergic disease in high-risk children: a randomized controlled trial. *J Allergy Clin Immunol* 2011; 128:360–365.
56. Osborn DA, Sinn J. Soy formula for prevention of allergy and food intolerance in infants. *Cochrane Database Syst Rev* 2006; (4):CD003741). doi: 10.1002/14651858.CD003741.pub4
57. Zeiger RS, Heller S. The development and prediction of atopy in high-risk children: follow-up at age seven years in a prospective randomized study of combined maternal and infant food allergen avoidance. *J Allergy Clin Immunol* 1995; 95:1179–1190.
58. Arshad SH, Bateman B, Sadeghnejad A, Gant C, Matthews SM. Prevention of allergic disease during childhood by allergen avoidance: the Isle of Wight prevention study. *J Allergy Clin Immunol* 2007; 119:307–313.
59. Brown SJ, McLean WH. Eczema genetics: current state of knowledge and future goals. *J Invest Dermatol* 2009; 129:543–552.
60. Dubrac S, Schmuth M, Ebner S. Atopic dermatitis: the role of Langerhans cells in disease pathogenesis. *Immunol Cell Biol* 2010; 88:400–409.
61. Palmer CN, Irvine AD, Terron-Kwiatkowski A, et al. Common loss-of-function variants of the epidermal barrier protein filaggrin are a major predisposing factor for atopic dermatitis. *Nat Genet* 2006; 38:441–446.
62. Smith FJ, Irvine AD, Terron-Kwiatkowski A, et al. Loss-of-function mutations in the gene encoding filaggrin cause ichthyosis vulgaris. *Nat Genet* 2006; 38:337–342.
63. Flohr C, England K, Radulovic S, et al. Filaggrin loss-of-function mutations are associated with early-onset eczema, eczema severity and transepidermal water loss at 3 months of age. *Br J Dermatol* 2010; 163:1333–1336.
64. Brown SJ, Irvine AD. Atopic eczema and the filaggrin story. *Semin Cutan Med Surg* 2008; 27:128–137.
65. Howell MD, Kim BE, Gao P, et al. Cytokine modulation of atopic dermatitis filaggrin skin expression. *J Allergy Clin Immunol* 2007; 120:150–155.
66. Perry TT, Conover-Walker MK, Pomes A, Chapman MD, Wood RA. Distribution of peanut allergen in the environment. *J Allergy Clin Immunol* 2004; 113:973–976.
67. Dubrac S, Schmuth M, Ebner S. Atopic dermatitis: the role of Langerhans cells in disease pathogenesis. *Immunol Cell Biol* 2010; 88:400–409.
68. Strid J, Thomson M, Hourihane J, Kimber I, Strobel S. A novel model of sensitization and oral tolerance to peanut protein. *Immunology* 2004; 113:293–303.
69. Strid J, Hourihane J, Kimber I, Callard R, Strobel S. Disruption of the stratum corneum allows potent epicutaneous immunization with protein antigens resulting in a dominant systemic Th2 response. *Eur J Immunol* 2004; 34:2100–2109.
70. Strid J, Hourihane J, Kimber I, Callard R, Strobel S. Epicutaneous exposure to peanut protein prevents oral tolerance and enhances allergic sensitization. *Clin Exp Allergy* 2005; 35:757–766.
71. Poole JA, Barriga K, Leung DY, et al. Timing of initial exposure to cereal grains and the risk of wheat allergy. *Pediatrics* 2006; 117:2175–2182.
72. Koplin JJ, Osborne NJ, Wake M, et al. Can early introduction of egg prevent egg allergy in infants? A population-based study. *J Allergy Clin Immunol* 2010; 126:807–813.
73. Katz Y, Rajuan N, Goldberg MR, et al. Early exposure to cow's milk protein is protective against IgE-mediated cow's milk protein allergy. *J Allergy Clin Immunol* 2010; 126:77–82.
74. Perkin MR, Strachan DP. Which aspects of the farming lifestyle explain the inverse association with childhood allergy? *J Allergy Clin Immunol* 2006; 117:1374–1381.
75. Levy Y, Broides A, Segal N, Danon YL. Peanut and tree nut allergy in children: role of peanut snacks in Israel? *Allergy* 2003; 58:1206–1207.
76. Learning Early About Peanut Allergy [LEAP] (2007) *The LEAP Study*. Available at www.leapstudy.co.uk (Last accessed July 12, 2013).
77. EAT: enquiring about tolerance. Available at www.eatstudy.co.uk. (Last accessed March 22, 2012).
78. Saarinen UM, Kajosaari M. Does dietary elimination in infancy prevent or only postpone a food allergy? A study of fish and citrus allergy in 375 children. *Lancet* 1980; 1:166–167.
79. Strachan DP. Family size, infection and atopy: the first decade of the "hygiene hypothesis". *Thorax* 2000; 55(Suppl. 1):S2–S10.
80. Eggesbo M, Botten G, Stigum H, Nafstad P, Magnus P. Is delivery by cesarean section a risk factor for food allergy? *J Allergy Clin Immunol* 2003; 112:420–426.
81. Bager P, Wohlfahrt J, Westergaard T. Caesarean delivery and risk of atopy and allergic disease: meta-analyses. *Clin Exp Allergy* 2008; 38:634–642.
82. Bager P, Wohlfahrt J, Westergaard T. Caesarean delivery and risk of atopy and allergic disease: meta-analyses. *Clin Exp Allergy* 2008; 38:634–642.
83. Waser M, Michels KB, Bieli C, et al. Inverse association of farm milk consumption with asthma and allergy in rural and suburban populations across Europe. *Clin Exp Allergy* 2007; 37:661–670.
84. Sudo N, Sawamura S, Tanaka K, et al. The requirement of intestinal bacterial flora for the development of an IgE production system fully susceptible to oral tolerance induction. *J Immunol* 1997; 159:1739–1745.

85. Boyle RJ, Tang ML. The role of probiotics in the management of allergic disease. *Clin Exp Allergy* 2006; 36:568–576.
86. Kukkonen K, Savilahti E, Haahtela T, et al. Probiotics and prebiotic galacto-oligosaccharides in the prevention of allergic diseases: a randomized, double-blind, placebo-controlled trial. *J Allergy Clin Immunol* 2007, 119:192–198.
87. Pelucchi C, Chatenoud L, Turati F, et al. Probiotics supplementation during pregnancy or infancy for the prevention of atopic dermatitis: a meta-analysis. *Epidemiology* 2012; 23(3):402–414.
88. Kalliomaki M, Salminen S, Poussa T, Arvilommi H, Isolauri E. Probiotics and prevention of atopic disease: 4-year follow-up of a randomised placebo-controlled trial. *Lancet* 2003; 361:1869–1871.
89. Boyle RJ, Robins-Browne RM, Tang ML. Probiotic use in clinical practice: what are the risks?. *Am J Clin Nutr* 2006; 83:1256–1264.
90. Heinrich J, Holscher B, Bolte G, Winkler G. Allergic sensitization and diet: ecological analysis in selected European cities. *Eur Respir J* 2001; 17:395–402.
91. Anandan C, Nurmatov U, Sheikh A. Omega 3 and 6 oils for primary prevention of allergic disease: systematic review and meta-analysis. *Allergy* 2009; 64:840–848.
92. Peat JK, Mihrshahi S, Kemp AS, et al. Three-year outcomes of dietary fatty acid modification and house dust mite reduction in the Childhood Asthma Prevention Study. *J Allergy Clin Immunol* 2004; 114:807–813.
93. Kull I, Bergstrom A, Lilja G, Pershagen G, Wickman M. Fish consumption during the first year of life and development of allergic diseases during childhood. *Allergy* 2006; 61:1009–1015.
94. Almqvist C, Garden F, Xuan W, et al. Omega-3 and omega-6 fatty acid exposure from early life does not affect atopy and asthma at age 5 years. *J Allergy Clin Immunol* 2007; 119:1438–1444.
95. Anandan C, Nurmatov U, Sheikh A. Omega 3 and 6 oils for primary prevention of allergic disease: systematic review and meta-analysis. *Allergy* 2009; 64:840–848.
96. Palmer DJ, Sullivan T, Gold MS, et al. Effect of n-3 long chain polyunsaturated fatty acid supplementation in pregnancy on infants' allergies in first year of life: randomised controlled trial. *BMJ* 2012; 344:e184.
97. Hypponen E, Laara E, Reunanen A, Jarvelin MR, Virtanen SM. Intake of vitamin D and risk of type 1 diabetes: a birth-cohort study. *Lancet* 2001; 358:1500–1503.
98. Milner JD, Stein DM, McCarter R, Moon RY. Early infant multivitamin supplementation is associated with increased risk for food allergy and asthma. *Pediatrics* 2004; 114:27–32.
99. Wjst M. Another explanation for the low allergy rate in the rural Alpine foothills. *Clin Mol Allergy* 2005; 3:7.
100. Hypponen E, Sovio U, Wjst M, et al. Infant vitamin D supplementation and allergic conditions in adulthood: Northern Finland birth cohort 1966. *Ann N Y Acad Sci* 2004; 1037:84–95.
101. Camargo Jr CA, Clark S, Kaplan MS, Lieberman P, Wood RA. Regional differences in EpiPen prescriptions in the United States: the potential role of vitamin D. *J Allergy Clin Immunol* 2007; 120:131–136.
102. Vassallo MF, Banerji A, Rudders SA, et al. Season of birth and food allergy in children. *Ann Allergy Asthma Immunol* 2010; 104:307–313.
103. Nwaru BI, Ahonen S, Kalia M, et al. Maternal diet during pregnancy and allergic sensitization in the offspring by 5 yrs of age: a prospective cohort study. *Pediatr Allergy Immunol* 2010; 21:29–37.
104. Kull I, Bergstrom A, Melen E, et al. Early-life supplementation of vitamins A and D, in water-soluble form or in peanut oil, and allergic diseases during childhood. *J Allergy Clin Immunol* 2006; 118:1299–1304.
105. Allan K, Kelly FJ, Devereux G. Antioxidants and allergic disease: a case of too little or too much?. *Clin Exp Allergy* 2010; 40:370–380.
106. Shaheen SO, Newson RB, Henderson AJ, et al. Umbilical cord trace elements and minerals and risk of early childhood wheezing and eczema. *Eur Respir J* 2004; 24:292–297.
107. Visness CM, London SJ, Daniels JL, et al. Association of obesity with IgE levels and allergy symptoms in children and adolescents: results from the National Health and Nutrition Examination Survey 2005–2006. *J Allergy Clin Immunol* 2009; 123:1163–1169.
108. Turcanu V, Maleki SJ, Lack G. Characterization of lymphocyte responses to peanuts in normal children, peanut-allergic children, and allergic children who acquired tolerance to peanuts. *J Clin Invest* 2003; 111:1065–1072.

39 Diets and Nutrition

Marion Groetch

The Elliot and Roslyn Jaffe Food Allergy Institute, Division of Allergy and Immunology, Department of Pediatrics, Icahn School of Medicine at Mount Sinai, New York, NY, USA

Key Concepts

- Food Allergen Labeling and Consumer Protection Act of 2004 (FALCPA)—FALCPA mandates the labeling of all food ingredients derived from commonly allergenic foods in the United States.
- World Allergy Organization (WAO) Diagnosis and Rationale for Action against Cow's Milk Allergy (DRACMA) Guidelines—consensus guidelines for the management of cow's milk allergy.
- Dietary reference intakes (DRI)—a set of reference values of nutrient intakes that not only prevent nutritional deficiencies, but also reduce the risk of chronic disease.
- Allergen avoidance is currently the cornerstone of food allergy management.
- The ability to accurately identify food allergens on product labels is fundamental to the success of allergen avoidance.
- Comprehensive nutrition education should include how to avoid the allergen and how to safely and appropriately substitute for eliminated foods and the nutrients in those foods.
- Children with food allergies may be at greater risk of inadequate growth and suboptimal nutrition and therefore require more stringent monitoring of growth and nutritional status.

Introduction

At this time there are no available prophylactic agents that have been consistently shown to prevent IgE-mediated reactions to food [1–3]. Therapeutic options that target specific foods or block the allergic response are under investigation but continue to require further study to assess safety and efficacy [4, 5]. Although hopeful treatment options are being explored, dietary avoidance continues to be the mainstay for the prevention of food-allergic reactions. The increasing prevalence of atopic disease presents a growing need for healthcare professionals who can effectively manage the dietary needs of those with food hypersensitivity.

As food elimination diets pose a challenge to providing a nutritionally balanced diet, it is essential that they are prescribed only when needed for the treatment of a properly diagnosed food allergy or for diagnostic purposes for a defined period of time. It may seem an easy task to eliminate a single allergen from the diet. However, the elimination of a single allergen, such as milk protein, makes it necessary to avoid many common foods including not only milk, butter, cheese, yogurt, and ice cream, but also numerous manufactured products such as many breads, cookies, cakes, crackers, cereals, processed meats, and cold cuts that may also contain milk protein as an ingredient. Additionally, the prescription of an elimination diet places a great burden on patients and their families. The social, psychological, financial, and nutritional impact of such a dietary prescription must be measured against the necessity or potential benefit of treatment. The time required for meal planning and food preparation may be greatly increased. Eating out in restaurants or friends' homes may become difficult or impossible, which may impact the socialization of the individual. Moreover, there are costs associated with the purchase of specialty allergen-free foods. Anxiety issues may arise about food and eating situations in general. In children, the acquisition of feeding skills may be delayed when food elimination diets present challenges to finding safe and appropriate textures required in developing oral motor feeding skills. Finally,

Food Allergy: Adverse Reactions to Foods and Food Additives, Fifth Edition. Edited by Dean D Metcalfe, Hugh A Sampson, Ronald A Simon and Gideon Lack.

food elimination diets may impact nutrient intake, and great care must be taken to ensure that the restricted diet continues to provide adequate nutrition. Comprehensive education should include not only how to avoid specific allergens, but also how to safely and appropriately substitute for eliminated foods and the nutrients inherent in those foods.

Label reading

Fundamental to the success of any elimination diet is the ability to accurately identify food allergens on product labels. The United States (US) National Institute of Allergy and Infectious Diseases Food Allergy Guidelines suggests that those with food allergy receive education and training on how to interpret ingredient lists on food labels and how to recognize labeling of the food allergens used as ingredients in foods [3]. Allergen labeling laws are country specific. Table 39.1 lists those foods, by country, considered "major allergens," hence requiring full disclosure on product labels.

In the United States, the Food Allergen Labeling and Consumer Protection Act of 2004, or FALCPA, mandates that food products clearly list on the package label, in plain English language, ingredients derived from commonly allergenic foods. Conventional food products, including those imported for sale in the United States, dietary supplements, infant formulas, and medical foods are all affected by FALCPA; raw agricultural commodities (meats, fruits, and vegetables) and medications are not. FALCPA requires any regulated product manufactured for sale in the United States (even those manufactured outside the country) to comply with the labeling law [6].

The ingredients subject to FALCPA, identified as the major food allergens, are those derived from these eight major food allergens:

- Milk
- Egg
- Soybean
- Wheat (but not other gluten-containing grains)
- Peanut
- Tree nut
- Fish
- Crustacean shellfish

Additionally, manufacturers must list the specific tree nut (almond, Brazil nut, cashew, hazelnut, pecan, pistachio, walnut, etc.), fish (salmon, tuna, cod, etc.), or crustacean shellfish (crab, lobster, shrimp, etc.) used as an ingredient. Mollusks (clam, muscles, oyster, scallops, etc.) are not considered major food allergens under FALCPA [6]. And while wheat is subject to full disclosure under FALCPA, other gluten-containing grains are not, which may pose a problem to individuals who are clinically reactive to other gluten-containing grains such as barley, rye, or other hybrid strains.

Prior to January 2006, ingredients could be listed by their scientific or usual name, such as casein, albumin, or whey, without any reference to the source of the ingredient, making identification of allergens difficult for the consumer. The plain language stipulation requires the presence of a major food allergen to be listed on the product label in one of the following ways:

1. In the ingredient list, for example, milk, egg, or soy.

2. Parenthetically in the ingredient list following the food protein derivative, for example, casein (milk).

3. Immediately below the ingredient list in a "contains" statement, for example, *Contains: wheat* [6, 7].

Table 39.1 Food allergen labeling major allergens by country.

Country	United States	Canada	European Union	Australia & New Zealand
Major allergens	Milk	Milk	Milk	Milk
	Egg	Egg	Egg	Egg
	Wheat	Gluten-containing grains	Gluten-containing grains	Gluten-containing grains
	Soy	Soy	Soy	Soy
	Peanut	Peanut	Peanut	Peanut
	Tree nuts	Tree nuts	Tree nuts	Tree nuts
	Fish	Fish	Fish	Fish
	Crustacean Shellfish	Crustacean shellfish	Crustacean shellfish	Crustacean shellfish
	Sulfites are not covered under FALCPA but they are covered under the Code of Federal Regulations in amounts of >10 mg/kg in the finished food (including sulfites in alcoholic beverages).	Mollusks	Mollusks	Sesame
		Sesame	Sesame	
		Mustard	Mustard	
		Sulfites >10 mg/kg	Lupine	
			Celery	
			Sulfites >10 mg/kg	

FALCPA, Food Allergen Labeling and Consumer Protection Act of 2004.

Foods and ingredients requiring full disclosure and considered major allergens based on legal standards of country/countries represented.

Only one of these methods is required and therefore consumers should be cautioned to avoid looking only for "contains" statements. However, if a "contains" statement is used and multiple major allergens are present in a product, they must all be listed in the "contains" statement even if one or more of the allergens were listed elsewhere on the label. For example, if casein, egg white, and almond are listed in the ingredient list, a "contains" statement would be necessary as casein was not identified as milk. The "contains" statement must, however, list all of the ingredients derived from major allergens; therefore, the following statement must be included on the label: *"Contains milk, egg, and almond"* [8].

Additionally, a major food allergen may not be omitted from the product label if it is only an incidental ingredient such as in a spice, flavoring, coloring, or additive, or used merely as a processing aid in a product [6]. Consumers should be aware that these regulations apply only to ingredients derived from the foods that are considered the major allergens. An individual with sensitivity to an ingredient not covered under FALCPA, such as mustard, garlic, or sesame would still need to call the manufacturer to ascertain if mustard, garlic, sesame, or sesame oil was included as an ingredient in a spice or natural flavoring of a product.

While it is likely that thresholds exist below which the vast majority of allergic individuals would not react, there is no consensus established on thresholds for many allergens at this time [7, 9, 10]. In addition, variability in individual threshold doses occurs as some people are clearly more sensitive than others to the same food allergen. This makes it difficult to determine whether an ingredient with a very low risk of allergenicity should be included on a product label. So while an ingredient may be derived from an allergenic source, it may contain insignificant amounts of the allergenic protein. One example would be lecithin, which may be derived from soy, but is generally tolerated by most individuals with soy allergy due to the low levels of allergenic protein and the minute amount of ingredient use in any given product. Another example is kosher gelatin, derived from fish, which has a very low relative allergenicity [7, 9]. In the United States, soy lecithin and gelatin derived from fish must be fully disclosed as soy and fish (more specifically, as the species of fish), respectively, on product labels. Currently, FALCPA allows for highly refined vegetable oils derived from major food allergens (including soy and peanut) to be exempt from the labeling requirement since highly refined oils have almost complete removal of allergenic protein and have not been shown to pose a risk to human health [6–8].

In European countries, the EU directive 2003/89/EC requires that 14 common food allergens be clearly identified on the ingredient label of all packaged foods. The 14 allergens required to be fully disclosed on package labels in the European Union are the following:

- Milk
- Egg
- Peanut
- Tree nuts
- Lupine
- Fish
- Crustacean shell fish
- Mollusks
- Soybean
- Gluten (wheat, rye, barley, oat, spelt, kamut, and their hybrid strains)
- Celery
- Mustard
- Sesame
- Sulfur dioxide and sulfites at concentrations of 10 mg/kg or 10 mg/l expressed as SO_2 or more.

Very similar to the US labeling laws, all intentional sources of the 14 common allergens, regardless of whether or not the ingredient is part of a compound ingredient, must be identified on the ingredient label. The EU directive applies to all prepackaged food but does not apply to foods sold loose or foods prepacked for direct sale such as freshly made bread or cakes sold in supermarkets in which they have been packaged for hygienic purposes, foods sold in restaurants, or fancy confectionery products [7, 11].

FALCPA and the EU directive do not yet address the issue of cross-contact, which is the presence of unintentional ingredients in manufactured products. Products may unintentionally come in contact with a potential allergen during customary methods of growing and harvesting crops, or from the use of shared storage, transportation, or production equipment, which may lead to significant levels of allergens in the product without any identification on the label. Many manufacturers address this issue of unintentional ingredients with precautionary labeling such as "may contain (allergen)" or "produced in a facility that also produces (allergen)." These statements, which are voluntary and unregulated, are appearing on more and more food product labels making the addition of many manufactured foods in the diet of individuals with food allergies quite difficult [12]. The voluntary nature of these labels means the absence of a precautionary statement does not necessarily mean there is no risk of cross-contact with the product. Furthermore, precautionary labeling is unregulated meaning it is not possible to assess the degree of risk based on the type of precautionary label used. So while "may contain peanut" certainly sounds riskier than "manufactured in a facility that manufactures peanuts," this is not necessarily the case [13]. The US Food Allergy Guidelines suggest advising our patients to avoid products that carry a precautionary statement for their allergen [3]. Regarding products without precautionary labeling, calling the manufacturer to discuss cross-contact risk may be prudent depending on the allergen and the patient's sensitivity [12]. For a more detailed discussion on precautionary labels and the potential presence of hidden allergens in foods, see Chapter 25.

Food preparation safety

Individuals with food allergies must be diligent about risk assessment of all food purchased and consumed. Cross-contamination also occurs outside of the manufacturing industry. It may occur in the home during food preparation as well as while eating out. Meals for the family member with allergies should be prepared first, covered, and removed from the cooking area. Then the other foods for the home may be prepared. The food preparation should be done in a clean environment with clean utensils, cooking surfaces, and cooking equipment. Those with food allergies are especially at risk while dining out since restaurants are not required to list ingredients and the servers are not typically well informed regarding the ingredients in a dish. Cross-contact is common such as when the same grill is used to make a cheese burger that was used for a plain hamburger, or the French fries might have been cooked in the same fryer as the coconut shrimp. The same tongs may be used to assemble the green salad as is used to assemble the salad with walnuts. Certain restaurants would be considered higher risk for those with certain food allergies. For instance, for those with peanut, tree nut, or soy allergy, Asian restaurants may pose greater risk due to the high occurrence of these foods in the kitchen and cooking equipment and utensils are not frequently washed between preparations of different orders. Another example would be a seafood restaurant for those with fish allergy. Cross-contact may be a risk even if a non-seafood dish is ordered. Additionally, sensitive individuals have been exposed through inhalation of cooking vapors [14]. Consumers should be taught to speak directly to the food service or restaurant manager to inquire about ingredients and cross-contact risk. They should feel confident that the restaurant staff understands the severity of their food allergy as well as how to prepare a safe meal and be willing to leave the restaurant if they do not feel confident that a safe meal can be prepared.

Resources

Beyond label reading, families must learn to manage the food allergy in all aspects of daily living. The Consortium of Food Allergy Research (CoFAR) has developed an extensive food allergy education program, which has been validated to show high rates of satisfaction and effectiveness with parents in a longitudinal study [15]. The program contains fact sheets on various food-allergic disorders, allergen avoidance sheets, and handouts on numerous food allergy management topics for patients such as eating in restaurants, avoiding cross-contact, cooking without allergens, managing food allergies in schools and camps, introducing foods to children with allergies, nutrition, label reading, food allergy prevention, and more. The website also contains an 8-minute food allergy management video. These excellent, patient educational materials are free and downloadable at www.cofargroup.org.

Food Allergy Research & Education or FARE (www.foodallergy.org) is a nonprofit organization whose mission is to raise public awareness, to provide advocacy and education, and to advance research on behalf of those affected by food allergies and anaphylaxis. Their medical advisory board ensures accuracy of information provided. FARE is a valuable resource for patients with food allergies and their families providing a wealth of information and resources including conferences, newsletters, recipes, cookbooks, videos, and DVDs including a comprehensive food allergy school education program. This program is a multimedia resource for school nurses and administrators to conduct in-service training on how to safely and effectively manage food allergies and anaphylaxis in the school environment.

Nutrition

The nutrient needs of each individual must be determined and a plan devised to meet those needs within the context of the allergen-restricted diet. In general, there is no good evidence describing altered nutritional needs in individuals with food allergies compared to their nonallergic peers. An exception would be the patient with severe atopic dermatitis who may have increased energy and protein needs due to loses through the compromised skin barrier and energy required for repair [16, 17]. Other altered nutritional states such as increased protein needs for individuals whose food allergies contribute to protein losing enteropathy may be more apparent. In general, however, the food-allergic individual is at greater nutritional risk primarily due to the restrictions in the diet.

Dietary reference intakes

The Food and Nutrition Board of the National Academy of Science establishes *dietary reference intakes* or the DRIs. The DRIs contain four distinct nutrient-based reference values: estimated average requirement (EAR), recommended dietary allowance (RDA), adequate intake (AI), and tolerable upper intake level (UL). DRIs are established for vitamins, minerals, energy, and macronutrients such as dietary fat, fatty acids, protein, amino acids, carbohydrates, sugars, and dietary fibers and provide reference values of nutrient intakes that not only prevent nutritional deficiencies, but also reduce the risk of chronic diseases such as osteoporosis, cancer, and cardiovascular disease.

Recommended dietary allowance

The RDA is the average daily dietary nutrient intake level sufficient to meet the nutrient requirement of nearly all healthy individuals (97–98%) in a particular life stage and gender group [18].

Adequate intake

The AI is the recommended average daily intake level based on observed or experimentally determined approximations or estimates of nutrient intake by a group (or groups) of apparently healthy people that are assumed to be adequate. The AI is used when an RDA cannot be determined and when sufficient scientific evidence is not available to derive an EAR. The AI is set at a level thought to meet or exceed the needs of virtually all members of a life stage and gender group. Therefore, in assessing individuals, if intake usually meets or exceeds the AI, a conclusion can be made that dietary intake is adequate. On the other hand, if intake regularly falls below the AI, prevalence of inadequacy cannot be determined as AI is set to meet or *exceed* the needs of most people [18, 19].

Tolerable upper intake level

The UL is the highest average daily nutrient intake level that is likely to pose no risk of adverse health effects to almost all individuals in the general population. As intake increases above the UL, the potential risk of adverse effects also increases [18].

Estimate average requirement

The EAR is the average daily nutrient intake level estimated to meet the requirement of half the healthy individuals in a particular life stage and gender group. The EAR exceeds the requirements of half the group and falls below the requirements of the other half as the EAR is actually the median requirement rather than the average [18, 19].

Estimated energy requirement (EER), defined below, is a reference value used specifically for energy needs.

Energy

The EER is the average dietary energy intake that is predicted to maintain energy balance in a healthy adult for a defined age, gender, weight, height, and level of physical activity consistent with good health. In children and pregnant or lactating women, the EER includes the needs associated with the deposition of tissues or the secretion of milk at rates consistent with good health. There is no established RDA for energy because energy intakes exceeding the EER would be expected to result in excessive weight gain. EER can be calculated using the equations provided in the DRI reports and can be found at www.nap.edu.

In individuals with food allergy, dietary boredom and severely restrictive diets may contribute to inadequate energy intake. Additionally, certain food-allergic disorders, such as eosinophilic gastrointestinal disorders, may negatively affect appetite or contribute to early satiety, hence impacting adequate energy intake [20, 21].

Energy is provided in the diet through three major classes of substrates or macronutrients, which are proteins, carbohydrates, and fats. Alcohol, another source of energy in the diet, will not be addressed here.

Protein

Many commonly allergenic foods are also excellent sources of protein: these include milk, egg, soy, fish, peanut, and tree nuts. Diets must be carefully planned to meet protein needs when high-quality protein sources are eliminated from the diet. The Food and Nutrition Board has set acceptable macronutrient distribution ranges (AMDR) for protein (and all macronutrients), which have been provided in Table 39.2. An AMDR is defined as "a range of intakes for a particular energy source that is associated with a reduced risk of chronic disease while providing adequate intake of essential nutrients" [18]. Dietary protein needs may also be estimated using the DRI, which can be found in Table 39.3.

In assessing adequacy of protein in the diet, quality and quantity of dietary protein needs to be considered as well as total energy intake as dietary protein recommendations are based on the assumption that energy intake is adequate [18]. Amino acids liberated from dietary proteins are oxidized for energy, incorporated into protein in the body, or used for the formation of other nitrogen-containing compounds. There is an interrelation between

Table 39.2 Acceptable macronutrient distribution range.[a]

Age	Carbohydrate	Protein	Fat	EFA n-3	EFA n-6
Children					
1–3 yr	45–65	5–20	30–40	0.6–1.2	5–10
4–18 yr	45–65	10–30	25–35	0.6–1.2	5–10
Adults	45–65	10–35	20–35	0.6–1.2	5–10

Source: Dietary reference intakes for energy, carbohydrate, fiber, fat, fatty acids, cholesterol, protein, and amino acids (2002/2005). The entire report is available at www.nap.edu.

AMDR, acceptable macronutrient distribution range; EFA, essential fatty acid; RDA, recommended dietary allowance; AI, adequate intake

[a]AMDR is the range of intake for a particular energy source, expressed as a percentage of total caloric intake that is associated with reduced risk of chronic disease while providing intakes of essential nutrients.

For infants, AMDR have not been established due to insufficient data regarding adverse effects of excess intakes but an RDA or AI has been established for these nutrients.

Table 39.3 Dietary reference intakes for dietary protein.

Age/life stage (group)	RDA (g/kg body weight/day)
Infants	
0–6 mo	1.5[a]
7–12 mo	1.5
Children	
1–3 yr	1.1
4–13 yr	0.95
14–18 yr	0.85
Adults	
18 yr	0.80
Pregnancy	1.1
Lactation	1.1

Source: Dietary reference intakes for energy, carbohydrate, fiber, fat, fatty acids, cholesterol, protein, and amino acids (2002/2005). The entire report is available at www.nap.edu.
[a]Adequate intake.

Table 39.4 Dietary reference intakes for dietary fat and EFAs in infants.

Age	Omega-3 EFA AI (g/day)	Omega-6 EFA AI (g/day)	Total fat AI (g/day)
Infant			
0–6 mo	0.5	4.4	31
7–12 mo	0.5	4.6	30

Source: Dietary reference intakes for energy, carbohydrate, fiber, fat, fatty acids, cholesterol, protein, and amino acids (2002/2005). The entire report is available at www.nap.edu.
EFA, essential fatty acid; AI, adequate intake.

energy needs and protein needs. If energy intake is insufficient, free amino acids will be oxidized for energy, allowing for less available amino acids for anabolic and synthetic pathways [22].

The quality of dietary protein will also impact nitrogen balance. Proteins are composed of amino acids and those amino acids that cannot be biosynthesized by enzymatic pathways are termed indispensable. These indispensable amino acids (IAAs) must be provided through the diet. An estimated 65–70% of protein needs should be of high biological value meaning those that contain a full complement of all IAAs. Animal products are considered high biological value proteins, although they are not necessary to provide optimal proteins. Most alternative sources from plants, legumes, grains, nuts, seeds, and vegetables do not contain a full complement of IAAs and therefore greater dietary planning will be required as plant foods are generally lower in protein content and one or more amino acids. Ensuring a mixture of plant foods eaten throughout the day is required to provide the complementary amino acids necessary.

Fat

Dietary fats provide energy and serve as a carrier for the absorption of fat-soluble vitamins. Adequate fat in the diet is also necessary to provide the fatty acids that are considered essential for human health. While too much fat can negatively impact health, a certain amount of fat is essential. The type of fat as well as the total amount of fat consumed will determine whether fat intake is appropriate and healthful.

Table 39.2 provides the AMDR of dietary fat as a percentage of total energy intakes. An AMDR for infants has not been established but the AI for total fat for infants 0–6 months of age is 31 g/day and for infants 7–12 months of age is 30 g/day and can be found in Table 39.4 [18]. Intakes below 20% of total caloric intake increase risk of hypocaloric, vitamin E deficient, and essential fatty acid (EFA) deficient diets while intakes greater than 35% (except in children younger than 3 years) are not recommended as they will likely increase intake of saturated fat and calories.

Dietary fats are largely present in the triacylglycerol (triglyceride) form, which consists of three fatty acids and a glycerol molecule. Fatty acids can be either saturated, polyunsaturated, monounsaturated, or present as trans fatty acids. Although some trans fatty acids occur naturally, they are predominantly present in our food supply through hydrogenated oils in margarines, cookies, cakes, crackers, and other snack foods. Saturated fatty acids are found in full fat dairy products, fatty meats, and tropical oils such as coconut and palm kernel oil. Individuals should consume predominantly polyunsaturated and monounsaturated fat sources since there is no required dietary role for saturated and trans fatty acids.

Unsaturated fatty acids can have either one (monounsaturated or MUFA) or more (polyunsaturated or PUFA) double bonds on the carbon chain. PUFAs are further categorized on the basis of the location of the first double bond. Human cells can introduce double bonds in all positions on the fatty acid chain except the omega-3 (n-3) and the omega-6 (n-6) positions hence the n-3 α-linolenic acid (ALA) and the n-6 linoleic acid (LA) are considered essential and must be provided through the diet. EFA are metabolized to their long chain metabolites, arachidonic acid, and dihomo-g-linolenic acid from LA, and eicosapentaenoic acid and docohexaenoic acid from ALA. These long chain metabolites form precursors to respective prostaglandins, thromboxanes, and leukotrienes that regulate a large number of vital functions in the body, including blood pressure, blood clotting, blood lipid levels, the immune response, and the inflammation response to injury and infection [22, 23].

EFA deficiency is rare and the challenge to all people including those with food allergies is finding a healthy balance between the two EFAs. There has been an increased interest in n-3 fatty acids as several lines of research have suggested that a high ratio of n-6 to n-3 fatty acids may contribute to a number of chronic diseases [24]. LA or n-6 fatty acid is generally provided abundantly in the diet and found in a wide variety of vegetable oils including safflower, sunflower, soy, grapeseed, and corn oils. ALA is less abundantly found and the sources tend to be from more commonly allergenic foods. Dietary sources that provide 10% or more of the RDA/AI for ALA or n-3 fatty acids are fish, fish oils, canola or rapeseed oil, soybean oil, flaxseed, pumpkin seeds, walnuts, and wheat germ [22].

The FNB has set AMDR for dietary fat and EFAs for individuals 1 year of age and older, which can be found in Table 39.2. There is no determined AMDR for dietary fat or EFAs for infants up to 12 months of age, but the AI is set to meet the requirement for neural development and growth and can be found in Table 39.3 [18]. AIs for the EFAs, which vary by age group and sex, as well as during pregnancy and lactation, can be accessed in the DRI reports at www.nap.edu [18].

Dietary fat is an important source of energy, supports the transport of fat-soluble vitamins, and provides the two fatty acids that are essential in the human diet. Maintaining a healthy balance of dietary fats including n-3 to n-6 fatty acids may pose a challenge to those with food allergies as the primary sources or n-3 fatty acids are from commonly allergenic foods. For individual with food allergies, and especially children with food allergies, adequate fat intake may be compromised due to dietary restrictions. The addition of vegetable oils to the allergen-restricted diet may be required to meet fat and EFA needs. The amount and type of oil required will need to be individualized based on current dietary intake and degree and type of dietary restrictions.

Carbohydrates

Carbohydrates make up the remaining energy sources and are an important supply of numerous micronutrients. The AMDR for carbohydrate is between 45% and 65% of total caloric intake [18]. The RDA is based on carbohydrates role as the primary source of energy for the brain and is set at 130 g/day for children and adults 1 year of age or older. The AI established for infants 0–6 months and for infants 7–12 months is 60 and 95 g of carbohydrates daily, respectively [18]. Grains, fruits, and vegetables provide dietary carbohydrates. Foods with added sugars also contribute carbohydrates and additional energy, but are of little further nutritional benefit and should be limited to no more than 25% of total energy intake [18]. Adequate carbohydrate intake prevents ketosis and excessive intake of dietary fats while contributing to AI of dietary fiber. Individuals with grain allergies may have an especially difficult time ingesting sufficient carbohydrates and dietary fiber.

Micronutrients

Variety in the diet contributes to adequacy of all nutrients provided. When a food group is eliminated, many nutrients provided by that food group must now be provided by other dietary sources. While it is important to ensure an appropriate intake of all essential nutrients, certain nutrients will be at greater risk of insufficiency depending on the food allergen. Table 39.6 lists the specific nutrients provided by a food or food group. Patients eliminating foods from their diet should, at minimum, be screened for adequacy of those nutrients lost to the elimination diet. Alternative dietary sources of these nutrients are provided in Tables 39.7 and 39.8.

When dietary modifications are inadequate to meet vitamin, mineral, and trace element needs, appropriate supplementation may be considered. Healthcare professionals should be aware that dietary supplements may contain allergenic ingredients and they should be chosen carefully with consideration for safe ingredients as well as risk assessment of potential cross-contact during manufacturing.

Pediatric nutrition

A special focus on the nutritional status of children with food allergies is warranted as food allergy and multiple food allergies are more prevalent in the pediatric population. Salman et al. reviewed nutrient intakes of children with food allergies and noted that several nutrients including calcium, vitamin D, vitamin E, iron, and zinc were insufficiently provided [25]. There are numerous reports of poor growth in children with milk allergy or multiple food allergies [26–28]. Christie et al. reported children with cow's milk allergy (CMA) or two or more food allergies were shorter, based on height-for-age percentiles than those without allergy or only one food allergy. Furthermore, children with CMA or multiple food allergies consumed dietary calcium less than age- and gender-specific recommendations compared with children without CMA and/or one food allergy [26]. Vitamin D deficiency in children in the United States and other developed nations in general has been reported with increasing frequency over the last 30 years [29, 30]. Furthermore, children on milk-free diets have been shown to have significantly lower intakes of energy, fat, protein, calcium, and riboflavin [31].

Since children with food allergies are at greater risk of inadequate growth and suboptimal nutrition, physicians may need to screen these patients more carefully, and refer them for nutritional counseling at the first signs of growth faltering, rather than take a "wait and see" position. Interventions aimed at meeting the distinct nutritional needs of children are imperative as poor nutrition may adversely affect growth and development, and nutrition counseling may significantly improve nutritional intake. The US Food Allergy Guidelines recommend nutrition counseling and close growth monitoring for all children with food allergies [3].

Growth in the pediatric population is a sensitive indicator of the provision of adequate energy and protein. Individual micronutrient deficiencies may not be reflected in growth alone, certainly not in the short term, and therefore the measurement and assessment of growth is only one aspect of the nutrition assessment. In addition to growth, the nutrition-focused physical assessment, biochemical indices, clinical diagnoses, and dietary intake including the frequency, amount and type of feeding, allergies and intolerances, food aversions and preferences the use of supplemental formula, dietary supplements, and medications must all be taken into consideration in the nutrition assessment.

Pediatricians generally track a patient's growth from birth and therefore have the best information regarding the child's growth patterns. A child's current weight gives an incomplete picture. Current weight needs to be compared to reference standards as well as to typical growth patterns for that child. Plotting a child's weight history on the appropriate growth chart provides a way to assess individual growth velocity and compare the growth of that child with a healthy reference population. In the United States, there are two sets of growth curves available. The World Health Organization (WHO) charts describe children raised in optimal environmental and health conditions, including 100% being breastfed until 12 months of age and exclusive or predominant breastfeeding until 4 months of age. The Centers for Disease Control (CDC) charts are a growth reference, not a standard, and describe the growth of children in the United States during a specific period of time (1963–1994). The U.S. CDC recommends that clinicians in the United States use the 2006 WHO international growth charts, rather than the CDC growth charts, for children younger than 24 months (available at https://www.cdc.gov/growthcharts) [32]. The 2.3rd and 97.7th percentiles (or ±2 standard deviations) are to be used with the WHO charts to screen for abnormal or unhealthy growth. The CDC growth charts should be used for children 2–19 years of age and the 5th and 95th percentiles are to be used with the CDC growth charts to screen for abnormal or unhealthy growth, although additional screening criteria are also used to assess for overweight. The recommendation to use the 2006 WHO international growth charts for children younger than 24 months is based on several considerations including the recognition that breastfeeding is the recommended standard for infant feeding. In the United Kingdom, the UK Department of Health has recommended use of the WHO growth standards for children 2 weeks to 5 years in combination with the UK birth weight charts [32].

Physical growth is an important indicator of health and adequate nutrition in infants and children. Clinicians should know how to interpret growth on these charts. Practitioners should be aware that healthy breastfed infants typically gain weight faster than formula-fed infants during the first 3 months of life. This is reflected in the WHO growth curve so a formula-fed infant may be perceived to have poor growth at this stage. On the other hand, the healthy breastfed infant gains weight more slowly during 3–18 months of age, so will maintain his growth curve percentile on the WHO chart but decrease in percentages on the CDC chart. This is a normal pattern of growth for breastfeeding infants so fewer US children will be identified as underweight using the WHO charts. This is important to prevent overdiagnosis of underweight, which may subject families to unnecessary interventions (such as weaning or supplemental feedings), stress, and potential damage to the parent–child feeding relationship [32].

While weight is the most sensitive measure of adequate energy intake and is affected earlier and to a greater extent than stature by dietary inadequacies, stature can be delayed due to dietary protein inadequacy or chronic energy deficits. Children younger than 2 years should have their length measured in the supine position and plotted on the WHO growth curve. Children 2 years of age or older should have a standing height measured and plotted on the CDC growth curve for children 2–20 years of age. A supine length is actually greater than a standing height; therefore, if a child is measured standing but plotted on the wrong growth chart, he will appear to be shorter. Accuracy in measurement is imperative for these assessment tools to be useful. In a randomized-controlled intervention trial of 878 children in 55 pediatric facilities, the reported accuracy of growth measurements was only 30% [33]. Body mass index (BMI), defined as weight in kilograms divided by the square of height in meters, may be used after 2 years of age on the CDC growth curves and is helpful as it takes into consideration weight for height. The CDC defined underweight in children as a BMI of less than the 5th percentile. Children are considered to be overweight when their BMI is between the 85th and 94th percentile and obese when their BMI is greater than the 95th percentile [34].

When to refer a patient to a registered dietitian for nutritional assessment is a frequent question. The consequences of inadequate nutrition due to allergen-restricted diets in the pediatric population warrant closer monitoring of growth by pediatricians since this population is at greater risk of growth failure that may be corrected with dietary intervention. Significant changes in growth velocity are not expected as normal development typically follows predictable increases in both height and weight. The effects of chronic undernutrition in children affect not only growth, but also include decreased school performance, delayed bone age, and increased susceptibility to infections [18]. Chronic undernutrition (energy, protein, and essential fatty acids) and micronutrient deficiencies (vitamin C, alpha tocopherol, beta carotene, zinc, and selenium) may impair skin repair in children with atopic dermatitis [17, 35, 36]. Children should be referred upon diagnosis of any food allergy but especially when initiating milk or wheat avoidance or when two or more foods are being eliminated. The US Food Allergy Guidelines recommend nutritional counseling and close growth monitoring for all children with food allergy [3].

Lastly, while the pediatric population has specific nutritional needs related to adequate growth and development, any individual on a long-term elimination diet will benefit from nutritional counseling with scheduled follow-up visits to assess intake and ensure nutritional adequacy and complete allergen elimination.

Food allergens

As previously stated, eight foods are responsible for 90% of all food-allergic disorders worldwide [5]. These foods are milk, egg, soy, wheat, peanut, tree nuts, fish, and shellfish. In adults, the most common allergens are peanut, tree nut, fish, and shellfish. In children, the most common allergens are milk, egg, soy, wheat, and peanut with a large percentage of children developing clinical tolerance to milk, egg, wheat, and soy during childhood.

Cow's milk protein

Cow's milk protein allergy (CMA) usually begins in infancy and affects approximately 2–5.9% of the infant population [37]. Patients with CMA may develop gastrointestinal symptoms (32–60% of cases), skin symptoms (5–90% of cases), and anaphylaxis (0.8–9% of cases). CMA is responsible for up to 13% of fatal food-induced anaphylaxis [38]. CMA affects predominantly the pediatric population. Although previous studies indicated CMA typically resolves by 5 years of age, more recent research indicates that tolerance to cow's milk may not be acquired until much later. This may extend the period of time the patient is at risk of nutritional inadequacy due to milk avoidance. Nonetheless, approximately 80% of children with CMA will develop clinical tolerance by 16 years of age [39].

The breastfed infant with CMA may benefit from maternal avoidance of milk protein from the diet, since immunologically recognizable proteins from the maternal diet can be found in breast milk [40, 41]. The American Academy of Pediatrics (AAP) also advises vitamin D supplementation (400 IU) shortly after birth for all breastfed infants and infants who take less than 32 ounces of formula per day [37]. Over 90% of infants with CMA tolerate extensively hydrolyzed milk protein-based infant formulas and for those who continue to exhibit symptoms, an amino acid-based formula may be warranted. Both extensively hydrolyzed and amino acid-based formulas are considered hypoallergenic [40]. To be considered hypoallergenic, preclinical studies must demonstrate with a 95% confidence interval that 90% of infants with documented CMA will not react with defined symptoms to the formula under double blind, placebo-controlled conditions [40]. Soy formula may be an alternative to cow's milk formula although soy formula is not hypoallergenic. Many infants (85–90%) with IgE-associated CMA may tolerate soy formula and those infants who do not show hypersensitivity to soy when it is initially introduced usually continue to tolerate it very well [40]. The AAP suggests that soy formula may be suitable for infants with IgE-mediated CMA, especially after 6 months of age [37]. For infants with non-IgE-mediated milk protein allergy such as proctocolitis or enterocolitis syndrome, the prevalence of hypersensitivity to both soy and milk may be greater so a hypoallergenic formula would therefore be the first recommendation [40]. The World Allergy Organization (WAO) has developed guidelines for the Diagnosis and Rationale for Action against Cow's Milk Allergy (DRACMA) [37]. These guidelines provide substitute formula recommendations for infants with CMA who are not being exclusively breastfed depending on the present symptom(s) and/or the specific diagnosed food-allergic disorder. The DRACMA guidelines are provided in Table 39.5 [37]. Partially hydrolyzed cow's milk formulas are not considered hypoallergenic and are not a suitable option for infants with CMA. Additionally, alternative mammalian milks such as goat's or sheep's

Table 39.5 DRACMA formula recommendations for infants with cow's milk allergy.

Symptoms or allergic disorder	First formula recommendation	Second formula recommendation	Third formula recommendation
Low risk of anaphylaxis	Extensively hydrolyzed casein	Amino acid based	Soy
High risk of anaphylaxis	Amino acid based	Extensively hydrolyzed casein	Soy
Non-IgE (FPIES or proctocolitis)	Extensively hydrolyzed casein	Amino acid based	–
Eosinophilic esophagitis	Amino acid based	–	–
Heiner syndrome	Amino acid based	Extensively hydrolyzed casein	Soy

DRACMA, Diagnosis and Rationale for Action against Cow's Milk Allergy; FPIES, food protein-induced enterocolitis syndrome.

milk are not suitable, because up to 92% of individuals with CMAs will also react to these mammalian milks [40].

Transitioning an infant from a complete formula to a milk product generally occurs around 1 year of age or ideally when at least two-thirds of the total daily caloric intake comes from a varied solid food diet since a wide variety of foods will contribute to micronutrient adequacy. Additional criteria for the milk-allergic child must be considered, as the alternative milk source (soy, rice, oat, almond, coconut, hemp) may not provide needed nutrients, even if enriched. Furthermore, a varied dietary intake for children with multiple food allergies may not be possible. If soy is tolerated, enriched soymilk may present an appropriate alternative and will provide dietary calcium, vitamin D, and protein sources. For children with concomitant milk and soy allergy, other alternative enriched beverages may provide calcium and vitamin D, but may be very low in protein, fat, and other nutrients. The DRACMA guidelines recommend continuing on breast milk (with maternal calcium supplementation) or a substitute formula until 2 years of age to meet nutritional needs [37].

The nutritional impact of a milk allergy is great since milk is an excellent source of protein, calcium, vitamin D, phosphorus, vitamin A, vitamin B12, and riboflavin. Furthermore, cow's milk is not only a good source of calcium and vitamin D, but it is the primary source as well as a major contributor of protein in the diet of children. Milk protein is also an ingredient in many manufactured food products so there are convenience and social burdens placed on the milk-allergic individual. Table 39.6 lists nutrients supplied by cow's milk in the diet. Possible alternative dietary sources for these nutrients can be found in Tables 39.7 and 39.8.

Baked milk and egg

Up to 75% of children with CMA may tolerate extensively heated (baked) milk [42]. Tolerance of baked milk appears to be a marker of transient IgE-mediated CMA, whereas reactivity to baked milk may indicate a more persistent phenotype. Those patients who are proven to tolerate baked milk (by physician supervised oral food challenge) may include these ingredients in the diet. The inclusion of baked milk in the diet of those who tolerate it appears to accelerate the development of tolerance to unheated milk [42]. Additionally, it can improve the nutritional quality of the diet as well as open up a greater range of food products that contain baked milk ingredients. Similarly, baked egg may be tolerated by 75% of those with egg allergy and may also be included in the diets of those who tolerated it (as proven by physician supervised oral food challenge) [1, 43]. Patients should be educated as to how to

Table 39.6 Nutrient content of commonly allergenic foods.

Allergenic food	Nutrients
Milk	Protein, fat (for infants and young children), vitamin A, vitamin D, riboflavin, pantothenic acid, vitamin B12, calcium
Egg	Protein, vitamin B12, riboflavin, pantothenic acid, biotin, selenium
Soy	Protein, riboflavin, thiamine, phosphorus, folate, calcium, magnesium, iron, zinc, pyridoxine
Wheat	Thiamine, riboflavin, niacin, iron, and folate (if fortified)
Peanut	Protein, vitamin E, niacin, magnesium, manganese

Table 39.7 Dietary sources of vitamins.

Vitamin	Dietary sources
Vitamin A	Retinol: liver, egg yolk, fortified milk, cheese, butter, margarine Carotene: deep orange fruits and vegetables such apricot, cantaloupe, papaya, peach, mango, carrot, pumpkin, sweet potato; deep green leafy vegetables such as spinach, kale, collard greens; broccoli, Brussels sprouts, cauliflower, cabbage
Vitamin D	Vitamin D fortified milk and orange juice, fortified alternative milk beverages (soy, rice, oat, almond, hemp, coconut, etc.), liver, fatty fish and fish liver oils. Some, but not all, ready to eat cereals and yogurts are also fortified.
Vitamin E	Polyunsaturated vegetable oils (sunflower, safflower, canola, corn, olive), nuts, seeds, green leafy vegetables, wheat germ
Biotin	Liver, egg yolk, green leafy vegetables, peanuts
Thiamine	Pork, whole and enriched grains and cereals, legumes, potatoes
Riboflavin	Milk and dairy products, some fortified/enriched alternative milk beverages (soy, rice, oat, almond, hemp, coconut) organ meats, whole and enriched grains and cereals
Niacin	Meat, fish, poultry, whole and enriched grains and cereals, nuts and legumes
Pyridoxine (B6)	Fish, organ meats, meats, potatoes, bananas, enriched grains and cereals, chick peas
Cyanocobalamin (B12)	Animal products (meats, fish, poultry, milk and dairy products, eggs); fortified cereals, fortified alternative milk beverages (soy, rice, oat, almond, hemp, coconut)
Folic acid	Liver, green leafy vegetables, oranges, legumes, seeds, enriched grains and cereals, wheat germ
Pantothenic acid	Egg, meats, milk, broccoli, kale, mushrooms, sweet potatoes, avocado, lentils, whole grains
Biotin	Liver, cooked egg, pork, salmon, nuts, legumes, yeast

Sources: From Reference 16, Office of Dietary Supplements. National Institute of Health. Available at http://ods.od.nih.gov/, and United States Department of Agriculture's Nutrient Data Lab. Available at http://ndb.nal.usda.gov/

Table 39.8 Dietary sources of minerals and trace elements.

Mineral or trace element	Dietary sources
Calcium	Milk and dairy products, fish with bones, dark green leafy vegetables, legumes, almonds, calcium fortified orange juice, calcium fortified tofu, calcium fortified/enriched alternative milk beverages (soy, rice, oat, almond, hemp, coconut)
Iron	Heme sources: Red meats, fish, poultry, shellfish Non-heme sources: dried fruits, legumes, whole and enriched grains and cereals
Magnesium	Nuts, legumes, whole grains, wheat bran and wheat germ
Manganese	Nuts, seeds, whole grains, wheat germ, tea
Selenium	Seafood, meats, eggs, sunflower seed, brazil nuts, Whole grains, plants (depends on soil content)
Zinc	Red meat, seafood (particularly oysters and also crab, lobster), beans, wheat germ

Sources: From Reference 16, Office of Dietary Supplements. National Institute of Health. Available at http://ods.od.nih.gov/, and United States Department of Agriculture's Nutrient Data Lab. Available at http://ndb.nal.usda.gov/

include these ingredients in the diet. Caution should be used when selecting products with baked ingredients as it is easy to overlook unbaked ingredients, for instance, in an iced cookie or cupcake that contains baked milk in the cookie or cake but unbaked milk in the icing or frosting. Additionally, some flavoring is topically applied in manufacturing after the product is baked. For instance, a cheese cracker may have the cheese baked into the cracker or the cheese flavor (with an unbaked milk ingredient) sprayed on after the product is baked.

Wheat allergy

The wheat-allergic patient must avoid all wheat-containing products resulting in the elimination of many processed and manufactured products. Wheat is a component of most commercial bread, cereal, pasta, crackers, cookies, and cakes. Those with wheat allergy should be aware that wheat starch is commonly used as a minor ingredient in other commercial food products such as condiments and marinades, cold cuts, soups, soy sauce, some low or non-fat products, hard candies, licorice, and jelly beans.

Nutritionally, wheat contributes necessary carbohydrates, the major source of energy in the diet, as well as many micronutrients such as thiamine, niacin, riboflavin, iron, and folate. Whole grain wheat products also contribute fiber to the diet. Four servings of wheat-based products such as whole grain and enriched cereals or breads generally provide greater than 50% of the RDA/AI for carbohydrate, iron, thiamine, riboflavin, and niacin for individuals 1 year of age and older as well as a significant source of vitamin B6 and magnesium. Elimination of wheat products from the diet may have great nutritional impact and care should be taken to offer tolerated whole and enriched wheat-free grain substitutes. Table 39.6 lists the major nutrients provided by wheat in the diet. Alternative sources of these nutrients may be found in Tables 39.7 and 39.8.

Many alternative flours are available to patients with wheat allergy, including rice, corn, oat, barley, buckwheat, rye, amaranth, millet, sorghum, and quinoa. Cereal grain proteins may be cross-reactive and therefore those with wheat allergy may test positive on prick skin testing to other grains as well. It has been reported that 20% of individuals with grain allergy may be clinically reactive to another grain; therefore, use of these products should be individualized and based on tolerance as determined by the patient's allergist or the diet history [44]. If a patient has tolerance to alternative grains, these flours may improve the nutritional quality, variety, and convenience of the wheat-restricted diet; not only are these flours commercially available, but there are now many wheat- and gluten-free products made from these flours. Many of the gluten-free flours and products are not well fortified so choosing those that are whole grain or have better fortification will improve the nutritional quality of the diet and provide better sources of iron, thiamine, riboflavin, niacin, and zinc.

Egg allergy

Egg allergy is typically transient with many children developing tolerance to egg protein by 3–5 years of age [5, 45]. Egg avoidance requires the same diligence as milk avoidance since egg is a common ingredient in manufactured products. Egg protein may be present in pasta, casseroles, baked goods, ice creams, candies, marshmallows, lollipops, and meat-based dishes such as meatballs or meatloaf. Egg whites and shells may also be used as a clarifying agent in soup stocks, consommés, wine, alcohol-based drinks, and coffee drinks.

Eggs contribute protein, vitamin B12, riboflavin, pantothenic acid, biotin, and selenium in the diet. Many foods supply the nutrients found in eggs. Egg in the diet does not usually account for a large percentage of daily dietary intakes; therefore, replacing lost nutrients may be easier for the egg-allergic individual than for the milk-allergic individual. Table 39.6 shows the major nutrients provided by egg in the diet. Alternative sources of these nutrients may be found in Tables 39.7 and 39.8.

Egg is a common ingredient in the Western diet and patients with egg allergy will need to learn how to replace egg in recipes so that they may continue to enjoy traditional foods. Many commercial egg substitutes are not suitable for the egg-allergic individual as they contain egg protein. The CoFAR website provides handouts, including one on how to substitute common allergens (milk, egg, wheat) when cooking at home (www.cofargroup.org).

Soybean allergy

Soybean protein is present in our food supply in a variety of forms and can be found in a surprising array of products including baked goods, cereals, crackers, canned tuna and soups, reduced-fat peanut butter, prebasted meat products, cold cuts, and hotdogs. Soy protein may be found in many vegetarian-based products and is often the base for hydrolyzed vegetable or hydrolyzed plant protein. Studies show that the vast majority of soy-allergic individuals tolerate soy oil and soy lecithin [9]. This is an important piece of knowledge, since soy oil and soy lecithin are pervasive in processed foods and avoidance of these two soy-derived ingredients eliminates an extensive list of processed or manufactured foods that might otherwise be safe. Highly refined soy oil is exempt from allergen labeling, but soy lecithin is not, and therefore products that contain soy lecithin with a "contains soy" statement may in fact be safe for consumption by many soy-allergic consumers. Patients should never assume that a product is safe, however, and should first call the manufacturer to determine whether any other soy protein ingredients are contained in a product, especially if a vague ingredient term such as natural flavoring is listed.

While soy itself contains a number of vital nutrients including protein, thiamine, riboflavin, pyridoxine, folate, calcium, phosphorus, magnesium, iron, and zinc, generally it is not a major component of the diet, and therefore the nutrients lost due to soy elimination may easily be replaced. The result of eliminating many manufactured foods with soy as an ingredient, however, will impact the variety of manufactured products available for consumption. Table 39.6 lists the major nutrients provided by soy in the diet. Alternative sources of these nutrients may be found in Tables 39.7 and 39.8.

Peanut allergy

Recent studies indicate that the prevalence of peanut allergy has doubled among children younger than 5 years in the last decade [46]. While food-induced anaphylaxis can be caused by any food allergen, the most common cause of fatal anaphylaxis is peanut ingestion [3].

Peanuts have become popular ingredients in our food; however, it is easier to avoid foods that contain peanut than it is to avoid, say milk or wheat, in the typical Western diet. Furthermore, avoidance of peanuts in the diet does not pose any specific nutritional risk as long as the remaining diet is varied, although peanuts are a good source of protein, fat, vitamin E, niacin, magnesium, manganese, and chromium. Peanuts are a common ingredient in cereal, crackers, cookies, candy, and frozen desserts. Peanut butter or peanut flour can be found in unexpected places such as in chili, stew, and pasta sauce where it may be added as a thickener. Peanut butter is sometimes used as an ingredient in egg rolls to seal the roll before frying. Peanut flours may also be used in protein bars and other high protein products. Individuals with peanut allergy need to take additional precautions when eating in restaurants. Certain ethnic cuisines such as Asian and African are considered high risk as peanut and tree nuts are pervasive ingredients and often cooking utensils and woks are merely wiped clean before preparing the next dish, potentially leaving enough residual protein to cause a reaction. Ice cream parlors are also considered high risk for those with peanut and tree nut allergies due to the likelihood of cross-contact. Ice cream scoopers are used for all flavors of ice cream including those flavors, which contain nuts. Using a clean scooper does not alleviate the risk as a previous scooper may already have contaminated the nut-free flavors. For more details on hidden peanut allergen and cross-reactive food proteins, see Chapter 25.

Highly refined peanut oil has been shown to be safe for those with peanut allergy and is not considered an allergen under FALCPA. Cold pressed, expressed, or expelled oils may contain sufficient protein to cause an allergic reaction [47]. Individuals with peanut allergy may choose to avoid peanut oil as information on how the oil was processed may not always be available and the variety of alternative vegetable oils is vast.

Tree nut allergy

Tree nuts (almond, Brazil nut, cashew, chestnut, filbert/hazelnut, macadamia, pecan, pine nut, pistachio, and walnut) are added to numerous products, similar to those products containing peanut. If a tree nut is including in manufactured product, the specific tree nut must be listed on the product label. Artificial nuts can be made from peanuts that are flavored with a flavoring made from a tree nut such as walnut or pecan, and therefore are not safe. Tree nut oils may be added to lotions and soaps and other cosmetic products. Lotions, soaps, shampoos, and cosmetic products are not covered under the food allergen labeling laws so these labels must be read very carefully for those with a tree nut allergy. Additionally, marinades and some brands of barbeque sauce are now adding tree nut oils and flavoring to their products.

Clinical reactions to tree nuts can be severe and cross-reactivity among the nuts is relatively high with 37% of patients with an allergy to one tree nut having IgE binding and clinical reactivity to another tree nut. Patients are often advised to avoid all tree nuts if one is proven to be allergic to one tree nut due to the high risk of cross-reactivity, the potential for severe reactions, and the risk of cross-contact in handling. However, if a specific tree nut had previously been eaten and tolerated, the patient may be advised to proceed with caution but to always ascertain the safety of the tree nut first from a cross-contact perspective [44].

Coconut and the following tree nuts also require disclosure on food labeling by United States law: beech nut, *Ginkgo*, shea nut, butter nut, hickory, chinquapin, lychee nut, and pili nut. Coconut allergy in patients with tree nut allergy is rare and coconut is generally not restricted in the diets of those with tree nut allergies. However, while rare, reactions to coconut have occurred and are most likely due to clinical cross-reactive proteins with walnut protein [48]. Including coconut in the diet of those allergic to tree nuts is likely safe, but should be individualized by the patient's allergist. The risk of allergic reaction to these other less common tree nuts has not been extensively studied. Nutmeg is not a nut and is safe to include in the diet of those with tree nut allergies.

Fish allergy

Fish is an excellent source of dietary protein and in some cultures, the primary source. Fish and more specifically the individual fish species must be listed on the food ingredient label and may no longer be "hidden" in a product. Those with fish allergies should be aware that fish is a common ingredient in Worcestershire sauce, surimi, and other imitation shellfish. The major allergens responsible for cross-reactivity among species of fish are parvalbumins. IgE binding to multiple fish species in patients with fish allergy is often the case and while clinical cross-reactivity occurs, isolated allergy to a single species of fish also occurs [44]. It has been estimated that approximately 50% of individuals with fish allergy are at risk of reacting to at least one other fish species [44].

Shellfish allergy

Allergic reactions to shellfish are the most common form of food allergy in adults, affecting 2% of the population. Shellfish represent a high risk for cross-reactivity, with a potential for severe reactions. Those who are allergic to a specific species of shellfish have a 75% risk of reacting to another species of shellfish. [44]. Crustacean shellfish (shrimp, lobster, crab, and crawfish) are considered major allergens in the United States and European Union, and therefore must be listed on the product label even if it is a minor ingredient such as a flavoring. Mollusks (clams, mussels, oysters, scallops, and squid) are not considered major allergens under FALCPA. Although shellfish are not commonly used as a hidden ingredient in a product, those with an allergy to clam, for instance, may need to call the manufacturer to determine whether clam was used in seafood flavoring. Those with shellfish allergy should avoid seafood restaurants because cross-contact is likely even if a non-shellfish dish is ordered. Also, some sensitive individuals may react to aerosolized shellfish protein through cooking vapors. There have been reported cases of fatal reactions caused by inhalation of shrimp protein from cooking fumes [14].

Sesame seed allergy

While sesame seed is not considered a major allergen in the United States, it is in the European Union and allergic reactions to sesame seed protein appear to be growing in prevalence in many countries, including the United States. Allergic reactions to sesame have been reported to be severe with respiratory symptoms and anaphylactic shock not uncommon. Sesame oil is a crude oil and not highly refined, and therefore may contain significant amounts of sesame protein. In a recent study by Morisset et al., five of six patients with sesame allergy were positive on double-blind, placebo-controlled food challenge to sesame oil and two of these patients experienced anaphylactic reactions. Of note, these subjects reacted to only a few milligrams of sesame protein in the sesame oil, but when challenged to sesame protein in crushed sesame seeds, the threshold for reaction was 100 mg–7 g of sesame protein. The authors contend that the considerable increase in allergenicity of the sesame protein in sesame oil may be due to the interaction between sesame allergens and the lipid matrix [49].

Food ingredients that contain sesame seed protein are sesame seeds, tahini (sesame seed paste), sesame oil, and sesame flour. Products to be aware of that may contain sesame seed protein are breads, bread crumbs and breading, hummus, halvah, falafel, high protein energy bars and snacks, vegetarian burgers and cold cuts, salad dressings and marinades, some herbal drinks, and certain brands of cereals (e.g., Kashi brand cereals) which routinely use sesame flour as part of their grain mixture. Cross-contact with sesame may occur in manufacturing and most especially in bakeries and bagel shops as well as pizza parlors.

Summary

Dietary management of food allergy requires extensive education regarding the elimination of the allergenic food as well as how to replace the nutrients usually provided by the food or foods to be eliminated. At their initial visit to the allergist's office, patients diagnosed with food allergy must absorb an overwhelming amount of new information. They must understand their emergency action plans, how to use their emergency medications and maintenance medications for chronic atopic disease, as well as the concept of dietary avoidance. Dietary issues may not be discussed extensively at the initial assessment and questions may arise after the patient has gone home and no longer has access to accurate information. Ideally, a patient with food allergies should be referred for dietary counseling upon diagnosis [3]. In the pediatric population, growth should be closely monitored and pediatricians have a specific responsibility in assessing growth and referring patients to a registered dietitian for evaluation if dietary inadequacies are suspected [3]. Success in dietary management depends on the practitioner's ability to educate the patient on dietary avoidance as well as how to substitute safe and appropriate foods to meet nutritional needs.

References

1. Nowak-Wegrzyn A, Sampson HA. Future therapies for food allergies. *J Allergy Clin Immunol* 2011; 127(3):558–573.
2. Nowak-Wegrzyn A. Immunotherapy for food allergy. *Inflamm Allergy Drug Targets* 2006; 5(1):23–34.
3. NIAID-Sponsored Expert Panel; Boyce JA, Assa'ad A, Burks AW, et al. Guidelines for the diagnosis and management of food allergy in the United States: report of the NIAID-sponsored expert panel. *J Allergy Clin Immunol* 2010; 126(6 Suppl):S1–S58.
4. Sicherer SH. Food allergy. *Mt Sinai J Med* 2011; 78(5):683–696.
5. Sicherer SH, Sampson HA. Food allergy. *J Allergy Clin Immunol* 2010; 125(2 Suppl 2):S116–S125.
6. U.S. FDA. *Food Allergen Consumer Protection Act of 2004*. Available at http://www.fda.gov/Food/GuidanceRegulation/GuidanceDocumentsRegulatoryInformation/Allergens/ucm106890.htm (Last accessed 12 June 2013).
7. Taylor SL, Hefle SL. Food allergen labeling in the USA and Europe. *Curr Opin Allergy Clin Immunol* 2006; 6(3):186–190.
8. U.S. FDA. *Questions and Answers Regarding Food Allergens including the Food Allergen Consumer Protection Act of 2004*, Edition 3. Available at http://www.fda.gov/Food/GuidanceRegulation/GuidanceDocumentsRegulatoryInformation/Allergens/ucm059116.htm (Last accessed 12 June 2013).
9. Taylor SL, Hefle SL, Bindslev-Jensen C, et al. Factors affecting the determination of threshold doses for allergenic foods: how much is too much? *J Allergy Clin Immunol* 2002; 109(1):24–30.
10. Taylor SL, Moneret-Vautrin DA, Crevel RW, et al. Threshold dose for peanut: risk characterization based upon diagnostic oral challenge of a series of 286 peanut-allergic individuals. *Food Chem Toxicol* 2010; 48(3):814–819.
11. MacDonald A. Better European food labelling laws to help people with food intolerances. *Matern Child Nutr* 2005; 1(3):223–224.
12. Ford LS, Taylor SL, Pacenza R, et al. Food allergen advisory labeling and product contamination with egg, milk, and peanut. *J Allergy Clin Immunol* 2010; 126:384–385.
13. Hefle SL, Furlong TJ, Niemann L, Lemon-Mule H, et al. Consumer attitudes and risks associated with packaged foods having advisory labeling regarding the presence of peanuts. *J Allergy Clin Immunol* 2007; 120(1):171–176.
14. Munoz-Furlong A. Daily coping strategies for patients and their families. *Pediatrics* 2003; 111(6 Pt 3):1654–1661.
15. Sicherer SH, Vargas PA, Groetch ME, et al. Development and validation of educational materials for food allergy. *J Pediatr* 2012; 160(4):651–656.
16. Mofidi S. Nutritional management of pediatric food hypersensitivity. *Pediatrics* 2003; 111(6 Pt 3):1645–1653.
17. Blass SC, Goost H, Tolba RH, et al. Time to wound closure in trauma patients with disorders in wound healing is shortened by supplements containing antioxidant micronutrients and glutamine: a PRCT. *Clin Nutr* 2012; 31:469–475.
18. Trumbo P, Schlicker S, Yates AA, Poos M, Food and Nutrition Board of the Institute of Medicine, The National Academies, et al. Dietary reference intakes for energy, carbohydrate, fiber, fat, fatty acids, cholesterol, protein and amino acids. *J Am Diet Assoc* 2002; 102(11):1621–1630.
19. Barr SI, Murphy SP, Poos MI. Interpreting and using the dietary references intakes in dietary assessment of individuals and groups. *J Am Diet Assoc* 2002; 102(6):780–788.
20. Pentiuk SP, Miller CK, Kaul A. Eosinophilic esophagitis in infants and toddlers. *Dysphagia* 2006; 22:44–48.
21. Feuling MB, Noel RJ. Medical and nutrition management of eosinophilic esophagitis in children. *Nutr Clin Pract* 2010; 25(2):166–174.
22. Shils M, Shike M, Ross A et al. *Modern Nutrition in Health and Disease*, 10th edn. Philadelphia, PA: Lippincott Williams & Wilkins, 2006.
23. *Effects of Omega-3 Fatty Acids on Lipids and Glycemic Control in Type II Diabetes and the Metabolic Syndrome and on Inflammatory Bowel Disease, Rheumatoid Arthritis, Renal Disease, Systemic Lupus Erythmatosus, and Osteoporosis*. Evidence report/technology assessment No. 89. Prepared by Southern California/RAND Evidence-based Practice Center, under contract No. 290-02-0003. AHRQ publication No. 04-E012-2. Rockville, MD: Agency for healthcare Research and Quality, March 2004.
24. James MJ, Gibson RA, Cleland LG. Dietary polyunsaturated fatty acids and inflammatory mediator production. *Am J Clin Nutr* 2000; 71(1 Suppl):343S–348S.
25. Salman S, Christie L, Burks AW. Dietary intakes of children with food allergies: comparison of the food guide pyramid and the recommended dietary allowances. *J Allergy Clin Immunol* 2002; 109:S214.
26. Christie L, Hine RJ, Parker JG, et al. Food allergies in children affect nutrient intake and growth. *J Am Diet Assoc* 2002; 102(11):1648–1651.
27. Flammarion S, Santos C, Guimber D, et al. Diet and nutritional status of children with food allergies. *Pediatr Allergy Immunol* 2011; 22(2):161–165.
28. Vieira MC, Morais MB, Spolidoro JV, et al. A survey on clinical presentation and nutritional status of infants with suspected cow' milk allergy. *BMC Pediatr* 2010; 10:25.
29. Harnack LJ, Steffen L, Zhou X, et al. Trends in vitamin D intake from food sources among adults in the Minneapolis-St Paul, MN, metropolitan area, 1980–1982 through 2007–2009. *J Am Diet Assoc* 2011; 111(9):1329–1334.
30. Hewison M. Vitamin D and immune function: an overview. *Proc Nutr Soc* 2012; 71:50–61.

31. Henriksen C, Eggesbo M, Halvorsen R, et al. Nutrient intake among two-year-old children on cows' milk-restricted diets. *Acta Paediatr* 2000; 89(3):272–278.
32. Grummer-Strawn LM, Reinold C, Krebs NF; Centers for Disease Control and Prevention (CDC). Use of World Health Organization and CDC growth charts for children aged 0–59 months in the United States. *MMWR Recomm Rep* 2010; 59(RR-9):1–15.
33. Lipman TH, Hench KD, Benyi T, et al. A multicentre randomised controlled trial of an intervention to improve the accuracy of linear growth measurement. *Arch Dis Child* 2004; 89(4):342–346.
34. Barlow SE; Expert Committee. Expert committee recommendations regarding the prevention, assessment, and treatment of child and adolescent overweight and obesity: summary report. *Pediatrics* 2007; 120(Suppl 4):S164–S192.
35. McDaniel JC, Massey K, Nicolaou A. Fish oil supplementation alters levels of lipid mediators of inflammation in microenvironment of acute human wounds. *Wound Repair Regen* 2011; 19(2):189–200.
36. Lu Y, Tian H, Hong S. Novel 14,21-dihydroxy-docosahexaenoic acids: structures, formation pathways, and enhancement of wound healing. *J Lipid Res* 2010; 51(5):923–932.
37. Fiocchi A, Brozek J, Schunemann H, et al. World Allergy Organization (WAO) Diagnosis and Rationale for Action against Cow's Milk Allergy (DRACMA) Guidelines. *Pediatr Allergy Immunol* 2010; 21(Suppl 21):1–125.
38. Bock SA, Munoz-Furlong A, Sampson HA. Further fatalities caused by anaphylactic reactions to food, 2001–2006. *J Allergy Clin Immunol* 2007; 119(4):1016–1018.
39. Skripak JM, Matsui EC, Mudd K, et al. The natural history of IgE-mediated cow's milk allergy. *J Allergy Clin Immunol* 2007; 120(5):1172–1177.
40. American Academy of Pediatrics. Committee on nutrition. Hypoallergenic infant formulas. *Pediatrics* 2000; 106(2 Pt 1):346–349.
41. Du Toit G, Lack G. Can food allergy be prevented? The current evidence. *Pediatr Clin North Am* 2011; 58(2):481–509.
42. Kim JS, Nowak-Wegrzyn A, Sicherer SH, et al. Dietary baked milk accelerates the resolution of cow's milk allergy in children. *J Allergy Clin Immunol* 2011; 128(1):125–131.
43. Nowak-Wegrzyn A, Fiocchi A. Rare, medium, or well done? The effect of heating and food matrix on food protein allergenicity. *Curr Opin Allergy Clin Immunol* 2009; 9(3):234–237.
44. Sicherer SH. Clinical implications of cross-reactive food allergens. *J Allergy Clin Immunol* 2001; 108(6):881–890.
45. Sampson HA. Update on food allergy. *J Allergy Clin Immunol* 2004; 113(5):805–819.
46. Branum AM LS. *Food allergy among U.S. children: trends in prevalence and hospitalizations*. NCHS data brief, No. 10. Hyattsville, MD: National Center for Health Statistics, 2008.
47. Crevel RWR, Kerkhoff MAT, Konig MMG. Allergenicity of refined vegetable oils. *Food and Chemical Toxicology* 2000; 38(4):385–393.
48. Teuber SS, Peterson WR. Systemic allergic reaction to coconut (*Cocos nucifera*) in 2 subjects with hypersensitivity to tree nut and demonstration of cross-reactivity to legumin-like seed storage proteins: new coconut and walnut food allergens. *J Allergy Clin Immunol* 1999; 103(6):1180–1185.
49. Morisset M, Moneret-Vautrin DA, Kanny G, et al. Thresholds of clinical reactivity to milk, egg, peanut and sesame in immunoglobulin E-dependent allergies: evaluation by double-blind or single-blind placebo-controlled oral challenges. *Clin Exp Allergy* 2003; 33(8):1046–1051.

40 Food Toxicology

Steve L. Taylor

Food Allergy Research and Resource Program, Department of Food Science and Technology, University of Nebraska–Lincoln, Lincoln, NE, USA

Key Concepts

- Food intoxications are caused by chemicals in foods including both synthetic and naturally occurring substances.
- The central axiom of toxicology is that all chemicals are toxic; it is the dose that makes the poison.
- Certain naturally occurring constituents (e.g., the toxins in poisonous mushrooms) and contaminants (e.g., the algal toxins causing paralytic shellfish poisoning and ciguatera poisoning) can be particularly hazardous to consumers causing serious and acute symptoms if ingested.
- Food additives do not typically elicit toxic reactions in consumers if ingested and used in accordance with governmental regulations, and ingested in doses consistent with those practices.
- Lactose intolerance results from a deficiency of β-galactosidase in the small intestine so that ingestion of milk sugar or lactose elicits acute gastrointestinal complaints including flatulence, abdominal pain, and frothy diarrhea.

Food toxicology could be defined as the science that establishes the basis for judgments about the safety of foodborne chemicals. The central axiom of toxicology as set forth by Paracelsus in the 1500s states "Everything is poison. Only the dose makes a thing not a poison." Thus, all chemicals in foods, whether natural or synthetic, inherent, adventitious, or added, are potentially toxic. The vast majority of foodborne chemicals are not hazardous because the amounts of each foodborne chemical in the typical diet are not sufficient to cause injury. The degree of risk posed by exposure to any specific foodborne chemicals is determined by the dose, duration, and frequency of exposure (and especially in the case of allergies, the degree of sensitivity of the individual). The age-old wisdom about the benefits of eating moderate amounts of a varied diet protects most consumers from any harm. Foodborne chemicals that are considered to be toxicants are those chemicals where the dose, duration, and frequency of exposure can, in at least some circumstances, be sufficient to elicit adverse reactions. Unusual dietary practices can sometimes result in intoxications from chemicals that would normally be considered safe and desirable. For example, polar explorers experienced toxic responses to excessive intake of vitamin A as the result of consuming large amounts of polar bear liver. More recently, the ingestion of copious quantities of water in a misguided radio contest resulted in the death of a contestant.

Acute adverse reactions to foods can occur through many mechanisms including infections (viral, bacterial, parasitic), various intoxications and allergies, and intolerances. Food allergies are the major focus of this book. Other medical conditions including some food intoxications can cause symptoms resembling food allergies. These other conditions must be considered and eliminated in diagnosing food allergy.

Toxic reactions to food encompass all food-associated illnesses that are caused by chemicals in food, although foodborne chemicals vary greatly in toxicity. All consumers are susceptible to most food intoxications, although differences will exist primarily related to the dose of exposure and body weight (infants vs. adults). Food allergy can be viewed as a category of food intoxication that affects only certain individuals in the population. Other categories of food intoxications, such as metabolic food disorders, also affect only certain individuals in the population. This chapter will focus on some of the more common types of acute foodborne intoxications including the most common

Food Allergy: Adverse Reactions to Foods and Food Additives, Fifth Edition. Edited by Dean D Metcalfe, Hugh A Sampson, Ronald A Simon and Gideon Lack.

metabolic food disorders. Some of the selected examples have certain manifestations in common with food allergies and intolerances and are thus of some importance in the differential diagnosis of food allergies.

Intoxications caused by synthetic chemicals in foods

Most of the synthetic chemicals in foods including food additives, agricultural chemical residues, and chemicals migrating from packaging materials have been rigorously tested for toxicity. These synthetic chemicals are typically safe under normal circumstances of exposure, although adverse reactions can occur from misuse, either intentional or accidental. In most situations, the concentrations of chemicals in these categories are well below any levels that might be associated with adverse reactions. The focus here will be on a few additional food additives, agricultural chemical residues, packaging migrants, and other man-made chemicals that can occur in foods at concentrations sufficient to cause concern.

Food additives

These examples were chosen because some of the manifestations are similar to symptoms that can occur during IgE-mediated allergic reactions.

Niacin

Excessive consumption of niacin (nicotinic acid), which is part of the B vitamin complex, can cause an acute onset of flushing, pruritus, rash, and burning or warmth in the skin especially on the face and upper trunk [1]. Gastrointestinal discomfort is noted by some patients. Outbreaks have sporadically occurred from the excessive enrichment of grain products as the result of inaccurate or inadequate labeling of food ingredient containers. Such episodes are rare because the amount of niacin required to elicit such symptoms is at least 50 times the recommended dietary allowance [2]. The symptoms of niacin intoxication are self-limited and without sequelae. More commonly, these symptoms occur when niacin is used for its cholesterol-lowering effects as a pharmaceutical. Niacin may also contribute to the adverse effects attributed to overconsumption of certain energy drinks that contain a variety of substances including ethanol, caffeine, taurine, niacin, and others that may act in combination [3].

Sorbitol and other polyhydric alcohols

Sugar alcohols, such as sorbitol, are widely used sweeteners in dietetic food products. They are especially common in candy and chewing gum because they are noncariogenic. Diarrhea can result from the excessive consumption of sugar alcohols [4]. Sorbitol and other sugar alcohols are not as easily absorbed as sugar. Because of their slow absorption, these sweeteners can cause an osmotic-type diarrhea if excessive amounts are ingested. For adults, symptoms can occur if more than 20 g of these sweeteners per day are ingested [4]. Infants are susceptible to lower doses. The illness is self-limited.

Toxic oil poisoning

In 1981 and 1982, an epidemic occurred in Spain linked to the ingestion of unlabeled, illegally marketed cooking oils [5]. Over 20 000 cases and approximately 300 deaths were recorded in this epidemic [6]. The illicit cooking oil contained oils from both plant and animal sources but some of the oils were denatured and intended for industrial rather than food uses. The causative toxins in the oils remain unknown, although fatty acid esters of 3-(N-phenylamino)-1,2-propanediol (PAP) resulting from the denaturation process are suspected to be at least partially responsible [6].

The clinical manifestations of this illness involved multiple organ systems [5, 6]. In the first few days after ingestion of the oil, patients experienced fever, chills, headache, tachycardia, cough, chest pain, and pruritus. Physical examinations revealed various skin exanthema, splenomegaly, and generalized adenopathy. Pulmonary infiltrates were noted in 84% of patients probably as the result of increased capillary permeability. The intermediate phase of the illness tended to begin in the second week and persist through the eighth week post-ingestion. GI symptoms, primarily abdominal pain, nausea, and diarrhea, predominated. Clinical examination revealed marked eosinophilia in 42% of patients, high IgE levels, thrombocytopenia, abnormal coagulation patterns, and evidence of hepatic dysfunction with abnormal enzymes. Some patients became jaundiced, and many had hepatomegaly. The late phase of the illness developed in 23% of cases and began after 2 months of illness. This phase was characterized initially by neuromuscular and joint involvement. Later, patients developed vasculitis and a scleroderma-like syndrome. Patients complained of intense muscular pain, edema, and progressive muscular weakness. Muscular atrophy was apparent in some patients. Neurological involvement included depressed deep tendon reflexes, anesthesia, and dysesthesia. Respiratory problems developed due to neuromuscular weakness and progressed to pulmonary hypertension and thromboembolic phenomena. The scleroderma-like symptoms included Raynaud's phenomenon, sicca syndrome, dysphagia, and contractures due to thickening collagen in the skin. Vascular lesions were noted in all organs apparently resulting from endothelial proliferation and thrombosis. All patients in the late group had antinuclear antibody and many had antibodies against smooth muscle and skeletal muscle [7].

The pathological and clinical features are consistent with an autoimmune mechanism for this illness. Since the precise causative agents and the mechanism have not been delineated, a recurrence is not impossible. Also, the toxin, if present in small amounts in other foods, may be producing or aggravating other clinical conditions.

Agricultural chemicals

A wide diversity of chemicals is used in modern agricultural practices. Residues of these chemicals can occur in raw and processed foods, although federal regulatory agencies evaluate the use and safety of such chemicals. The major categories of agricultural chemicals would include insecticides, herbicides, fungicides, fertilizers, and veterinary drugs including antibiotics.

Insecticides

Insecticides are added to foods to control the extent of insect contamination. The major categories of insecticides include organochlorine compounds (DDT, chlordane, and others, many of which are now banned), organophosphate compounds (e.g., parathion and malathion), carbamate compounds (e.g., carbaryl and aldicarb), botanical compounds (e.g., nicotine and pyrethrum), and inorganic compounds (e.g., arsenicals).

The exceedingly low residue levels of insecticides found in most foods are not particularly hazardous especially on an acute basis. Large doses of insecticides can be toxic to humans. For example, the organophosphates and carbamates are cholinesterase inhibitors and act as neurotoxins by blocking synaptic nerve transmission. Several reasons exist for the low degree of hazard posed by insecticide residues in foods: (1) the level of exposure is very low; (2) some insecticides are not very toxic to humans; (3) some insecticides decompose rapidly in the environment; and (4) many different insecticides are used, which limits exposure to any one particular insecticide.

No food poisoning incidents have ever been attributed to the proper use of insecticides on foods. However, problems have occasionally arisen from the inappropriate use of certain insecticides [8]. Several incidents of aldicarb intoxication have occurred as a result of misuse of this pesticide in the production of watermelons and hydroponic cucumbers [9, 10]. The watermelon episode was the largest known outbreak of pesticide poisoning in North America [9]. Symptoms of aldicarb intoxication include nausea, vomiting, diarrhea, and mild neurological manifestations such as dizziness, headache, blurred vision, and loss of balance [9, 10]. Many other episodes of pesticide intoxications have resulted from the misuse of pesticides including contamination of foods during storage and transport, the use of pesticides in food preparation due to their mistaken identity as common food ingredients such as sugar and salt, and their misuse in agricultural practice as in the examples noted above [8].

Herbicides

Herbicides are applied to control the growth of weeds. Among the more important herbicides are chlorophenoxy compounds (e.g., 2,4-D), dinitrophenols (e.g., dinitro-ortho-cresol), bipyridyl compounds (e.g., paraquat), substituted ureas (e.g., monuron), carbamates (e.g., propham), and triazines (e.g., simazine). Generally, herbicide residues in foods are not a hazard to consumers. No food poisoning incidents have resulted from the proper use of herbicides on food crops. The lack of hazard from herbicide residues is associated with the low level of exposure, their low degree of toxicity to humans and selective toxicity toward plants, and the use of many different herbicides, which limits exposure to any particular herbicide.

Since most herbicides are selectively toxic to plants, they pose little hazard to humans in the amounts normally used for weed control. The bipyridyl compounds, including paraquat and diquat, are an exception. These nonselective herbicides are rather toxic to humans and tend to exert their toxic effects on the lung [11, 12]. However, no food poisoning incidents have ever been attributed to inappropriate use of the bipyridyl compounds.

Fungicides

Fungicides are used to prevent the growth of molds on food crops. Important fungicides include captan, folpet, dithiocarbamates, pentachlorophenol, and the mercurials. The hazards from foodborne fungicides are miniscule because exposure is quite low, most fungicides do not accumulate in the environment, and fungicides are typically not very toxic.

Exceptions are the mercurial compounds and hexachlorobenzene. The mercurials are often used to treat seed grains to prevent mold growth during storage. These seed grains are usually colored pink and are clearly intended for planting rather than consumption. However, on several occasions, consumers have eaten these treated seed grains and developed mercury poisoning [8]. Although some severe episodes have resulted in deaths, mild cases of mercury intoxication can be manifested in GI symptoms such as abdominal cramps, nausea, vomiting, and diarrhea and dermal symptoms such as acrodynia and itching [8]. Hexachlorobenzene caused one of the most massive outbreaks of pesticide poisoning in recorded history affecting over 3000 individuals in Turkey from 1955 through 1959 [13]. Hexachlorobenzene-treated seed grain was consumed rather than planted resulting in severe symptoms including 10% mortality rate, porphyria cutanea tarda, ulcerated skin lesions, alopecia, porphyrinuria, hepatomegaly, thyroid enlargement, and a 10% mortality rate [13].

Fertilizers

The commonly used fertilizers are combinations of nitrogen and phosphorus compounds. Nitrogen fertilizers are oxidized to nitrate and nitrite in the soil. Both nitrate and nitrite are hazardous to humans if ingested in large amounts. Infants are particularly susceptible to nitrate and nitrite intoxication. Some plants, such as spinach, can accumulate nitrate to hazardous levels if allowed to grow on overly fertilized fields. Because nitrite is more toxic than nitrate, the situation can be worsened if nitrate-reducing bacteria are allowed to proliferate on these foods.

Acute nitrite intoxications have occurred. In low doses, the symptoms include flushing of the face and extremities, GI discomfort, and headache; in larger doses, cyanosis, methemoglobinemia, nausea, vomiting, abdominal pain, collapse, and death can occur. For example, nitrite-induced illnesses resulted from the improper storage of carrot juice that allowed the proliferation of nitrate-reducing bacteria causing the accumulation of hazardous levels of nitrite [14].

Veterinary drugs and antibiotics

Food-producing animals can be treated with a variety of veterinary drugs especially antibiotics. Residues in foods are typically quite low. Acute food poisoning incidents have not occurred as a result of properly used veterinary drugs and antibiotics. Penicillin is probably one of the major concerns because of the potential for allergic reactions to penicillin residues. However, the likelihood of allergic reactions to the very low levels of penicillin residues found in foods is quite remote [15].

Chemicals migrating from packaging materials and containers

Chemicals migrating from packaging materials into foods and beverages are not a significant source of chemical exposure. A variety of chemicals, including plastics monomers, plasticizers, stabilizers, printing inks, and others, do migrate at extremely low levels into foods. These chemicals do not often create any known hazards for consumers. Lead, copper, and tin are perhaps the main concerns associated with packaging materials. The storage of acidic foods in inappropriate containers can result in the leaching of toxic heavy metals, such as zinc. Contact of acidic beverages with copper can also release potentially hazardous levels of copper into the beverage.

Lead

Lead (Pb) exposure from foods has always been a comparatively moderate contributor to overall environmental lead exposure. The migration of Pb from Pb-soldered cans was previously a source of some concern. However, Pb-soldered cans have been successfully phased out of use in the United States. The main issue with Pb contamination remains the occasional use of Pb-based glazes on pottery or paint on glassware that may come in contact with acidic foods or beverages. Pb is a well-known toxicant that can affect the nervous system, the kidney, and the bone.

Tin

Tin plate is commonly used in the construction of metal cans for foods. The inner surfaces of these cans are lined with a lacquer material when cans are used for acidic foods or beverages. Acute tin intoxication has occurred from the inappropriate placement of tomato juice or fruit cocktail in unlined cans. Since tin is poorly absorbed, the primary symptoms are bloating, nausea, abdominal cramps, vomiting, diarrhea, and headache occurring 30 minutes to 2 hours after consumption of the acidic product.

Copper

Copper poisoning, characterized primarily by nausea and vomiting, most commonly occurs from faulty check valves in soft drink vending machines. The check valves prevent contact between the acidic, carbonated beverage and the copper tubing that delivers the water or ice in the machine. Several outbreaks of copper poisoning have resulted from such occurrences. Copper poisoning results in acute gastroenteritis.

Zinc

Zinc intoxication typically results from the unwise storage of acidic foods or beverages in galvanized containers. Zinc is a potent emetic. The symptoms of zinc intoxication include irritation of the mouth, throat, and abdomen; nausea and vomiting; dizziness; and collapse.

Industrial chemicals

Industrial and/or environmental pollutants often migrate into foods in small amounts. On rare occasions, hazardous levels of such chemicals enter the food supply often with devastating consequences.

Polychlorinated biphenyls and polybrominated biphenyls

The contamination of foods with polychlorinated biphenyls (PCBs) and polybrominated biphenyls (PBBs) has occurred on several occasions. PCBs and PBBs are quite persistent in the environment and are considered to be toxic pollutants from industrial practices. PBBs are commonly used as fire retardants, while PCBs are frequently used in transformer fluid. PCBs and PBBs are not worrisome acute toxicants in foods. However, since they are lipid-soluble, the potential exists for chronic effects. The most infamous incident involved the accidental contamination of dairy feed in Michigan with PBBs. This incident resulted in the destruction of many cows and their milk. Leaking transformers have contributed to the contamination of feeds with PCBs that led to the destruction of chickens, eggs, and egg-containing food products.

Mercury

Minamata disease, due to mercury (Hg) intoxication, is the classic example of the contamination of foods by industrial pollutants [16]. An industrial firm located on the shores of Minamata Bay in Japan dumped Hg-containing wastes into the bay where bacteria converted the inorganic Hg into highly toxic methylmercury. Fish in the Bay became contaminated with the methylmercury. Over 1200 cases of Hg intoxication occurred among consumers of Minamata Bay fish [16]. The symptoms included tremors and other neurotoxic effects and kidney failure.

Intoxications caused by naturally occurring chemicals in foods

The naturally occurring chemicals in foods are less frequently tested for their potential toxic effects than synthetic chemicals. While the vast majority of naturally occurring chemicals in foods are safe under the normal circumstances of exposure, some potentially hazardous situations do exist. Those naturally occurring chemicals with significant pharmacological activity including the vasoactive amines, methylxanthines, ethanol, and myristicin are covered elsewhere. However, naturally occurring chemicals in foods can elicit a wide variety of adverse reactions including both acute and chronic intoxication. Naturally occurring toxicants could be defined as those naturally occurring chemicals in foods that might be hazardous under typical circumstances of exposure. Naturally occurring chemicals in foods are more likely to be hazardous under typical circumstances of exposure than are synthetic chemicals. Although chronic illnesses, such as cancer, are undeniably important, this chapter will focus exclusively on acute intoxications caused by natural, foodborne toxicants.

Naturally occurring contaminants

Naturally occurring contaminants can be produced in foods as the result of contamination by bacteria, molds, algae, and insects. The chemicals produced from these biological sources can remain in foods even after the living organism has been removed or destroyed. Naturally occurring contaminants are not always present in foods and can be avoided, if contamination is prevented. Such contaminants represent the most important and potentially hazardous chemicals of natural origin existing in foods. The bacterial and insect toxins will not be discussed in detail. The bacterial toxins cause very familiar diseases including staphylococcal food poisoning and botulism. The insect toxins have not been studied to any extent, and their impact on human health is uncertain.

The toxicants produced by algal species that bioaccumulate in seafoods are among the most common causes of foodborne illness of chemical etiology. These algal toxicants are involved with several of the seafood poisonings including ciguatera poisoning and paralytic shellfish poisoning. Mycotoxins produced by foodborne molds are a source of considerable toxicological concern and occur at low levels rather frequently in certain stored foods. Several of the mycotoxins will be discussed in some detail because they are confirmed to be involved in acute foodborne illness. A bigger concern with the mycotoxins is their potential involvement with chronic toxicity. The chronic toxicity of mycotoxins will not be described here because it is unlikely to be relevant to the investigation of allergic reactions.

Ciguatera poisoning

Ciguatera poisoning results from the ingestion of fish that have fed on toxic dinoflagellate algae. Ciguatera poisoning is the most common cause of acute foodborne disease of chemical etiology reported to the Centers for Disease Control [17, 18]. This foodborne illness is common throughout the Caribbean, South Pacific, and Indian Ocean areas, but is now encountered around the world due to the improved distribution of fish. In the United States, the illness occurs most frequently in Florida, Hawaii, and the Virgin Islands. The fish most commonly implicated in cases of ciguatera poisoning are large tropical and semitropical reef fishes such as grouper, barracuda, sea bass, Spanish mackerel, snappers, and sea perches, although as many as 400 different fish species have been implicated in this illness.

With the tropical and semitropical reef fishes, the fish acquire the toxic agent(s) by feeding on smaller fishes that acquire the toxin from the poisonous planktonic algae [17]. Several species of dinoflagellate algae, primarily *Gambierdiscus* spp., appear to be able to produce toxins of the type associated with ciguatera poisoning [17]. Multiple, related toxins are involved in ciguatera poisoning [17, 19]. Lipid-soluble ciguatoxins are heat-stable, polyether compounds that have ionophoric properties selectively opening the voltage-sensitive sodium channels of the neuromuscular junction [19]. The toxins accumulate in the liver and viscera of the fish, but enough can enter the muscle tissues to result in ciguatera poisoning among humans ingesting these fish [17]. Larger fish pose a greater risk than smaller fish. The symptoms of ciguatera poisoning tend to be somewhat variable perhaps confirming the role of several different dinoflagellate algae and several different toxins in this syndrome. GI and neurological manifestations are the predominant symptoms associated with ciguatera poisoning, although in some cases, the GI symptoms predominate, while in other cases, the neurological symptoms predominate. The GI symptoms include nausea, vomiting, diarrhea, and abdominal cramps. The neurological symptoms include dysesthesia, paresthesia, especially in the perioral region and extremities, pruritus, vertigo, muscle weakness, malaise, headache, and myalgia. A peculiar reversal of hot and cold sensations occurs in about 65% of all patients [20]. In severe cases, the neurological manifestations can progress to delirium, pruritus, dyspnea, prostration, brachycardia, and coma [20]. Many patients recover within a few days or weeks, although treatment is difficult and deaths from cardiovascular collapse have been encountered in about 0.1% of cases [21].

Paralytic shellfish poisoning

Paralytic shellfish poisoning results from the ingestion of molluscan shellfish, such as clams, mussels, cockles, and scallops, that have become poisonous by feeding on toxic dinoflagellate algae [22]. Paralytic shellfish poisoning occurs worldwide but is commonly encountered along the Pacific and North Atlantic coasts of North America, the coastal areas of Japan, and the coasts of Chile and Argentina [22]. Several species of toxic dinoflagellate algae have been implicated in paralytic shellfish poisoning; *Alexandrium catanella* (formerly *Gonyaulax catanella*) and *A. tamarensis* are two of the most common ones. "Blooms" of the toxic dinoflagellates are sporadic, so most shellfish will be hazardous only during the times of the blooms. While most shellfish species clear the toxins from their system within a few weeks after the end of the dinoflagellate bloom, a few species, such as the Alaskan butter clam, seem to retain the toxin for long periods [23]. The toxins involved in paralytic shellfish poisoning are known as saxitoxins [22]. Saxitoxins are neurotoxins that bind to and block the sodium channels in nerve membranes [22]. The saxitoxins are heat-stable, so processing and cooking have no affect on the toxicity of the shellfish.

Through the blocking of nerve transmission, the saxitoxins are very potent neurotoxins. The symptoms of paralytic shellfish poisoning include a tingling sensation and numbness of the lips, tongue, and fingertips followed by numbness in the legs, arms, and neck, ataxia, giddiness, staggering, drowsiness, incoherent speech progressing to aphasia, rash, fever, and respiratory and muscular paralysis [22]. Death from respiratory failure occurs frequently, usually within 2–12 hours depending upon the dose ingested. No antidotes are known, although prognosis is good if the victim survives the first 24 hours of the illness.

Amnesic shellfish poisoning

Amnesic shellfish poisoning was first recognized following an outbreak in Canada in late 1987 [24]. Amnesic shellfish poisoning was associated with the ingestion of mussels from Prince Edward Island, which resulted in over 100 cases and at least 4 deaths [24]. The source of the toxin was a planktonic algae, *Nitzschia pungens*, which was blooming in an isolated area of Prince Edward Island at the time of the outbreak [25]. The toxin involved was identified as domoic acid, a neuroexcitatory amino acid [25,26]. Amnesic shellfish poisoning is characterized by GI symptoms and unusual neurological abnormalities [25,26]. The GI symptoms, which occurred within the first 24 hours, were vomiting, abdominal cramps, and diarrhea. The neurological symptoms, which had onset within 48 hours, were severe incapacitating headaches, confusion, loss of short-term memory, and, in a few cases, seizures and coma. Severely affected patients who did not die experienced prolonged neurologic sequelae including memory deficits and motor or sensorimotor neuronopathy or axonopathy [25,26].

Diarrhetic shellfish poisoning

Diarrhetic shellfish poisoning is primarily associated with the ingestion of clams that have become toxic through the ingestion of toxic dinoflagellate algae of the genus *Dinophysis* and *Prorocentrum* [27]. No confirmed outbreaks have occurred in North America but outbreaks have occurred primarily in Japan and Europe [27]. The toxins responsible for diarrhetic shellfish poisoning are polyether compounds: okadaic acid and its derivatives, the dinophysis toxins [27]. The symptoms include diarrhea, nausea, vomiting, and abdominal cramps [27].

Pufferfish poisoning

Pufferfish poisoning occurs primarily in Japan and China, the only parts of the world where pufferfish are frequently consumed. While about 30 species of pufferfish are found worldwide, most species are not toxic. The most hazardous pufferfish belong to the genus, *Fugu*, which are considered in Japan and China to be delicacies. The toxin in pufferfish is a potent neurotoxin called tetrodotoxin [28]. For many years, the toxin was thought to be produced by the fish, but evidence now exists that marine bacteria may be the original source of the toxin [29]. Tetrodotoxin is heat-stable and, like saxitoxin, acts by blocking the sodium channels in nerve cell membranes. The symptoms of tetrodotoxin poisoning usually begin with a tingling sensation of the fingers, toes, lips, and tongue, followed by nausea, vomiting, diarrhea, and epigastric pain [28]. Twitching, tremors, ataxia, paralysis, and death often ensue [28]. The fatality rate is about 60% in untreated cases. Most of the tetrodotoxin accumulates in the liver, viscera, and roe of the pufferfish. Careful cleaning of the fish, before ingestion of the edible muscle, is required to safeguard against tetrodotoxin intoxication.

Mycotoxins

Mycotoxins are produced by a wide variety of molds that can grow and produce toxins on a wide variety of foods

[30]. Most of the known mycotoxins have been recognized because of their toxicity to domestic animals fed moldy feed grains. However, a few mycotoxins are noteworthy because they are known hazards for humans.

Ergotism

Ergotism was the first recognized mycotoxin-associated illness. The responsible mold is *Claviceps purpurea*, which can infect the grains of rye, wheat, barley, and oats. The last recorded outbreak of ergotism occurred in Europe in 1951. Ergotism is caused by a group of toxins known as the ergot alkaloids. Ergotism is manifested in two forms: gangrenous ergotism and convulsive ergotism. Gangrenous ergotism, also known as Saint Anthony's fire, is characterized by a burning sensation in the feet and hands followed by progressive restriction of blood flow to the hands and feet resulting ultimately in gangrene and loss of limbs. Convulsive ergotism is characterized by hallucinations leading to convulsive seizures and sometimes death. Modern agricultural practices and grain milling procedures have virtually eliminated ergotism as a concern.

Alimentary toxic aleukia

Alimentary toxic aleukia (ALA) was observed in Russia during World War II and was associated with the consumption of over-wintered millet that contained trichothecene mycotoxins. Trichothecenes are a group of mycotoxins produced by molds of the genus, *Fusarium*. ALA occurs in four stages. In the first stage, affected individuals experience burning sensations in the mouth, throat, and esophagus followed 1–3 days later by diarrhea, nausea, and vomiting. The GI symptoms cease after about 9 days. The second stage of ALA begins during the second week and lasts through the second month. This stage involves bone marrow destruction, leukemia, agranulocytosis, anemia, and loss of platelets. Small hemorrhages begin to appear at the end of this stage. The third stage of ALA lasts for 5–20 days and involves total loss of bone marrow with necrotic angina, sepsis, total agranulocytosis, moderate fever, larger hemorrhages on the skin, and the appearance of necrotic skin lesions. Bronchial pneumonia usually develops along with abscesses and hemorrhages in the lungs. The fourth stage of ALA is death, which occurred in about 80% of cases within 3 months of the onset of symptoms. Due to the circumstances at the time of this outbreak, the identification of the exact species of *Fusarium* and the trichothecenes responsible for ALA were not accomplished. The level of contamination of the millet with trichothecenes was not determined.

Fusarium molds are very common on grain crops worldwide. Trichothecene mycotoxins continue to occur at low levels in many cereal foods. However, no acute illnesses in humans including ALA have been attributed to trichothecene intoxication since the original outbreak. The effects of ingestion of low levels of toxic trichothecenes on humans remain uncertain.

Naturally occurring constituents

Many fungi, some plants, and a few animals contain hazardous levels of various naturally occurring toxicants. Such fungi, plants, and animals should not be eaten, but are accidentally or intentionally consumed on occasion resulting in foodborne illness. Furthermore, many plants and animals contain levels of naturally occurring toxicants that are probably not hazardous to humans ingesting typical amounts of these foods. The ingestion of abnormally large quantities of such foods and their naturally occurring toxicants is potentially hazardous. Some naturally occurring toxicants are inactivated or removed during processing or preparation of foods prior to consumption. The failure to adhere to such processing and preparation practices can result in foodborne illness.

Poisonous animals

Very few animal species are poisonous, although several species of poisonous fish and other marine animals are known to exist. Pufferfish is the best known example, although the toxin in pufferfish may actually emanate from bacteria [28, 29].

Animal tissues and products also contain very few naturally occurring toxicants that could cause adverse reactions if ingested in abnormally large quantities. Fat-soluble vitamins, most notably vitamin A, serve as an example. Cases of vitamin A intoxication have occurred in polar explorers ingesting polar bear liver and in infants resulting from feeding diets rich in vitamin A (e.g., chicken livers and fortified milk) and carotenoids (e.g., pureed carrots), while also administering daily vitamin supplements [31].

Poisonous plants

Many poisonous plants exist in nature [32]. Classic examples would include water hemlock and nightshade that were used in centuries past to poison one's enemies. While consumers purchasing foods from commercial sources can usually avoid the ingestion of poisonous plants, intoxications occur among individuals who have harvested their own foods in the wild. For example, an elderly couple succumbed after mistaking foxglove for comfrey while harvesting herbs for tea; foxglove contains digitalis. In another example, a team member in a desert survival course died after eating a salad prepared in part from a *Datura* species, jimsonweed. Jimsonweed contains tropane alkaloids including atropine. While atropine is a useful pharmaceutical agent, its ingestion from natural sources in uncontrolled doses can be fatal. Atropine has potent anticholinergic properties, and individuals ingesting jimsonweed and other plants containing tropane alkaloids suffer neurotoxic effects. Many more such examples could be provided.

More rarely, intoxications from poisonous plants occur with products purchased from commercial sources. In one well-investigated outbreak, a commercial herbal tea was contaminated with *Senecio longilobus*, a well-known poisonous plant [33]. The herbal tea, called gordolobo yerba, was sold to the Mexican-American population in Arizona, and promoted as a cure for colic, viral infections, and nasal congestion in infants. Several infants died from the ingestion of this contaminated herbal tea. *Senecio* and many other plants contain a group of chemicals known as pyrrolizidine alkaloids. The pyrrolizidine alkaloids can cause both acute and chronic symptoms. Chronic low doses produce liver cancer and cirrhosis. The acute symptoms associated with the contaminated herbal tea included ascites, hepatomegaly, veno-occlusive liver disease, abdominal pain, nausea, vomiting, headache, and diarrhea [33]. Death resulted from liver failure.

Occasionally, intoxications from poisonous plants occur from the intentional addition of such materials to foods. The intentional addition of marijuana to bakery items is the most common example.

Many plant-derived foods contain naturally occurring toxicants at doses that are not hazardous, at least on an acute basis, unless large quantities of the food are eaten. Examples would include solanine and chaconine in potatoes, oxalates in spinach and rhubarb, furan compounds in mold-damaged sweet potatoes, and cyanogenic glycosides in lima beans, cassava, and many fruit pits [34].

The cyanogenic glycosides, for example, can release cyanide from enzymatic action occurring during the storage and processing of the foods, or on contact with stomach acid. Commercial varieties of lima beans contain minimal amounts of these cyanogenic glycosides having a hydrogen cyanide (HCN) yield of 10 mg per 100 g of lima beans (wet weight). The lethal oral dose of cyanide for humans is 0.5 mg/kg, so a 70 kg adult would need to ingest 35 mg of cyanide, an amount that would require the ingestion of at least 350 g of lima beans. Such levels of consumption are quite unlikely, and human illnesses from cyanide intoxication from lima bean ingestion have not been reported. Wild varieties of lima beans contain much higher levels of the cyanogenic glycosides (up to 300 mg HCN/100 g) and would likely be hazardous to consume. Cyanide intoxications have occurred in Africa and South America due to the consumption of cassava, which is sometimes ingested in large quantities due to a lack of other foods [34]. Cyanide intoxication has also occurred from the ingestion of fruit pits, especially by the grinding of pits with the fruit in food processors during the preparation of jams and wines. The symptoms of cyanide intoxication include a rapid onset of peripheral numbness and dizziness, mental confusion, stupor, cyanosis, twitching, convulsions, coma, and death.

Many toxic constituents of plants are inactivated or removed during processing and preparation. For example, raw soybeans contain trypsin inhibitors, lectins, amylase inhibitors, saponins, and various antivitamins. Fortunately, these toxicants are inactivated during the heating and fermentation processes used with soybeans. Failure to remove or inactivate these toxicants can result in foodborne illness. For example, raw kidney beans contain lectins, which are typically inactivated during cooking. In the United Kingdom, immigrants who did not appreciate the importance of thorough cooking of kidney beans have ingested undercooked kidney beans leading to the onset of nausea, vomiting, abdominal pain, and bloody diarrhea from the lectins.

Poisonous mushrooms

Many species of mushrooms are poisonous. The harvesting of mushrooms in the wild can be a hazardous practice. Intoxications occur each year in the United States from the ingestion of poisonous mushrooms. Poisonous mushrooms contain a variety of naturally occurring toxicants, which can be classified into Groups I–VI [35].

The Group I toxins are the most hazardous and include amatoxin and phallotoxin. Amatoxin is produced by *Amanita phalloides*, the death cap mushroom. Amatoxin poisoning occurs in three stages. The first stage involves abdominal pain, nausea, vomiting, diarrhea, and hyperglycemia beginning 6–24 hours after ingestion of the mushrooms. A short period of remission then occurs. The third and often fatal stage involves severe liver and kidney dysfunction, hypoglycemia, convulsions, coma, and death. Death resulting from hypoglycemic shock occurs 4–7 days after the onset of symptoms.

The Group II toxins are hydrazines; gyromitrin is the best known example. Gyromitrin is produced by *Gyromitra esculenta* or false morel mushrooms. The symptoms elicited by ingestion of these mushrooms include a bloated feeling, nausea, vomiting, watery or bloody diarrhea, abdominal pain, muscle cramps, faintness, and ataxia occurring with a 6–12 hour onset time.

The Group III toxins are characterized by muscarine and affect the autonomic nervous system. Muscarine is found in fly agaric (*Amanita muscaria*) sometimes in association with the Group I toxins. Symptoms include perspiration, salivation, lacrimation with blurred vision, abdominal cramps, watery diarrhea, constriction of the pupils, hypotension, and a slowed pulse occurring rapidly following the ingestion of the poisonous mushrooms.

The Group IV toxins cause symptoms only when ingested with alcoholic beverages. Coprine, a Group IV toxin produced by *Coprinus atramentarius*, is the best example. Symptoms include flushing of the neck and face, distension of the veins in the neck, swelling and tingling of the hands, metallic taste, tachycardia, and hypotension progressing to nausea and vomiting. Symptoms begin within 30 minutes of ingestion of the mushrooms and can last for up to 5 days.

The Group V and VI toxins act primarily on the central nervous system causing hallucinations. The Group V toxins include ibotenic acid and muscimol and cause dizziness, drowsiness followed by hyperkinetic activity, confusion, delirium, incoordination, staggering, muscular spasms, partial amnesia, a coma-like sleep, and hallucinations beginning 30 minutes to 2 hours after ingestion. Fly agaric is a good source of the Group V toxins.

The Group VI toxins include psilocybin and psilocin. The symptoms of the Group VI toxins include pleasant or aggressive mood, anxiety, unmotivated laughter and hilarity, compulsive movements, muscle weakness, drowsiness, hallucinations, and sleep. The Group VI toxins are found in Mexican mushrooms, *Psilocybe mexicana*. Symptoms usually begin 30–60 minutes after ingestion of the mushrooms and recovery is often spontaneous in 5–10 hours. When the dose of the Group VI toxins is high, prolonged and severe sequelae, even death, can occur.

Metabolic food disorders

Like food allergies, metabolic food disorders affect only certain individuals in the population. These individuals display increased sensitivity to certain chemicals in foods because they lack an enzyme necessary to metabolize that particular chemical or because they have a genetic abnormality that makes them especially susceptible to the toxic effects of a particular foodborne chemical. The best examples of metabolic food disorders are lactose intolerance and favism.

Lactose intolerance

Lactose intolerance is associated with an inherited deficiency in the amount of the enzyme, β-galactosidase, in the small intestine [36, 37]. β-Galactosidase is needed for the hydrolysis of the milk disaccharide, lactose, into its constituent monosaccharides, glucose and galactose. While glucose and galactose can be absorbed and used for metabolic energy, lactose cannot be absorbed without prior hydrolysis. If the activity of β-galactosidase is insufficient, the lactose from milk or dairy products will be incompletely hydrolyzed. Undigested lactose will pass into the colon where the large numbers of bacteria will convert it to CO_2, H_2, and H_2O. The symptoms associated with lactose intolerance are abdominal cramps, flatulence, and frothy diarrhea.

Almost all individuals are born with sufficient levels of β-galactosidase activity. However, with increasing age, the levels of enzyme activity diminish. At some point, the levels of β-galactosidase activity may be insufficient to handle the load of lactose ingested in the diet. Symptoms of lactose intolerance can begin to appear in the early teen years and often worsen with advancing age. Many lactose-intolerant individuals can tolerate some lactose in their diets, often as much as the amount found in an 8-oz glass of milk [38]. The degree of tolerance may lessen with advancing age.

Lactose intolerance is an inherited trait. It affects only about 6–12% of all Caucasians, but ultimately affects 60–90% of some ethnic groups including Black Americans, Native Americans, Hispanics, Asians, Jews, and Arabs [36].

Lactose intolerance is treated with dairy product avoidance diets, although some dairy products can usually be ingested without harm. Lactose-intolerant individuals can often safely consume yogurt if the yogurt contains live bacterial cultures with β-galactosidase [36]. Lactose-hydrolyzed milk is also available in many markets.

Favism

Favism is caused by the ingestion of fava beans or the inhalation of pollen from the *Vicia faba* plant by individuals with a deficiency of the enzyme, glucose-6-phosphate dehydrogenase (G6PDH), in their erythrocytes [39, 40]. Erythrocyte G6PDH deficiency is the most common enzyme deficiency in the world, affecting perhaps 100 million individuals. Erythrocyte G6PDH deficiency is most prevalent among Kurds, Iraqis, Iranians, Sardinians, Cypriot Greeks, Black Americans, and some African populations. This deficiency is virtually unknown in northern Europeans, North American Indians, and Eskimos. G6PDH is a critical enzyme which is essential for the maintenance of adequate levels of the reduced form of glutathione (GSH) and nicotinamide dinucleotide phosphate (NADPH) in erythrocytes. GSH and NADPH protect the erythrocyte membrane from oxidation. Fava beans contain two potent, naturally occurring oxidants, vicine and convicine. These oxidants can damage the erythrocyte membranes in G6PDH-deficient individuals, but not normal persons. Exposure to fava beans in sensitive individuals results in acute hemolytic anemia. The typical symptoms are pallor, fatigue, dyspnea, nausea, abdominal and/or back pain, fever, and chills. In a few severe cases, hemoglobinuria, jaundice, and renal failure may occur. Favism is not a common malady in the United States because fava beans are rarely ingested here. Favism occurs primarily in the Mediterranean area, the Middle East, China, and Bulgaria where the genetic trait is fairly prevalent and fava beans are more frequently consumed. G6PDH deficiency is often unrecognized in these patients until ingestion of fava beans leads to symptomatic and sometimes severe hemolysis [37, 38].

References

1. Press E, Yeager L. Food "poisoning" due to sodium nicotinate. Report of an outbreak and a review of the literature. *Am J Public Health Nations Health* 1962; 52:1720–1728.
2. Burkhalter J, Shore M, Wollstadt L, et al. Illness associated with high levels of niacin in cornmeal—Illinois. *CDC Morb Mortal Wkly Rep* 1981; 30(1):11–12.
3. Wolk BJ, Ganetsky M, Babu KM. Toxicity of energy drinks. *Curr Opin Pediatr* 2012; 24:243–251.
4. Taylor SL, Byron B. Probable case of sorbitol-induced diarrhea. *J Food Prot* 1984; 47:249.
5. Kilbourne EM, Rigau-Perez JG, HeathJr CW, et al. Clinical epidemiology of toxic oil syndrome: manifestations of a new illness. *N Engl J Med* 1983; 309:1408–1414.
6. Gelpi E, de la Paz MP, Terracini B, et al. The Spanish toxic oil syndrome 20 years after onset: a multidisciplinary review of scientific knowledge. *Environ Health Perspect* 2002; 110:457–464.
7. Rodriguez M, Nogura AE, Del Villaras S, et al. Toxic synovitis from denatured rapeseed oil. *Arthritis Rheum* 1982; 25:1477–1480.
8. Ferrer A, Cabral R. Toxic epidemics caused by alimentary exposure to pesticides. *Food Addit Contam* 1991; 8:755–776.
9. Goldman LR, Beller M, Jackson RL. Aldicarb food poisonings in California, 1985–1988; toxicity estimates for humans. *Arch Environ Health* 1990; 45:141–147.
10. Goes EA, Savage EP, Gibbons G, Aaronson M, Ford SA, Wheeler HW. Suspected foodborne carbamate pesticide intoxication associated with ingestion of hydroponic cucumbers. *Am J Epidemiol* 1980; 111:254–260.
11. Taylor SL, Nordlee JA, Kapels LM. Foodborne toxicants affecting the lung. *Pediatr Allergy Immunol* 1991; 3:180–187.
12. Gawarammana IB, Buckley NA. Medical management of paraquat ingestion. *Br J Clin Pharmacol* 2011; 72:745–752.
13. Schmid R. Cutaneous porphyria in Turkey. *N Engl J Med* 1960; 268:397–398.
14. Keating JP, Lell ME, Straus AW, Zarkowsky H, Smith GE. Infantile methemoglobinemia caused by carrot juice. *N Engl J Med* 1973; 288:825–826.
15. Dewdney JM, Edwards RG. Penicillin hypersensitivity—is milk a significant hazard?: a review. *J R Soc Med* 1984; 77:866–877.
16. Ekino S, Susa M, Nimomiya T, Imamura K, Kitamura T. Minamata disease revisited: an update on the acute and chronic manifestations of methyl mercury poisoning. *J Neurol Sci* 2007; 262:131–144.
17. Dickey RW, Plakas SM. Ciguatoxin: a public health perspective. *Toxicon* 2010; 56:123–136.
18. Farstad DJ, Chow T. A brief case report and review of ciguatera poisoning. *Wilderness Environ Med* 2001; 12:263–269.
19. Paredes I, Rietjens IM, Vieites JM, Carbado AG. Update of risk assessment of main marine biotoxins in the European Union. *Toxicon* 2011; 58:336–354.
20. Russell FE, Egen NB. Ciguatoxic fishes, ciguatoxin (CTX) and ciguatera poisoning. *J Toxicol Toxin Rev* 1991; 10:37–62.
21. Mines D, Stahmer S, Shephard SM. Poisonings—food, fish, shellfish. *Emerg Med Clin North Am* 1997; 13:157–177.
22. Etheridge SM. Paralytic shellfish poisoning: seafood safety and human health perspective. *Toxicon* 2010; 56:108–122.
23. Gessner BD, Middaugh JP. Paralytic shellfish poisoning in Alaska: a 20-year retrospective analysis. *Am J Epidemiol* 1995; 141:766–770.
24. Perl TM, Bedard L, Kosatsky T, Hockin JC, Todd ECD, Remis RS. An outbreak of toxic encephalopathy caused by eating mussels contaminated with domoic acid. *N Engl J Med* 1990; 322:1775–1780.
25. Lefebvre KA, Robertson A. Domoic acid and human exposure risks: a review. *Toxicon* 2010; 56:218–230.
26. Kumar KP, Kumar SP, Nair GA. Risk assessment of the amnesic shellfish poison, domoic acid, on animals and humans. *J Environ Biol* 2009; 30:319–325.
27. Rossini GP, Hess P. Phycotoxins: chemistry, mechanism of action and shellfish poisoning. *EXS* 2010; 100:65–122.
28. Hwang DF, Noguchi T. Tetrodotoxin poisoning. *Adv Food Res* 2007; 52:141–236.
29. Miyazawa K, Noguchi T. Distribution and origin of tetrodotoxin. *J Toxicol Toxin Rev* 2001; 20:11.
30. Richard JL. Some major mycotoxins and their mycotoxicoses—an overview. *Int J Food Microbiol* 2007; 119:3–10.
31. Food and Nutrition Board, Institute of Medicine. *Dietary Reference Intakes—A Risk Assessment Model for Establishing Upper Intake Levels for Nutrients*. Washington, DC: National Academies Press, 1998.
32. Smith RA. Poisonous plants. In: Hui YH, Gorham JR, Murrell KD, Cliver DO (eds), *Foodborne Disease Handbook: Diseases Caused by Hazardous Substances*, vol. 3. New York: Marcel Dekker, 1994; pp. 187–226.
33. Huxtable RJ. Herbal teas and toxins: novel aspects of pyrrolizidine poisoning in the United States. *Perspect Biol Med* 1980; 24:1–14.
34. Beier RC, Nigg HN. Toxicology of naturally occurring chemicals in foods. In: Hui YH, Gorham JR, Murrell KD, Cliver DO (eds) *Foodborne Disease Handbook: Diseases Caused by Hazardous Substances*, vol. 3. New York: Marcel Dekker, 1994; pp. 1–186.
35. SpoerkeJr DG. Mushrooms: epidemiology and medical management. In: Hui YH, Gorham JR, Murrell KD, Cliver DO (eds) *Foodborne Disease Handbook: Diseases Caused by Hazardous Substances*, vol. 3. New York: Marcel Dekker, 1994; pp. 433–462.

36. Stear GIJ, Horsburgh K, Steinman HA. Lactose intolerance—a review. *Curr Allergy Clin Immunol* 2005; 18:114–119.
37. Lomer MC, Parkes GC, Sanderson JD. Review article: lactose intolerance in clinical practice—myths and realities. *Aliment Pharmacol Ther* 2008; 27:93–103.
38. Savaiano DA, Boushey CJ, McCabe SB. Lactose intolerance symptoms assessed by meta-analysis: a grain of truth that leads to exaggeration. *J Nutr* 2006; 136:1107–1113.
39. Marquardt RR, Wang N, Arbid MS. Pyrimidine glycosides. In: D'Mello JPF (ed.) *Handbook of Plant and Fungal Toxicants*. Boca Raton FL: CRC Press, 1997; pp. 139–155.
40. Schuurman M, Van Waardenburg D, Da Costa J, Niemarkt H, Leroy P. Severe hemolysis and methemoglobinemia following fava bean ingestion in glucose-6-phosphate dehydrogenase deficiency: case report and literature review. *Eur J Pediatr.*2009; 168:779–782.

41 Seafood Toxins

Soheil Chegini[1], Sarah J. Austin[2], & Dean D. Metcalfe[2]

[1]Exton Allergy & Asthma Associates, Exton, PA, USA
[2]Laboratory of Allergic Diseases, Division of Intramural Research, National Institute of Allergy and Infectious Diseases, National Institutes of Health, Bethesda, MD, USA

Key Concepts

- Seafood poisoning is uncommon in non-endemic regions, but may be responsible for adverse reactions to seafood.
- Marine toxins produce syndromes with primarily acute gastrointestinal and neurological manifestations that frequently masquerade as allergic reactions.
- Seafood poisoning may result in similar symptoms in several individuals who shared the seafood and display an "endemic" nature.
- The absence of a prior history of allergy to seafood and its subsequent tolerance point away from an allergic etiology and suggest poisoning.
- Knowledge of specific seafood toxic syndromes is necessary to consider them in the differential diagnosis and obtain the appropriate history and collect specimens to confirm the diagnosis and institute the correct treatment.

Introduction

Fish and shellfish are nutritious foods that constitute desirable components of a healthy diet. However, seafood, including fish, shrimps, lobsters, crabs, mussels, and clams, are among the most frequent causes of food allergy [1]. The differential diagnosis of seafood allergy is extensive and includes true hypersensitivity reactions to the seafood, allergic reactions to non-seafood components, reactions to toxins within the seafood, and adverse reactions to food contaminants such as antibiotic residues. Other diagnostic considerations include adverse reactions to associated food additives such as sulfites or monosodium glutamate (MSG) (Table 41.1) [2].

While IgE-mediated seafood allergy is reviewed in other chapters within this text, we focus here on the various types of seafood poisoning, with special emphasis on important aspects of the clinical picture, the marine species most commonly involved, and their general geographic distribution. The aim is to provide information that we hope will be helpful in recognizing these reactions, making the correct diagnosis, and differentiating such reactions from seafood allergy. Current knowledge on mechanisms of toxicity and methods of detection and quantification of various seafood toxins are reviewed and general treatment and preventive measures are discussed.

Background

Scombroid and ciguatera fish poisoning, paralytic shellfish poisoning (PSP), puffer fish poisoning (PFP), and various forms of neurotoxic shellfish poisoning, all result from toxins found in the seafood itself. Poisoning by such toxins primarily results in acute gastrointestinal and neurological manifestations. These reactions frequently masquerade as allergic reactions on presentation to emergency departments and urgent care clinics [3–5]. Similarly, bacteria and bacterial toxins in the setting of seafood ingestion may cause gastrointestinal and systemic symptoms that can also be confused with food allergy.

Fish poisoning can be classified into two categories based on the presence or absence of a toxin at the time of capture. In ciguatera and puffer fish poisoning the toxin is present in the live fish, whereas in scombroid poisoning, the substance provoking the reaction is produced by contaminating bacteria only after capture of the fish. PFP is associated with a high rate of mortality, as opposed to scombroid and ciguatera reactions, which are self-limiting illnesses that

Food Allergy: Adverse Reactions to Foods and Food Additives, Fifth Edition. Edited by Dean D Metcalfe, Hugh A Sampson, Ronald A Simon and Gideon Lack.

Table 41.1 Differential diagnosis of seafood-associated poisoning.

- **A.** Seafood poisons
  - **1.** Fish poisoning
    - **a.** Ciguatera
    - **b.** Scombroid (histamine)
    - **c.** Tetrodon (puffer fish) poisoning
  - **2.** Shellfish poisoning
    - **a.** Paralytic
    - **b.** Neurotoxic
    - **c.** Amnesic
    - **d.** Diarrhetic
    - **e.** Azaspiracid
- **B.** Infections and bacterial intoxications
  - **1.** Bacterial toxins
    - **a.** *Clostridium botulinum*
    - **b.** *Staphylococcus aureus*
  - **2.** Bacterial infections
    - **a.** *Vibrio cholerae*
    - **b.** *Vibrio parahemolyticus*
    - **c.** *Vibrio vulnificus*
  - **3.** Viral infections
    - **a.** Norwalk and Norwalk-like enteric viruses

resolve spontaneously in the majority of cases. PFP may be severe and life threatening, but other shellfish poisonings are usually transient, self-limited, and rarely fatal. Treatment is primarily supportive.

In the United States, seafood poisoning, principally scombroid and ciguatera fish poisoning (CFP) (Table 41.2), is responsible for about 4% of all reported foodborne disease outbreaks and less than 1% of foodborne illnesses reported by the Centers for Disease Control [11–13] (Table 41.3). This is significantly smaller than the 17.8% reported for the period 1978–1987 [6]. In Australia from 1995 to 2000, CFP and scombroid poisoning were responsible for 11% and 3% of all foodborne outbreaks, respectively [14]. Worldwide, ciguatera is the most frequently reported poisoning associated with seafood [15].

National surveillance data on seafood-related poisoning in the United States is based on outbreaks of acute foodborne disease reported by state health departments to the CDC. Since 1978 an average of about 20 outbreaks of scombroid poisoning has been reported annually, involving over 100 cases. CFP ranks second with approximately 15 outbreaks each year and over 60 cases. PSP has been the most commonly reported poisoning due to shellfish in the United States, with an average of one outbreak and 9 cases annually. Only three outbreaks of PFP affecting seven individuals and eight outbreaks of neurotoxic shellfish poisoning (NSP) with 32 individuals were reported over a period of 32 years (Table 41.2). However, these figures are likely to underrepresent the true incidence of seafood poisoning, since some cases remain undiagnosed and many are not reported to health authorities. For instance, even in the endemic area of Queensland, Australia, it has been estimated that only about 20% of ciguatera cases are reported to the local database [16].

The bulk of shellfish-associated illness is infectious in nature, which can be either bacterial or viral, with the Norwalk virus likely to account for most cases of gastroenteritis. Ingestion of contaminated shellfish results in a wide variety of symptoms, depending on the toxins present, their concentrations in the shellfish, and the amount of contaminated shellfish consumed. Five different types of shellfish poisoning have been identified including PSP, NSP, diarrhetic shellfish poisoning (DSP), amnesic shellfish poisoning (ASP), and azaspiracid shellfish poisoning (AZP). Except for ASP, which is caused by the diatomean toxin, domoic acid (DA), all of these syndromes and CFP are caused by dinoflagellate toxins. Dinoflagellates are unicellular biflagellates that belong to the ancient eukaryotic lineage, Alveolata. Approximately, 2000 species of dinoflagellates exist and most of these are marine species that are most commonly known for their capacity to form harmful algal blooms (HABs). Fewer than 100 dinoflagellate species produce toxins. However, toxins can be mass produced due to the extraordinary potential of dinoflagellates to proliferate and the concentration of toxins increases within marine organisms that ingest dinoflagellates, and then within higher organisms that in turn ingest these lower organisms [17]. Toxins responsible for the clinical manifestations are generally produced in the warmer summer months and are then concentrated in filter-feeding bivalve mollusks such as clams and mussels. Only about 30 dinoflagellates and a few diatom species are known to cause human illness, and fewer still are potentially lethal [18].

Generally, marine toxins do not alter the appearance, taste, or smell of seafood and are not inactivated by heat or gastric acid. Anthropogenic eutrophication has been incriminated in the higher frequency of HABs and increased production of biotoxins by marine dinoflagellates [19]. Case frequency of CFP recorded by the South Pacific Epidemiological and Health Information Service (SPEHIS) seems to correlate with environmental variables such as southern oscillation index (SOI) and sea surface temperature (SST) [20, 21]. However, the incidence of shellfish poisoning appears to be declining, most likely because of careful monitoring, beach closures, and improved public awareness. It is recommended that the public should avoid collecting shellfish from areas where red tides are known to occur and refrain from consumption of suspect shellfish that should be submitted to health authorities for investigation [22].

Seafood poisoning is largely a regional problem and cases are usually concentrated in endemic areas. However, poisonings associated with imported seafood are an exception, since they occur sporadically and do not follow geographic

Table 41.2 Epidemiology of seafood poisoning in the United States from 1978 through 2009.

	Scombroid		Ciguatera		PFP		NTSP		PSP	
Year	*Outbreaks*	*Cases*	*Outbreaks*	*Cases*	*Outbreaks*	*Cases*	*Outbreaks*	*Cases*	*Outbreaks*	*Cases*
1978	7	30	19	56					4	10
1979	14	134	21	91					1	3
1980	28	151	15	52					5	116
1981	9	93	30	219						
1982	18	58	8	37					1	5
1983	13	271	13	43						
1984	12	53	18	78						
1985	14	56	26	104					2	3
1986	20	60	18	70	1	3	1	3		
1987	22	98	11	35						
1988	16	65	4	8					1	6
1989	17	80	19	66						
1990	11	194	11	44					2	24
1991	17	40	7	50					2	35
1992	15	135	1	8						
1993	5	21	13	44						
1994	21	83	11	54					3	29
1995	16	91	10	27					1	7
1996	19	55	9	32						
1997	22	92	18	65					2	4
1998	29	182	19	87					1	6
1999	30	97	15	53					1	3
2000	37	136	19	67			1	3	4	12
2001	36	187	26	88			2	4		
2002	16	60	22	79					2	25
2003	43	219	19	62					1	2
2004	33	104	10	31					2	4
2005	26	115	10	38			1	4		
2006	32	113	10	45	1	2	2	15		
2007	20	74	14	84	1	2	1	3	1	4
2008	12	55	15	104					1	3
2009	7	32	10	36						
Sum	637	3234	471	1957	3	7	8	32	37	301
Average Annual	20	101	15	61	<0.1	0.2	0.3	1	1	9

Source: Compiled from References 6–10.
Number of outbreaks and cases reported to the Centers for Disease Control and Prevention (CDC).

patterns. At present, well over half the seafood supply in the United States is imported. As reef fish are increasingly exported from tropical areas, seafood poisoning has become a more widespread problem. Most current health risks associated with seafood contamination originate in the environment and should be dealt with by the control of harvest or at the point of capture by application of the principles of hazard analysis and critical control point (HACCP). Some seafood poisonings, although not yet a problem in the United States, could become more common in the United States as international tourism increases and seafood from different regions of the world becomes available. Thus, knowledge about these clinical syndromes is helpful.

Some marine toxins are allelopathic, functioning in nature to inhibit the growth of other microalgae as an adaptive mechanism. Animals may have evolved to acquire toxicity by sequestration of toxic compounds from their food source, which provides protection from predators that have thus learned to avoid them. More recently, two new classes of marine toxins that can cause human disease were discovered: azaspiracid and spirolides. The sources of these toxins have also been identified in phytoplanktons that have widespread presence in Atlantic waters.

Aquaculture is gaining an ever-increasing importance in the production of seafood, which introduces new challenges to health care and the practicing physician.

Table 41.3 Relative contribution of outbreaks and cases associated with seafood toxins to the foodborne diseases in the United States and U.S. territories (2001–2008).

	Outbreaks								Illnesses							
	2001–2005		2006		2007		2008		2001–2005		2006		2007		2008	
	Mean annual total		Total		Total		Total		Mean annual total		Total		Total		Total	
Etiology	No.	%[a]	No.	%[a]	No.	%[a]	No.	%[a]	No.	%[a]	No.	%[a]	No.	%[a]	No.	%[a]
Scombroid toxin/histamine	30	3 (4)	32	3 (4)	20	2 (3)	12	1 (2)	117	0 (1)	113	0 (1)	74	0	55	0
Ciguatoxin	17	1 (2)	10	1	14	1 (2)	14	1 (2)	59	0	45	0	84	0 (1)	81	0
Neurotoxic shellfish poison	1	0	2	0	1	0	–	0	2	0	15	0	3	0	–	–
Puffer fish tetrodotoxin	–	–	1	0	1	0	–	0	–	–	2	0	2	0	–	–
Paralytic shellfish poison	1	0	–	–	1	0	1	<1	2	0	–	–	4	0	3	0
All seafood toxins	49	4 (6)	45	4 (5)	37	3 (5)	27	3 (4)	180	1	175	1	167	1	139	1
All known causes	758	64	884	70	698	64	666	64	18,981	74	22,510	81	15,477	73	18,240	79
All causes	1,179	100	1,270	100	1,097	100	1,034	100	25,702	100	27,634	100	21,244	100	23,152	100

Source: Compiled from References 11–13.

[a]The Percentage of outbreaks and cases was calculated based on all reported to the Centers for Disease Control and Prevention (CDC). The figures in parenthesis reflect the percentage of seafood toxin-related outbreaks and cases with a defined etiology.

Use of algicides, antibiotics, and antiparasitic compounds that leave detectable residues in farm-raised seafood is a potential human health hazard. Genetic engineering and neoantigens incorporated into seafood or introduced into other food from a marine origin can present an alternative source of antigen that could potentially lead to allergic sensitization.

Common intoxications associated with fish

Scombroid (histamine) poisoning

A constellation of gastrointestinal, neurological, cardiovascular, and cutaneous symptoms such as nausea, vomiting, diarrhea, abdominal cramping, throbbing headache, palpitations, flushing, tingling, burning, itching, hypotension, urticaria and angioedema characterize scombroid fish poisoning. In severe cases and in persons with asthma, bronchospasm may develop. The most frequent symptoms are tingling and burning sensations around the mouth, gastrointestinal complaints, and skin rash. Patients sometimes describe a peppery or bitter taste to the fish, but often the fish tastes completely normal. In general, the onset of symptoms is rapid, usually within 10–30 minutes following ingestion of the contaminated fish. Physical signs may include a diffuse blanching erythema, tachycardia, wheezing, and hypotension or hypertension. Immediate reactions may be indistinguishable from anaphylaxis and scombroid poisoning is often misdiagnosed as an allergic reaction [2–5].

Scombroid intoxication results from ingestion of fish containing high levels of free histamine. Since histamine is resistant to heat, cooking the fish and even high temperatures used in canning processes will not prevent scombroid poisoning [23]. Because the symptoms are usually self-limited and resolve in the vast majority of cases within 4–10 hours without any sequelae, there is often no need for specific treatment. However, H1 and H2 antihistamines ameliorate the symptoms in severe cases [24]. The mildness and transient nature of scombroid poisoning contribute to underreporting of the disease.

Initially, the disease was associated with consumption of scombroid fish. Scombroid means like mackerel (*Scomber*). Fish belonging to the Scombroidea family found in temperate and tropical waters include tuna, mackerel, bonito, and saury. More recently, non-scombroid species have been identified as causing this intoxication, including mahi-mahi, bluefish, jack, mackerel, amberjack, herring, sardine, and anchovy. Some of these species constitute highly commercialized marine products and have been among the most valuable resources of the canning industry [23]. In the United States between 1978 and 2009, scombroid poisoning owing to mahi-mahi, tuna, and bluefish accounted for the majority of the cases reported to CDC [6–10].

The histamine is not present when the fish are caught, but is later produced during spoilage by decarboxylation of free histidine, which is naturally present at high levels in species of fish implicated in scombroid poisoning [25]. The production of histamine is due to the action of histidine decarboxylase, an enzyme produced by bacteria growing on the fish. The enteric bacteria *Morganella morganii, Klebsiella pneumonias*, and *Hafnia alvei* are most frequently implicated. These organisms are not considered as natural flora of living fish and contamination probably occurs during catching and handling [27]. This reaction occurs optimally between 20°C and 30°C and is prevented by refrigeration or chemical decontamination. Experimental studies have shown that histamine formation is negligible in fish stored at 0°C [25, 26].

Even though histamine levels may not be correlated with any obvious signs of decomposition, histamine content may be used as an index of spoilage in certain fish. Fresh fish normally contain histamine levels of 10 ppm or 1 mg/100 g of fish flesh. Laboratory confirmation of scombroid poisoning is based on demonstrating elevated histamine levels of 0.50 ppm in the muscle tissue of incriminated fish using an enzyme-linked immunosorbent assay (ELISA) [28, 29].

Although histamine was first suggested as the causative toxin over 50 years ago, it was not until 1991 that urinary excretion of histamine, in quantities exceeding those required to produce toxicity, was documented *in vivo* in humans in association with the clinical syndrome [30]. Subsequently, elevated plasma histamine levels were demonstrated in patients with scombroid poisoning [31]. Various hypotheses have been put forward to explain why histamine consumed in spoiled fish is more toxic than pure histamine taken orally. One idea postulates a role for other heat-stable substances produced in fish by putrefactive bacteria that inhibit the metabolism of histamine by intestinal flora and permit absorption of a more substantial portion of the ingested histamine. A second hypothesis suggests that urocanic acid, another imidazole compound derived from histidine in spoiling fish, may induce mast cell degranulation, and endogenous histamine release may augment the exogenous histamine consumed in spoiled fish [32].

Scombroid poisoning is preventable by proper handling and prompt refrigeration of fish at the time of capture and during subsequent storage, processing, and distribution until it is preserved or cooked. Fish should be chilled rapidly to temperatures below 10°C within 4 hours after capture and stored at 0–4°C to keep bacterial numbers and histamine levels low. Despite the huge expansion in trade in recent years, great progress has been made in ensuring the quality and safety of fish products. This is largely the result of the introduction of international standards of food hygiene and the application of HACCP principles [25, 32].

Ciguatera

CFP is a clinical syndrome that presents after consumption of ciguatoxic fish with characteristic gastrointestinal, neurological, and occasionally, cardiovascular symptoms [33]. The onset of the symptoms ranges between 30 minutes and 12 hours after ingestion of contaminated fish, depending on the severity of intoxication. Nausea, vomiting, watery diarrhea, and abdominal pain usually develop within 3–6 hours and typically last 12–24 hours. Neurological symptoms develop over 24 hours and tend to be the most distinctive and enduring. They include paresthesias that initially involve the lips, tongue, and throat, which later may extend to the extremities, hypoesthesia, dysesthesias, pruritus, generalized weakness, and anxiety. Cold allodynia (burning dysesthesia or sensation of heat upon touching cold water or objects) is almost pathognomonic for ciguatera and is often incorrectly referred to as "temperature reversal" [16]. Paresthesias do not follow dermatome patterns [34]. Neurological symptoms are often aggravated by alcohol consumption, stress, and physical activity [35]. Other less common symptoms include diaphoresis, chills, dizziness, headache, blurred vision, prostration, myalgias, dry mouth, taste disturbances or a metallic taste, and pain or a loose sensation in the teeth. Weakness may last for 1–7 days. Mean duration of acute illness is typically 8.5 days, although it is not unusual for neurological symptoms such as paresthesias or cold allodynia to periodically reoccur for a month or longer. Diminished or increased reflexes and dilated pupils may also be noted which usually resolve in 2–3 days. Cardiovascular symptoms are found in 10–15% of cases, most commonly in individuals previously exposed to the toxin but, when present, bradycardia or hypotension may require urgent management. In cases of severe intoxication, seizures, coma, and respiratory paralysis may occur and which, in the absence of adequate life support, may be fatal [33, 34]. CFP is usually a self-limiting disease, but symptoms may be extremely debilitating, resulting in extended periods of disability.

Some estimates place the annual number of ciguatera cases at 50,000 worldwide [35]. This poisoning spans the globe and generally is observed in warm waters between latitudes within 35° of the equator [36]. It is the most common type of fish poisoning in the Caribbean. In the United States during the period from 1978 through 2004, 390 outbreaks of CFP involving 1576 persons were reported to CDC. No ciguatera-related deaths were reported [7–10]. In Hawaii, the average annual incidence of CFP was 8.7/100000 based on 150 outbreaks involving 462 individuals that were reported to the State Department of Health during a 5-year interval from January 1984 through December 1988 [37]. These figures, however, are substantially higher than the CDC statistics which accounted for only 77 outbreaks and 295 cases in the United States during that period. Of the 189 outbreaks and 774 cases between 1998 and 2008, 110 outbreaks and 337 cases were reported from Hawaii and 53 outbreaks and 278 cases from Florida [10]. Reported outbreaks in other states have been related, in most cases, to a travel to the endemic areas, or from eating fish caught in endemic ciguatera areas; and there is concern that many cases are not recognized by mainland United States physicians. Despite its exceedingly low incidence outside endemic areas, as the domestic fish industry expands its sources of supply, the diagnosis of this "tropical" disease must also be considered in areas where coral reef fish are not native [36].

Ciguatoxins (CTX) are a group of lipid-soluble toxins responsible for ciguatera. CTX are produced by *Gambierdiscus toxicus*, a marine dinoflagellate that usually grows attached to dead coral and is ingested by small herbivores off the reef [38]. These polyether toxins are among the most potent natural substances known [39]. CTX activate voltage-gated sodium channels (VGSCs), causing cell membrane excitability and instability [40]. *In vitro* studies suggest that CTX causes a nerve conduction block after initial neural stimulation [41]. When ingested by certain subtropical and tropical finfish, they accumulate in their tissues. Biotransformation of CTX in fish increases their polarity and thus their toxicity. Thus, the toxins and their metabolites are concentrated when carnivorous reef fish (e.g. barracuda, grouper, and amberjacks) prey on smaller herbivorous fish. The toxic effect is amplified in large predatory fish that become the most toxic to humans at the end of the food chain [39]. Factors influencing the concentration of CTX that accumulate in fish include the rate of dietary intake, the efficiency of assimilation, the degree and nature of any toxin biotransformation, the rate of depuration, and the rate of growth of fish. More than 400 species of fish can be vectors of CTX, but generally only a relatively small number of species of reef fish belonging to the family, Carrangidae are regularly incriminated in CFP. The fish most commonly implicated include amberjack, snapper, grouper, barracuda, and goatfish. The toxin may be most concentrated in the head, liver, intestines, testes, ovaries, and roe [36].

Maitotoxins (MTX) are water-soluble polyether phytotoxins also produced by *Gambierdiscus toxicus*, which are distinct from CTX and have slightly higher potency than CTX when administered parenterally. Experimental intraperitoneal injection of MTX to mice or rats induces severe pathological changes involving the stomach, heart, and lymphoid tissues [42]. MTX have low oral bioavailability and do not tend to accumulate in fish flesh; consequently they are unlikely to play a significant role in causing human illness. To date, no compelling evidence exists to support a role for water-soluble toxins, including MTX, in CFP [16].

Only certain genetic strains produce CTX, and environmental triggers for increasing toxin production are unknown [43]. However, there is concern as to whether disruptions in the reef ecosystem may shift the balance toward a higher rate of toxin-producing *G. toxicus* and an increased incidence of CFP [44].

CTX are heat stable, so are not inactivated by either cooking or freezing. They are not affected by gastric acid and are harmless to the fish itself. Since CTX are odorless, colorless, and tasteless, ciguateric fish look, taste, and smell normal, and detection of toxins in fish remains a problem. CTX in fish can be screened using a high-throughput *in vitro* assay to detect the specific activating effects of CTX on VGSCs in mouse neuroblastoma cells. This methodology allows discrimination between algal toxins that affect VGSCs and can distinguish CTX from brevetoxins (BTX), tetrodotoxins (TTX) and saxitoxins (STX). Subsequently, in fish samples that screen positive, liquid chromatography–mass spectrometry (LC–MS) is used to confirm the molecular presence of CTX and establish their concentration [33].

The diagnosis of CTX ingestion is based on a history of recent consumption of potentially ciguateric fish, clinical findings, and by the detection of toxin in samples of fish. Thus, any uneaten portions of fish should be saved in a freezer and submitted to state or local public health officials when suspected cases are reported to assist with the investigation and control of a possible outbreak [33].

There is no immunity and no known antidote for CTX poisoning. Intravenous mannitol may be effective in reducing the associated neurological and muscular symptoms if administered early in the course, within 48–72 hours of the onset of the illness. Otherwise, treatment is primarily supportive and for relief of symptoms. To prevent CTX poisoning, persons living in or traveling to areas where ciguatera toxin is endemic should follow these general precautions [33]: (1) Avoid consuming large, predatory reef fish, especially barracuda and amberjack; (2) Avoid eating the head, viscera, or roe of any reef fish; and (3) Avoid eating fish caught at sites with known ciguatera toxins.

Puffer fish (tetrodon) poisoning

Symptoms begin with paresthesias 10–45 minutes after ingestion, initially usually a stinging of the lips, tongue, and inner surface of the mouth. Common symptoms that follow include headache, light-headedness, dizziness, vomiting, diaphoresis, pallor, weakness, malaise, and feelings of doom [45]. Some patients may experience a floating sensation, salivation, muscle twitching, and pleuritic chest pain. Depending on the amount of TTX ingested, the patient may experience ataxia, dysphagia, aphonia, and convulsions. Severe poisoning is indicated by hypotension, bradycardia, depressed corneal reflexes, and fixed dilated pupils. An ascending paralysis may develop and death can occur within 6–24 hours secondary to respiratory muscle paralysis [6]. Petechial hemorrhage, blistering and desquamation, and hematemesis have also been reported. Prognosis is good if the patient survives the first 24 hours [46].

Diagnosis is based on clinical symptoms and a history of recent consumption of suspect fish. Treatment is supportive, including active airway management and ventilatory and circulatory support as needed. To minimize the amount of toxin absorbed, gastric lavage and activated charcoal may be beneficial soon after the ingestion. PFP is rare in the United States but more common in Japan. The institution of strict public health measures has reduced the fatality rate [47, 48]. Untreated, the mortality rate is high and approaches 60% [46–48].

PFP results from the ingestion of certain fish species belonging to the order *Tetraodontidae*. These include ocean sunfishes, porcupine fishes, and fugu, which are among the most poisonous of all marine life [49]. These fish have their name because they characteristically inflate to several times normal size by swallowing air or water when threatened. The liver, gonads, intestines, and skin of these fish contain TTX; but the flesh is edible if cleaned and prepared properly, and considered a delicacy by some people. Strict public health standards, including training and certification of fugu chefs, have decreased the incidence of PFP but it has not eliminated the risk associated with consumption of fugu. All puffer species in US waters have been implicated in fatalities and it would seem prudent to consider them potentially toxic [42].

TTX is a guanidinium-containing heat-stable alkaloid that blocks VGSCs with high affinity and specificity. It binds to the neurotoxin receptor site 1, in the outer vestibule of the conducting pore and blocks Na^+ conductance and neuronal transmission [50]. TTX is also present in several other marine and terrestrial species such as snails, starfish, blue-ringed octopus and horseshoe crab, as well as some newts and toads [49]. TTX concentration in puffer fish fluctuates drastically with the reproductive cycle, reaching a peak around the spawning season, and is considerably higher in the female than the male [51]. It is not present in cultured puffer fish, nor is it found in all puffer fish of the same species caught in the wild. These observations and the marked individual, regional, and seasonal variability in TTX concentration suggest that all TTX-bearing animals do not themselves produce the toxin, but accumulate it through the food chain, which starts from marine bacteria. This hypothesis was confirmed when the natural source of TTX was identified in marine *Vibrio, Pseudoalteromonas, Nocardiopsis,* and *Shewanella* species that are part of microflora in the puffer fish and other TTX bearing animals, and it was proven the fish itself merely accumulated the toxin in its tissue [49, 51]. The consumption of as little as 10 g of the toxic tissue may be fatal and 1–4 mg of TTX constitutes a lethal dose for humans [6]. A standard method for determining TTX in food is the mouse bioassay (MBA). This is a procedure in which mice are injected with toxin extracts, and their responses are compared with known amounts of toxin. LC–MS is the alternative methodology to determine TTX concentration. An inhibition-type ELISA has been adapted for rapid detection of TTX, which is relatively inexpensive, sensitive, and selective. The more recent methodology is based on the antibody-based inhibition assay that utilizes surface plasmon resonance (SPR) sensors and can reproducibly quantify TTX in aqueous buffer samples [52].

Common intoxications associated with shellfish

Paralytic shellfish poisoning

PSP, which is caused by STX and its analogs known collectively as "saxitoxins" (STXs), is the best known of shellfish poisonings and causes the most severe symptoms. It is a serious illness in which neurological symptoms predominate. The first and most consistent symptoms are numbness, tingling, and/or burning of the lips, tongue, and throat that begin within 30 minutes of ingestion. Paresthesias spread to the face and neck and often to the fingertips and toes. This precedes muscular weakness that affects the upper and lower limbs and in more severe cases is followed by dysphonia, dysphagia, and ataxia. Paralysis may follow within 2–12 hours, and may persist for as long as 72 hours. The sensation of floating in air, dizziness, weakness, drowsiness, headache, salivation, intense thirst, and throat tightness are commonly described. Diaphoresis, nausea, vomiting, diarrhea, tachycardia, and temporary blindness may also occur. Reflexes may be normal or absent, and most patients remain calm and conscious throughout. Death can result from paralysis of the respiratory muscles within 2–24 hours, depending on the dose. Prognosis is good for individuals surviving past 12 hours. The duration of the illness may be from a few hours to a few days, but muscular weakness can occasionally persist for weeks following recovery [22, 53].

Diagnosis is based on characteristic symptoms and on a history of recent ingestion of shellfish. Treatment is symptomatic. Gastric emptying has been advocated by some authors as an early treatment and activated charcoal has generally been recommended to help block further absorption of the toxins. Airway management and ventilatory support is the mainstay of treatment. Fluid therapy facilitates renal excretion of the toxin and intravenous administration of sodium bicarbonate may be beneficial to correct possible acidosis. Since the half-life of elimination of the toxin from the body is about 90 minutes, 9 hours should be adequate in most cases for physiological reduction of toxin concentration to relatively harmless levels. There is no known immunity to PSP and the second attack may be more severe than the first [53].

In the United States, PSP is a problem primarily in the New England states and in Alaska, California, and Washington. Most disease incidents involve mussels and clams gathered and eaten by recreational collectors, often from closed areas, reflecting the effectiveness of current testing and control measures for commercially produced shellfish. The CDC listed 37 outbreaks involving 301 people with four fatal cases during 1978–2009 suggesting a mortality rate of 2% [6–13]. A recent PSP outbreak involved 21 cases in southeast Alaska during May to June 2011 that represented a considerable increase over the numbers reported in recent years (≤10 cases annually in Alaska since 1998), but none was fatal [54, 55]. Historically, the case-fatality rate was quoted at about 8.5%, but at present it is probably 1% in developed countries [55]. Although PSP is an extremely dangerous disease that can cause death, there is reason to believe that mild cases due to consumption of marginally toxic clams by recreational diggers are never reported to health authorities or are misdiagnosed. Of the 21 cases of PSP that were identified in southeast Alaska during May to June of 2011, a total of 17 were unreported and were identified through active case finding by epidemiologists among persons with PSP symptoms who had not sought care. This underscores the fact that the overall burden of PSP is underestimated through standard reporting.

The first case of PSP was described in 1793 as poisoning by mussels in explorers of the coastline of British Columbia [56]. The primary sources of STX include three morphologically distinct genera of saltwater dinoflagellates: *Alexandrium* spp., *Pyrodinium* spp., and *Gymnodinium* spp. [57]. Subsequently, several cyanobacteria genera were also identified that produce saxitoxin analogs. Dinoflagellates are marine eukaryotes and cyanobacteria are freshwater prokaryotes. Genes involved in STX syntheses have been identified in cyanobacteria but not in dinoflagellates [58]. However, the analysis of putative eukaryotic homologues of cyanobacterial STX synthesis genes indicated that the STX synthesis pathway was likely assembled independently using some evolutionarily related proteins in dinoflagellates. This suggests that STX production in these two ecologically distinct groups may confer an evolutionary advantage [59]. Bivalve mollusks such as mussels, clams, and oysters, assimilate and temporarily store STXs, a complex of neurotoxins produced by dinoflagellates and thus they function as vectors for the toxins.

The STXs are a family of water-soluble alkaloids consisting of various sulfonated and hydroxylated derivatives that contain the basic structure of a tetrahydropurine skeleton and two guanidinium groups. They are among the most potent neurotoxins known. More than 57 STX analogs have been described which include STX, neosaxitoxin, gonyautoxins and their derivatives [58]. The positively charged guanidinium group of the toxins binds specifically to a negatively charged site of the VGSC on the extracellular side of the plasma membrane of nerve and muscle cells, thus blocking the transmembrane flow of Na^+ and resulting in paralysis [57]. STX has also been found to bind to calcium and potassium channels and to affect the function of enzymes such as neuronal nitric oxide synthase [60].

Most shellfish contain a mixture of several STX analogs, depending on the species of algae, geographic area, and type of marine animal involved. Biotransformation of the toxin results in generation of more toxic forms. The higher the net charge, the greater is the toxicity. The potency of STX is expressed in mouse units per milligram (MU/mg). One MU is the amount of toxin required to kill a mouse weighing 20 g in 15 minutes after intraperitoneal injection and is equivalent to 0.18 mg STX. Toxicity of the STX is generally expressed in terms of STX equivalents per 100 g of shellfish meat. There is great variation in individual susceptibility and children are thought to be more susceptible. As little as 120–180 mg of STX can induce moderate symptoms in adults, and fatalities have been associated with levels of 0.3–12 mg [22]. Although normal steaming or boiling will not inactivate the toxins, exposure of toxic shellfish to high temperatures (e.g. in the sterilization step of the canning process) substantially reduces STX concentrations [61].

The MBA has been the classical method for analysis of STX, which is rather insensitive with a detection limit of only 40 mg STX eq/100 g shellfish tissue [62]. High-performance liquid chromatography (HPLC) is quite rapid and has been considered as an optional assay, with detection limits generally an order of magnitude lower [63]. Other alternatives to animal assays for marine toxins utilize cell-based assays with neuroblastoma cell lines or biosensors [64].

In the United States, the toxigenic dinoflagellates causing PSP are *Alexandrium catenella* and *Alexandrium tamarense*; the first being most dominant on the West Coast and the second on the East Coast [65]. When dinoflagellates proliferate or "bloom," they often give the water a red or reddish-brown discoloration, giving rise to a "red tide." Outbreaks of PSP tend to cluster from shortly before, up to several weeks after, the appearance of red tide [66]. Some *Alexandrium* species do not produce toxins and thus not all red tides are caused by toxic algae [67]. Conversely, shellfish may also become toxic in the absence of red tide [34]. Anthropogenic eutrophication has been incriminated in a rising number of red tides or harmful algal blooms and increased production of biotoxins by marine dinoflagellates [19].

STX persist in shellfish for varying periods, depending on the shellfish and the tissue involved [65]. Mussels become highly toxic within a few hours to a few days of the onset of a red tide, but lose their toxin rapidly. Clams and oysters generally do not become as toxic as mussels. They require more time to accumulate high levels of toxins and longer to cleanse themselves. The Alaska butter clam, once contaminated, may never be safe for consumption as it retains paralytic shellfish toxins for years. Sea scallops can take up large amounts of STX, even in the absence of algal blooms, but generally do not pose a threat because their adductor muscle, the only part of the scallop that is usually consumed, does not accumulate toxins. Gastropods can also accumulate significant amounts of STX and in Spain, levels as high as 44 ppm have been recorded in the meat of abalone. Even though paralytic shellfish toxins have been reported in the viscera of rock lobsters and crabs, STX do not appear to accumulate in significant amounts in muscle tissue. Similarly, they can accumulate up to 50 ppm in intestine, liver, and gills of Atlantic mackerel, but not to any extent in muscle. Therefore, crustaceans and finfish do not appear to present a threat of PSP unless consumed whole or unless livers are consumed [22].

Seafood containing STX looks and tastes normal and cooking or steaming only partially destroys the toxins. The most effective way of protecting consumers is to establish and maintain comprehensive monitoring programs for toxic algal blooms and toxins in shellfish in all growing areas [68,69]. To further minimize the risk of PSP, the public should avoid collecting shellfish from areas of known red tides and refrain from consuming suspect shellfish. In addition, since the toxins are water soluble, they can dissolve and concentrate in the cooking broth, which should be discarded after cooking or steaming [22].

Neurotoxic shellfish poisoning

NSP is characterized by both gastrointestinal and neurological symptoms. The illness resembles a mild case of ciguatera poisoning or PSP, but with neuroexcitation rather than flaccid paralysis. The onset is rapid and symptoms occur within 3 hours following the ingestion of contaminated shellfish. Symptoms include numbness of the lips, tongue, and throat; and paresthesias, initially circumoral, which then spread to other parts of the body, "temperature reversal," myalgias, vertigo, headache, nausea, vomiting, diarrhea, and abdominal pain. Less commonly, victims may experience a feeling of inebriation, burning pain in the rectum, dysphagia, ataxia, tremor, decreased reflexes, mydriasis, and bradycardia. The intoxication is usually self-limited and resolves spontaneously within a few hours. Treatment is supportive and generally all patients recover within a few days with no after effects. No fatalities have been reported. From 1978 through 2009, eight outbreaks involving 32 individuals were reported to the CDC [6–10]. The diagnosis can be confirmed by detection of the causative toxins, BTX, in the urine of the patients and in extracts of the leftover food or shellfish collected from the same location.

BTX can aerosolize by surf and wave action along the beach during red tides. Irritant toxin aerosols produce a syndrome characterized by conjunctival irritation, sneezing, and rhinorrhea that resembles an allergic response. Shortness of breath, non-productive cough, and wheezing due to bronchospasm are also triggered in individuals with underlying asthma or chronic obstructive pulmonary disease. The syndrome is self-limited and treatment of the bronchospastic episodes due exposure to aerosolized toxins is symptomatic. In September 2007, a red tide was discovered when local health authorities investigated clustering of upper and lower respiratory symptoms among workers of a dredging company, stationed at the beach and on a ship 3 miles off the northeast Florida coast. The most prevalent symptoms were cough, throat and eye irritation, sneezing, and sniffling. Symptoms occurred more frequently among workers at the beach than those on the ship since beach surf results in BTX aerosolization. This was an unusual presentation, since human respiratory symptoms preceded the observation of dead fish and detection of a brevetoxin odor that indicated a red tide bloom in the proximity which was subsequently confirmed by water sampling [70].

Karenia brevis is the dinoflagellate that synthesizes BTX, a group of more than 10 related lipid soluble cyclic polyethers that are responsible for clinical manifestations of NSP. They bind with high affinity to a specific site of VGSCs that enhances Na^+ influx. This results in depolarization of nerve membranes and spontaneous firing that manifests as neuroexcitation. The major BTX produced by *K. brevis* in red tides is PbTx-2, with lesser amounts of PbTx-1, which are more toxic than all of their derivatives. Filter-feeding bivalve mollusks, such as oysters, clams, and mussels, that consume *K. brevis* concentrate the toxins in various organs and become toxic to humans but remain unaffected. They are active *in vivo* in the nanomolar to picomolar concentration range. Due to their lipid solubility, BTX pass through cell membranes including the blood–brain barrier. BTX are rapidly absorbed and distributed throughout the body, and are metabolized in the liver [71]. In coastal areas affected by *K. brevis*, red tide-aerosolized BTX concentrations can reach levels that activate VGSCs on lower airway cholinergic nerve fibers, resulting in contraction of bronchial smooth muscle and symptoms indistinguishable from asthma [72].

Traditionally, there have been three distinct methodologies for the assessment of BTX in environmental and biological samples including the MBA, ELISA, and LC–MS. The BTX congener profile in *K. brevis* blooms depends on environmental conditions, as well as the stage and age of the red tide bloom. Analytic results will vary depending on the detection method used and the medium sampled (seawater vs. shellfish). LC–MS is the only test capable of confirming the presence of a specific toxin, while ELISA and the MBA measure the overall toxin concentration without indication of a specific toxin [71].

NSP in the United States is generally associated with the consumption of shellfish harvested along the coast of the Gulf of Mexico from Florida to Texas, and, sporadically, along the southern Atlantic coast. This is identical with the geographic distribution of *K. brevis* blooms or "red tides." These red tides occur in many areas within the Gulf of Mexico and may result in massive fish kills. The earliest record of fish kills, later attributed to a *K. brevis* bloom, was in 1844 off the West Coast of Florida, where they still occur frequently, but may be carried north to the Gulf Stream, affecting the coastline of adjacent states. Red tides occur throughout the world and NSP outbreaks are regularly observed in association with blooms [71].

K. brevis blooms are usually initiated on the continental shelf or at the shelf edge, over 40 miles offshore, rather than near the shore where they produce the most deleterious effects. Bloom initiation is characteristically associated with intrusion of deeper, offshore waters that are nutrient-rich onto the shelf. Once dense blooms move inshore, they cannot be sustained without maintaining a minimum nutrient level. Thus, human inputs of nutrients could be responsible for extending the duration and impacts of red tides when blooms enter the nearshore waters [73]. Concern has been raised that human activity may increase the frequency of harmful algal blooms and disseminate *K. brevis* and other toxic phytoplanktons to non-indigenous waters and result in globalization [74, 75].

K. brevis is well adapted and is able to outcompete or otherwise exclude other phytoplankton species. Low concentrations of the organism occur in offshore waters throughout the year and can be detected microscopically. Typically, in late summer and fall when nutrients are abundant, and physical, chemical, and biological conditions are favorable, *K. brevis* grows rapidly, gradually building high densities that in 2–8 weeks reach bloom concentrations ($1–25 \times 10^5$ cells/L). During severe blooms, fish die rapidly from the neurotoxic effects and do not survive to accumulate high toxin concentrations in their tissues. However, fish exposed to sublethal concentrations may accumulate these toxins. Such bioaccumulation in fish eaten by marine mammals, such as dolphins and manatees, results in their demise due to BTX exposure and may also affect human health [76].

Chlorophyll in *K. brevis* results in discoloration of surface water at 10–100 mg/m^3 and is a good surrogate for biomass. It can be detected by satellite color sensors at densities three orders of magnitude less than when water discoloration is visible to human eye, at about 10^6 cells/L. However, it cannot detect deep patches or distinguish *K. brevis* from other algae, which limit the utility of this technology as an early warning system for a ban on shellfish harvest and beach closure. Local authorities may close shellfish harvesting to industries and the public. The basis for closure is the occurrence of more than 5000 *K. brevis* cells per liter of seawater. The small number of cases of NSP testifies to the effectiveness of the surveillance and closure systems [77].

Amnesic shellfish poisoning

ASP presents initially with vomiting, diarrhea, and abdominal cramps within 24 hours post-ingestion of contaminated shellfish. In some cases, varying degrees of neurological dysfunction follow within 48 hours, including confusion, loss of memory, and disorientation. Other neurological symptoms are headache, hyporeflexia, hemiparesis, ophthalmoplegia, and abnormalities of arousal ranging from agitation to coma, seizures, and myoclonus, especially affecting the face. The acute symptoms are milder compared with PSP. Loss of short-term memory is unique among the marine poisonings, hence the name ASP. It is the most persistent symptom and can be permanent [78].

The syndrome was first described in a series of outbreaks in individuals that had eaten mussels cultivated in the river estuaries of Prince Edward Island in Canada from November through December 1987 [79]. In this cohort, the acute symptoms included vomiting (76%), abdominal cramps (50%), diarrhea (4%), severe headache (43%), and loss of short-term memory (25%). Gastrointestinal symptoms were present in all but 7 of the 107 cases. Onset of symptoms after mussel ingestion ranged from 15 minutes to 38 hours, with a median of 5.5 hours. Nineteen patients (18%) were hospitalized, of whom 12 required intensive care because of seizures, coma, profuse respiratory secretions, or unstable blood pressure. Severity of the disease and permanent neurological sequelae, especially cognitive dysfunction, are associated with age over 60 years, male sex and with pre-existing illnesses, as well as the amount of mussels consumed. Three elderly patients died directly and one died indirectly from the intoxication. Neuropathological studies in these four fatal cases showed neuronal necrosis in the hippocampus and amygdala [80]. The clinical records of 14 more severely affected patients that displayed neurological manifestations were reviewed. All 14 patients reported confusion and disorientation within 1.5–48 hours after ingestion and exhibited a variety of neurological abnormalities including coma, mutism, seizures, purposeless chewing and grimacing, and uncontrolled crying or aggressiveness. In neuropsychological testing performed in those 14 patients several months after the acute episode, 12 had severe anterograde memory deficits, with relative preservation of other cognitive functions. Eleven of the 14 individuals had clinical and electromyographic evidence of pure motor or sensory motor neuronopathy or axonopathy. The maximal neurological deficits were seen 4 hours post-ingestion in the least affected patients and 72 hours in those most affected, with maximal improvement within 24 hours to 12 weeks post-ingestion. Acute coma was associated with the slowest recovery. Seizures ceased by 4 months but were frequent up to 8 weeks [80]. Relative preservation of intellect and higher cortical function appears to distinguish ASP from Alzheimer's disease, and the absence of confabulation with well-preserved frontal lobe function differentiates it from Korsakoff's syndrome.

In mussels left uneaten by the patients, as well as mussels harvested later from the same estuaries, the toxic agent was isolated and identified as DA. Its concentration ranged from 31 to 128 mg/100 g of mussel meat that suggested an estimated ingestion of 60–290 mg of DA per patient [78].

Diagnosis is based on a recent history of shellfish ingestion and is made on clinical grounds. It is confirmed by demonstration of DA in shellfish samples. At this point, the treatment of ASP is symptomatic and supportive. Seizures respond well to parenteral benzodiazepins and phenobarbital. There is no antidote and immunity does not develop.

The source of DA in the Prince Edward Island outbreak was subsequently identified as the phytoplanktonic diatom *Pseudo-nitzschia multiseries*, formerly known as *Nitzschia pungens* [80]. ASP is the only shellfish poisoning caused by diatoms. Ten isomers of DA (isodomoic acids) have been identified in marine samples, but are minor constituents in ASP relative to DA [81, 82]. DA is a potent neurotoxin that accumulates in mussels and clams that feed on toxic planktons during a bloom. On the Pacific Coast, DA is produced by *P. multiseries* and two other species *P. australis* and *P. pseudodelicatissima* that bloom in late summer and fall. DA is water soluble and heat stable, similar in structure and function to another excitatory neurotoxin known as kainic acid (KA), which is found in the Japanese seaweed, *Digenea simplex*. DA and KA both appear to produce neurotoxic effects by activating the glutamate receptors. These receptors are ligand-gated, voltage-dependent Ca^{2+} channels that are activated by glutamic acid, mediating a fast excitatory synaptic transmission in the mammalian central nervous system (CNS). Persistent activation of KA receptors results in elevated levels of intracellular calcium (Ca^{2+}) that causes neurotoxicity with subsequent lesions in areas of the brain where glutaminergic pathways are heavily concentrated. The observations that the glutamate receptors are present within the cardiac conducting system, intramural ganglia, and cardiac nerve fibers could explain some of the clinical manifestations such as the arrhythmia described with DA intoxication in humans. Hence individuals with premorbid cardiac conditions may be at higher risk of the toxic effects of these excitatory compounds [82, 83].

DA poisoning first became a noticeable problem in the West Coast of the United States in September 1991 when it was reported that brown pelicans had died after eating anchovies in Monterey Bay off the coast of California. It was subsequently found that the death of these pelicans was due to the bloom of *P. multiseries* that produced high levels of DA [84]. Since this time and through December 2004, 29 cases of ASP were reported to the CDC, all of which occurred in November 1991 and were caused by razor clams harvested in Washington. No fatalities were reported in the United States. However, the mortality rate was 3.7% in the 1987 Canadian outbreak [85].

Traditionally an MBA has been used for the detection of DA. There are several other methods used to detect DA in seawater and shellfish such as HPLC, ELISA, and a receptor binding assay (RBA). The RBA measures the competitive displacement of radiolabeled KA bound to a cloned glutamate receptor (GluR6) by DA in a sample. RBA has a larger working range whereas an enzyme immunoassay (EIA) is more sensitive. The detection limit and working range are 3.1 and 5–100 μg/L for the RBA and 0.01 and 0.15–15 μg/L for the EIA, respectively. RBA and EIA yield statistically equivalent results for detection of DA in seawater [86].

In Canada, to prevent future outbreaks of ASP, sacks of mussels are labelled with respect to time and place of harvesting. In addition, both water column and shellfish are monitored for the presence of *Pseudo-nitzschia* and DA, respectively [69,87,88]. On the Pacific Coast, DA poisoning has been a serious problem affecting razor clams and Dungeness crabs in Washington and oysters, bay and razor clams, and mussels in Oregon. Authorities in Washington, Oregon, and California now randomly analyze samples of commercially harvested or cultivated shellfish for DA. States in the northeastern United States also monitor shellfish for DA, which is present at low levels that do not necessitate quarantine.

Diarrhetic shellfish poisoning

DSP is the mildest and most benign of the toxic shellfish poisonings. Clinical features are generally limited to the gastrointestinal tract. Diarrhea is the dominant symptom and present in 92% of cases. Other common symptoms include nausea (80%), vomiting (79%), abdominal pain and cramps (53%). Chills, fever, or headache may also be present in up to 10% of cases. The symptoms usually manifest in a period ranging from 30 minutes to 6 hours after ingestion of contaminated shellfish and persist on average for 36 hours. No known fatalities have occurred, and total recovery is expected within 3 days. Due to the transient nature of the illness and its spontaneous resolution, often patients do not seek medical attention, however the duration could be shortened with charcoal, which reduces the bioavailability of the toxins and its repeated administration interrupts their enterohepatic recirculation. Treatment, if required, is limited to the alleviation of symptoms [89].

DSP is associated with the consumption of mussels, scallops, clams, and oysters contaminated with biotoxins produced by toxic marine dinoflagellates during their blooms in the summer. *Dinophysis* and *Prorocentrum* species have been identified as the source of DSP toxins that are heat stable and not denatured by normal cooking. Although to date there has been no documented DSP outbreak in the United States, toxin-producing *Dinophysis* species are present in the U.S. waters and in 1990 caused an outbreak in eastern Canada. The disease occurs worldwide in temperate waters. It is common in Japan, where over 200 cases are reported annually and has become a public health problem in Europe. Sporadic outbreaks have also been documented in Southeast Asia, Scandinavia, Western Europe, Chile, Australia, New Zealand, and eastern Canada. DSP is caused primarily by the lipophilic, high molecular weight polyether, okadaic acid (OA) and derivatives, the dinophysistoxins (DTXs) [89, 90]. Other minor toxins isolated from dinoflagellates and shellfish in association with DSP are pectenotoxins (PTX) and yessotoxin (YTX) [90].

OA is a highly selective inhibitor of serine/threonine protein phosphatases 1 and 2A that causes dramatic increases in phosphorylation of proteins which regulate metabolic processes in eukaryotic cells. Accumulation of phosphorylated proteins leads to calcium influx, which increases paracellular permeability of the intestinal epithelial lining, raises the intracellular cAMP level and stimulates prostaglandin production, which together results in secretory diarrhea [91, 92]. DTX are structurally related to OA and cause highly similar pathologic changes in intestinal mucosa that appear within 5 minutes of dosing and resolve completely within 2 days. PTX, although non-diarrheagenic, are potently cytotoxic [93]. YTX is a weak cytotoxin, and is not orally lethal to mice. It does not cause accumulation of intestinal fluid or inhibit protein phosphatase and has no diarrheagenic or hemolytic effects, suggesting that it should not be classed as a DSP toxin. OA and its derivatives can act as a potent tumor promoter and PTX can contribute to carcinogenesis in animals. For that reason, it has been postulated that shellfish consumption might be a risk factor for colorectal cancer [94, 95]. The DSP toxins, particularly OA and some DTX, are potent microalgal inhibitors. They are probably an evolutionary adaptive mechanism and are produced by toxic dinoflagellates to create a survival advantage against other competing microalgae [96].

An MBA is a standard method for DSP surveillance but is non-specific and lacks sensitivity. HPLC and LC–MS are alternative techniques and have a low detection limit and are in agreement [97, 98]. There is also a rapid screening method for OA based on its ability to inhibit protein phosphatase coupled with the use of fluorescent substrates. At present, for the U.S. consumer, the risk of DSP is limited to imported products and should be controlled by import regulations that permit import of shellfish only from countries that test it for the presence of toxins.

Azaspiracid shellfish poisoning

Azaspiracids (AZA) are a group of structurally novel polyether marine toxins that contain a unique azaspiro ring assembly. AZA were found to be responsible for outbreaks resembling DSP associated with consumption of contaminated shellfish in Europe. The first outbreak was reported in November 1995 in the Netherlands following the consumption of mussels harvested on the west coast of Ireland and initially was mistaken for DSP but was subsequently proven to be azaspiracid shellfish poisoning (AZP). Since then, outbreaks have been reported in other European countries, including France, Italy, Ireland, Norway, and the United Kingdom [99]. The onset is 12–24 hours after consumption of mussels and the symptoms of the illness include severe diarrhea, vomiting, nausea, abdominal cramps, headaches, and chills, which resolve in 2–5 days [100]. Scallops have been also reported to cause AZP and toxin levels exceeding safety levels have been detected in crabs harvested in Norway. However, no associated cases of human disease apparently have been reported [101, 102]. In July 2008, the first United States case of AZP was reported, which affected two individuals who consumed a pre-package frozen meal of mussels harvested in Ireland. Subsequent FDA investigation confirmed AZP as the etiology by determining AZA levels that approached or exceeded the regulatory threshold in some of the product packages [103].

To date, 24 different AZA have been described, and their toxicity is not affected by heat or freezing. The causative organism is *Protoperidinium crassipes*, a dinoflagellate found in North Atlantic waters. While AZA was initially classified as a DSP toxin, it was subsequently reclassified into a new poisoning category known as AZP. AZA has a number of unique properties that set it apart from the "classic" DSP toxins, OA, DTX, and YTX. In animal experiments, AZA administered orally induces pronounced neurotoxic effects and causes necrosis in the lamina propria of the small intestine, liver, and lymphoid tissues in the Peyer's patches, spleen, and thymus, whereas toxic effects of OA are limited to the gastrointestinal mucosa [104].

A liquid chromatography–multiple tandem mass spectrometry method for determination of AZA is capable of detecting each of the 10 AZA and is far more sensitive than the MBA [105]. Tissue recovery of AZA is very slow following exposure and long depuration suggests that AZA is more dangerous than the other shellfish toxins [105, 106].

Conclusions

This review presents the more common clinical syndromes which have been mistaken for allergic reactions and are produced by the ingestion of natural seafood toxins. For the practicing allergist, knowledge of this wide array of toxic syndromes is important for the proper differential diagnosis of seafood allergy (Table 41.4). A careful history and physical examination are essential to establish the diagnosis on clinical grounds, which can be confirmed by detection of toxins either in remnants of the seafood or in specimens collected from the patient. The history should

Table 41.4 Summary of common toxic syndromes associated with naturally occurring toxins in seafood.

Type of poisoning	Type of toxins	Source	Symptom onset	Clinical syndrome
Scombroid	Histamine	Tuna, mahi-mahi, bonita, marlin, bluefish, wahoo, mackerel, and salmon	Minutes to 4 hours	Severe headache, dizziness, nausea, vomiting, flushed skin, urticaria, and wheezing
Ciguatera	Ciguatoxins	Coral reef fish: amberjack, snappers, grouper, goat fish, barracuda, sea bass, surgeon fish, ulua, and papio	30 minutes–4 hours	Abdominal pain, diarrhea, vomiting, paresthesias, cold-to-hot sensory reversal, weakness, and myalgias
Puffer fish poisoning	Tetradotoxin	Ocean sunfishes, porcupine fishes, and fugu	10–45 minutes	Paresthesias headache, vomiting, diaphoresis, and respiratory paralysis
Paralytic shellfish	Saxitoxins	Mussels, clams, and oysters	5–30 minutes	Vomiting, diarrhea, facial paresthesias, and respiratory paralysis
Neurotoxic shellfish	Brevetoxins	Mussels and clams	30 minutes–3 hours	Diarrhea, vomiting, abdominal pain, myalgias, paresthesias, and ataxia
Amnesic shellfish	Domoic acid	Mussels, clams, crabs, and anchovies	15 minutes–38 hours	Vomiting, diarrhea, headache, myoclonus, loss of short-term memory, seizures, coma, and hemiparesis
Diarrhetic shellfish	Okadaic acid, dinophysistoxins, pectenotoxins, yessotoxin	Mussels, clams, and scallops	30 minutes–6 hours	Diarrhea, nausea, vomiting, and abdominal pain

include symptoms and their severity, time of onset with respect to ingestion of seafood, number and frequency of reactions, whether others became ill, previous history of food allergy, types of marine species ingested and where they were captured, and the quantity of food consumed and the way in which it was prepared. Whether the food was eaten at a restaurant, the patient was travelling, alcohol was consumed, or medications were taken by the patient should be recorded.

Presence of similar symptoms in other individuals who shared the seafood meal and the "endemic" nature of the syndrome are paramount in alerting the physician to possible seafood poisoning. The absence of prior reactions to the same seafood and its subsequent tolerance without symptoms point away from an allergic etiology and should be considered as corroborative evidence in support of a toxic syndrome. Since histamine mediates the symptoms of both scombroid and type I hypersensitivity reactions, clinical manifestations of scombroid poisoning may be virtually indistinguishable from seafood allergy. History of a "peppery" taste and type of fish consumed, as well as suspected improper refrigeration, are helpful in reaching the proper diagnosis.

Neurological symptoms associated with an allergic reaction are the result of hypoperfusion of the CNS and correlate with the severity of cardiovascular involvement and hypotension in anaphylaxis. This may help the physician to distinguish ciguatera, PSP, NSP, and ASP, where neurological impairment is commonly present in the absence of hypotension. In ciguatera poisoning, knowledge of the type of fish and whether it is imported from or consumed in endemic areas, such as Caribbean, Hawaii, and Pacific Islands, will provide clinical information to differentiate it from seafood allergy. The same is true in cases of PFP and in shellfish poisoning, where knowledge of the location where the seafood was caught aides in proper diagnosis.

The seasonal association with algal blooms and presence of high levels of biotoxins or toxic algae that are reported by authorities surveying coastal waters should increase the index of suspicion for physicians practicing in endemic areas. In the majority of these toxic syndromes, the causative toxin does not alter the taste and appearance of the seafood and is not inactivated by normal cooking.

Treatment is supportive, with active early respiratory support, especially in cases where neurological involvement could lead to respiratory paralysis. Upper respiratory reactions in individuals with no history of atopy and exacerbation of chest symptoms in asthmatics are caused by aerosolized NSP toxins. These irritant reactions are usually associated with a red tide and should not be mistaken for allergic respiratory symptoms.

Most current health risks associated with seafood contamination originate in the environment and should be dealt with by control of the harvest or at the point of capture. The most effective way of protecting consumers is to establish and maintain comprehensive monitoring programs for toxic algae and toxins in shellfish in all growing areas. Developing a better understanding of factors that promote harmful algal blooms and lead to production of toxins by marine algae is crucial to control human exposure and deleterious environmental effects. Further research is needed in most areas of seafood poisoning. Easy, accurate, and cost-effective methods for detection of toxins in seafood, monitoring shellfish for viral and bacterial contamination, and surveillance of coastal waters for harmful marine algae and their toxins are needed. Knowledge gained from research on the mechanism of action of marine toxins should lead to more specific treatment modalities that would limit morbidity and mortality of seafood intoxications. The following general preventive measures could greatly reduce the incidence of poisoning outbreaks that are associated with seafood:

1. Avoid eating raw seafood.
2. Avoid eating lightly steamed and undercooked shellfish.
3. Adhere to the public health agency guidelines on harvesting, processing, and consumption of shellfish and avoid shellfish from areas of frequent red tides.
4. Promptly refrigerate the catch of sport fishermen.
5. Avoid eating large, predatory reef fish usually implicated in ciguatera poisoning, especially barracuda, amberjack, and snapper.
6. Avoid reef fish caught in ciguatera endemic areas, especially the head, viscera, and roe.
7. Promptly report the suspected outbreaks of seafood poisoning to local health departments.
8. Submit leftover seafood or uncooked portions of the fish or shellfish to local health departments for analysis to establish nature and amount of contaminating toxin.
9. Finally, the informed physician can be of great help in public health prevention through public education and involvement with the local and public agencies that deal with these health issues.

Acknowledgment

This work was in part supported by the Division of Intramural Research, NIAID, NIH.

References

1. Sicherer SH, Sampson HA. Food allergy. *J Allergy Clin Immunol* 2006; 117:S470–S475.
2. Chegini S, Metcalfe DD. Contemporary issues in food allergy: seafood toxin-induced disease in the differential diagnosis of allergic reactions. *Allergy Asthma Proc* 2005; 26:183–190.

3. Ohnuma S, Higa M, Hamanaka S, Matsushima K, Yamamuro W. An outbreak of allergy-like food poisoning. *Intern Med* 2001; 40:833–835.
4. Sanchez-Guerrero IM, Vidal JB, Escudero AI. Scombroid fish poisoning: a potentially life-threatening allergic-like reaction. *J Allergy Clin Immunol* 1997; 100:433–434.
5. O'Connor MM, Forbes GM. Scombroid poisoning: not fish allergy. *Aust N Z J Med* 2000; 30:520.
6. Ahmed FE (ed.). Naturally occurring fish and shellfish poisons [Chapter 4]. *Seafood Safety*, Washington, DC: National Academy Press, 1991: 87–110.
7. Bean NH, Griffin PM, Goulding JS, Ivey CB. Foodborne disease outbreaks, 5-year summary, 1983–1987. *MMWR CDC Surveill Summ* 1990; 39:15–57.
8. Bean NH, Goulding JS, Lao C, Angulo FJ. Surveillance for foodborne disease outbreaks, United States, 1988–1992. *MMWR CDC Surveill Summ* 1996; 45:1–66.
9. Olsen SJ, MacKinnon LC, Goulding JS, Bean NH, Slutsker L. Surveillance for foodborne disease outbreaks—United States, 1993–1997. *MMWR CDC Surveill Summ* 2000; 49:1–51, see also 262.
10. Centers for Disease Control and Prevention. Foodborne Outbreak Online Database (FOOD). http://www.cdc.gov/foodborneoutbreaks/
11. Ayers LT, Williams IT, Gray S, Griffin PM. Surveillance for foodborne disease outbreaks—United States, 2006. *Morb Mortal Wkly Rep* 2009; 58:609–615.
12. Boore A, Herman KM, Perez AS, et al. Surveillance for foodborne disease outbreaks—United States, 2007. *Morb Mortal Wkly Rep* 2010; 59:973–979.
13. Gould LH, Nisler AL, Herman KM, et al. Surveillance for foodborne disease outbreaks—United States, 2008. *Morb Mortal Wkly Rep* 2011; 60:1197–1202.
14. Dalton CB, Gregory J, Kirk MD, et al. Foodborne disease outbreaks in Australia, 1995 to 2000. *Commun Dis Intell Q Rep* 2004; 28:211–224.
15. Isbister GK, Kiernan MC. Neurotoxic marine poisoning. *Lancet Neurol* 2005; 4:219–228.
16. Lewis RJ. Ciguatera: Australian perspectives on a global problem. *Toxicon* 2006; 48:799–809.
17. Kellmann R, Stüken A, Orr RJ, Svendsen HM, Jakobsen KS. Biosynthesis and molecular genetics of polyketides in marine dinoflagellates. *Mar Drugs* 2010; 8:1011–1048.
18. Arnott GH. Toxic marine microalgae: a worldwide problem with major implications for seafood safety. *Adv Food Safety* 1998; 1:24–34.
19. Viviani R. Eutrophication, marine biotoxins, human health. *Sci Total Environ* 1992;(Suppl.):631–662.
20. Derne B, Fearnley E, Goater S, Carter K, Weinstein P. Ciguatera fish poisoning and environmental change: a case for strengthening health surveillance in the Pacific? *Pac Health Dialog* 2010; 16:99–108.
21. Llewellyn LE. Revisiting the association between sea surface temperature and the epidemiology of fish poisoning in the South Pacific: reassessing the link between ciguatera and climate change. *Toxicon* 2010; 56:691–697.
22. Lehane L. *Paralytic Shellfish Poisoning: A Review*. Canberra, Australia: National Office of Animal and Plant Health Agriculture, Fisheries and Forestry, 2000.
23. Merson MH, Baine WB, Gangarosa EJ, Swanson RC. Scombroid fish poisoning. Outbreak traced to commercially canned tuna fish. *J Am Med Assoc* 1974; 228:1268–1269.
24. Lange WR. Scombroid poisoning. *Am Fam Physician* 1988; 37:163–168.
25. Hungerford JM. Scombroid poisoning: a review. *Toxicon* 2010; 56:231–243.
26. Lukton A, Olcott HS. Content of free imidazole compounds in the muscle tissue of aquatic animals. *Food Res* 1958; 23:611–618.
27. Taylor SL. Histamine food poisoning: toxicology and clinical aspects. *CRC Crit Rev Toxicol* 1986; 17:91–128.
28. Centers for Disease Control [CDC]. Scombroid fish poisoning—Illinois, South Carolina. *Morb Mortal Wkly Rep* 1989; 38:140–142.
29. Hughes JM, Potter ME. Scombroid-fish poisoning. From pathogenesis to prevention. *N Engl J Med* 1991; 324:766–768.
30. Morrow JD, Margolies GR, Rowland J, Roberts LJ. Evidence that histamine is the causative toxin of scombroid fish poisoning. *N Engl J Med* 1991; 324:716–720.
31. Bedry R, Gabinski C, Paty MC. Diagnosis of scombroid poisoning by measurement of plasma histamine. *N Engl J Med* 2000; 342:520–521.
32. Lehane L, Olley J. Histamine fish poisoning revisited. *Int J Food Microbiol* 2000; 58:1–37.
33. Friedman MA, Fleming LE, Fernandez M, et al. Ciguatera fish poisoning: treatment, prevention and management. *Mar Drugs* 2008; 6:456–479.
34. Hughes JM, Merson MH. Fish and shellfish poisoning. *N Engl J Med* 1976; 295:1117–1120.
35. Lange WR. Ciguatera fish poisoning. *Am Fam Physician* 1994; 50:579–584.
36. Rakita RM. Ciguatera poisoning. *J Travel Med* 1995; 2:252–254.
37. Gollop JH, Pon EW. Ciguatera: a review. *Hawaii Med J* 1992; 51:91–99.
38. Bagnis R, Chameau S, Chungue E, et al. Origins of ciguatera fish poisoning: a new dinoflagellate *Gambierdiscus toxicus* Adachi and Fukuyo, definitely involved as a causal agent. *Toxicon* 1980; 18:199–208.
39. Dickey RW, Plakas SM. Ciguatera: a public health perspective. *Toxicon* 2010; 56:123–136.
40. Lewis RJ, Holmes MJ. Origin and transfer of toxins involved in ciguatera. *Comp Biochem Physiol C* 1993; 106:615–628.
41. Bidard JN, Vijuerben HPM, Frelin C, et al. Ciguatoxin is a novel type of Na^+ channel toxin. *J Biol Chem* 1984; 359:8353–8357.
42. Escobar LI, Salvador C, Martinez M, Vaca L. Maitotoxin, a cationic channel activator. *Neurobiology* 1998; 6:59–74.
43. Lehane L, Lewis RJ. Ciguatera: recent advances but the risk remains. *Int J Food Microbiol* 2000; 61:91–125.
44. Van Dolah FM. Marine algal toxins: origins, health effects, and their increased occurrence. *Environ Health Perspect* 2000; 108:133–141.
45. Noguchi T, Arakawa O. Tetrodotoxin—distribution and accumulation in aquatic organisms, and cases of human intoxication. *Mar Drugs* 2008; 6:220–242.

46. Lange WR. Puffer fish poisoning. *Am Fam Physician* 1990; 42:1029–1033.
47. J Field. Puffer fish poisoning. *J Accid Emerg Med* 1998; 15:334–336.
48. CDC. Tetradotoxin poisoning associated with eating puffer fish transported from Japan—California, 1996. *Morb Mortal Wkly Rep* 1996; 45:389–391.
49. Noguchi T, Onuki K, Arakawa O. Tetrodotoxin poisoning due to pufferfish and gastropods, and their intoxication mechanism. *ISRN Toxicology* 2011:276939. doi:10.5402/2011/276939
50. Fozzard HA, Lipkind GM. The tetrodotoxin binding site is within the outer vestibule of the sodium channel. *Mar Drugs* 2010; 8:219–234.
51. Noguchi T, Arakawa O. Tetrodotoxin—Distribution and accumulation in aquatic organisms, and cases of human intoxication. *Mar Drugs* 2008; 6:220–242.
52. Taylor DA, Vaisocherova H, Deeds J, DeGrasse S, Jiang S. Tetrodotoxin detection by a surface plasmon resonance sensor in pufferfish matrices and urine. *J Sensors* 2011:601704. doi:10.1155/2011/601704
53. Etheridge SM. Paralytic shellfish poisoning: seafood safety and human health perspectives. *Toxicon* 2010; 56:108–122.
54. McLaughlin JB, Fearey DA, Esposito TA, Porter KA. Paralytic shellfish poisoning—southeast Alaska, May–June 2011. *Morb Mortal Wkly Rep* 2011; 60:1554–1556.
55. Gessner BD, Middaugh JP. Paralytic shellfish poisoning in Alaska: a 20-year retrospective analysis. *Am J Epidemiol* 1995; 141:766–770.
56. Kao CY. Paralytic shellfish poisoning [Chapter 4]. In: Falconer IR (ed.), *Algal Toxins in Seafood and Drinking Water*. London and New York: Academic Press, 1993; pp. 75–86.
57. Hall S, Strichartz G, Moczydlowski E, et al. The saxitoxins: sources, chemistry, and pharmacology [Chapter 3]. In: Hall S, Strichartz G (eds) *Marine Toxins: Origin, Structure and Molecular Pharmacology*. Washington, DC: American Chemical Society Symposium Series, 1990; pp. 29–65.
58. Wiese M, D'Agostino PM, Mihali TK, Moffitt MC, Neilan BA. Neurotoxic alkaloids: saxitoxin and its analogs. *Mar Drugs* 2010; 8:2185–2211.
59. Hackett JD, Wisecaver JH, Brosnahan ML, et al. Evolution of saxitoxin synthesis in cyanobacteria and dinoflagellates. *Mol Biol Evol* 2012; 30:70–78.
60. Llewellyn LE. Saxitoxin, a toxic marine natural product that targets a multitude of receptors. *Nat Prod Rep* 2006; 23:200–222.
61. Leftley JW, Hannah F. Phycotoxins in seafood. In: Watson DH (ed.), *Natural Toxicants in Food*. Sheffield: Sheffield Academic, 1998; pp. 182–224.
62. Hungerford JM, Weckell MM. Analytical methods for marine toxins. In: Tu AT (ed.) *Handbook of Natural Toxins, Food Poisoning*, vol. 7. New York: Marcel Dekker Inc., 1992; pp. 416–473.
63. Ben-Gigirey B, Rodríguez-Velasco ML, Otero A, Vieites JM, Cabado AG. A comparative study for PSP toxins quantification by using MBA and HPLC official methods in shellfish. *Toxicon* 2012; 60:864-873.
64. Humpage AR, Magalhaes VF, Froscio SM. Comparison of analytical tools and biological assays for detection of paralytic shellfish poisoning toxins. *Anal Bioanal Chem* 2010; 397:1655–1671.
65. Taylor SL. Marine toxins of microbial origin. *Food Tech* 1988; 42:94–98.
66. Dale B, Yentsch CM. Red tide and paralytic shellfish poisoning. *Oceanus* 1978; 21:41–49.
67. Scholin CA, Anderson DM. Population analysis of toxic and non-toxic Alexandrium species using ribosomal RNA signature sequences. In: Smayda TJ, Shimizu Y (eds), *Toxic Phytoplankton Blooms in the Sea*. Amsterdam, The Netherlands: Elsevier, 1993; pp. 95–102.
68. Food and Drug Administration [FDA]. Natural toxins [Chapter 6]. *Fish and Fishery Products Hazards and Controls Guide*, 2nd edn. Washington, DC: Department of Health and Human Services, Public Health Service, Food and Drug Administration, Center for Food Safety and Applied Nutrition, Office of Seafood, 1998; pp. 65–72.
69. Regulation (EC) No 853/2004 of the European Parliament and of the Council of 29 April 2004 laying down specific hygiene rules for food of animal origin. *Offic J Eur Union* L 226:22–82.
70. Reich A, Blackmore C, Lazensky R, Geib K. Illness associated with red tide—Nassau County, Florida, 2007. *Morb Mortal Wkly Rep* 2008:57; 717–720.
71. Watkins SM, Reich A, Fleming LE, Hammond R. Neurotoxic shellfish poisoning. *Mar Drugs* 2008; 6:431–455.
72. Shimoda T, Krzanowski Jr J, Nelson R, et al. In vitro red tide toxin effects on human bronchial smooth muscle. *J Allergy Clin Immunol* 1988; 81:1187–1191.
73. Tester PA, Steidinger KA. Gymnodynium breve red tide: initiation, transport, and consequences of surface circulation. *Limnol Oceanogr* 1997; 42:1052–1075.
74. Carlton JT, Geller JB. Ecological roulette: the global transport of nonindigenous marine organisms. *Science* 1993; 261:78–82.
75. Anderson DM, Burkholder JM, Cochlan WP, et al. Harmful algal blooms and eutrophication: examining linkages from selected coastal regions of the United States. *Harmful Algae* 2008; 8:39–53.
76. Pierce RH, Henry MS. Harmful algal toxins of the Florida red tide (*Karenia brevis*): natural chemical stressors in South Florida coastal ecosystems. *Ecotoxicology* 2008; 17:623–631.
77. Food and Drug Administration [FDA]. Natural toxins [Chapter 6]. *Fish and Fishery Products Hazards and Controls Guidance*, 4th edn. FDA, 2011; pp. 99–112.
78. Todd ECD. Amnesic shellfish poisoning—a new seafood toxin syndrome. In: Graneli E, Sundstrom B, Edler L, Anderson DM (eds) *Proceedings of the 4th International Conference on Toxic Marine Phytoplankton*. Amsterdam, The Netherlands: Elsevier, 1989; pp. 504–508.
79. Perl TM, Bedard L, Kosatsky T, et al. An outbreak of toxic encephalopathy caused by eating mussels contaminated with domoic acid. *N Engl J Med* 1990; 322:1775–1780.
80. Teitelbaum JS, Zatorre RJ, Carpenter S, et al. Neurologic sequelae of domoic acid intoxication due to the ingestion of contaminated mussels. *N Engl J Med* 1990; 322:1781–1787.

81. Subba RD, Quilliam M, Pocklington R. Domoic acid—a neuro-toxic amino acid produced by the marine diatom *Nitzschia pungens* in culture. *Can J Fish Aquat Sci* 1988; 45:2076–2079.
82. Jeffery B, Barlow T, Moizer K, et al. Amnesic shellfish poison. *Food Chem Toxicol* 2004; 42:545–557.
83. Pulido OM. Domoic acid toxicologic pathology: a review. *Mar Drugs* 2008; 6:180–219.
84. Walz PM, Garrison DL, Graham WM, et al. Domoic acid—producing diatom blooms in Monterey Bay, California: 1991–1993. *Nat Toxins* 1994; 2:271–279.
85. Jeffery B, Barlow T, Moizer K, Paul S, Boyle C. Amnesic shellfish poison. *Food Chem Toxicol* 2004; 42:545–557.
86. He Y, Fekete A, Chen G, et al. Analytical approaches for an important shellfish poisoning agent: domoic Acid. *J Agric Food Chem* 2010; 58:11525–11533.
87. Lefebvre KA, Robertson A. Domoic acid and human exposure risks: a review. *Toxicon* 2010; 56:218–230.
88. Washington State Department of Health. *Establishing Tolerable Dungeness Crab (Cancer Magister) and Razor Clam (Siliqua Patula) Domoic Acid Contaminant Levels.* Olympia, WA: Office of Environmental Health Assessment, 1996.
89. Whittle K, Gallacher S. Marine toxins. *Br Med Bull* 2000; 56:236–253.
90. Goto H, Igarashi T, Yamamoto M, et al. Quantitative determination of marine toxins associated with diarrhetic shellfish poisoning by liquid chromatography coupled with mass spectrometry. *J Chromatogr A* 2001; 907:181–189.
91. Vale C, Botana LM. Marine toxins and the cytoskeleton: okadaic acid and dinophysistoxins. *FEBS J* 2008; 275:6060–6066.
92. Tripuraneni J, Koutsouris A, Pestic L, et al. The toxin of diarrheic shellfish poisoning, okadaic acid, increases intestinal epithelial paracellular permeability. *Gastroenterology* 1997; 112:100–108.
93. Burgess V, Shaw G. Pectenotoxins—an issue for public health: a review of their comparative toxicology and metabolism. *Environ Int* 2001; 27:275–283.
94. Quilliam MA. Phycotoxins. *J AOAC Int* 1999; 82:773–781.
95. Manerio E, Rodas VL, Costas E, Hernandez JM. Shellfish consumption: a major risk factor for colorectal cancer. *Med Hypotheses* 2008; 70:409–412.
96. Windust AJ, Wright JLC, McLachlan JL. The effects of the diarrhetic shellfish poisoning toxins, okadaic acid and dinophysistoxin-1, on the growth of microalgae. *Mar Biol* 1996; 126:19–25.
97. Paz B, Daranas AH, Norte M, Riobó P, Franco JM, Fernández JJ. Yessotoxins, a group of marine polyether toxins: an overview. *Mar Drugs* 2008; 6:73–102.
98. Louppis AP, Badeka AV, Katikou P, Paleologos EK, Kontominas MG. Determination of okadaic acid, dinophysistoxin-1 and related esters in Greek mussels using HPLC with fluorometric detection, LC–MS/MS and mouse bioassay. *Toxicon* 2010; 55:724–733.
99. Twiner MJ, Rehmann N, Hess P, Doucette GJ. Azaspiracid shellfish poisoning: a review on the chemistry, ecology, and toxicology with an emphasis on human health impacts. *Mar Drugs* 2008; 6:39–72.
100. CDR. Food poisoning caused by shellfish contaminated by marine algal toxins. *Commun Dis Rep CDR Wkly* 2001; 11:19.
101. James KJ, Fidalgo Saez MJ, Furey A, Lehane M. Azaspiracid poisoning, the food-borne illness associated with shellfish consumption. *Food Addit Contam* 2004; 21:879–892.
102. Food Safety Authority of Ireland (FSAI). *Risk Assessment of Azaspiracids in Shellfish*, August 2006. A Report of the Scientific Committee of the Food Safety Authority of Ireland, Dublin, Ireland.
103. Klontz KC, Abraham A, Plakas SM, Dickey RW. Mussel-associated azaspiracid intoxication in the United States. *Ann Intern Med* 2009; 150:361.
104. Ito E, Satake M, Ofuji K, et al. Multiple organ damage caused by a new toxin azaspiracid, isolated from mussels produced in Ireland. *Toxicon* 2000; 38:917–930.
105. Lehane M, Fidalgo Saez MJ, Magdalena AB, et al. Liquid chromatography—multiple tandem mass spectrometry for the determination of ten azaspiracids, including hydroxyl analogues in shellfish. *J Chromatogr A* 2004; 1024: 63–70.
106. Furey A, O'Doherty S, O'Callaghan K, Lehane M, James KJ. Azaspiracid poisoning (AZP) toxins in shellfish: toxicological and health considerations. *Toxicon* 2010; 56:173–190.

42 Neurologic Reactions to Foods and Food Additives

Richard W. Weber
Denver School of Medicine, University of Colorado, Denver, CO, USA

Key Concepts

- Dietary factors have been suspected or demonstrated in several conditions with neurological manifestations, the most prominent being migraine and epilepsy.
- Dietary migraine is a bona fide entity, with both pharmacologic and immunologic mechanisms involved in subsets of migraineurs.
- The benefit of ketogenic diets for epilepsy management is well established, but the manner in which they operate remains uncertain.
- Food-induced anaphylaxis may present with neurological manifestations in one quarter of cases.
- Neurological complications associated with gluten sensitivity are of unclear etiology.

The impact of foods or food additives on neurological functioning has received varying attention, ranging from case reports to placebo-controlled double-blind challenges. Signs and symptoms range from those that are purely subjective to those that may be validated by objective findings. Syndromes such as food-induced migraine and epilepsy will be addressed in this chapter.

Migraine headache

In 1962, the Ad Hoc Committee on the Classification of Headache defined migraine as recurrent attacks of headache, widely varied in intensity, frequency, and duration. The attacks are commonly unilateral in onset; are usually associated with anorexia and, sometimes, with nausea and vomiting; in some are proceeded by, or associated with, conspicuous sensory, motor, and mood disturbances; and are often familial [1]. Classic migraine presents with a prodromal aura prior to headache onset, frequently a visual disturbance such as scintillating scotomata, whereas common migraine lacks such a prodrome. Complicated migraine has more significant neurological dysfunction such as transient hemiplegia.

Migraine headache occurs in 5–30% of the general population, with a familial predisposition in 60–80% of cases, affecting females threefold more than males. A 1992 survey of 20 468 individuals revealed that 5.7% of males and 17.6% of females suffered one or more migraines per year, with highest prevalence between 35–45 years of age [2]. In the US population, 8.7 million females and 2.6 million males suffer from migraine with moderate-to-severe disability. A 1992 Minnesota study estimated migraine prevalence as high as 40% [3].

Precipitating factors of migraine include stress, bright lights or loud sounds, physical exertion, fasting, and foods. Menses or oral contraception use may precipitate headaches, but migraine frequently improves during pregnancy. Electroencephalogram (EEG) abnormalities are minimal and more common in childhood migraine, with epileptiform discharges noted in 18 of 100 patients [4]. With no definitive confirmatory laboratory tests, the diagnosis is based primarily on history. Other migraine-mimicking conditions need to be excluded: aneurysm, temporal arteritis, carcinoid, pheochromocytoma, brain tumor, arteriovenous malformation, glaucoma, mastocytosis, and carotid, or vertebrobasilar vascular insufficiency.

Theories of migraine etiology

There is no consensus on the primary etiology of migraine. The pulsatile nature of the headache supports a vascular theory wherein aura was explained by intracerebral vasoconstriction and following headache by post-vasodilatation inflammation. This theory was supported by evidence of

Food Allergy: Adverse Reactions to Foods and Food Additives, Fifth Edition. Edited by Dean D Metcalfe, Hugh A Sampson, Ronald A Simon and Gideon Lack.

cerebral hypoperfusion [5]. The neurogenic theory suggests a defective neuronal response to neurotransmitters with vascular changes secondary to neuronal impulses and vasoactivity of such neurotransmitters as substance P [6]. Moskowitz and Macfarlane emphasized that several levels of pathophysiologic triggering and potentiating factors may consolidate neurogenic and vasogenic elements in migraine headache [7]. It has been proposed that ionic and metabolic cortical mechanisms release nociceptive substances that stimulate trigeminovascular sensory fibers. These impulses cause pain and release vasoactive neuropeptides like substance P and neurokinin A, inducing vasodilatation and protein extravasation, causing further nociceptive substance release and sensory nerve ending sensitization. The large number of dural mast cells has been implicated in this process [7]. The marked female predominance and exacerbation by menses and contraceptive hormonal therapy reinforce the importance of hormonal issues in migraine. One study of 200 migraineurs revealed hormonal factors as important triggers in 54% of women [8]. Therefore, the great variety of therapeutic modalities may be explained by the complexity of initiating and potentiating elements in the migraine reaction.

Diet manipulation in migraine

Diets may play a role in migraine severity by limiting precursor availability for the generation of vasoactive mediators or nociceptor transmitters. Carbohydrate-rich, protein–tryptophan-low diets have been attempted to modify migraine headaches. If platelet serotonin is a precipitator of the vasoconstrictory phase of migraine, a restricted dietary intake of serotonin and its precursor tryptophan may lower levels within platelets, alleviating migraine headaches. However, increased brain serotonin levels may improve migraine through the antinociceptive system. Insulin release induced by carbohydrate-rich meals would increase tryptophan availability to the brain, with subsequent increased serotonin synthesis. Hasselmark and coworkers tried such a diet for 50 days after 30 days of routine diet in 10 migraineurs, with seven completing the study [9]. While three of four with classic migraine had a marked improvement in headache frequency, no common migraineurs noted benefit, and there were no differences in platelet serotonin uptake. The authors felt that the benefit could be due to, either a decrease in the ingestion of migraine-precipitating foods, or increased brain serotonin levels. Drummond observed the effects of acute dietary tryptophan depletion on induction of motion sickness [10]. He compared 37 controls with 39 migraineurs, who as a group are susceptible to motion sickness. Tryptophan depletion raised dizziness, nausea, and illusion of motion in the controls to levels approaching that of the migraineurs, in whom depletion had little effect. It was postulated that migraineurs have chronically low central serotonin levels, or that serotonergic receptors may be less sensitive in migraineurs than controls.

In a double-blind, cross-over study, Harel and coworkers examined the benefit in adolescent migraine of dietary supplementation with fish oil rich in very-long-chain omego-3 polyunsaturated fatty acids versus olive oil placebo [11]. Headache frequency and severity were reduced compared to baseline by both fish oil and olive oil ($p < 0.0001$ and $p < 0.01$–0.03, respectively). Reductions were between 65% and 87% for severity, duration, and frequency for both treatments. The authors felt both oils were active, thus the magnitude of the improvement arguing against placebo effect.

Association of food allergy and migraine

Food allergy is self-reported more commonly in migraineurs than those with nonmigrainous headache or without headache [12]. Pinnas and Vanselow reported that the allergy–migraine association is more than a hundred years old: in 1885, Trousseau had included periodic headache in the allergic diathesis; Tileston in 1918 likened migraine to asthma; and the following year, Pagniez considered migraine as a manifestation of anaphylaxis [13]. In 1921, Brown linked attacks to milk, egg, fish, beef, pork, and chocolate [14]. In 1927, Vaughan reported that 10 of 33 migraine patients studied showed specific food triggers [15]. These were identified by skin testing followed by elimination and rechallenge of the incriminated foods. Except for a solitary blinded challenge, these were open challenges. Eyermann reported that 69% of headache patients improved on an elimination diet [16]. Forty-four subjects had headaches with suspected foods, beginning 3–6 hours after ingestion. The diet was directed by skin test results, but even 53% of nonresponders had positive tests, suggesting over-interpretation of the skin tests. Also, many of the patients did not have accepted criteria for migraine headache. Balyeat and Rinkel stated that of 202 consecutive migraine patients managed with food skin testing and elimination diets, 120 had 60% or greater improvement, with only 12% of the patients demonstrating little or no improvement [17]. In 1932, DeGowin reported results in 60 migraine patients with prick or intradermal skin tests to foods [18]. Elimination diets in 42 patients brought about complete relief in 14 and partial relief in another 19; incidence of headache on the reintroduction of foods was not reported.

These early studies suggested that food allergy, as determined by skin tests, was a significant cause of migraine headache. They are flawed by being open studies and susceptible to expectation bias and placebo effect. Thereafter, mainstream migraine opinion moved away from the causative role of allergy. Nonetheless, in 1952 Unger and Unger entitled a paper "Migraine Is an Allergic Disease" [19]. Of interest, the preceding article in that issue was captioned "Is Migraine an Allergic Disease?" [20]. Therein, Schwartz detailed his extensive epidemiological work in Denmark, involving 241 asthmatics, 200 nonallergic controls, and their 3815 relatives spanning four generations. He found no difference in the frequency of migraine in relatives of asthmatics and normal controls, since commented that migraine was so common, and it was not unexpected to find it in allergic kindreds.

Unger and Unger investigated 55 patients with skin tests, elimination diets, food diaries, and the "feeding test" to identify migraine-provoking foods [19]. All foods ingested for 24 hours before the onset of migraine were recorded. The patients were challenged with one or two portions of the suspected food after 2 weeks on an elimination diet, and all symptoms recorded for the next 24 hours. Thirty-five of 55 patients achieved complete relief of migraine symptoms, 9 had no improvement, and 11 had partial benefit. Food skin testing was unhelpful, identifying a provoking food only five times. The onset of the headache could be delayed 3–6 hours after ingestion of the provoking agent.

Open studies over the next 25 years supported the value of elimination diets in migraine with little insight into mechanisms. Grant in 1979, reported remarkable results in 60 patients placed on a strict lamb-and-pear elimination diet [21]. Of an initial group of 126 migraineurs, 35 discontinued the diet, and data was reported on only 60. After 5 days of the diet, foods were reintroduced singly, with symptoms and pulse rate monitored up to 1.5 hours. All patients improved, with complete resolution in 51 (85%). Foods found to provoke symptoms for each patient ranged from 1 to 30, with a mean of 10. No blinded challenges were performed, and these results undoubtedly reflect substantial placebo effect. The use of the pulse test has no documented validity and could lead to unnecessary elimination of numerous foods. The 31 patients who continued the diet but were not included in the data analysis presumably had less striking results.

Monro and coworkers reported 47 migraineurs managed with elimination and rotation diets [22]. Twenty-three of 36 patients completing the diet phase identified provoking foods. Subsequently, the radioallergosorbent test (RAST) to a battery of foods found migraine provokers to have higher RAST titers than foods not producing headaches. In follow up, these authors presented nine migraine patients with reproducible food sensitivity documented by elimination diets with open challenges [23]. High-dose oral cromolyn blocked headache in five patients while placebo did not. In 1983, Ratner and associates reported the benefit of a strict milk-protein-free diet for lactase-deficient classic migraineurs [24]. Eighteen of 19 deficient patients improved on the diet; one lactase-deficient patient and seven lactose tolerant patients did not benefit. Hughes and colleagues reported 19 of 21 migraine patients placed on a weeklong "semi-elemental" diet had a marked reduction of headache severity [25]. These unblinded studies suggested that a large percentage of migraineurs could benefit from elimination of specific foods, and the more stringent the diet, the more likely the success.

There are few studies using double-blind placebo control (DBPC) challenges that are necessary to clarify issues in an area where cause and effect are assessed by subjective symptomatology. A preliminary report by Vaughan and colleagues in 1983 linked the value of food skin tests and DBPC food capsule challenges in adult migraine patients [26]. Also that year, Egger and associates studied 99 children with weekly migraine maintained for 3–4 weeks on an "oligoantigenic" diet: lamb or chicken; rice or potato; apple or banana; brassica (turnip); and water plus vitamin supplements [27]. If no benefit was derived, the alternate foods were given. Those improving had daily-reintroduced foods in normal portions: those identifying a provoking food entered a DBPC challenge phase. Eighty-eight completed the diet, and 78 recovered fully, four were greatly improved, and six received no benefit. Of the 82 who were improved, 74 had migraines with one or more foods, with median onset of headache 2 days after reintroduction of the responsible food. DBPC food challenges were performed with 40 children. Twenty-six responded to the active agent alone, two to the placebo, four to both, and eight to neither ($p < 0.001$). Skin prick testing identified all of the precipitants in only three patients. Eighty-nine percent of the children completing the diet phase recovered completely, and in 29.5% of those children, at least one provocative food was verified on DBPC challenge.

Another DBPC study by Atkins and coworkers was negative [28]. They studied 36 children with a battery of 20 food skin prick tests. Sixteen suspected a food or additive, and two had a positive skin test. Foods suggested by the patients were studied with a total of 19 DBPC challenges: none provoked a migrainous attack. Twenty patients could not identify any precipitants, and only five had more than two headaches per week. These five were placed on an elimination diet and two became free of headache, which did not recur on resumption of a normal diet. The outcome differences between these two studies may be explained by protocol design and patient selection. Egger placed all the patients on the elimination diet, probably dealt with a more severely affected group, and challenged with larger amounts of foods over several days. This more prolonged challenge might lead to more false-positives because of the spontaneous recurring nature of migraine. Because headache may be delayed in onset, patients may not identify such agents, and testing only history-suspected items would falsely lower the response rate.

Mansfield, Vaughan, and coworkers evaluated 43 consecutive migraine adult patients referred from a neurology clinic [29]. Eighty-three food skin prick tests were performed, and positive foods were eliminated from the diet for 1 month. Those patients with negative skin tests were placed on a wheat, corn, milk, and egg elimination diet. Patients with two-thirds or greater reduction in headache frequency underwent a series of single-blind challenges with 8 g of desiccated food or similar number of placebo capsules. Positive challenges were followed by DBPC challenges. Thirteen of 43 (30%) had the dietary two-thirds reduction. Of seven who underwent DBPC challenges, no patient responded to placebo, five had migraine with the active challenge, and two were without headache for either challenge.

Vaughan and associates studied a further 104 adult migraine subjects in another DBPC protocol [30–32]. All patients had neurology-verified migraine and headache frequency of at least three per month on a regular diet. Skin prick tests were performed with 83 foods, and all foods suggested by skin tests and/or history, as well as wheat, corn, milk, and egg were eliminated for 1 month. Patients with a greater than 50% reduction in headache frequency were studied further. Foods were reintroduced in an open fashion and eaten three times daily. Identification of at least one provoking food led to the DBPC phase. Desiccated foods were given in capsules three times daily, with a 4-day randomized challenge sequence of two placebo (P) and two active (A) days. Since Egger had reported that some patients only reacted on the second day of challenge with larger amounts of the incriminated food [27], the active days followed each other, giving challenge sequences of AAPP, PAAP, or PPAA. A positive challenge was headache occurring on both days or on the second challenge day, and any response to placebo was ruled a negative challenge.

Forty patients (38.5%) had a greater than 50% reduction in migraine frequency, with eight becoming headache-free. Twenty-seven of 36 undergoing open challenges could identify at least one precipitant, with a range of 1–4. Of 24 patients with DBPC challenges, 15 had migraine on both active days and two on the second day only. Three reported headache on placebo and four had no migraine at all. Therefore, over one-third of 104 consecutive adult migraine patients had improvement on an elimination diet, and 17 of 104 (16%) had reproducible DBPC demonstration of food-induced migraine. In contrast to Vaughan's earlier study, but agreeing with Egger's study, food skin testing was not helpful [26, 27]. Skin tests were positive for less than half of the documented food triggers (Table 42.1). The skin test neither consistently identified migraine-provoking foods nor identified migraineurs more likely to benefit from dietary manipulation.

Table 42.1 Value of double-blind food challenges and skin tests in migraineurs.

Patient #	Positive open challenges	Skin test results	Positive double-blind challenges
1	Egg	1+	Egg
	Milk	0	
	Wheat	1+	
2	Coffee	2+	Coffee
	Maple syrup	ND	
3	Wheat	3+	Wheat
4	Black-eyed peas	4+	Black-eyed peas
	Pinto beans	3+	
5	Egg	1+	Egg
	Chocolate	0	
6	Egg	0	Egg
	Milk	0	
7	Wheat	0	Wheat
	Cheese	0	
8	Wheat	0	Wheat
9	Wheat	0	Wheat
	Chocolate	0	
10	Milk	0	Milk
	Wheat	0	
	Chocolate	0	
	Cheese	0	
11	Cheese	0	Cheese
	Chocolate	0	
12	Corn	0	Corn
	Wheat	0	
13	Coffee	0	Coffee
14	Cheese	0	Cheese
	Chocolate	0	
15	Corn	0	Corn
	Soy	0	
16	Wheat	0	Wheat
	Egg	0	

Source: From References 31–33.

Pharmacologic triggering agents

In 1925, Curtis-Brown had proposed that defective protein metabolism was responsible for migraine headache, leading to "protein poisoning" [33]. Migraine could thus occur on the first exposure, and patients could improve on restrictive diets. While there was no support for this theory, it did suggest that food intolerance in migraine patients could be due to pharmacologic action of a constituent.

In the 1960s, severe pounding headache was described in patients on monoamine oxidase inhibitors when ingesting foods containing tyramine. Hanington noted that such foods were frequently incriminated by migraine sufferers as causing their headaches [34]. A double-blind challenge in 45 migraine patients showed an 80% response of headache to 125 mg of tyramine, and an 8% response to placebo [35]. While other following studies confirmed tyramine sensitivity in migraineurs, another series of papers could not demonstrate a significant role for tyramine. In a DBPC trial, Moffett and coworkers studied eight presumed tyramine-sensitive migraine patients, another 10 migraineurs without this history, and seven patients with migraine and epilepsy [36]. The presumed sensitive patients had symptoms as often on placebo as with tyramine, one patient with epilepsy had a tyramine-induced headache, and none of the other migraineurs had headache. Forsythe and Redmond, in a blinded challenge, used 100 mg tyramine and found that 12 of 61 children reacted; a second group of 38 children had only five reactors to tyramine [37]. Ziegler and Stewart reported 49 of 80 patients had symptoms with neither 200 mg of tyramine nor placebo, 12 with both, 11 with placebo alone, and only eight with tyramine alone [38]. Tyramine-free diets have failed to affect headache frequency [39].

Traditional provokers of migraine such as chocolate, cheeses, and red wine may not contain tyramine, but rather phenylethylamine [40]. This vasoactive amine crosses the blood–brain barrier and can cause changes in cerebral blood flow. Five of six patients with histories of chocolate-induced migraine developed headaches within 8 hours of an open challenge of 100 g of chocolate [41]. Sandler and associates studied 36 single-blind patients who believed that chocolate precipitated headache [42]. They received either 3 mg phenylethylamine or placebo: 18 patients reported headache with the amine, whereas six reported headache with placebo, a statistically significant difference. However, Schweitzer and coworkers analyzed a number of chocolate varieties and found about 150-fold less phenylethylamine than in the preparations tested by Sandler [43]. They concluded, either chocolate-induced migraine was not due to phenylethylamine or migraine sufferers were sensitive to extremely low levels of this substance. Another DBPC study of 25 patients with a history of chocolate- or cocoa-induced migraine found: eight patients had headache with only chocolate, five with only placebo, one with both, and 11 with neither [44]. Fifteen patients underwent repeat challenges with different chocolate and placebo preparations: five had migraine with chocolate alone, only two repeating the same result as the first trial. The authors believed that chocolate alone was rarely a precipitant of migraine.

Twenty-eight chronic headache patients adhered to a histamine-free diet avoiding alcoholic beverages, fish, cheeses, sausages, and pickled cabbage for months [45]. After 4 weeks, four lost their headaches, 15 had greater than 50% improvement, and nine had no change; after 1 year, eight of nine continued to be improved. Salfield and coworkers randomized 39 migrainous children to either a high-fiber diet or a low vasoactive amine diet [46]. There was no influence of dietary vasoamines because both groups improved equally, with significant decreases in headache, reinforcing the need for double-blind studies. While there probably are patients sensitive to substances such as tyramine and phenylethylamine, it is difficult to demonstrate appreciable reactors in controlled settings. Lai and associates performed clinical assessments and EEG on 38 patients with diet-induced migraine [47]. After a control day, the patients were challenged with a combination of red wine, chocolate, and sharp cheddar cheese: 16 developed headache, four with scotomata. Abnormalities in the EEG were demonstrated but generally did not separate headache responders from nonresponders. All of the patients with headache showed photic driving of the EEG, while only 64% of the nonresponders did so ($p < 0.01$); the significance of this finding is uncertain.

Nitrites added to meats as coloring agents, are incriminated in hot dog or cured meat headache. High concentrations of nitrites are found in hot dogs, bacon, ham luncheon meats, smoked fish, and some imported cheeses; it is common to find levels much higher than the FDA-recommended levels of 200 ppm. The headache usually begins within minutes or hours after ingestion, is bitemporal or bifrontal, and is pulsatile 50% of the time [48]. The mechanism is unclear.

Migraineurs commonly identify alcohol as a precipitant, headache usually appearing within 30–45 minutes after consumption, similar to the timing of cutaneous vasodilatation. Alcohol has little to no effect on cerebral blood flow; therefore, intracerebral vasodilatation is not the mechanism of alcohol headache. Depression of brain serotonin turnover by high levels of alcohol may play a role, considering the role of serotonin metabolism postulated in migraine [6, 40]. Red wine is incriminated more often than other forms of alcohol. Littlewood and associates assembled 19 migraineurs who believed that red wine but not other forms of alcohol provoked headache [49]. Chilled red wine and vodka with similar alcohol content were consumed in a blinded fashion, and the incidence of headache compared. The tyramine content of the wine was 2 mg/L and that ingested less than 1 mg. The wine produced significantly more headaches than the vodka. The authors concluded, alcohol and tyramine were not responsible for the migraine headaches, rather other ingredients such as phenolic flavonoids found in higher quantities in red than white wine.

The "Chinese restaurant syndrome" induced by monosodium glutamate (MSG) is comprised of headache, facial tightness, warmth across the shoulders, and also dizziness, nausea, and abdominal cramps [40, 50]. Approximately 30% of people ingesting Chinese food have symptoms, usually beginning 20 minutes after ingestion. Thresholds vary from 1.5 to 12 gm, commonly below 3 gm, the amount found in a portion of wonton soup. Symptoms are presumed to be due to central nervous system (CNS) neuroexcitatory effects.

Since its introduction in 1981, the artificial sweetener aspartame has provoked numerous reports of adverse reactions. A large number included headache or were of a neurologic or behavioral nature [51]. In 1987, a DBPC crossover study in 40 subjects reporting aspartame-induced headaches showed no differences in headache induction between the sweetener and placebo [52]. One year later a 13-week study demonstrated differing results [53]. Twenty-five subjects began, but only eleven completed the protocol of a 4-week baseline followed by randomized sequential 4-week periods with either aspartame 300 mg q.i.d. or placebo, with 1-week washouts. Headaches occurred twice as frequently on aspartame as on placebo or during the baseline period ($p < 0.02$). The differences were due to a marked increase of headaches in 4 of the 11 subjects. Ironically, two patients have been reported with headache triggered by aspartame contained in their migraine medication [54]. Another commonly used sweetener, sucralose, has also been reported to induce migraine [55].

Mediators and immunologic mechanisms in migraine

Immunologic studies have been generally unrewarding in migraine. Medina and Diamond reported no differences in total IgE between migraineurs and the normal population [39]. Merrett and colleagues examined IgE levels in 74 adults with dietary migraine, 45 with nondietary migraine, 29 with cluster headache, and 60 with normal controls [56]. They found no differences in specific and total IgE in the groups except for a higher total IgE in the cluster headache patients, which they attributed to a higher percentage of smokers. Specific IgE for cheese, milk, and chocolate showed no difference between dietary and nondietary migraine. While consensus holds that specific IgG has no clinical value in the assessment of immediate hypersensitivity reactions to foods, several reports have assessed their relevance in food-related migraine [57]. Arroyave Hernández and associates compared a battery of 108 food-IgG ELISA tests in patients with migraine and a control group without headache and found increased positives in the migraineurs, and that elimination diets based on the laboratory results improved the migraines [58]. Alpay and colleagues reported in 2010 a double-blind randomized cross-over trial of provocative versus elimination diets individualized to 30 common migraine patients based on results of 266 food-IgG assays [59]. Mitchell and coworkers obtained IgG ELISA assays for 113 foods in 167 food-intolerant migraineurs and placed half on an elimination diet based on the ELISA results, and the other half on a sham diet [60]. At week 4 of the 12-week trial, headaches were reduced in the true elimination group, but disability and impact on daily life were not different between groups.

Pradalier and coworkers reported that 20 consecutive patients with common migraine (11 with food-induced migraine and nine without) had mid-duodenal biopsies examined for lamina propria IgE, IgG, IgA, or IgM containing plasmocytes [61]. There were no differences between the two groups for histologic appearance, total plasmocytes, or subsets. Ratner and associates have linked dietary migraine with lactase deficiency, and represented data on elevated IgM in 11 such migraine patients [62]. Martelletti and coworkers, using a C1q binding assay, showed increased circulating immune complexes in 21 food-induced migraine patients (29% versus 10% in the control group) [63]. They also demonstrated that activated T cells showed an increase at 4 hours after challenge followed by a decrease at 72 hours [64].

Three studies have examined mediator release in dietary migraine. Three patients in the Mansfield adult migraine study had repeat challenges with histamine plasma levels [29]. Headache was provoked only with the active challenge and was associated with increases in the histamine levels coinciding with or preceding the onset of the headache. Placebo challenge on two revealed no or little change in histamine. Steinberg and colleagues reported a case of beef-induced migraine in a young woman [65]. There was a threefold increase in histamine and an increase of a PGF2α metabolite coinciding with the onset of the headache. Increased intracerebral blood flow was demonstrated with Xenon computerized tomography and Doppler ultrasonography. Skin prick test and RAST to beef were negative.

Olson and colleagues reported serial histamine and prostaglandin D (PGD) levels during DBPC challenges in five patients with food-induced migraine [66]. Placebo challenges produced no changes; with active challenge, all five had a 3 to 38-fold increase in plasma histamine as well as increase in PGD_2 before or coinciding with the onset of symptoms. A second increase in the PGD_2 was noted 4 to 6 hours after ingestion, without a concomitant rise in histamine. This discordance suggests the late recruitment of non-basophil inflammatory cells. Skin tests in this group were all negative.

Summary

There is a wealth of clinical data supporting that dietary migraine is a bona fide entity, with both pharmacologic and immunologic mechanisms involved in subsets (Table 42.2). These are not mutually exclusive conditions. What the exact pathophysiology is remains unclear, although the release of immediate hypersensitivity mediators has been demonstrated. The variable results of immediate skin testing suggest while some reactions may be IgE mediated, many are probably pseudoallergic or anaphylactoid. Why release of these mediators causes

Table 42.2 Incriminated agents in dietary migraine.

Presumed pharmacologic action
Tyramine
Phenylethylamine
Phenolic flavonoids
Ethanol
Nitrites
Caffeine
Monosodium glutamate
Aspartame
Sucralose
Immunologic or uncertain action
Food proteins

migraine in susceptible persons and not more traditional allergic manifestations is unclear.

The exact frequency of dietary migraine is not settled. Studies suggest that 15% may have reproducible triggers under controlled situations, but twice that number may benefit from dietary restriction. While the majority of headache patients believe that there are connections between food intake and their headaches, fewer than half have this relationship addressed by their physicians, and fewer modify their dietary practices [67]. Such patients should be evaluated by appropriate history and physical examination and the exclusion of migraine-mimicking conditions. Once bona fide migraine has been established, and pharmacological control achieved, it is reasonable to pursue possible dietary triggers. Global dietary restrictions are not indicated. Although history may identify a number of triggers, some patients with reproducible headaches on DBPC challenges could not separate the causative agents during a normal diet.

Food skin testing will present both false-positives and false-negatives, and should not be relied on alone, and IgE RAST is of little additional value, and the role of food-specific IgG remains to be better delineated. This leaves the prospect of food diaries and elimination diets. For patients with infrequent migraines, a diary listing foods ingested in the previous 48 hours to a headache may be useful. A diet eliminating wheat, corn, milk, and egg may be helpful for a period of 2 to 4 weeks. Patients benefiting should reintroduce foods singly and for three consecutive days. Foods not provoking symptoms should be returned freely to the diet. Suspect foods should be eliminated and rechallenged. In patients with numerous suspected positives, it is wise to perform challenges under blinded conditions to remove expectation or anxiety as confounding factors, to avoid unnecessary restriction of the diet. Consulting with a nutritionist is warranted for patients who have multiple documented triggers.

Epilepsy

Epilepsy was historically compared to the similarly episodic syndromes of anaphylaxis and atopic disorders. Schwartz, in his monumental epidemiological study of asthma and atopy in 4256 probands and relatives in Denmark, also collected data on migraine and epilepsy [68]. He found very few cases of epilepsy in the kindreds, and no evidence for any genetic correlation between epilepsy and the atopic disorders. Nonetheless, there have been a number of reports linking food allergy and epilepsy. In 1927, Ward and Patterson food skin tested 1000 epileptics and 100 controls, finding patient reactivity between 37% and 67%, and only 8% reactivity in the controls [69].

In 1951, Dees and Lowenbach reported on 37 children with epilepsy who were treated with antiallergic therapy, environmental avoidance measures, and elimination diets as well as anticonvulsant therapy [70]. Twenty-two met criteria for "allergic epilepsy": personal and family history of allergy, blood eosinophilia, positive skin tests, and no organic disease of the CNS. The remainder had possible allergic disease, but did not meet all criteria, half had eosinophilia. Twenty of the "allergic" group and 13 of the "nonallergic" group had positive food skin tests. The predominant EEG finding was occipital dysrhythmia (73% of both groups), a rhythm the authors reported to be present in some allergic children without overt seizure disorder. Thirteen in the allergic group were treated with allergen immunotherapy as well as the dietary and medical manipulations. Convulsions were controlled in 18 of 22 allergic children and 6 of 15 "nonallergic" children; anticonvulsant therapy could be stopped in 13 of the former and one of the latter group. The authors felt that epilepsy could be on an allergic basis, and therefore could be controlled with appropriate antiallergic therapy. They did not provide any indication of how many epileptic children were surveyed to arrive at their study group; so it is difficult to place this observation in proper perspective.

Egger and colleagues in their assessment of food factors in migraine had several patients who had epilepsy and or behavioral problems that appeared to respond to the oligoantigenic diet [27]. They further investigated children who either had difficult-to-control epilepsy, either alone or associated with migraine [71]. None of 18 with epilepsy alone improved on the oligoantigenic diet, while 40 of 45 with both epilepsy and migraine reported improvement of one or more symptoms. In follow up ranging from 7 months to 3 years, 25 patients had complete control of their epilepsy. Thirty-two patients had seizure during reintroduction of incriminated foods. In double-blind challenges of 16 children, seven reacted to the suspected food only, none to placebo only, and one to both. Pelliccia and colleagues have reported a total of four cases of cow's intolerance where partial idiopathic epilepsy was improved, both clinically and with EEG findings, with cow's milk-free diets, with recurrence, and with reintroduction [72,73].

There is a variant of reflex epilepsy where it is not the food ingested which is the precipitant of the seizure, but rather the act of eating itself. This entity is called "eating epilepsy," and while quite rare, appears to be more common in kindreds in Sri Lanka and the Indian subcontinent [74–76]. The seizure type is usually complex partially, does not occur with all meals, and usually happens at home. Many episodes are linked to the ingestion of rice, but since this is a staple of the diet, it is likely that this is not truly specific [74]. It has been postulated that stimulation of areas of the brain that receive sensory input during eating may lower the seizure threshold [77]. A report of two patients localized the seizure focus to the suprasylvanian and temporolimbic regions, respectively [78].

Diet manipulation in epilepsy

It was observed that many epilepsy patients were free of seizures while fasting, the benefit persisting after return to a normal diet. It was suggested that this effect was due to ketonemia, and a "ketogenic" high-fat, low-carbohydrate diet was proposed for treatment. The diet was rigid, unpalatable, and difficult to maintain, requiring strict nutritional supervision [79, 80]. It appeared useful, especially in younger age children whose seizures were not responsive to antiepileptic medications. Kinsman and associates showed benefit from the diet in 58 epileptic children requiring multiple medications [80]. Seizure control improved in 67%, with reduced medication in 64%, greater alertness in 36%, and improved behavior in 23%. Seventy-five percent of these improved patients were able to maintain the diet, at least 18 months. A medium chain triglyceride diet was found to be more ketogenic than the fat in the traditional diet, and felt to be more palatable; Sills and colleagues reported on their success with such a diet in 50 epileptic children [79]. Eight achieved complete control of seizures, four without medication, four had seizures reduced by 90%, and 10 by 50–90%. Extra dosing of the medium-chain triglycerides at bedtime was useful for control of nocturnal seizures. The diet appears to work in a variety of epileptic syndromes, and the response is not predicted by age, syndrome, or etiology [81]. Making the diet easier and more palatable appears to be successful, as is the use of the Atkins diet [82, 83]. Gradual introduction of the diet appears to be both better tolerated and effective [84]. The mechanisms remain unclear. Possibilities include alterations in acid–base balance, water and electrolyte distribution, or lipid concentrations, and direct action of ketone bodies [85,86]. Increased flux through the inhibitory neurotransmitter, γ-aminobutyric acid (GABA) shunt, induced by the diet may have a protective effect [86]. Experimental models have shown increased plasma levels of linoleate and α-linoleate decrease seizure susceptibility either directly or through promoting ketosis [87].

Epilepsy and migraine

The link between migraine and epilepsy is apparent, but the nature of the relationship is unclear. Wilson addressed several overlapping issues [88]. If attacks and auras are brief, especially if the attacks are stereotyped, a diagnosis of epilepsy is preferred; if attacks with prodrome are longer, and if the impact on consciousness is primarily confusion, migraine may be more likely. Therapeutic trials of migraine prophylaxis and antiepileptic drugs may help clarify the diagnosis. Several migraine–epilepsy syndromes have been identified: seizures with typical migraine prodrome; migraine with later development of epilepsy; alternating hemiplegic migraine. In the first case, impairment of cerebral blood flow associated with migraine may precipitate the seizure. In the next, repeated ischemic insult may lead to an epileptogenic focus. Despite such cases, the relationship between epilepsy and migraine remains obscure. Can one condition trigger the other, in a dually susceptible individual, or is epilepsy an epiphenomenon in a vascular disease?

Summary

While the role of food is important in provoking attacks of migraine, less is known concerning dietary factors in epilepsy. The efficacy of ketogenic diets is well established, but the manner in which they operate remains uncertain. That bona fide anaphylactoid reactions could trigger convulsions in susceptible patients appears likely, but DBPC studies are absent, and would be helpful in validating the clinical observations to date. And certainly, mediator release studies are needed.

Vertigo

In 1976, Dunn and Snyder reported 33 pediatric cases of benign paroxysmal vertigo, a syndrome of sporadic brief episodes of disequilibrium, nystagmus, and/or vomiting [89]. During infancy, this often manifested by paroxysmal torticollis. While food allergy was considered in all, in only four cases was it likely. Three children had histories suggestive of milk allergy: attacks were eliminated by removing milk from the diet, and with vertigo reappearing with milk challenges. In another chocolate was suspected, but could not be challenge-confirmed. Unstated is whether these were open or blinded challenges. At best, a tenth of the cases had evidence for a food etiology.

In 1923, Duke postulated a food cause for adult vertigo or Meniere's syndrome [90]. Five cases of Meniere's improved on elimination diets. There are no well-performed double-blind studies. Older reports are limited to the suspect nonreproducible technique of provocation–neutralization. In 2000, Derebery surveyed 137 Meniere's patients: 113 revealed they underwent allergen immunotherapy and/or elimination diet [91]. An analysis of pre- and post-treatment symptoms revealed improved frequency and severity of vertigo, tinnitus, and unsteadiness ($p < 0.005$–0.001). Unfortunately, diagnosis of food allergy was by both skin testing and provocation–neutralization, and those that received diet manipulations were not segregated from those that received immunotherapy. Also, a quarter of the patients acknowledged not following the diet, 30% "sometimes," and about 45% followed the diet "almost always." So this survey, at best, suggests there may be an association between diet and vertigo. Whether a food role can be substantiated in this area will require appropriately controlled studies.

Hemiplegia

Several case reports exist of transient neurological deficits following presumed allergic reaction to foods. Cooke reported transient third cranial nerve palsy associated with hemiparesis, followed by an episode of contralateral blindness and paresthesia in a food allergic patient [92]. Symptoms resolved with avoidance of beef and pork, and challenges were not performed. In 1951, Staffieri and colleagues reported a case of right-sided hemiplegia immediately following a meal, and associated with angioedema, urticaria, purpura, and peripheral eosinophilia ranging from 34% to 40% [93]. A wheat elimination diet was attended within a few days by resolution of the symptoms. To rule out coincidence, a total of four presumed single-blind wheat challenges were performed over 4 months, resulting initially in headache, with purpura and angioedema, and ultimately in the skin manifestations alone. Passive transfer of skin sensitizing antibodies was not successful. Such reports are fascinating, presumably reflecting that anaphylactic reactions may be attended by edema anywhere to include the central and peripheral nervous systems. Reinforcing this concept is a report of 55 cases of anaphylaxis in 50 children by Dibs and Baker, where neurologic symptoms were manifest in 26% [94]. Symptoms included aura, irritability, lethargy, disorientation, dizziness, tremor, syncope, and seizure.

Gluten sensitivity and neurological abnormalities

As reviewed by Wills and Unsworth, several case reports have described neurological complications with gluten sensitivity: cerebellar ataxia, myoclonus, epilepsy, neuropathy, and dementia [95]. Interestingly, there is a dichotomy between celiac disease patients and those with dermatitis herpetiformis: two series have failed to find any increased neurological problems in the latter [96, 97]. While previous reports had not shown a benefit of gluten dietary elimination in neurological symptoms, Cicarelli and colleagues did so in a series of 176 gluten-sensitive patients and 52 age-matched controls [98]. Increased occurrence of headache, dysthymia, cramps, and weakness in the patients compared to the controls was reduced in those patients adhering to a strict gluten-free diet, with no impact on occurrence of paresthesia or hyporeflexia. A constellation of celiac disease, epilepsy, and occipital lobe calcifications has been described in Italians [99]. Three additional Australian patients of non-Mediterranean extraction have been reported with biopsy documented celiac disease, bilateral occipital–parietal, bilateral cortical calcification, epilepsy, and visual disturbances [100]. Occipital lobe epilepsy was simple-partial, complex-partial, and secondarily generalized; visual disturbances included blurred vision, colored dots, and visual hallucinations. Jacob and colleagues reported two cases of optic neuritis with acute transverse myelitis with biopsy and serology documented celiac disease [101]. The neurologic complications associated with gluten sensitivity remain of uncertain etiology, with direct neurotoxic effects, autoimmune injury, or resultant metabolic deficiency from malabsorption all being possible mechanisms.

References

1. Ad Hoc Committee on the Classification of Headache. Classification of headache. *Arch Neurol* 1962; 6:173–176.
2. Stewart WF, Lipton RB, Celentano DD, Reed ML. Prevalence of migraine headache in the United States: relation to age, income, race, and other sociodemographic factors. *J Am Med Assoc* 1992; 267:64–69.
3. Stang PE, Yanagihar PA, Swanson JW, et al. Incidence of migraine headache: a population-based study in Olmstead County, Minnesota. *Neurology* 1992; 42:1657–1662.
4. Millichap JG. Recurrent headaches in 100 children. Electroencephalographic abnormalities and response to phenytoin (Dilantin). *Childs Brain* 1978; 4:95–105.
5. Woods RP, Iacoboni M, Mazziotta JC. Brief report: bilateral spreading cerebral hypoperfusion during

spontaneous migraine headache. *N Engl J Med* 1994; 331:1689–1692.

6. Zeigler DK, Murrow RW. Headache. In: Joynt RJ (ed.), *Clinical Neurology*, vol. 2, revised edition. Philadelphia, PA: JB Lippincott Co, 1988; pp. 1–49.
7. Moskowitz MA, Macfarlane R. Neurovascular and molecular mechanisms in migraine headaches. *Cerebrovasc Brain Metab Rev* 1993; 5:159–177.
8. Fukui PT, Goncalves TR, Strabelli CG, et al. Trigger factors in migraine patients. *Arq Neuropsiquiatr* 2008; 66:494–499.
9. Hasselmark L, Malmgren R, Hannerz J. Effect of a carbohydrate-rich diet, low in protein-tryptophan, in classic and common migraine. *Cephalalgia* 1987; 7:87–92.
10. Drummond PD. Effect of tryptophan depletion on symptoms of motion sickness in migraineurs. *Neurology* 2005; 65:620–622.
11. Harel Z, Gascon G, Riggs S, Vaz R, Brown W, Exil G. Supplementation with omega-3 polyunsaturated fatty acids in the management of recurrent migraines in adolescents. *J Adolesc Health* 2002; 31:154–161.
12. Schéle R, Ahlborg B, Ekbom K. Physical characteristics and allergic history in young men with migraine and other headaches. *Headache* 1978; 18:80–86.
13. Pinnas JL, Vanselow NA. Relationship of allergy to headache. *Res Clin Stud Headache* 1976; 4:85–95.
14. Brown TR. Role of diet in etiology and treatment of migraine and other types of headache. *J Am Med Assoc* 1921; 77:1396–1400.
15. Vaughan WT. Allergic migraine. *J Am Med Assoc* 1927; 88:1383–1386.
16. Eyermann CH. Allergic headache. *J Allergy* 1930; 2:106–112.
17. Balyeat RM, Rinkel HJ. Further studies in allergic migraine: based on a series of two hundred and two consecutive cases. *Ann Intern Med* 1931; 5:713–728.
18. DeGowin EL. Allergic migraine: a review of sixty cases. *J Allergy* 1932; 3:557–566.
19. Unger AH, Unger L. Migraine is an allergic disease. *J Allergy* 1952; 23:429–440.
20. Schwartz M. Is migraine an allergic disease? *J Allergy* 1952; 23:426–428.
21. Grant EC. Food allergies and migraine. *Lancet* 1979; 1:966–969.
22. Monro J, Carini C, Brostoff J, et al. Food allergy in migraine: study of dietary exclusion and RAST. *Lancet* 1980; 2:1–4.
23. Monro J, Carini C, Brostoff J. Migraine is a food-allergic disease. *Lancet* 1984; 2:719–721.
24. Ratner D, Shoshani E, Dubnov B. Milk protein-free diet for nonseasonal asthma and migraine in lactase-deficient patients. *Isr J Med Sci* 1983; 19:806–809.
25. Hughes EC, Gott PS, Weinstein RC, et al. Migraine: a diagnostic test for etiology of food sensitivity by a nutritionally supported fast and confirmed by long term report. *Ann Allergy* 1985; 55:28–32.
26. Vaughan TR, Mansfield LE, Haverly RW, Chamberlin WM, Waller SF. The value of cutaneous testing for food allergy in the diagnostic evaluation of migraine headache [Abstract]. *Ann Allergy* 1983; 50:362.
27. Egger J, Wilson J, Carter CM, Turner MW. Is migraine food allergy? A double-blind controlled trial of oligoantigenic diet treatment. *Lancet* 1983; 2:865–868.
28. Atkins FM, Ball BD, Bock A. The relationship between the ingestion of specific foods and the development of migraine headaches in children [Abstract]. *J Allergy Clin Immunol* 1988; 81:185.
29. Mansfield LE, Vaughan TR, Waller SF, Haverly RW, Ting S. Food allergy and adult migraine: double blind and mediator confirmation of an allergic etiology. *Ann Allergy* 1985; 55:126–129.
30. Vaughan TR, Stafford WW, Miller BT, Weber RW, Tipton WR, Nelson HS. Food and migraine headache (MIG): a controlled study [Abstract]. *Ann Allergy* 1986; 56:522.
31. Weber RW, Vaughan TR. Food and migraine headache. *Immunol Allergy Clin N Am* 1991; 11:831–841.
32. Vaughan TR. The role of food in the pathogenesis of migraine headache. *Clin Rev Allergy* 1994; 12:167–180.
33. Curtis-Brown R. A protein poison theory: its application to the treatment of headache and especially migraine. *Br Med J* 1925; 1:155–157.
34. Hanington E. Preliminary report on tyramine headache. *Br Med J* 1967; 2:550–551.
35. Smith I, Kellow AH, Hanington E. A clinical and biochemical correlation between tyramine and migraine headache. *Headache* 1970; 10:43–51.
36. Moffett A, Swash M, Scott DF. Effect of tyramine in migraine: a double-blind study. *J Neurol Neurosurg Psychiatry* 1972; 35:496–499.
37. Forsythe WI, Redmond A. Two controlled trials of tyramine in children with migraine. *Dev Med Child Neurol* 1974; 16:794–799.
38. Zeigler DK, Stewart R. Failure of tyramine to induce migraine. *Neurol* 1977; 27:725–726.
39. Medina JL, Diamond S. The role of diet in migraine. *Headache* 1978; 18:31–34.
40. Raskin NH. Chemical headaches. *Ann Rev Med* 1981; 32:63–71.
41. Peatfield RC, Hampton KK, Grant PJ. Plasma vasopressin levels in induced migraine attacks. *Cephalalgia* 1988; 8:55–57.
42. Sandler M, Youdim MBH, Hanington E. A phenylethylamine oxidising defect in migraine. *Nature* 1974; 250:335–337.
43. Schweitzer JW, Friedhoff AJ, Schwartz R. Letter: Chocolate, beta-phenylethylamine and migraine re-examined. *Nature* 1975; 257:256.
44. Moffett AM, Swash M, Scott DF. Effect of chocolate in migraine: a double-blind study. *J Neurol Neurosurg Psychiatry* 1974; 37:445–448.
45. Wantke F, Götz M, Jarisch R. Histamine-free diet: treatment of choice for histamine-induced food intolerance and supporting treatment for chronic headaches. *Clin Exp Allergy* 1993; 23:982–985.
46. Salfield SA, Wardley BL, Houlsby WT, et al. Controlled study of exclusion of dietary vasoactive amines in migraine. *Arch Dis Child* 1987; 62:458–460.

47. Lai C-W, Dean P, Ziegler DK, Hassanein RS. Clinical and electrophysiological responses to dietary challenge in migraineurs. *Headache* 1989; 29:180–186.
48. Henderson WR, Raskin NH. "Hot-dog" headache: individual susceptibility to nitrite. *Lancet* 1972; 2:1162–1163.
49. Littlewood JT, Glover V, Davies PTG, Gibb C, Sandler M, Rose FC. Red wine as a cause of migraine. *Lancet* 1988; 1:558–559.
50. Yang WH, Drouin MA, Herbert M, Mao Y, Karsh J. The monosodium glutamate symptom complex: assessment in a double-blind, placebo-controlled, randomized study. *J Allergy Clin Immunol* 1997; 99:757–762.
51. Centers for Disease Control. Evaluation of consumer complaints related to aspartame use. *Morb Mortal Wkly Rep* 1984; 33:605–607.
52. Schiffman SS, Buckley CE III, Sampson HA, et al. Aspartame and susceptibility to headache. *N Engl J Med* 1987; 317:1181–1185.
53. Koehler SM, Glaros A. The effect of aspartame on migraine headache. *Headache* 1988; 28:10–14.
54. Newman LC, Lipton RB. Migraine MLT-down: an unusual presentation of migraine in patients with aspartame-triggered headaches. *Headache* 2001; 41:899–901.
55. Bigal ME, Krycmchantowski AV. Migraine triggered by sucralose—a case report. *Headache* 2006; 46:515–517.
56. Merrett J, Peatfield RC, Rose FC, Merrett TG. Food related antibodies in headache patients. *J Neurol Neurosurg Psychiatry* 1983; 46:738–742.
57. Teuber SS, Porch-Curren C. Unproven diagnostic and therapeutic approaches to food allergy and intolerance. *Curr Opin Allergy Clin Immunol* 2003; 3:217–221.
58. Arroyave Hernández CM, Echavarría Pinto M, Hernández Montiel HL. Food allergy mediated by IgG antibodies associated with migraine in adults. *Rev Alerg Mex* 2007; 54:162–168.
59. Alpay K, Ertas M, Orhan EK, Üstay DK, Lieners C, Baykan B. Diet restriction in migraine, based on IgG against foods: a double-blind, randomised cross-over trial. *Cephalalgia* 2010; 30:829–837.
60. Mitchell N, Hewitt C, Jayakody S, et al. Randomised controlled trial of food elimination diet based on IgG antibodies for the prevention of migraine like headaches. *Nutrition J* 2011; 10:85–93.
61. Pradalier A, De Saint Maur P, Lamy F, Launay JM. Immunocyte enumeration in duodenal biopsies of migraine without aura patients with or without food-induced migraine. *Cephalalgia* 1994; 14:365–367.
62. Ratner D, Eshel E, Shneyour A, Teitler A. Elevated IgM in dietary migraine with lactase deficiency. *Isr J Med Sci* 1984; 20:717–719.
63. Martelletti P, Sutherland J, Anastasi E, Di Mario U, Giacovazzo M. Evidence for an immune-mediated mechanism in food-induced migraine from a study on activated T-cells, IgG_4 subclass, anti-IgG antibodies and circulating immune complexes. *Headache* 1989; 29:664–670.
64. Martelletti P. T cells expressing IL-2 receptor in migraine. *Acta Neurol* 1991; 13:448–456.
65. Steinberg M, Page R, Wolfson S, Friday G, Fireman P. Food induced late phase headache [Abstract]. *J Allergy Clin Immunol* 1988; 81:185.
66. Olson GC, Vaughan TR, Ledoux RA, et al. Food induced migraine: search for immunologic mechanisms [Abstract]. *J Allergy Clin Immunol* 1989; 83:238.
67. Guarnieri P, Radnitz C, Blanchard EB. Assessment of dietary risk factors in chronic headache. *Biofeedback Self Regul* 1990; 15:15–25.
68. Schwartz M. Heredity in bronchial asthma: a clinical and genetic study of 191 asthma probands and 50 probands with baker's asthma. *Acta Allergol Suppl* 1952; 2:1–288.
69. Ward RF, Patterson HA. Protein sensitization in epilepsy: a study of one thousand cases and one hundred normal controls. *Arch Neurol Psych* 1927; 17:427–443.
70. Dees SC, Lowenbach H. Allergic epilepsy. *Ann Allergy* 1951; 9:446–458.
71. Egger J, Cater CM, Soothill JF, Wilson J. Oligoantigenic diet treatment of children with epilepsy and migraine. *J Pediatr* 1989; 114:51–58.
72. Pelliccia A, Lucarelli S, Frediani T, et al. Partial cryptogenic epilepsy and food allergy/intolerance. A causal or a chance relationship? Reflections on three clinical cases. *Minerva Pediatr* 1999; 51:153–157.
73. Frediani T, Pelliccia A, Aprile A, Ferri E, Lucarelli S. Partial idiopathic epilepsy: recovery after allergen-free diet. *Pediatr Med Chir* 2004; 26:196–197.
74. Ahuja GK, Pauranik A, Behari M, Prasad K. Eating epilepsy. *J Neurol* 1988; 235:444–447.
75. Senanayake N. Familial eating epilepsy. *J Neurol* 1990; 237:388–391.
76. Senanayake N. 'Eating epilepsy'—a reappraisal. *Epilepsy Res* 1990; 5:74–79.
77. Fiol ME, Leppik IE, Pretzel K. Eating epilepsy: EEG and clinical study. *Epilepsia* 1986; 27:441–446.
78. Labate A, Colosimo E, Gambardella A, et al. Reflex periodic spasms induced by eating. *Brain Dev* 2006; 28:170–174.
79. Sills MA, Forsythe WI, Haidukewych D, Macdonald A, Robinson M. The medium chain triglyceride diet and intractable epilepsy. *Arch Dis Child* 1986; 61:1168–1172.
80. Kinsman SL, Vining EPG, Quaskey SA, Mellits D, Freeman JM. Efficacy of the ketogenic diet for intractable seizure disorders: review of 58 cases. *Epilepsia* 1992; 33:1132–1136.
81. Mackay MT, Bicknell-Royle J, Nation J, Humphrey M, Harvey AS. The ketogenic diet in refractory childhood epilepsy. *J Paedietr Child Health* 2005; 41:353–357.
82. Kossoff EH, Krauss GL, McGrogan JR, Freeman JM. Efficacy of the Atkins diet as therapy for intractable epilepsy. *Neurology* 2003; 61:1789–1791.
83. Pfieffer HH, Thiele EA. Low-glycemic-index treatment: a liberalized ketogenic diet for treatment of intractable epilepsy. *Neurology* 2005; 65:1810–1812.
84. Bergqvist AV, Schall JI, Gallagher PR, Cnaan A, Stallings VA. Fasting versus gradual initiation of the ketogenic diet: a prospective, randomized clinical trial of efficacy. *Epilepsia* 2005; 46:1810–1819.

85. Papandreou D, Pavlou E, Kalimeri E, Mavromichalis I. The ketogenic diet in children with epilepsy. *Br J Nutr* 2006; 95:5–13.
86. Freeman JM, Kossoff EH, Hartman AL. The ketogenic diet: one decade later. *Pediatrics* 2007; 119:535–543.
87. Cunnane SC, Musa K, Ryan MA, Whiting S, Fraser DD. Potential role of polyunsaturates in seizure protection achieved with the ketogenic diet. *Prostaglandins Leukot Essent Fatty Acids* 2002; 67:131–135.
88. Wilson J. Migraine and epilepsy. *Develop Med Child Neurol* 1992; 34:645–647.
89. Dunn DW, Snyder CH. Benign paroxysmal vertigo of childhood. *Am J Dis Child* 1976; 130:1099–1100.
90. Duke WW. Meniere's syndrome caused by allergy. *J Am Med Assoc* 1923; 81:2179–2181.
91. Derebery MJ. Allergic management of Meniere's disease: an outcome study. *Otolaryngol Head Neck Surg* 2000; 122:174–182.
92. Cooke RA. Allergic neuropathies. In: Cooke RA (ed.), *Allergy in Theory and Practice*. Philadelphia, PA: WB Saunders Co, 1947; pp. 325–336.
93. Staffieri D, Bentolila L, Levit L. Hemiplegia and allergic symptoms following ingestion of certain foods. *Ann Allergy* 1952; 10:38–39.
94. Dibs SD, Baker MD. Anaphylaxis in children: a 5-year experience. *Pediatrics* 1997; 99(1):E7.
95. Wills AJ, Unsworth DJ. The neurology of gluten sensitivity: separating the wheat from the chaff. *Curr Opin Neurol* 2002; 15:519–523.
96. Reunala T, Collin P. Diseases associated with dermatitis herpetiformis. *Br J Dermatol* 1997; 136:315–318.
97. Wills AJ, Turner B, Lock RJ, et al. Dermatitis herpetiformis and neurological dysfunction. *J Neurol Neurosurg Psychiatry* 2002; 72:259–261.
98. Cicarelli G, Della Rocca G, Amboni M, et al. Clinical and neurological abnormalities in adult celiac disease. *Neurol Sci* 2003; 24:311–317.
99. Gobbi G, Bouquet F, Greco L, et al. Coeliac disease, epilepsy, and cerebral calcification. *Lancet* 1992; 340:439–443.
100. Pfaender M, D'Souza WJ, Trost N, Litewka L, Paine M, Cook M. Visual disturbances representing occipital lobe epilepsy in patients with cerebral calcifications and coeliac disease: a case series. *J Neurol Neurosurg Psychiatry* 2004; 75:1623–1625.
101. Jacob S, Zarei M, Kenton A, Allrogen H. Gluten sensitivity and neuromyelitis optica: two case reports. *J Neurol Neurosurg Psychiatry* 2005; 76:1028–1030.

43 Experimental Approaches to the Study of Food Allergy

M. Cecilia Berin & Madhan Masilamani
Pediatric Allergy and Immunology, Icahn School of Medicine at Mount Sinai, New York, USA

Key Concepts

- Animal models of IgE-mediated anaphylaxis in response to oral challenge with common food allergens have been developed in rodents, pigs, and dogs.
- Adjuvant-free models of allergic sensitization to foods are emerging.
- Reductionist systems can be used to perform mechanistic studies with human cells and tissues.

Animal models of IgE-mediated food allergy

Our understanding of the mechanisms of sensitization and tolerance to food allergens is limited by our ability to rigorously test the contribution of these mechanisms in human subjects. For this purpose, animal models are needed that appropriately mimic the human response to food allergens. In such a model, exposure of a susceptible animal to a relevant food allergen would lead to sensitization, such that subsequent oral exposure to that allergen would lead to the generation of acute symptoms that reflect the human response to food allergens. Those symptoms could involve the skin, respiratory tract, gastrointestinal tract, or lead to systemic anaphylaxis. The factors that determine host susceptibility to allergic sensitization to foods in humans are not clearly understood. The role of animal models is to elucidate pathways that may contribute to susceptibility in humans. Experimental animal models and clinical or translational studies using human specimens should ideally be used together in order to make progress in understanding mechanisms of food allergic disease and to develop new therapeutic approaches. A summary of mouse models of IgE-mediated food allergy are presented in Table 43.1.

Oral sensitization to food allergens

In mice, as in humans, the normal response to antigens delivered by the oral route is that of immune tolerance. In mice this is an active immune response mediated by regulatory T cells [1]. Although it has been reported that mice can develop allergic sensitization to peanut through a single high-dose exposure by the gastric route [2], most models require the use of an experimental adjuvant to break oral tolerance. The most widely used adjuvant for oral sensitization is cholera toxin, which was described to induce IgE and prime for systemic anaphylaxis by Snider and colleagues [3]. Gastric administration together with cholera toxin has been used to sensitize mice to peanut, egg, milk, soy, shrimp tropomyosin, and a number of other foods or purified food allergens [4–7]. This is associated with the development of an allergen-specific antibody response of multiple isotypes, including IgE. Although strain differences have been reported in oral sensitization using cholera toxin, most common strains of mice can be sensitized to generate an allergen-specific IgE response. Where strain differences become important is in the susceptibility to systemic anaphylaxis upon oral challenge. Anaphylaxis upon oral challenge is consistently observed only in the C3H strain of mouse. Both C3H/HeJ mice carrying a mutation in TLR4 and C3H/HeOuJ mice carrying a normal TLR4 are susceptible [8], indicating that TLR4 is not the primary factor in this susceptibility. Although Balb/c mice do not exhibit signs of systemic anaphylaxis in response to oral challenge, mediators such as histamine released locally (measured in fecal extracts) or mucosal mast cell protease released into the circulation indicate that there is a local hypersensitivity response to allergen challenge

Food Allergy: Adverse Reactions to Foods and Food Additives, Fifth Edition. Edited by Dean D Metcalfe, Hugh A Sampson, Ronald A Simon and Gideon Lack.

Table 43.1 Mouse models of IgE-mediated food allergy.

Route of sensitization	Adjuvant	Strain	Antigen(s)	Route of challenge	Outcome
Oral	Cholera toxin	C3H	Peanut[a], β-lactoglobulin, α-lactalbumin, ovalbumin, ovomucoid	Oral	Systemic anaphylaxis
Oral	Cholera toxin	C3H	Peanut, casein, heated milk, or egg allergens	IP, IV	Systemic anaphylaxis
Oral	Cholera toxin	C3H, Balb/c, C57BL/6	Peanut, ovalbumin	IP	Systemic anaphylaxis
Oral	SEB	C3H, Balb/c	Peanut, ovalbumin	Oral	Systemic anaphylaxis
Oral	Cholera toxin	Balb/c	Peanut, ovalbumin	Oral	Local (MMCP-1 release, fecal histamine)
Cutaneous	none	Balb/c	Hazelnut, cashew, whey, ovalbumin	Oral	Systemic anaphylaxis
Cutaneous	Cholera toxin	C3H/HeJ	α-lactalbumin, casein	Oral (ALA), IP (casein)	Systemic anaphylaxis
IP	Alum	Balb/c	Ovalbumin, peanut	Oral (repeated)	Diarrhea, inflammation

SEB, staphylococcal enterotoxin B; IP, intraperitoneal; IV, intravenous.
[a]Mixed reports on the efficacy of peanut to induce systemic anaphylaxis by the oral route.

[9, 10]. Although common strains of mice including Balb/c and C57BL/6 are resistant to systemic symptoms of anaphylaxis upon oral challenge, they will undergo anaphylaxis when systemically challenged by the intraperitoneal or intravenous route [11, 12].

In addition to strain dependence of induction of anaphylaxis by the oral route, the nature of the allergen plays a critical role in determining the outcome of challenge. Not all antigens can elicit anaphylaxis by the oral route, despite their capacity to sensitize and generate an IgE response. This has been shown for the individual milk proteins. The whey proteins α-lactalbumin and β-lactoglobulin will induce systemic anaphylaxis in sensitized C3H/HeJ mice after oral challenge, whereas casein requires systemic challenge to induce anaphylaxis [13]. All three milk allergens generate a robust allergen-specific IgE response, but it is the trafficking of antigen across the intestinal epithelium that determines this ability to trigger reactions by the oral route. Casein is taken up by M cells overlying Peyer's patch, but is not readily absorbed across villus enterocytes. Heating of antigens including β-lactoglobulin, α-lactalbumin, ovalbumin, and ovomucoid renders them unable to induce anaphylaxis by the oral route. Their retained capacity to trigger reactions by the systemic route indicates that this is not due to destruction of epitopes, but was shown to be due to altering the uptake across the intestinal epithelium [13, 14].

Symptoms elicited after oral or systemic allergen challenge of mice orally sensitized using cholera toxin adjuvant affect the skin (edema around the eyes and snout), the respiratory tract (wheezing, labored respiration), the gastrointestinal tract (diarrhea in severe cases), and the systemic circulation (shock that can be measured by drop in body temperature and increase in hematocrit). These symptoms are mediated primarily by IgE and mast cells [11, 15], although a minor role for IgG antibodies and macrophages has also been demonstrated in systemically challenged mice [9, 15]. Platelet activating factor and histamine are the major factors that drive anaphylaxis in mice [16].

A second adjuvant that has been used to break oral tolerance in mice and lead to allergic sensitization is staphylococcal enterotoxin B (SEB), a toxin derived from *Staphylococcus aureus*. As with cholera toxin, repeated gastric administration of SEB together with ovalbumin or peanut leads to allergen-specific IgE antibodies and anaphylaxis affecting multiple organ systems upon oral rechallenge with allergen alone [17].

The mechanism by which cholera toxin or SEB break tolerance and promote allergic sensitization centers on gastrointestinal dendritic cells (DCs). Cholera toxin induces a change in the phenotype of the normally tolerogenic $CD103^+$ DC that migrates to the mesenteric lymph node (MLN) and drives a Th2-dominated immune response [18]. This induction of Th2 responses is mediated in part by upregulation of OX40L on DCs. SEB has been shown to induce the upregulation of TIM-4 on DCs that also drives a Th2 cytokine response from naïve T cells [19].

It is not clear what factors might be driving this process of sensitization in human disease. Cholera toxin is an experimental tool that is useful for probing immune pathways that can lead to allergic sensitization, but is unlikely to play a role in human allergic disease. Exposure to SEB is more likely to occur in humans, although there is no evidence for an association between exposure to SEB and development of food allergy. However, there may be microbial or environmental factors that drive this sensitization pathway and contribute to the development of food allergy in human disease. One factor that has been shown to play a role in both murine models and in human subjects is treatment with antacids that promote the development of allergic sensitization to food allergens [20, 21].

The mechanism of this enhanced sensitization was shown to be in part due to alum ingredients of oral antacids that can provide adjuvant activity [22].

Alternative routes of sensitization to food allergens

The default response of the gastrointestinal tract to antigens is one of tolerance. Allergic sensitization could be a result of a breach of this tolerance, or potentially by exposure to food allergens through a route that is not inherently tolerogenic. The impact of route of exposure to the milk allergen α-lactalbumin was studied in mice, with the finding that allergic sensitization predisposing to anaphylaxis upon oral rechallenge could be induced by exposure through the skin, the respiratory tract, and the sublingual route [23]. However, this was dependent on the presence of adjuvant, indicating that like the gastric route, none of these alternative routes were found to be inherently sensitizing. Contrary to these findings, adjuvant-free sensitization to food allergens has been described for hazelnut, cashew, and whey milk proteins [24–26] using exposure through the skin. This model requires prolonged exposure of the skin to allergen through occlusive dressings. Allergic sensitization through the skin has also been described after minor damage to the skin (induced by tape-stripping), activating immune pathways that drive a Th2-polarizing T cell response [27, 28]. It was reported that the rate of use of peanut oil-containing creams was elevated in children with peanut allergy [29], leading to the hypothesis that skin exposure to food allergens may be clinically relevant. Mutations in the filaggrin gene that encodes for a protein contributing to skin barrier function are associated with elevated risk for peanut allergy in humans [30], which supports the concept that exposure to foods through the skin may be highly relevant to human disease. Mice deficient in the filaggrin gene are also more susceptible than controls to allergic sensitization through the skin [31].

Modeling gastrointestinal manifestations of food allergy

In addition to models of systemic anaphylaxis, mouse models have been developed to study gastrointestinal manifestations of food allergy. Most of the studies utilizing this model have used the model antigen ovalbumin [32, 33], but peanut has also been used to drive gastrointestinal symptoms [34]. Mice are primed by systemic immunization with antigen plus alum, followed by repeated high-dose oral challenges with antigen given 2–3 days apart. After a minimum of three oral challenges, mice develop an acute severe diarrhea response that is mediated by IgE and mast cells, through the release of serotonin and platelet activating factor [33]. Symptoms are associated with a Th2-biased inflammation of the small intestine, and the cytokines IL-4 and IL-13 produced by T cells and mast cells are required for generation of symptoms although do not directly participate in the acute diarrhea response to allergen [34, 35]. Intestinal epithelial cells regulate these gastrointestinal manifestations of food allergy through the release of chemokines and cytokines that orchestrate the T cell response to allergens in the gastrointestinal tract [12, 36].

Large animal models of food allergy

Nonrodent models of food allergy have been developed that feature symptoms that may be more closely related to human food-allergic reactions than rodent models. Although these large animal models are unlikely to be used widely for mechanistic studies, they offer a unique opportunity to test potential therapeutics in a nonrodent model prior to human trials. Dogs, like humans, develop spontaneous allergic disease, most commonly atopic dermatitis. It was found that 32.7% of dogs with allergic skin disease seen at a veterinary dermatology practice had food hypersensitivity, indicating a similar association of atopic dermatitis and food hypersensitivity in dogs as has been described in humans [37]. A colony of spontaneous food-allergic dogs (maltese/beagle cross) has been described [38, 39]. These dogs have hypersensitivity to soy and corn, manifesting as pruritic skin disease, otitis, and colitis that resolves in response to a restricted diet and recurs upon food challenge.

Experimental food allergy in dogs has also been described. Dogs in an atopic spaniel/basenji dog colony have been shown to develop allergy to peanut, tree nuts, soy, wheat, barley, and milk when immunized with allergen extracts in alum at birth [40, 41]. The sensitized dogs were described as undergoing severe gastrointestinal and systemic symptoms after allergen challenge, and were treated with epinephrine, diphenhydramine, and intravenous fluids postchallenge. This dog model was used to show that immunotherapy of allergic dogs with peanut plus heat-killed *Listeria monocytogenes* in incomplete Freund's adjuvant could improve symptom scores in peanut-allergic dogs [40].

Experimental approaches using human specimens

Animal models of food allergy have contributed substantially to our understanding of disease pathology. However, translation of this knowledge gained from animal models into useful human applications requires experimentation in human systems. Laboratory research on human food allergy is restricted to the availability of limited amounts of human specimen. Relatively noninvasive patient samples that are available for study are saliva [42], serum, peripheral blood, stool [43], and breast milk [44]. Various tools and experimental technologies are available for researchers to study food allergy with human samples.

Assessment of B cell responses

Allergen-specific IgE and IgG4

Clinical reactivity to food allergens is driven by serum antibodies, as demonstrated by classic passive sensitization experiments performed by Prausnitz and Küstner showing that a wheal and flare reaction to ingested fish could be induced in a nonallergic individual by local injection of serum from an allergic donor [45]. B cell responses to food allergen can be investigated *in vitro* by quantifying allergen-specific antibodies in serum. Although the presence of IgE does not necessarily indicate clinical reactivity or severity of reactions, the level of allergen-specific IgE is predictive of the likelihood of developing clinical symptoms upon ingestion. For example, in peanut allergy, more than 95% of subjects with specific IgE of >14 kUA/L against peanut (using the ImmunoCAP™ assay from Phadia/Thermo Fisher Scientific) will react to oral food challenge with peanut [46, 47]. Based on this *in vitro* assay and established predictive curves, individuals can be categorized as "likely" allergic to milk, egg, and peanut. In addition to IgE, plasma allergen-specific IgG4 levels can also influence the allergic responses, presumably by functioning as blocking antibodies. It has been shown that children with positive oral food challenge to egg have an elevated IgE/IgG4 ratio toward egg proteins [48]. A rise in serum allergen-specific IgG4 is associated with the development of clinical tolerance during immunotherapy to foods [49]. However, IgG4 values alone are not a good predictor of clinical reactivity. Allergen-specific IgA levels in saliva have also been shown to be associated with the development of clinical tolerance [42], and therefore obtaining a quantitative measure of multiple allergen-specific isotypes in serum or saliva may provide a more complete picture of the immune response to any given food allergen. The ratio of allergen-specific to total IgE may also influence clinical reactivity. ImmunoCAP technologies can be used to detect total and allergen-specific IgE, IgG4, and IgA in serum.

Additional information about the nature of the IgE response to food allergens can be obtained by component-resolved diagnostics or molecular allergy diagnosis [50]. This refers to the measurement of IgE antibodies to individual allergens, either as panels of selected antigens run as ImmunoCAP assays, or microarrays with greater than 100 components per chip. The latter technology is referred to as immuno solid phase allergen chip (ISAC, from Thermo Scientific). This technology involves the detection of IgE or IgG4 against multiple allergens in a chip using a very small volume of serum (approximately 30–50 μL). In addition to measuring antibody binding to the most clinically relevant allergen within a food, profiling of reactivity to large numbers of allergens offers the opportunity to examine patterns of antibody binding to protein families. These assays are potentially useful for discriminating between true primary sensitization to foods and cross-reactivity due to sensitization to related antigens.

Peptide microarray for epitope detection

In addition to measuring IgE levels to various allergens, determination of specific antigenic determinants in a particular allergen is also informative in designing therapies. Recognition of epitopes may be more informative than IgE levels against the whole allergen. Patients with persistent food allergy have been shown to recognize more allergen epitopes than those with transient food allergy [51, 52]. Peptide microarrays have been developed for large-scale epitope mapping with the aim of understanding the molecular basis of the clinical reactivity [53]. Immunodominant and allergenic B cell epitopes of milk, peanut, and several other food allergens have been described using this technology [53–55]. The technique utilizes overlapping 15–20mer peptides covering the full length of an allergen printed on a glass slide. Printed slides are incubated with patient serum and subsequently labeled with biotinylated antihuman IgE detection antibodies and fluorescently labeled dendrimers to amplify the signal. One added advantage to this technique is the ability to detect multiple antibody isotypes concurrently, allowing for tracking epitope-specific IgE together with regulatory isotypes such as IgG4 and IgA. This may be particularly relevant for monitoring the immune response to immunotherapy. A disadvantage of peptide microarray is that it does not detect conformational epitopes that may also contribute to clinical reactivity.

Functional tests of allergen-specific IgE

Factors affecting the function of IgE that are not routinely reflected in solid phase binding assays include affinity and specific activity (ratio of specific to total IgE). Modification of microarray assays to include a competition step to remove low-affinity binding IgE antibodies has shown that patients that had outgrown their milk allergy or those that were tolerant to heated forms of milk had lower affinity IgE antibodies [56]. Therefore factors that take into account affinity and competition with other IgE antibodies may be more useful assays of allergic sensitization to foods. The functionality of allergen-specific IgE can be tested indirectly by mediator release assay using RBL-2H3 cells [48]. Humanized RBL-2H3 cells stably transfected with the α, β, and γ chains of the human FcεRI receptor are passively sensitized by incubating with patients' serum. Stimulation of the cells with a range of dilutions of the allergen leads to degranulation that can be measured by the release of β-hexosaminidase. Alternatively, human peripheral blood mononuclear cells (PBMCs) can be passively sensitized with the serum of sensitized individuals after stripping of surface IgE from basophils with lactic acid, and subsequent basophil activation measured as outlined below [14].

Flow cytometry allows for simultaneously detecting multiple immune parameters from a limited volume of blood. The basophil activation test has been shown to be a useful assay for predicting clinical reactivity and in immunotherapy trials appear to correlate with loss of clinical reactivity [57, 58]. This technique is based on the detection of CD63, a marker for secretory granules that move to the surface of basophils during degranulation. As little as 500 μL of blood per test condition is sufficient for this assay. Whole blood is incubated with specific allergen, followed by fixing, staining, and acquisition by flow cytometry.

A multicolor gating strategy is required to identify the basophils. Basophils are characterized as CD123$^+$ CD203$^+$ HLA-DR^{lo} lineage (CD3, CD14, CD19, and CD41a)^{neg} and FcεRI/surface IgE$^+$. CD123 is a receptor for IL-3, which is necessary for the survival of basophils. CD203 is a basophil-specific ectoenzyme that is a marker for basophil activation. However, there are reports that CD203c is expressed on mast cells, activated B cells, and plasma cells and also in some myeloid derived cells. There are commercially available basophil activation kits using as few as two antibodies (for diagnostic purposes), but it is preferred to use a full panel of antibodies to unambiguously identify basophils.

Assessment of allergen-specific T cell responses

T cell responses to allergen can be phenotyped using multicolor flow cytometry by assessing the expression of various surface markers, intracellular cytokine expression, and proliferation (by expression of Ki-67 or carboxyfluorescein succinimidyl ester [CFSE]-dilution). Prior to the widespread availability of multicolor flow cytometry, phenotyping of food allergen-specific T cell responses was dependent on growing T cell lines from peripheral blood, which could introduce artifact into the system. Using CFSE to detect proliferating cells, it was found that the phenotype rather than the presence of allergen-specific T cells was associated with clinical reactivity. There was an increased expression of Th2 cytokines in allergic individuals compared to healthy controls or those that had outgrown their allergy [59]. This approach was also used to demonstrate that regulatory CD4$^+$ T cells expressing Foxp3 and CD25 were increased in children who were tolerant to extensively heated milk and who were believed to be on their way to complete milk tolerance [60].

Even relatively short-term cultures of 5 to 7 days have been criticized as potentially introducing artifact into the system, and therefore alternative approaches to identify allergen-specific T cells have been utilized. Short-term (6–16 hours) culture is sufficient to observe upregulation of CD154 (CD40 ligand) by allergen-specific T cells, and this approach has been used to demonstrate that the phenotype of allergen-specific Th2 cells differs depending on the clinical manifestation of food allergy [61]. Permeabilization and detection of intracellular CD154 is commonly used for this assay [62, 63]. The use of allergen-specific class II tetramers allows for bypassing *in vitro* culture, but requires relatively large volumes of blood because of the low precursor frequency in untouched PBMCs. This also requires knowledge of T cell epitopes across different HLA alleles. Ara h 1-specific tetramers have been used to identify Ara h 1-specific T cells in peanut-allergic individuals, with a frequency of approximately 9 per million CD4$^+$ T cells [64]. This low precursor frequency highlights the importance of being able to accurately identify allergen-specific T cells within the large pool of T cells specific for other antigens.

Identification of T cell epitopes of allergens is generating a lot of interest, not only for designing allergen-specific tetramers, but also for therapeutic purposes. T cell epitopes are smaller than B cell epitopes and mostly lack the ability to cross-link IgE receptors on mast cells and basophils. Once the T cell epitopes of the allergen are known, it is possible to design immunotherapy or a T cell vaccine to specifically skew or suppress the T cell response toward that epitope and thereby influence the humoral immune response without the risk of activating allergic effector cells. Various algorithms have been developed to predict MHC binding of T cell epitopes known as *in silico* analyses [65, 66]. T cell epitope mapping has been performed by culturing PBMCs from allergic individuals with overlapping short peptides from peanut allergens and assessment by proliferation assays, cytokine detection, or tetramer-guided epitope mapping (TGEM) approach [64, 67]. Because MHC class II molecules exhibit very high polymorphisms, each peptide may have different binding avidities for different alleles. Humans have three MHC class II molecules (HLA-DR, DP, and DQ, each with their own polymorphic alleles) providing a significant diversity of peptide binding. Therefore, any results obtained from a specific T cell line or a clone that is restricted to a particular allele of HLA is true only for that MHC/T cell combination. Therefore polymorphisms in HLA haplotypes necessitates that the T cell epitope repertoire must be generated from a diverse sample of patients containing MHC class II types relevant to the population of interest.

Reductionist approaches to studying the human gastrointestinal tract

One of the benefits of using mouse models of experimental food allergy is access to the gastrointestinal tract to examine the contribution of mucosal handling of food allergens to clinical reactivity [13, 14]. Some components of the gastrointestinal mucosa, such as the epithelial barrier or gastric and duodenal digestion, can be modeled using *in vitro* model systems with human cells.

Resistance to degradation by gastrointestinal enzymes is a common feature of food allergens, as antigens must reach the mucosal immune system in a form that can be presented by antigen presenting cells during the sensitization phase, or can cross-link IgE on mast cells or basophils in the effector phase. Most studies on susceptibility to digestion use static *in vitro* digestion assays with proteolytic enzymes at a pH modeling gastric and then duodenal digestion [68]. These assays will provide information about the relative digestibility of simple proteins, but do not take into account the complexity of the processing of food that occurs in the mouth, stomach, and intestine. Factors including lipids from the food itself or from gastrointestinal secretions can significantly alter the susceptibility of foods to digestion. Dynamic digestion models also incorporate factors such as mixing, diffusion of acid and enzymes, shear stress, viscosity, and removal of digestion products [69]. The immunogenicity of the digestion products can be sampled over time and tested with SDS-PAGE and antibodies from sensitized individuals.

The interaction of food allergens with intestinal epithelial cells can be modeled using human intestinal epithelial cell lines that can be grown as polarized monolayers. These include T84, Caco-2, some HT-29 subclones, and HCA-7 cells. Caco-2 cells are the most commonly used. When grown on porous transwells, they will form a monolayer with tight junctions that prevent the passive transport of macromolecules. Protein antigens are transported across these monolayers by a transcellular transport mechanism, initiated by fluid phase endocytosis at the apical membrane. The basolateral media can be sampled over time and tested for the presence of antigens capable of triggering allergic effector cells, for example, passively sensitized basophils from human PBMC [14, 70]. These approaches are useful for understanding how antigen processing can influence uptake of immunoreactive antigens from the intestinal lumen.

Humanized mouse models

Humanized mouse models have been developed that bring together the individual advantages of studying mouse models and human specimens. Extensively immunodeficient mice (NOD/SCID/γ-chain deficient mice) can be reconstituted with PBMCs from human donors. Although graft-versus-host disease (GVHD) develops in these mice by approximately 4 weeks after engraftment, they can be utilized before this time to study *in vivo* responses of human immune cells to antigen. Mice engrafted with PBMCs from patients with sensitization to birch or grass pollen, or hazelnut, develop allergen-specific human IgE when cells are coadministered with the allergen [71]. Rectal or oral allergen challenge of the recipient mice results in localized changes in the colonic mucosa that are visible by endoscopy, and these changes are mediated by IgE and human basophils. Although the use of this model has been limited to date, this is a promising approach for the study of human cells in an *in vivo* setting. Caveats include the onset of GVHD, and the fact that mouse target tissues may not be responsive to all factors (i.e., some cytokines) produced by human cells. The use of hematopoietic stem cells rather than PBMCs for engraftment avoids the GVHD, but loses the mature allergen-specific T cell phenotype of the patient.

Conclusions

In our quest to understand individual susceptibility to the development of food allergy and to understand the basis of food allergenicity, we have a number of experimental tools at our disposal. Mouse models are by nature artificial, and no model of spontaneous food allergy has been described to date although adjuvant-free systems utilizing skin sensitization have been described. However, *in vivo* models provide the opportunity to do mechanistic studies that are not possible using specimens from human subjects. Ideally, animal models should be used together with patient specimens and *in vitro* human model systems where possible to validate the results. Although the use of immunodeficient mice reconstituted with human leukocytes is an approach still in its infancy, it may become a powerful tool to study human cells in a physiological context.

References

1. Hadis U, Wahl B, Schulz O, et al. Intestinal tolerance requires gut homing and expansion of FoxP3+ regulatory T cells in the lamina propria. *Immunity* 2011; 34(2):237–246.
2. Proust B, Astier C, Jacquenet S, et al. A single oral sensitization to peanut without adjuvant leads to anaphylaxis in mice. *Int Arch Allergy Immunol* 2008; 146(3):212–218.
3. Snider DP, Marshall JS, Perdue MH, Liang H. Production of IgE antibody and allergic sensitization of intestinal and peripheral tissues after oral immunization with protein Ag and cholera toxin. *J Immunol* 1994; 153(2):647–657.
4. Li XM, Serebrisky D, Lee SY, et al. A murine model of peanut anaphylaxis: T- and B-cell responses to a major peanut allergen mimic human responses. *J Allergy Clin Immunol* 2000; 106(1 Pt. 1):150–158.
5. Li XM, Schofield BH, Huang CK, Kleiner GI, Sampson HA. A murine model of IgE-mediated cow's milk hypersensitivity. *J Allergy Clin Immunol* 1999; 103(2 Pt. 1):206–214.
6. Gizzarelli F, Corinti S, Barletta B, et al. Evaluation of allergenicity of genetically modified soybean protein extract in a

murine model of oral allergen-specific sensitization. *Clin Exp Allergy* 2006; 36(2):238–248.

7. Reese G, Viebranz J, Leong-Kee SM, et al. Reduced allergenic potency of VR9–1, a mutant of the major shrimp allergen Pen a 1 (tropomyosin). *J Immunol* 2005; 175(12):8354–8364.
8. Berin MC, Zheng Y, Domaradzki M, Li XM, Sampson HA. Role of TLR4 in allergic sensitization to food proteins in mice. *Allergy* 2006; 61(1):64–71.
9. Smit JJ, Willemsen K, Hassing I, et al. Contribution of classic and alternative effector pathways in peanut-induced anaphylactic responses. *PLoS One* 2011; 6(12):e28917.
10. Adel-Patient K, Bernard H, Ah-Leung S, Creminon C, Wal JM. Peanut- and cow's milk-specific IgE, Th2 cells and local anaphylactic reaction are induced in Balb/c mice orally sensitized with cholera toxin. *Allergy* 2005; 60(5):658–664.
11. Sun J, Arias K, Alvarez D, et al. Impact of CD40 ligand, B cells, and mast cells in peanut-induced anaphylactic responses. *J Immunol* 2007; 179(10):6696–6703.
12. Blazquez AB, Mayer L, Berin MC. Thymic stromal lymphopoietin is required for gastrointestinal allergy but not oral tolerance. *Gastroenterology* 2010; 139(4):1301–1309.
13. Roth-Walter F, Berin MC, Arnaboldi P, et al. Pasteurization of milk proteins promotes allergic sensitization by enhancing uptake through Peyer's patches. *Allergy* 2008; 63(7):882–890.
14. Martos G, Lopez-Exposito I, Bencharitiwong R, Berin MC, Nowak-Wegrzyn A. Mechanisms underlying differential food allergy response to heated egg. *J Allergy Clin Immunol* 2011; 127(4):990–997.e2.
15. Arias K, Chu DK, Flader K, et al. Distinct immune effector pathways contribute to the full expression of peanut-induced anaphylactic reactions in mice. *J Allergy Clin Immunol* 2011; 127(6):1552–1561.e1.
16. Arias K, Baig M, Colangelo M, et al. Concurrent blockade of platelet-activating factor and histamine prevents life-threatening peanut-induced anaphylactic reactions. *J Allergy Clin Immunol* 2009; 124(2):307–314.
17. Ganeshan K, Neilsen CV, Hadsaitong A, Schleimer RP, Luo X, Bryce PJ. Impairing oral tolerance promotes allergy and anaphylaxis: a new murine food allergy model. *J Allergy Clin Immunol* 2009; 123(1):231–238.e4.
18. Blazquez AB, Berin MC. Gastrointestinal dendritic cells promote Th2 skewing via OX40L. *J Immunol* 2008; 180(7):4441–4450.
19. Yang PC, Xing Z, Berin CM, et al. TIM-4 expressed by mucosal dendritic cells plays a critical role in food antigen-specific Th2 differentiation and intestinal allergy. *Gastroenterology* 2007; 133(5):1522–1533.
20. Untersmayr E, Scholl I, Swoboda I, et al. Antacid medication inhibits digestion of dietary proteins and causes food allergy: a fish allergy model in BALB/c mice. *J Allergy Clin Immunol* 2003; 112(3):616–623.
21. Scholl I, Untersmayr E, Bakos N, et al. Antiulcer drugs promote oral sensitization and hypersensitivity to hazelnut allergens in BALB/c mice and humans. *Am J Clin Nutr* 2005; 81(1):154–160.
22. Brunner R, Wallmann J, Szalai K, et al. The impact of aluminium in acid-suppressing drugs on the immune response of BALB/c mice. *Clin Exp Allergy* 2007; 37(10):1566–1573.
23. Dunkin D, Berin MC, Mayer L. Allergic sensitization can be induced via multiple physiologic routes in an adjuvant-dependent manner. *J Allergy Clin Immunol* 2011; 128(6):1251–1258.
24. Birmingham NP, Parvataneni S, Hassan HM, et al. An adjuvant-free mouse model of tree nut allergy using hazelnut as a model tree nut. *Int Arch Allergy Immunol* 2007; 144(3):203–210.
25. Gonipeta B, Parvataneni S, Tempelman RJ, Gangur V. An adjuvant-free mouse model to evaluate the allergenicity of milk whey protein. *J Dairy Sci* 2009; 92(10):4738–4744.
26. Parvataneni S, Gonipeta B, Tempelman RJ, Gangur V. Development of an adjuvant-free cashew nut allergy mouse model. *Int Arch Allergy Immunol* 2009; 149(4):299–304.
27. Oyoshi MK, Larson RP, Ziegler SF, Geha RS. Mechanical injury polarizes skin dendritic cells to elicit a T(H)2 response by inducing cutaneous thymic stromal lymphopoietin expression. *J Allergy Clin Immunol* 2010; 126(5):976–984. e1–e5.
28. Strid J, Sobolev O, Zafirova B, Polic B, Hayday A. The intraepithelial T cell response to NKG2D-ligands links lymphoid stress surveillance to atopy. *Science* 2011; 334(6060):1293–1297.
29. Lack G, Fox D, Northstone K, Golding J. Factors associated with the development of peanut allergy in childhood. *N Engl J Med* 2003; 348(11):977–985.
30. Brown SJ, Asai Y, Cordell HJ, et al. Loss-of-function variants in the filaggrin gene are a significant risk factor for peanut allergy. *J Allergy Clin Immunol* 2011; 127(3):661–667.
31. Oyoshi MK, Murphy GF, Geha RS. Filaggrin-deficient mice exhibit TH17-dominated skin inflammation and permissiveness to epicutaneous sensitization with protein antigen. *J Allergy Clin Immunol* 2009; 124(3):485–493.e1.
32. Kweon MN, Yamamoto M, Kajiki M, Takahashi I, Kiyono H. Systemically derived large intestinal CD4(+) Th2 cells play a central role in STAT6-mediated allergic diarrhea. *J Clin Invest* 2000; 106(2):199–206.
33. Brandt EB, Strait RT, Hershko D, et al. Mast cells are required for experimental oral allergen-induced diarrhea. *J Clin Invest* 2003; 112(11):1666–1677.
34. Wang M, Takeda K, Shiraishi Y, et al. Peanut-induced intestinal allergy is mediated through a mast cell-IgE-FcepsilonRI-IL-13 pathway. *J Allergy Clin Immunol* 2010; 126(2):306–316.e1–e12.
35. Brandt EB, Munitz A, Orekov T, et al. Targeting IL-4/IL-13 signaling to alleviate oral allergen-induced diarrhea. *J Allergy Clin Immunol* 2009; 123(1):53–58.
36. Blazquez AB, Knight AK, Getachew H, et al. A functional role for CCR6 on proallergic T cells in the gastrointestinal tract. *Gastroenterology* 2010; 138(1):275–284.e1–e4.
37. Chesney CJ. Food sensitivity in the dog: a quantitative study. *J Small Anim Pract* 2002; 43(5):203–207.

38. Jackson HA, Jackson MW, Coblentz L, Hammerberg B. Evaluation of the clinical and allergen specific serum immunoglobulin E responses to oral challenge with cornstarch, corn, soy and a soy hydrolysate diet in dogs with spontaneous food allergy. *Vet Dermatol* 2003; 14(4):181–187.
39. Jackson HA, Hammerberg B. Evaluation of a spontaneous canine model of immunoglobulin E-mediated food hypersensitivity: dynamic changes in serum and fecal allergen-specific immunoglobulin E values relative to dietary change. *Comp Med* 2002; 52(4):316–321.
40. Frick OL, Teuber SS, Buchanan BB, Morigasaki S, Umetsu DT. Allergen immunotherapy with heat-killed Listeria monocytogenes alleviates peanut and food-induced anaphylaxis in dogs. *Allergy* 2005; 60(2):243–250.
41. Teuber SS, Del Val G, Morigasaki S, et al. The atopic dog as a model of peanut and tree nut food allergy. *J Allergy Clin Immunol* 2002; 110(6):921–927.
42. Kulis M, Saba K, Kim EH, et al. Increased peanut-specific IgA levels in saliva correlate with food challenge outcomes after peanut sublingual immunotherapy. *J Allergy Clin Immunol* 2012; 129(4):1159–1162.
43. Li H, Nowak-Wegrzyn A, Charlop-Powers Z, et al. Transcytosis of IgE-antigen complexes by CD23a in human intestinal epithelial cells and its role in food allergy. *Gastroenterology* 2006; 131(1):47–58.
44. Jarvinen KM, Suomalainen H. Leucocytes in human milk and lymphocyte subsets in cow's milk-allergic infants. *Pediatr Allergy Immunol* 2002; 13(4):243–254.
45. Cohen SG, Zelaya-Quesada M. Prausnitz and Kustner phenomenon: the P–K reaction. *J Allergy Clin Immunol* 2004; 114(3):705–710.
46. Caubet JC, Sampson HA. Beyond skin testing: state of the art and new horizons in food allergy diagnostic testing. *Immunol Allergy Clin North Am* 2012; 32(1):97–109.
47. Sampson HA. Utility of food-specific IgE concentrations in predicting symptomatic food allergy. *J Allergy Clin Immunol* 2001; 107(5):891–896.
48. Caubet JC, Bencharitiwong R, Moshier E, Godbold JH, Sampson HA, Nowak-Wegrzyn A. Significance of ovomucoid- and ovalbumin-specific IgE/IgG(4) ratios in egg allergy. *J Allergy Clin Immunol* 2012; 129(3):739–747.
49. Jones SM, Pons L, Roberts JL, et al. Clinical efficacy and immune regulation with peanut oral immunotherapy. *J Allergy Clin Immunol* 2009 ; 124(2):292–300.e1–e97.
50. Shreffler WG. Microarrayed recombinant allergens for diagnostic testing. *J Allergy Clin Immunol* 2011; 127(4):843–849; quiz 850–851.
51. Jarvinen KM, Beyer K, Vila L, Chatchatee P, Busse PJ, Sampson HA. B-cell epitopes as a screening instrument for persistent cow's milk allergy. *J Allergy Clin Immunol* 2002; 110(2):293–297.
52. Jarvinen KM, Beyer K, Vila L, Bardina L, Mishoe M, Sampson HA. Specificity of IgE antibodies to sequential epitopes of hen's egg ovomucoid as a marker for persistence of egg allergy. *Allergy* 2007; 62(7):758–765.
53. Lin J, Bardina L, Shreffler WG, et al. Development of a novel peptide microarray for large-scale epitope mapping of food allergens. *J Allergy Clin Immunol* 2009; 124(2):315–322.e1–e3.
54. Shreffler WG, Beyer K, Chu TH, Burks AW, Sampson HA. Microarray immunoassay: association of clinical history, in vitro IgE function, and heterogeneity of allergenic peanut epitopes. *J Allergy Clin Immunol* 2004; 113(4):776–782.
55. Vereda A, Andreae DA, Lin J, et al. Identification of IgE sequential epitopes of lentil (Len c 1) by means of peptide microarray immunoassay. *J Allergy Clin Immunol* 2010; 126(3):596–601.e1.
56. Wang J, Lin J, Bardina L, et al. Correlation of IgE/IgG4 milk epitopes and affinity of milk-specific IgE antibodies with different phenotypes of clinical milk allergy. *J Allergy Clin Immunol* 2010; 125(3):695–702.e1–e6.
57. Wanich N, Nowak-Wegrzyn A, Sampson HA, Shreffler WG. Allergen-specific basophil suppression associated with clinical tolerance in patients with milk allergy. *J Allergy Clin Immunol* 2009; 123(4):789–794.e20.
58. Patil SU, Shreffler WG. Immunology in the clinic review series; focus on allergies: basophils as biomarkers for assessing immune modulation. *Clin Exp Immunol* 2012 ; 167(1): 59–66.
59. Turcanu V, Maleki SJ, Lack G. Characterization of lymphocyte responses to peanuts in normal children, peanut-allergic children, and allergic children who acquired tolerance to peanuts. *J Clin Invest* 2003; 111(7):1065–1072.
60. Shreffler WG, Wanich N, Moloney M, Nowak-Wegrzyn A, Sampson HA. Association of allergen-specific regulatory T cells with the onset of clinical tolerance to milk protein. *J Allergy Clin Immunol* 2009; 123(1):43–52.e7.
61. Prussin C, Lee J, Foster B. Eosinophilic gastrointestinal disease and peanut allergy are alternatively associated with IL-5+ and IL-5(-) T(H)2 responses. *J Allergy Clin Immunol* 2009; 124(6):1326–1332.e6.
62. Van Hemelen D, Oude Elberink JN, Bohle B, Heimweg J, Nawijn MC, van Oosterhout AJ. Flow cytometric analysis of cytokine expression in short-term allergen-stimulated T cells mirrors the phenotype of proliferating T cells in long-term cultures. *J Immunol Methods* 2011; 371(1–2):114–121.
63. Campbell JD, Buchmann P, Kesting S, Cunningham CR, Coffman RL, Hessel EM. Allergen-specific T cell responses to immunotherapy monitored by CD154 and intracellular cytokine expression. *Clin Exp Allergy* 2010; 40(7):1025–1035.
64. DeLong JH, Simpson KH, Wambre E, James EA, Robinson D, Kwok WW. Ara h 1-reactive T cells in individuals with peanut allergy. *J Allergy Clin Immunol* 2011; 127(5):1211–1218.e3.
65. Nielsen M, Lund O, Buus S, Lundegaard C. MHC class II epitope predictive algorithms. *Immunology* 2010; 130(3):319–328.
66. Wang P, Sidney J, Kim Y, et al. Peptide binding predictions for HLA DR, DP and DQ molecules. *BMC Bioinformatics* 2010; 11:568.
67. Glaspole IN, de Leon MP, Rolland JM, O'Hehir RE. Characterization of the T-cell epitopes of a major peanut allergen, Ara h 2. *Allergy* 2005; 60(1):35–40.

68. Mandalari G, Adel-Patient K, Barkholt V, et al. In vitro digestibility of beta-casein and beta-lactoglobulin under simulated human gastric and duodenal conditions: a multi-laboratory evaluation. *Regul Toxicol Pharmacol* 2009; 55(3):372–381.
69. Wickham M, Faulks R, Mills C. In vitro digestion methods for assessing the effect of food structure on allergen breakdown. *Mol Nutr Food Res* 2009; 53(8):952–958.
70. Bernasconi E, Fritsche R, Corthesy B. Specific effects of denaturation, hydrolysis and exposure to Lactococcus lactis on bovine beta-lactoglobulin transepithelial transport, antigenicity and allergenicity. *Clin Exp Allergy* 2006; 36(6):803–814.
71. Weigmann B, Schughart N, Wiebe C, et al. Allergen-induced IgE-dependent gut inflammation in a human PBMC-engrafted murine model of allergy. *J Allergy Clin Immunol* 2012; 129(4):1126–1135.

44 Food Allergy: Psychological Considerations and Quality of Life

Ma. Lourdes B. de Asis[1] & Ronald A. Simon[2,3]

[1]Allergy and Asthma Consultants of Rockland and Bergen West Nyack, NY, USA
[2]Division of Allergy, Asthma and Immunology Scripps Clinic, San Diego, CA, USA
[3]Department of Molecular and Experimental Medicine Scripps Research Institute, La Jolla, CA, USA

Key Concepts

- Food allergic patients and their families are subject to increased anxiety, vigilance, and social limitation, which leads to diminished quality of life (QOL). A greater number of food allergies, history of an anaphylactic episode, and presence of comorbid allergic conditions such as asthma and atopic dermatitis are associated with poorer QOL.
- Diagnostic and therapeutic measures such as food challenges and epinephrine autoinjector prescriptions have been shown to improve QOL and decrease anxiety levels. Practitioners should also be alert to the presence of comorbid psychological disorders, such as maladaptive anxiety in patients and families and consider referral for psychologic/psychiatric evaluation.
- Many patients who attribute multiple physical and psychologic symptoms to food allergy/sensitivity without scientific basis after appropriate allergy evaluation may have an underlying psychiatric disorder. The most commonly reported disorders are anxiety, depression, somatoform disorder, and panic disorder.
- The key features differentiating the person with food aversion or food sensitivity from the person with a true food allergy are: (i) the absence or inconsistent finding of recognized signs and symptoms, physical findings, and laboratory evaluation supportive of an allergic, toxic, enzymatic, or pharmacological reaction to a specific food and (ii) the inability to reproduce symptoms or physical changes under adequately controlled double-blind food challenge conditions.
- Single-blinded placebo-controlled (SBPC) challenges may be performed to confirm neuropsychological complaints associated with food ingestion.
- There are four elements necessary to accomplish this type of challenge: (i) a single substance (food/additive/substance, etc.); (ii) that produces a consistent reaction (even totally subjective); (iii) with a known amount; and (iv) in a set time frame.
- Direct cause and effect relationship between food allergy, intestinal inflammation, and increased intestinal permeability in autism spectrum disorders (ASDs) have yet to be proven. Available research does not support the use of casein-free and/or gluten-free diets as a primary treatment for these patients. These unproven treatments contribute to poor nutrition, further social isolation, and divert efforts from more useful treatments.
- Patients with complaints of multiple food intolerance/sensitivities, as frequently seen in multiple chemical sensitivity (MCS)/idiopathic environmental intolerance (IEI) syndromes have frequently been shown to have underlying somatoform, depression, or panic disorders.

Introduction

Food is central to our physical and social development from our earliest memory as individuals and as a society. Since childhood, the sight, smell, and taste of food are inextricably linked to experiences that shape our personalities and how we relate to the world. It is therefore small wonder that food is involved in numerous psychological and somatic disorders with psychological overtones such as anorexia, bulimia, obesity, and many others [1]. Food-related behavior has not only been the means of expression of psychological disorder, but food itself has also been implicated in the causation and exacerbation of emotional and psychological problems. In food-allergic patients, the anxiety and limitations imposed by their condition have been recognized to have significant impact on quality of life (QOL). There has also been increased interest in the psychological response to the restrictions on diet and

Food Allergy: Adverse Reactions to Foods and Food Additives, Fifth Edition. Edited by Dean D Metcalfe, Hugh A Sampson, Ronald A Simon and Gideon Lack.

lifestyle required of patients and their families and how these effects can be mitigated.

This chapter addresses these issues and provides the practicing allergist with an approach to managing and counseling patients with documented food allergies as well as psychogenic food reactions. It also examines the current literature on the association between perceived food sensitivity and psychological disorders, such as autism, anxiety, and somatoform disorder. Increasing recognition of psychological and psychosocial factors in food allergy confirms Pearson's observation [2] that effective communication (and coordination) between patients, families, and the medical practitioner is a key component in management.

Psychological impact and quality of life

The most common abnormal psychological responses to physical illness include denial, anxiety, anger, depression, and dependency. These psychological states are a reaction to loss of health. The extent of psychopathology and impaired somatic functioning depends on the degree to which emotional issues related to the illness are resolved [3]. A recent review and meta-analysis examining the association between psychosocial factors and allergic disease reported a bidirectional association, with psychological distress and poor social support having a negative impact on the prognosis of allergic disease, and the presence of allergic disease having a negative effect on future mental health [4]. Surveys on the association of self-reported food and nonfood allergies and psychological disorders found a link with psychological disorders such as depression, anxiety, substance abuse, bipolar disorder, social phobia, and panic disorder/agoraphobia [5]. In asthma patients, anxiety and depression have been found to influence perception of and response to symptoms, reduce treatment adherence, increase hospitalization, and reduce QOL [6]. Food allergy carries with it the additional psychological burden of dietary restriction, vigilance, and continuous anxiety regarding the consequences of accidental exposure, which has been shown to affect the QOL of patients and their families.

The concept of health-related quality of life (HRQOL) developed in the 1980s, and has since grown to include aspects of overall QOL that influence physical, social, and psychological well-being. Numerous generic and disease-specific measures have been used to assess HRQOL in food-allergic patients and their families and these consistently show decreased QOL compared to healthy controls and even compared to patients with other allergic and nonallergic disease. Flokstra-de Blok et al. [7] measured the generic HRQOL of children, adolescents, and adults with food allergy compared to the general population and other similarly aged patients with asthma, irritable bowel syndrome (IBS), diabetes mellitus and rheumatoid arthritis (RA). They found that food-allergic adolescents and adults reported more pain, poorer overall health, more limitations in social activities, and less vitality than the general population. The HRQOL of food-allergic adults and adolescents was poorer compared to patients with diabetes, but was better when compared to patients with asthma, IBS, and RA. Ostblom and colleagues [8] found that children with food allergies had lower HRQOL scores for physical functioning and role/social limitations compared with allergic children without food allergies. In particular, children with lower airway symptoms related to food allergy had lower scores on self-esteem, parental impact-time, and family cohesion. Coexisting atopic disease such as asthma and atopic dermatitis was found to negatively impact HRQOL in food allergic children [9, 10]. Avery [11] compared the QOL scores of peanut-allergic children and children with insulin-dependent diabetes mellitus. They found that peanut-allergic children had poorer QOL and had more fear of adverse events, anxiety about eating, and felt more restricted regarding physical activities, but felt safer when they ate in familiar places or when carrying epinephrine kits.

Primeau et al. [12] performed one of the first studies examining the impact of peanut allergy on QOL and family relations in children and adults compared to patients of similar age group with a rheumatological disease. Peanut-allergic children, as reported by their parents, were found to have significantly more disruption in their daily activities and increased impairment of familial social interactions compared to the families of children with rheumatological disease. However, the families of peanut-allergic children scored better on mastery and coping mechanisms. The reverse was true of peanut-allergic adults who scored worse on mastery and coping mechanisms associated with their disease, but had less personal strain and familial disruption than adults with rheumatological disease. King et al. [13] reported that girls with peanut allergy had poorer physical HRQOL compared to their female siblings. They also found that mothers of peanut-allergic children reported poorer QOL compared to fathers and experienced more stress and anxiety. Bollinger and colleagues [14] studied the effects of food allergy on families and found that it had significant effect on meal preparation, family social activities, stress levels, and school attendance, with the number of allergic foods having a greater effect than the presence of comorbid conditions such as asthma and atopic dermatitis. A third of the study group reported significant impact on the child's school attendance and 10% home-schooled because of food allergy concerns. A recent large survey using the Food Allergy Quality of Life-Parental Burden (FAQL-PB) [15] demonstrated that social limitation resulting from their child's food allergy was a major cause for concern for parents. Parents who were more knowledgeable about food allergy; whose children had multiple food allergies or were allergic to egg, milk, or wheat; or who had an emergency department visit in the past year due to food allergy had poorer QOL. Despite their concern, parents of food-allergic children were found to underestimate their child's HRQOL impairment in the presence of nearly identical perceptions of disease severity [16], which calls attention for the need to include both the child's and the parents' perceptions in assessing impact on HRQOL.

Adolescents and young adults are particularly vulnerable and are a group known to be at high risk for fatal food-allergic reactions. Their risk-taking behaviors and coping mechanisms were examined by Sampson et al. [17], who found that a significant number of food-allergic teens and young adults engage in risk-taking behaviors such as ingesting potentially unsafe food and failure to "always" carry epinephrine. Participants in this study thought that educating other students about food allergy, wider meal selection, and having preselected staff members with whom to discuss meal selection would help them cope better at school. Resnick and colleagues [18] developed a food-allergy-specific HRQOL measure for adolescents (FAQL-Teen) and found that teens with a history of anaphylaxis, compared to those who had food allergy without a previous episode of anaphylaxis, had significantly lower QOL and that limitation on social activities, inability to eat what others are eating, and limited choice of restaurants were the areas that caused greatest concern for most adolescents with food allergy. van der Velde and colleagues [19] studied the discrepancy between adolescent self-reported HRQOL and parent-proxy-reported HRQOL as a possible contributor to family conflict resulting from teens' risk-taking behaviors and found that the teens' age (>15 years), poorer self-reported illness comprehension, and higher self-perceived disease severity were associated with teen–parent disagreement. A previous episode of anaphylaxis was also found by Herbert and Dahlquist [20] to be associated with perception of greater disease severity, increased worry, and increased parental overprotection in food-allergic young adults.

The reaction and knowledge of the public, friends, extended family, and other social contacts influence the patient's and family's QOL, and impact the management of food allergy. If a food-allergic child or young adult feels that their friends do not give importance to asking about ingredients when eating out, they may be less vigilant [21]. Lieberman and colleagues [22] report frequent and repetitive bullying and harassment of pediatric patients with food allergy by classmates, teachers, school staff, and siblings. Verbal teasing and taunting were more common, but 57% described physical events such as being touched by an allergen, having an allergen thrown or waved at them, and even intentional contamination of their food with an allergen. Psychological distress as a result of these episodes was frequent. While food allergy in a child can promote greater family cohesion [9, 14], lack of social support and cooperation among family members can create tension and potentially damage relationships [23].

Psychosocial support of patients and families with food allergy

The first step in the management of food-allergic patients is obtaining an accurate diagnosis. Aside from identifying the problem and guiding therapy, diagnosis also reduces anxiety and improves QOL. Knibb et al. [24] demonstrated improved QOL and anxiety levels in mothers and children after food allergy challenge, irrespective of the challenge outcome and in spite of persistence of coexisting food allergies in the children. Once the diagnosis is established, education of the patient and their family regarding avoidance of the allergic food, and treatment of anaphylactic reactions can be conducted [25]. Avoidance measures and the vigilance required may initially lead to diminished QOL and increased stress levels [12, 14]. However, increased anxiety levels may be necessary and protective [11] if it encourages patients and families to comply with avoidance measures and management plans. High levels of anxiety motivate parents to gain information and support but should eventually diminish when they have management strategies in place, such as obtaining an epinephrine injector prescription [26].

The development and validation of disease-specific HRQOL measures applicable to all age groups and parents/caregivers has provided an important means of assessing the global impact of food allergy on patients and families' lives [27]. Questionnaires currently validated and used for research and clinical evaluation include the FAQL-PB [28], which examines parental burden; the FAQLQ-Parent Form (FAQL-PF) [29], which examines the Impact of food allergy from the child's perspective ages 0–12; the FAQL-Teen [18], which evaluates the impact of food allergy on adolescents and young adults; the FAQLQ-Child Form (FAQLQ-CF) [30] for food-allergic children aged 8–12 years; the FAQLQ-Teenager Form (FAQL-TF) for teens aged 13–17 years [31]; and the FAQLQ-Adult Form (FAQLQ-AF) [32] for food-allergic patients over 17 years of age. The wider use and availability of these food-allergy-disease-specific QOL questionnaires aid the practitioner's ability to provide a more integrated approach to treatment and evaluating outcomes.

The areas of day-to-day life in which food allergy has the greatest impact on QOL for patients and families are social limitation due to food restriction and increased vigilance associated with the patient's condition. A greater number of allergic foods, history of an anaphylactic episode, and comorbid allergic disease such as asthma and atopic dermatitis are also associated with poorer QOL in food-allergic patients and families. Families with younger children, particularly mothers, are at higher risk for stress and anxiety. Diagnostic and therapeutic measures such as food challenges and epinephrine auto-injector prescriptions have been shown to improve QOL and decrease anxiety levels [24, 26]. A study of group intervention in the form of half-day workshops for parents and children was shown to improve parent-perceived competence in coping with food allergy and parent-perceived burden [33].

Recommendations for reducing patient and parental anxiety include ongoing education and the development of realistic management plans, which provide reassurance that by adhering to the recommended plan, accidental reactions can be avoided and that should they occur they are usually mild [34]. Management and avoidance plans should be in the form of concrete, clear, and concise materials [35]. Children and families can be empowered and reassured by educating them to understand the relative risks of their food allergy and by providing them with communication skills through role-play (e.g., checking labels, asking about ingredients, ordering at a restaurant, being offered food). It is important to enlist parents as allies and advocates in managing the child's food allergy and reinforce their capacity to ensure safety, model healthy coping, and promote healthy coping in their child [36]. Educating extended family, especially siblings, friends, school personnel, and the wider community on the necessity of constant vigilance and the recognition and treatment of possible anaphylaxis is key to promoting safety and improved social interaction [37]. Educational awareness and training in the school setting, as well as having management plans in place, are necessary to reduce parental anxieties and improve school attendance.

Since food allergy is a chronic, often lifelong condition, guidance for patients and parents of food-allergic children should be ongoing and not limited to a single discussion. Professional support and communication should continue as parental and child roles change with time (e.g., parents must learn the best way to influence the child's behavior at different ages, how best to advocate as the child progresses through school, transition from parental to self-management in adolescents) [38]. Practitioners should also be alert to the presence of comorbid psychological disorders, such as excessive or maladaptive anxiety in these patients and their families, which add to the psychological distress already present, lead to restrictions in lifestyle that are unrealistic and unfounded, and obstruct appropriate therapeutic interventions. It is clear that caring for food-allergic patients and their families not only requires thorough diagnosis and management of the allergic disease, but also psychosocial support of the accompanying QOL and psychological effects, which should include evaluation and treatment by a psychologist or psychiatrist, if indicated. Some early signs of psychological disorders include persistent pain, lack of energy, palpitations, dizziness, digestive complaints, and other physical symptoms with no medical explanation; excessive irritability or restlessness; insomnia or excessive sleeping; and persistent feelings of anxiety or sadness, which may interfere with work or daily activities and disrupt relationships.

Food allergy and psychological disorders

It is recognized that the experience and expression of illness reflects the interaction between the physical and psychological states of an individual, such that an individual's mental state can influence physiological changes, including the reactivity of the immune system [39, 40]. Psychologically mediated allergic changes can be classified into a nonspecific autonomic nervous system response to emotional arousal, such as an asthma attack due to fright or violent emotion and changes due to suggestion or conditioning to specific stimuli [41]. It has been reported that nasal, eye, and airway symptoms, as well as changes in eosinophil levels, nasal secretion, bronchoconstriction, and gastrointestinal (GI) and skin blood flow can be experimentally induced by suggestion alone [42, 43]. These findings emphasize the importance of performing diagnostic tests, particularly challenge/provocation procedures, under blinded, placebo-controlled conditions.

In 1984, the Royal College of Physicians and the British Nutrition Program formed a joint committee to address the public's concern about food processing and food allergies. In their report [44], they defined two main disorders: food intolerance, or adverse physical reaction to a specific food or food ingredient that is reproducible under blinded challenge conditions; and food aversion, or "pseudo-food allergy," as Pearson called it [41], which includes psychological avoidance of food and psychogenic physical reactions to food due to emotions associated with the food rather than a physical response to the food itself, which is not reproducible in a blinded challenge. Food allergy is classified under food intolerance or adverse reaction with characteristic clinical and immunological abnormalities that may be immediate IgE-mediated or non-IgE-mediated.

The key features differentiating the person with food aversion or food sensitivity, as they are currently called, from the person with a true food allergy or adverse food reaction are: (i) the absence or inconsistent finding of recognized signs and symptoms, physical findings, and laboratory evaluation supportive of an allergic, toxic, enzymatic, or pharmacological reaction to a specific food and (ii) the inability to reproduce symptoms or physical changes under adequately controlled double-blind food challenge conditions. The DBPCFC in an appropriate clinical setting is the gold standard in the diagnosis of food allergy and is the best method to avoid patient and observer bias [45,46].

Autism spectrum disorders

Autism spectrum disorders (ASDs) are a group of developmental disorders characterized by significant impaired development in social interaction and verbal/nonverbal communication, and restricted repetitive repertoire of behavior and interests [1]. Immunological abnormalities, gluten sensitivity, and food allergy have been proposed to play a role in the pathogenesis and management of autism [47]. However, evidence supporting the beneficial effects of dietary manipulation on behavior and cognition in children with ASDs has consisted mainly of anecdotal reports and small trials.

Studies by Sponheim [48], Renzoni et al. [49], and Pavone et al. [50] were unable to demonstrate improvement in behavior with a gluten-free diet, or any association between autism and food allergy or celiac disease (CD). Lymphocytic infiltration in the upper and lower GI tract [51], immune activation [52], and abnormal lymphocytic responses to dietary antigens [53] have been reported in children with autism, but the relevance of these findings to cognitive function or to development of autism is still unclear. A 2010 consensus report published by a multispecialty panel generated evidence-based recommendations on the evaluation, diagnosis, and management of gastrointestinal disorders in ASDs. Among them: that available research does not support the use of casein-free diet, gluten-free diet, or combined casein-free, gluten-free (CSGF) diet as a primary treatment for individuals with ASDs; that immunologic aberrations have been reported in individuals with ASDs, but a direct cause-and-effect relationship between immune dysfunction and ASDs have yet to be proven; and that at present, there are inadequate data to establish a causal role for intestinal inflammation, increased intestinal permeability, immunologic abnormalities, or food allergies in ASDs [54].

Given the lack of hard evidence supporting the benefits of dietary manipulation in preventing or treating autistic patients [55], implementation of rigorous elimination diets should be undertaken with great caution. Such unproven measures divert the autistic patient's family from more useful treatments and contribute to poor nutrition and further social isolation in families already facing great difficulties.

Celiac disease and psychiatric disorders

CD, or gluten-sensitive enteropathy, is a chronic disease of the small intestinal mucosa with intermittent diarrhea, abdominal pain, distension, and irritability induced by gliadin, the prolamin protein of wheat [56]. Aside from the resulting weight loss and malabsorption, neurological and psychiatric illnesses have also been reported in patients with CD [57, 58].

A high prevalence of anxiety, depression, and disruptive behavioral disorders has been reported in adults and adolescents with CD [59–61]. The prevalence of these disorders has been attributed to the reduction in the QOL due to chronic disease in these patients [59, 60] and serotonergic dysfunction due to impaired availability of tryptophan related to either malabsorption or impaired transport [62]. Hallert and Sedvall [63] reported significant increases in monoamine metabolites and tryptophan in the cerebrospinal fluid in patients with CD after being on a gluten-free diet for 1 year. Addolorato et al. [59] studied 35 patients with CD, anxiety, and depression for 1 year on a gluten-free diet. They reported a significant decrease in anxiety state to values similar to controls after 1 year on the gluten-free diet without significant reduction in depression. They attributed these findings to the fact that anxiety in CD patients is predominantly reactive, and related to poor QOL due to chronic illness, whereas depression is a characteristic of CD. They recommend that patients with CD obtain psychological support to improve compliance to treatment and limit related disease complications. Pynnonen [64] also reported significant improvement in depressive symptoms in adolescents with CD after 3 months on a gluten-free diet. Hallert [63] studied 12 patients with CD and depression and reported no improvement in depressive symptoms after 1 year on a gluten-free diet despite improvement in small intestinal biopsies. However, he reported significant reduction in depression as evaluated by the MMPI after 6 months on oral pyridoxine (vitamin B6) therapy (80 mg/day). Their findings suggest that the metabolic effects of pyridoxine deficiency may influence central nervous mechanisms regulating mood in CD.

CD patients are at higher risk for depression and anxiety; however, studies have found no increased risk of schizophrenia in comparison with the general population [65]. Screening and psychosocial support are advised to improve patient compliance and QOL.

Somatoform disorders

In 1984, Rix and colleagues [66] studied the psychiatric characteristics of 19 patients who believed they had allergies to multiple foods but were subsequently found not to be allergic on skin testing and double-blind provocation. These patients attributed to food allergy a variety of symptoms, such as lethargy, head pain or tightness, abdominal discomfort, nausea, depression, and irritability, among others. The authors found this group to be almost identical, in terms of psychiatric symptoms, with a group of new psychiatric patients who attended an outpatient clinic. The majority of these patients had depressive neurotic complaints, which under current classification criteria would be categorized under the somatoform disorders.

The characteristic feature of the somatoform disorders is the presence of multiple physical symptoms that cannot be explained by a medical condition or by another mental disorder, and which cause significant social or occupational dysfunction [1]. Somatization disorder, conversion disorder, pain disorder, hypochondriasis, and body dysmorphic disorder are included in this category.

Somatization disorder is of special interest because food intolerance is a common complaint in these patients. Patients with this disorder complain of numerous physical problems over several years, with onset before age 30. These complaints cannot be fully explained by any known medical condition, or if they occur in the presence of a medical condition, the resulting functional impairment is in excess of what would be expected.

Criteria for diagnosis require that the patient report at least four pain symptoms, two GI symptoms (which may include multiple food intolerance), one sexual symptom, and one pseudoneurological symptom. Patients with this disorder have increased suggestibility and are more likely to complain of multiple problems [67]. Other studies [68–70] have also found increased frequency of somatoform disorders, depression, and anxiety in community samples of professionals and students reporting intolerance to foods not confirmed by allergy skin testing or oral challenge.

Patients with somatoform disorders are the most frequently encountered type of patient who present with an unconfirmed food allergy and nonspecific symptoms. They present a special challenge to the physician and require extra effort and support in terms of time, education, and attempts to build rapport, since most patients will reject a psychiatric referral if they do not have a good relationship with their physicians and if they feel that their emotional and physical problems are not taken seriously.

Panic disorder and environmental intolerance

Self-reported multiple food intolerances/sensitivities have also been reported to be frequently associated with IEI, formerly called MCS [66, 71, 72]. IEI is a clinical description for a cluster of symptoms of unknown etiology that have been attributed by patients to multiple environmental exposures when other medical explanations have been excluded. There are no specific physical or laboratory findings. There is substantial heterogeneity in exposure, illness history, and presentation among persons with this diagnosis [73]. Other terms for IEI are cerebral allergy, chemically induced immune dysregulation, total allergy syndrome, and ecological illness [74].

The most common complaints are fatigue, headache, nausea, malaise, pain, mucosal irritation, disorientation, and dizziness, which are mostly nonspecific. No gross or microscopic evidence of inflammation or other objective signs of pathology have been associated with IEI. As in somatoform disorders, these patients have multiple chronic symptoms and have previously consulted with numerous physicians and other health-care professionals without satisfaction nor any finding of underlying immunological, autoimmune, or any physical disease to explain their symptoms [75]. Patients attribute their illness to exposure to a combination of environmental chemicals, multiple foods, and drugs. A unique feature of IEI is the general absence of a dose–response curve in the provocation of symptoms [76].

Evidence is growing in support of a causal role of underlying psychiatric illness, specifically somatoform [77, 78], depression, and panic disorder in IEI [79–82]. IEI and panic disorder share common symptoms such as chest tightness, breathlessness, and palpitations; apprehension; and avoidance of situations that have been associated with onset of symptoms. Panic attacks may temporarily occur with nonnoxious stimuli that are then associated with symptoms by the patient and are subsequently considered the cause of the symptoms. Placebo-controlled studies using saline infusions [83], carbon dioxide inhalation [84], and provocative challenges [85] note that these approaches provoke symptoms suggestive of panic disorder and anxiety syndrome with hyperventilation in IEI patients. The association of hypocarbia with reproduction of symptoms suggests that anxiety-driven hyperventilation resulting in hypocarbia may be contributing to IEI symptom production. Evidence for a common neurogenetic basis linking IEI and panic disorders was reported by Binkley and colleagues [86] in a study of 11 IEI patients who were found to have a significantly increased prevalence of cholecystokinin B (CCK-B) receptor alleles, which are known to be associated with panic disorder, compared to age-, sex-, and ethnic-background-matched controls.

Approach to the patient with psychological symptoms attributed to food allergy

Epidemiological research has found a large discrepancy between the high prevalence of self-reported food allergy symptoms in the general population and the low prevalence of actual food allergy as documented by skin testing and oral challenges. Up to 20% of the population report some form of food intolerance or food allergy, whereas the prevalence of documented immunological food reactions is around 2% [87, 88]. As previously discussed, many patients who attribute their symptoms to food allergy without scientific basis after appropriate allergy evaluation may have an underlying psychiatric disorder. The most commonly reported disorders are somatoform disorder, anxiety, depression, or panic disorder. The stigma placed on psychiatric disorders in our society makes it more acceptable to attribute symptoms to an organic cause, such as allergy, rather than psychiatric etiology. Physicians may contribute to this perception by paying selective attention to physical symptoms. Patients may also be hesitant to reveal psychological issues if they sense that the doctor has negative attitudes toward psychiatric problems or is uncomfortable dealing with emotional distress [89]. Every effort should therefore be made to maintain good rapport and communication with these patients. It is important that they feel that their physician takes them and their symptoms seriously.

When taking the history, psychosocial cues from the patient such as description of symptoms worsening around stressful situations should be noted and explored if the patient is willing. Physicians should be alert to the presence of paroxysmal episodes of symptoms which involve a combination of physical and psychological symptoms (palpitations, nausea, sweating, tension, fear), since they may be suggestive of a panic or anxiety disorder. Multiplicity of symptoms is also suggestive of a psychiatric disorder. A linear association has been found between the number and severity of somatic complaints such as myalgia, tiredness, and pain, changes in sleep and energy levels, and psychological distress [90].

The Patient Health Questionnaire Somatic, Anxiety, and Depressive Symptom Scales (PHQ-SADS) (Figure 44.1) is a brief, self-administered measure developed for use in the primary care setting that allows clinicians to quickly and efficiently screen patients at risk for depression, anxiety, and somatization disorders [91]. Use of these measures in patients with self-reported but unconfirmed food allergies/intolerance at higher risk for these mental disorders will facilitate referral for psychiatric evaluation and intervention.

The importance of performing blinded placebo-controlled challenges, as opposed to open challenges, to evaluate suspected psychogenic food reactions cannot be stressed enough due to the multiple, nonspecific character of these complaints, the increased suggestibility in the majority of these patients, and to avoid patient and observer bias. It is also important to perform only investigations that the physicians feel is warranted based on the history and physical examination, as further investigations may serve only to reinforce the patient's belief in an organic pathology and to delay appropriate treatment [92].

Although DBPC challenges are the gold standard in the diagnosis of food allergy and should be performed whenever feasible, SBPC challenges may also be performed to confirm neuropsychological complaints associated with food ingestion, as long as guidelines are followed. The Scripps Clinic has had a very positive experience with an SBPC challenge protocol and has found it to be highly effective in screening patients with psychogenic food reactions and in overcoming patients' belief system that there is a cause-and-effect relationship between exposure to the substance and onset of symptoms. There are four elements necessary to accomplish this type of challenge: (i) a single substance (food/additive/substance, etc.), (ii) that produces a consistent reaction (even totally subjective), (iii) with a known amount, (iv) in a set time frame. While we anticipated multiple reactions to both placebo and active challenges, we have found that under direct observation, in a "laboratory" environment, with multiple placebo challenges spread within the active challenges, with a placebo always given first and last, and with the patient having no knowledge as to the time of the final challenge, only rarely do reactions occur to any of the challenges.

Part of the discussion of negative challenge results should include an explanation that the patient's symptoms may be due to a "conditioned reflex" association. This type of association may have been established when the patient experienced symptoms that coincidentally occurred in the presence of the suspected substance. The patient may then have mistaken a temporal association between substance exposure and onset of symptoms with a cause-and-effect association.

Repeated episodes of substance exposure paired with symptom onset reinforce this association. After a sufficient period, whenever the patient believes he or she has been exposed to the food or substance, symptoms are triggered. As previously mentioned, the patient should not be told that they were "imagining" or "making up" their symptoms. They should be informed that they were in fact experiencing symptoms, but these symptoms were not caused by exposure to the suspected substance. Most patients will accept and be reassured by explanations that an allergic etiology is not involved in their symptoms and that there is no serious organic pathology found on evaluation.

When the physician feels he or she does not have the expertise to manage more serious psychiatric disorders or to address psychosocial issues, a referral to a psychiatrist with an interest in patients who present with somatic complaints would be appropriate. The manner in which the referral is made is crucial to the success of future treatment, because patients may be reluctant or even hostile to the idea of seeing a psychiatrist. Insensitively handled psychiatric referrals will add to the patient's distress and loss of confidence in orthodox medicine and may lead them to seek help from unorthodox practitioners instead [94].

Patients may be more receptive to accept psychologically based treatment if they are reminded of the complex interactions between psychological, social, and physical influences, and if there is a discussion of how psychological issues can contribute to symptoms [89].

Close liaison and communication between the referring physician and the treating psychiatrist is important to enhance communication between the physicians and the

PATIENT HEALTH QUESTIONNAIRE (PHQ-SADS)

This questionnaire is an important part of providing you with the best health care possible. Your answers will help in understanding problems that you may have. Please answer every question to the best of your ability

A. During the last 4 weeks, how much have you been bothered by any of the following problems?	**Not bothered (0)**	**Bothered a little (1)**	**Bothered a lot (2)**
1. Stomach pain	☐	☐	☐
2. Back pain	☐	☐	☐
3. Pain in your arms, legs, or joints (knees, hips, etc.)	☐	☐	☐
4. Feeling tired or having little energy	☐	☐	☐
5. Trouble falling or staying asleep, or sleeping too much	☐	☐	☐
6. Menstrual cramps or other problems with your periods	☐	☐	☐
7. Pain or problems during sexual intercourse	☐	☐	☐
8. Headaches	☐	☐	☐
9. Chest pain	☐	☐	☐
10. Dizziness	☐	☐	☐
11. Fainting spells	☐	☐	☐
12. Feeling your heart pound or race	☐	☐	☐
13. Shortness of breath	☐	☐	☐
14. Constipation, loose bowels, or diarrhea	☐	☐	☐
15. Nausea, gas, or indigestion	☐	☐	☐

PHQ-15 Score ☐ = _____ + _____

B. Over the last 2 weeks, how often have you been bothered by any of the following problems?	**Not at all (0)**	**Several days (1)**	**More than half the days (2)**	**Nearly every day (3)**
1. Feeling nervous anxiety or on edge	☐	☐	☐	☐
2. Not being able to stop or control worrying	☐	☐	☐	☐
3. Worrying too much about different things	☐	☐	☐	☐
4. Trouble relaxing	☐	☐	☐	☐
5. Being so restless that it is hard to sit still	☐	☐	☐	☐
6. Becoming easily annoyed or irritable	☐	☐	☐	☐
7. Feeling afraid as if something awful might happen	☐	☐	☐	☐

GAD-7 Score ☐ = _____ + _____ + _____

Figure 44.1 The Patient Health Questionnaire Somatic, Anxiety, and Depressive Symptom Scales (PHQ-SADS).

C. Questions about anxiety attacks.

	NO	YES
a. In the last 4 weeks, have you had an anxiety attack — suddenly feeling fear or panic?....................................	☐	☐
If you checked "NO", go to question E.		
b. Has this ever happened before?...........................	☐	☐
c. Do some of these attacks come suddenly out of the blue — that is, in situations where you don't expect to be nervous or uncomfortable?...	☐	☐
d. Do these attacks bother you a lot or are you worried about having another attack?..	☐	☐
e. During your last bad anxiety attack, did you have symptoms like shortness of breath, sweating, or your heart racing, pounding or skipping?..	☐	☐

D. Over the last 2 weeks, how often have you been bothered by any of the following problems?	**Not at all (0)**	**Several days (1)**	**More than half the days (2)**	**Nearly every day (3)**
1. Little interest or pleasure in doing things......................	☐	☐	☐	☐
2. Feeling down, depressed, or hopeless........................	☐	☐	☐	☐
3. Trouble falling or staying asleep, or sleeping too much...	☐	☐	☐	☐
4. Feeling tired or having little energy............................	☐	☐	☐	☐
5. Poor appetite or overeating...	☐	☐	☐	☐
6. Feeling bad about yourself — or that you are a failure or have let yourself or your family down.......................	☐	☐	☐	☐
7. Trouble concentrating on things, such as reading the newspaper or watching television.............................	☐	☐	☐	☐
8. Moving or speaking so slowly that other people could have noticed? Or the opposite – being so fidgety or restless that you have been moving around a lot more than usual...	☐	☐	☐	☐
9. Thoughts that you would be beter off dead of or hurting yourself in some way...	☐	☐	☐	☐

PHQ-9 Score ☐ = _____ + _____ + _____

E. If you checked off any problems on this questionnaire, how difficult have these problems made it for you to do your work, take care of things at home, or get along with other people?

Not difficult at all	Somewhat difficult	Very difficult	Extremely difficult
☐	☐	☐	☐

Developed by Drs. Robert L. Spitzer, Janet B.W. Williams, Kurt Kroenke and colleagues, with an educational grant from Pfizer Inc. No permission required to reproduce, translate, display or distribute. http://www.phqscreeners.com/pdfs/05_PHQ-SADS/English.pdf

Figure 44.1 *(Continued)*

patient. These patients present a special challenge to the allergy specialist, and it is our task to counsel them with compassion and guide them toward more appropriate and effective therapy for their problem.

References

1. American Psychiatric Association. *DSM-IV Diagnostic and Statistical Manual of Mental Disorders*, 4th edn. Washington, DC: American Psychiatric Association, 2000.
2. Pearson DJ. Psychologic and somatic interrelationships in allergy and pseudoallergy. *J Allergy Clin Immunol* 1986; 1:351–359.
3. Stoudemire A, Fogel BS, Greenberg DB (eds). *Psychiatric Care of the Medical Patient*. New York: Oxford University Press, 2000; pp. 4–5.
4. Chia Y, Hamer M, Steptoe A. A bidirectional relationship between psychosocial factors and atopic disorders: a systematic review and meta-analysis. *Psychosom Med* 2008; 70: 102–116.
5. Scott KM, Von Korff M, Ormel J, et al. Mental disorders among adults with asthma: results from the world mental health surveys. *Gen Hosp Psychiatry* 2007; 29(2):123–133.
6. Patten SB, Williams JV. Self-reported allergies and their relationship to several axis I disorders in a community sample. *Int J Psychiatry Med* 2007; 37:11–22.
7. Flokstra-de Blok BM, Dubois AE, Vlieg-Boerstra BJ, et al. Health-related quality of life of food allergic patients: comparison with the general population and other diseases. *Allergy* 2010; 65:238–244.
8. Ostblom E, Egmar AC, Gardulf A, Lilja G, Wickman M. The impact of food hypersensitivity reported in 9-year-old children by their parents on health-related quality of life. *Allergy* 2008; 63:211–218.
9. Sicherer SH, Noone SA, Munoz-Furlong A. The impact of childhood food allergy on quality of life. *Ann Allergy Asthma Immunol* 2001; 87:461–464.
10. Marklund B, Ahlstedt S, Nordstrom G. Health-related quality of life in food hypersensitive school children and their families: parents' perceptions. *Health Qual Life Outcomes* 2006; 4:48.
11. Avery NJ, King RM, Knight S, Hourihand JO. Assessment of quality of life in children with peanut allergy. *Pediatr Allergy Immunol* 2003; 14:378–382.
12. Primeau MN, Kagan R, Joseph L, et al. The psychological burden of peanut allergy as perceived by adults with peanut allergy and parents of peanut allergic children. *Clin Exp Allergy* 2000; 30:1135–1143.
13. King RM, Knibb RC, Hourihane JO. Impact of peanut allergy on quality of life, stress, and anxiety in the family. *Allergy* 2009; 64:461–468.
14. Bollinger ME, Dahlquist LM, Mudd K, et al. The impact of food allergy on the daily activities of children and their families. *Ann Allergy Asthma Immunol* 2006; 96:415–421.
15. Springston EG, Smith B, Shulruff J, et al. Variations in quality of life among caregivers of food allergic children. *Ann Allergy Asthma Immunol* 2010; 105:287–294.
16. van der Velde JL, Flosktra-de Blok BM, Dunngalvin A, Hourihane JO, Duiverman EJ, Dubois AE. Parents report better health-related quality of life for their food-allergic children than children themselves. *Clin Exp Allergy* 2011; 41(10):1431–1439.
17. Sampson MA, Munoz-Furlong A, Sicherer SH. Risk-taking and coping strategies of adolescents and young adults with food allergy. *J Allergy Clin Immunol* 2006; 117:1440–1445.
18. Resnick ES, Pieretti MM, Maloney J, et al. Development of a questionnaire to measure quality of life in adolescents with food allergy: the FAQL-teen. *Ann Allergy Asthma Immunol* 2010; 105:364–368.
19. van der Velde JL, Florkstra-de Blok BM, Hamp A, Knibb RC, Duiverman EJ, Dubois AE. Adolescent–parent disagreement on health-related quality of life of food-allergic adolescents: who makes the difference? *Allergy* 2011; 66(12):1580–1589.
20. Herbert LJ, Dahlquist M. Perceived history of anaphylaxis and parental overprotection, autonomy, anxiety, and depression in food allergic young adults. *J Clin Psychol Med Settings* 2008; 15:261–269.
21. Lyons AC, Forde EM. Food allergy in young adults: perceptions and psychological effects. *J Health Psychol* 2004; 9:497–504.
22. Lieberman JA, Weiss C, Furlong TJ, Sicherer M, Sicherer SH. Bullying among pediatric patients with food allergy. *Ann Allergy Asthma Immunol* 2010; 105:282–286.
23. Mandell D, Curtis R, Gold M, Hardie S. Anaphylaxis: how do you live with it?. *Health Soc Work* 2005; 30:325–335.
24. Knibb RC, Ibrahim NF, Stiefel G, et al. The psychological impact of food diagnostic challenges to confirm the resolution of peanut or tree nut allergy. *Clin Exp Allergy* 2012; 42(3):451–459.
25. Munoz-Furlong A. Daily coping strategies for patients and their families. *Pediatrics* 2003; 111:1654–1661.
26. Cummings AJ, Knibb RC, Erlewyn- Lajeunesse M, King RM, Roberts G, Lucas JS. Management of nut allergy influences quality of life and anxiety in children and their mothers. *Pediatr Allergy Immunol* 2010; 21:586–594.
27. Lieberman JA, Sicherer SH. Quality of life in food allergy. *Curr Opin Allergy Clin Immunol* 11:236–242.
28. Cohen BL, Noone S, Munoz-Furlong A, Sicherer SH. Development of a questionnaire to measure quality of life in families with a child with food allergy. *J Allergy Clin Immunol* 2004; 114:1159–1163.
29. DunnGalvin A, Flokstra-de Blok BM, Burks AW, et al. Food Allergy QoL questionnaire for children aged 0–12 years: content, construct, and cross-cultural validity. *Clin Exp Allergy* 2008; 38:977–986.
30. Flokstra-de Blok BMJ, DunnGalvin A, Ving-Boersta BJ, et al. Development and validation of the self-administered Food Allergy Quality of Life Questionnaire for children. *Clin Exp Allergy* 2009; 39:127–137.
31. Flokstra-de Blok BMJ, DunnGalvin A, Ving-Boersta BJ, et al. Development and validation of the self-administered Food Allergy Quality of Life Questionnaire for adolescents. *J Allergy Clin Immunol* 2008; 122(1):139–144.
32. Flokstra-de Blok BM, DunnGalvin A, Ving-Boersta BJ, et al. Development and validation of the self-administered Food

Allergy Quality of Life Questionnaire-Adult Form (FAQLQ-AF). *Allergy* 2009; 64:1209–1217.
33. Lebovidge JS, Timmons K, Rich C, et al. Evaluation of a group intervention for children with food allergy and their parents. *Ann Allergy Immunol* 2008; 101:170–165.
34. Clark AT, Ewan PW. Good prognosis, clinical features, and circumstances of peanut and tree nut reactions in children treated by a specialist allergy center. *J Allergy Clin Immunol* 2008; 122:286–289.
35. Vargas PA, Sicherer SH, Christie L. Developing a food allergy curriculum for parents. *Ped Allergy Immunol* 2011; 22:575–582.
36. Monga S, Manassis K. Treating anxiety in children with life-threatening anaphylactic conditions. *J Am Acad Child Adolesc Psych* 2006; 45:1007–1010.
37. Cummings AJ, Knibb RC, King RM, Lucas JS. The psychosocial impact of food allergy and food hypersensitivity in children, adolescents and their families: a review. *Allergy* 2010; 65:933–945.
38. Manassis K. Managing anxiety related to anaphylaxis in childhood: a systematic review. *J Allergy* 2012; 2012:316296.
39. Crayton JW. Adverse reactions to food: relevance to psychiatric disorders. *J Allergy Clin Immunol* 1986; 78:243–250.
40. Keller SE, Weiss JM, Schleifer SJ, et al. Suppression of immunity by stress: effects of a graded series of stressors on lymphocyte stimulation in the rat. *Science* 1981; 213:1397–1400.
41. Pearson DJ. Pseudo food allergy. *BMJ* 1986; 292:221–222.
42. Horton DJ, Sude WL, Kinsman RA, et al. Bronchoconstrictive suggestions in asthma: a role for airways hyperreactivity and emotions. *Am Rev Respir Dis* 1978; 117:1029–1038.
43. Graham DR, Wolf S, Wolff H. Changes in tissue sensitivity associated with varying life situations and emotions: their relevance to allergy. *J Allergy* 1950; 21:478–486.
44. Food intolerance and food aversion. A joint report of the Royal College of Physicians and the British Nutrition Foundation. *J R Coll Physicians Lond* 1984; 18(2):83–123.
45. Atkins FM. A critical evaluation of clinical trials in adverse reactions to foods in adults. *J Allergy Clin Immunol* 1986; 78:174-181.
46. Metcalfe DD, Sampson HA. Workshop on experimental methodology for clinical studies of adverse reactions to foods and food additives. *J Allergy Clin Immunol* 1990; 86:421–442.
47. Coleman M. Autism: non-drug biologic treatments. In: Gilbert C (ed.) *Diagnosis and Treatment of Autism*. New York: Plenum Press, 1989; pp. 219–235.
48. Sponheim E. Gluten-free diet in infantile autism. A therapeutic trial. *Tidsskr Nor Laegeforen* 1991; 111:704–707.
49. Renzoni E, Beltrami V, Sestani P, et al. Brief report: allergological evaluation of children with autism. *J Autism Dev Disord* 1995; 25:327–333.
50. Pavone L, Fiumara A, Bottaro G, et al. Autism and coeliac disease: failure to validate the hypothesis that a link might exist. *Biol Psychiatr* 1997; 42:72–75.
51. Ashwood P, Anthony A, Pellicer AA, et al. Intestinal lymphocyte populations in children with regressive autism: evidence for extensive mucosal immunopathology. *J Clin Immunol* 2003; 23:504–517.
52. Ashwood P, Anthony A, Torrente F, Wakefield AJ. Spontaneous mucosal lymphocyte cytokine profiles in children with autism and gastrointestinal symptoms: mucosal immune activation and reduced counter regulatory interleukin-10. *J Clin Immunol* 2004; 24:664–673.
53. Jyonouchi H, Geng L, Ruby A, Zimmerman-Bier B. Dysregulated innate immune responses in young children with autism spectrum disorders: their relationship to gastrointestinal symptoms and dietary intervention. *Neuropsychobiology* 2005; 51:77–85.
54. Buie T, Campbell DB, Fuchs III GJ, et al. Evaluation, diagnosis, and treatment of gastrointestinal disorders in individuals with ASDs: a consensus report. *Pediatrics* 2010; 125:S1–S18.
55. Millward C, Ferriter M, Calver S, Connel-Jones G. Gluten- and casein-free diets for autistic spectrum disorder. *Cochrane Database Syst Rev* 2008; 2:CD003498.
56. Corrazza GR, Gasbarrini G. Coeliac disease in adults. *Bailiere Clin Gastroenterol* 1995; 9:329–350.
57. Smith DF, Gerdes LU. Meta-analysis on anxiety and depression in adult celiac disease. *Acta Psychiatr Scand* 2012; 125(3):189–193.
58. Hauser W, Janke KH, Klump B, Gregor M, Hinz A. Anxiety and depression in adult patients with celiac disease on a gluten-free diet. *World J Gastroenterol* 2010; 16:2780–2787.
59. Addorato G, Stefanini GF, Capristo E, et al. Anxiety and depression in adult untreated celiac subjects and in patients affected by inflammatory bowel disease: a personality trait or a reactive illness? *Hepatogastroenterology* 1996; 43:1153–1157.
60. Hallert C, Astrom J, Sedvall G. Psychic disturbances in adult coeliac disease. III. Reduced central monoamine metabolism and signs of depression. *Scand J Gastroenterol* 1982; 17:25–28.
61. Pynnonen PA, Isometsa ET, Aronen ET, et al. Mental disorders in adolescents with celiac disease. *Psychosomatics* 2004; 45:325–335.
62. Hernanz A, Polanco I. Plasma precursor amino acids of central nervous system monoamines in children with coeliac disease. *Gut* 1991; 32:1478–1481.
63. Hallert C, Sedvall G. Improvement in central monoamine metabolism in adult coeliac patients starting a gluten-free diet. *Psychol Med* 1983; 13(2):267–271.
64. Pynnonen PA, Isometsa ET, Verkasalo MA, et al. Gluten-free diet may alleviate depressive and behavioural symptoms in adolescents with celiac disease: a follow-up case-series study. *BMC Psychiatry* 2005; 5:14.
65. West J, Loran RF, Hubbard RB, Card TR. Risk of schizophrenia in people with celiac disease, ulcerative colitis, and Crohn's disease: a general population-based study. *Alimen Pharmacol Ther* 2006; 23:71–74.
66. Rix KJ, Pearson DJ, Bentley SJ. A psychiatric study of patients with supposed food allergy. *Br J Psych* 1984; 145:121–126.
67. Woodruff R, Clayton P, Guze S. Hysteria-studies of diagnosis, outcome, and prevalence. *J Am Med Assoc* 1971; 215:425–428.
68. Vatn MH, Grimstad IA, Thorsen L, et al. Adverse reactions to food: assessment by double-blind placebo-controlled food challenge and clinical, psychosomatic and immunological analysis. *Digestion* 1995; 56:419–426.
69. Knibb RC, Armstrong A, Booth DA, et al. Psychological characteristics of people with perceived food intolerance in a community sample. *J Psychosom Res* 1999; 57:545–554.
70. Bell IR, Schartz GE, Peterson JM, Amend D. Symptom and personality profiles of young adults from a college student

population with self-reported illness from foods and chemicals. *J Am Coll Nutr* 1993; 12:693–702.
71. Bell IR, Schwartz GE, Amend D, et al. Sensitization to early life stress and response to chemical odors in older adults. *Biol Psychiatr* 1994; 35:857–863.
72. Ross GH. Clinical characteristics of chemical sensitivity: an illustrative case history of asthma and MCS. *Environ Health Perspect* 1997; 105:437–441.
73. Sparks PJ. Idiopathic environmental intolerances: overview. *Occup Med* 2000; 15:497–695.
74. Green MA. "Allergic to everything": 20th century syndrome. *J Am Med Assoc* 1985; 253:842.
75. Brodsky CM. "Allergic to everything": a medical subculture. *Psychosomatics* 1983; 24:731–742.
76. Terr AI. Clinical ecology in the workplace. *J Occup Med* 1989; 31:257–261.
77. Black DW, Rathe A, Goldstein RB. Environmental illness: a controlled study of 26 subjects with "20th century disease". *J Am Med Assoc* 1990; 204:3166–3170.
78. Bailer J, Witthoft M, Paul C, et al. Evidence for overlap between idiopathic environmental intolerance and somatoform disorders. *Psychosom Med* 2005; 67:921–929.
79. Simon G, Daniell W, Stockbridge H, et al. Immonologic, psychological and neuropsychological factors in multiple chemical sensitivity: a controlled study. *Ann Intern Med* 1993:119:97–103.
80. Black DW, Rathe A, Golstein RB. Environmental illness: a controlled study of 26 subjects with "20th century disease". *J Am Med Assoc* 1990; 264:3166–3170.
81. Dietel A, Jordan L, Muhlinghaus T, et al. Psychiatric disorders of environmental outpatients—results of the standardized psychiatric interview (CIDI) from the German multi-center study on Multiple Chemical Sensitivity (MCS). *Psychother Psychosom Med Psychol* 2006; 56:162–171.
82. Papo D, Eberlein-Konig B, Berresheim HW, et al. Chemosensory function and psychological profile in patients with multiple chemical sensitivity: comparison with odor-sensitive and asymptomatic controls. *J Psychosom Res* 2006; 60:199–209.
83. Binkley KE, Kutcher S. Panic response to sodium lactate infusion in patients with multiple chemical sensitivity syndrome. *J Allergy Clin Immunol* 1997; 99:570–574.
84. Poonal N, Antony MM, Binkley KE, et al. Carbon dioxide inhalation challenges in idiopathcic environmental intolerance. *J Allergy Clin Immunol* 2000; 105:358–363.
85. Leznoff A. Provocative challenges in patients with multiple chemical sensitivity. *J Allergy Clin Immunol* 1997; 99:438–442.
86. Binkley K, King N, Poonal N, et al. Idiopathic environmental intolerance: increased prevalence of panic disorder-associated cholecystokinin B receptor allele 7. *J Allergy Clin Immunol* 2001; 107:887–890.
87. Young E, Patel S, Stoneham M, et al. The prevalence of reaction to food additives in a survey population. *J Coll Phys* 1987; 721:214–247.
88. Young E, Stoneham MD, Petruckevitch A, et al. A population study of food intolerance. *Lancet* 1994; 343:1127–1130.
89. Howard LM, Wessely S. Psychiatry in the allergy clinic: the nature and management of patients with non-allergic symptoms. *Clin Exp Allergy* 1995; 25:503–514.
90. Bass C, Benjamin S. The management of chronic somatisation. *Br J Psychiatr* 1993; 162:472–480.
91. Kroenke K, Spitzer RL, Williams JB, Lowe B. The patient health questionnaire somatic, anxiety, and depressive symptom scales: a systematic review. *Gen Hosp Psych* 2010; 32:345–359.
92. Buchwald A, Rudick Davis D. The symptoms of major depression. *J Abn Psychol* 1993; 102:197–205.
93. Cohen BL, Noone S, Munoz-Furlong A, Sicherer SH. Development of a questionnaire to measure quality of life in families with a child with food allergy. *J Allergy Clin Immunol* 2004; 114:1159–1163.
94. Coleman MT, Newton KS. Supporting self-management in patients with chronic illness. *Am Fam Phy* 2005; 72:1503–1510.

45 Foods and Rheumatologic Diseases

Lisa K. Stamp[1] & Leslie G. Cleland[2]

[1]Department of Medicine, University of Otago, Christchurch, New Zealand
[2]Rheumatology Unit, Royal Adelaide Hospital, Adelaide, Australia

Key Concepts

- There is little convincing evidence for RA occurring as a result of food allergy.
- Patients with RA commonly associate certain foods with increased joint symptoms, although in many cases this is not confirmed by formal assessments.
- Individual patients with RA may have an improvement in disease control on elimination of certain foods from the diet.
- Prolonged periods of fasting or hypocaloric diets should be avoided due to potential adverse outcomes.
- In patients with RA, long-term dietary supplementation with n-3 fatty acids is associated with improvements in disease activity when combined with DMARD therapy.

Introduction

Food has been linked to joint symptoms in three ways. Firstly, primary food allergy can be associated with self-limited arthralgia (joint pain) and/or arthritis (joint inflammation) in addition to the other manifestations of allergy such as urticaria [1]. Secondly, reactive arthritis may be associated with a preceding gastrointestinal infection acquired from eating contaminated food. Thirdly, patients with primary inflammatory arthritis often report a link between certain foods and joint symptoms. The causal link between diet and inflammatory arthritis is strongest for gout [2]. However, patients with other forms of inflammatory arthritis such as rheumatoid arthritis (RA) sometimes report an association between their symptoms and food. The frequency with which RA occurs as a consequence of true food allergy is uncertain. Notwithstanding, certain foods seem to have a significant impact on disease activity for some individuals with RA and elimination of particular foods may benefit some patients. However, there is no easy way to predict who will respond to dietary avoidance strategies. There is more robust evidence for the benefits of dietary supplementation with omega-3 fatty acids in RA. The focus of this chapter is the relationship between foods and RA.

Rheumatoid arthritis

RA is a chronic condition which affects 1–2% of the general population. The hallmark of RA is inflammation of synovial lining of joints. Early in the disease, inflammation results in joint pain, swelling, and stiffness. Over time, the joints become damaged with erosion of bone and cartilage by inflamed synovial tissue, which leads to joint deformities and functional impairment.

Disease classification criteria for RA rest on the pattern of joint involvement, presence of rheumatoid factor (RF) and antibodies against cyclic citrullinated peptide (CCP), and elevated inflammatory markers (e.g., C-reactive protein (CRP) and erythrocyte sedimentation rate (ESR)).

The aims of management in RA are reduction of symptoms, prevention of joint damage, and preservation of function. Pharmacological therapies, which are the mainstay of treatment, can be broadly classified into three groups:

1. Nonsteroidal, anti-inflammatory drugs (NSAIDs) which act rapidly to reduce pain but have no beneficial effect on long-term disease progression;
2. Corticosteroids which rapidly control inflammation and may reduce joint erosion, but are associated with many unwanted effects;

Food Allergy: Adverse Reactions to Foods and Food Additives, Fifth Edition. Edited by Dean D Metcalfe, Hugh A Sampson, Ronald A Simon and Gideon Lack.

3. Disease modifying antirheumatic agents (DMARDs) (e.g., methotrexate, tumor necrosis factor blockers), which lack a direct analgesic effect but reduce disease activity thereby preventing joint destruction and improving functional outcomes.

In addition to these standard therapies, patients frequently request information regarding alternative and/or complementary therapies, including dietary therapies for management of their disease. Up to 75% of RA patients believe food influences their symptoms and it has been reported that as many as 50% try dietary manipulation in an attempt to control their symptoms [3]. By contrast, relatively few physicians would regard diet as contributing to the etiology of RA or as having a significant role in the management of RA.

Diet in the etiology of RA

A number of genetic factors have been shown to predispose to RA. As heritability is well short of 100%, it follows that environmental factors contribute substantially to etiology. A decreased risk of developing RA has been reported with high consumption of fish, a rich source of omega-3 fatty acids [4]. Consumption of β-cryptoxanthin (a carotenoid found in fruit and vegetables) has also been associated with reduced risk for RA [5]. Some, but not all, studies have reported an increased risk of developing RA with high red meat consumption [6–8] and caffeine intake [9–11].

Evidence for a RA-like illness as a result of food allergy is sparse. Panush described two patients who developed subjective and objective evidence of a nonerosive, RF-negative, palindromic inflammatory arthritis after exposure to shrimp and nitrites [12].

Genetics in the etiology of RA—the potential interaction with food

Twin studies provide a means for assessing the relative extent of contributions by genetic and environmental factors to multifactorial diseases. In RA, the concordance rate in monozygotic twins is reported to be 12% [13] to 15% [14]. Quantitative genetic analysis using the data from both of these cohorts has demonstrated that the "heritability" or extent to which liability to RA is explained by genetic variation in the population is about 60% [15].

Human leukocyte antigen (HLA) class II alleles are among the most important genetic contributors to RA. HLA antigens are surface membrane molecules that play a central role in specific immunity through their ability to present peptide fragments that have been processed by antigen-presenting cells (APCs). HLA-DR molecules are strongly expressed on APCs. They present peptides derived from both endogenous and exogenous antigens to CD4+ve T cells. The strongest allelic associations in RA are with subtypes of HLA-DR4 and HLA-DR1, in particular HLA-DR*0401, -*0404, and -*0101. These HLA-DR specificities are determined by the HLA-DRβ1 locus and have a conserved amino acid sequence in the third hypervariable region of the DRβ chain, known as the "shared epitope." It is this "shared epitope" portion that is thought to confer the risk of RA [16]. The canonical feature of the shared epitope is a positively charged pocket with neutral and positively charged amino acids elsewhere in the groove. This configuration is favorable for presentation of peptide fragments with appropriately located negative charge. The "shared epitope" provides a potential mechanism whereby an individual may inherit a susceptibility to RA. According to this scenario, when a predisposed person meets a potentially pathogenic antigen in an appropriate immunological context (with endogenous and exogenous co-stimulatory molecules signaling a "danger" context), a pathogenic immune response may occur directed against either exogenous and endogenous antigens or both. From the perspective of a possible allergic component to RA, it is notable that the HLA-DR4 alleles have been associated with atopy. While food is an abundant source of exogenous antigens, presentation of peptides within the specialized immunological tissues of the gut mucosa generally evokes immunological tolerance rather than responsiveness because "danger signals" that promote the latter are typically lacking.

Food allergy/intolerance in RA

A number of case reports link symptom severity with certain foods in RA (Table 45.1). In all of these reports patients responded with an improvement in arthritic symptoms on elimination of the offending food from the diet. Van der Laar et al. reported on two patients with RA who had raised serum IgE concentrations to several foods, which reduced after elimination of the foods from the diet. This was accompanied by an improvement in clinical symptoms and a reduction in mast cells in both the synovial membrane and proximal small intestine [25]. Liden et al. found that 64 out of 241 RA patients reported food intolerance, in particular to cow's milk protein, meat, and wheat gluten. Joint and muscle symptoms were the second most frequent symptoms associated with food intolerance occurring in 35%. Despite this there was no association between rectal mucosal reactivity to cow's milk protein or gluten and self-reported adverse effects to these foods [26]. While a number of patients describe food-related

Table 45.1 Reports of food allergy/intolerance in RA.

Case summary	Allergen	Effect of removal of putative food allergen from diet	Effect of reintroduction of putative food allergen from diet	Reference
RF-positive RA, extra-articular manifestations, ↑ESR, ↑IgE	Cereals (SPT-positive)	Remission	Recurrence of symptoms	[17]
Erosive RF-negative RA, 11 years duration	Milk and cheese	Significant improvement with ↓ESR, able to stop prednisone	Recurrence of symptoms within 24 hours of reintroduction of dairy products IgE antibodies to milk and cheese became positive during rechallenge	[18]
Active RA, 35 years duration	Corn	Improved, ↓ESR, able to stop DMARDs	Recurrence of symptoms	[19]
RF-negative arthritis elbow and tenosynovitis	Milk (RAST-positive for cow's milk)	Improved	Recurrence of symptoms	[20]
Spondylitis	Milk and wheat (serum-specific IgE positive for milk and wheat)	Marked improvement	Recurrence of symptoms	[20]
RF-positive inflammatory arthritis	Milk (↑IgG anti-milk antibodies)	Improved	Challenges with milk resulted in deterioration of symptoms	[21]
Juvenile RA, 6 years duration, RF negative	Cow's milk (lactose intolerant) (IgG and IgM anti-milk antibodies)	Marked improvement	Multiple challenges resulted in recurrence of symptoms	[22]
Monoarthritis form of juvenile chronic arthritis, ANA negative	Milk	Improved, but not resolved	Swelling of the affected joint after milk challenge After 2 years patient asymptomatic and tolerating milk	[23]
RA 8 years duration	Animal products	Improved	Swelling and tenderness of affected joints	[24]

RF, rheumatoid factor; ESR, erythrocyte sedimentation rate; ANA, antinuclear antibody.

aggravation of symptoms, this often is not substantiated by more formal assessment [12].

The concept of food allergy/intolerance in RA has led to studies examining the effects of dietary manipulation on disease activity in RA. Dietary manipulation can be divided into two categories—exclusion diets where foods thought to increase symptoms are removed from the diet and supplementation diets where foods that improve symptoms are added to the diet. In RA, exclusion diets have been shown to be of some value in individual patients only. In comparison, supplementation of the diet with omega-3 fatty acids have been shown to benefit groups of patients in randomized controlled trials. In this section we review the evidence for exclusion diets in RA.

Elemental diets

Elemental diets are designed to provide foods in their simplest forms, (e.g., proteins as amino acids, carbohydrates as glucose or small saccharides, fats as medium chain triglycerides). Such diets are thought to be hypoallergenic and thereby provide a means for determining whether food allergy/intolerance has a role in RA. In a prospective, double-blind, controlled study in 20 patients with active RA, patients received either an elemental diet or a control diet consisting of well mixed and blended soup which contained milk, meat, corn, and wheat for 3 weeks. In the fourth week of the study all patients returned to their normal diet. While 3 out of 10 patients in the elemental group and 2 out of 7 patients in the control group improved, overall there was no significant difference between the two groups [27]. In a larger study, 4 weeks of an artificial elemental peptide diet was compared to normal diet in 30 patients. While there were improvements in pain and health assessment questionnaire (HAQ) scores at 4 weeks, these improvements were lost by 3 months [28]. Similar findings with individual patient improvement, particularly in the more subjective aspects of disease assessment, have been reported [29].

While individual patients may benefit from such elemental diets there is insufficient evidence to support their routine use in the management of RA. Furthermore, the benefits appear to be short-lived once patients return to a normal diet and the long-term sustainability of such diets is questionable.

Elimination diets

Elimination diets remove foods that are thought to be allergenic or "arthritogenic" in the case of RA, from the diet. An elimination diet needs to be continued for at least 3 weeks and is usually followed by gradual reintroduction of potentially offending foods. Such a diet trial is considered to be positive if elimination of those potentially allergenic foods from the diet results in clinical improvement with a subsequent deterioration after reintroduction. However, such studies are usually single-blind as patients are aware of what they eat and a double-blind placebo controlled food challenge is the only validated test for the diagnosis of food allergy/intolerance.

As with elemental diets, elimination diets have been reported to be of some benefit in individual patients with RA. One such elimination diet, The Dong Diet, contains little meat except occasional fish and chicken, no herbs or spices, dairy products, additives or preservatives, and no alcohol. The Dong Diet was created by Dr Dong after his personal experience of remission of arthritis with such a diet and gained widespread popularity among patients [30]. However, a 10-week, double-blind, controlled study of the Dong Diet in 33 patients with RA showed no overall benefit, although 2 out of 11 patients did improve while on the Dong Diet with subsequent deterioration after return to normal diet [31].

To achieve an even more restrictive diet, van der Laar et al. used artificial foods in order to remove potential allergens from the diet. Ninety-four patients with RA consumed their normal diet for 4 weeks and were then assigned to either an "allergen free" (free of all potentially allergenic foods, additives, and preservatives) or "allergen restricted" diet (contained milk proteins and yellow azo colorings) for 4 weeks, followed by a return to normal diet for the final 4 weeks of the study. Out of 94 patients, 78 completed the study and while there were subjective improvements in both groups, there was no difference between the two diets [32].

The withholding or stopping of DMARD therapy for the purposes of studying the effects of dietary manipulation would no longer be considered ethical. Therapy in the twenty-first century is far more intensive than even 10 years ago, thus there would be few patients with RA neither receiving nor requiring DMARD therapy. However, in the early 1980s Darlington et al. examined the effects of an elimination diet in 53 RA patients receiving no DMARD treatment [33]. During the first week of the study, patients were only allowed foods thought very unlikely to cause symptoms. In the ensuing 5 weeks, other foods considered more likely to cause symptoms such as cereals, were gradually reintroduced. During the study there were significant improvements in pain, swollen joint count, and ESR. Interestingly, 9 out of 10 patients with a family history of atopy had a good response to the diet as compared to 24 out of 34 patients with no family history of atopy ($p < 0.05$) [33]. While these results are encouraging, patients who do not require DMARD therapy are likely to have milder disease and the results of dietary studies in these patients may not be generalizable to those with more active or severe disease.

Compliance with such restrictive diets may be problematic, especially in the long term. In a dietary study of patients with RA, only 52% of the patients completed the study, and only 3 out of 27 patients adhered to the diet for 10 months [34].

These studies demonstrate that individual patients may respond to dietary manipulation and that compliance with dietary therapy is a major limiting factor in many cases. Determining an appropriate diet for an individual might be expected to result in clinical improvements and increased compliance. Skin prick test (SPT) of potential allergens is one means of determining if an allergy exists. In an attempt to "individualize" dietary manipulation, Karatay et al. studied 20 patients with RA who had a positive SPT for at least one food and 20 RA patients with negative SPT. All patients had clinically inactive disease at study entry. Patients underwent an elimination diet for 12 days in which the most common allergenic foods were avoided. This was followed by a 12-day "challenge phase" during which SPT-positive foods were added and finally a 12-day "re-elimination" phase whereby the SPT-positive foods were removed. In the SPT-negative group, corn, which is reported to be a common allergenic food in RA, and rice which is not thought to be an allergenic food, were added in increasing amounts. At the end of the challenge phase, swollen and tender joint counts, pain, patient, and physician global assessment, morning stiffness, ESR, and CRP all increased significantly in the SPT-positive group. In the SPT-negative group only pain and patient global assessment increased during the "challenge phase." This increase in disease activity was observed in 72% of SPT-positive patients compared to 17% of SPT-negative patients during the "challenge phase" and continued in all but one patient during the "re-elimination" phase [35]. The authors concluded that food allergy may be a triggering factor in RA and that an individualized avoidance diet may be helpful in some patients. SPT may not be practical for many patients; thus in patients who believe their arthritis is due to or worsened by a particular food, objective measures of disease activity should be undertaken before and after one or more cycles of removal of the putative "food allergen." The resulting evidence may then be used by both the patient and physician to determine whether long-term avoidance of the "food allergen" is warranted.

Vegetarian and vegan diets

Vegan and vegetarian diets have been the subject of a number of studies in patients with RA. In the largest study, 66 patients with active RA were randomized to either a gluten-free vegan diet or a well-balanced, nonvegetarian diet for 12 months. Only 58% of the vegan diet group and 89% of the control group completed at least 9 months of the study. At 12 months, 41% of the vegan group and 4% of the control group achieved an ACR20 response. Radiographic progression was similar in both groups. In those patients on the study diet who achieved the ACR20 response, a significant reduction in serum IgG-anti-gliadin antibodies and IgG-β-lactoglobulin antibodies was observed. The authors suggest a diminished immune response to exogenous food antigens may have had a role in the observed clinical benefits [36].

Other studies of vegetarian/vegan diets have been preceded by a period of fasting. In a 13-month prospective, single-blind trial, 27 patients with active RA were randomized to a 7- to 10-day fast followed by gradual reintroduction of foods, which were eliminated if they resulted in symptom deterioration. During the first $3^1/_2$ months, a gluten-free vegan diet was allowed with subsequent introduction of milk-based products and gluten. Twenty-six matched control patients with active RA continued their normal diet. In the diet group, improvements were noted as early as 1 month with significant reductions in tender and swollen joint counts, duration of morning stiffness, ESR, and CRP. The improvements persisted throughout the duration of the study [37]. Of note, 37% of patients in the diet group and 35% in the control group withdrew. Disease flare was the cause for withdrawal in 4 out of 10 patients in the diet group and 7 out of 9 in the control group while one patient in the diet group was unable to tolerate the diet. Importantly some patients were consuming cod liver oil prior to and during the study, although the exact numbers and doses are not revealed. As discussed below, cod liver oil is rich in omega-3 fatty acids which have been shown to provide a benefit in patients with RA. In those patients taking the cod liver oil supplement, it is possible that the change in diet produced a more significant alteration in the ratio of dietary omega-3/omega-6 fatty acids, in favor of the less inflammatory omega-3 fats, thereby contributing to at least some of the observed benefits. Out of the 27 patients in the diet group who identified foods that exacerbated their symptoms, 10 were studied further. Of these 10 patients, 8 were classified as responders and 2 as nonresponders to the dietary regimen. However, in 9 out of 10 patients, there was no associated antibody activity to the suspected foods. Only one patient who suspected meat aggravated his arthritis symptoms was found to have elevated concentrations of IgM anti-BSA antibody activity, which subsequently reduced dramatically during the study period in parallel with a reduction in disease activity [38].

It has been suggested that a vegan diet which is also low in all kinds of fats is more likely to provide benefit to RA patients. In an uncontrolled trial, 24 patients with active RA maintained such a diet for 4 weeks. Compliance was not a problem and improvements were observed in tender and swollen joint counts as well as pain scores. However, there was no improvement in duration of morning stiffness, ESR, or CRP [39]. Further, longer-term, double-blind controlled studies of this diet are required.

Overall vegetarian/vegan diets may be of benefit in some RA patients. However, restrictive diets are problematic with regard to compliance and there currently is no way to predict which patients will respond.

Fasting

Total and subtotal fasting preceded some studies of vegetarian/vegan diets. In most cases improvements were observed during the fasting period, but rapidly disappeared on reintroduction of food [37, 40–42]. Patients with RA frequently lose weight during periods of active disease. However, even patients with well-controlled disease have a lower body cell mass compared to healthy controls [43]. Rheumatoid cachexia is a term used to describe the severe loss of body cell mass that may occur [44] despite adequate protein and calorie intake and is associated with increased resting energy expenditure and protein catabolism as well as reduced physical activity. Diets which restrict protein and calorie intake may further compound this loss of body cell mass and should be avoided. In this regard, fasting which can only be maintained for short periods may be detrimental. Given the benefits of fasting are modest and short-lived when compared with the chronic nature of RA, fasting is an impractical approach to the management of RA.

Potential mechanisms of food intolerance/allergy RA

A number of potential mechanisms have been postulated in those patients who respond to elimination of suspected food allergens.

Disease and psychological factors

Patients who are willing to undertake dietary studies, particularly diets that involve fasting or are severely restrictive may differ from the general RA population. Patients participating in a study of fasting/vegetarian diet have been reported to believe more in "alternative" treatments and less in "standard" medical treatments, have a higher perceived ability to control their own health and a lower perception that chance affected their health and response to treatment than non-study participants. Furthermore, study participants who responded to the diet believed less in ordinary medical treatment than the nonresponders [45]. While these data suggest that psychological factors do indeed play a role, one would not usually expect clinical improvements to last for such an extended period of time (12 months) if this was the sole explanation.

Patients who are prepared to take part in dietary studies have been reported to have shorter disease duration and less steroid and DMARD therapy suggesting milder disease compared to a group of non-study participants [45].

Weight loss

In the majority of dietary studies in RA, weight loss has been observed despite the dietary protocols aiming to be isocaloric. In general, weight loss per se has not been associated with improved disease control [33, 37]. However, significant associations between reduction in body mass index and reduction in swollen joint count [46] and between weight loss and improved grip strength [29] have been reported. Analysis of data from three studies of lacto-vegetarian, vegan, or Mediterranean diets suggests that weight loss per se does contribute to the observed improvements in disease control [47].

Alterations in proinflammatory cytokines

A number of proinflammatory cytokines including interleukin (IL)-1, IL-6, and tumor necrosis factor (TNF) are important in the inflammation and tissue destruction observed in RA. A significant reduction in IL-6, along with a decrease in ESR and CRP has been observed after a 7-day fast in 10 patients with RA [48].

Biological therapies that block TNF or IL-1β activities have been shown to reduce disease activity and prevent joint damage in RA [49, 50]. In RA patients challenged with foods which had previously resulted in a positive SPT, serum TNF and IL-1β concentrations increased along with an increase in clinical disease activity [51] suggesting that food allergy may be a triggering rather than a causative factor in RA.

Alterations in dietary fatty acid composition

Dietary polyunsaturated fatty acids (PUFA) are subject to remodeling and incorporated into cell membrane phospholipids. The C20 PUFAs are released from cell membranes by phospholipase A_2 and can be metabolized to inflammatory lipid mediators known as eicosanoids (prostaglandins (PG) and leukotrienes (LT)). The omega-6 fatty acid, linoleic acid (LA) is converted to arachidonic acid (AA), the precursor for the proinflammatory eicosanoids PGE_2, PGI_2, thromboxane $(TX)A_2$, and $(LT)B_4$ (Figure 45.1). In comparison, the omega-3 fatty acid, α-linoleic acid (ALA), can be converted in a limited way to eicosapentaneoic acid (EPA). EPA is a substrate inhibitor of AA metabolism to eicosanoids and EPA itself can be converted to the three series eicosanoids (PGE_3, TXA_3, PGI_3, LTB_5), which are generally less inflammatory than the AA-derived eicosanoids (Figure 45.1). The limited conversion of ALA to EPA within the context of a Western diet has led to the use of dietary supplements of EPA-rich fish oils as a means of achieving anti-inflammatory effects. Alteration of dietary fatty acids may therefore modulate inflammatory disease expression (discussed further in section of omega-3 fatty acids).

After a one-week fast, the relative proportion of both AA and EPA has been shown to increase in serum and platelets. Although the increase in AA and EPA was small in neutrophils, there was a reduction in LTB_4 release from stimulated neutrophils *ex vivo* [41]. While plasma AA concentrations have been shown to decrease in patients on a vegan diet, concentrations returned to baseline values when the diet was changed to lacto-vegetarian. In comparison, EPA decreased with both the vegan and lacto-vegetarian diets [52]. However, fatty acid concentrations were no different between diet responders and nonresponders, suggesting that other mechanisms must be responsible for the observed benefits of such diets [52].

Alterations in intestinal microbial flora

The intestine is a rich source of microbes and the balance of microbes present contributes to an individual's overall health. Changes in intestinal microbial flora are believed to contribute to many chronic diseases [53]. Patients with RA have a high carriage rate of *Clostridium perfringens* compared to healthy controls and patients with active RA had significantly higher *Clostridia* counts compared to those with inactive disease [54]. Genetic variations in the way individuals respond to normal gut flora may also contribute. *Proteus mirabilis*, a normal bowel commensal, contains an amino acid sequence similar to that found in the "shared epitope" and patients with RA have higher titres of antibodies directed against this sequence compared to healthy controls [55]. Patients with active RA have higher concentrations of anti-*Proteus* antibodies compared to patients with inactive-RA, healthy controls, and healthy HLA-identical same-sexed siblings [56].

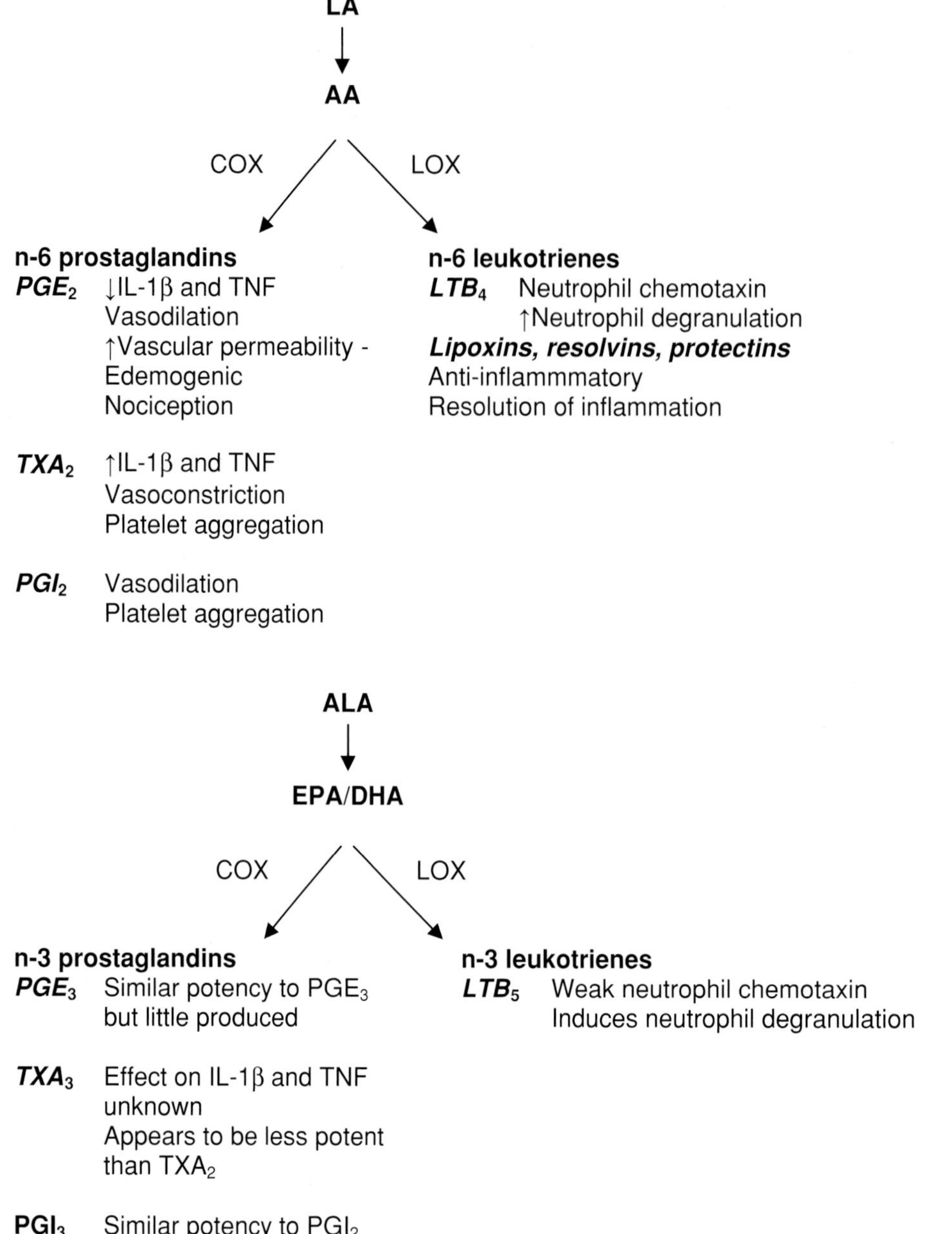

Figure 45.1 Metabolism of LA and ALA.

The diet can have a significant impact on fecal microbial flora and may thus provide a mechanism for alterations in disease activity. In RA patients who fasted for 7–10 days followed by 1-year vegetarian diet, there was a significant reduction in anti-*Proteus* antibodies, which was greater in those patients who responded to the dietary therapy. Furthermore, a correlation was seen between reduced antibody levels and the extent of reduction in disease activity [57]. Alterations in fecal microbial flora which correlate with improvements in disease activity have also been observed in patients on a vegan diet, although individual organisms could not be identified with the method employed [58]. However, in a more recent study, neither fasting for 8 days nor a 2-week vegetarian Mediterranean diet altered fecal bacterial counts despite a significant reduction in the DAS28 score in the fasting group [59].

Altered intestinal permeability and gut antigen handling

The gastrointestinal epithelium is a complex structure which allows entry of essential nutrients while at the same time providing a critical barrier which prevents antigens in the lumen gaining access to the circulation. Abnormal intestinal permeability may have a role in the pathogenesis of autoimmune disorders [60]. In a study of five patients with RA, fasting decreased intestinal permeability and was accompanied by improved disease control. When patients were commenced on a lacto-vegetarian diet, intestinal permeability and disease activity both increased [61]. Although limited, such data suggest that alterations in intestinal permeability, which allows increased entry of "arthritogenic" pathogens may have a role in RA.

In addition to providing a physical barrier, the gut has a highly developed immune system (mucosa associated lymphoid tissue (MALT)), that protects the host from potentially harmful pathogens, while simultaneously "tolerating" or allowing entry of "beneficial" antigens. MALT has a preference for production of IgA, in particular, secretory IgA, which is released into the gut lumen where it binds and prevents antigens from attaching to intestinal cells and gaining entry. In patients with RA and healthy controls, short-term fasting has been reported to enhance mucosal antigen-specific B cell responses but not systemic immune responses [62]. Thus activation of the mucosal immune system may not be reflected in the serum. In comparison to healthy controls, patients with RA had significantly increased concentrations of IgM in jejunal fluid. While there was an increase in IgA and IgG concentrations this did not reach statistical significance. The activities of jejunal IgA, IgM, and IgG antibodies against a variety of different food antigens were also increased. The authors suggest that mucosal immune activation is important in the pathogenesis of RA, at least in some patients, and that apparent food intolerance may reflect the additive effect of hypersensitivity reactions [63].

Dietary omega-3 supplementation and RA

Omega (n)-3 fatty acids, which are abundant in fish and fish oils, have been shown to have a beneficial effect in patients with both early [64] and long-standing RA when combined with standard DMARD therapies [65]. For maximal benefits of n-3 supplementation to be achieved, the background diet should be low in competitor n-6 fatty acids [66]. Only one study has examined the effects of a diet containing hypoallergenic foods as well as being high in mono- and PUFA and low in saturated fatty acids. In this 24-week, double-blind, randomized, controlled study, 50 patients with RA were randomized to the experimental diet or a balanced control diet. In the experimental diet group, modest improvements were observed in all clinical variables although only ESR and tender joint count improved significantly [67]. The relative contributions of fatty acids and hypoallergenic foods to the outcomes could not be distinguished.

Like most of the DMARDs, there is a latent period of 6–12 weeks before benefits of n-3 supplements are observed and it is important that patients appreciate the lack of immediate effect when they commence n-3 supplements. The latent period can be shortened with use of higher doses [68–71].

Dietary supplementation with n-3 fatty acids has been shown reduce NSAID requirements [72, 73]. NSAIDs are associated with gastrointestinal toxicity and may contribute to an increase in risk of cardiovascular disease. Furthermore, NSAIDs alter the ratio of TXA_2/PGE_2 in favor of TXA_2, which increases monocyte production of the proinflammatory cytokines IL-1β and TNF [74]. Thus the reduction in NSAID requirement associated with n-3 supplementation has a number of additional benefits including reduction in cardiovascular and gastrointestinal risk and potentially less joint damage.

The dose of n-3 fatty acids (EPA + DHA) required for the anti-inflammatory effect is 2.7 gm/day, which equates to at least nine standard fish oil capsules daily. Perhaps a more efficient way of ingesting sufficient n-3 fatty acids is through bottled fish oil. Fifteen milliliters of fish oil, taken on fruit juice is for many patients easier to consume than large numbers of capsules and is significantly cheaper (~45c/day compared to ~$3.00/day for capsules). EPA + DHA comprise approximately 30% w/w of standard fish oil. Double and triple strength fish oils are now available in capsules and double strength bottled fish is also available. The fatty acids excluded from fish oil in EPA + DHA concentrates, are harmless nutrients, and unless a patient is fat intolerant, the extra expense involved is considerable relative to the convenience of smaller capsule numbers or lower volumes of medicinal fish oil required to achieve an anti-inflammatory dose of EPA + DHA.

Anti-inflammatory mechanisms of n-3 fatty acids

Fish and fish oils are rich in the n-3 long chain fatty acids EPA (20:5 n-3) and DHA (22:5 n-3). EPA and DHA can be incorporated into cell membranes and tissues and may displace the n-6 derived AA (20:4 n-6). These n-3 and n-6 fatty acids are released from cell membranes and are metabolized by cyclooxygense or lipoxygenase and the terminal synthases to the eicosanoids and leukotrienes respectively (Figure 45.1). In general the n-6 derived eicosanoids (PGE_2, TXA_2, PGI_2, LTB_4) are more pro-inflammatory than their n-3 derived counterparts (PGE_3, TXA_3, PGI_3, LTB_5). In humans, dietary supplementation with n-3 fatty acids has been shown to reduce production of PGE_2 [75, 76], TXA_2 [76], and LTB_4 [77] and increase production of TXA_3 [78] and LTB_5 [79]. DHA can be converted to C22 oxylipids, which also have anti-inflammatory properties. n-3 fatty acids have also been shown to decrease production of IL-1β and TNF-α in both healthy subjects and patients with RA [70, 75, 76, 80, 81].

EPA and DHA can be metabolized by multiple lipoxygenases to trihydroxymetabolites, known as lipoxins, resolvins, and protectins, which have been shown to be active in resolving inflammation in animal models [82]. The potential importance of these mediators, derived from EPA and DHA, for the control of human inflammatory diseases remains to be established.

Matrix metalloproteinases (MMPs) have a pivotal role in cartilage degradation and bone erosion in RA. *In vitro* studies have demonstrated that n-3 fatty acids can suppress MMP expression and reduce proteoglycan degradation in IL-1 stimulated bovine chondrocytes [83]. Thus n-3 fatty acids may have the ability to reduce cartilage damage in inflamed joints.

As discussed above, HLA-DR is strongly expressed on APCs and present antigen to T cells. *In vitro*, the n-3 fatty acids EPA and/or DHA reduce monocyte expression of HLA-DR and HLA-DP molecules [84] and reduce the ability of monocytes to present antigen to autologous lymphocytes [85]. In RA, one could speculate that n-3 fatty acids may inhibit APC function and suppress pathogenic T cell activation, thereby reducing disease activity.

Cardiovascular risk in RA and the benefits of n-3 supplements

Patients with RA have an increased risk of death with a standardized mortality ratio of ~2 and most excess deaths are attributable to cardiovascular and cerebrovascular diseases [86]. There is no increase in traditional cardiovascular risk factors in patients to explain the observed increase [87]. The inflammatory process as well as use of NSAIDs may contribute to the increase in risk [88]. In both primary and secondary prevention studies, n-3 fatty acid supplementation has been shown to reduce cardiovascular mortality [89]. To date there have been no studies examining whether n-3 fatty acid supplementation reduces cardiovascular morbidity and mortality in RA. However, a recent study has shown that patients with early RA taking n-3 fatty acid supplementation have lower triglycerides, increased "good" HDL cholesterol, lower CRP, less NSAID use, greater disease suppression, and reduced platelet synthesis of TXA_2 compared to patients not taking fish oil [64]. All of these factors would be expected to reduce cardiovascular risk.

Potential side effects of n-3 supplements

The most common adverse effects of n-3 fatty acid supplements are a fishy after-taste, gastrointestinal upset, and nausea. In general, these adverse effects are mild and can be controlled by taking the supplement with food. Fish can contain toxins, including methylmercury, polychlorinated biphenyls, and dioxins which would accumulate in humans who consume contaminated fish on a regular basis. These toxins are in general reduced to acceptable limits in readily available commercial fish oils during processing.

Probiotics for the treatment of arthritis

Probiotics are live microorganisms that can confer health benefits when administered in adequate amounts. While probiotics may be widely used, the evidence for benefit based on randomized controlled clinical trials is small and their use is the subject of ongoing evaluation.

In studies of patients with arthritis results vary depending on the specific probiotic administered. For example, *Lactobacillus rhamnosus* has been reported to have no effect on disease activity in a small study of 21 patients with RA, while *Bacillus coagulans* GBI-30 supplements led to improvements in pain and patient global scores in 45 patients with RA, compared to placebo [90]. Thus, while theoretical considerations and empirical data provide some support for use of probiotics in RA, the evidence is not sufficient to recommend routine use.

Summary

Dietary restriction may prove useful in controlling RA in suitably motivated patients. Difficulties encountered in sustaining exclusion and other rigorous diets militate against a general application. By contrast, dietary fish in appropriate doses is relatively easy to take as a dietary additive. The preferred method is to take bottled fish oil on juice with the two-glass technique (quickly swallow 15 mL of fish oil layered on juice, then begin slowly sipping a juice chaser immediately, followed by food). This is the least expensive and most convenient way to achieve an anti-inflammatory dose of fish oil, since the equivalent dose of capsules is 14×1000 mg capsules. The symptomatic benefits of fish oil are delayed until the second or third month of treatment and include reduced reliance on NSAIDs, which carry risk for serious gastrointestinal and cardiovascular events. Fish oil in the long term also improves disease control and remission rates with DMARD therapy. There are thus two contrasting approaches, which are not mutually exclusive: elimination of candidate food allergens and arthritogens, while maintaining balance in the diet otherwise, and ingestion of increased amounts of the n-3 fatty acids EPA and DHA in essentially pharmacological, anti-inflammatory doses as a dietary supplement.

The latter approach is generally applicable, while the former in practice may be best applied in those who are well disposed to dietary avoidance strategies.

Appendix

ACR 20 response: [91]

20% improvement in five out of the seven core set variables, first two required
tender joint count;
swollen joint count;
acute phase reactant;
patient's pain;
patient's global assessment of disease activity;
physician's global assessment of disease activity;
physical disability.

Disease Activity Score (DAS) 28: [92]

$$\begin{aligned}\text{DAS28} = {} & (0.56\sqrt{(28\ \text{tender joint count})} \\ & + 0.28\sqrt{(28\ \text{swollen joint count})} \\ & + 0.70 \times \ln(\text{ESR}))1.08 + 0.16\end{aligned}$$

References

1. Golding D. Is there an allergic synovitis? *J Royal Soc Med* 1990; 83:312–314.
2. Choi H, Liu S, Curhan G. Intake of purine-rich foods, protein, and dairy products and relationship to serum levels of uric acid. *Arthritis Rheum* 2005; 52(1):283–289.
3. Salminen E, Heikkila S, Poussa T, et al. Female patients tend to alter their diet following the diagnosis of rheumatoid arthritis and breast cancer. *Preventative Med* 2002; 34(5):529–535.
4. Shapiro JA, Koepsell TD, Voigt LF, Dugowson CE, Kestin M, Nelson JL. Diet and rheumatoid arthritis in women: a possible protective effect of fish consumption. *Epidemiology* 1996; 7(3):256–263.
5. Pattison D, Symmons D, Lunt M, et al. Dietary β-cryptoxanthin and inflammatory polyarthritis: results from a population-based prospective study. *Am J Clin Nutr* 2005; 82: 451–455.
6. Pattison D, Symmons D, Lunt M, et al. Dietary risk factors for the development of inflammatory polyarthritis: evidence for a high level of red meat consumption. *Arthritis Rheum* 2004; 50(12):3804–3812.
7. Grant W. The role of red meat in the expression of rheumatoid arthritis. *Br J Nutr* 2000; 84:589–595.
8. Pedersen M, Stripp C, Klarlund M, Olsen S, Tjonneland A, Frisch M. Diet and risk of rheumatoid arthritis in a prospective cohort. *J Rheumatol* 2005; 32(7):1249–1252.
9. Mikuls T, Cerhan J, Criswell L, et al. Coffee, tea, and caffeine consumption and risk of rheumatoid arthritis. *Arthritis Rheum* 2002; 46(1):83–91.
10. Heliovaara M, Aho K, Knekt P, Impivaara O, Reunanen A, Aromaa A. Coffee consumption, rheumatoid factor, and the risk of rheumatoid arthritis. *Ann Rheum Dis* 2000; 59: 631–635.
11. Karlson E, Mandl L, Aweh G, Grodstein F. Coffee consumption and risk of rheumatoid arthritis. *Arthritis Rheum* 2003; 48(11):3055–3060.
12. Panush RS. Food induced (allergic) arthritis: clinical and serological studies. *J Rheumatol* 1990; 17(3):291–294.
13. Aho K, Koskenvuo M, Tuominen J, Kaprio J. Occurrence of rheumatoid arthritis in a nationwide series of twins. *J Rheumatol* 1986; 13(5):899–902.
14. Silman A, MacGregor A, Thomson W, et al. Twin concordance rates for rheumatoid arthritis: results from a nationwide study. *Br J Rheumatol* 1993; 32:903–907.
15. MacGregor A, Snieder H, Rigby A, et al. Characterizing the quantitative genetic contribution to rheumatoid arthritis using data from twins. *Arthritis Rheum* 2000; 43(1): 30–37.
16. Gregersen P, Silver J, Winchester R. The shared epitope hypothesis: an approach to understanding the molecular genetics of susceptibility to rheumatoid arthritis. *Arthritis Rheum* 1987; 30(11):1205–1213.
17. Lunardi C, Bambara L, Biasi D, et al. Food allergy and rheumatoid arthritis. *Clin Exp Rheumatol* 1988; 6:423–425.
18. Parke AL, Hughes GRV. Rheumatoid arthritis and food: a case study. *Br Med J* 1981; 282:2027–2029.
19. Williams R. Rheumatoid arthritis and food: a case study [Letter]. *Br Med J* 1981; 283:563.
20. Pacor M, Lunardi C, Di Lorenzo G, Biasi D, Corrocher R. Food allergy and seronegative arthritis: a report of two cases. *Clin Rheumatol* 2001; 20:279–281.
21. Panush RS, Stroud RM, Webster EM. Food-induced (allergic) arthritis: inflammatory arthritis exacerbated by milk. *Arthritis Rheum* 1986; 29(2):220–226.
22. Ratner D, Eshel E, Vigder K. Juvenile rheumatoid arthritis and milk allergy. *J Royal Soc Med* 1985; 78:410–413.
23. Schrander J, Marcelis C, de Vries R, Van Santen-Hoeufft H. Does food intolerance play a role in juvenile chronic arthritis? *Br J Rheumatol* 1997; 36:905–908.
24. Kutlu A, Öztürk S, Taşkapan O, Önem Y, Kiralp M, Özçakar L. Meat-induced joint attacks, or meat attacks the joint: rheumatism versus allergy. *Nutr Clin Prac* 2010; 25(1):90–91.
25. van der Laar MA, Aalbers M, Bruins F, van Dinther-Janssen A, van der Korst JK, Meijer C. Food intolerance in rheumatoid arthritis. II. Clinical and histologic aspects. *Ann Rheum Dis* 1992; 51:303–306.
26. Liden M, Kristjannsson G, Valtysdottir S, Venge P, Hallgren R. Self-reported food intolerance and mucosal reactivity after rectal food protein challenge in patients with rheumatoid arthritis. *Scand J Rheumatol* 2010; 39:292–298.
27. Haugen M, Kjeldsen-Kragh J, Forre O. A pilot study of the effect of an elemental diet in the management of rheumatoid arthritis. *Clin Exp Rheumatol* 1994; 12:275–279.
28. Holst-Jensen SE, Pfeiffer-Jensen M, Monsrud M, et al. Treatment of rheumatoid arthritis with a peptide diet: a randomized, controlled trial. *Scand J Rheumatol* 1998; 27: 329–336.

29. Kavanagh R, Workman E, Nash P, Smith M, Hazleman B, Hunter J. The effects of elemental diet and subsequent food reintroduction on rheumatoid arthritis. *Br J Rheumatol* 1995; 34:270–273.
30. Ziff M. Diet in the treatment of rheumatoid arthritis. *Arthritis Rheum* 1983; 26(4):457–461.
31. Panush R, Carter R, Katz P, Kowsari B, Longley S, Finnie S. Diet therapy for rheumatoid arthritis. *Arthritis Rheum* 1983; 26(4):462–471.
32. van der Laar MA, van der Korst JK. Food intolerance in rheumatoid arthritis. I. A double blind, controlled trial of the clinical effects of elimination of milk allergens and azo dyes. *Ann Rheum Dis* 1992; 51:298–302.
33. Darlington LG, Ramsey NW, Mansfield JR. Placebo-controlled, blind study of dietary manipulation therapy in rheumatoid arthritis. *Lancet* 1986; 1:236–238.
34. Beri D, Malaviya AN, Shandilya R, Singh RR. Effect of dietary restrictions on disease activity in rheumatoid arthritis. *Ann Rheum Dis* 1988; 47(1):69–72.
35. Karatay S, Erdem T, Kiziltunc A, et al. General or personal diet: the individualized model for diet challenges in patients with rheumatoid arthritis. *Rheumatol Int* 2006; 26: 556–560.
36. Hafstrom I, Ringertz B, Spangberg A, et al. A vegan diet free of gluten improves the signs and symptoms of rheumatoid arthritis: the effects on arthritis correlate with a reduction in antibodies to food antigens. *Rheumatology* 2001; 40(10):1175–1179.
37. Kjeldsen-Kragh J, Borchgrevink C, Mowinkel P, et al. Controlled trial of fasting and one-year vegetarian diet in rheumatoid arthritis. *Lancet* 1991; 338(8772):899–902.
38. Kjeldsen-Kragh, Hvatum M, Haugen M, Forre O, Scott H. Antibodies against dietary antigens in rheumatoid arthritis patients treated with fasting and one-year vegetarian diet. *Clin Exp Rheumatol* 1995; 13:167–172.
39. McDougall J, Bruce B, Spiller G, Westerdahl J, McDougall M. Effects of a very low-fat vegan diet in subjects with rheumatoid arthritis. *J Altern Complement Med* 2002; 8(1): 71–75.
40. Skoldstam L, Larsson L, Lindstrom F. Effects of fasting and lactovegetarian diet on rheumatoid arthritis. *Scand J Rheumatol* 1979; 8:249–255.
41. Hafstrom I, Ringertz B, Gyllenhammar H, Palmblad J, Harms-Ringdahl M. Effects of fasting on disease activity, neutrophil function, fatty acid composition, and leukotriene biosynthesis in patients with rheumatoid arthritis. *Arthritis Rheum* 1988; 31(5):585–592.
42. Uden A-M, Trang L, Venizelos N, Palmblad J. Neutrophil functions and clinical performance after total fasting in patients with rheumatoid arthritis. *Ann Rheum Dis* 1983; 42:45–51.
43. Walsmith J, Abad L, Kehayias J, Roubenoff R. Tumor necrosis factor-α is associated with less body mass in women with rheumatoid arthritis. *J Rheumatol* 2004; 31(1):23–29.
44. Rall L, Roubenoff R. Rheumatoid cachexia: metabolic abnormalities, mechanisms and interventions. *Rheumatology* 2004; 43:1219–1223.
45. Kjeldsen-Kragh J, Haugen M, Forre O, Laache H, Malt UF. Vegetarian diet for patients with rheumatoid arthritis: can the clinical effects be explained by the psychological characteristics of the patients? *Br J Rheumatol* 1994; 33: 569–575.
46. Hansen GV, Nielsen L, Kluger E, et al. Nutritional status of Danish rheumatoid arthritis patients and effects of a diet adjusted in energy intake, fish-meal, and antioxidants. *Scand J Rheumatol* 1996; 25(5):325–330.
47. Skoldstam L, Brudin L, Hagfors L, Johansson G. Weight reduction is not a major reason for improvement in rheumatoid arthritis from lacto-vegetarian, vegan or Mediterranean diets. *Nutr J* 2005; 4:15–21.
48. Fraser D, Thoen J, Djoseland O, Forre O, Kjeldsen-Kragh J. Serum levels of interleukin-6 and dehydroepiandrosterone sulphate in response to either fasting or a ketogenic diet in rheumatoid arthritis patients. *Clin Exp Rheumatol* 2000; 18: 357–362.
49. Keystone EC, Kavanagh AF, Sharp J, et al. Radiographic, clinical, and functional outcomes of treatment with Adalimumab (a human anti-tumor necrosis factor monoclonal antibody) in patients with active rheumatoid arthritis receiving methotrexate therapy. *Arthritis Rheum* 2004; 50(5):1400–1411.
50. Dayer J-M, Feige U, Edwards C, Burger D. Anti-interleukin-1 therapy in rheumatic diseases. *Curr Opin Rheumatol* 2001; 13: 170–176.
51. Karatay S, Erdem T, Yildirim K, et al. The effect of individualized diet challenges consisting of allergenic foods on TNF-α and IL-1β levels in patients with rheumatoid arthritis. *Rheumatology* 2004; 43:1429–1433.
52. Haugen MA, Kjeldsen-Kragh J, Bjerve KS, Hostmark AT, Forre O. Changes in plasma phospholipid fatty acids and their relationship to disease activity in rheumatoid arthritis patients treated with a vegetarian diet. *Br J Nutr* 1994; 72(4):555–566.
53. Hawrelak J, Meyers S. The causes of intestinal dysbiosis: a review. *Altern Med Rev* 2004; 9(2):180–197.
54. Shinebaum R, Neumann VC, Cooke EM, Wright V. Comparison of faecal florae in patients with rheumatoid arthritis and controls. *Br J Rheumatol* 1987; 26:329–333.
55. Wilson C, Ebringer A, Ahmadi K, et al. Shared amino acid sequences between major histocompatibility complex class II glycoproteins, type XI collagen and *Proteus mirabilis* in rheumatoid arthritis. *Ann Rheum Dis* 1995; 54:216–220.
56. Deighton C, Gray J, Bint A, Walker D. Anti-*Proteus* antibodies in rheumatoid arthritis same-sexed sibships. *Br J Rheumatol* 1992; 31:241–245.
57. Kjeldsen-Kragh J, Rashid T, Dybwad A, et al. Decrease in anti-*Proteus mirabilis* but not anti-*Escherichia coli* antibody levels in rheumatoid arthritis patients treated with fasting and a one year vegetarian diet. *Ann Rheum Dis* 1995; 54:221–224.
58. Peltonen R, Nenonen M, Helve T, Hanninen O, Toivanen P, Eerola E. Faecal microbial flora and disease activity in rheumatoid arthritis during a vegan diet. *Br J Rheumatol* 1997; 36:64–68.

59. Michalsen A, Riegert M, Ludtke R, et al. Mediterranean diet or extended fasting's influence on changing the intestinal microflora, immunoglobulin A secretion and clinical outcome in patients with rheumatoid arthritis and fibromyalgia: an observational study. *BMC Complement Altern Med* 2005; 5: 22–31.
60. Arrieta M, Bistritz L, Meddings J. Alterations in intestinal permeability. *Gut* 2006; 55:1512–1520.
61. Sundqvist T, Lindstrom F, Magnusson K, Skoldstam L, Stjernstrom I, Tagesson C. Influence of fasting on intestinal permeability and disease activity in patients with rheumatoid arthritis. *Scand J Rheumatol* 1982; 11:33–38.
62. Trollmo C, Verdrengh M, Tarkowski A. Fasting enhances mucosal antigen specific B cell responses in rheumatoid arthritis. *Ann Rheum Dis* 1997; 56:130–134.
63. Hvatum M, Kanerud L, Hallgren R, Brandtzaeg P. The gut-joint axis: cross reactive food antibodies in rheumatoid arthritis. *Gut* 2006; 55:1240–1247.
64. Cleland L, Caughey G, James M, Proudman S. Reduction of cardiovascular risk factors with long-term fish oil treatment in early rheumatoid arthritis. *J Rheumatol* 2006; 33(10):1973–1979.
65. Stamp LK, James M, Cleland L. Diet and rheumatoid arthritis: a review of the literature. *Semin Arthritis Rheum* 2005; 35:77–94.
66. Adam O, Beringer C, Kless T, et al. Anti-inflammatory effects of a low arachidonic acid diet and fish oil in patients with rheumatoid arthritis. *Rheumatol Int* 2003; 23:27–36.
67. Sarzi-Puttini P, Comi D, Boccassini L, et al. Diet therapy for rheumatoid arthritis. A controlled double-blind study of two different dietary regimens. *Scand J Rheumatol* 2000; 29(5):302–307.
68. Cleland LG, French JK, Betts WH, Murphy GA, Elliott MJ. Clinical and biochemical effects of dietary fish oil supplements in rheumatoid arthritis. *J Rheumatol* 1988; 15(10):1471–1475.
69. Volker D, Fitzgerald P, Major G, Garg M. Efficacy of fish oil concentrate in the treatment of rheumatoid arthritis. *J Rheumatol* 2000; 27(10):2343–2346.
70. Kremer JM, Lawrence DA, Jubiz W, et al. Dietary fish oil and olive oil supplementation in patients with rheumatoid arthritis. *Arthritis Rheum* 1990; 33(6):810–819.
71. Leeb B, Sautner J, Andel I, Rintelen B. Intravenous application of omega-3 fatty acids in patients with active rheumatoid arthritis. The ORA-1 trial. An open pilot study. *Lipids* 2006; 41(1):29–34.
72. Skoldstam L, Borjesson O, Kjallman A, Seiving B, Akesson B. Effect of six months of fish oil supplementation in stable rheumatoid arthritis. A double-blind, controlled study. *Scand J Rheumatol* 1992; 21(4):178–185.
73. Kjeldsen-Kragh J, Lund JA, Riise T, et al. Dietary omega-3 fatty acid supplementation and naproxen treatment in patients with rheumatoid arthritis. *J Rheumatol* 1992; 19(10): 1531–1536.
74. Penglis P, Cleland LG, Demasi M, Caughey GE, James MJ. Differential regulation of prostaglandin E_2 and thromboxane A_2 production in human monocytes: implications for the use of cyclooxygenase inhibitors. *J Immunol* 2000; 165:1605–1611.
75. Endres S, Ghorbani R, Kelley V, et al. The effect of dietary supplementation with n-3 polyunsaturated fatty acids on the synthesis of interleukin-1 and tumor necrosis factor by mononuclear cells. *N Engl J Med* 1989; 320(5):265–271.
76. Caughey GE, Mantzioris E, Gibson RA, Cleland LG, James MJ. The effect on human tumor necrosis factor-α and interleukin-1β production of diets enriched in n-3 fatty acids from vegetable oil or fish oil. *Am J Clin Nutr* 1996; 63:116–122.
77. Lee TH, Hoover RL, Williams JD, et al. Effect of dietary enrichment with eicosapentaenoic and docosahexaenoic acids on in vitro neutrophil and monocyte and leucocyte leukotriene generation and neutrophil function. *N Engl J Med* 1985; 312(19):1217–1224.
78. Fischer S, Weber P. Thromboxane A_3 is formed in human platelets after dietary eicosapentaenoic acid. *Biochem Biophys Res Comm* 1983; 116(3):1091–1099.
79. Sperling RI, Benincaso A, Knoell C, Larkin J, Austen K, Robinson D. Dietary omega-3 polyunsaturated fatty acids inhibit phosphoinositide formation and chemotaxis in neutrophils. *J Clin Invest* 1993; 91:651–660.
80. Molvig J, Pociot F, Worsaae H, et al. Dietary supplementation with omega-3 polyunsaturated fatty acids decreases mononuclear cell proliferation and interleukin-1β content but not monokine secretion in healthy and insulin-dependent diabetic individuals. *Scand J Immunol* 1991; 34(4):399–410.
81. Meydani SN, Endres S, Woods M, et al. Oral (n-3) fatty acid supplementation suppresses cytokine production and lymphocyte proliferation: comparison between young and older women. *J Nutr* 1991; 121(4):547–555.
82. Charles N, Serhan C, Nan Chiang N, Van Dyke T. Resolving inflammation: dual anti-inflammatory and pro-resolution lipid mediators. *Nat Rev Immunol* 2008; 8:349–361.
83. Curtis C, Rees S, Little C, et al. Pathological indicators of degradation and inflammation in human osteoarthritis cartilage are abrogated by exposure to n-3 fatty acids. *Arthritis Rheum* 2002; 46(6):1544–1553.
84. Hughes DA, Southon S, Pinder A. (n-3) Polyunsaturated fatty acids modulate the expression of functionally associated molecules on human monocytes in vitro. *J Nutr* 1996; 126:603–610.
85. Hughes DA, Pinder AC. n-3 Polyunsaturated fatty acids inhibit the antigen-presenting function of human monocytes. *Am J Clin Nutr* 2000; 71(Suppl.):357S–360S.
86. Wolfe F, Mitchell D, Sibley J, et al. The mortality of rheumatoid arthritis. *Arthritis Rheum* 1994; 37(4):481–494.
87. Solomon D, Curhan G, Rimm E, Cannuscio C, Karlson E. Cardiovascular risk factors in women with and without rheumatoid arthritis. *Arthritis Rheum* 2004; 50(11):3444–3449.
88. van Doornum S, Jennings G, Wicks I. Reducing the cardiovascular disease burden in rheumatoid arthritis. *Med J Aust* 2006; 184(6):287–290.
89. Wang C, Harris WS, Chung M, et al. n-3 Fatty acids from fish or fish-oil supplements, but not α-linoleic acid, benefit

cardiovascular disease outcomes in primary- and secondary-prevention studies: a systematic review. *Am J Clin Nutr* 2006; 84:5–17.

90. Mandel D, Eichas K, Holmes J. Bacillus coagulans: a viable adjunct therapy for relieving symptoms of rheumatoid arthritis according to a randomized, controlled trial. *BMC Complement Altern Med* 2010; 10(1).

91. Felson D, Anderson J, Boers M, et al. The American College of Rheumatology preliminary definition of improvement in rheumatoid arthritis. *Arthritis Rheum* 1995; 38:727–735.

92. Prevoo M, van't Hof M, van Leeuwen M, Van de Putte L, Van Riel P. Modified disease activity scores that include twenty-eight-joint counts. *Arthritis Rheum* 1995; 38(1):44–48.

46 Approaches to Therapy in Development

Anna Nowak-Węgrzyn[1,3] & Hugh A. Sampson[2,3]

[1]Division of Pediatric Allergy and Immunology
[2]Translational Biomedical Sciences
[3]Jaffe Food Allergy Institute Department of Pediatrics, Icahn School of Medicine at Mount Sinai, New York, NY, USA

Key Concepts

- Current management of food allergy relies on strict dietary avoidance, nutritional counseling, and emergency treatment of adverse reactions.
- Immunotherapy for food allergy remains an investigational procedure.
- Novel immunotherapeutic approaches for food allergy that are antigen-specific include oral, sublingual, and epicutaneous immunotherapy (desensitization) with native food allergens, and mutated recombinant proteins of reduced IgE-binding ability, co-administered within heat-killed *Escherichia coli.*
- Diets including baked milk or egg are tolerated by the majority (>70%) of the milk- and egg-allergic children and appear to accelerate development of tolerance to unheated milk and egg compared to strict dietary avoidance of these foods.
- Nonspecific immunotherapeutic approaches in clinical trials include monoclonal anti-IgE antibodies, which may increase the threshold dose for food allergen in food-allergic adults, and a Chinese herbal formulation, FAHF-2.

Food allergy has become a major public health problem in modern societies with a Western lifestyle [1, 2]. Strict dietary avoidance, nutritional counseling, and emergency treatment of adverse reactions remain the cornerstones of therapy [3]. Here we focus on novel approaches to therapy for IgE-mediated food allergy. First attempts to orally desensitize food-allergic patients were reported more than 100 years ago [4], but to date there are no therapies proven to accelerate the development of oral tolerance or to provide effective protection from accidental exposures [5]. Among the most promising allergen-specific approaches are oral, sublingual, and epicutaneous immunotherapy (desensitization) with native food allergens, and mutated recombinant proteins of reduced IgE-binding ability, coadministered within heat-killed *Escherichia coli* to generate maximum immune response (Figure 46.1). In most children with milk and egg allergy, diets including baked milk or egg are well tolerated, and appear to accelerate resolution of milk and egg allergy in an allergen-specific approach. Nonspecific approaches in clinical trials include monoclonal anti-IgE antibodies, which may increase the threshold dose for food allergen in food-allergic adults, and a Chinese herbal formulation, FAHF-2.

Immunotherapeutic approaches for treating food allergy

Food-allergic patients can be classified into three basic phenotypes: transient food-allergic, persistent food-allergic, and pollen-food (oral allergy) syndrome (Table 46.1) [1]. Each of these forms of IgE-mediated food allergy is the result of a different immunologic mechanism and therefore likely to require different approach to bring about resolution. Novel therapies primarily target foods that induce severe anaphylaxis (peanut, tree nuts, shellfish) or are most common in children, such as cow's milk and hen's egg.

Allergen-specific immunotherapy

Baked milk and egg diet

Children with transient egg and milk allergy generate IgE antibodies directed primarily against conformational epitopes that are altered during extensive heating or food processing [6, 7]. Two large clinical trials investigated the

Food Allergy: Adverse Reactions to Foods and Food Additives, Fifth Edition. Edited by Dean D Metcalfe, Hugh A Sampson, Ronald A Simon and Gideon Lack.

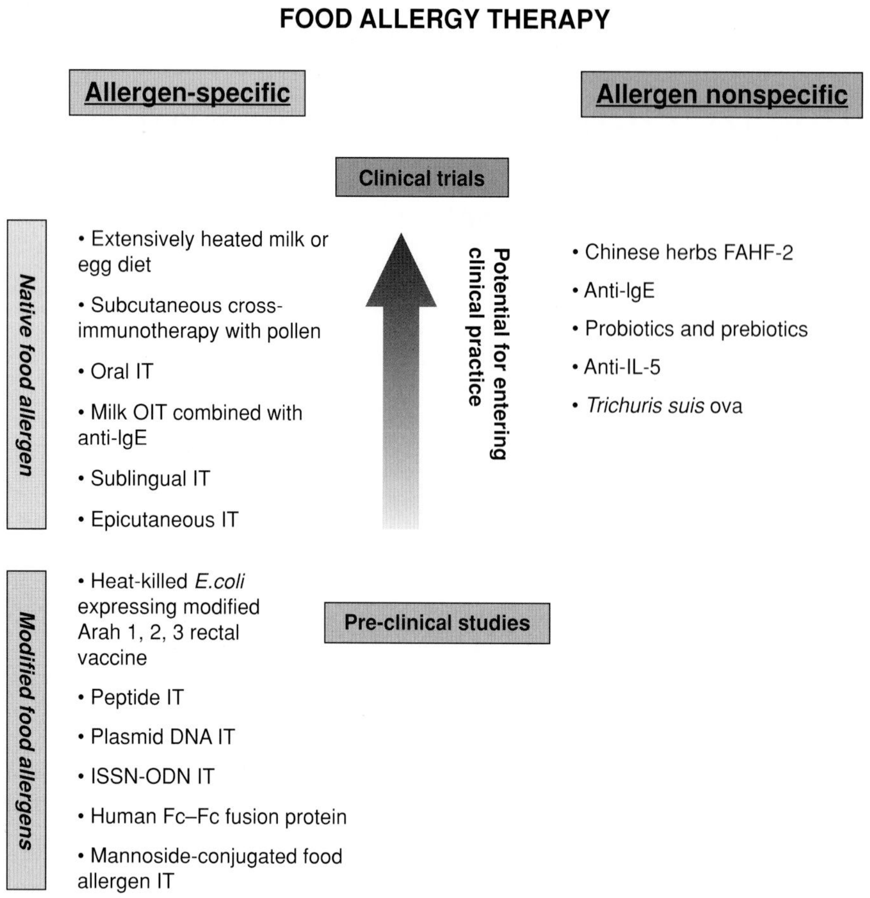

FOOD ALLERGY THERAPY

Allergen-specific

Allergen nonspecific

Clinical trials

Native food allergen

- Extensively heated milk or egg diet
- Subcutaneous cross-immunotherapy with pollen
- Oral IT
- Milk OIT combined with anti-IgE
- Sublingual IT
- Epicutaneous IT

Potential for entering clinical practice

- Chinese herbs FAHF-2
- Anti-IgE
- Probiotics and prebiotics
- Anti-IL-5
- *Trichuris suis* ova

Modified food allergens

- Heat-killed *E.coli* expressing modified Arah 1, 2, 3 rectal vaccine
- Peptide IT
- Plasmid DNA IT
- ISSN-ODN IT
- Human Fc–Fc fusion protein
- Mannoside-conjugated food allergen IT

Pre-clinical studies

Figure 46.1 Approaches to food allergy immunotherapy. Reprinted from Reference 5 with permission.

Table 46.1 Phenotypes of food allergy.

	Transient food allergy	Persistent food allergy	Pollen-food allergy syndrome
Onset	Infancy–early childhood	Infancy–early childhood	Older children–young adults
Frequency	Approximately 75% of milk- or egg-allergic children	Approximately 25% of milk- or egg-allergic children, 80–90% of peanut- or tree-nut-allergic children	Approximately 25–75% among pollen-allergic subjects
Natural history	Usually resolves by school age (3–7 years)	Persists into adolescence and adulthood	Unclear, fluctuation of symptoms due to pollen seasons
Sensitization route	Oral or epicutaneous	Oral or epicutaneous	Respiratory sensitization to pollen followed by reactions to cross-reactive foods
Typical foods	Cow's milk, hen's egg, wheat, soybean	Peanut, tree nuts, fish, shellfish	Fruits (e.g., apple, peach) and vegetables (carrot, celery)
Clinical characteristics	Tolerance to baked milk or egg	Reactivity to baked milk or egg, anaphylaxis to trace amounts of food	Reactions to raw fruits and vegetables, tolerance to cooked fruits and vegetables
Laboratory characteristics	Peak lifetime-specific IgE level less than 50 kU_A/l; IgE to conformational epitopes of milk and egg	Peak lifetime-specific IgE level more than 50 kU_A/l for milk, egg, wheat, soybean, and peanut; IgE to high number of sequential epitopes, increased binding affinity to sequential epitopes	High pollen IgE levels; IgE to conformational epitopes highly cross-reactive with pollen allergens, e.g., Bet v 1
Management	Baked milk and egg diet	Strict avoidance; consider future therapies	IT with cross-reacting pollen or avoidance of raw fruits/vegetables

IT, immunotherapy.

tolerance to extensively heated (baked into other products) milk and egg in children [8, 9]. In both studies approximately 80% of children tolerated baked milk and egg products during a physician-supervised OFC.

Children who reacted to baked milk had significantly greater milk and casein-specific IgE-antibody levels and basophil reactivity *in vitro* following casein stimulation compared to the baked-milk-tolerant children [10]. Baked-milk-tolerant children had a significantly greater median percentage of circulating casein-specific Foxp3(+) CD25(+)CD27(+) T cells (T_{regs}) compared to baked milk-reactive subjects [11]. A higher frequency of casein-specific T_{regs} correlated with a phenotype of mild transient milk allergy (baked-milk-tolerant) and favorable prognosis.

Children ingesting baked egg or milk were followed every 3–6 months. Food-specific IgG_4 antibodies increased, SPT wheal sizes decreased, and there was a trend for decreasing food-specific IgE antibodies; findings similar to those observed in food oral immunotherapy (OIT). Baked-milk-reactive children had more reactions treated with epinephrine during the OFC than children tolerant to baked milk, but reactive to unheated milk, and a very low rate of progression to tolerating baked milk. In contrast, the majority (61%) of children initially reactive to baked egg eventually tolerated baked egg [12]. Compared to the children who continued strict dietary avoidance according to the current standard of care, children ingesting baked milk or egg accelerated their tolerance to unheated milk and egg [13]. A large trial is ongoing to further explore the effects of introducing progressively higher doses of less-extensively heated milk protein on the development of tolerance to unheated milk.

Subcutaneous peanut immunotherapy

Subcutaneous immunotherapy (SCIT) has been established as an effective treatment for environmental and venom allergies for the past 100 years. In a proof-of-concept study, aqueous peanut extract SCIT was administered to peanut-allergic adults. Three SCIT-treated subjects had a 67–100% decrease in symptoms during double-blind, placebo-controlled food challenges (DBPCFCs), and a 2- to 5-log reduction in end-point peanut-SPT at the end of SCIT, while placebo-treated subjects had no change [14]. Due to a pharmacy error, one placebo-treated subject died of anaphylaxis following administration of a dose of peanut extract, resulting in the termination of the study. In a follow-up study, six subjects were treated with a maintenance dose of 0.5 mL of 1:100 weight/volume peanut extract, and six were followed as untreated controls [15]. Following 12 months, all 6 SCIT-subjects tolerated an increased peanut dose during OFC and had decreased sensitivity on titrated peanut SPT, whereas untreated controls had no improvement. However, adverse reactions proved to be unacceptable: anaphylaxis occurred with 23% of the doses administered during the rush phase and an average of 9.8 epinephrine injections were given per subject treated with SCIT. Only 3 of 6 subjects achieved the target maintenance dose due to adverse reactions; an average of 12.6 epinephrine injections per subject was given during the maintenance phase. This study demonstrated that food-SCIT induced desensitization, but the high rate of unpredictable, severe adverse reactions discouraged further evaluation of this form of therapy.

Immunotherapy with pollen for the cross-reactive food

The concept of cross-immunotherapy has been applied to the pollen–food allergy syndrome (PFAS), also referred to as oral allergy syndrome (OAS). Subjects treated with pollen SCIT or sublingual immunotherapy (SLIT) experience variable effects on oral symptoms and SPT to plant foods [16–18]. An open trial of birch-SCIT in 49 birch pollen-allergic adults with apple PFAS reported a complete resolution of apple-induced oral symptoms in 84% of SCIT subjects compared to no benefit in controls ($p < 0.001$), and a reduction in raw apple SPT in 88% of SCIT subjects after 12 months [16]. Eighteen months after discontinuing SCIT, over 50% of subjects tolerated apple. Trials in which oral allergy symptoms to apple and other raw foods were diagnosed with DBPCFCs support a beneficial effect of birch-SCIT in a subset of subjects [18–20]. Birch pollen-extract-SLIT in adults with birch rhinitis was less effective than SCIT and did not significantly reduce apple PFAS [21]. A small clinical study reported a desensitizing effect of continued oral intake of raw fruits causing oral symptoms in pollen-allergic individuals, who over time experienced decreased clinical symptoms [22].

Oral immunotherapy

Successful oral desensitization in a teenage boy with severe egg allergy was first reported in 1908 [4]. A century later, OIT emerged as the most actively investigated therapeutic approach for food allergy. While results suggest that a majority of food-allergic patients can be desensitized with OIT, no studies have proven the development of permanent oral tolerance. Few trials to date have established patient reactivity prior to therapy and/or included a placebo control.

Oral tolerance versus desensitization

The goal of food allergy therapy is oral tolerance, defined as the ability to ingest the food without symptoms despite prolonged periods of avoidance or irregular intake. The mechanism of permanent oral tolerance likely involves the initial development of T_{regs} and immunologic deviation away from the pro-allergic T_h2 response, followed by anergy at later stages [23]. In contrast, in a "desensitized state", protection depends on the regular ingestion of the food; when dosing is interrupted or discontinued, the protective effect may be lost or significantly decreased. In addition, augmentation factors such as viral infection, exercise, or menstrual period may trigger reactions to the previously tolerated maintenance dose. Immunologic changes accompanying oral desensitization include decreased reactivity of mast cells and basophils, increased food-specific serum and salivary IgG_4 and IgA antibodies, and eventually decreased serum food-specific IgE antibodies [24]. There is also an early (following 1 week of high dose desensitization after pretreatment with anti-IgE antibody) decrease in milk-specific $CD4^+$ T cells that return over the ensuing 3–4 months and is characterized by a shift from interleukin-4 to interferon-γ secretion [25].

The permanence of protection may be tested with intentional interruption of dosing for at least 4–12 weeks followed by a tolerance OFC [26–28]. Early studies showed that a subset of food-allergic subjects could be "desensitized" to milk, egg, fish, fruit, peanut, and celery [29–31]. Some subjects who tolerated a maintenance dose, even for a significant period of time, redeveloped allergic symptoms if the food was not ingested on a regular basis, highlighting a concern that permanent tolerance was not achieved [27, 28].

OIT dosing

During OIT, food is mixed with a vehicle and ingested in gradually increasing doses. Dose escalations typically occur in a controlled setting, whereas daily regular ingestion of tolerated doses during the build-up and maintenance phases occurs at home.

Milk OIT

In the first large OIT trial, 45 children (median age 2.5 years, range 0.6–12.9 years) with challenge-proven IgE-mediated cow's milk or egg allergy were randomly assigned to OIT ($n = 25$) or an elimination diet as a control group ($n = 20$) [26]. OIT with fresh cow's milk or lyophilized egg was given at home daily. Following a median 21 months, children in the OIT group were placed on an elimination diet for 2 months prior to a tolerance OFC to determine oral tolerance. At the tolerance OFC, there was no difference between the two groups: nine of 25 (36%) OIT-group showed permanent tolerance compared to seven of 20 (35%) control children. An additional three OIT-treated children (12%) tolerated milk while on active therapy and four children (16%) tolerated increased amounts of milk/egg compared to baseline. Allergen-specific IgE decreased significantly in children who developed natural tolerance during the elimination diet ($p < 0.05$) as well as in those treated with OIT ($p < 0.001$).

In a milk OIT trial, 20 children with IgE-mediated milk allergy, 6–17 years of age, were randomized to milk or placebo OIT [32]. Dosing occurred in three phases: the build-up in-office day (initial dose, 0.4 mg of milk protein; final dose, 50 mg), daily doses with 8 weekly in-office dose increases to a maximum of 500 mg, and continued daily maintenance doses at home for 3–4 months. Twelve patients in the OIT and seven in the placebo group completed the treatment. The median milk threshold dose in both groups was 40 mg at the baseline DBPCFC. Following OIT, the median threshold dose in the OIT group was 5140 mg (range 2540–8140 mg) compared to 40 mg in the placebo-group ($p = 0.0003$). Milk-specific IgE levels did not change in either group, whereas milk-IgG_4 levels increased significantly in the OIT group. In a follow-up, open-label study, 15 children (6–16 years old) were treated for 3–17 months [33]. Fourteen children were able to significantly escalate daily doses by a median (range) of ninefold (2- to 32-fold), with a maximum median (range) tolerated daily dose of 7 g (1–16 g). Follow-up OFCs were timed according to the success of home dosing and were conducted within 13–75 weeks of open-label dosing. Six children tolerated 16 g, and seven reacted at 3–16 g.

Milk OIT combined with pretreatment with omalizumab

The combination of anti-IgE and specific allergen immunotherapy has been successfully applied to environmental aeroallergens [34]. A small, uncontrolled phase I trial utilizing omalizumab with OIT enrolled 11 children with milk allergy, median age 8 years (range, 7–17 years). At entry, the median serum milk-IgE was 50 kU_A/l; range, 41.6–342 kU_A/l. Nine weeks after the start of omalizumab, oral cow's milk desensitization was started. Rush oral desensitization occurred on the first day, starting with 0.1 mg of milk powder and increasing doses every 30 minutes to a maximum dose of 1000 mg (cumulative dose, 1992 mg). One subject discontinued the study because of abdominal pain. Nine of the 10 remaining subjects reached the 1000 mg dose on the first day of desensitization. Milk-OIT continued with weekly increases over 7–11 weeks. Nine of the 10 patients reached the maximum daily dose of 2000 mg milk (the primary end point of the study); one subject reached a daily dose of 1200 mg when the omalizumab was stopped at week 16. Daily milk OIT continued at home for 8 more weeks following discontinuation of omalizumab. All nine patients who had reached a daily dose of 2000 mg passed the DBPCFC with a 7250 mg cumulative dose of milk protein and an open challenge. All nine patients continued with daily milk ingestion >8000 mg/day [35]. A large randomized study of anti-IgE and milk OIT in children and adults with milk allergy is currently ongoing.

Peanut OIT

A number of peanut OIT trials in young children with peanut allergy have been completed to date [36–38] (Table 46.2). In one study, 39 children (median age 57.5 months; range 12–111 months; 64% male) were enrolled in an open-label, uncontrolled trial of peanut OIT [36]. Pretherapy OFCs were not performed. All children completed the initial day escalation phase up to 50 mg, although 36 experienced some allergic symptoms. During the build-up phase, children ingested peanut flour daily; doses increased by 25 mg every 2 weeks until 300 mg was reached. Following 4–22 months of maintenance, 27 of 29 children tolerated 3.9 g of peanut during OFC. Ten (25%) children withdrew following the initial day escalation. Six withdrew for personal reasons and four withdrew because of ongoing allergic reactions to the OIT. Three had gastrointestinal complaints, and one had asthma. Twenty-nine subjects completed all three phases of the study and peanut challenges.

By 6 months, titrated SPT and basophil activation decreased significantly. Peanut-specific IgE antibody concentrations decreased by 12–18 months whereas peanut-specific IgG_4 antibody concentrations increased significantly. In a subset of patients studied, serum factors inhibited IgE-peanut complex formation in an IgE-facilitated allergen-binding assay and secretion of IL-10, IL-5, IFN-γ, and TNF-α from peanut-stimulated peripheral blood mononuclear cells *in vitro* increased over a period of 6–12 months. Peanut-specific forkhead box protein-3 (Fox P3)-positive T_{regs} increased until 12 months and decreased thereafter, and T-cell microarrays showed downregulation of genes in the apoptotic pathways.

In a German study, 23 children (median (range) age 5.6 years, (3.2–14.3) with severe peanut allergy confirmed by DBPCFC received OIT with roasted peanut [37]. The median (range) peanut-specific IgE was 95.6 kU_A/L (3–2071). Following the baseline DBPCFC, a rush OIT was initiated in the hospital with increasing doses of crushed roasted peanuts, 2–4 times per day for up to 7 days. The starting dose was equal to approximately 1% of the threshold dose during the baseline peanut challenge. If a protective dose of at least 500 mg peanut was not achieved, children continued with a long-term build-up protocol using biweekly dose increases up to the maintenance dose of at least 500 mg peanut. Following 8 weeks of maintenance therapy, therapy was discontinued for 2 weeks before conducting the final DBPCFC. After a median of 7 months, 14 of 23 (60%) children reached the protective dose of 500 mg of peanut. At the final DBPCFC, children tolerated a median of 1000 mg (range, 250–4000 mg) compared with a median 190 mg (range, 20–1000 mg) of peanut during the baseline DBPCFC. There was a significant increase in peanut-specific serum IgG_4 and a decrease in peanut-induced IL-5, IL-4, and IL-2 production by PBMCs *in vitro* following OIT.

Egg OIT

In a recent multicenter randomized clinical trial 55 children with egg allergy, median age 7 years (range, 5–11 years) received either egg-white powder OIT with a maintenance dose goal of 2 g (n = 40) or placebo (n = 15) [28]. Intention-to-treat analysis was used to assess all clinical outcomes. Five children in the OIT group and two in the placebo group withdrew from the study prior to the first OFC. All remaining children underwent an OFC with 5 g of egg-white powder at 10 months. Twenty-two children (55%) in the OIT group passed the challenge compared with none in the placebo group. The study was unblinded after the OFC at 10 months. The OIT group continued on maintenance dosing and the placebo group continued complete egg avoidance until the second challenge with 10 g of egg-white powder at 22 months (one OIT patient withdrew prior to the second OFC). Thirty children (75%) in the OIT group passed the 22 month OFC, and the one eligible child in the placebo group (egg-white-specific IgE <2 kU_A/l) failed the challenge. The other children in the placebo group were considered still allergic to egg (egg-white-specific IgE ≥2 kU_A/L).

The children who passed the 22-month OFC stopped OIT for 2 months. Eleven of 29 children (27.5% of the original 40 on OIT) who underwent the OFC at 24 months passed, demonstrating sustained unresponsiveness. Egg was introduced into the diet without restrictions in these children. Laboratory markers associated with sustained unresponsiveness (tolerance) at the 24-month OFC included increased egg-white-specific IgG4 and small skin prick test wheal diameter, but not egg-white-specific IgE or basophil activation.

Similar findings were reported in several observational studies although egg OIT was not found to expedite the natural acquisition of tolerance in one randomized but unblinded study [26, 46–48].

Patterns of response to food oral immunotherapy

Distinct patterns of response to OIT emerge from the published studies [27, 32, 36, 37, 49] (Figure 46.2). Approximately 10–20% fail the initial rush/escalation phase (desensitization failure) and withdraw due to significant adverse reactions. About 10–20% fail to achieve the full planned maintenance dose (partial desensitization). Overall, approximately 50–77% tolerated the maintenance dose. The majority of children tolerated >5 g of the food

Table 46.2 Clinical trials in specific-food oral immunotherapy.

Study	Subjects	Success rate[a]	Immunologic changes	Side effects/comments
Mixed foods OIT				
Patriarca et al. (2003) [39]; open-label clinical trial	Milk ($n = 29$), egg ($n = 15$), fish ($n = 11$), orange ($n = 2$), and other	45/54 (83.3%)	After 18 months: SPT negative in 78%, food-IgE decreased and food-IgG_4 increased	51% of patients experienced urticaria, emesis, diarrhea, or abdominal pain. Protocol stopped in 19% due to side effects; no differences between children and adults
Morisset et al. (2007) [31]; randomized clinical trial	$n = 141$; mean age, milk: 2.2 years; egg: 3.5 years, milk ($n = 57$), egg ($n = 84$)	Milk: 89%, egg: 69%	SPT sizes and specific IgE levels significantly decreased in children that became tolerant	Only children tolerating 60 mL of milk or 965 mg raw egg white at baseline OFC were included (milder clinical phenotype)
Staden et al. (2007) [26]; randomized clinical trial	Milk ($n = 14$), egg ($n = 11$), control group ($n = 20$)	Permanent tolerance 9/25 (36%); tolerant with regular intake 3/25 (12%); desensitization 4/25 (16%)	Food-IgE decreased both in children who became tolerant during the elimination diet ($p < 0.05$) and those on OIT ($p < 0.001$)	The first study to test the permanence of the therapeutic effect following a 2-month period of complete avoidance of the food. The spontaneous resolution rate of food allergy in the control group was comparable, 7/20 (35%) to OIT-treated group 9/25 (36%)
Cow's milk OIT				
Meglio et al. (2004) [40]	$n = 21$, age: 5–10 years	15/21 (71.4%)	SPT to BLG and CS decreased at 6 months ($p < 0.001$), milk-IgE levels not different	3/21 reacted to minimal dose of milk; 3/21 tolerated only 40–80 mL milk/day; 15/21 tolerated 200 mL milk/day for 6 months; side effect rate 13/21
Skripak et al. (2008) [32]; randomized, placebo-controlled clinical trial Narisety et al. (2009) [33]; open-label follow-up study	$n = 20$; active to placebo 2:1 ratio; age 6–17 years	19 subjects completed treatment; post-OIT, the median cumulative dose of milk inducing a reaction in the active group increased from 40 mg to 5140 mg; there was no change in the placebo group, $p = 0.0003$	Milk-IgE levels did not change in either group. Milk-IgG levels increased significantly in the OIT group, with a predominant milk-IgG_4 increase	The median frequency of side effects was 35% in the active group compared to 1% in the placebo group **Blinded study**: Mild oral pruritus median 16% doses/child Gastrointestinal median 2% doses/child Epinephrine: 0.2% of total doses; two doses during build up and two doses during home maintenance (in four subjects) **Open-label home study:** 1–3 months: 2.5–96.4% of doses per subject; >3 months: 0–79%/subject Percentage of total doses with reactions: Oral pruritus: 17% Gastrointestinal: 3.7% Respiratory: 0.9% Cutaneous: 0.8% Multisystem: 5.5% Epinephrine: six reactions in four subjects. One subject developed EoE.

Longo et al. (2008) [41]; randomized clinical trial	$n = 60$; active treatment $n = 20$; untreated comparison $n = 30$; mean age 7.9 years (5–17)	After 1 year 11/30 (36%) tolerated 150 mL milk on daily basis; 16/30 tolerated 5–150 mL milk. None of the children in the comparison group tolerated >150 mL of milk during the final food challenge, $p < 0.001$	Reduction in milk-specific IgE in 15/30 subjects treated with milk-OIT	Three children (10%) discontinued the study due to significant respiratory or abdominal side effects; 17/30 children reported side effects at home treated with: oral steroids (17), nebulized epinephrine (six), and intramuscular epinephrine (one). Six comparison subjects had symptoms upon accidental milk ingestion
Combination milk OIT therapies				
Keet et al. (2012) [42]; randomized clinical trial comparing milk OIT and SLIT	$n = 30$, 6–17 years	1/10 in the SLIT group, 6/10 subjects in the SLIT/OITB group, and 8/ 10 subjects in the OITA group passed the 8 g challenge ($p = 0.002$, SLIT vs. OIT)	Titrated CM skin prick tests, basophil CD63 and CD203c expression decreased; CM–IgG4 increased in all groups; CM–IgE and spontaneous histamine release decreased in only the OIT group	After screening DBPCFC and initial SLIT escalation, subjects continued SLIT escalation to 7 mg daily *or* began OIT to either 1000 mg (the OITB group) or 2000 mg (the OITA group) of milk protein. OFC to 8 g of milk protein was done after 12 and 60 weeks of maintenance. If the 60-week OFC was asymptomatic, IT was stopped, OFC repeated 1 and 6 weeks later. OIT caused more systemic side effects than SLIT. After avoidance, six of 15 subjects (3/6 subjects in the OITB and 3/8 subjects in the OITA group) regained reactivity, two after only 1 week
Nadeau et al. (2011) [35]; small phase 1 trial, uncontrolled open-label study of rapid milk oral desensitization combined with omalizumab	$n = 11$, 7–17 years	9/10 tolerated 1000 mg milk protein on initial rush day; one subject dropped out due to gastrointestinal symptoms; nine subjects who reached a daily dose of 2000 mg passed the DBPCFC and an open challenge	Following a week of milk OIT, the CD4(+) T-cell response to milk was reduced. Following 3 months of daily milk OIT, the CD4(+) T-cell response returned, with a shift from IL-4 to IFN-γ. Milk-IgE decreased; milk-IgG4 increased 15-fold	Following 9 weeks of omalizumab, milk-OIT begun. Omalizumab was discontinued at week 16; milk-OIT was continued DBPCFC was performed after 24 weeks. The mean frequency for total reactions reported by week 24 was 1.6%; most were mild; 0.3% were moderate; 0.1% severe
Peanut OIT				
Jones et al. (2009) [36]; open-label study	$n = 39$; median age at enrollment: 57.5 months (range, 12–111 months)	Open-label study, follow-up 30 months. 29/39 subjects completed (74%), 27 (27/35; 77%) ingested 3.9 g peanut protein during the final OFC	*6 months*: titrated SPT and activation of basophils significantly decreased. *12–18 months:* peanut-IgE decreased, IgG_4 increased. Serum factors inhibited IgE-peanut complex formation in an IgE-facilitated allergen-binding assay. In a subset of subjects, secretion of IL-10, IL-5, IFN-γ, and TNF-α from PBMCs increased over a period of 6–12 months. Peanut-specific FoxP3 (+) T_{reg} cells increased until 12 months, decreased thereafter. T-cell microarrays: downregulation of genes in apoptotic pathways	Withdrawals: four subjects due to the side effects (10%); six due to personal reasons. Most side effects resolved spontaneously or with antihistamines. *Build-up phase:* Mild/moderate reactions (% of total doses): [43, 44, 45] Oropharyngeal: 69% Skin: 62% Nausea or pain: 44% Diarrhea/emesis: 21% Wheezing: 18% *Maintenance phase:* (% total doses) Upper respiratory: 29% Skin: 24% Any treatment: 0.7% of doses Epinephrine: two subjects (one dose each)

(*continued*)

Table 46.2 *(Continued)*

Study	Subjects	Success rate[a]	Immunologic changes	Side effects/comments
Clark et al. (2009) [38]	$n = 4$; case series; ages 9–13 years	Open label; follow-up 6 weeks on maintenance dose 800 mg peanut flour; all subjects tolerated significantly more peanut during a final open OFC than during the baseline DBPCFC	No information	Peanut OIT was well tolerated; no epinephrine used for treatment of adverse reactions
Blumchen et al. (2010) [37]	$n = 23$; age, 3.2–14.3 years	After the rush phase, patients tolerated a median 0.15 g peanut. 22/23 patients continued with the long-term protocol. After a median 7 months, 14 (63%) patients reached the protective dose 0.5–2 g peanut. At the final DBPCFC, patients tolerated a median 1 g (range, 0.3–4 g) in comparison with 0.2 g peanut at the DBPCFC pre-OIT (range, 0.02–1 g), $p = 0.002$	Peanut-specific serum IgG(4) increased whereas peanut-specific IL-5, IL-4, and IL-2 production by PBMCs decreased following OIT	In 2.6% of 6137 total daily doses, mild to moderate side effect; in 1.3%, lower respiratory symptoms occurred. OIT was discontinued in four of 22 (18%) subjects because of adverse events. No epinephrine was used for treatment of reactions
Egg OIT				
Buchanan et al. (2007) [46]; open label	$n = 7$; mean age 4 years (subjects with history of egg-induced anaphylaxis were excluded)	4/7 (57%)	Egg-white-IgG increased significantly from baseline to 24 months ($p = 0.002$). Five subjects showed decreased egg-white-IgE	Four subjects tolerated 24 months egg OFC. Two (50%) reacted to a tolerance OFC 3 months after treatment was stopped
Burks and Jones (2008) [47]; open-label follow-up study of egg OIT in children with nonanaphylactic egg allergy	$n = 21$	19/21		Two of 21 did not achieve the maintenance dose of 300 mg of egg daily. These two subjects were withdrawn from the study because of almost daily allergic side effects, including pruritus, urticaria, and abdominal pain
Vickery et al. (2010) [48]; open label	$n = 8$; median age 5 years (range, 3–13 years)	6/8	EW SPT wheal and ovomucoid IgE decreased, whereas ovomucoid-IgG4 increased during OIT. Transient increases were seen in egg-induced OL-10 and TGF-β levels; the ratio of T_h1:T_h2 cytokine production was decreased	All six children who achieved the median maintenance dose of 2400 mg developed clinical tolerance to egg over a median 33 months of treatment. Individualized dosing regimens may be necessary to achieve a full therapeutic effect in some patients
Burks (2012) [28]; multicenter double-blind placebo controlled clinical trial	$n = 55$ active −40 placebo −15	10 mo challenge: 55% active group passed; 0% placebo passed 22 mo challenge: 75% active group passed (desensitized) 24 mo challenge (6–8 weeks off OIT): 28% active group passed (sustained unresponsiveness)	Small wheal diameters on skin-prick testing and increases inegg-specific IgG4 antibody levels were associated with passing the oral food challenge at 24 months.	The results of this clinical trial raise concerns about the long-term protection (sustained unresponsiveness) afforded by OIT. It remains to be determined whether a higher maintenance dose and longer duration of OIT might improve the rates of sustained unresponsiveness

CM, cow's milk; SPT, skin prick test; BLG, β-lactoglobulin; CS, casein; EoE, eosinophilic esophagitis; DBPCFC, double-blind, placebo-controlled food challenge; OFC, oral food challenge; IT, immunotherapy; PBMC, peripheral blood mononuclear cells.

[a]Success rate defined as regular ingestion of the tested food for at least 6 months.

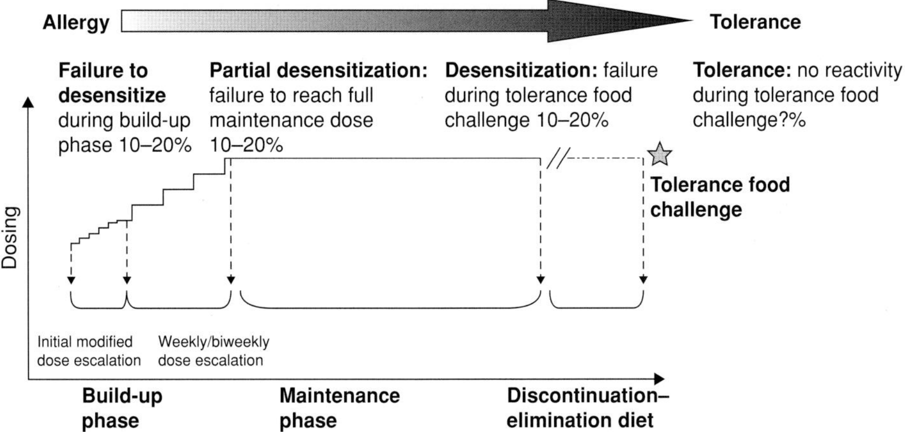

Figure 46.2 Patterns of responses to the food oral immunotherapy. Reprinted from Reference 5 with permission.

while on therapy [48]. It is unclear whether desensitization failure is associated with the most severe food allergy phenotype, as opposed to successful desensitization that may be associated with a milder, transient phenotype and higher chances of spontaneous resolution of food allergy. Despite these encouraging results, three recent meta-analyses of the published literature all concluded that current evidence is inadequate to recommend OIT in clinical practice and called for well-done, large-scale double-blind controlled studies [43, 44, 50].

Sublingual immunotherapy

SLIT represents another approach to desensitization induction, discussed in detail in Table 46.3. Case reports of successful SLIT have been reported for milk, kiwi, hazelnut, peach, and peanut [45, 51–54, 55]. In SLIT, food allergen extract is kept in the mouth for 2–3 minutes and then spit out. The starting dose is usually 100- to 1000-fold lower than in OIT, but SLIT is generally better-tolerated than OIT and the rate of systemic adverse reactions is lower, but the degree of desensitization appears to be less than with OIT.

Head-to-head comparison: milk OIT versus milk SLIT

Thirty children (aged 6–17 years) with milk allergy were randomized to SLIT or SLIT followed by OIT [42]. After screening DBPCFC and initial SLIT escalation, subjects either continued SLIT escalation to 7 mg daily or began OIT to either 1000 mg (the OITB-group) or 2000 mg (the OITA-group) of milk protein. They were challenged with 8 g of milk protein after 12 and 60 weeks of maintenance. After therapy, 1 of 10 subjects in the SLIT group, 6 of 10 subjects in the SLIT/OITB group, and 8 of 10 subjects in the OITA group passed the 8 g challenge ($p = 0.002$, SLIT vs. OIT). After discontinuing SLIT, 6 of 15 subjects (3 of 6 subjects in the OITB group and 3 of 8 subjects in the OITA group) again reacted to milk challenge, two after only 1 week. Systemic reactions were more common during OIT than during SLIT. By the end of therapy, titrated milk SPT and basophil CD63 and CD203c expression decreased and milk-specific IgG_4 levels increased in all groups, whereas milk-specific IgE and spontaneous histamine release decreased only in the OIT group. In this trial, milk OIT was more efficacious for desensitization to milk than SLIT alone but was accompanied by more systemic side effects.

Preliminary data on food OIT and SLIT suggest a beneficial treatment effect, although significant adverse reactions in the former are common. Before these treatments can be used in clinical practice, additional studies are needed to determine optimal maintenance doses and duration, degree of protection, efficacy for different ages, severity and type of food allergies responsive to treatment, and the need for patient protection during home administration [50, 44, 56, 57]. Combination approaches including pretreatment with anti-IgE, SLIT induction to OIT and multi-food immunotherapy based on the individual food allergy profiles need to be investigated to determine the optimal regimens for individual patients.

Epicutaneous immunotherapy (EPIT)

An alternative route of allergen delivery is via epicutaneous patch. In the mouse model, T cells purified from mesenteric lymph nodes (MLNs) of mice orally immunized with ovalbumin transferred allergic skin inflammation to naive recipients that were cutaneously challenged with ovalbumin. These results indicated that cutaneous exposure to food antigens can reprogram gut-homing effector T cells in LNs to express skin-homing receptors [58]. Epicutaenous administration of peanut in sensitized mice resulted in decreased eosinophilia and decreased expression of T_h2 cytokines in the esophageal tissue, decreased serum peanut-specific IgE, and increased peanut-specific $IgG_{2,}$ suggesting that epicutaneous antigen delivery could reduce the GI side effects of OIT [59].

Table 46.3 Clinical trials in specific-food SLIT.

Food/Study	Subjects	Success rate^	Immunologic changes	Side effects/comments
MILK DeBoissieu and Dupont (2006) [45]; open-label pilot study	$n = 8$, children	7/8; following 6 months of milk SLIT, the threshold dose of milk increased from a mean of 39 mL at baseline to 143 mL ($p < 0.01$)	Not studied	Following baseline milk OFC, SLIT started with 0.1 mL of milk for 2 weeks, increasing by 0.1 mL every 15 days until 1 mL/day. One child dropped out due to gastrointestinal side effects
HAZELNUT Enrique et al. (2005), (2008) [51, 52]; randomized DBPC trial	$n = 23$, adults, (54.5% with allergy symptoms to hazelnut	50% of SLIT-subjects tolerated 20 g of hazelnut during follow-up DBPCFC, versus 9% in the placebo group	Levels of serum hazelnut IgG_4 and total serum IL-10 increased only in the SLIT-group, but there were no differences in hazelnut-IgE levels pre- and post-SLIT	All SLIT subjects reached the max dose with a 4-day rush protocol, followed by a daily maintenance dose (188.2 μg of Cor a 1 and 121.9 μg of Cor a 8, major hazelnut allergens). After 5 months, the mean threshold dose of hazelnut increased from 2.3 g to 11.6 g in the active group ($p = 0.02$) compared to 3.5–4.1 g in placebo (nonsignificant)
PEACH *(Pru p 3)* Fernandez-Rivas et al. (2009) [53]; randomized DBPC trial	$n = 37$, adults	In the SLIT-treated subjects ($n = 37$), the threshold doses of Pru p 3 for local reactions (usually oral pruritus) during a DBPCFC were nine times higher and for systemic reactions (usually transient gastrointestinal discomfort or mild rhinitis) were three times higher following 6 months of SLIT compared to pre-SLIT threshold doses. In contrast, the placebo-treated subjects experienced no significant changes in their threshold doses of Pru p 3	Specific IgE to recombinant Pru p 3 increased both in the active ($p < 0.001$) and placebo ($p = 0.03$) groups, although the increase remained only significant at 6 months in the active group (active 4.2, $p < 0.001$; placebo 4.0, $p = 0.08$, *T*-test). IgG_4 to native Pru p 3 increased significantly in the active group ($p = 0.007$) but not in the placebo group ($p = 0.2$)	Peach SLIT was well tolerated
PEANUT Kim (2011) [54]; DBPC study	$n = 18$, 1–11 years old	At post-treatment DBPCFC, the SLIT-group ingested 20 times more peanut than the placebo-group; median, 1710 mg vs. 85 mg; $p = 0.011$	SPT wheals ($p = 0.020$) and basophil peanut responsiveness decreased. Peanut-IgE increased over 4 months ($p = 0.002$) and decreased over subsequent 8 months ($p = 0.003$); peanut-IgG_4 increased ($p = 0.014$). Salivary peanut IgA increased in SLIT-subjects and correlated positively with DBPCFC outcome [24]	6 months dose escalation and 6 months maintenance dosing were followed by peanut DBPCFC. Dosing side effects were primarily oropharyngeal and resolved without treatment. SLIT may be better tolerated by patients

In a small clinical pilot study, 18 cow's-milk-allergic children (mean age 3.8 years, range 10 months to 7.7 years) were randomized 1:1 to receive active EPIT or placebo [60]. CMA was confirmed by baseline OFC and the threshold dose of milk was established. Children applied 1 mg skimmed milk powder or 1 mg glucose as placebo on the skin under patch for 48 hours three times per week for 3 months. EPIT-children had a trend toward increased threshold doses at the follow-up milk OFC, from a mean of 1.8 mL at baseline to 23.6 mL at 3 months; there was no change in the placebo group. There were no significant changes in milk-specific IgE levels from baseline to 3 months in either group. The most common side effects were local pruritus and eczema at the site of EPIT application. There were no severe systemic reactions; however, one child had repeated episodes of diarrhea following EPIT. EPIT warrants further evaluation for food allergy.

Immunotherapy with modified recombinant engineered food proteins

Risk of an immediate allergic reaction during immunotherapy can be decreased by altering IgE antibody-binding sites (epitopes) with point mutations introduced by site-directed mutagenesis or protein polymerization [61] (Table 46.4).

Table 46.4 Modified recombinant allergen immunotherapy for food allergy evaluated in pre-clinical studies in murine models.

Therapy	Mechanism of action	Effects	Comments
Heat-killed bacteria mixed with or containing modified peanut proteins Li et al. (2003) [62]	Upregulation of T_h1 and T- regulatory cytokine responses	Protection against peanut anaphylaxis in mice, lasting up to 10 weeks after treatment	Concern for toxicity of bacterial adjuvants, excessive T_h1 stimulation, and potential for autoimmunity; heat-killed *E. coli* expressing modified peanut allergens administered rectally viewed as the safest approach for future human studies; a phase 1 pilot study in adults completed
Peptide immunotherapy Li et al. (2001) [63]	Overlapping peptides (10–20 amino acids) covering entire protein sequence. Binding to mast cells eliminated, T-cell responses preserved	Protection against peanut anaphylaxis	Improved safety profile compared with conventional IT, does not require identification of IgE-binding epitopes
Plasmid DNA immunotherapy Li et al. (1999) [64]	Prolonged humoral and cellular responses due to CpG motifs in the DNA backbone	Protection against peanut anaphylaxis in AKR/J, but induction of anaphylaxis in C3H/HeJ (H-2^K) mice; no effect on peanut-IgE levels	Serious concerns regarding: (1) safety due to strain-dependent effects; (2) excessive T_h1 stimulation and autoimmunity
Immunostimulatory sequences immunotherapy (ISS-ODN) Srivastava et al. (2001) [65]	Potent T_h1-skewing via activation of antigen-presenting cells, natural killer cells, and B cells; increased T_h1 cytokines	Protection against peanut sensitization	Not shown to reverse established peanut allergy, concern for excessive T_h1 stimulation and autoimmunity
Engineered recombinant peanut immunotherapy Srivastava et al. (2002) [61]	Binding to mast cells eliminated/markedly decreased, T-cell responses comparable to native peanut	Protection against peanut anaphylaxis	Improved safety compared with conventional IT, requires identification of IgE-binding sites
Human immunoglobulin Fc–Fc fusion protein Zhang et al. (2004) [66], Kepley et al. (2004) [67], Zhu (2005) [68]	Fusion protein cross-links the high-affinity FcεRI and low-affinity FCγRIIb receptors on mast cells and basophils	Fusion protein inhibits degranulation of mast cells and basophils	A human Fc–Fel d 1 fusion protein inhibited Fel d 1-mediated degranulation in purified human basophils from cat-allergic patients and blocked allergic responses in a mouse model. A similar approach can be utilized for food allergy
Sugar-conjugated BSA Zhou et al. (2010) [69]	Mannoside-conjugated BSA (Man_{51}-BSA) targeted lamina propria dendritic cells expressing SIGNR-1 and promoted CD4+ type 1 T_{reg} cells	Mice sensitized with Man_{51}-BSA were protected from anaphylaxis due to BSA and Man_{51}-BSA	Sugar-modified food allergens might be used to induce oral tolerance by targeting SIGNR-1 and lamina propria dendritic cells

IT, immunotherapy.

Modified allergens may be combined with bacterial adjuvants (such as heat-killed *Listeria monocytogenes* (HKLM) or heat-killed *E. coli,* (HKE)) to enhance the T_h1 skewing [70]. A nonpathogenic strain of *E. coli* expressing the modified peanut proteins was used as an adjuvant, and the vaccine was administered rectally [62]. Peanut-allergic C3H/HeJ mice received 0.9 (low dose), 9 (medium dose), or 90 (high dose) μg of heat-killed *E. coli* expressing modified proteins Ara h 1-3 (HKE-MP123), HKE-containing vector (HKE-V) alone, or vehicle alone weekly for 3 weeks per rectum. Mice were challenged with peanut 2 weeks following the final vaccine dose, and then at monthly intervals for 2 months more. After the first peanut challenge, all three doses of HKE-MP123 and the HKE-V-treated groups had reduced severity of anaphylaxis ($p < 0.01$, 0.01, 0.05, 0.05, respectively) compared with the sham-treated group. However, only the medium- and high-dose HKE-MP123-treated mice remained protected for up to 10 weeks following treatment. Peanut-IgE levels were lower in all HKE-MP123-treated groups ($p < 0.001$). *In vitro*, peanut-stimulated splenocytes from the high-dose HKE-MP123-treated mice produced significantly less IL-4, IL-13, IL-5, and IL-10. IFN-γ and TGF-β synthesis were significantly increased compared with sham-treated mice at the time of the final challenge. A Phase 1 clinical safety study has been completed in 10 adult subjects with peanut allergy. Doses were increased rapidly to maintenance for a total duration of 20 weeks. Unexpectedly, five of the subjects experienced adverse symptoms including two that required epinephrine for anaphylactic symptoms. Subjects reacting to EMP-123 did not have IgE antibodies that bound modified or unmodified epitopes differently than the five subjects who experienced no symptoms, so the cause of their adverse allergic reactions is not clear. There was a significant decrease in end point skin test titration after 20 weeks, but no significant change in serum peanut-specific IgE or IgG4. In future studies, probiotic bacteria might be used as bacterial adjuvants to avoid the concerns of excessive T_h1 stimulation by killed pathogenic bacteria [71, 72].

Other antigen-specific approaches

A number of additional approaches to food allergy have been evaluated in animal studies, as outlined in Table 46.4, including peptide immunotherapy, immunization with pDNA, CpG immunotherapy, human immunoglobulin Fc–Fc fusion proteins [63–65, 68, 69, 73–76].

Allergen-nonspecific therapy

A number of novel therapies that are not specific for individual allergens have been evaluated in clinical studies including anti-IgE therapy, FAHF-2, probiotics, and *Trichuris suis* therapy. Additional pre-clinical approaches include probiotic bacteria transfected with IL-10 and IL-12 and toll-like receptors [71, 72, 77] (Table 46.5).

Humanized monoclonal anti-IgE

Humanized monoclonal mouse anti-IgE IgG_1-antibodies bind to the constant region (third domain of the Fc region) of IgE-antibody molecules and prevent IgE from binding to high-affinity $Fc_\varepsilon RI$ receptors expressed on mast cells and basophils and to low-affinity $Fc_\varepsilon RII$ receptors expressed on B cells, dendritic cells, and intestinal epithelial cells. With the decrease in free IgE due to anti-IgE therapy, the expression of $Fc_\varepsilon RI$ receptors on mast cells and basophils is down-regulated, resulting in decreased activation and release of histamine and other inflammatory mediators [88]. In addition, anti-IgE appears to inhibit IgE-facilitated antigen uptake by B cells and antigen-presenting cells, which would inhibit IgE-antibody synthesis.

A multicenter clinical trial tested humanized monoclonal anti-IgE antibody (Hu-901) in 84 peanut-allergic adults [78] (Table 46.5). Peanut allergy was confirmed by DBPCFC. Subjects were randomized 3:1 to receive either Hu-901 at 150, 300, or 450 mg doses or placebo subcutaneously monthly for four doses. Peanut OFCs were repeated within 2–4 weeks following the fourth anti-IgE dose. In the highest anti-IgE dose (450 mg) group, the threshold dose increased significantly from one-half of a peanut kernel (178 mg) to nine peanut kernels (2805 mg). Approximately 25% of subjects treated with the highest dose of Hu-901 showed no change in their threshold dose suggesting that a subset of patients may not benefit from the anti-IgE therapy or may require higher doses for protection. A controlled trial of a different anti-IgE antibody molecule (omalizumab [Xolair®]) in peanut-allergic children was terminated prematurely due to the occurrence of two severe allergic reactions during the pretherapy screening peanut challenge that raised serious safety concerns [89].

Traditional Chinese medicine

Traditional Chinese Medicine (TCM) has utilized herbs for many centuries, although not for food allergies. The initial study of TCM tested an herbal formula (FAHF-1) containing 11 herbs in peanut-allergic mice [90]. Herbs included in FAHF-1 were used for treating parasitic infections, gastroenteritis, and asthma by TCM. FAHF-1 protected peanut-allergic mice against anaphylaxis. It reduced mast cell degranulation, histamine release, peanut-specific serum IgE levels, and peanut-induced *in vitro* lymphocyte proliferation, as well as the synthesis of IL-4, IL-5, and IL-13, but not interferon-γ. FAHF-1 had no toxic effects on the liver or kidneys.

A nine-herb formula, FAHF-2 completely blocked anaphylaxis during peanut OFC up to 5 months following

Table 46.5 Allergen-nonspecific therapy for food allergy.

Therapy	Mechanism of action	Effects	Comments
Clinical trials			
Monoclonal anti-IgE Leung et al. (2003) [78]	Binds to circulating IgE, prevents IgE deposition on mast cells, blocks degranulation, interferes with the IgE-facilitated antigen presentation by B- and dendritic cells.	Improves symptoms of asthma and allergic rhinitis, protection against peanut anaphylaxis in 75% of treated patients (highest dose group).	Subcutaneous at monthly or 2-week intervals, unknown long-term consequences of IgE depletion; may be combined with specific-food OIT [35]
Chinese herbs FAHF-2 Wang et al. (2010), Patil et al. (2011) [79, 80]	*Upregulation of T_h1 cytokines:* IFN-, IL-12 *Downregulation of T_h2 cytokines:* IL-4, IL-5, IL-13, decreased allergen-IgE and T cell proliferation to peanut	Reverses allergic inflammation in the airways, protects mice from peanut-induced anaphylaxis for prolonged periods of time	Oral, generally safe and well tolerated; current studies focus on identification of the crucial active herbal components in the nine-herb formula and establishing optimal dosing in human phase 1 and 2 trials
Probiotics and prebiotics	Increased IgA and IL-10, suppression of TNF-α, reduced casein-induced T-cell activation and circulating soluble-CD4, and toll-like receptor 4 signaling	Prenatal, maternal, and postnatal infant supplementation for 6 months decreased AD prevalence at 2 and 7 years of age. [81] In 830 healthy-term infants at low risk for atopy [82] cumulative prevalence of AD at 1 year of age was 5.7% in infants fed with the cow's-milk-based formula with prebiotic compared to 9.7% infants in the control group not fed prebiotic ($p = 0.04$).	Generally safe, well-tolerated and cost-effective.
Trichuris suis ova therapy Summers et al. (2005) [83, 84]	Stimulation of IL-10 synthesis	In a mouse model of food allergy protection against food-IgE sensitization and anaphylaxis. [85]	Safe and afforded clinical improvement in Crohn's disease and ulcerative colitis; no beneficial effect in adults with allergic rhinitis. [86] High prevalence of GI side effects. [87]
Pre-clinical (murine models)			
Lactococcus lactis transfected with IL-10 Frossard et al. (2007) [71]	Decreased serum IgE and IgG_1; increased gut IgA, increased gut and serum IL-10	Pretreatment of young mice prior to sensitization with β-lactoglobulin in the presence of cholera toxin protected against anaphylaxis on the oral food challenge	Probiotic bacteria may be applied to delivery of engineered allergens in humans due to superior safety.
L. lactis transfected with IL-12 and β-lactoglobulin Cortes-Perez et al. (2009) [72]	Decreased IgG_1 in serum and BAL; decreased IL-4 and increased IFN-γ production by β-lactoglobulin stimulated splenocytes	Intranasal co-administration of live *L. lactis* transfected with IL-12 and β-lactoglobulin inhibited allergic reactions in mice	Probiotic bacteria engineered to deliver IL-12 and food allergen may be useful for preventing IgE sensitization to food.
Toll-like receptor 9 agonist Zhu et al. (2007) [77]	Induction of mucosal and systemic Th1 responses; decreased peanut-specific IgE and IgG_2	Oral administration of TLR-9-agonists decreased gastrointestinal inflammation and protected mice from peanut anaphylaxis	Protective effect observed during sensitization as well as in already sensitized mice.

therapy [91]. This protection was mediated by interferon-γ produced by CD8+ T cells [92, 93]. Each individual herb provided some degree of protection, but none of them offered protection that was equivalent to the complete FAHF-2, suggesting synergy among the herbs. In mice with peanut anaphylaxis, reduction of peripheral blood basophils began after 1 week of treatment and continued for at least 4 weeks post therapy. The number and FcεRI expression of peritoneal mast cells were also significantly decreased 4 weeks post therapy. FAHF-2-treated MC/9 cells showed significantly reduced IgE-induced FcεRI expression, FcεRI γ mRNA subunit expression, proliferation, and histamine release on challenge. Fraction-2 from FAHF-2 inhibited RBL-2H3 cell and human mast cell degranulation. Three compounds from fraction 2-berberine, palmatine, and jatrorrhizine inhibited RBL-2H3 cell degranulation via suppressing spleen tyrosine kinase phosphorylation [94]. In addition, in a mouse model of multiple food allergy, FAHF-2 prevented peanut-, egg-, and fish-induced anaphylaxis [95].

A Phase 1, randomized, DBPC dose escalation study in 19 subjects (12–45 years) with peanut and tree nut allergy recently reported that FAHF-2 was safe and well tolerated [79]. Serum IL-5 levels decreased in the active treatment group following 7 days of treatment with FAHF-2. *In vitro*, synthesis of IL-5 decreased, whereas interferon-γ and IL-10 increased in allergen-stimulated PBMCs cultured with FAHF-2. A phase 2 extended safety and efficacy trial in subjects 12–45 years with peanut, tree nut, sesame, fish, or shellfish allergy is ongoing [80].

Conclusions

Food allergy is an increasingly prevalent problem in Westernized countries and there is an unmet medical need for an effective therapy for food allergy. Among the plethora of novel approaches, the strategies most likely to advance into clinical practice in the more immediate future include the Chinese herbal formula FAHF-2 and OIT alone or in combination with anti-IgE antibody. However, these approaches have to be further validated in large clinical trials before advancing into clinical practice. Diets containing extensively heated (baked) milk and egg represent an alternative approach to food OIT and are already changing the paradigm of strict dietary avoidance for milk- and egg-allergic children.

References

1. Sicherer SH, Sampson HA. Food allergy: recent advances in pathophysiology and treatment. *Annu Rev Med* 2009; 60:261–277.
2. Branum AM, Lukacs S. *Food Allergy Among US Children: Trends in Prevalence and Hospitalizations*. Hyattsville, MD: National Center for Health Statistics, 2008.
3. Boyce J, Assa'ad A, Burks AW, et al. Guidelines for the diagnosis and management of food allergy in the United States: summary of the NIAID-sponsored expert panel report. *J Allergy Clin Immunol* 2010; 126(6 Suppl.):S1–S58.
4. Schofield AT. A case of egg poisoning. *Lancet* 1908; 1:716.
5. Nowak-Wegrzyn A, Sampson HA. Future therapies for food allergies. *J Allergy Clin Immunol*, 2011; 127(3):558–573; quiz 574–575.
6. Cooke SK, Sampson HA. Allergenic properties of ovomucoid in man. *J Immunol* 1997; 159(4):2026–2032.
7. Chatchatee P, Järvinen KM, Bardina L, et al. Identification of IgE- and IgG-binding epitopes on alpha(s1)-casein: differences in patients with persistent and transient cow's milk allergy. *J Allergy Clin Immunol* 2001; 107(2):379–383.
8. Nowak-Wegrzyn A, Bloom KA, Sicherer SH, et al. Tolerance to extensively heated milk in children with cow's milk allergy. *J Allergy Clin Immunol* 2008; 122(2):342–347.
9. Lemon-Mulé H, Sampson HA, Sicherer SH, et al. Immunologic changes in children with egg allergy ingesting extensively heated egg. *J Allergy Clin Immunol* 2008; 122(5):977–983.
10. Wanich N, Nowak-Wegrzyn A, Sampson HA, et al. Allergen-specific basophil suppression associated with clinical tolerance in patients with milk allergy. *J Allergy Clin Immunol* 2009; 123(4):789–794.
11. Shreffler WG, Wanich N, Moloney M, et al. Association of allergen-specific regulatory T cells with the onset of clinical tolerance to milk protein. *J Allergy Clin Immunol* 2009; 123(1):43–52.
12. Leonard SA, Sampson HA, Sicherer SH, et al. Dietary baked egg accelerates resolution of egg allergy in children. *J Allergy Clin Immunol* 2012; 130(2):473–480.e1.
13. Kim JS, Nowak-Węgrzyn A, Sicherer SH, et al. Dietary baked milk accelerates the resolution of cow's milk allergy in children. *J Allergy Clin Immunol* 2011; 128(1):125–131.
14. Oppenheimer JJ, Nelson HS, Bock SA, et al. Treatment of peanut allergy with rush immunotherapy. *J Allergy Clin Immunol* 1992; 90(2):256–262.
15. Nelson HS, Lahr J, Rule R, et al. Treatment of anaphylactic sensitivity to peanuts by immunotherapy with injections of aqueous peanut extract. *J Allergy Clin Immunol* 1997; 99(6 Pt. 1):744–751.
16. Asero R. Effects of birch pollen-specific immunotherapy on apple allergy in birch pollen-hypersensitive patients. *Clin Exp Allergy* 1998; 28:1368–1373.
17. Asero R. How long does the effect of birch pollen injection SIT on apple allergy last? *Allergy* 2003; 58(5):435–438.
18. Bolhaar ST, Tiemessen MM, Zuidmeer L, et al. Efficacy of birch-pollen immunotherapy on cross-reactive food allergy confirmed by skin tests and double-blind food challenges. *Clin Exp Allergy* 2004; 34(5):761–769.
19. Alonso R, Enrique E, Pineda F, et al. An observational study on outgrowing food allergy during non-birch pollen-specific, subcutaneous immunotherapy. *Int Arch Allergy Immunol* 2007; 143(3):185–189.
20. Bucher X, Pichler WJ, Dahinden CA, et al. Effect of tree pollen specific, subcutaneous immunotherapy on the oral allergy syndrome to apple and hazelnut. *Allergy* 2004; 59(12):1272–1276.
21. Kinaciyan T, Jahn-Schmid B, Radakovics A, et al. Successful sublingual immunotherapy with birch pollen has limited effects on concomitant food allergy to apple and the immune response to the Bet v 1 homolog Mal d 1. *J Allergy Clin Immunol* 2007; 119(4):937–943.
22. Kopac P, Rudin M, Gentinetta T, et al. Continuous apple consumption induces oral tolerance in birch-pollen-associated apple allergy. *Allergy* 2012; 67(2):280–285.
23. Vickery BP, Scurlock AM, Jones SM, et al. Mechanisms of immune tolerance relevant to food allergy. *J Allergy Clin Immunol* 2011; 127(3):576–584.
24. Kulis M, Saba K, Kim EH, et al. Increased peanut-specific IgA levels in saliva correlate with food challenge outcomes after peanut sublingual immunotherapy. *J Allergy Clin Immunol* 2012; 129(4):1159–1162.
25. Bedoret D, Singh AK, Shaw V, et al. Changes in antigen-specific T-cell number and function during oral

desensitization in cow's milk allergy enabled with omalizumab. *Mucosal Immunol* 2012; 5(3):267–276.

26. Staden U, Rolinck-Werninghaus C, Brewe F, et al. Specific oral tolerance induction in food allergy in children: efficacy and clinical patterns of reaction. *Allergy* 2007; 62(11):1261–1269.
27. Rolinck-Werninghaus C, Staden U, Mehl A, et al. Specific oral tolerance induction with food in children: transient or persistent effect on food allergy? *Allergy* 2005; 60(10):1320–1322.
28. Burks AW, Jones SM, Wood RA, et al. Oral immunotherapy for treatment of egg allergy in children. *N Engl J Med* 2012; 367(3):233–243.
29. Patriarca C, Romano A, Venuti A, et al. Oral specific hyposensitization in the management of patients allergic to food. *Allergol Immunopathol (Madr)* 1984; 12(4):275–281.
30. Patriarca G, Schiavino D, Nucera E, et al. Food allergy in children: results of a standardized protocol for oral desensitization 1. *Hepatogastroenterology* 1998; 45(19):52–58.
31. Morisset M, Moneret-Vautrin DA, Guenard L, et al. Oral desensitization in children with milk and egg allergies obtains recovery in a significant proportion of cases. A randomized study in 60 children with cow's milk allergy and 90 children with egg allergy. *Allerg Immunol(Paris)* 2007; 39(1):12–19.
32. Skripak JM, Nash SD, Rowley H, et al. A randomized, double-blind, placebo-controlled study of milk oral immunotherapy for cow's milk allergy. *J Allergy Clin Immunol* 2008; 122(6):1154–1160.
33. Narisety SD, Skripak JM, Steele P, et al. Open-label maintenance after milk oral immunotherapy for IgE-mediated cow's milk allergy. *J Allergy Clin Immunol* 2009; 124(3):610–612.
34. Kuehr J, Brauburger J, Zielen S, et al. Efficacy of combination treatment with anti-IgE plus specific immunotherapy in polysensitized children and adolescents with seasonal allergic rhinitis. *J Allergy Clin Immunol* 2002; 109(2):274–280.
35. Nadeau KC, Schneider LC, Hoyte L, et al. Rapid oral desensitization in combination with omalizumab therapy in patients with cow's milk allergy. *J Allergy Clin Immunol* 2011; 127(6):1622–1624.
36. Jones SM, Pons L, Roberts JL, et al. Clinical efficacy and immune regulation with peanut oral immunotherapy. *J Allergy Clin Immunol* 2009; 124(2):292–300, 300.e1–e97.
37. Blumchen K, Ulbricht H, Staden U, et al. Oral peanut immunotherapy in children with peanut anaphylaxis. *J Allergy Clin Immunol* 2010; 126(1):83–91.
38. Clark AT, Islam S, King Y, et al. Successful oral tolerance induction in severe peanut allergy. *Allergy* 2009; 64(8):1218–1220.
39. Patriarca G, Nucera E, Roncallo C, et al. Oral desensitizing treatment in food allergy: clinical and immunological results. *Aliment Pharmacol Ther* 2003; 17(3):459–465.
40. Meglio P, Bartone E, Plantamura M, et al. A protocol for oral desensitization in children with IgE-mediated cow's milk allergy. *Allergy* 2004; 59(9):980–987.
41. Longo G, Barbi E, Berti I, et al. Specific oral tolerance induction in children with very severe cow's milk-induced reactions. *J Allergy Clin Immunol* 2008; 121(2):343–347.
42. Keet CA, Frischmeyer-Guerrerio PA, Thyagarajan A, et al. The safety and efficacy of sublingual and oral immunotherapy for milk allergy. *J Allergy Clin Immunol* 2012; 129(2):448–455, 455.e1–e5.
43. Fisher HR, du Toit G, Lack G. Specific oral tolerance induction in food allergic children: is oral desensitisation more effective than allergen avoidance?: a meta-analysis of published RCTs. *Arch Dis Child* 2011; 96(3):259–264.
44. Brozek JL, Terracciano L, Hsu J, et al. Oral immunotherapy for IgE-mediated cow's milk allergy: a systematic review and meta-analysis. *Clin Exp Allergy* 2012; 42(3):363–374.
45. De Boissieu D, Dupont C. Sublingual immunotherapy for cow's milk protein allergy: a preliminary report. *Allergy* 2006; 61(10):1238–1239.
46. Buchanan AD, Green TD, Jones SM, et al. Egg oral immunotherapy in nonanaphylactic children with egg allergy. *J Allergy Clin Immunol* 2007; 119(1):199–205.
47. Burks AW, Jones SM. Egg oral immunotherapy in non-anaphylactic children with egg allergy: follow-up. *J Allergy Clin Immunol* 2008; 121(1):270–271.
48. Vickery BP, Pons L, Kulis M, et al. Individualized IgE-based dosing of egg oral immunotherapy and the development of tolerance. *Ann Allergy Asthma Immunol* 2010; 105(6):444–450.
49. Staden U, Blumchen K, Blankenstein N, et al. Rush oral immunotherapy in children with persistent cow's milk allergy. *J Allergy Clin Immunol* 2008; 122(2):418–419.
50. Sheikh A, Nurmatov U, Venderbosch I, et al. Oral immunotherapy for the treatment of peanut allergy: systematic review of six case series studies. *Prim Care Respir J* 2012; 21(1):41–49.
51. Enrique E, Pineda F, Malek T, et al. Sublingual immunotherapy for hazelnut food allergy: a randomized, double-blind, placebo-controlled study with a standardized hazelnut extract 2. *J Allergy Clin Immunol* 2005; 116(5):1073–1079.
52. Enrique E, Malek T, Pineda F, et al. Sublingual immunotherapy for hazelnut food allergy: a follow-up study. *Ann Allergy Asthma Immunol* 2008; 100(3):283–284.
53. Fernandez-Rivas M, Garrido Fernández S, Nadal JA, et al. Randomized double-blind, placebo-controlled trial of sublingual immunotherapy with a Pru p 3 quantified peach extract. *Allergy* 2009; 64(6):876–883.
54. Kim EH, Bird JA, Kulis M, et al. Sublingual immunotherapy for peanut allergy: clinical and immunologic evidence of desensitization. *J Allergy Clin Immunol* 2011; 127(3):640–646.e1.
55. Kerzl R, Simonowa A, Ring J, et al. Life-threatening anaphylaxis to kiwi fruit: protective sublingual allergen immunotherapy effect persists even after discontinuation. *J Allergy Clin Immunol* 2007; 119(2):507–508.
56. Thyagarajan A, Varshney P, Jones SM, et al. Peanut oral immunotherapy is not ready for clinical use. *J Allergy Clin Immunol* 2010; 126(1):31–32.
57. Fisher HR, Toit GD, Lack G. Specific oral tolerance induction in food allergic children: is oral desensitisation more effective than allergen avoidance?: A meta-analysis of published RCTs. *Arch Dis Child* 2010; 96(3):259–264.
58. Oyoshi, MK, Elkhal A, Scott JE, et al. Epicutaneous challenge of orally immunized mice redirects antigen-specific gut-homing T cells to the skin. *J Clin Invest* 2011; 121(6):2210–2220.

59. Mondoulet L, Dioszeghy V, Ligouis M, et al. Epicutaneous immunotherapy on intact skin using a new delivery system in a murine model of allergy. *Clin Exp Allergy* 2009; 40(4):659–667.
60. Dupont C, Kalach N, Soulaines P, et al. Cow's milk epicutaneous immunotherapy in children: a pilot trial of safety, acceptability, and impact on allergic reactivity. *J Allergy Clin Immunol* 2010; 125(5):1165–1167.
61. Srivastava KD, Li XM, King N, et al. Immunotherapy with modified peanut allergens in a murine model of peanut allergy. *J Allergy Clin Immunol* 2002; 109:S287.
62. Li XM, Srivastava K, Grishin A, et al. Persistent protective effect of heat-killed *Escherichia coli* producing "engineered," recombinant peanut proteins in a murine model of peanut allergy. *J Allergy Clin Immunol* 2003; 112(1):159–167.
63. Li S, Li XM, Burks AW, et al. Modulation of peanut allergy by peptide-based immunotherapy. *J Allergy Clin Immunol* 2001; 107:S233.
64. Li XM, Huang CK, Schofield BH, et al. Strain-dependent induction of allergic sensitization caused by peanut allergen DNA immunization in mice. *J Immunol* 1999; 160:1378–1384.
65. Srivastava K, Li XM, Bannon GA, et al. Investigation of the use of ISS-linked Ara h2 for the treatment of peanut-induced allergy [Abstract]. *J Allergy Clin Immunol* 2001; 107:S233.
66. Zhang K, Kepley CL, Terada T, et al. Inhibition of allergen-specific IgE reactivity by a human Ig Fcgamma-Fcepsilon bifunctional fusion protein. *J Allergy Clin Immunol* 2004; 114(2):321–327.
67. Kepley CL, Taghavi S, Mackay G, et al. Co-aggregation of FcgammaRII with FcepsilonRI on human mast cells inhibits antigen-induced secretion and involves SHIP-Grb2-Dok complexes. *J Biol Chem* 2004; 279(34):35139–35149.
68. Zhu D, Kepley CL, Zhang K, et al. A chimeric human-cat fusion protein blocks cat-induced allergy. *Nat Med* 2005; 11(4):446–449.
69. Zhou Y, Kawasaki H, Hsu SC, et al. Oral tolerance to food-induced systemic anaphylaxis mediated by the C-type lectin SIGNR1. *Nat Med* 2010; 16(10):1128–1133.
70. Li XM, Srivastava K, Huleatt JW, et al. Engineered recombinant peanut protein and heat-killed Listeria monocytogenes coadministration protects against peanut-induced anaphylaxis in a murine model. *J Immunol* 2003; 170(6):3289–3295.
71. Frossard CP, Steidler L, Eigenmann PA. Oral administration of an IL-10-secreting *Lactococcus lactis* strain prevents food-induced IgE sensitization. *J Allergy Clin Immunol* 2007; 119(4):952–959.
72. Cortes-Perez NG, Ah-Leung S, Bermúdez-Humarán LG, et al. Allergy therapy by intranasal administration with recombinant *Lactococcus lactis* producing bovine beta-lactoglobulin. *Int Arch Allergy Immunol* 2009; 150(1):25–31.
73. Rupa P, Mine Y. Oral immunotherapy with immunodominant T-cell epitope peptides alleviates allergic reactions in a Balb/c mouse model of egg allergy. *Allergy* 2012; 67(1): 74–82.
74. Roy K, Mao HQ, Huang SK, et al. Oral gene delivery with chitosan–DNA nanoparticles generates immunologic protection in a murine model of peanut allergy. *Nat Med* 1999; 5(4):387–391.
75. Horner AA, Nguyen MD, Ronaghy A, et al. DNA-based vaccination reduces the risk of lethal anaphylactic hypersensitivity in mice. *J Allergy Clin Immunol* 2000; 106(2):349–356.
76. Salo DP, Ovcharenko FD, Kulish AA.Paligorskit as a gluing and solvent agent in tablets and granules. *Farm Zh* 1965; 20(5):9–13.
77. Zhu FG, Kandimalla ER, Yu D, et al. Oral administration of a synthetic agonist of Toll-like receptor 9 potently modulates peanut-induced allergy in mice. *J Allergy Clin Immunol* 2007; 120(3):631–637.
78. Leung DY, Sampson HA, Yunginger JW, et al. Effect of anti-IgE therapy in patients with peanut allergy. *N Engl J Med* 2003; 348(11):986–993.
79. Wang J, Patil SP, Yang N, et al. Safety, tolerability, and immunologic effects of a food allergy herbal formula in food allergic individuals: a randomized, double-blinded, placebo-controlled, dose escalation, phase 1 study. *Ann Allergy Asthma Immunol* 2010; 105(1):75–84.
80. Patil SP, Wang J, Song Y, et al. Clinical safety of Food Allergy Herbal Formula-2 (FAHF-2) and inhibitory effect on basophils from patients with food allergy: extended phase I study. *J Allergy Clin Immunol* 2011; 128(6):1259–1265.e2.
81. Kalliomaki M, Salminen S, Poussa T, et al. Probiotics and prevention of atopic disease: 4-year follow-up of a randomised placebo-controlled trial. *Lancet* 2003; 361(9372):1869–1871.
82. Gruber C, van Stuijvenberg M, Mosca F, et al. Reduced occurrence of early atopic dermatitis because of immunoactive prebiotics among low-atopy-risk infants. *J Allergy Clin Immunol* 2010; 126(4):791–797.
83. Summers RW, Elliott DE, Urban Jr JF, et al. Trichuris suis therapy in Crohn's disease. *Gut* 2005; 54(1):87–90.
84. Summers RW, Elliott DE, Urban Jr JF, et al. Trichuris suis therapy for active ulcerative colitis: a randomized controlled trial. *Gastroenterology* 2005; 128(4):825–832.
85. Bashir ME, Andersen P, Fuss IJ, et al. An enteric helminth infection protects against an allergic response to dietary antigen. *J Immunol* 2002; 169(6):3284–3292.
86. Bager P, Arnved J, Rønborg S, et al. Trichuris suis ova therapy for allergic rhinitis: a randomized, double-blind, placebo-controlled clinical trial. *J Allergy Clin Immunol* 2010; 125(1):123–130.
87. Bager P., Kapel C, Roepstorff A, et al. Symptoms after ingestion of pig whipworm Trichuris suis eggs in a randomized placebo-controlled double-blind clinical trial. *PLoS One* 2011; 6(8):e22346.
88. MacGlashan DW, Bochner BS, Adelman DC, et al. Down-regulation of Fc(epsilon)RI expression on human basophils during in vivo treatment of atopic patients with anti-IgE antibody. *J Immunol* 1997; 158:1438–1445.
89. Sampson HA, Leung DY, Burks AW,et al. A phase II, randomized, double-blind, parallel-group, placebo-controlled oral food challenge trial of Xolair (omalizumab) in peanut allergy. *J Allergy Clin Immunol* 2011; 127(5):1309–1310.e1.
90. Li XM, Zhang TF, Huang CK, et al. Food allergy herbal formula -1 (FAHF-1) blocks peanut-induced anaphylaxis in a murine model. *J Allergy Clin Immunol* 2001; 108:639–646.

91. Srivastava KD, Kattan JD, Zou ZM, et al. The Chinese herbal medicine formula FAHF-2 completely blocks anaphylactic reactions in a murine model of peanut allergy 1. *J Allergy Clin Immunol* 2005; 115(1):171–178.
92. Qu C, Srivastava K, Ko J, et al. Induction of tolerance after establishment of peanut allergy by the food allergy herbal formula-2 is associated with up-regulation of interferon-gamma. *Clin Exp Allergy* 2007; 37(6):846–855.
93. Srivastava KD, Qu C, Zhang T, et al. Food Allergy Herbal Formula-2 silences peanut-induced anaphylaxis for a prolonged posttreatment period via IFN-gamma-producing CD8+ T cells. *J Allergy Clin Immunol* 2009; 123(2):443–451.
94. Song Y, Qu C, Srivastava K, et al. Food allergy herbal formula 2 protection against peanut anaphylactic reaction is via inhibition of mast cells and basophils. *J Allergy Clin Immunol* 2010; 126(6):1208–1217.
95. Srivastava K, Bardina L, Sampson HA, et al. Efficacy and immunological actions of FAHF-2 in a murine model of multiple food allergies. *Ann Allergy Asthma Immunol* 2012; 108(5):351–358.e1.

Index

Food Allergy: Adverse Reactions to Foods and Food Additives, Fifth Edition. Edited by Dean D Metcalfe, Hugh A Sampson, Ronald A Simon and Gideon Lack.